AF342413

Daniel's Knee Injuries

Ligament and Cartilage Structure, Function, Injury, and Repair

Second Edition

Daniel's Knee Injuries

Ligament and Cartilage Structure, Function, Injury, and Repair

Second Edition

Editors

Robert A. Pedowitz, M.D., Ph.D.
Associate Professor
Chief, Sports Medicine
Department of Orthopaedics
University of California, San Diego
San Diego, California

John J. O'Connor, Ph.D., Hon. D.Sc.
Professor Emeritus
Department of Engineering Science
University of Oxford
Emeritus Fellow of St. Peter's College
Oxford, England

Wayne H. Akeson, M.D.
Professor Emeritus
Department of Orthopaedics
University of California, San Diego
Chief, Department of Orthopedics
VA San Diego Health Care System
San Diego, California

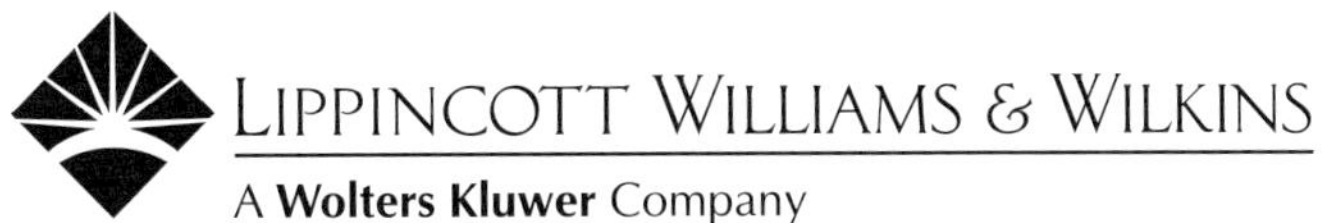

LIPPINCOTT WILLIAMS & WILKINS
A **Wolters Kluwer** Company
Philadelphia · Baltimore · New York · London
Buenos Aires · Hong Kong · Sydney · Tokyo

Acquisitions Editor: James Merritt
Developmental Editor: Michael Standen
Project Editor: Sheila Higgins
Manufacturing Manager: Benjamin Rivera
Cover Designer: Patty Gast
Compositor: Lippincott Williams & Wilkins Desktop Division
Printer: Edwards Brothers

© **2003 by LIPPINCOTT WILLIAMS & WILKINS**
530 Walnut Street
Philadelphia, PA 19106 USA
LWW.com

Library of Congress Cataloging-in-Publication Data
Daniel's knee injuries: ligament and cartilage structure, function, injury and repair /
  editors, Robert A. Pedowitz, John J. O'Connor, Wayne H. Akeson.
    p. ; cm.
  Rev. ed. of : Knee ligaments / editors, Dale M. Daniel, Wayne H. Akeson, John J. O'
Connor, 1990.
  Includes bibliographical references and index.
  ISBN 0-7817-1817-1
  1. Knee—Wounds and injuries.   2. Ligaments—Wounds and injuries.
3. Cartilage—Wounds and injuries.   4. Knee—Wounds and injuries—Patients—
Rehabilitation.   5. Ligaments—Wounds and injuries—Patients—Rehabilitation.
I. Title: Knee ligaments.   II. Daniel, Dale M., 1939–   III. Pedowitz, Robert A.
IV. O'Connor, John J. (John Joseph), 1934–   V. Akeson, Wayne H., 1928–
  [DNLM: 1. Knee Injuries.   2. Cartilage, Articular—injuries.   3. Ligaments,
Articular—injuries.WE 870 D184 2003]
RD561 .K577 2003
607.5′82044—dc21

2002035293

10 9 8 7 6 5 4 3 2 1

"Our study of knee ligaments begins with the patient. We identify problems. We go to the laboratory seeking solutions. We return to the patient." Of all the ways one might describe the ideal cycle of medical research, it is hard to improve on these simple statements, with which Dale Daniel opened the first edition of this book, *Knee Ligaments: Structure, Function, Injury, and Repair*. Nor is there a more fitting way to characterize his career than to say that the sequence of empirical observation, followed by carefully controlled experiment, and then by objective application to patient care, was the central principle of his approach to knee surgery. What Dale did not state, but clearly implied, was that we should remain critical as we apply what our research has taught us to the care of patients in the clinic, for the cycle does not end in the laboratory. Research can have its greatest effect only as an extension of, but not as a substitute for, clinical experience. Unless we close the cycle, neither experience nor experiment alone can achieve its greatest potential in building the scientific foundations of knee surgery.

Currently, few textbooks can withstand more than a few years on the shelf before the patina of obsolescence begins to accumulate. Continuing research and applied clinical orthopaedics are pushing us rapidly beyond the old paradigms. Since the first edition of this book, the variety of techniques for cartilage reconstruction and repair has virtually exploded. Ligament injuries are understood not only for their effect on joint laxity, but on biologic processes as well. Our understanding of anterior cruciate, posterior cruciate, and collateral ligament injuries has changed rather profoundly, and techniques for their repair and reconstruction have evolved considerably in the past 10 years. As the result of the continuing cycle of research and application, the time had come for a new edition of this text.

With Dale Daniel's death in 1995, the field of knee surgery lost one of its most trusted and enlightened scientists. Yet his approach to knee surgery remains an inspiration to us all. As long as we remain curious and critical, the fundamental lessons of his career will never lose their luster. We should all take the time to observe carefully, and in making our observations, to remain objective. Some investigators and clinicians use observation only for the purpose of confirming their own preconceived ideas. Too few have the discipline to hold doctrine in abeyance as they test the veracity of what they *think* they know. The discoveries of the past 10 years have elevated our perspective so that we see things quite differently than we did before. But for progress to continue we must continually challenge what is written. If we follow Dale's example, we will make our clinical observations objectively, with a good measure of skepticism about authority. This approach, which he exemplified so well, represents the most enlightened form of clinical practice in this or any other field of medicine.

Donald C. Fithian
John J. O'Connor
Wayne H. Akeson
Robert A. Pedowitz

Contents

Section IV: Special Clinical Issues

Contributing Authors

Wayne H. Akeson, M.D.
Professor Emeritus
Department of Orthopaedics
University of California, San Diego
Chief, Department of Orthopedics
VA San Diego Health Care System
San Diego, California

David Amiel, Ph.D.
Professor
Director, Connective Tissue Biochemistry
Department of Orthopaedics
University of California, San Diego
La Jolla, California

Christopher C. Annunziata, M.D.
Fellow in Sports Medicine
Department of Orthopedic Surgery
University of Pittsburgh Medical Center
Center for Sports Medicine
Pittsburgh, Pennsylvania

Elizabeth A. Arendt, M.D.
Associate Professor
Department of Orthopaedic Surgery
University of Minnesota
Department of Orthopaedic Surgery
Fairview University Medical Center
Minneapolis, Minnesota

Bruce D. Beynnon, Ph.D.
Director of Research
Department of Orthopaedics and Rehabilitation
University of Vermont
Burlington, Vermont

Richard A. Brand, M.D.
Clinical Professor
Department of Orthopaedic Surgery
University of Iowa
Iowa City, Iowa
Editor-in-Chief
Clinical Orthopaedics and Related Research
Philadelphia, Pennsylvania

Robert T. Burks, M.D.
Professor
Department of Orthopedic Surgery
University of Utah Medical Center
Salt Lake City, Utah

Henry G. Chambers, M.D.
Associate Clinical Professor
Department of Orthopaedics
University of California, San Diego
Chief of Staff
San Diego Children's Hospital
San Diego, California

Constance R. Chu, M.D.
Assistant Professor
Director of Cartilage Restoration Program
Department of Orthopaedic Surgery
University of Pittsburgh Medical Center
Pittsburgh, Pennsylvania

Brad S. Cohen, M.D.
Fellow
San Diego Sports Medicine & Orthopaedic Center
San Diego, California

Dale M. Daniel, M.D. (Deceased)
Associate Clinical Professor
Department of Orthopedic Surgery
Division of Orthopedics and Rehabilitation
La Jolla, California
Staff Surgeon
Kaiser Permanente Medical Center
San Diego, California

Scott F. Dye, M.D.
Associate Clinical Professor
Department of Orthopaedic Surgery
University of California, San Francisco
San Francisco, California

Jennifer Feikes, B.Sc, D.Phil.
Alumna
Department of Engineering Science
University of Oxford
Oxford Orthopaedic Engineering Centre
Nuffield Orthopaedic Centre
Headington, Oxford, England

Donald C. Fithian, M.D.
Assistant Clinical Professor
Department of Orthopaedics
University of California, San Diego
Director
San Diego Knee and Sports Medicine Fellowship
Southern California Permanente Medical Group
San Diego, California

Braden C. Fleming, Ph.D.
Research Assistant Professor
Department of Orthopaedics and Rehabilitation
McClure Musculoskeletal Research Center
University of Vermont
Burlington, Vermont

Cyril B. Frank, M.D., F.R.C.S.C.
Professor and Chief of Orthopaedics
Department of Surgery
Calgary Health Region
University of Calgary
Calgary, Alberta, Canada

T. Tadashi Funahashi, M.D.
Associate Clinical Professor
Department of Orthopedic Surgery
University of California at Irvine
Irvine, California
Regional Coordinator
Department of Orthopedic Surgery
Kaiser Permanente Southern California
Anaheim, California

J. Robert Giffin, M.D.
Fellow in Sports Medicine
Department of Orthopedic Surgery
Center for Sports Medicine
University of Pittsburgh Medical Center
Pittsburgh, Pennsylvania

Richie H.S. Gill, D.Phil.
Senior Research Fellow
Nuffield Department of Orthopedic Surgery
University of Oxford
Nuffield Orthopaedic Centre
Headington, Oxford, England

David H. Goltz, M.D.
Staff Physician
Department of Orthopaedic Surgery
Marin General Hospital
Greenbrae, California

Paul N. Grooff, M.D.
Associate Staff
Division of Radiology
The Cleveland Clinic Foundation
Cleveland, Ohio

Christopher D. Harner, M.D.
Medical Director
Department of Orthopaedics
Professor
UPMC Center for Sports Medicine
University of Pittsburgh
Pittsburgh, Pennsylvania

David A. Hart, Ph.D.
Calgary Foundation–Grace Glaum Professor
McCaig Centre for Joint Injury and Arthritis
*   Research*
University of Calgary
Calgary, Alberta, Canada

Diane C. Hillard-Sembell, M.D.
Department of Orthopaedic Surgery
Springfield Clinic
Springfield, Illinois

Tom Hogervorst, M.D., Ph.D.
Orthopaedic Surgeon
Department of Orthopaedic Surgery
Rode Kruis Ziekenhuis
Den Haag, The Netherlands

Adam H. Hsieh, Ph.D.
Postdoctoral Researcher
Department of Orthopaedic Surgery
University of California, San Francisco
San Francisco, California

Timothy J. Hunt, M.D.
Fellow
San Diego Sports Medicine & Orthopaedic
*   Center*
San Diego, California

Clemente Ibarra, M.D.
Chief
Orthopaedic Sports Medicine and Arthroscopy
Service
Orthopaedic Institute
National Center for Rehabilitation
Associate Professor of Sports Medicine
Universidad Nacional Autónoma de México
Mexico City, Mexico

Robert J. Johnson, M.D.
McClure Professor of Orthopaedic Surgery
Department of Orthopaedics and Rehabilitation
McClure Musculoskeletal Research Center
University of Vermont
Burlington, Vermont
Head, Sports Medicine
Department of Orthopaedics and Rehabilitation
Fletcher Allen Health Care
Colchester, Vermont

Monti Khatod, M.D.
Adult Reconstructive Fellow
Department of Orthopaedics
New England Baptist Hospital
Boston, Massachusetts

Choll W. Kim, M.D., Ph.D.
Assistant Professor
Department of Orthopaedics
University of California, San Diego
San Diego, California

Thomas E. Klootwyk, M.D.
Methodist Sports Medicine
Indianapolis, Indiana

Peter D. Laimins, M.D.
Assistant Clinical Professor
Department of Orthopaedics Surgery
USC School of Medicine
Los Angeles, California
Chief
Department of Orthopedic Surgery
Southern California Permanente Medical Group
Panorama City, California

Richard L. Lieber, M.D.
Professor
Departments of Orthopaedics and
Bioengineering
University of California, San Diego
La Jolla, California
Biomedical Engineer/Career Research Scientist
Veteran Affairs Medical Center
San Diego, California

William F. Luetzow, M.D.
Staff Physician
Department of Orthopaedic Surgery
San Diego Knee and Sports Medicine
Fellowship
El Cajon, California
Attending Physician
Department of Orthopedic Surgery
Kaiser Permanente
San Diego, California

Mark G. Luker, M.D.
Rocky Mountain Orthopaedic Assoc., P.C.
Grand Junction, Colorado

Eric C. McCarty, M.D.
Assistant Professor
Department of Orthopaedics and Rehabilitation
Vanderbilt University Medical Center
Nashville, Tennessee

John W. Miles III, M.D.
Clinical Instructor
Department of Orthopaedics
University of California, San Diego
La Jolla, California
Senior Staff
Department of Orthopedic Surgery
Sharp Memorial Hospital
San Diego, California

John J. O'Connor, Ph.D., Hon. D.Sc.
Emeritus Professor
Department of Engineering Science
University of Oxford
Emeritus Fellow of St. Peter's College
Oxford, England

William M. Ohara, M.D.
Kaiser Orthopedics
El Cajon, California

Elizabeth W. Paxton, M.A.
Research Scientist
Department of Orthopedics
Kaiser Permanente
El Cajon, California

Robert A. Pedowitz, M.D., Ph.D.
Associate Professor
Chief, Sports Medicine
Department of Orthopaedics
University of California, San Diego
San Diego, California

Scott E. Powell, M.D.
Assistant Clinical Professor
Department of Orthopedics
University of Southern California
Keck School of Medicine
Los Angeles, California
Department of Orthopedics
Kaiser Permanente
Panorama City, California

Per A. Renström, M.D., Ph.D.
Professor
Department of Orthopaedics
Section of Sports Medicine
Karolinska Hospital
Stockholm, Sweden

Donald L. Resnick, M.D.
Professor
Department of Radiology
University of California, San Diego
Chief of Osteoradiology Section
Veterans Affairs Medical Center
San Diego, California

Alan M. Reznik, M.D., M.B.A.
Associate Professor
Department of Orthopaedics and
  Rehabilitation
Yale University School of Medicine
Attending Physician
Department of Orthopedics
Hospital of Saint Raphael
New Haven, Connecticut

Raymond A. Sachs, M.D.
Kaiser Orthopedics
San Diego, California

Jean P. Schils, M.D.
Division of Radiology
Section of Musculoskeletal Radiology
The Cleveland Clinic Foundation
Cleveland, Ohio

Mark D. Shaieb, M.D.
Southern Orthopedic Specialists
Panama City, Florida

K. Donald Shelbourne, M.D.
Methodist Sports Medicine
Indianapolis, Indiana

Nigel G. Shrive, M.A., D.Phil., P.Eng.
Professor
Department of Civil Engineering
University of Calgary
Adjunct Professor
Department of Surgery
Foothills Hospital
Calgary, Alberta, Canada

Stephanie Silberberg, M.D.
Fellow in Sports Medicine
The Hughston Clinic, P.C.
Columbus, Georgia

Mary Lou Stone, R.P.T.
Clinical Specialist II and Research Therapist
Department of Orthopedics
Kaiser Permanente
San Diego, California

K-L. Paul Sung, Ph.D.
Professor
Departments of Orthopaedics and
  Bioengineering
University of California, San Diego
La Jolla, California

Marc F. Swiontkowski, M.D.
Professor and Chair
Department of Orthopaedic Surgery
University of Minnesota
Staff Surgeon
Department of Orthopaedic Surgery
Fairview University Medical Center
Minneapolis, Minnesota

James P. Tasto, M.D.
Clinical Professor of Orthopaedics
University of California, San Diego
San Diego Sports Medicine & Orthopaedic
  Center
San Diego, California

Glenn C. Terry, M.D.
The Hughston Clinic, P.C.
Columbus, Georgia

Gail M. Thornton, Ph.D., P.Eng.
Assistant Professor
Department of Mechanical Engineering
University of Alberta
Calgary, Alberta, Canada

Peter A. Torzilli, Ph.D.
Associate Professor
Department of Orthopaedics
Weill Medical College of Cornell University
Senior Scientist
Laboratory for Soft Tissue Research
Hospital for Special Surgery
New York, New York

Steven Tradonsky, M.D.
Clinical Instructor
Department of Orthopaedics
University of California, San Diego
Alvarado Hospital Medical Centre
San Diego, California

Albert M-H. Tsai, M.D.
Department of Orthopaedic Surgery
Southern California Permanente Medical
  Group
Fontana, California

Russell F. Warren, M.D.
Surgeon-in-Chief
Department of Surgery
Hospital for Special Surgery
Professor of Orthopaedic Surgery
Department of Orthopaedics
Weill Medical College of Cornell University
New York, New York

Edmond P. Young, M.D.
Kaiser Orthopedics
El Cajon, California

Amy B. Zavatsky, M.A., D.Phil.
University Lecturer
Department of Engineering Science
University of Oxford
Oxford, England

Preface

Knowledge has expanded markedly in our burgeoning field since publication of the first edition, *Knee Ligaments: Structure, Function, Injury, and Repair,* in 1990. Literally thousands of articles have been published that address relevant issues, from cell biology to long-term studies of the clinical outcome of knee ligament injuries. This second edition updates currently published knowledge in this field. The book is now appropriately titled *Daniel's Knee Injuries: Ligament and Cartilage Structure, Function, Injury, and Repair,* in honor of the clarity of vision and original contributions of the late Dale Daniel, who was the prime motivator of the original book.

The format of the current edition is modified a bit from the first, in an attempt to make the textbook current for students, researchers, and clinicians alike. We tried to integrate issues that directly impact decision-making for ligament injuries, such as evaluation and management of cartilage injury, meniscus injury, malalignment, and pediatric concerns. Our hope is that this book will help "bridge the gap" by providing clinical information that will stimulate investigators and help focus further research and by presentation of the basic scientific foundations and principles for improvement of clinical care.

Whereas the first edition focused primarily on the anterior cruciate ligament, the scope of the current text was expanded to include the basic science and clinical treatment of injuries of the posterior cruciate ligament and posterolateral corner as well as multiligament knee injuries and articular cartilage injuries. Considerable new information is available in these important and challenging areas.

Despite our very best conditioning and equipment improvements, we will never be able to completely eliminate severe knee ligament injuries from our active populations. Unfortunately, we are still a long way from having ideal management protocols that restore perfect knee function and eliminate adverse long-term sequelae. There is little doubt that advances in molecular and cellular biology, noninvasive diagnostic imaging, surgical technique, alternative graft development, and patient rehabilitation will improve the long-term outcome of these life-altering injuries. This textbook will provide useful information for clinicians and scientists as we look forward to the next decade of progress in the field.

Robert A. Pedowitz, M.D., Ph.D.
John J. O'Connor, Ph.D., Hon. D.Sc.
Wayne H. Akeson, M.D.

SECTION I

Structure

CHAPTER 1

Anatomy

Robert T. Burks and Mark G. Luker

MEDIAL KNEE ANATOMY

It is helpful to describe the supportive structures on the medial side of the knee as three layers (1) (Fig. 1.1). The most superficial is layer I, which is the extension of the deep fascia covering the quadriceps and continues on as the deep fascia of the leg (Fig. 1.2). This invests the sartorius and serves as that muscle's insertion. The discrete tendons of the underlying gracilis and semitendinosus are directly under this layer (Figs. 1.1–1.3). Layer II is the superficial medial collateral ligament (MCL). Layers I and II blend together approximately 1 to 2 cm anterior to the leading edge of the superficial MCL. These fibers join with fibers from the vastus medialis to form the medial patellar retinaculum (Fig. 1.1). Layer I completely covers the medial aspect of the knee and is infrequently torn with injury. This layer usually needs to be incised to find the underlying pathology when the medial structures are damaged. Incising layer I over the posterior aspect of the superficial MCL allows all three layers to be identified.

The gracilis and semitendinosus run between layers I and II and insert distal to the tibial tuberosity. They overlie the tibial attachment of the superficial MCL (Figs. 1.3, 1.4). Although these tendons have discrete insertions on the tibia, they also have attachments to the deep fascia near the medial gastrocnemius that need to be cut to harvest the tendons for use in knee reconstructive procedures.

Layer II is the superficial MCL, which originates at the medial femoral epicondyle. It runs approximately 10 to 11 cm to its tibial insertion, where it is covered by the gracilis and semitendinosus (2–5) (Figs. 1.4, 1.5). This has been called the MCL, the tibial collateral ligament, or the superficial medial ligament (1,6). Posterior to the long vertical fibers of the superficial MCL, layers II and III merge together and, along with the semimembranosus tendon and sheath, form the posteromedial corner

of the knee (Fig. 1.1). Warren et al. (5) demonstrated different strain patterns within the fibers of the superficial MCL when the knee was placed through a range of motion. They thought that the ligament should not be viewed as a single homogeneous unit, because its anterior fibers behaved differently from the more posterior fibers. Others have confirmed this idea and have shown that the anterior fibers tighten and have increased strain during the first 70° to 105° of flexion and that the more posterior fibers relax and have decreased strain (7,8) (Fig. 1.5). As the knee flexes, the femur moves posteriorly on the tibia, and the superficial MCL slides posteriorly over the proximal tibia, helping to maintain a more uniform fiber tension (2,3) (Figs. 1.4, 1.5). There can be no meniscal attachment to the superficial MCL in this arrangement, because it would preclude a change in position (9).

Layers II and III blend at the posteromedial corner of the knee. This area is confluent with the posterior edge of the superficial MCL, which runs obliquely to the tibia (Figs. 1.4–1.6) This was called the "posterior oblique ligament" by Hughston and Eilers (10) and referred to as the oblique portion of the tibial collateral ligament or, simply, the posteromedial corner (2,3, 5,11). Hughston and Eilers (10) reported that the ligament originates from the adductor tubercle, slightly posterior and proximal to the femoral epicondyle, and proposed it as a distinctly separable ligament. Warren and Marshall (1) were unable to identify a discrete separable ligament, and because the fibers are in the same layer as the superficial MCL, they preferred to call it the oblique fibers of the superficial medial ligament. This chapter describes the structure as the *oblique fibers of the superficial MCL*. The attachment sites of the fibers in this area move toward each other with increasing flexion and therefore relax (Figs. 1.5, 1.6). Hughston and Eilers (10) found this distance change to be 8 to 18 mm with knee flexion. The more posterior proximal fibers also move

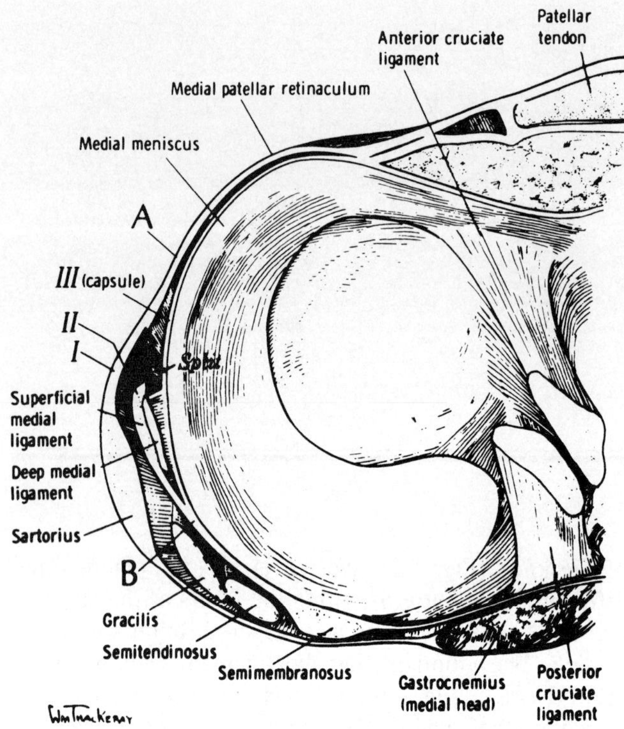

FIGURE 1.1. A transverse section at the joint line of a right knee illustrates the medial layers. Point *A* is the junction of layers I and II anteriorly, and point *B* is the merging of layers II and III posteriorly. (From Warren LF, Marshall JL. The supporting structures and layers on the medial side of the knee. *J Bone Joint Surg Am* 1979;61:56–62, with permission.)

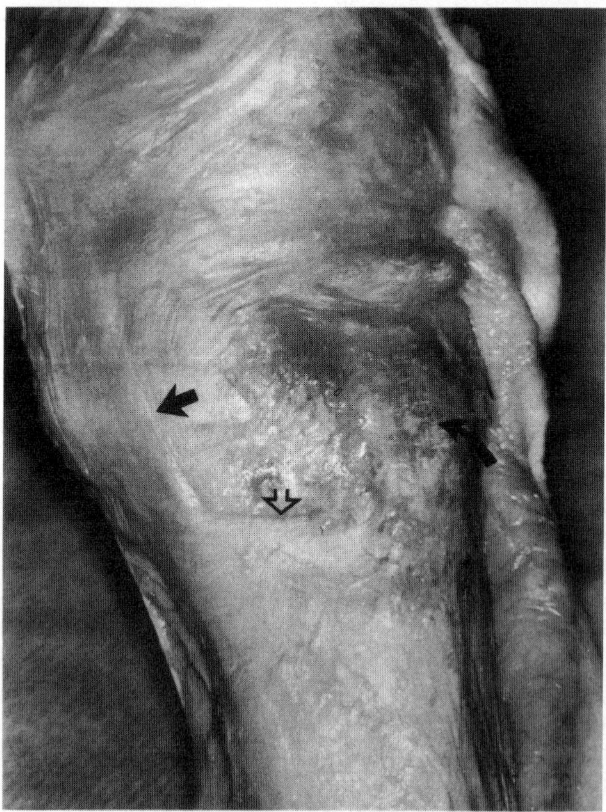

FIGURE 1.2. Skin reflection from a left knee to expose layer I. The *closed arrow* indicates the leading edge of the superficial medial collateral ligament. The *open arrow* indicates the top edge of the sartorius fibers in layer I. The *curved arrow* is on the tibial tubercle.

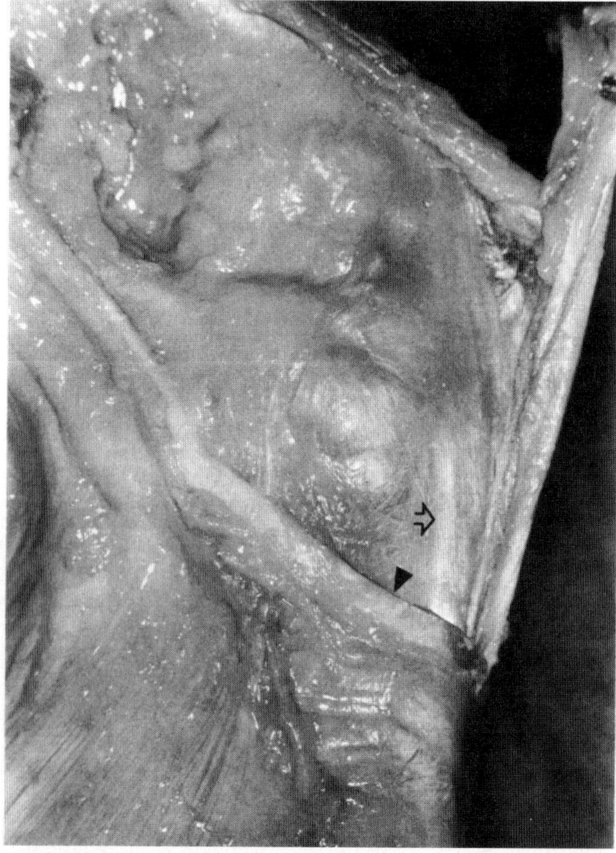

FIGURE 1.3. A left knee with layer I and the sartorius reflected anteriorly. The *arrowhead* indicates the gracilis tendon, and the *open arrow* indicates the posterior edge of the superficial medial collateral ligament.

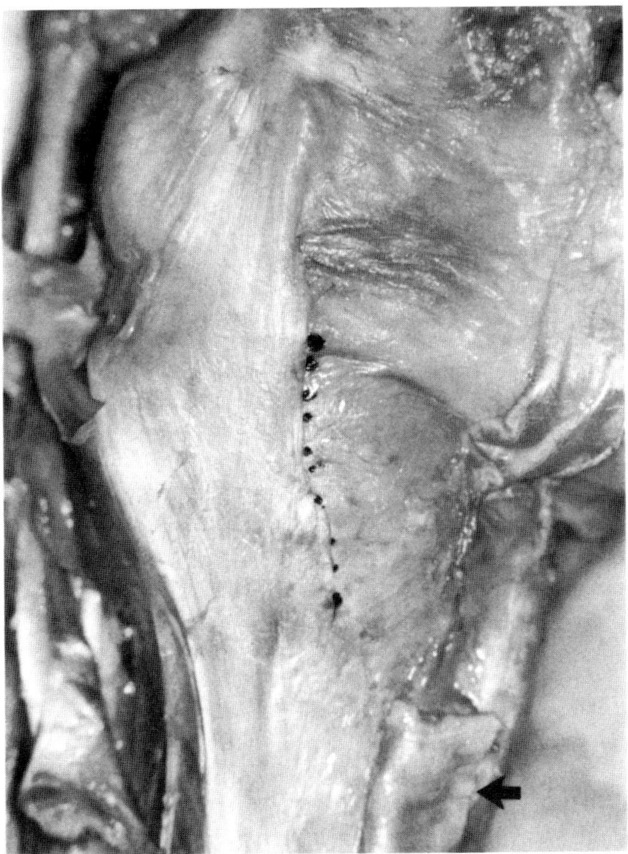

FIGURE 1.4. A left knee in full extension, with ink outlining the anterior edge of the superficial medial collateral ligament. The *closed arrow* indicates the cut edge of the pes tendons that have been folded back anteriorly to show their tibial attachments.

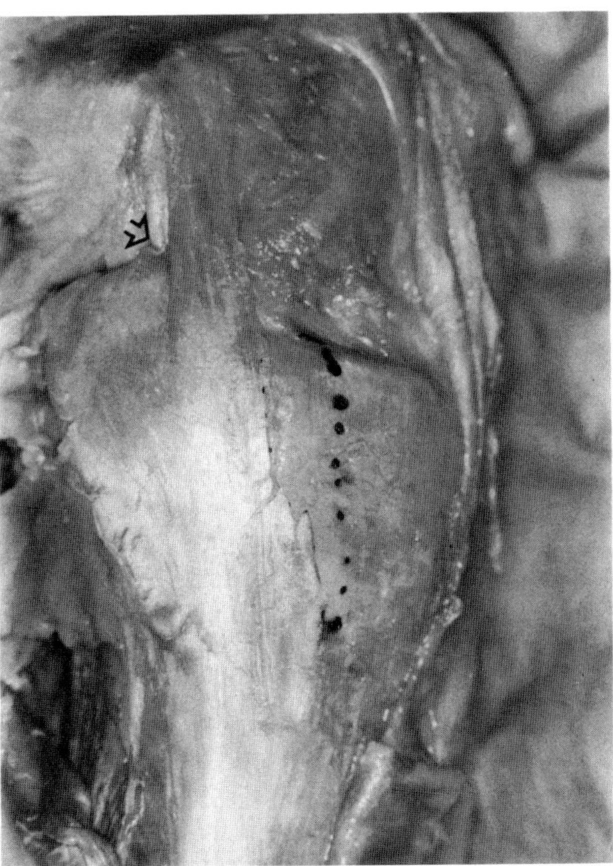

FIGURE 1.5. A left knee in 90° of flexion and some external tibial rotation, demonstrating the posterior displacement of the superficial medial collateral ligament (MCL) as shown by the distance of the ligament from the original ink line. The *open arrow* indicates the posterior oblique fibers folding deep to the superficial MCL.

underneath or deep to the more anterior fibers with knee flexion (8) (Figs. 1.4, 1.5). All investigators (1,2,3,10, 12) call attention to the fact that the oblique fibers are reinforced by the semimembranosus and its tendon sheath (Figs. 1.6, 1.7).

Layer III is the capsule of the knee joint, and it attaches primarily to the articular margins (1). It is thin anteriorly and provides little stability to the knee. The part of the capsule that holds the meniscal rim to the tibia is called the *coronary ligament*. It is short and holds the meniscus tighter in relation to the tibia than the femur. Beneath the superficial MCL, this layer is thickened and called the *deep MCL* or the *deep medial ligament* (5,6,13) (Figs. 1.4–1.7). The deep MCL may be divided into the meniscofemoral and meniscotibial ligaments, which run from the meniscus to the femur and from the meniscus to the tibia, respectively. The peripheral fiber system of the medial meniscus is intimately blended with this area, but many of the capsular fibers run uninterrupted from the

femur to the tibia (2,3,9,14). The capsule posterior to the oblique fibers of the superficial MCL is redundant with knee flexion. An arthrotomy to gain access to the posterior aspect of the knee should be made in this redundant capsule, avoiding the oblique fibers of the superficial MCL.

The semimembranosus and its tendon sheath are important contributors to the posteromedial corner anatomy (1,12,15,16). The tendon is described as having five arms of insertions (Fig. 1.7). The first is a direct attachment to the posteromedial tibia just below the joint line. The second direct attachment proceeds anteriorly just beneath the superficial MCL. A third arm, more from the tendon sheath, runs to blend with the posteromedial capsule. A fourth contributes substantially to the oblique popliteal ligament, which runs over the posterior surface of the joint line capsule. The fifth arm blends with the superficial MCL distally.

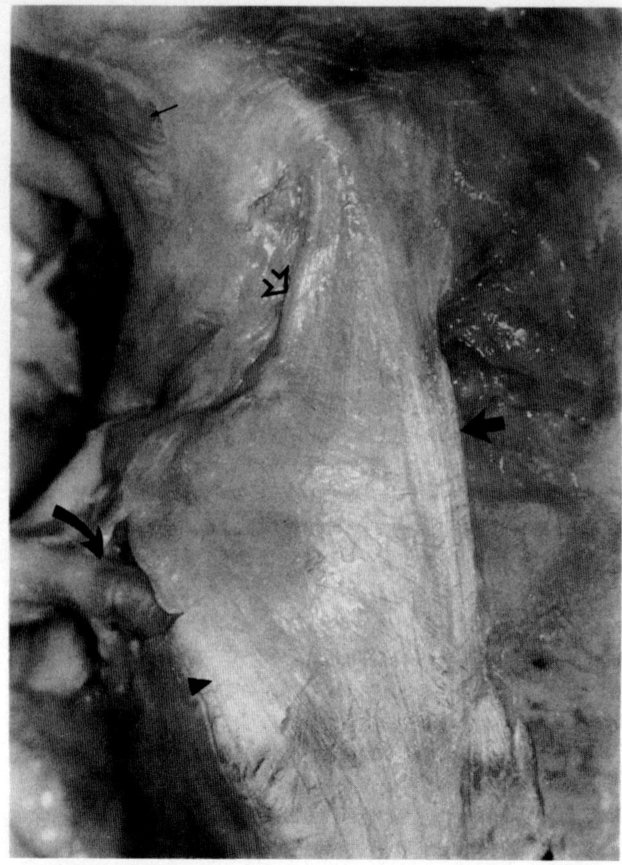

FIGURE 1.6. Close-up of the medial side of the left knee. The *open arrow* indicates the oblique fibers of the superficial medial collateral ligament (MCL). The *closed arrow* indicates the leading edge of the superficial MCL. The *arrowhead* points to the obliquely oriented fibers of the distal aspect of the superficial MCL and the area of contribution from the semimembranosus tendon sheath. The *curved arrow* is on the semimembranosus tendon (the sheath has been opened). The *small arrow* shows the adductor magnus tendon.

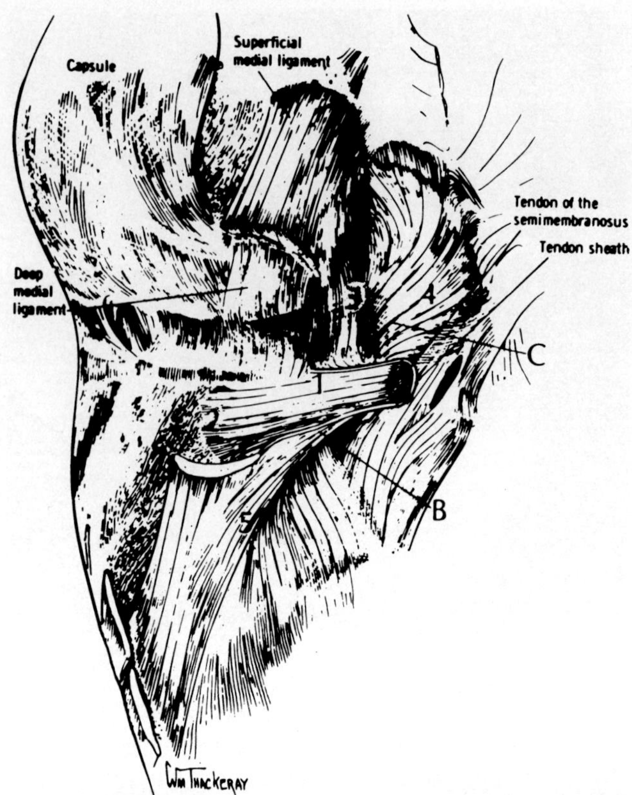

FIGURE 1.7. Five arms of the semimembranosus tendon and its sheath in a right knee. Points *1* and *2* are direct insertions of the tendon. Point *3* is the contribution of the sheath to the posterior oblique fibers. Points *4* and *C* are the oblique popliteal ligament. Points *5* and *B* are the fiber contribution to the distal superficial medial collateral ligament. Point *C* is the oblique popliteal ligament. (From Warren LF, Marshall JL. The supporting structures and layers on the medial side of the knee. *J Bone Joint Surg Am* 1979;61:56–62, with permission.)

LATERAL KNEE ANATOMY

Efforts to understand the functional anatomy of the lateral side of the knee have increasingly focused on the posterolateral corner of the knee (17–21). This is the *tendoligamentous complex*, sometimes referred to as the arcuate ligament complex (22–24). Several investigators have tried to organize the anatomic findings. Seebacher et al. (25) divided the lateral side of the knee into three layers (Fig. 1.8), as Warren and Marshall did on the medial side (1). Hughston et al. (24) divided it into three areas from anterior to posterior. Terry and LaPrade (19) emphasized a detailed understanding of the anatomy as viewed through three longitudinal intervals: a split in the iliotibial band, a division between the iliotibial band and the biceps, and the area between the peroneal nerve and the biceps tendon (Fig. 1.9). The emphasis here is on the

latter approach, focusing attention on the relationships between the structures of the posterolateral corner as seen at surgery.

Beneath the subcutaneous fat lies the deep fascia of the thigh and calf. It extends over the popliteal fossa and condenses in the iliotibial tract before continuing anteriorly to blend into the prepatellar bursa and the patellar retinaculum (25) (Fig. 1.9). Deep to this superficial layer are the retinaculum of the quadriceps, the lateral patellomeniscal ligament, and the lateral patellofemoral ligament.

The dense superficial layer of the iliotibial tract inserts distally at Gerdy's tubercle (Fig. 1.9). A longitudinal incision in this layer reveals its coronal plane communication with the intermuscular septum above the level of the supracondylar tubercle of the femur. Kaplan (26) first emphasized the stabilizing function of these firm attachments to the femur. Terry and LaPrade (19) called this

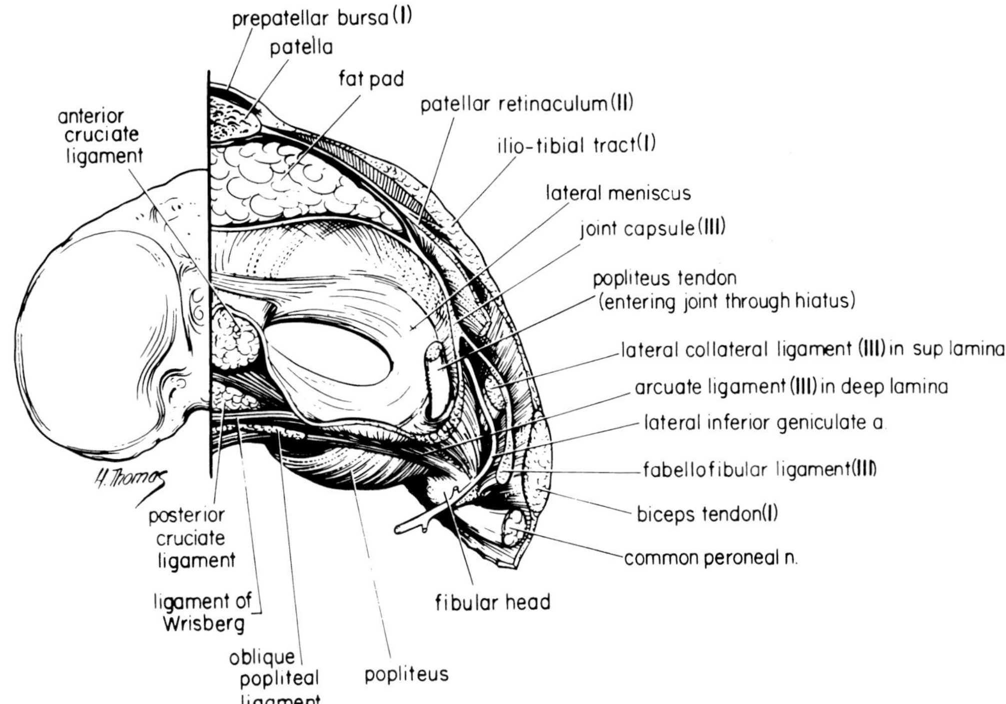

FIGURE 1.8. A view of a right knee after removal of the femur. Notice the division of the fabellofibular ligament and lateral collateral ligament from the arcuate ligament by the lateral inferior geniculate artery. I, first layer; II, second layer; III, third layer. (From Seebacher JR, Inglis AE, Marshall JL, et al. The structure of the posterolateral aspect of the knee. *J Bone Joint Surg Am* 1982;64:536–541, with permission.)

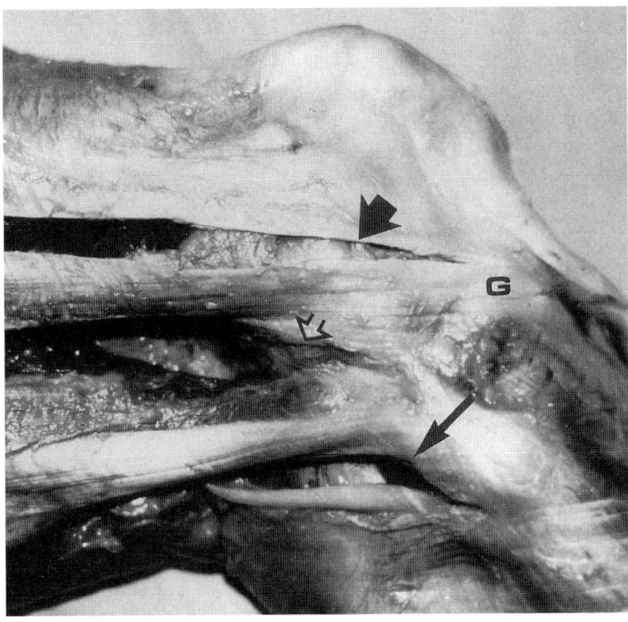

FIGURE 1.9. Lateral aspect of a right knee. The *wide arrow* indicates the split iliotibial band. The *open arrow* shows the interval between the iliotibial band and the short head of the biceps. The *thin arrow* indicates the biceps tendon–peroneal nerve interval, and Gerdy's tubercle *(G)* is shown.

communication the "deep layer" of the iliotibial tract and separated it from the "capsulo-osseous layer." Several investigators have emphasized the functional significance of this portion of the iliotibial tract that courses between attachments on the femur and tibia, considering it an *anterolateral ligament of the knee* (19,26,27).

Dissecting distally in this interval, the femoral attachments of the lateral capsule, lateral collateral ligament, and mid-third lateral capsular ligament can be inspected. After incising the capsule, the surgeon can visualize the lateral meniscus, popliteus tendon, and intracapsular elements of the popliteus complex (Fig. 1.10). An alternative exposure of this area requires reflection of a block of Gerdy's tubercle with the attached insertion of the iliotibial tract.

The lateral collateral ligament (LCL) originates on the lateral epicondyle. The lateral capsule (with the lateral and anterior expansions of the biceps insertion) invests the ligament and must be incised to find a distinct border of the ligament (Fig. 1.11). Most fibers insert on the lateral edge of the fibular head anterior to its apex, although a few lateral fibers extend distally and anteriorly to blend into the periosteum of the fibula and the fascia of the lateral compartment of the leg. The fibular insertion is best

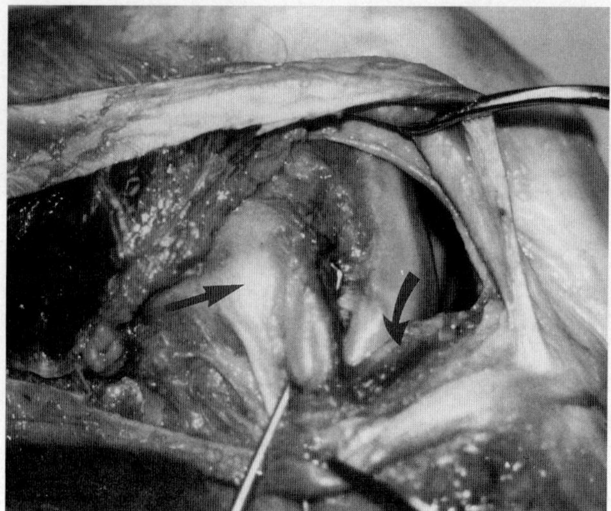

FIGURE 1.10. The split in the iliotibial band is retracted, and the lateral capsule is partially excised. The *straight arrow* points to the lateral epicondyle, and the *curved arrow* indicates the lateral meniscus. The probe passes over the lateral collateral ligament and beneath the popliteus tendon.

visualized by incising the anterior arm of the biceps insertion and entering the small bursa between the two structures (Fig. 1.11). Because of its location slightly behind the axis of rotation, the LCL is tightest in extension and relaxes in flexion, especially at angles greater than 30° (2,12,28,29). Once thought to play a minor role in varus stability, the LCL is now considered the primary restraint to varus stress (28,30).

Anterior to the LCL, the capsule condenses into the mid-third capsular ligament. This originates anterior to the lateral epicondyle and inserts on the tibia just distal to the articular surface from the anterior border of the popliteus hiatus to the posterior edge of Gerdy's tubercle (19). The meniscotibial portion of the ligament provides the attachment of the lateral meniscus to the tibia over this region. When the knee is flexed, the mid-third lateral capsular ligament conceals the femoral portion of the popliteus tendon; it must be incised to inspect that insertion and the articular surface.

The posterior border of the iliotibial tract and the anterior border of the short head of the biceps can be separated to inspect the ramifications of the biceps tendon and some of the posterior joint line structures. The biceps tendon has a complex insertion, up to 11 insertions and expansions have been identified (19,31). The main tendon of the long head has a large direct insertion on the posterolateral edge of the fibular head and a tendinous anterior arm that crosses lateral to the LCL, separated from it by a small bursa (Fig. 1.11). The short head also has a direct tendinous insertion on the fibular head, medial and posterior to the LCL insertion. It has muscular attachments to the posterior capsule and the tendon of

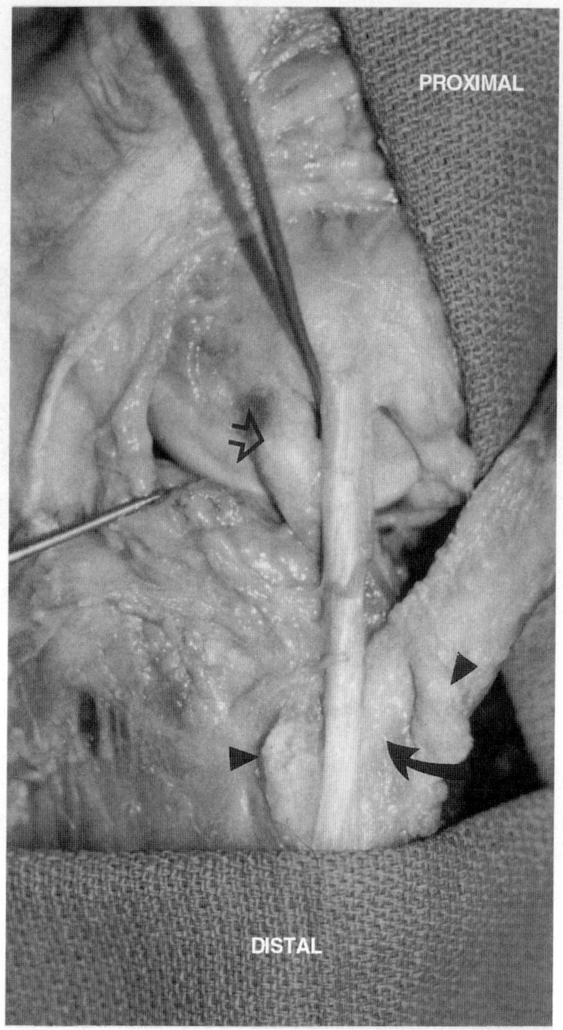

FIGURE 1.11. Lateral aspect of a flexed left knee. The large probe is at the origin of the lateral collateral ligament. The relation with the popliteus tendon *(open arrow)* can be seen. The *arrowheads* are on the cut and reflected anterior expansion of the biceps tendon. The direct tendinous insertion of the biceps is marked by the *curved arrow*.

the long head. Other fascial expansions from both heads course anteriorly and superiorly to augment the lateral and posterior capsule, invest the LCL, and blend with the iliotibial tract. These appear to reinforce the capsule and facilitate a dynamic tensioning mechanism for the structures of the posterolateral corner.

To expose the most posterior aspect of the posterolateral corner, a third interval may be developed by dissecting the peroneal nerve off the posterior edge of the biceps tendon (Fig. 1.9). This region is best understood when viewed from a more posterior perspective. Anterior retraction of the biceps and medial retraction of the gastrocnemius permits inspection of the posterior biceps tendon, arcuate ligament complex, fabellofibular ligament, popliteofibular ligament, popliteus muscle, and posterior capsule.

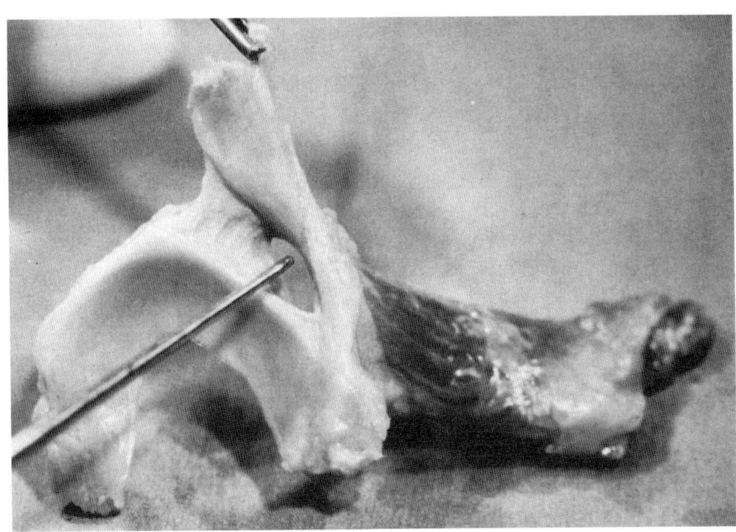

FIGURE 1.12. Lateral meniscus of a right knee. The forceps is on the popliteus tendon, and the tip of the probe shows the popliteal hiatus. The popliteomeniscal fascicles can be seen. (Courtesy of Tom Wickiewicz, M.D., Hospital for Special Surgery, New York, NY.)

The popliteus complex has been the subject of a number of investigations (18–21). It includes the muscle tendon unit and its attachments to the tibia, meniscus capsule, and fibula. The muscle originates from the posteromedial surface of the proximal tibial metaphysis and runs proximally and laterally. The tendon courses deep to the LCL and inserts in the popliteal groove on the lateral femoral condyle just distal to the LCL origin (Fig. 1.11). Superior and inferior popliteomeniscal fascicles bind the tendon to the lateral meniscus and define the borders of the hiatus (Fig. 1.12). Additional fibers blend medially with the arching fibers of the posterior capsule, and some insert directly on the proximal tibia. The popliteus complex is therefore firmly anchored to the posterior tibia just below the articular surface cartilage margin. The muscular portion of the popliteus appears to play a role in dynamic tensioning of the posterolateral corner attachments.

The popliteofibular ligament, a robust connection between the popliteus tendon and the posterosuperior fibula, makes an important contribution to the stabilizing function of the posterolateral structures (Figs. 1.13, 1.14). Although frequently overlooked in the past, it has been rediscovered. Watanabe et al. (21) identified it in 94% of 115 knees and called it the "origin from the fibular head" of the popliteus muscle. Maynard et al. (18) identified it in 20 of 20 knees and found its cross-sectional area was about equal to that of the LCL. Cutting studies show that it resists posterior translation, varus, and external rotation of the tibia with respect to the femur (20) (Fig. 1.15).

The popliteus muscle passes beneath two ligamentous structures originating from the fibular styloid before its tendon passes deep to the LCL. The fabellofibular ligament is a distinct fibrous connection between the styloid and the fabella and lateral gastrocnemius tendon (Fig. 1.16). It is superficial to and easily separated from the underlying capsular layer. The inferior lateral geniculate artery (ILGA) crosses over the popliteus, passes deep to the fabellofibular ligament, and separates it from the capsule and, in our opinion, the arcuate complex (Fig. 1.17). Seebacher et al. (25) and Kaplan (32) pointed out that the fabellofibular ligament may be attenuated when the fabella is not present; conversely, this ligament is usually robust when large fabella is present.

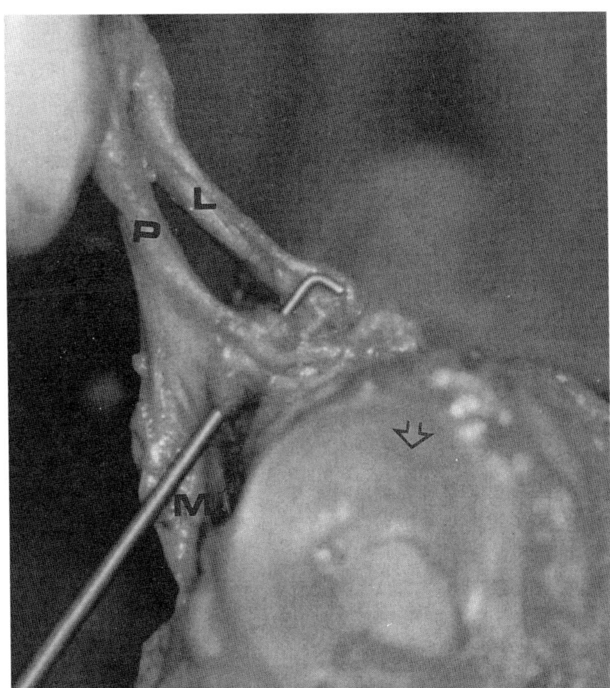

FIGURE 1.13. The left knee has all structures cut except the lateral collateral ligament (L) and popliteus tendon (P). The joint is distracted, and the popliteus muscle (M) can be seen. The open arrow is on the lateral meniscus. The probe is under the large popliteofibular ligament and shows the connection from the popliteus to the fibular head.

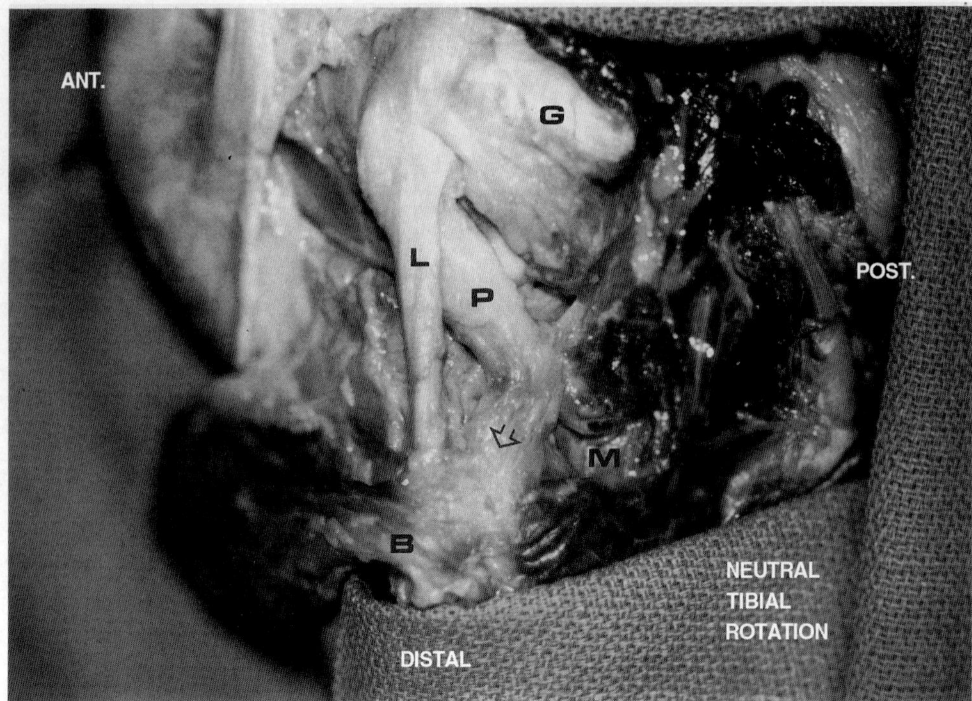

FIGURE 1.14. Lateral view of a left knee. The lateral collateral ligament *(L)*, lateral gastrocnemius tendon *(G)*, and reflected biceps insertion *(B)* are indicated. The popliteus tendon *(P)* and muscle *(M)* are indicated. The *open arrow* identifies the course and insertion of the popliteofibular ligament.

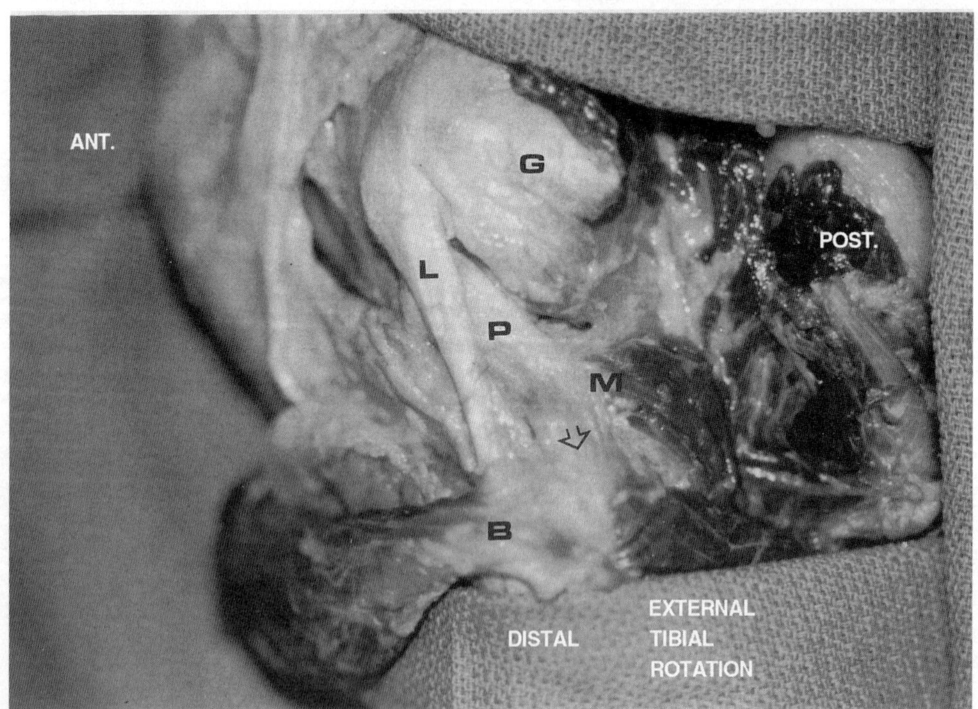

FIGURE 1.15. This is the same specimen as in Figure 1.14. The tibia is externally rotated, and notice that the course of the popliteofibular ligament is nearly parallel with the lateral collateral ligament.

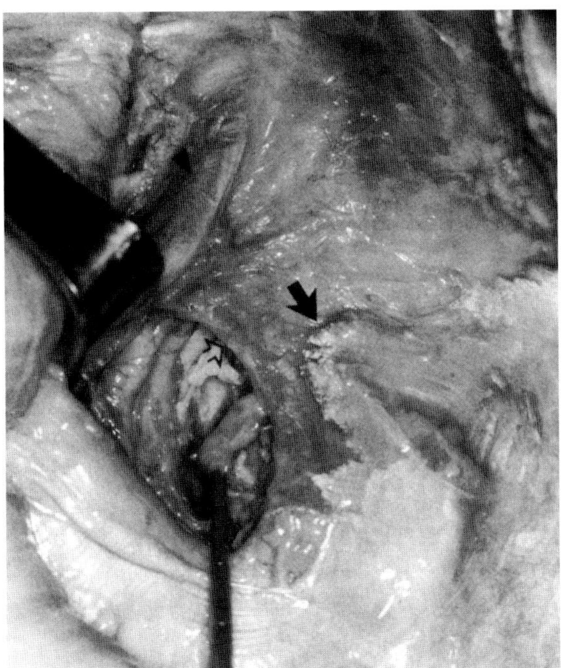

FIGURE 1.16. Lateral view of a right knee. The *closed arrow* is on the cut iliotibial band, and the *open arrow* shows the posterior edge of the fabellofibular ligament. The retractor is pulling the lateral head of the gastrocnemius posteriorly, and the probe is under the inferior lateral geniculate artery.

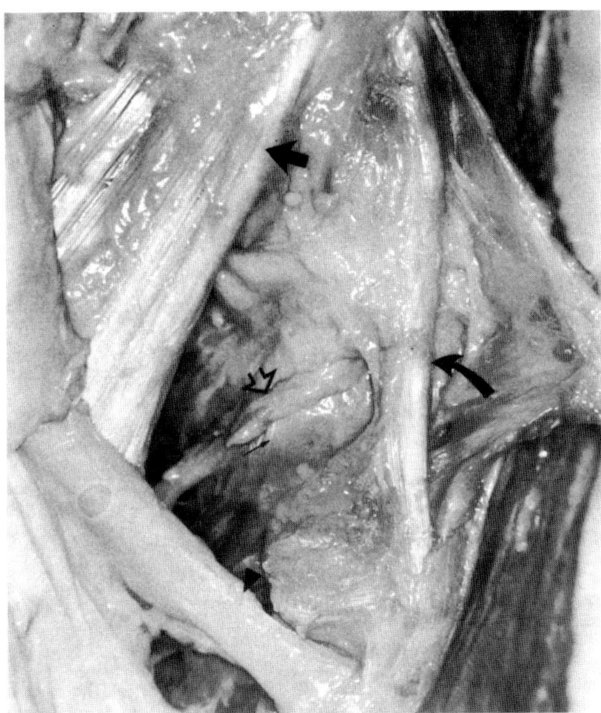

FIGURE 1.17. Posterolateral view of a right knee. The *curved arrow* is on the lateral collateral ligament, and the *open arrow* is on the inferior lateral geniculate artery. The vessel is superficial to the underlying arcuate ligament *(small arrow)*. The *arrowhead* shows the peroneal nerve, and the *closed arrow* is on the lateral head of the gastrocnemius.

Conversely, the arcuate ligament is not a single ligamentous structure but a complex of fibers that arch over the popliteus tendon and reinforce the posterior capsule. Terry et al. (27) tried to refine this concept, suggesting that the lateral limb of the arcuate ligament is a discrete band running from the styloid to the posterior capsule, superficial to the ILGA. They observed, however, that the size and caliber of this lateral limb varied significantly.

We have not found a substantive or consistent structure that correlates with this description.

Our dissections do demonstrate a significant lateral arch of fibers that arises from the fibular styloid, just superficial to the popliteofibular ligament (Figs. 1.17, 1.18). It crosses over the popliteus at the muscle tendon

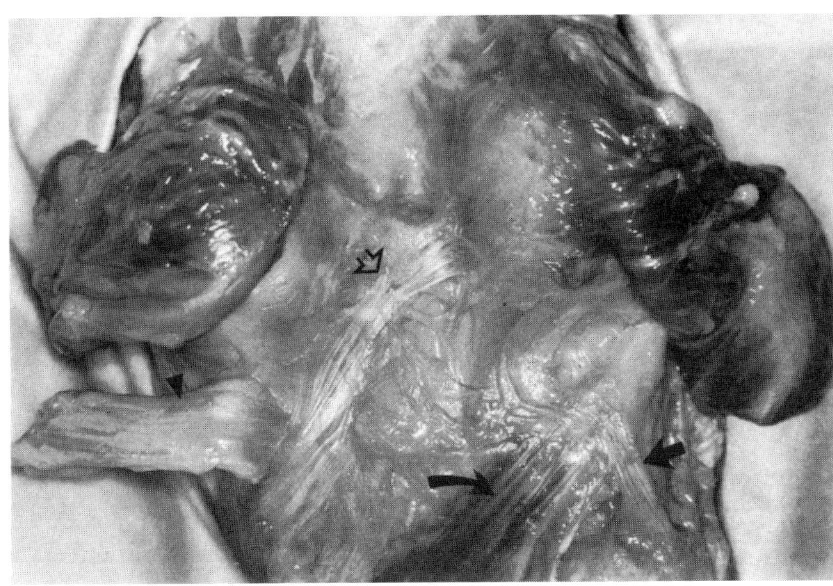

FIGURE 1.18. Posterior capsule of the right knee. The two heads of the gastrocnemius have been transected and placed medially and laterally. The *open arrow* is on the oblique popliteal ligament. The *arrowhead* is on the semimembranosus tendon. The *curved arrow* is on the popliteus muscle. The *closed arrow* is on the popliteofibular ligament.

junction, where it blends with the posterior capsule. These fibers are tightly applied to the popliteus and run deep to the ILGA. The medial part of the arch attaches firmly to the popliteus muscle, blends with the coronary ligament, and attaches directly to the tibia.

The superior attachment of the posterior capsule is proximal to the femoral condyles. Although relatively thin here, it is supported by the two heads of the gastrocnemius muscle. Inferiorly, there is a direct capsular attachment adjacent to the posterior cruciate ligament, but more laterally, the capsule blends with the popliteus muscle expansions to attach to the tibia. At the fibular styloid, the capsule is tethered by the popliteofibular ligament and attached near the base of the arcuate and fabellofibular ligaments (19). Medially, it is reinforced by the oblique popliteal ligament, which runs diagonally from the semimembranosus tendon sheath toward lateral head of the gastrocnemius and contributes fibers to the medial portion of the arcuate arch (Fig. 1.18).

CRUCIATE LIGAMENT ANATOMY

Histologic Anatomy

The anterior and posterior cruciate ligaments (ACL and PCL, respectively) are intracapsular but extrasynovial ligaments. These ligaments appear crossed (hence the term *cruciate*) on viewing the knee anteriorly or laterally (33). Most of the microscopic anatomy has been done on the ACL by Danylchuk et al. (34). The ligament is composed of collagen fibrils, 150 to 250 μm in diameter, which appear parallel under high magnification. These fibrils form fibers 1 to 20 μm in diameter, and most of these fibers run parallel to the long axis of the ligament. A large number of collagen fibers merge together to make the sub-

fascicular unit, which varies from 100 to 250 μm in diameter. A thin band of loose connective tissue called the endotenon surrounds the subfasciculus. In humans, the amount of endotenon is great, which makes the ligament appear to be made of bundles and less uniform. Three to 20 subfasciculi are bound together to form the collagen fasciculus, which ranges from 250 μm to several millimeters in diameter. The epitenon surrounds the fasciculus and is denser than the endotenon. Surrounding the entire ligament is the paratenon, which blends with the epitenon. The synovium then covers the ligament, making it extrasynovial (Fig. 1.19).

An important aspect of the cruciate anatomy is the change from flexible ligamentous tissue to rigid bone, mediated by a transitional zone of fibrocartilage and mineralized cartilage (35) (Fig. 1.20). This helps prevent stress concentration at the attachment site by allowing a gradual change in stiffness (35). Cooper and Misol (36) characterized four discrete regions in this transition. Zone I is composed of wavy collagen fibers. Zone II is the fibrocartilage zone, with chondrocytes being the predominant cell. In zone III, the ground substance becomes mineralized. In zone IV, the bone matrix collagen fibers blend with the mineralized fibrocartilage. A darkly stained line can be seen between zones II and III (Fig. 1.20).

Vascular Anatomy

The cruciate ligaments are covered by synovial folds that originate at the posterior inlet of the intercondylar notch and extend to the anterior tibial insertion of the ACL (35,37–39). It there joins with the synovium from the joint capsule distal to the fat pad. The predominant source of blood supply is the middle geniculate artery,

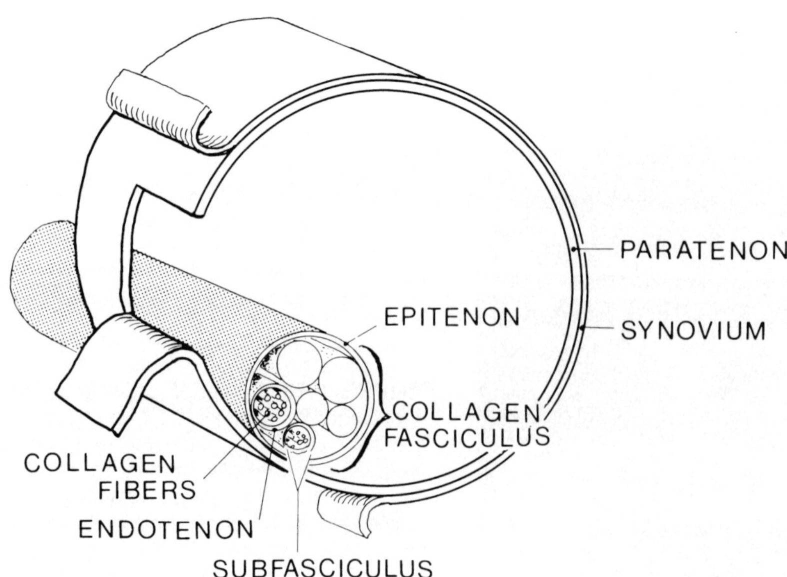

FIGURE 1.19. Diagrammatic view of a cruciate ligament down to the collagen fiber level.

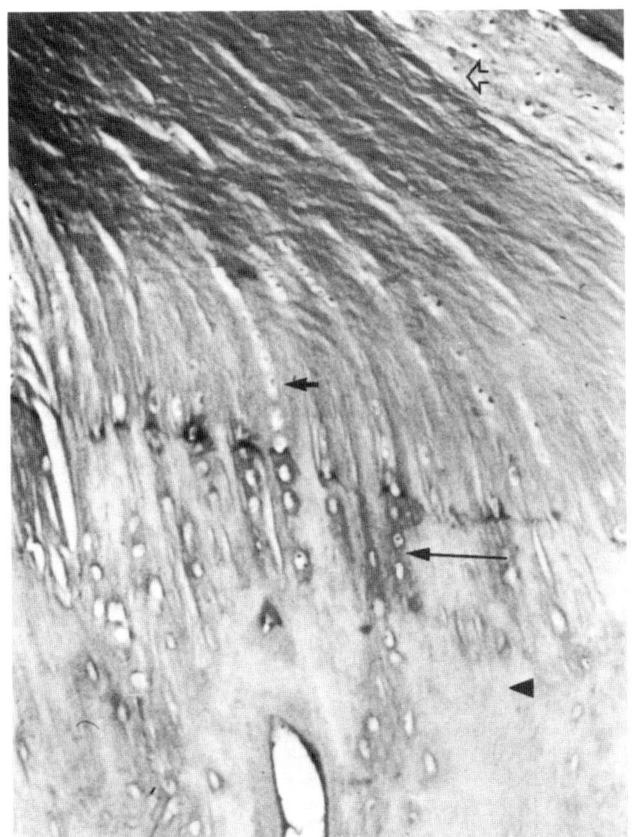

FIGURE 1.20. Anterior cruciate insertion. The *open arrow* is on the ligament (zone I). The *small closed arrow* is on zone II, the *long arrow* is on zone III, and the *arrowhead* is on zone IV. (Photomicrograph courtesy of Steven Arnoczky, M.D., Michigan State University, East Lansing, MI.)

which leaves the popliteal artery and directly pierces the posterior capsule (35,37–41). Figure 1.21 shows the vascularity of the ACL and the PCL. The cruciates have an arborization of the vessels that penetrates the ligament transversely. These vessels anastomose with endoligamentous vessels that lie parallel to the collagen bundles in the ligaments (35,38). The osseous attachments of the cruciates contribute little to their vascularity (37,38). There is a significant blood supply from the fat pad through the inferior medial and lateral geniculate arteries, which may play a more important role when the ligament is injured (37,42).

Neurologic Anatomy

Nerve fibers, which are of the size most consistent with transmitting pain, are readily visualized in the intrafascicular spaces occupied by the vessels (16,43). These are presumably terminal branches from the tibial nerve in the popliteal fossa (44). In 1984, Schultz et al. (45) investigated mechanoreceptors in cruciate ligaments and found a few thin axons in the substance of the ligaments and bundles of axons running on the surface of the ligament. Mechanoreceptors were identified in the ligament and were thought to be similar to Golgi tendon organs. They were mostly on the surface of the ligament, well beneath the synovial lining, and primarily at the insertion sites. They were postulated to respond as proprioceptors and to signal potentially injurious deformation of the ligaments and joint.

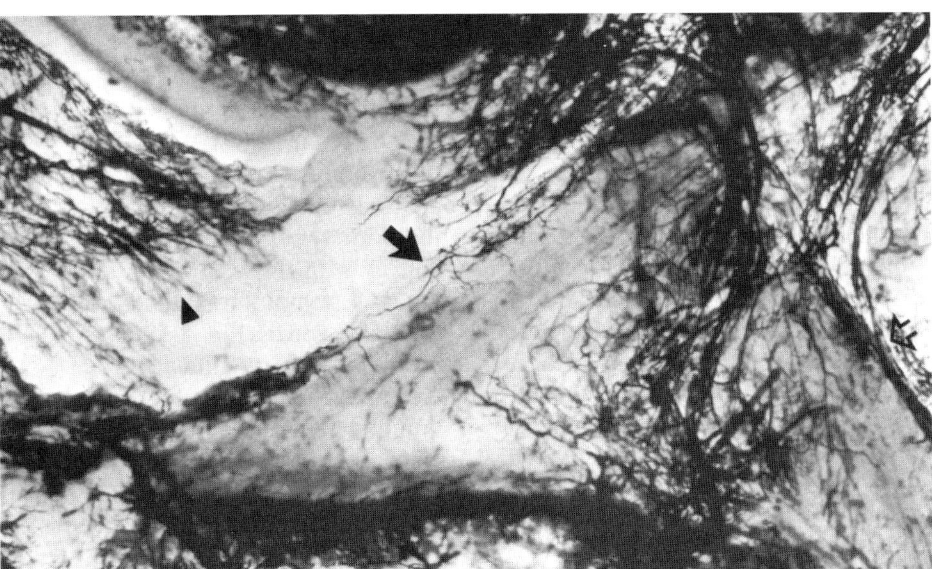

FIGURE 1.21. Photomicrograph of the vascularity to the cruciate ligaments. The *arrowhead* indicates the fat pad. The *closed arrow* is on the anterior edge of the anterior cruciate ligament, and the *open arrow* is on the posterior edge of the posterior cruciate ligament. (From Arnoczky SP. Anatomy of the anterior cruciate ligament. *Clin Orthop* 1983;172:19–25, with permission.)

Schutte et al. (16) studied the neuroanatomy of the human ACL and found three morphologic types of mechanoreceptors as well as free nerve endings. The three mechanoreceptors were Ruffini endings, which are slow adapting and respond to slight changes in ligament tension; a second type of Ruffini mechanoreceptor, which is also slow adapting, resembling a Golgi tendon organ; and a pacinian corpuscle, which is a rapidly adapting mechanoreceptor. Free nerve endings for transmitting pain were also identified but were far scarcer than the mechanoreceptors.

Insertion Site Anatomy

The bony attachments of the cruciates have been investigated by several researchers. In 1975, Girgis et al. (46) described the ACL and PCL attachments in detail. Later publications by Odensten and Gillquist (47) and Harner et al. (48) also addressed this issue. We have performed detailed dissections to illustrate the orientation and anatomy of both cruciate ligaments and for comparison with the prior studies.

The tibial attachment for the ACL is much larger than the femoral attachment and is oriented in the anteroposterior plane. Tibial ACL attachments are shown for the Odensten study (Fig. 1.22). The ACL tibial attachment fans out and forms a "foot" region that allows the ACL to tuck under the roof of the intercondylar notch with the knee in full extension (Fig. 1.23). This unique attachment of the ACL causes concern for ACL reconstruction tech-

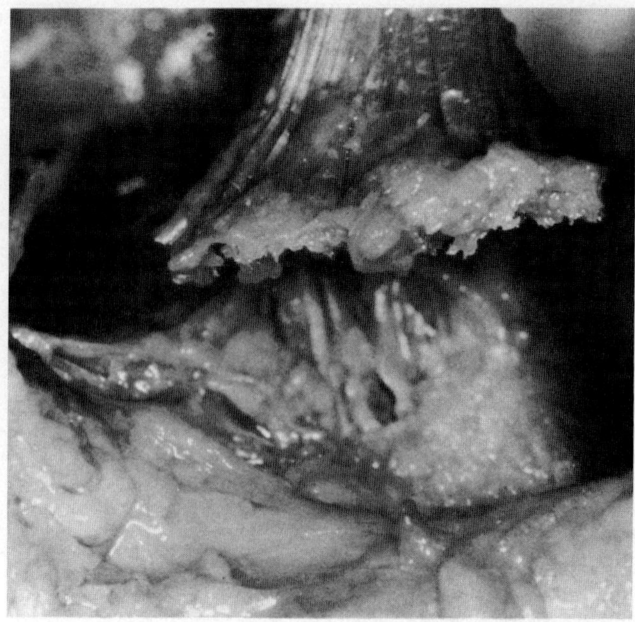

A

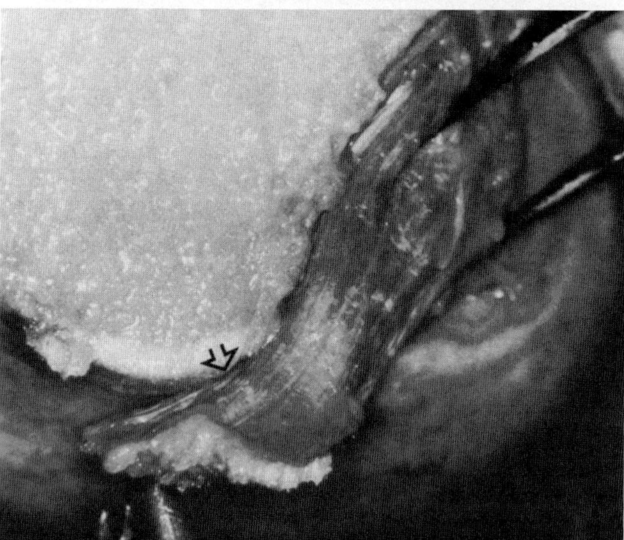

B

FIGURE 1.23. A: Anterior view of a right knee with tibial attachment of the anterior cruciate ligament avulsed from the tibia, demonstrating the "foot" region. **B:** Lateral view of the same knee with the anterior cruciate ligament held in the normal position for full knee extension. The *open arrow* is on the area of potential impingement.

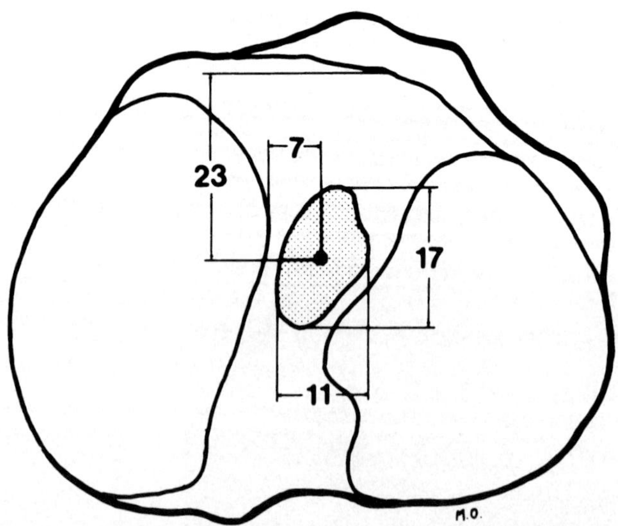

FIGURE 1.22. Tibial attachment of the anterior cruciate ligament, with measurements in millimeters as determined by Odensten. (From Odensten M, Gillquist J. Functional anatomy of the anterior cruciate ligament and a rationale for reconstruction. *J Bone Joint Surg Am* 1985;67:257–261, with permission.)

niques. If an anteriorly placed drill hole is used with a graft whose fibers do not process a foot-type region, the graft will be predisposed to impingement on the roof of the intercondylar notch. As shown in Figure 1.24, the borders of a straight graft material (dashed line) impinge on the notch with the knee in full extension. However, with the same starting point, the fibers of a normal ACL can slip under this point as a result of their sweeping nature. Morgan et al. (49) determined that at 90° of knee flexion

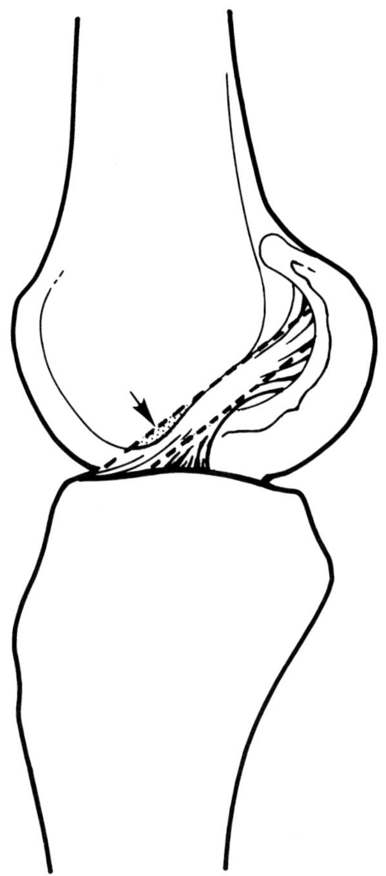

FIGURE 1.24. Replacement of an anterior cruciate ligament (ACL) "foot" region by a straight graft. If the anterior fibers of the ACL are used as a guide for the drill hole, the *dashed line* representing the anterior edge of the new graft is seen to intersect with the notch when the knee is in full extension. This dotted area *(arrow)* is the location of possible impingement.

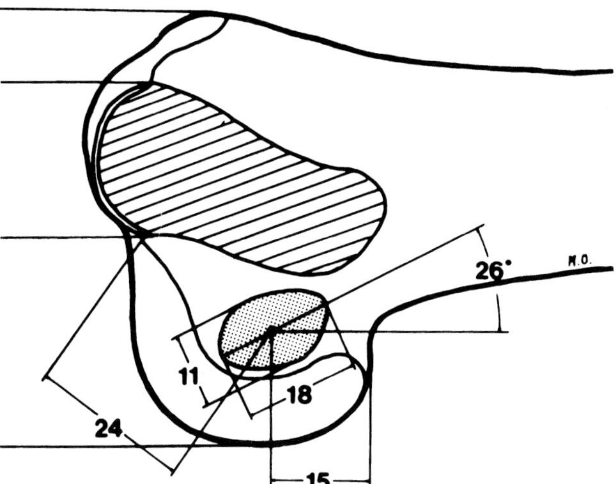

FIGURE 1.25. Femoral attachment of the anterior cruciate ligament as determined by Odensten. The measurements are in millimeters. (From Odensten M, Gillquist J. Functional anatomy of the anterior cruciate ligament and a rationale for reconstruction. *J Bone Joint Surg Am* 1985;67:257–261, with permission.)

and regardless of size, the center of a tibial tunnel should be 7 mm anterior to the anterior border of the PCL. This is within the ACL footprint but also keeps the tibial tunnel placed to avoid impingement. Jackson and Gasser (50) agree and feel this point is approximately 40% of the width of the tibia on a lateral view.

The femoral attachment of the ACL is smaller and located just in front of the "over the top" position (Fig. 1.25). Because of the different plane of attachment for the ACL here, this arrangement leads to the well-known twist of the ACL fibers when the knee moves from extension to flexion (46) (Fig. 1.26). There is also a twist of the ACL fibers in the coronal plane with external rotation of the fibers by approximately 90° as they approach the tibial surface (28). In 1986, van Rens et al. (51) reported that cutting of all ligaments in dogs except the ACL and letting the tibia hang free resulted in 180° derotation. There is a similar relationship in the human knee, which agrees

with the 90° twist of fibers described by Odensten and shown in Figure 1.27.

In the sagittal plane, the average angle between the long axis of the femur and the ACL with the knee flexed 90° is 28±4° (47). With the knee at 90° of flexion, the ACL runs approximately 35° to the tibia. At full extension, the angle is about 60° to the tibia (49). Because Blumensaat's line is approximately 30° to 40° to the long axis of the femur, the angles predict the ACL will run right along the roof of the notch in extension.

The PCL insertional anatomy in some ways is more complex and less well understood than that of the ACL. Most of the depictions are done from two-dimensional pictures that do not relate many of the nuances of the insertions. The femoral attachment is half-moon shaped with a very sharp, discrete posterior (or proximal) border (Figs. 1.28, 1.29). This insertion anatomy shows that no fibers of a reconstruction should ever be posterior to this line. The femoral attachment size is opposite to the ACL in that the femoral attachment is much larger than the tibial attachment (48). The superior (or anterior) border runs vertically and does not attach just to the inner wall of the medial femoral condyle, as frequently depicted in diagrams, but to the roof of the notch as well (Fig. 1.30). Another confusing issue is the ligament of Humphrey. This is the large ligament from the posterior horn of the lateral meniscus that travels anterior to the PCL to attach on the medial femoral condyle. If this is removed, the true PCL attachment appears a little less close to the articular surface at the middle aspect of the inner wall on the

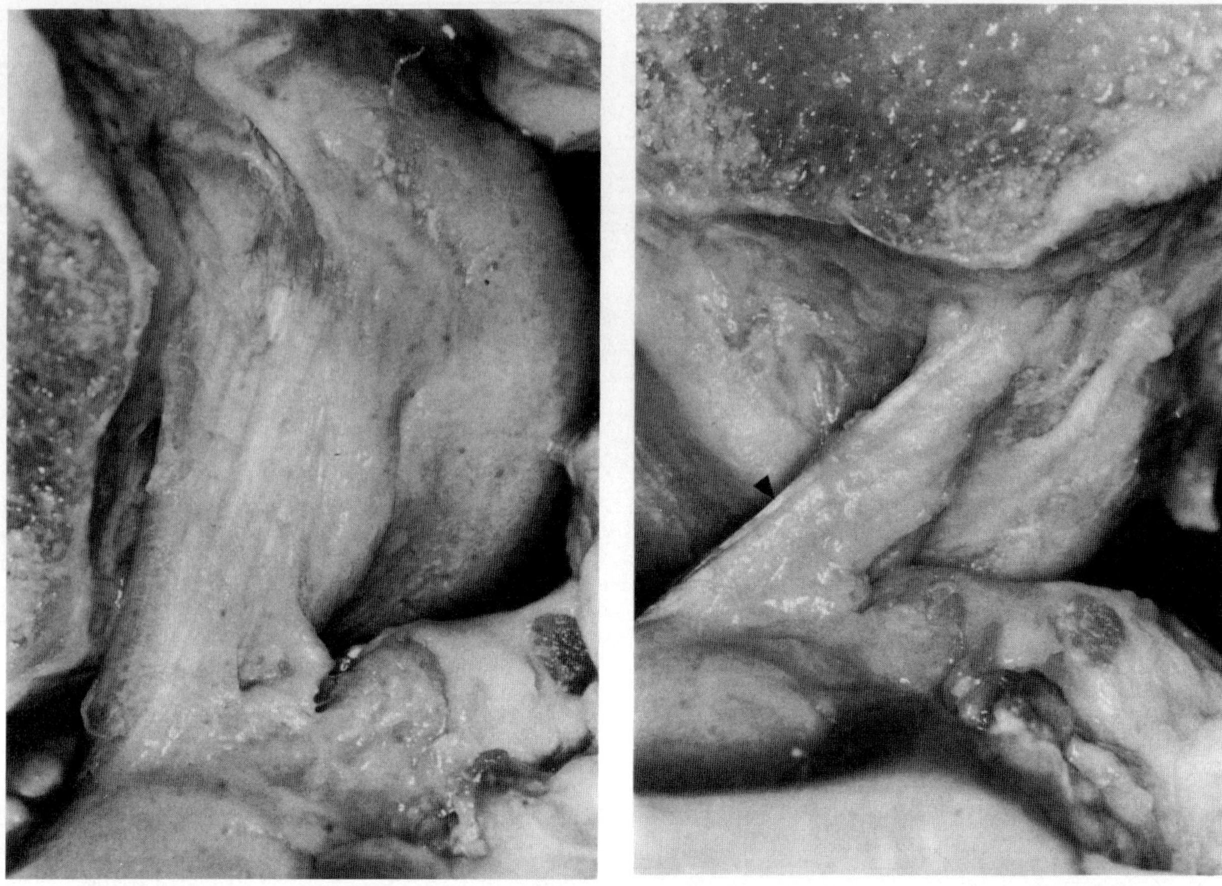

FIGURE 1.26. A: A right knee in full extension with the medial femoral condyle removed. **B:** The same knee in 90° of flexion, showing the twist of the anterior cruciate ligament fibers. The *arrowhead* indicates the anteromedial fibers, which are taut.

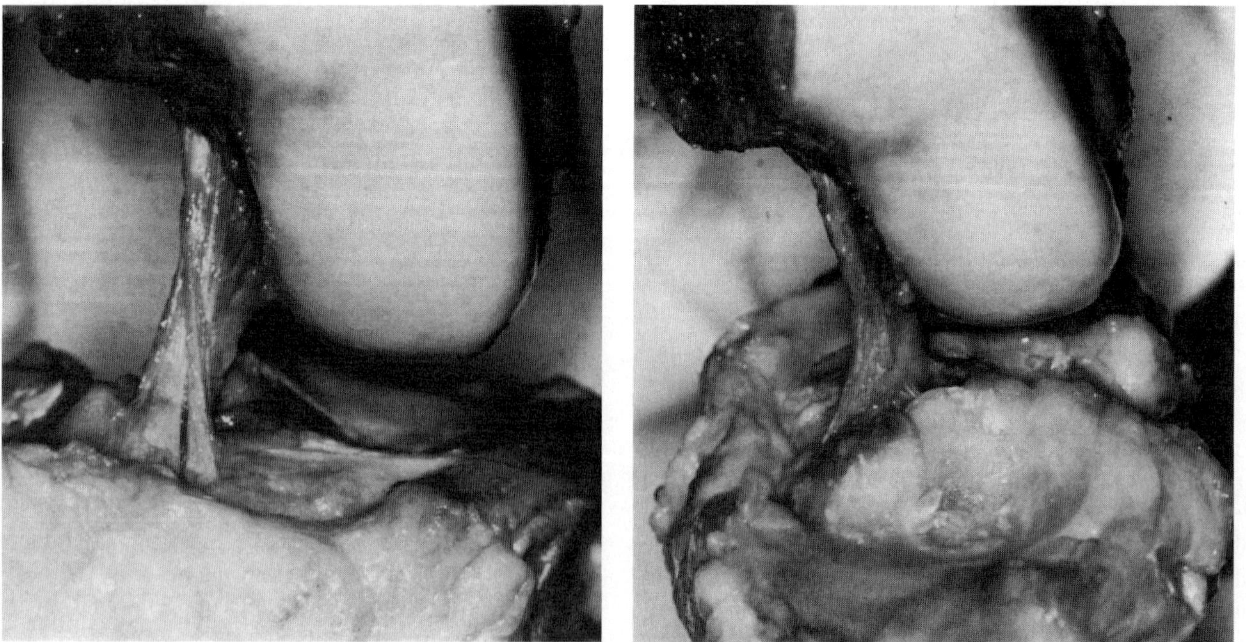

FIGURE 1.27. A: Anterior view of a left knee. The medial femoral condyle and all ligaments except the anterior cruciate ligament have been removed. The tibia is being held in its normal position. **B:** The same knee with the tibia allowed to rotate freely. Notice the 90° internal rotation of the tibia in relation to the femur.

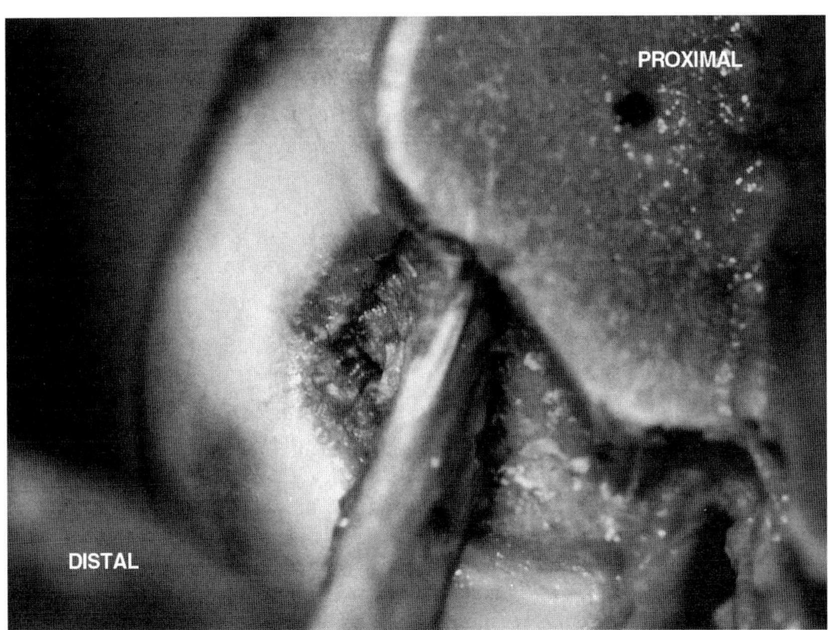

FIGURE 1.28. Left knee with the lateral femoral condyle removed. The tibial attachment of the posterior cruciate ligament has been moved anteriorly to show the posterior fiber attachment on the femur. Notice the very vertical line of posterior attachment when the knee is viewed at 90° of flexion.

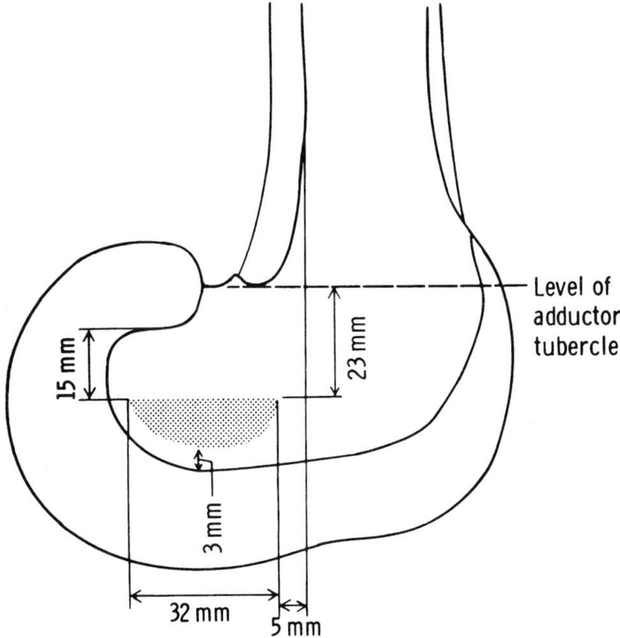

FIGURE 1.29. Femoral attachment of the posterior cruciate ligament. (From Girgis FG, Marshall JL, Al Monajem ARS. The cruciate ligaments of the knee joint: anatomical functional and experimental analysis. *Clin Orthop* 1975;106: 216–231, with permission.)

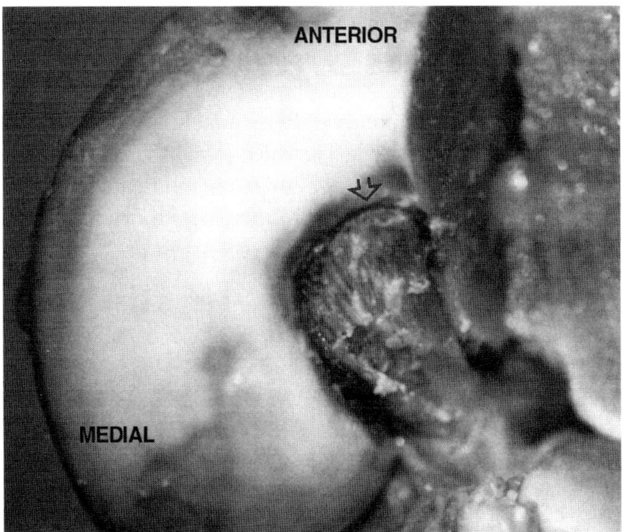

FIGURE 1.30. Left knee with the lateral femoral condyle removed. The *closed arrow* is at the top of the notch, showing the attachment of some of the fibers of the posterior cruciate ligament.

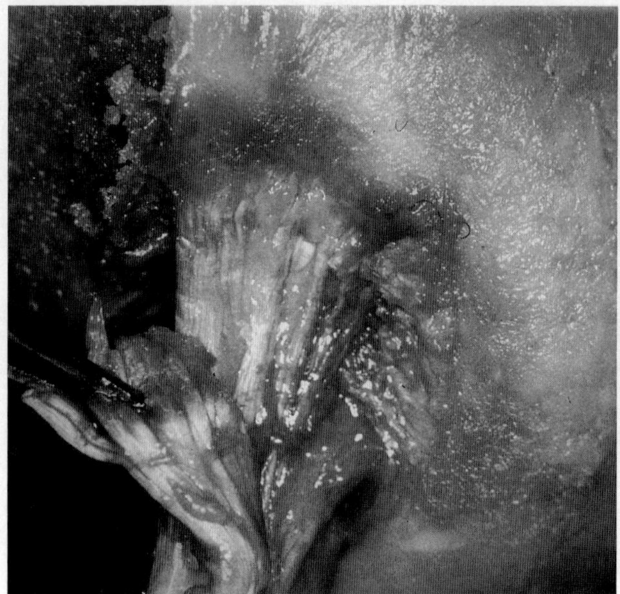

FIGURE 1.31. Right knee with the lateral femoral condyle removed. The forceps hold the ligament of Humphrey, which has been removed from the condyle.

medial femoral condyle. However, the attachment is still very close to the articular surface at the top of the notch (Fig. 1.31). Figure 1.32 is a dissection with the outline of the medial femoral condyle PCL attachments darkened with ink and the fibers cut. The ruler shows the general size of the attachment, and the two guide pins indicate how two femoral tunnels can be drilled to recreate a more anatomic femoral attachment during a PCL reconstruction.

The tibial attachment is rectangular and is at the most posterior and inferior aspect of the joint. It is still intraarticular, however, and lies in a sulcus between the medial and lateral plateaus (Fig. 1.33). A lateral radiograph of the PCL attachments outlined by wire is shown in Figure 1.34, which emphasizes the inferior location of the PCL tibial attachment.

Fiber Orientation

Many investigators have described anatomically separate bands in the ACL and the PCL (46,52,53). For the ACL, the bands are called *anteromedial* and *posterolateral*, with some including an intermediate band (54). The appearance of anatomically different bands may be caused by the increased amount of loose connective tissue (i.e., endotenon) that is seen in human cruciate ligaments (34,43). Although there is controversy about the anatomic division of the ligament, it seems agreed that the ACL has "functional bands" such that tension is variable among fiber bundles within the ligament during range of motion; the anteromedial band is tighter in flexion and the posterolateral band is tighter in extension (35,46,53) (Fig. 1.26).

Hughston et al. (55) refers to the PCL as having an anterolateral band and a posteromedial band. In extension, the posterior fibers are taut, whereas the bulk of the ligament is relaxed (46,55) (Fig. 1.35). This contributes to the well-known curve of the PCL seen on magnetic resonance imaging (MRI) as the ligament is traced from the tibia to the femur. This occurs because the knee is imaged in extension. Conversely, the more posterior fibers become lax in flexion, whereas the remainder (anterolateral) becomes taut.

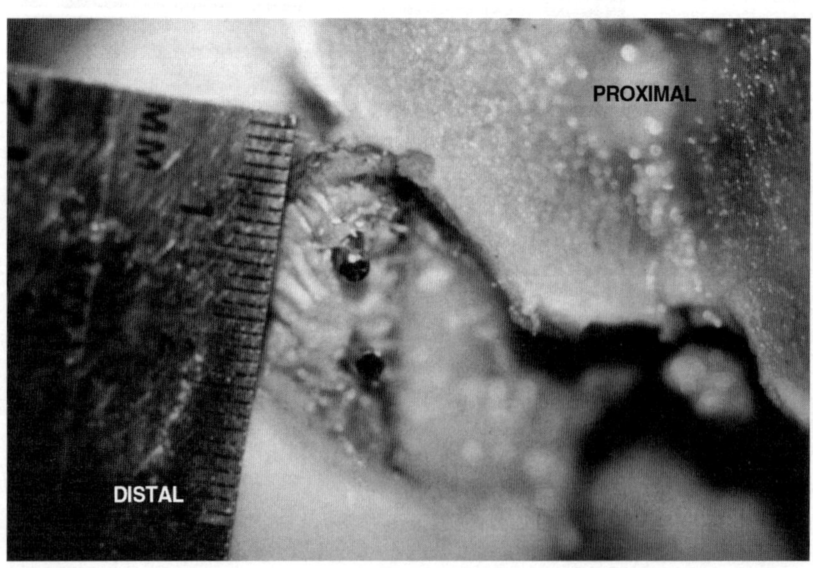

FIGURE 1.32. Left knee with the lateral femoral condyle removed. Two guide pins have been placed in the posterior cruciate ligament footprint. The ruler is a reference for overall size of the footprint. Each of the pins could be overdrilled for a two-tunnel posterior cruciate ligament reconstruction.

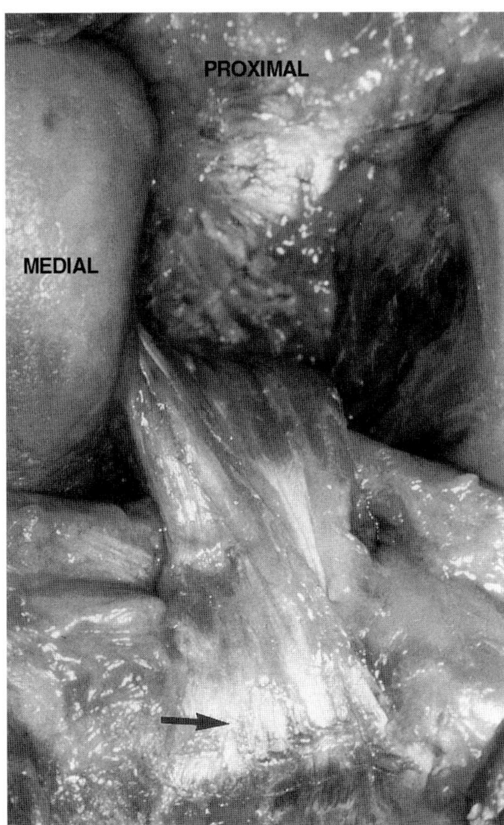

FIGURE 1.33. Posterior view of a right knee. The *arrow* is on the tibial attachment just above the posterior ridge.

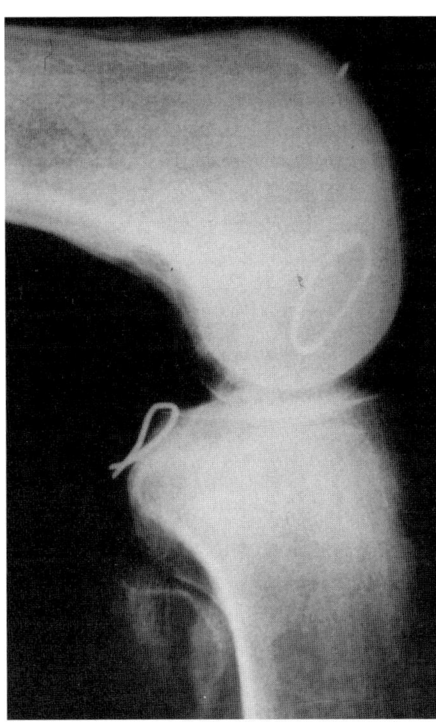

FIGURE 1.34. Lateral radiograph with the femoral and tibial attachments of the posterior cruciate ligament outlined with wire.

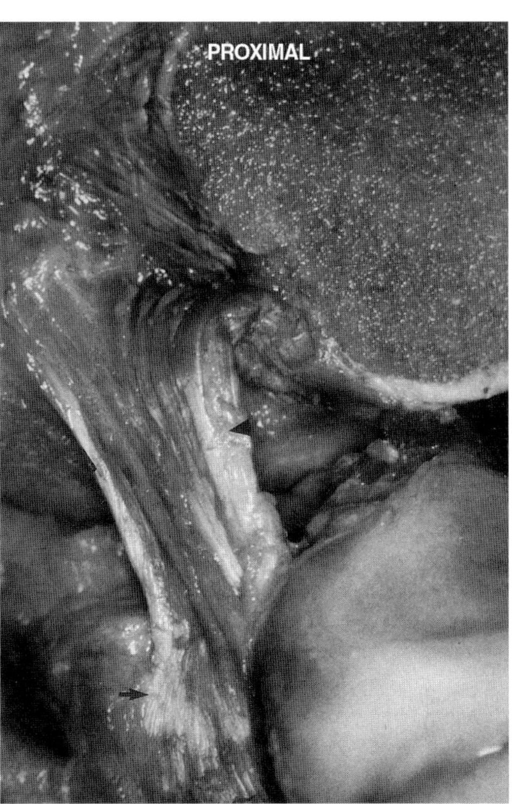

FIGURE 1.35. Right knee with the lateral femoral condyle removed. The tibial attachment fibers are shown by the *closed arrow*. The knee is in extension, and the tight posteromedial fibers *(small arrow)* and the loose anterolateral fibers *(arrowhead)* can be seen. These fibers show why the posterior cruciate ligament appears more curved in extension.

MENISCUS

The menisci are C-shaped wedges of fibrocartilage with direct tibial attachments at each horn. They are also attached to the articular margin of the tibia through coronary ligaments. Each has a thick periphery that tapers to a thin inner rim. The medial meniscus has a much thinner anterior horn region compared with the large posterior horn. The lateral meniscus is more uniform in dimension from anterior to posterior aspects. A study by Kohn and Moreno (56) nicely depicts the exact locations of attachment of the horns as shown in Figure 1.36. The posterior horn of the medial meniscus is directly behind the medial spine next to the posterior cruciate ligament. The anterior horn is flat and inserted into the anterior tibia off the articular margin. The anterior horn of the lateral meniscus blends with the tibial attachment of the ACL and attaches just anterior to the lateral spine. The posterior horn inserts off the posterior aspect of the lateral spine anterior to the PCL.

Although there is a "bare" area at the popliteal hiatus, the anteroinferior and posterosuperior popliteomeniscal

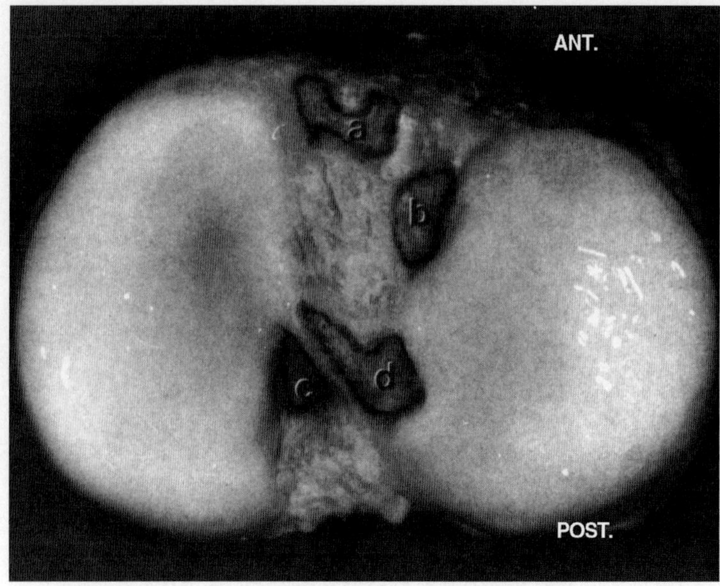

FIGURE 1.36. Right tibia viewed from the superior surface. The anterior *(a)* and posterior *(c)* medial meniscus attachments and the anterior horn *(b)* and posterior horn *(d)* of the lateral meniscus are shown.

fascicles are important attachments to the popliteus tendon (57–59) (Fig. 1.12). The lateral meniscus is not bound to the lateral collateral ligament (as the medial meniscus is bound to the deep medial collateral) and is therefore much more mobile in the anteroposterior direction on the tibia. Thompson et al. (60) used MRI images to determine that the mean medial meniscus excursion is about 5 mm in the anteroposterior plane in flexion and extension. The mean lateral meniscus excursion is about 11 mm. The relative motion of the anterior horn of each meniscus is greater than that of the posterior horn. The posterior horn of the lateral meniscus is connected to the medial femoral condyle by one or both of the meniscofemoral ligaments. The ligament of Humphrey anterior to the PCL and the ligament of Wrisberg courses posterior to the PCL.

The menisci are approximately 75% collagen, about 90% of which is type I collagen (61). The fibers are primarily oriented in a circumferential pattern and, because of their central bony attachments, effectively resist being displaced out of the joint when force is applied through the femur. This is what is known as resisting "hoop stress." Although most of the fibers are longitudinal, there are radially oriented fibers that tie these circumference fibers together and help prevent longitudinal splitting (62).

The vascular supply to the menisci comes primarily from the lateral and medial genicular vessels, including the superior and inferior branches (63). These give rise to a perimeniscal capillary plexus that supplies the peripheral border of the menisci (Fig. 1.37). The vascular penetration of the medial meniscus varies from 10% to 30% of

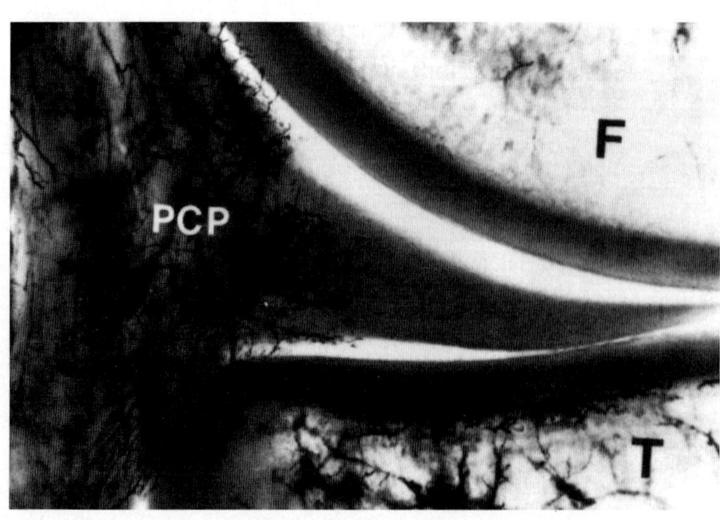

FIGURE 1.37. The perimeniscal capillary plexus *(PCP)*, femur *(F)*, and tibia *(T)* are shown. (From Arnoczky SP, Warren RF. Microvasculature of the human meniscus. *Am J Sports Med* 1982;10:90–95, with permission.)

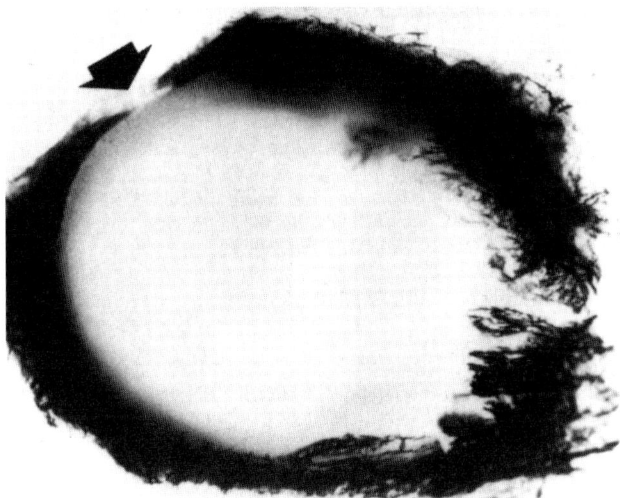

FIGURE 1.38. A superior view of a right lateral meniscus. The *arrow* is on the bare area of the hiatus. Notice the increased vascularity of the horn attachments. (From Arnoczky SP, Warren RF. Microvasculature of the human meniscus. *Am J Sports Med* 1982;10:90–95, with permission.)

the width of the body of the meniscus. The anterior and posterior horns receive a more extensive vascular supply. A small, 1- to 3-mm vascular synovial tissue fringe covers the periphery of the meniscus but does not contribute blood supply to the meniscus itself. The lateral meniscus is similar to the medial in many respects. The vascular penetration of the lateral meniscus is 10% to 25% of the width. This is altered in the posterolateral corner of the popliteal hiatus, where there is an avascular area in the peripheral wall immediately adjacent to the popliteal tendon (Fig. 1.38).

REFERENCES

1. Warren LF, Marshall JL. The supporting structures and layers on the medial side of the knee. *J Bone Joint Surg Am* 1979;61:56–62.
2. Brantigan OC, Voshell AF. The mechanics of the ligaments and menisci of the knee joint. *J Bone Joint Surg* 1941;23–44.
3. Brantigan OC, Voshell AF. The tibial collateral ligament: its function, its bursae, and its relation to the medial meniscus. *J Bone Joint Surg* 1943;25:121–131.
4. Reider B, Marshall JL, Koslin RT, et al. The anterior aspect of the knee joint. *J Bone Joint Surg Am* 1981;63:351–356.
5. Warren LF, Marshall JL, Girgis F. The prime static stabilizer of the medial side of the knee. *J Bone Joint Surg Am* 1974;56:665–674.
6. Kennedy JC, Fowler PJ. Medial and anterior instability of the knee. *J Bone Joint Surg Am* 1971;53:1257–1270.
7. Arms S, Boyle J, Johnson R, et al. Strain measurement in the medial collateral ligament of the human knee: an autopsy study. *J Biomech* 1983;16:491–496.
8. Bartel DL, Marshall JL, Schieck RA, et al. Surgical repositioning of the medial collateral ligament. *J Bone Joint Surg Am* 1977;59:107–116.
9. Müller W. *The knee: form, function, and ligament reconstruction.* Berlin: Springer-Verlag, 1983.
10. Hughston JC, Eilers AF. The role of the posterior oblique ligament in repairs of acute medial (collateral) ligament tears of the knee. *J Bone Joint Surg Am* 1973;55:923–940.
11. Last RJ. Some anatomical details of the knee joint. *J Bone Joint Surg Br* 1948;30:683–688.
12. Kaplan EB. Some aspects of the functional anatomy of the human knee joints. *Clin Orthop* 1962;23:18–29.
13. Slocum DB, Larson RL, James SI. Late reconstruction of ligamentous injuries of the medial compartment of the knee. *Clin Orthop* 1974;100:23–55.
14. Heller L, Langman J. The menisco-femoral ligaments of the human knee. *J Bone Joint Surg Br* 1964;46:307–313.
15. Hollinshead WJ. *Anatomy for surgeons: the back and limbs,* vol III. New York: Harper & Row, 1969.
16. Schutte MJ, Dabezies EJ, Zimmy MI, et al. Neural anatomy of the human anterior cruciate ligament. *J Bone Joint Surg Am* 1987;69:243–247.
17. Hughston JC, Norwood LA Jr. The posterolateral drawer test and external rotational recurvatum test for posterolateral rotary instability. *Clin Orthop* 1980;147:82–87.
18. Maynard MJ, Deng X, Wickiewicz TL, et al. The popliteofibular ligament. Rediscovery of a key element in posterolateral stability. *Am J Sports Med* 1996;24:311–316.
19. Terry G, LaPrade RF. The posterolateral aspect of the knee. *Am J Sports Med* 1996;24:732–739.
20. Veltri DM, Deng XH, Torzilli PA, et al. The role of the popliteofibular ligament in stability of the human knee. A biomechanical study. *Am J Sports Med* 1996;24:19–27.
21. Watanabe Y, Moriya H, Takahashi K, et al. Functional anatomy of the posterolateral structures of the knee. *Arthrosc Assoc North Am* 1993;9:57–62.
22. Baker CL, Norwood LA Jr, Hughston JC. Acute posterolateral rotary instability of the knee. *J Bone Joint Surg Am* 1983;65:614–618.
23. De Lee JC, Riley MB, Rockwood CA Jr. Acute posterolateral rotary instability of the knee. *Am J Sports Med* 1983;11:199–206.
24. Hughston JC, Andrews JR, Cross MJ, et al. Classification of knee ligament instabilities. Part II. The lateral compartment. *J Bone Joint Surg Am* 1976;58:173–179.
25. Seebacher JR, Inglis AE, Marshall JL, et al. The structure of the posterolateral aspect of the knee. *J Bone Joint Surg Am* 1982;64:536–541.
26. Kaplan EB. The iliotibial tract. *J Bone Joint Surg Am* 1958;40:817–832.
27. Terry GC, Hughston JD, Norwood LA. The anatomy of the iliopatellar band and iliotibial tract. *Am J Sports Med* 1986;14:39–45.
28. Noyes FR, Grood ES, Butler DL, et al. Clinical biomechanics of the knee: ligamentous restraints and functional stability. In: Funk FJ Jr, ed. *American Academy of Orthopedic Surgeons' symposium on the athlete's knee.* St. Louis: CV Mosby, 1980:1–35.
29. Wang CJ, Walker PS, Wolf B. The effects of flexion and rotation on the length patterns of the ligaments of the knee. *J Biomech* 1973;6:587–596.
30. Grood ES, Noyes FR, Butler DL, et al. Ligamentous and capsular restraints preventing medial and lateral laxity in intact human cadaver knees. *J Bone Joint Surg Am* 1981;63:1257–1269.
31. Marshall JL, Girgis FG, Zelko RR. The biceps femoris tendon and its functional significance. *J Bone Joint Surg Am* 1972;54:1444–1450.
32. Kaplan EB. The fabellofibular and short lateral ligaments of the knee joint. *J Bone Joint Surg Am* 1961;43:169–179.
33. Palmer I. On injuries to the ligaments of the knee joint: a clinical study. *Acta Chir Scand Suppl* 1938;53.
34. Danylchuck KD, Finlay JB, Kreck JP. Microstructural organization of human and bovine cruciate ligaments. *Clin Orthop* 1978;131:204–298.
35. Arnoczky SP. Anatomy of the anterior cruciate ligament. *Clin Orthop* 1983;172:19–25.
36. Cooper RR, Misol S. Tendon and ligament insertion: a light and electron microscopic study. *J Bone Joint Surg Am* 1970;52:1–20.
37. Arnoczky SP, Rubin RM, Marshall JL. Microvasculature of the cruciate ligaments and its response to injury. *J Bone Joint Surg Am* 1979;61:1221–1229.
38. Marshall JL, Arnoczky SP, Rubin RM, et al. Microvasculature of the cruciate ligaments. *Physician Sports Med* 1979;7:87–91.
39. Scapinelli R. Studies on the vasculature of the human knee joint. *Acta Anat* 1968;70:305–331.
40. Alm A, Stromberg G. Vascular anatomy of the patellar and cruciate ligaments: a microangiographic and histologic investigation in the dog. *Acta Chir Scand Suppl* 1974;44:25–35.
41. Arnoczky SP. Blood supply to the anterior cruciate ligament and supporting structures. *Orthop Clin North Am* 1985;16:15–28.

42. Arnoczky SP. The vascularity of the anterior cruciate ligament and associated structures. In: Jackson DW, Drez D Jr, eds. *The anterior cruciate deficient knee.* St. Louis: CV Mosby, 1987;27–54.
43. Kennedy JC, Alexander IJ, Hayes KC. Nerve supply of the human knee and its functional importance. *Am J Sports Med* 1982;10:329–335.
44. Kennedy JC, Weinberg HW, Wilson AS. The anatomy and functions of the anterior cruciate ligament. *J Bone Joint Surg Am* 1974;56:223–235.
45. Schultz RA, Miller DC, Kerr CS, et al. Mechanoreceptors in human cruciate ligaments. *J Bone Joint Surg Am* 1984;66:1072–1076.
46. Girgis FG, Marshall JL, Al Monajem ARS. The cruciate ligaments of the knee joint: anatomical functional and experimental analysis. *Clin Orthop* 1975;106:216–231.
47. Odensten M, Gillquist J. Functional anatomy of the anterior cruciate ligament and a rationale for reconstruction. *J Bone Joint Surg Am* 1985;67:257–261.
48. Harner CD, Xerogeanes JW, Livesay GA, et al. The human posterior cruciate ligament complex: an interdisciplinary study. Ligament morphology and biomechanical evaluation. *Am J Sports Med* 1995; 23:736–745.
49. Morgan CD, Kalman VR, Grawl D. Definitive landmarks for reproducible tibial tunnel placement in anterior cruciate ligament reconstruction. *Arthroscopy* 1995;11:275–288.
50. Jackson DW, Gasser SI. Tibial tunnel placement in ACL reconstruction. *Arthroscopy* 1994;10:124–131.
51. van Rens TJG, van den Berg AF, Huiskes R, et al. Substitution of the anterior cruciate ligament: long-term histologic and biomechanical study with autogenous pedicled grafts of the iliotibial band in dogs. *Arthroscopy* 1986;2:139–154.
52. Abbot LS, Saunders JB, De CM, et al. Injuries to the ligaments of the knee joint. *J Bone Joint Surg* 1944;26:503–521.
53. Furman W, Marshall JL, Girgis FG. The anterior cruciate ligament: a functional analysis based on postmortem studies. *J Bone Joint Surg Am* 1976;58:179–185.
54. Norwood LA, Cross MJ. Anterior cruciate ligament: functional anatomy of its bundles in rotary instabilities. *Am J Sports Med* 1979;7:23–26.
55. Hughston JC, Bowden JA, Andrews JR, et al. Acute tears of the posterior cruciate ligament. *J Bone Joint Surg Am* 1980;62:438–450.
56. Kohn D, Moreno B. Meniscus insertion anatomy as a basis for meniscus replacement: a morphologic cadaveric study. *Arthroscopy* 1995;11:96–103.
57. Cohn AK, Mains DB. Popliteal hiatus of the lateral meniscus. *Am J Sports Med* 1979;7:221–226.
58. Last RJ. The popliteus muscle and the lateral meniscus. *J Bone Joint Surg Br* 1950;32:93–99.
59. Simonian PT, Susmann PS, Wickiewicz TL, et al. Poplioteomeniscal fasciculi and the unstable lateral meniscus: clinical correlation and magnetic resonance diagnosis. *Arthroscopy* 1997;13:590–596.
60. Thompson WO, Thaete FL, Fu FH, et al. Tibial meniscal dynamics using three-dimensional reconstruction of magnetic resonance images. *Am J Sports Med* 1991;19:210–216.
61. Ingman AM, Ghosh P, Taylor TK. Variation of collagenous and non-collagenous proteins of human knee joint menisci with age and degeneration. *Gerontologia* 1974;20:212–233.
62. Bullough PG, Munuera L, Murphy J, et al. The strength of the menisci of the knee as it relates to their fine structures. *J Bone Joint Surg Br* 1970;52:564–567.
63. Arnoczky SP, Warren RF. Microvasculature of the human meniscus. *Am J Sports Med* 1982;10:90–95.

CHAPTER 2

The Knee as a Biologic Transmission

Scott F. Dye

The living human knee is one of the most complex, intellectually intriguing systems in the biologic realm. Composed of hundreds of billions of living cells, the knee is a system evolutionarily designed to accept, transfer, and dissipate the high loads between and among the femur, tibia, fibula, and patella that occur millions of times each year and still maintain tissue homeostasis (1). It is not surprising that such a system occasionally sustains damage requiring treatment during a lifetime of use. The wonder of the knee is that it maintains and repairs itself remarkably well, often without any modern therapeutic intervention and, in some cases, despite it.

The number of anatomic and functional asymmetries that characterize this joint is impressive. There is, for example, the osseous asymmetry of the cam-shaped femoral condyles on relatively flat tibial plateaus, as well as the longer lateral facet of the patella compared with the medial facet. Many soft tissue asymmetries have a cord-shaped lateral collateral ligament inserting roughly equally proximal and distal to the joint line, whereas the medial collateral ligament is broad and flat and inserts far distal to the joint line in a ratio of approximately 2:7 (Fig. 2.1). The popliteus tendon courses proximally to insert along with the origin of the lateral collateral ligament on the lateral femoral condyle. No such tendon–muscle system exists medially.

The functional kinematics of the knee are also asymmetric. From a sagittal perspective, the knee is neither a pure rolling nor gliding system from extension to flexion, but a combined rolling gliding motion instead occurs, with the point of femoral–tibial contact moving posteriorly in flexion (Fig. 2.2). Further kinematic asymmetry exists, with the femoral–tibial contact point moving posteriorly only 11 mm in the medial compartment compared with 24 mm in the lateral compartment (2). The menisci translate asymmetrically posteriorly in flexion along with the femoral–tibial contact point, but they move only about one-half that distance (i.e., 5 mm for the

medial meniscus and 10 mm for the lateral meniscus) (3). The naturally greater soft tissue constraints of the medial compartment are reflected in the higher rate of medial meniscal injury compared with that of the lateral meniscus. The medial meniscus is less tolerant of increases in anterior—posterior translation and rotation compared with the lateral meniscus, which has an evolutionary design for greater mobility.

Many of the asymmetries of design and function of the knee are explained by the concepts of Alfred Menschik of Vienna, who, according to Werner Müller (4), visualized the knee as a four-bar linkage mechanism (Fig. 2.3). The four bars in this concept represent the anterior cruciate ligament, the posterior cruciate ligament, and the unvarying bony distances between the origin and insertions of these two ligaments on the femur and tibia. The cam shape of the femoral condyles and relatively flat tibial plateaus, as well as the rolling and gliding kinematics, directly result from the mathematical assumption that the knee is a type of four-bar linkage mechanism. In a brilliant insight, equal to any in the field of functional joint morphology, Menschik realized that the asymmetries of the collateral ligament insertion sites could be explained and predicted by the application of a mathematical concept called the Burmester curve. The Burmester curve consists of two third-order derivative curves that together determine regions of relative isometry between the regions on the cam (femoral) side of the knee to the flat (tibial) side of a four-bar linkage such as the knee during the rolling-gliding motion that occurs with flexion and extension (Fig. 2.4). The Burmester curve concept provides a mathematical rationale for the asymmetries of collateral ligament morphology. If dynamic stability is to be provided to a four-bar rolling and gliding mechanism with living tissues such as fibroblasts, which cannot readily accept greater than minimal strain, the insertions must be asymmetric—as nature has developed and as the Burmester curve predicts. The rather surprising finding

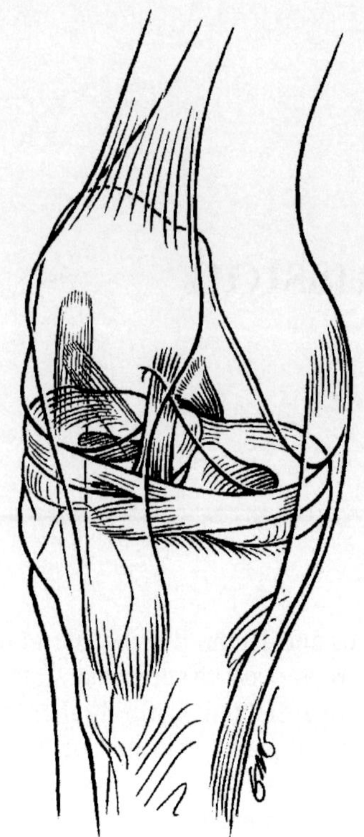

FIGURE 2.1. The knee is a biologic transmission composed of multiple asymmetric components.

was that these same sets of asymmetries of design and function can be found in virtually all living orders of tetrapods (i.e., vertebrates with four limbs). This finding implies that the asymmetric design of the knee is extremely ancient in origin and is profoundly functional over a broad range of biomechanical demands. This

observation can lead to a deeper intellectual and aesthetic appreciation of the design of the human knee.

The overall design of the knee, including cruciate ligaments, menisci, and asymmetric collateral ligaments, was well established by the time of *Eryops*—an amphibian thought to be an ancestor common to all living reptiles, birds, and mammals—more than 320 millions years ago (5). The patella is a relatively recent evolutionary development, appearing in the fossil record approximately 65 millions years ago, at the beginning of the Cenozoic era, with the ascendancy and diversification of mammals. The asymmetry of the larger lateral facet and asymmetric trochlea, as found in living humans, did not develop until approximately 3 millions years ago, when bipedalism was becoming established in hominid primates ancestral to modern humans.

As Larson observed, all of the specific asymmetries of the knee seem to be important for the overall function of the entire system (6). Evolutionary mechanisms seem to quickly delete any structural component that is not providing a function. A good example of this concept is that cetaceans (i.e., whales and dolphins) rapidly lost all remnants of the hind limbs of their tetrapod terrestrial ancestors. This "de-evolution" of the knee occurred in the Cenozoic era over a period of approximately 5 million years, rather rapidly from a geologic standpoint.

Concurrent with the evolution of structural characteristics, neurologic mechanisms have evolved to appraise central nervous system components of the biomechanical and biochemical conditions within the knee. My associates and I undertook a study to map the functional intraarticular sensory characteristics of the human knee by having the structures of my own knees palpated with-

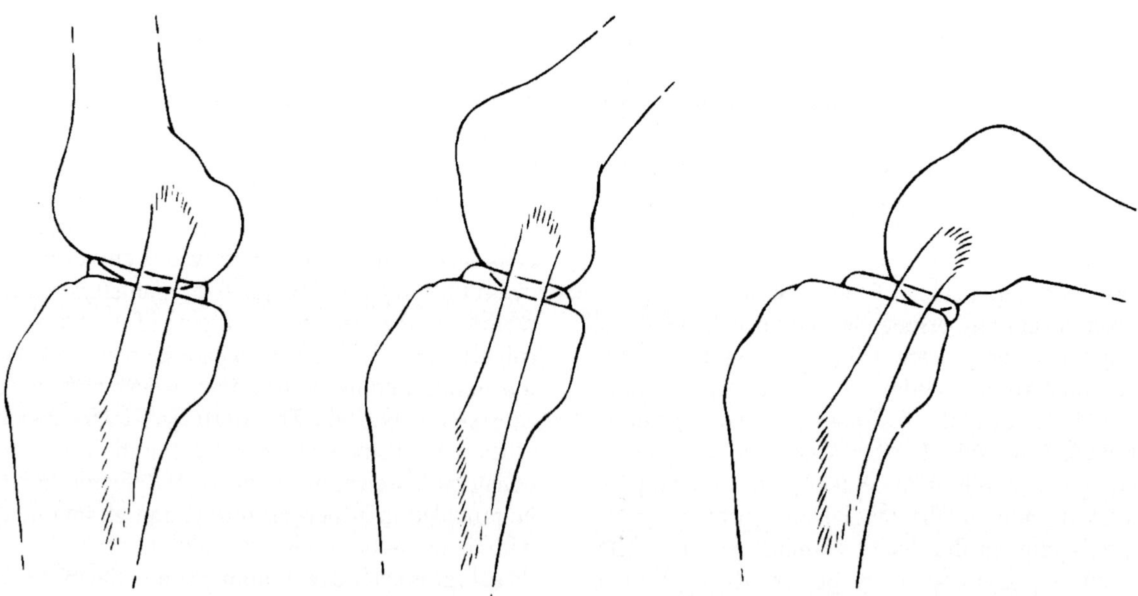

FIGURE 2.2. The functional kinematics of the knee result in posterior displacement of the femoral tibial contact point with flexion. (From Dye SF. An evolutionary perspective of the knee. *J Bone Joint Surg Am* 1987;7:976–983, with permission.)

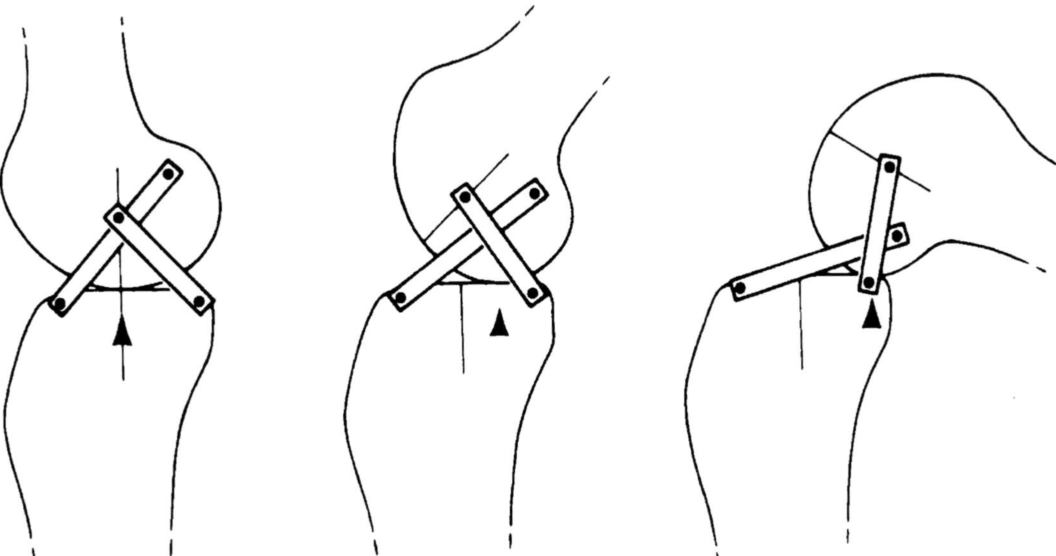

FIGURE 2.3. The knee can be conceived as a type of four-bar linkage mechanism determining the posterior displacement of the femoral tibial contact point from extension to flexion. (From Dye SF. An evolutionary perspective of the knee. *J Bone Joint Surg Am* 1987;7:976–983, with permission.)

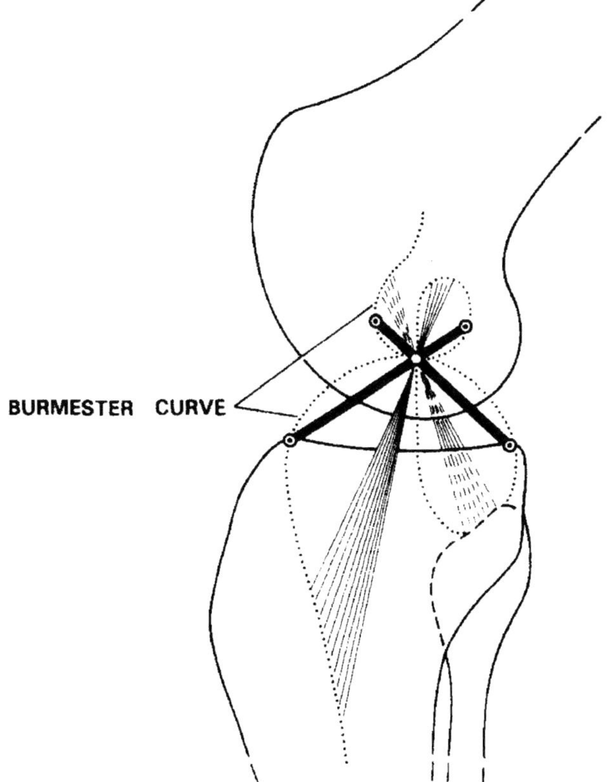

FIGURE 2.4. The Burmester curve is composed of two third-order derivative curves that predict regions of relative isometry between regions on the cam (femoral side) of the knee to that of the flat (tibial side) of the knee. The asymmetric origin insertions of the lateral and medial collateral ligaments are predicted by these areas of relative isometry. (From Dye SF. An evolutionary perspective of the knee. *J Bone Joint Surg Am* 1987;7:976–983, with permission.)

out intraarticular anesthesia (7). Perceived sensation was graded subjectively (scale of 0 for no sensation to 4 for severe pain) with a modifier for localization (A for accurate spacial localization with probing or B for inaccurate localization). Results are provided in Figure 2.5. Most intraarticular structures of the knee, with the exception of the patellar articular cartilage, are sensate. The synovium was particularly sensitive, even to light touch (<100 g of pressure through a probe footprint of 1×3 mm). The cruciate ligaments could be felt when probed and were painful to tugging at the origins and insertion sites, as were the menisci. This work, although from one individual, confirms that intraarticular ligaments and most other intraarticular components are sensate. We speculate that one of the causes for failure of ligamentous reconstructions in some patients may be the lack of restoration of neurosensory characteristics of the surgically created structures. Perhaps some improvements in ligamentous reconstructions about the knee and other joints may be derived from the development of successful techniques to safely restore normal neurosensory qualities to the ligaments.

The function of the knee or any joint can be defined as the capacity of that musculoskeletal system to safely generate, transmit, and dissipate loads while maintaining tissue homeostasis. This capacity can be represented in an easily understandable two-dimensional graph called the *envelope of function* (1). The envelope of function is a load and frequency distribution that defines a range of loading that is compatible with and probably inductive of overall tissue homeostasis of a given joint (Fig. 2.6). The area within the envelope of function can be defined as the

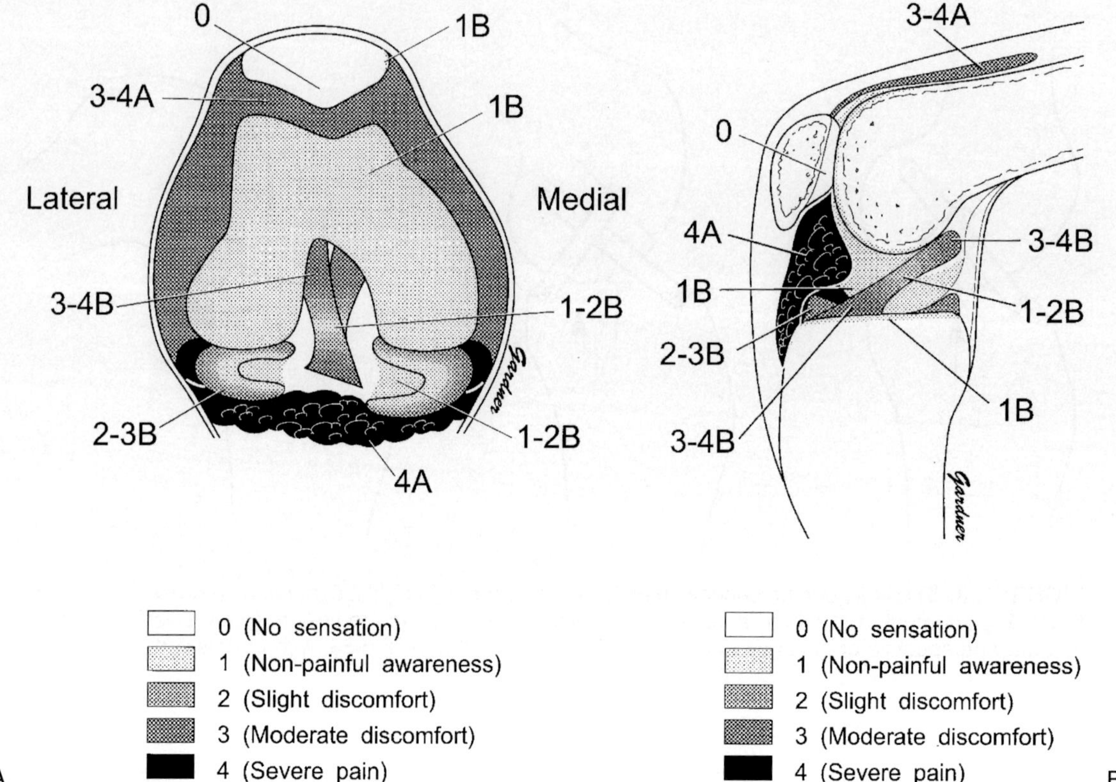

FIGURE 2.5. The conscious neurosensory findings for the intraarticular structures are schematically illustrated for a right knee. **A:** Coronal representation. **B:** Sagittal representation. 0, no sensation; 1, non-painful awareness; 2, slight discomfort; 3, moderate discomfort; 4, severe pain; A, accurate spatial localization; B, poorly localized sensation. (From Dye SF, Vaupel GL, Dye CC. Conscious neurosensory mapping of the internal structures of the human knee without intra-articular anesthesia. *Am J Sports Med* 1998;26:773–777, with permission.)

zone of homeostasis, or zone of homeostatic loading (Fig. 2.7). Loads greater than this but insufficient to cause macrostructural damage can be defined as the *zone of supraphysiologic overload*. An example of such loading is a runner who increases running from 5 to 10 miles per day and who then develops painful increased osseous remodeling of the tibia (i.e., early stages of a stress fracture). Treatment of such a patient consists of decreasing the loading and frequency of loading sufficiently to allow the patient's genetically controlled biologic processes of molecular and cellular restoration to proceed without subversion. Decreasing loading to within the patient's envelope of function allows healing to occur. If sufficiently high loads are applied across a joint, overt macrostructural failure of one or more components may result (e.g., rupture of an anterior cruciate ligament, fracture of a tibial plateau).

The shape of the envelope of function of an individual joint or musculoskeletal system is determined by specific anatomic, kinematic, physiologic, and treatment factors (1). *Anatomic factors* include the micromorphology and macromorphology and associated biomechanical characteristics of all components that comprise a joint, includ-ing ligaments, tendons, articular cartilage, menisci, retinaculum, muscles, nerves, vessels, and bone. Mere restoration of normal structural and biomechanical characteristics of a knee with an injured anterior cruciate ligament is insufficient to restore the envelope of function, as Daniel et al. showed in their landmark study (8). The patients with reconstructed anterior cruciate ligaments who were allowed to return to high-stress sports had greater degenerative changes identified by radiography and technetium scintigraphy than patients who did not have surgery but decreased the loading across their joints. The early development of degenerative changes, despite restoration of biomechanical characteristics (i.e., normal KT-1000 arthrometer data), in Daniel's patients is explained by the lack of full restoration of the envelope of function (Fig. 2.8).

Kinematic factors determine the motion of a joint under load and include the osseous morphology, pattern of sequential tightening of ligaments, and function of the highly complex neuromuscular systems that dynamically keep control of the joint. They comprise the neurosensory and proprioceptive systems, including the cerebrum, cerebellum, basal ganglia, and spinal cord mechanisms,

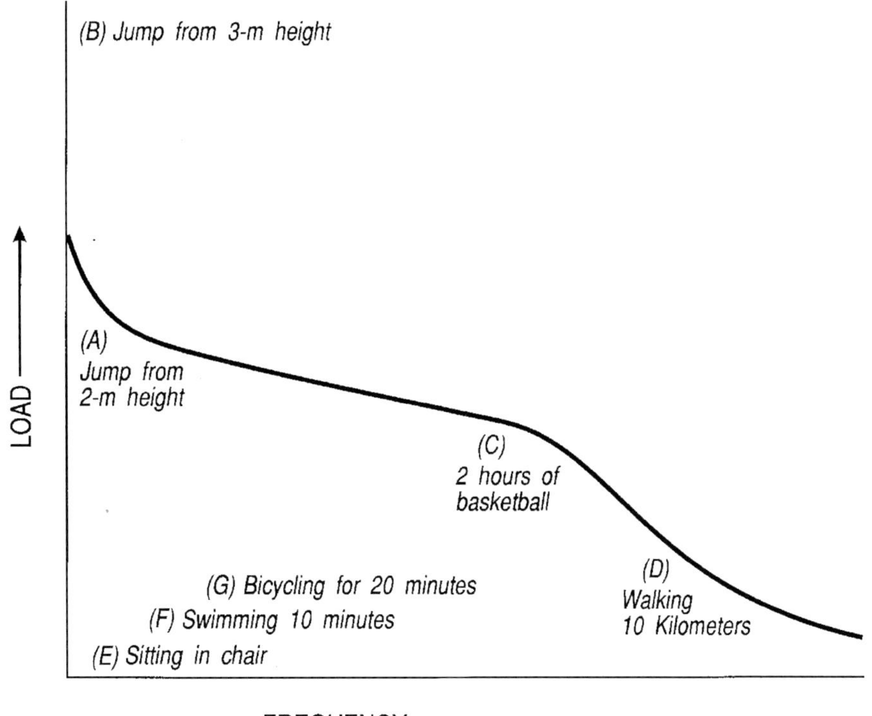

FIGURE 2.6. The graph represents the envelope of function for an athletically active, young adult. The letters represent the loads associated with different activities. All loading examples, except *B*, are within the envelope for this particular knee. The shape of the envelope of function represented is an idealized model. The actual loads transmitted across an individual knee under these different conditions vary because of multiple complex factors, including a dynamic center of gravity, the rate of load application, and the angles of flexion and rotation. The limits of the envelope of function for the joint of an actual patient are probably more complex. *(A)* Jump from a 2-m height. *(B)* Jump from a 3-m height. *(C)* Two hours of basketball. *(D)* Walking 10 km. *(E)* Sitting in a chair. *(F)* Swimming for 10 minutes. *(G)* Bicycling on an exercise bike for 20 minutes. (From Dye SF. The knee as a biologic transmission with an envelope of function. *Clin Orthop* 1996;325:10–18, with permission.)

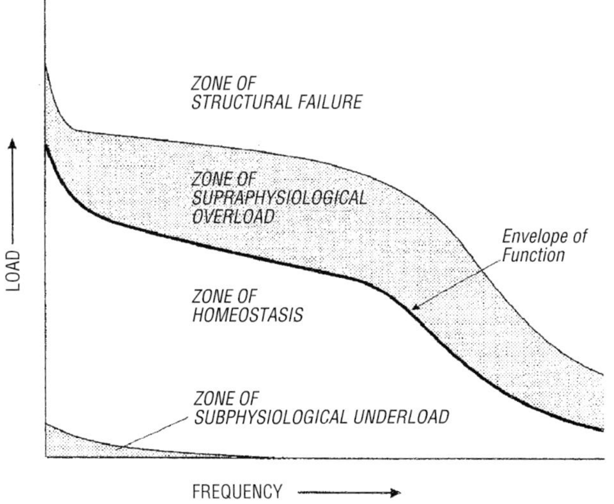

FIGURE 2.7. Graph showing the four different zones of loading across a joint. The area within the envelope of function is the zone of homeostasis. The region of loading greater than that within the envelope of function but insufficient to cause macrostructural damage is the zone of supraphysiologic overload. The region of loading great enough to cause macrostructural damage is the zone of structural failure. The region of decreased loading over time resulting in a loss of tissue homeostasis is the zone of subphysiological underload. (From Dye SF. The knee as a biologic transmission with an envelope of function. A theory. *Clin Orthop* 1996;325:13, with permission.)

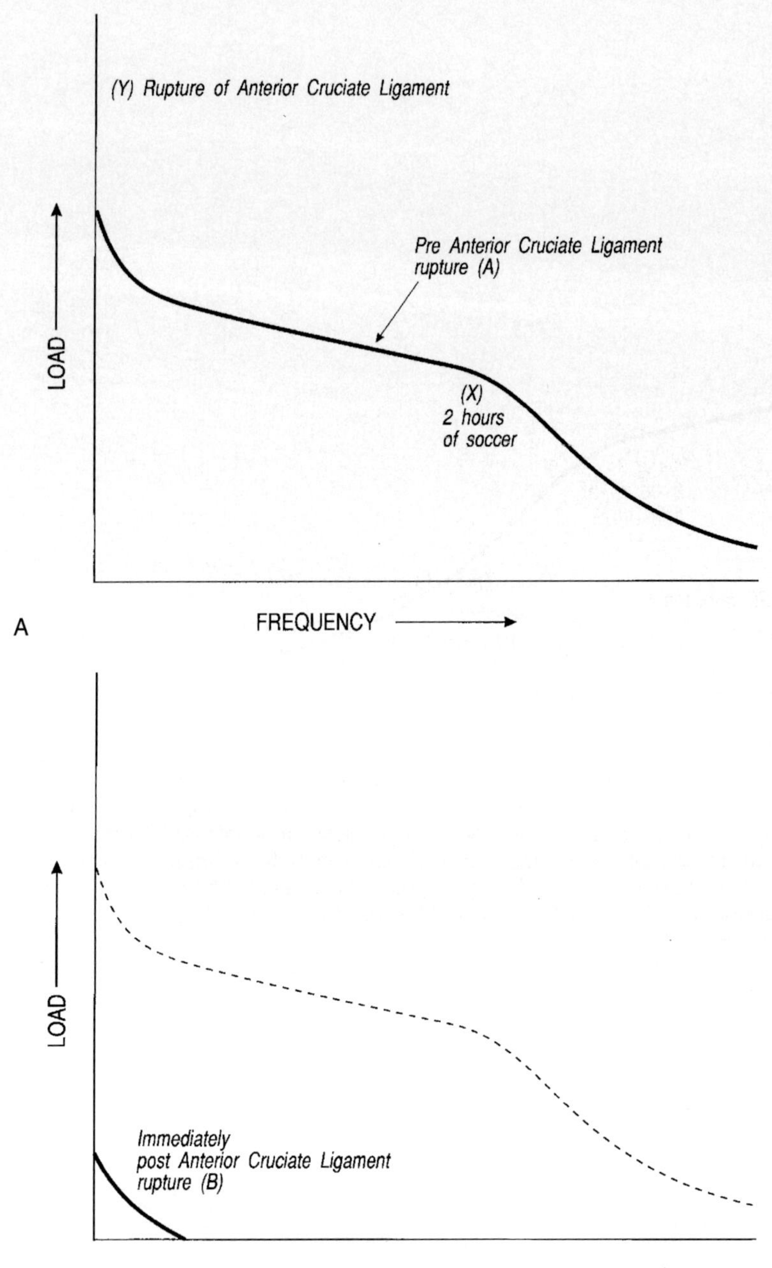

FIGURE 2.8. The dynamic character of the envelope of function is represented for a knee that sustains a rupture of the anterior cruciate ligament. **A:** Preinjury envelope of function. Loading *(X)* represents 2 hours of soccer and is within this knee's preinjury envelope. The loading event *(Y)* represents a single load great enough to cause an acute rupture of the anterior cruciate ligament. **B:** The envelope of function immediately after rupture of the anterior cruciate ligament.

which control the specific and exact temporal sequencing of millions of motor units. Degradation of any of these neuromuscular components (e.g., postoperative muscular atrophy, lack of neurosensory restoration of a reconstructed ligament) can negatively affect the capacity of the entire joint to safely transmit loads, which is reflected in a diminished envelope of function.

Physiologic factors are biochemical and molecular processes that maintain tissue homeostasis and restore tissue homeostasis after mechanical injury or other perturbations. The potency of these systems is unique to each individual. Loading within the envelope of function for a given joint allows the systems to proceed at their most efficient rate. Major surgical intervention, such as reconstruction of the anterior cruciate ligament, represents a significant but reversible physiologic perturbation of the knee. Restoration of joint homeostasis, as documented by normal postoperative technetium scintiscans, is possible after such surgery and associated incremental rehabilitation. Some individuals, however, may have a genetic tendency for development of early degenerative changes, and they are likely to develop osteoarthrosis despite what might have been done for them therapeutically.

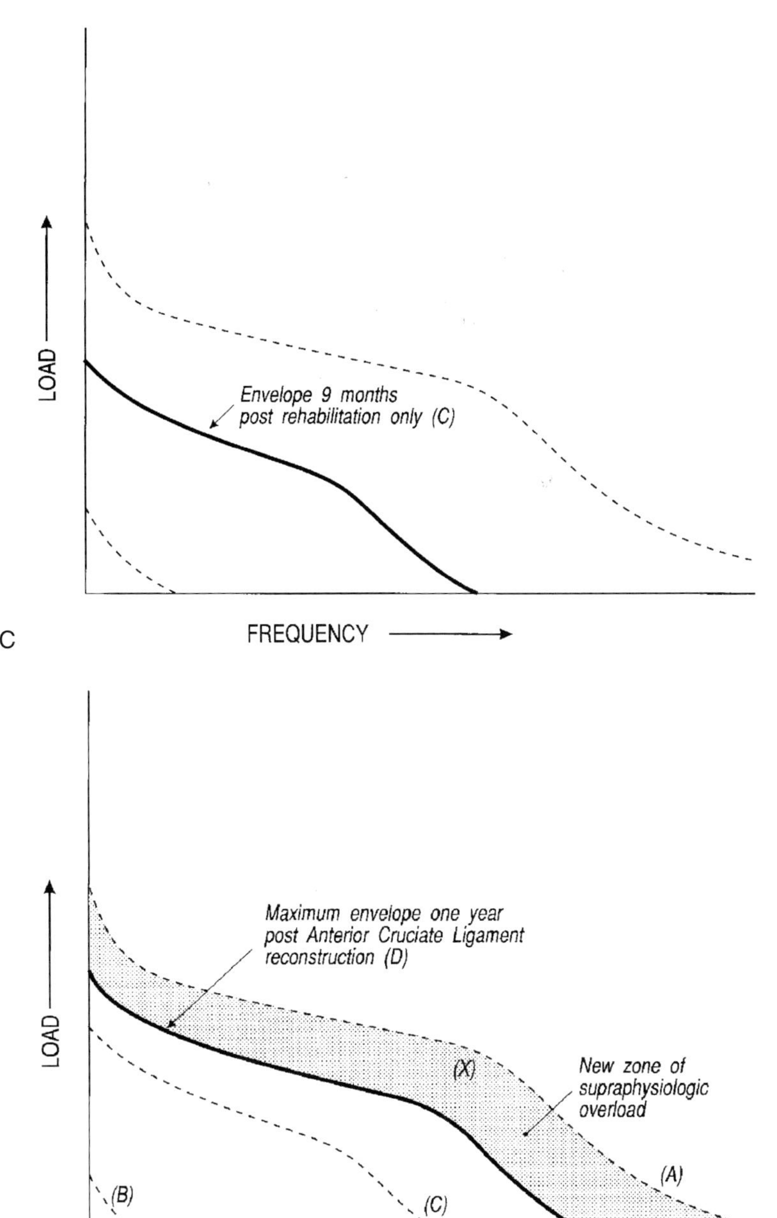

FIGURE 2.8. *Continued.* **C:** The envelope of function 9 months after treatment with a rehabilitation program alone. This envelope has broadened sufficiently to include most activities of daily living and certain low-impact sports, such as bicycling. **D:** The envelope of function 1 year after anterior cruciate ligament reconstructive surgery and postoperative rehabilitation. The envelope in this case has not been fully restored to the preinjury status. The area between the postsurgical and preinjury envelopes represents a zone of supraphysiologic overload, potentially extending to a zone of structural failure. If the patient returns to previous high-impact loading *(X)*, which is now out of the postsurgical envelope of function, the knee would be at risk for early degenerative changes and even for structural failure of the graft. (From Dye SF. The knee as a biologic transmission with an envelope of load acceptance. A theory. *Clin Orthop* 1996;325:1–9, with permission.)

Treatment factors, including operative and nonoperative factors, may also contribute to the restoration of the envelope of function of a given joint after injury. Nonoperative factors include load restriction (i.e., safely protecting the involved joint by loading within its diminished envelope of function); antiinflammatory therapy, including nonsteroidal antiinflammatory medications and tissue cooling; and rehabilitation, including muscle strengthening, stretching, and endurance enhancement, as well as proprioceptive enhancements, including the use of braces and taping. Operative factors include reconstruction of a torn ligament, meniscus repair, articular cartilage surgery, and synovectomy.

The goal of any therapy for the knee and other musculoskeletal systems should be to maximize the envelope of function for that joint or system as safely and predictably as possible (1,9). Current techniques of reconstruction of the anterior cruciate ligament combined with incremental rehabilitation have been shown to produce near normalcy (9,10). However, full and complete restoration to the preinjury state is rarely achieved (11). Future advances in the treatment of injuries, such as rupture of the anterior cruciate ligament or tears of menisci, will depend on better methods of recreating internal structures and on improvements in neuromuscular restoration and enhanced physiologic healing of all components of the living knee transmission system (7,12,13).

REFERENCES

1. Dye SF. The knee as a biologic transmission with an envelope of function. *Clin Orthop* 1996;325:10–18.
2. Shapeero LG, Dye SF, Lipton ML, et al. Functional dynamics of the knee joint by ultrafast cine-CT. *Invest Radiol* 1988;23:118–123.
3. Thompson WO, Thaete FL, Fu FH, et al. Tibial meniscal dynamics using three-dimensional reconstruction of magnetic resonance images. *Am J Sports Med* 1991;19:210–216.
4. Müller WM. *The knee: form, function, and ligament reconstruction.* Berlin: Springer-Verlag, 1983:8–75.
5. Dye SF. An evolutionary perspective of the knee. *J Bone Joint Surg* 1987;7:976–983.
6. Larson RL. The knee—the physiological joint. *J Bone Joint Surg Am* 1983;65:143–144.
7. Dye SF, Vaupel GL, Dye CC. Conscious neurosensory mapping of the internal structures of the human knee without intra-articular anesthesia. *Am J Sports Med* 1998;26:773–777.
8. Daniel DM, Stone ML, Dobson BE, et al. Fate of the ACL-injured patient—a prospective outcome study. *Am J Sports Med* 1994;22:632–644.
9. Dye SF, Wojtys EM, Fu FH, et al. Factors contributing to function of the knee joint after injury or reconstruction of the anterior cruciate ligament. *J Bone Joint Surg Am* 1998;80:1380–1393.
10. Dye SF, Chew MH. Restoration of osseous homeostasis after anterior cruciate ligament reconstruction. *Am J Sports Med* 1993;21:748–750.
11. Frank CB, Jackson DW. The science of reconstruction of anterior cruciate ligament. *J Bone Joint Surg Am* 1997;79:1556–1577.
12. Dye SF. The future of anterior cruciate ligament restoration. *Clin Orthop Rel Res* 1996;325:130–139.
13. Dye SF. Overview of biological intervention in sports medicine. *Sports Med Arthrosc Rev* 1998;6:69–73.

CHAPTER 3

Ligament Biochemistry and Physiology

Monti Khatod and David Amiel

Clinical outcome measures represent the ultimate test of innovations in treatment of ligament injuries. But clinical observations leading to improved therapies cannot occur in a vacuum. Rather, the theoretic basis for clinical innovations aimed at improving outcomes in this field must rest on the foundation provided by a clear understanding of connective tissue biology and mechanics. The required elements of that understanding must embrace tissue structure and function as well as the underlying cell biology. For these reasons, this chapter and several that follow review the current understanding of basic and applied research relating to ligament injury, repair, and reconstruction.

For many years, tendons and ligaments have been classified together as dense, regularly arranged connective tissue (1–3). Although tendons and ligaments are composed primarily fibrillar collagens, they have entirely different functions. Tendons are a conduit, connecting muscle to bone and thereby allowing movement of a joint complex through muscle contraction or relaxation. Ligaments are short bands of fibrous tissue that bind bone to bone and provide support for internal organs. In concert with the bony geometry and the dynamic effects of muscle and tendon (4,5), ligaments limit and guide joint motion.

Collagen is the single most abundant animal protein in mammals, accounting for up to 30% of all proteins (6). Collagen molecules assemble into characteristic fibers responsible for the functional integrity of tissues such as bone, cartilage, skin, ligament, and tendon (7). They contribute a structural framework for most organs. Crosslinks between adjacent molecules are a prerequisite for the collagen fibers to withstand the physical stresses to which they are exposed. A variety of human conditions, normal and pathologic, involve the ability of tissues to repair and regenerate their collagenous framework. Many disabling conditions result from changes in the nature and organization of collagen (6).

STRUCTURE

The histology of periarticular tendons and ligaments is a much-neglected area of investigation. Although many histology texts combine these two tissues as "dense, regular connective tissue" (8–11), certain ligaments and tendons are sufficiently characteristic to be distinguishable from each other based on their histologic appearance (Fig. 3.1).

The following histologic analysis describes some of the basic differences among a variety of tendons and ligaments. The variables considered are collagen bundle width, cell morphology, and size, as well as *crimp*. Crimp is a feature of tendons and ligaments; it represents a regular sinusoidal pattern in the matrix. The periodicity and amplitude of crimp appear to be structure-specific features, and they are best evaluated under polarized light. A simple functional explanation for this accordion-like pattern in the matrix is that it provides a "buffer" in which slight longitudinal elongation may occur without fibrous damage. It also provides a mechanism for control of tension and acts as a "shock absorber" along the length of the tissue. When physiologic mechanical limits of this crimp are exceeded, however, irreversible damage occurs and the physical properties of the tissue are changed (12).

Although tendons and ligaments have crimping within their fascicles, there appear to be differences in the crimp pattern between these two structures (13). In the canine anterior cruciate ligament (ACL) and patellar tendon, two patterns of crimping are observed. The centrally located fascicles in the ACL are straight or undulated in a planar wave pattern (Fig. 3.2), whereas those located at the periphery are arranged in a helical wave pattern (Fig. 3.3). In the patellar tendon, all the fascicles are found to undulate in the helical wave pattern.

The following histologic description refers to rabbit tendons and ligaments unless otherwise specified. Microscopic examination of patellar tendon sections that have

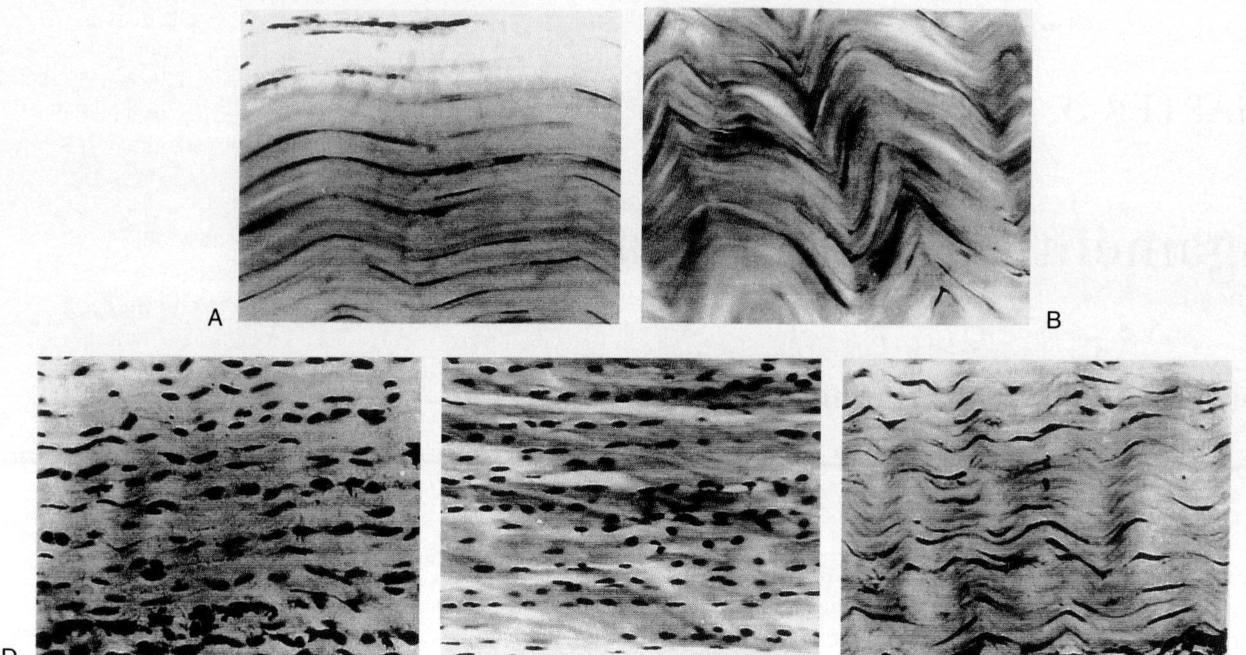

FIGURE 3.1. Mid-substance frozen sections of various tendons and ligaments (hematoxylin and eosin stain, original magnification ×250). **A:** Patellar tendon. **B:** Achilles tendon. **C:** Posterior cruciate ligament. **D:** Anterior cruciate ligament. **E:** Medial collateral ligament. (From Amiel D, Frank CB, Harwood FL, et al. Tendons and ligaments: a morphological and biochemical comparison. *J Orthop Res* 1984:1: 257, with permission.)

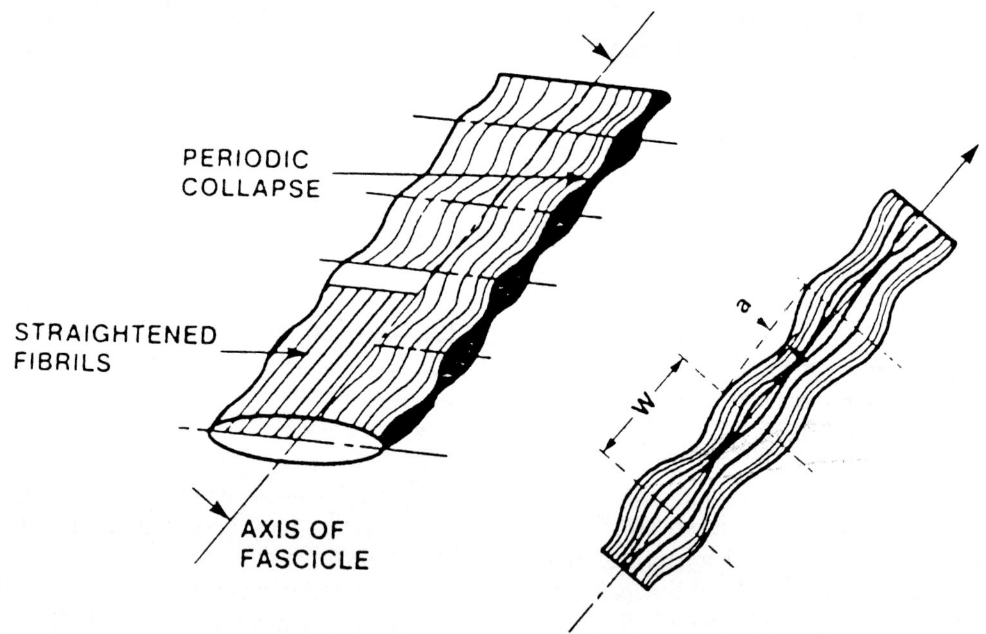

FIGURE 3.2. Schematic diagram of the collagenous fascicles shows the planar waveform model. (From Yahia LH, Drouin G. Microscopical investigation of canine anterior cruciate ligament and patellar tendon: collagen fascicle morphology and architecture. *J Orthop Res* 1989;7:243–251, with permission.)

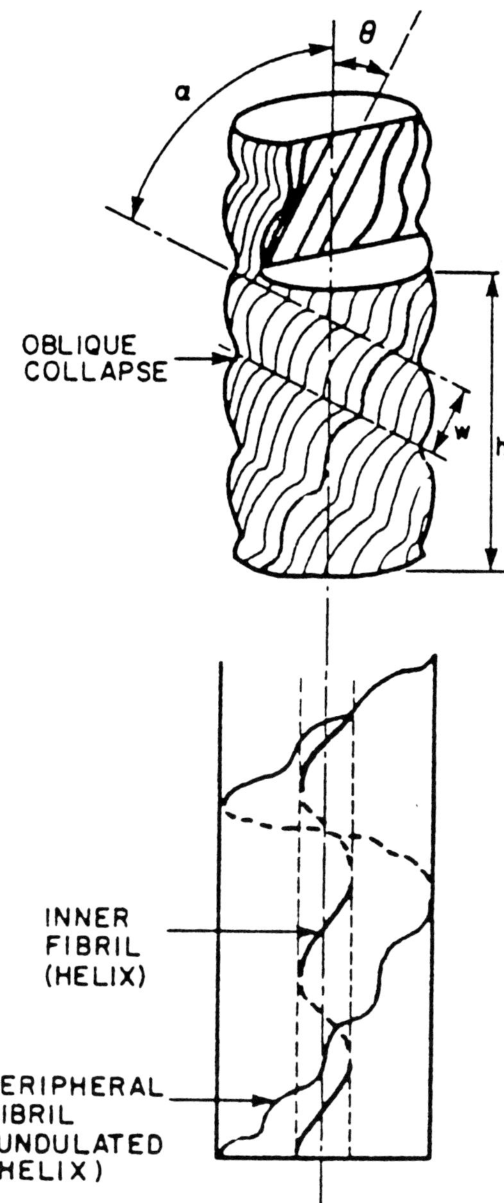

FIGURE 3.3. Schematic diagram of the collagenous fascicle shows the helical wave form model. θ, helix angle; α, inclination angle; w, wavelength; h, apparent half-pitch. (From Yahia LH, Drouin G. Microscopical investigation of canine anterior cruciate ligament and patellar tendon: collagen fascicle morphology and architecture. *J Orthop Res* 1989;7:243–251, with permission.)

been stained with hematoxylin and eosin or evaluated directly under polarized light reveals the presence of longitudinally oriented bundles of collagenous tissue. These bundles are approximately 20 µm wide and have the characteristic crimp pattern of regular connective tissue. In patellar tendon, the crimp period is approximately 120 µm long, with a corresponding amplitude of about 15 µm. On either side of the bundles or fascicles are spindle-shaped fibroblasts that are approximately 25 µm long.

They are aligned longitudinally. Cytoplasm is indistinct, and only nuclei can be seen. More cellular areas within areolar connective tissue are observed. These sites, which are actually investing layers of tissue, are called *peritendineum* (Fig. 3.4) and have been previously described as a site of reserve cells (14). They also mark the site of nerve and blood supply to the tendon.

Rabbit Achilles tendon demonstrates cell morphology, cell size, bundle width, and crimp period that are similar to those of patellar tendon. The crimp amplitudes of these tissues are different, with the Achilles tendon having almost three times (40 µm) the wave height relative to the patellar tendon. This difference may be related to an increased margin of shock absorbance for the Achilles tendon.

Histologic assessment of the ACL demonstrates longitudinally oriented bundles of collagen with a width of about 20 µm as seen in the patellar tendon. The crimp period in the ACL, however, is considerably shorter (45 to 60 µm), and the amplitude is less than 5 µm. Fibroblasts are located on either side of the collagenous bundles, but the ligament is considerably more cellular than the tendon (Fig. 3.5). ACL fibroblasts are round to ovoid and are substantially different in appearance from the fibroblasts in the patellar tendon. They are about 5 to 8 µm in diameter and 12 to 15 µm in length. Cells are arranged longitudinally along the borders of the fascicles. Like the patellar tendon, groups of cells, which concentrate in areolar connective tissue, are observed (Fig. 3.5). They may be the ligamentous correlates to the peritendineum areas.

The medial collateral ligament (MCL) of the knee is notable for rod-shaped and spindle-shaped cells that are intermediate in length compared with patellar tendon and ACL cells. The MCL has cells that are 15 µm long and 25 µm wide. The crimp period measures approximately 45 µm, with a 10-µm amplitude, and the collagen bundle width is approximately 20 µm, as seen in the other structures discussed. Measurements of cell size, shape, crimp specifics, and bundle width of the tendons and ligaments are provided in Table 3.1.

These substantial differences in morphology and ultrastructure may reflect the functional and environmental differences between these two periarticular ligaments, the ACL and MCL. The cellular morphologic characteristics of the MCL are those of all fibroblasts, whereas the ACL cellular characteristics are similar to fibrocartilage cells. These observations led to a series of profound and important questions concerning the differences in function, homeostasis, and repair between the ACL and MCL.

The biochemical parameters used to assess the constitutional properties of collagenous tissue include collagen structure and type, collagen reducible and nonreducible crosslink analysis, and proteoglycan content. The value of each of these variables is related to its importance in the study of soft tissue injury and healing and study of the response to exercise and the deleterious effects of immo-

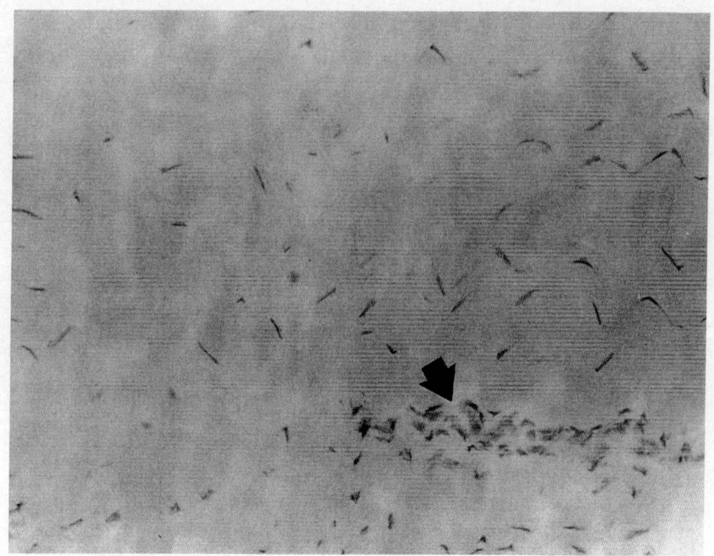

FIGURE 3.4. Histology of normal patellar tendon (hematoxylin and eosin stain, original magnification ×50). Notice the spindle-shaped fibroblasts, coarse fibrillar crimp, and peritendineum (*arrow*).

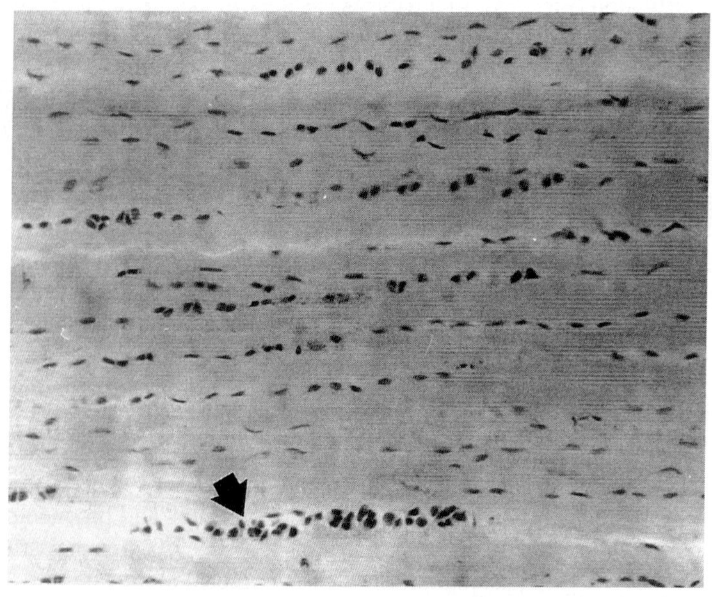

FIGURE 3.5. Histology of a normal anterior cruciate ligament (hematoxylin and eosin stain, original magnification ×50). Notice the rounded fibroblasts, fine fibrillar crimp, and cluster of potential reserve cells (*arrow*).

TABLE 3.1. *Summary of histologic observations of rabbit periarticular connective tissue*

Tissue width	Collagen bundle (μm)	Crimp period (μm)	Crimp amplitude (μm)	Cell shape	Cell size (μm × μm)
Patellar tendon	20	120	15	Spindle	3–5 × 15
Achilles tendon	20	120	40	Spindle	3–5 × 15
Anterior cruciate ligament	20	45–60	<5	Round to Ovoid	5–8 × 12–15
Medial collateral ligament	20	45	10	Rod to Spindle	3–5 × 15

From Amiel D, Kleiner JB. Biochemistry of tendon and ligament. In: Nimni ME, Olsen B, eds. *Collagen biotechnology,* vol III. Cleveland: CRC Press, 1988, with permission.

bilization. A more complete understanding of these problems could improve various treatment modalities and place them on firm scientific ground. This is particularly the case because most investigations of tissue injury and healing involve skin, not tendons or ligaments (15–17).

Collagen is the major protein in ligaments and tendons, and it is not a single entity. At least 19 different types of collagen have been described (Table 3.2). All the collagen molecules participate in supramolecular aggregates that are stabilized in part by interactions between triple-helical domains. They form a wide range of structures. The remainder of this chapter is devoted to the current understanding of collagen structure, typing, function, biosynthesis, metabolism, and crosslinking.

The collagen triple helix is characterized by the intertwining of three helical polypeptides forming a coiled—coiled structure. This triple-helical structure is well described. Each polypeptide forms a left-handed helix in which every third residue comes into the center of the superhelix shifted by 30° from the preceding central residue of the same chain. This results in the formation of a right-handed superhelix. Steric reasons impose that the

TABLE 3.2. *Types and characteristics of known collagens*

Type	Subgroup	Chain	Characteristics	Localization (reference)
I	Fibrillar	$\alpha_1(1)$, $\alpha_2(1)$	Hybrid composed of two kinds of chains; most abundant; low in hydroxylysine and glycolysate hydroxylysine	Bone, tendon, skin, dentin, ligament, fascia, uterus, and artery
Type I trimer	Fibrillar	$\alpha_1(I)$	Increased content of 3- and 4-hydroxyproline and hydroxylysine	Fetal tissues, inflammatory and neoplastic states
II	Fibrillar	$\alpha_1(II)$	Abundant; relatively high in hydroxylysine and glycosylated hydroxylysine	Hyaline cartilage, vitreous humor
III	Fibrillar	$\alpha_1(III)$	High in hydroxylysine-containing interchain disulfide bonds	Skin, artery, uterus
IV	Sheet forming	$\alpha_1(IV)$, $\alpha_2(IV)$	High in hydroxylysine and glycosylated hydroxylysine; may contain large globular regions	Basement membranes; glomerular basement membrane (18)
V	Fibrillar	$\alpha_1(V)$, $\alpha_2(V)$, $\alpha_3(V)$	Similar to type IV	Most interstitial tissue
VI	Beaded filament	$\alpha_1(VI)$, $\alpha_2(VI)$, $\alpha_3(VI)$	Microfibrils	Most interstitial tissue
VII	Anchoring fibril	$\alpha_1(VII)$	Long chain; 90% triple helical (62)	Dermoepidermal junction (18)
VIII	Sheet forming	$\alpha_1(VIII)$	Small helix linked in tandem	Some endothelium
IX	FACIT	$\alpha_1(IX)$, $\alpha_2(IX)$, $\alpha_3(IX)$	Minor cartilage protein; contains attached glycosaminoglycan	Hyaline cartilage, vitreous humor (18)
X	Sheet forming	$\alpha_1(X)$	Short chain; homotrimer	Hypertrophic mineralizing cartilage
XI	Fibrillar	$\alpha_1(XI)$, $\alpha_2(XI)$, $\alpha_3(XI)$	Associated with type I collagen	Bone and placenta
XII	FACIT	$\alpha_1(XII)$	Contains only two triple helical domains; homotrimer	Embryonic skin and tendon (18)
XIII	Transmembrane	$\alpha_1(XIII)$	Several forms by alternative splicing (63)	Endothelial cells, bone, cartilage, skin (64)
XIV	FACIT	$\alpha_1(XIV)$	Homotrimer	Fetal skin and tendon (18)
XV	Multiplexin	$\alpha_1(XV)$	Several sites for *N*-linked glycosylation and glycosaminoglycan attachment	Heart and skeletal muscle, placenta (40)
XVI	FACIT	$\alpha_1(XVI)$	Interact with fibrillar collagens and other matrix constituents	Most interstitial tissue
XVII	Transmembrane	$\alpha_1(XVII)$	Bullous pemphigoid antigen (BPAG2) (38)	Liver and kidney
XVIII	Multiplexin	$\alpha_1(XVIII)$	Similar to type XV	Basement membrane of muscle and other interstitial tissues (31)
XIX	FACIT	$\alpha_1(XIX)$	Similar to XVI with unique carboxyl terminus	

FACIT, fibril-associated collagens with interrupted triple helices.

center of the helix be occupied only by glycyl residues (18). Glycine is the smallest amino acid and permits the close packing necessary for the assembly of the superhelices (19). The amino acid sequences of triple-helical domains are characterized by the repetition of triplets Gly-X-Y. Any other amino acid sequence would perturb the triple-helical conformation (20). Proline and hydroxyproline follow each other relatively frequently, and the Gly-Pro-Hyp sequence makes up about 10% of the molecule (6). Proline and hydroxyproline are cyclic imino acids whose structure presumably imparts rigidity to the final triple-helix configuration (19). These superhelices, known as α chains, have a molecular mass of about 100 kd and contain approximately 1,000 amino acids for the interstitial collagen types I, II, and III. There are 3.27 residues per turn, with a distance of 0.201 nm between residues and a relative twist of 100° (6).

This triple-helical structure provides two properties that are crucial to the functioning of the various collagen molecules. First, the triple-helical domains may serve as molecular rods that can physically separate globular domains in a protein. Second, the amino acids in the X and Y position have their side chains pointing outward from the helix. This offers an exceptional potential for lateral interactions, particularly with other triple helices (18). The triple-helical sequences are rigid and inextensible, thereby providing high tensile strength. Within the superfamily of collagens, multiple distinct subgroups exist. The lengths and the number of triple-helical domains within nonfibrillar collagens are frequently quite different from those of triple-helical domains in fibrillar collagens. The non–triple-helical domains that separate (interrupt) triple-helical domains in nonfibrillar collagens represent regions of relative flexibility (21). Nineteen unique collagen types have been described in the literature. To facilitate their understanding, the distinct collagen types have been subgrouped by structure. This structural grouping may also have implications on functional differences; however, the functions of many of the more recently discovered collagens have not been elucidated.

TYPES OF COLLAGEN

Collagens Participating in Quarter-Staggered Fibrils

The presence of striated fibrils in extracellular matrix (ECM) was recognized in the very first electron microscopy observations of collagen-containing tissues (22). It is now understood that lateral interaction between homologous regions within the triple-helical domains is the basis for fibril formation. The molecules are staggered by approximately 67 nm (18). The banding pattern of collagen fibrils is very similar from tissue to tissue, reflecting the presence of quarter-staggered collagen molecules (i.e., fibrillar collagens). There are, however,

important differences in the three-dimensional packing of the molecules and important variations in the diameters of the fibrils. These differences can be explained in part by the existence of several distinct but structurally homologous collagen molecules involved in fibril formation. These collagen types are referred to as the *fibrillar collagens*, and their genes are derived from a single ancestral gene (23). Collagen types I, II, III, V, and XI are all considered fibrillar collagens that form quarter-staggered fibrils. Although the collagen molecules are able to form fibrils by themselves, they appear to participate in heterotypic fibrils *in vivo* (24–27). Collagen fibrils may be described as molecular alloys (18).

Fibril-Associated Collagens with Interrupted Triple Helices

The structure of fibril-associated collagens with interrupted triple helices (FACITs) can be divided into three main functional regions. One region comprises one or two triple-helical domains and serves for the interaction and adhesion of these molecules to the fibrils. A second region, comprising another triple-helical domain, serves as a rigid arm that projects out from the fibril. A third region, which does not include triple helices, may serve for interaction with other matrix elements or with cells. The various triple-helical domains are separated (or interrupted) by short non–triple-helical domains (18). Collagen types IX, XII, XIV, XVI, and XIX appear to belong to this subgroup (28,29), but only by virtue of intermittent sequence homology within the noncollagenous amino terminus; the arrangement of two 2–amino acid imperfections in the last triple-helical subdomain; and a highly conserved Cys-Xaa₄-Cys motif near the carboxyl terminus have types XVI and XIX been included in this subgroup (30,31). No information exists on the relation of types XVI or XIX with the fibrillar or other collagen molecules (30), and these types may compose a unique subgroup in and of themselves.

Type IX collagen is the best described of this group (32). The role of collagen type IX has been described in ECMs containing type II collagen: to serve as a means of attachment of new functionality to the fibrils (18). Type XII collagen was discovered by using cDNA clones of homologs of type IX collagen in ECM containing type I collagen (33). According to these findings, type XII collagen is associated with type I collagen much the same way as type IX collagen is associated with type II collagen.

Collagens Forming Sheets

Basement membranes, Descemet's membrane, worm cuticle, and sponge organic skeleton are examples of protein sheets created by this group of collagen molecules

(18). Type IV collagen is involved with basement membrane formation. A fine network of cords is laced together and entraps large, associated molecules (34). Descemet's membrane, which separates the corneal endothelial cells from the stroma, consists of stacks of hexagonal collagen lattices made of type VIII collagen (35). Nodes interconnected by rodlike structures with a dumbbell appearance build the type VIII lattice (18). The amino acid sequence, gene structure, and molecular organization of type X collagen is extremely similar to those of type VIII collagen, and it has a very restricted pattern of distribution. Type X collagen is synthesized primarily by hypertrophic chondrocytes during the process of endochondral ossification (18).

Collagen Forming Beaded Filaments

Type VI collagen is the major constituent of beaded filaments. It has been shown by rotary shadowing electron microscopy analysis that two molecules aggregate in a head-to-tail orientation to form a dimer (32). Two dimers assemble into tetramers, which form linear aggregates. These aggregates are described as beaded filaments with repeats of approximately 110 nm. This assembly requires interactions between triple helices and globular domains. The function of type VI collagen is still a matter of speculation. It may play a role as an interface between the main collagen fibril network and the cell (18).

Collagen Forming Anchoring Fibrils

Collagen type VII, which is synthesized by keratinocytes, is assembled first into antiparallel dimers that overlap by 60 nm (36). During this process, an amino-terminal noncollagenous domain appears to be cleaved. The dimers then aggregate laterally in a nonstaggered fashion. By triple-helix to triple-helix interaction, type VII collagen becomes the main constituent of anchoring fibrils (18).

Collagens with Transmembrane Domains

Type XIII and XVII collagens possess a transmembrane domain (29,37,38). The mouse BPAG2 protein, identified as collagen type XVII, is predicted to be a cell membrane protein. Type XVII functions as a hemidesmosomal collagen at the cutaneous basement membrane zone with an extracellular collagenous region, which may serve as an attachment site to the other components of the basement membrane zone, including integrins or lamina lucida proteins (38).

Collagen Multiplexins

Type XV and XVIII form a new subgroup of collagens, called multiplexins (for protein with *multiple* triple-helix domains and *in*terruptions) (21). Comparison of the α_1(XV) and α_1(XVIII) sequences reveals a striking similarity (21). Both collagen types are characterized by extensive interruptions in their triple-helical collagenous sequences (21,39–41). RNA studies reveal that type XV collagen may be distributed in a tissue-specific pattern resembling that of type I collagen (39). Both collagen types have many interruptions in their rigid triple-helical domains, providing for a high level of flexibility (21).

BIOSYNTHESIS AND DEGRADATION

For the organism to develop an extracellular network of collagen fibers, the cells involved in the biosynthetic process must first synthesize a precursor known as procollagen. This molecule is later enzymatically trimmed of its nonhelical ends, giving rise to a collagen molecule that spontaneously assembles into fibers in the extracellular space. Procollagen molecules have been identified as precursors of the three interstitial collagens (types I, II, and III). Several of the N- and C-terminal peptides (i.e., propeptides) have been characterized and their primary sequences determined.

Gene Expression

Fiber-forming collagens, types I, II, III, V, and XI, exhibit lengthy, uninterrupted collagenous domains and are first synthesized as biosynthetic precursors (i.e., procollagens). Gene cloning experiments have demonstrated that the group I collagen genes are evolutionarily related, for they share a common ancestral gene structure. Human chromosome 17 contains the coding information for the α_1 chain of type I collagen, and chromosome 7 codes for its complementary α_2 chain. A comparison of the five fibrillar collagens described shows that, with one exception (types III and α_2[V] are located on chromosome 2), all other genes are located on different chromosomes.

The genes coding for fiber forming collagens are large, about 10 times the size of their functional mRNA. Many of the coding sequences (exons) are 54 base pairs (bp) long and are separated from each other by large intervening sequences (introns) that range in size from about 80 to 2,000 bp. The gene itself contains 38,000 bp and is very complex. The finding that most exons of these genes have identical lengths suggests that the ancestral gene for collagen was assembled by multiple duplications of single genetic units containing an exon of 54 bp (Fig. 3.6). It is likely that a primordial exon this size could have encoded for a Gly-Pro-Pro tripeptide repeated six times. Such a polypeptide of 18 amino acids probably had the minimum length needed to form a stable triple-helical structure.

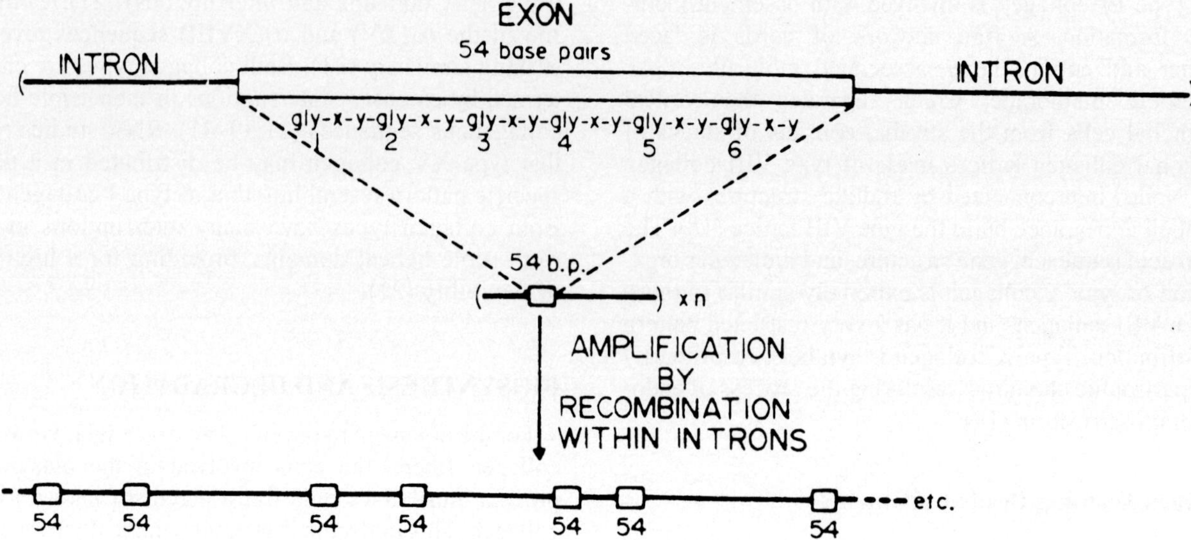

FIGURE 3.6. Assembly of the ancestral collagen gene. The collagen gene is made up of multiple units containing 54 base pairs, each of which corresponds to sequences of 18 amino acids. (From Amiel D, Nimni ME. The collagen in normal ligaments. *Iowa Orthop J* 1993;13:49–55, with permission.)

Translational, Cotranslational, and Early Posttranslational Events

After the gene is transcribed, it is spliced to remove introns and yield a functional mRNA that contains about 3,000 bases. Specific mRNA for each chain and collagen type are translocated to the cytoplasm and translated into proteins in the rough endoplasmic reticulum on membrane-bound polysomes. As the collagen polypeptide is synthesized in the rough endoplasmic reticulum, it is modified in important ways. Two major constituents of collagen are the modified amino acids hydroxyproline and hydroxylysine. Neither amino acid, however, can be directly incorporated into proteins. Instead, proline and lysine are incorporated and then modified by two hydroxylating enzymes, prolyl-hydroxylase and lysyl-hydroxylase. These enzymes require ferrous iron, ascorbate, and α-ketoglutarate for their activity. The degree of hydroxylation differs from tissue to tissue and depends on the availability of substrate, rate of synthesis, turnover, and the time during which the molecule remains in the presence of the hydroxylating enzymes. The time required for the synthesis of a complete pro α chain is about 6.7 minutes.

As lysyl residues in the newly synthesized pro α chains are hydroxylated, sugar residues are added to the resulting hydroxylysyl groups. Two specific enzymes, a galactosyltransferase and glucosyltransferase, catalyze glycosylation. After the translation, modifications, and additions are completed, the individual pro α chains become properly aligned for the triple helix to form.

Intracellular Translocation of Procollagen and Extrusion into the Extracellular Space

The procollagen molecule, now detached from the ribosome, emerges from the endoplasmic reticulum and

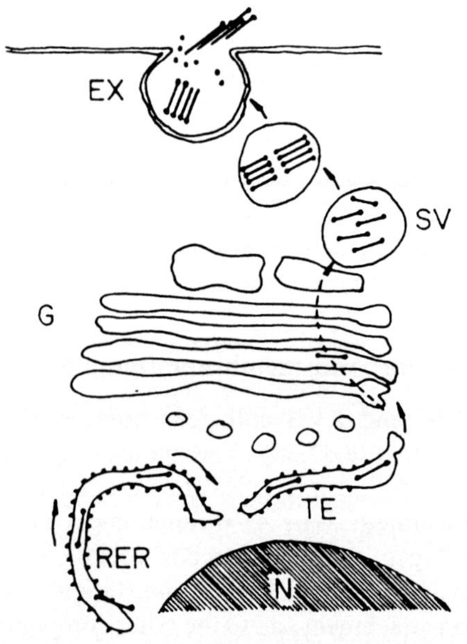

FIGURE 3.7. Procollagen transcription occurs in the nucleus *(N)*. Procollagen then moves through the cisternae of the rough endoplasmic reticulum *(RER)* and through a transitional endoplasm *(TE)* to the Golgi apparatus *(G)*, where it is packaged into secretory vesicles *(SV)* before extrusion by exocytosis *(EX)*. (From Amiel D, Nimni ME. The collagen in normal ligaments. *Iowa Orthop J* 1993;13:49–55, with permission.)

moves toward the Golgi apparatus through the microsomal lumen. In the Golgi, the C-terminal, mannose rich, carbohydrate extensions are remodeled; the molecules are packaged into vesicles, and subsequently carried toward the cellular membrane (Fig. 3.7).

The small aggregates of oriented procollagen molecules are probably trimmed of their nonhelical amino and carboxyl extensions by specific peptidases when they reach the extracellular space. In the case of type I collagen, the first peptidase to act seems to be the amino protease; this is followed by a carboxyprotease. In type II collagen the sequence of removal may be reversed.

Lysyl Oxidase Recognition

Recently formed microfibrils seem to be recognized by the enzyme lysyl oxidase, which converts certain peptide-bound lysines and hydroxylysines to aldehydes. The enzyme is an extracellular amine oxidase, which has been purified from a variety of connective tissues. It requires Cu^{2+} and probably requires pyridoxal as cofactors; molecular oxygen seems to be the cosubstrate and hydrogen acceptor. It is irreversibly inhibited by the lathyrogen β-amino propionitrile (BAPN), a substance found in the flowering sweet-pea, *Lathyrus odoratus*. This enzyme exhibits maximal activity when acting on collagen fibrils rather than on monomeric collagen (Fig. 3.8).

Fibrillogenesis

The tendency of collagen molecules to form macromolecular aggregates is well known. This tendency is common with most fibrous proteins that form filaments with helical symmetry and occupy equivalent or quasi-equivalent positions.

The exact mode in which the collagen molecules pack into microfibrils (precursors of the larger fibrils) remains a subject for speculation. A five-stranded microfibril was first suggested to account for such a substructure, one that would satisfy the condition that adjacent molecules were equivalently related by a quarter-staggered pattern.

When monomeric collagen is heated to 37°C, it progressively polymerizes, generating a turbidity curve that reflects the presence of intermediate aggregates. The lag phase (i.e., persistence of monomers), the nucleation and appearance of turbidity (i.e., microfibrils), and the rapid increase in turbidity (i.e., fiber formation) have been equated to how the cell may handle this process.

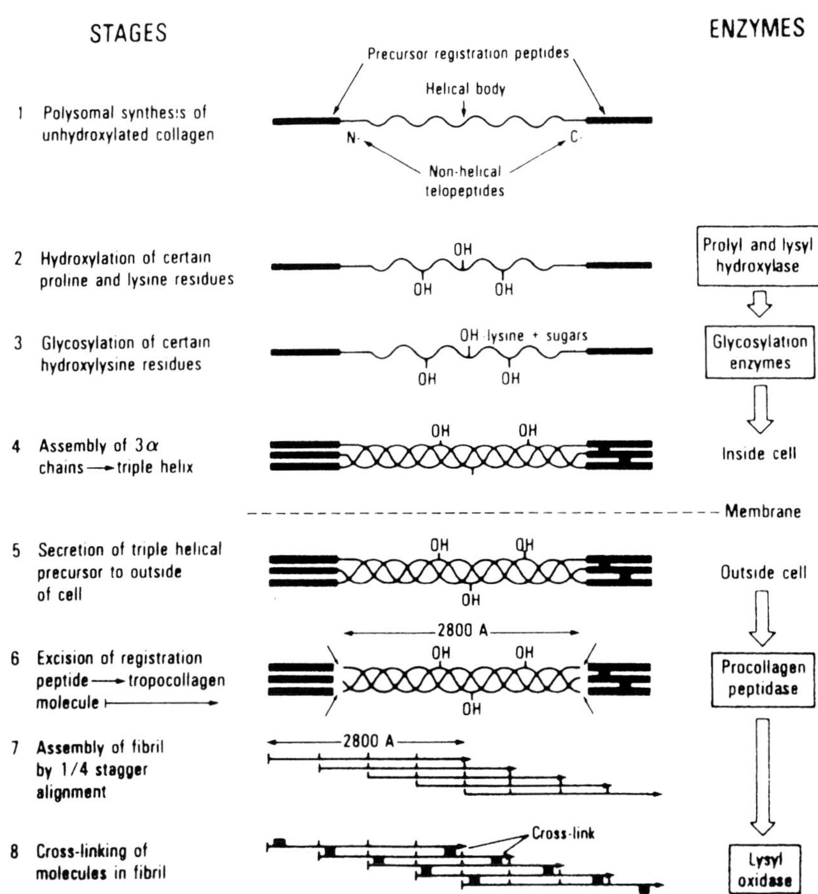

FIGURE 3.8. The enzymatic stages in maturation of collagen. Several enzymatic steps are necessary for the creation of the final collagen molecule and its maturation into a collagen fibril. These enzymatic steps take place partly within the cell and partly outside the cell. Even those steps that occur inside the cell are posttranslational; they are not directly under genetic control. However, they are essential for proper development of the final structure. Defects in many of the steps have been identified in a variety of heritable disorders of connective tissues. The final aggregation of collagen into a structure that becomes crosslinked is essential to produce the requisite tensile stress-resistant properties characteristic of mature connective tissue. (From Levine CI. Diseases of the collagen molecule. *J Clin Pathol* 1978;12:82, with permission.)

Metabolism

Because of its triple-helical structure stabilized by hydrogen bonds, the collagen molecules are quite resistant to enzymatic degradation in their native configuration. They can be degraded by collagenases. These enzymes interact tightly with the collagen fibers and appear to remain bound to the macromolecular aggregate during the degradation process. Approximately 10% of the collagen molecules found in reconstituted collagen fibrils are accessible for binding. This is in close agreement with the theoretic number of molecules estimated to be near the surface of the fiber. Bacterial and mammalian collagenases have been described. Mammalian collagenases display a great deal of specificity, cleaving bands between Gly-Leu or Gly-Ile. Collagen from older individuals is more resistant to enzymatic digestion.

Crosslinking

Structural collagen obtains its stability from its unique molecular coil configuration, the quarter-staggered packing of tropocollagen units (42), and its ability to form covalent intramolecular and intermolecular crosslinks (43–49). The former occur between α chains of the same tropocollagen molecule, and the latter occur between adjacent tropocollagen molecules. Crosslinks are key to tensile strength characteristics and resistance to chemical or enzymatic breakdown. Their absence causes the collagen fibers to be extremely weak and friable. The classic manifestation of this problem is lathyrism, which is induced in animals ingesting the common sweet pea. Curvature of the spine, rupture of the aorta, and fragile skin are common consequences (50). These compounds are potent inhibitors of lysyl oxidase, an enzyme of vital importance in the creation of crosslinks (51).

The crosslinks result from enzyme-mediated reactions involving mainly lysine and hydroxylysine. These molecules have secondary amine groups on terminal projections extending laterally from the α chain that are available for crosslinking reactions. Intramolecular crosslinks occur by the enzyme lysyl oxidase to form an aldol condensation product. Intermolecular crosslinks characteristically form in the reaction of allysine with lysine or hydroxylysine to form a Schiff base. These aldol condensation and Schiff-base reaction products possess double bonds that apparently are reduced to more stable forms *in vivo* with the passage of time. In addition to lysinonorleucine (a compound first identified in elastin), other bimolecular Schiff bases of importance in ligaments are hydroxylysinonorleucine (HLNL) and dihydroxylysinonorleucine (DHLNL). Although these hydroxylysine-containing crosslinks are the most prevalent intermolecular crosslinks in native insoluble collagen, other more complex combinations also exist, including histidinohydroxymerodesmosine (HHMD), a tetramolecular crosslink. Identifying the "reducible" crosslinks is done by using the presence of the double bond of the unsaturated compound to label the crosslink with tritium. Typically, this is done by reducing the aldol condensation product (i.e., δ-semialdehyde) with tritium-labeled sodium borohydride. The reduced product is thereby labeled with tritium and can be detected after acid hydrolysis and column chromatography.

The type of intermolecular collagen reducible crosslinks present in patellar and Achilles tendon differs considerably from those in the MCL and ACL (52). The tendinous tissue has a considerably different collagen reducible crosslink elution profile from that of ligamentous tissue. The reducible crosslinks studied include DHLNL, HLNL, and HHMD. The relative concentrations of the crosslinks can be expressed as ratios for the tendinous and ligamentous tissues (Table 3.3). The ligaments are seen to have 12 to 17 times the DHLNL/HLNL ratio as the tendons, and 3 to 4 times the [DHLNL + HLNL]/HHMD ratio. The ACLs were observed to have the highest ratio of these crosslinks.

In addition to the reducible collagen crosslinks, isolation of a naturally fluorescing, nonreducible, crosslinking amino acid has been identified as pyridinoline (53–55). It has been observed, in order of increasing concentration, in tendon, ligament, and hyaline cartilage. A threefold to fivefold difference in its concentration is seen between rabbit ACL and patellar tendon, with an intermediate concentration in the MCL. Pyridinoline may be an age-related transformation of the reducible crosslink, DHLNL, to a more stable, nonreducible crosslink. This may explain why the concentration of reducible, keto-imine crosslinks decreases with age in connective tissue (56).

TABLE 3.3. *Reducible crosslink distribution*

Tissue	DHLNL/HLNL	(DHLNL + HLNL)/HHMD
Patellar tendon	0.16 ± 0.06	1.47 ± 0.23
Achilles tendon	0.15 ± 0.04	1.32 ± 0.06
Anterior cruciate ligament	2.77 ± 0.73	4.64 ± 0.73
Medial collateral ligament	1.86 ± 0.17	3.17 ± 0.37

DHLNL, dihydroxylysinonorleucine; HLNL, hydroxylysinonorleucine; HHMD, histidinohydroxymerodesmosine.

From Amiel D, Kleiner JB. Biochemistry of tendon and ligament. In: Nimni ME, Olsen B, eds. *Collagen biotechnology,* vol III. Cleveland: CRC Press, 1988, with permission.

TABLE 3.4. *Biochemical properties of tendons and ligaments*

Tissue	Total collagen (mg/g dry tissue)	Type of collagen			Glycosaminoglycan content (mg hexosamine/g dry tissue)
		I	II	III	
Patellar tendon	867.2 ± 8.9	>95	—	<5	3.92 ± 0.16
Achilles tendon	868.2 ± 10.2	>95	—	<5	2.75 ± 0.20
Anterior cruciate ligament	802.6 ± 9.8	88 ± 2	—	12 ± 2	9.89 ± 0.56
Medial collateral ligament	797.1 ± 11.1	91 ± 2	—	9 ± 2	4.56 ± 0.26

From Amiel D, Frank CB, Harwood FL, et al. Tendons and ligaments: a morphological and biochemical comparison. *J Orthop Res* 1984:1:257, with permission.

PROTEOGLYCANS

Proteoglycans are macromolecules that consist of a protein core to which at least one extended polysaccharide chain (glycosaminoglycan [GAG]) is covalently linked (57). On a dry-weight basis, the proteoglycans of a tendon constitutes less than 1% of the total tissue and comprises an only slightly higher amount in ligaments. Water, however, comprises 60% to 80% of the total wet weight, and a significant part of that water is associated with the proteoglycans. Proteoglycans and water provide lubrication and spacing that are crucial to the gliding function at intercept points where fibers cross in tissue matrices (58).

Aggrecan, a proteoglycan that possesses more than 100 chondroitin sulfate and keratan sulfate chains, is a major component of ligament and tendon. Aggrecan is also characterized by its ability to interact with hyaluronic acid to form large proteoglycan aggregates. The high anionic charge on the individual aggrecan molecules endowed by the sulfated glycosaminoglycan chains and localization within the matrix endowed by aggregate formation are essential for aggrecan function (59).

One of the other major proteoglycans in tendon is a small molecule named decorin (57). Decorin is associated with the surface of collagen fibrils in tendon, and it is possible that this proteoglycan is involved in the regulation of fibril diameter *in vivo* (57). However, it has been found that even within tendons, the proteoglycan and collagen content of the tensional regions differs from that in compressive regions. In the compressive region, around the bones of a joint, some type II collagen is expressed by the tendon, as well as a 5- to 10-fold higher proteoglycan content than in the tensional region. Most of the increased proteoglycan content is of the large (M_r >10^6) proteoglycan type (57,60). These large proteoglycans are the same types that provide compressive stiffness to cartilage (61).

Hyaluronic acid, chondroitin-4-sulfate, and dermatan sulfate represent most of the GAGs present. Except for hyaluronic acid, the GAGs are covalently linked to proteins to create aggregate molecules of massive molecular weight. They are highly negatively charged and possess a large number of hydroxyl groups. These hydroxyl groups attract water through hydrogen binding, contributing important features to the collagen-fiber-proteoglycan interaction, and may correlate with some of the differences in mechanical properties between tendon and ligament. The concentration of GAGs present in the rabbit ligamentous tissue studied differs significantly from that present in tendinous tissue. The ACLs have the highest proportion of GAGs, two to four times the amount observed in the tendons. The MCL also demonstrates a higher GAG concentration than the tendons (52) (Table 3.4).

REFERENCES

1. Bloom W, Fawcett DW, eds. *A textbook of histology,* 8th ed. Philadelphia: WB Saunders, 1962.
2. Copenhaver WM, Bunge RP, Bune MP, eds. *Bailey's textbook of histology,* 16th ed. Baltimore: Williams & Wilkins, 1971.
3. Ham AW, ed. *Histology,* 6th ed. Philadelphia: JB Lippincott, 1974.
4. Noyes FR, Grood ES, Butler DL, et al. Clinical biomechanics of the knee: ligament restraints and functional stability. In: *American Academy of Orthopaedic Surgeons' symposium on the athlete's knee. Surgical repair and reconstruction.* St. Louis: CV Mosby, 1980.
5. Palmer I. On injuries to the ligaments of the knee joint. *Acta Chir Scand Suppl* 1938;53:1.
6. Amiel D, Nimni ME. The collagen in normal ligaments. *Iowa Orthop J* 1993;13:49–55.
7. Nimni ME, Harkness RD. Molecular structures and functions of collagen. In: Nimni ME, ed. *Collagen: biochemistry.* Boca Raton, FL: CRC Press, 1988.
8. Amenta P, ed. *Histology,* 3rd ed. New Hyde Park, NY: New York Medical Examination Publishing Company, 1983.
9. Bailey FR. In: Kely DE, Wook RL, Enders AC, eds. *Bailey's textbook of microscopic anatomy,* 18th ed. Baltimore: Williams & Wilkins, 1984:172.
10. Leeson CR. In: Leeson CR, Leeson TS, eds. *Textbook of histology,* 5th ed. Philadelphia: WB Saunders, 1985:97.
11. Snell RS, ed. *Clinical and functional histology for medical students,* 1st ed. Boston: Little Brown, 1984.
12. Viidik A. Simultaneous mechanical and light microscopic studies of collagen fibers. *Z Anat Entwicklungsgesch* 1972;136:204.
13. Yahia LH, Drouin G. Microscopical investigation of canine anterior cruciate ligament and patellar tendon: collagen fascicle morphology and architecture. *J Orthop Res* 1989;7:243–251.
14. Leeson TS, Leeson CR, eds. *A brief atlas of histology.* Philadelphia: WB Saunders, 1979.
15. Clore JN, Cohen K, Diegelmann RF. Quantitation of collagen types I and III during wound healing in rat skin. *Proc Soc Exp Biol Med* 1979;161:337.
16. Dunphy JE. *Wound healing.* New York: Medcom Press, 1974.
17. Gay S, Viljanto J, Rackallio J, et al. Collagen types in early phases of wound healing in children. *Acta Chir Scand* 1978;144:205.

18. Van Der Rest M, Garrone R. Collagen family of proteins, *FASEB J* 1991;5:2815–2823.
19. Amiel D, Billings E, Akeson WH. Ligament structure, chemistry, and physiology. In: Daniel DM, Akeson WH, O'Conner JJ, eds. *Knee ligaments: structure, function, injury, and repair.* New York: Raven Press, 1990.
20. Ramchandran GN, Reddi AH, eds. *Biochemistry of collagen.* New York: Plenum, 1976.
21. Oh SK, Kamagata Y, Muragaki Y, et al. Isolation and sequencing of cDNAs for proteins with multiple domains of Gly-Xaa-Yaa repeats identify a distinct family of collagenous proteins. *Proc Natl Acad Sci U S A* 1994;91:4229–4233.
22. Schmitt FO. Electron microscope investigations of the structure of collagen. *J Cell Comp Physiol* 1942;20:11–33.
23. Vuorio E, de Crombrugghe B. The family of collagen genes. *Annu Rev Biochem* 1990;59:837–872.
24. Henkel W, Glanvill RW. Covalent crosslinking between molecules of type I and type III collagen. *Eur J Biochem* 1982;122:205–213.
25. Birk DE, Fitch JM, Babiarz JP, et al. Collagen type I and V are present in the same fibril in the avian corneal stroma. *J Cell Biol* 1988;106:999–1008.
26. Keene DR, Sakai LY, Bachinger HP, et al. Type III collagen can be present on banded collagen fibrils regardless of fibril diameter. *J Cell Biol* 1987;105:2393–2402.
27. Mendler M, Eich-Bender SG, Vaughan L, et al. Cartilage contains mixed fibrils of collagen types II, IX, and XI. *J Cell Biol* 1989;108:191–197.
28. Gordon MK, Olsen BR. The contribution of collagenous proteins to tissue-specific matrix assembly. *Curr Opin Cell Biol* 1990;2:833–838.
29. Grassel S, Timpl R, Tan EML, et al. Biosynthesis and processing of type XVI collagen in human fibroblasts and smooth muscle cells. *Eur J Biochem* 1996;242:576– 584.
30. Pan TC, Zhang RZ, Mattei MG, et al. Cloning and chromosomal location of human α1(XVI) collagen. *Proc Natl Acad Sci U S A* 1992;89:6565–6569.
31. Myers JC, Li D, Bageris A, et al. Biochemical and immunohistochemical characterization of human type XIX defines a novel class of basement membrane zone collagens. *Am J Pathol* 1997;151:1729–1740.
32. Mayne R, Burgeson RE, eds. *Structure and function of collagen types.* Orlando: Academic Press, 1987.
33. Gordon MK, Gerecke DR, Olsen BR. Type XII collagen: distinct extracellular matrix component discovered by cDNA cloning. *Proc Natl Acad Sci U S A* 1987;84:6040– 6044.
34. Timpl R. Structure and biological activity of basement membrane protein. *Eur J Biochem* 1989;190:487–502.
35. Sawada H, Konomi H, Hirosawa K. Characterization of the collagen in the hexagonal lattice of Descemet's membrane: its relation to type VIII collagen. *J Cell Biol* 1990;110:219–227.
36. Regauer S, Seiler GR, Barrandon Y, et al. Epithelial origin of cutaneous anchoring fibrils. *J Cell Biol* 1990;111:2109–2115.
37. Pihlajaniemi T, Rehn M. Two new collagen subgroups: membrane-associated collagens and types XV and XVIII. *Prog Nucleic Acid Res Mol Biol* 1995;50:225–262.
38. Li K, Tania K, Tan EML, et al. Cloning of type XVII collagen. Complementary and genomic DNA sequences of mouse 180 kD bullous pemphigoid antigen (BPAG2) predict an interrupted collagenous domain, a transmembrane segment and unusual features in the 5′ end of the gene and 3′ untranslated region of the mRNA. *J Biol Chem* 1993;268:8825–8834.
39. Myers JC, Kivirikko S, Gordon MK, et al. Identification of a previously unknown human collagen chain, α1(XV) characterized by extensive interruptions in the triple-helical region. *Proc Natl Acad Sci U S A* 1992;89:10144–10148.
40. Kivirikko S, Heinamaki P, Rehn M, et al. Primary structure of the α1 chain of human type XV collagen and exon-intron organization in the 3′ region of the corresponding gene. *Biol Chem* 1994;269:4773–4779.
41. Rehn M, Pihlajaniemi T. α1(XVIII), a collagen chain with frequent interruptions in the collagenous sequence, a distinct tissue distribution, and homology with type XV collage. *Proc Natl Acad Sci U S A* 1994;89:6565–6569.
42. Petruska JA, Hodge AJ. A subunit model for the tropocollagen macromolecule. *Proc Natl Acad Sci U S A* 1964;51:871.
43. Bailey AJ. The nature of collagen. In: Florkin M, Stots E, eds. *Comprehensive biochemistry,* vol 26B. Amsterdam: Elsevier, 1968.
44. Bailey AJ, Robins SP, Balian G. Biological significance of the intermolecular cross-links of collagen. *Nature* 1974;251:105.
45. Gallop PM, Blumenfeld OO, Henson E, et al. Isolation and identification of -amino aldehydes in collagen. *Biochemistry* 1968;7:2409.
46. Mechanic GL. An automated scintillation counting system for continuous analysis: cross-links of (^{3}H)NaBH$_4$ reduced collagen. *Ann Biochem* 1974;62:349.
47. Paz MA, Henson EH, Rombauer R, et al. Alpha-amino alcohols as products of a reductive side reaction of denatured collagen with sodium borohydride. *Biochemistry* 1970;9:2123.
48. Tanzer ML. Crosslinking of collagen. *Science* 1973;180:561.
49. Traub W, Piez KA. The chemistry and structure of collagen. *Adv Protein Chem* 1971;25:243.
50. Bornstein P. The biosynthesis of collagen. *Annu Rev Biochem* 1974;43:567.
51. Narayanan AS, Siegal RC, Marin GR. On the inhibition of lysyl oxidase by β aminoprioitride. *Biochem Biophys Res Commun* 1972;46:745.
52. Amiel D, Frank CB, Harwood FL, et al. Tendons and ligaments: a morphological and biochemical comparison. *J Orthop Res* 1984;1:257.
53. Eyre DR, Oguchi H. Collagens: their measurement, properties and a proposed pathway of formation. *Biochem Biophys Res Commun* 1980;92:403.
54. Fujimoto D. Isolation and characterization of a fluorescent material in bovine Achilles tendon collagen. *Biochem Biophys Res Commun* 1977;76:1124.
55. Fujimoto D, Moriguschi T. Pyridinoline, a non-reducible cross-link of collagen. *J Biochem* 1978;83:863.
56. Tanzer ML. Cross-linking. In: Ramuchandran GN, Reddi AH, eds. *Biochemistry of collagen.* New York: Plenum, 1976:137.
57. Blevins FT, Djurasovic M, Flatow EL, et al. Biology of the rotator cuff tendon. *Orthop Clin North Am* 1997;28:1–16.
58. Ogston AG. The biological functions of the glycosaminoglycans. In: Balasz EA, ed. *Chemistry and molecular biology of the intercellular matrix,* vol 3. London: Academic Press, 1970.
59. Roughley PJ, Lee ER. Cartilage proteoglycans: structure and potential functions. *Microsc Res Tech* 1994;28:385–397.
60. Berenson MC, Blevins FT, Plaas AHK, et al. Proteoglycans of human rotator cuff tendons. *J Orthop Res* 1996;14:518–525.
61. Vogel KG, Sandy JD, Pogany G, et al. Aggrecan in bovine tendon. *Matrix Biol* 1994;14:171–179.
62. Bentz H, Morris NP, Murray LW, et al. Isolation and partial characterization of a new human collagen with an extended triple-helical structural domain. *Proc Natl Acad Sci U S A* 1983;80:3168–3172.
63. Shows TB, Tikka L, Byers MG, et. al. Assignment of the human collagen alpha 1 (XIII) chain gene *(COL13A1)* to the q22 region of chromosome 10. *Genomics* 1989;5:128–133.
64. Sandberg M, Tamminen M, Hirvonen H, et al. Expression of mRNAs coding for the alpha 1 chain of type XIII collagen in human fetal tissues: comparison with expression of mRNAs for collagen types I, II, and III. *J Cell Biol* 1989;109:1371–1379.

CHAPTER 4

Effects of Anatomic and Developmental Variation on Evaluation and Treatment of Knee Conditions

Glenn C. Terry and Stephanie Silberberg

Understanding knee function requires an in-depth awareness of the importance of each of the anatomic components of the physiologic joint and how they interact with each other. The physiologic joint consists of long bones, sesamoids, articular cartilage, menisci, the anterior and posterior ligaments (ACL and PCL), capsular ligaments (medial and lateral), musculotendinous units, synovial layers, bursae, and the nervous system components (1). A baseline understanding of these normal anatomic structures must be combined with some awareness of the effect of congenital, developmental, and acquired knee disorders and variations in anatomy that can affect accurate diagnosis of knee conditions.

Anatomic variations can be divided into congenital, developmental, and acquired conditions. Examples of congenital issues include a congenital knee dislocation (2–4), the nail-patella syndrome (5), congenital patella dislocation (6), congenital absence of the ACL (7,8) or PCL (9), a discoid meniscus (10), intercalary bone defects (11), and congenital defects of development that may create long-term disorders (e.g., congenital tendency to osteoarthrosis) (12).

There is considerable overlap between the developmental and acquired abnormalities that can affect the knee. Examples of developmental issues include genu varum and valgum and their effect on acquired unicompartmental osteoarthritis, as well as Blount's disease, the extreme form of genu varum in children (13–16). Other causes of lower extremity malalignment that have developmental basis may be a consequence of femoral anteversion (17,18) or excessive foot pronation (19,20).

An acquired problem can also predispose abnormal development over time. For example, a traumatic event with a ring closure of the epiphyseal plate on a long bone can create a genu varum or valgus deformity. Genu valgum can occur as a consequence of a long-bone fracture, such as the tibia, in a child with an intact fibula; overstimulation of the tibia by the fracture combined with the tethering effect of the intact, more slowly growing fibula can create a genu valgum deformity that can affect the knee (21–23).

The recurvatum knee is another example of a developmental cause of knee difficulty. Even though it may not specifically increase injury potential, it does pose difficulties in accurate diagnosis of instability. The physiologic reverse pivot shift can be demonstrated frequently in a knee with increased recurvatum, which can complicate the evaluation of a knee with an acute ligament injury (24). The loose capsular attachments to the menisci in the recurvatum knee can increase the normal meniscal excursion, predisposing the meniscus to an increased risk for injury (2,3,6,25). Another unusual but important disorder is the congenital absence of the ACL and of the PCL. Treatment is conservative and depends on recognition of the condition, followed by counseling and therapy. Surgical treatment, if required, should be well planned because adaptive bone changes make appropriate drill hole placement problematic (4,7–9).

The relatively tight-ligament knee that demonstrates a mild degree of genu varum may never hamper the athlete's function, but it may increase his or her risk for developing medial compartment gonarthrosis with aging. Torsional abnormalities of the tibia and femur can also cause osteoarthritis of the knee (26,27).

It is easy to see how an underlying anatomic or developmental abnormality may predispose further problems and, in some cases, lead to surgical treatment. It is also important for the surgeon to recognize an underlying developmental problem, because inadequate management could lead to iatrogenic disability. For example, the knee with a loose patella retinaculum should have increased medial and lateral mobility of the patella. If this knee undergoes a lateral release, there may be an increased risk for postoperative medial patella subluxation as an iatrogenic, acquired effect of inappropriate treatment (28,29).

In some cases, there is an important relationship between a developmental condition and the management of an acute knee injury. Examples include torn discoid lateral meniscus and stenotic intercondylar notch in a patient with a torn anterior cruciate ligament. In the first example, the stress-relieving function of a discoid meniscus is so important that subtotal meniscectomy can dramatically increase the stress on the compartment treated, making long-term symptom relief impossible in some cases (10,30–32). The lateral geniculate artery penetrates the discoid lateral meniscus further than it does the normal lateral meniscus; therefore, significant hemarthrosis is a possibility after saucerizing a tear of a discoid lateral meniscus. Failure to recognize the relationship of the stenotic intercondylar notch may increase the risk for a recurrent ACL tear after reconstruction if inadequate notchplasty is performed. A notch width of less than 15 mm has five times the probability of an ACL tear (33,34).

Knee sesamoids play an important role in knee function, but it may be difficult to distinguish a small posterior sesamoid (i.e., fabella) from a loose body in some cases. The patella itself is the largest sesamoid of the knee. A congenitally dislocated patella can adversely affect its deceleration function. When the static restraints of the patella have been loosened as a result of lower extremity malalignment, recurrent lateral subluxation may result as a developmental problem (35). Excessive tightness of the patellar restraints can predispose the knee to patella infera (i.e., patella baja) as an acquired problem related to posttraumatic or iatrogenic scarring (e.g., fibrosis) (36).

Another condition that can affect the patella is a developmental accessory ossification center of the superior lateral portion of the patella (37). This can become symptomatic from overuse or from a traumatic event, in which case it acts as an ununited fracture (38).

Acquired "sesamoids" can appear in the patellar tendon as a result of the fragmentation of the growth plate that occurs in Osgood-Schlatter disease (39). These ossicles can become symptomatic, create a chronic patellar tendonitis, and irritate the deep infrapatellar tendon bursa (40,41). Sinding-Larsen-Johansson disease is another traction tendonitis associated with fragmentation of the patella's inferior pole and is similar in symptoms to Osgood-Schlatter disease (42).

The most common posterior site for a sesamoid is in the lateral head of the gastrocnemius tendon: the fabella (43). The fabella has been identified on 17% of radiographs. The relation of the fabella to a more atavistic knee in being more susceptible to development of osteoarthritis has been questioned in the literature. Hypertrophy of the fabella, as well as osteophyte formation of the fabella, may require surgical treatment in cases of unicompartmental osteoarthritis and in patients with total-knee replacements. A less common knee sesamoid is the chymelia, which is embedded in the popliteus tendon. It can be mistaken for a calcific-popliteus tendonitis.

The articular cartilage can also be involved in developmental and acquired difficulties. Osteochondritis dissecans (44) and the susceptibility of articular cartilage to isolated chondral fracture in the third and fourth decades are examples of acquired difficulties (45). Developmental conditions such as ochronosis (46), gout (46), and pseudogout (46) and their effect on articular cartilage over time may be considered congenital problems of articular cartilage. Multiple epiphyseal dysplasia and its relation to an increased incidence of osteoarthritis is an example of a congenital defect affecting articular cartilage, because it is passed as an autosomal dominant trait (12).

Synovial folds and bursal thickenings also warrant discussion. Failure of the suprapatellar plica pouch to develop into the medial and lateral components produces a persistent connection between the medial and lateral plicae. This condition may be aggravated by repetitive microtrauma or by an acute traumatic event, creating a fibrotic lesion of the plica fold. The thickened plica can abrade articular cartilage and interfere with patellofemoral contact, creating significant dysfunction of the knee (47,48). Fat pad hypertrophy can create a similar problem, with the potential for impingement and ongoing significant fat pad symptoms (49).

In children, overproduction of joint fluid may occur, and the subsequent collection of fluid in the semimembranosus medial gastrocnemius bursa may be diagnosed as a baker's cyst (50). In a child, this collection of fluid is contained in the normal semimembranosus and medial gastrocnemius bursae. These are normal structures in children and should be treated conservatively in most cases (51).

Congenital and developmental neurologic disorders can affect the structure and the function of the lower extremities. For example, peroneal nerve palsy, equinus, and cavus foot are associated with Charcot-Marie-Tooth disease (52). Profound dysfunction may be observed after polio infection (53,54), central nervous system stroke (55), or cerebral palsy (56). Neuropathic, or Charcot, joints are associated with diabetes mellitus, syphilis, and congenital insensitivity to pain (57); these conditions are extremely important considerations for surgical decision making.

In summary, comprehensive management of knee disorders requires appreciation of the interplay between physical examination, arthroscopic evaluation, and the congenital and development conditions that may predispose to or modulate disease. Such a perspective should help optimize our treatment decisions.

REFERENCES

1. Terry GC. Office evaluation and management of the symptomatic knee. *Orthop Clin North Am* 1988;19:699–713.
2. Bensahel H, Monte Dal A, Hjelmstedt A, et al. Congenital dislocation of the knee. *J Pediatr Orthop* 1989;9:174–177.
3. Johnson E, Audell R, Oppenheim WL. Congenital dislocation of the knee. *J Pediatr Orthop* 1987;7:194–200.
4. Ooishi T, Sugioka Y, Matsumoto S, et al. Congenital dislocation of the knee. Its pathologic features and treatment. *Clin Orthop* 1993;287:187–192.
5. Guidera KJ, Satterwhite Y, Ogden JA, et al. Nail patella syndrome: a review of 44 orthopaedic patients. *J Pediatr Orthop* 1991;11:737–742.
6. Drennan JC. Congenital dislocation of the knee and patella. *Instr Course Lect* 1993;42:517–524.
7. Thomas NP, Jackson AM, Aichroth PM. Congenital absence of the anterior cruciate ligament. *J Bone Joint Surg Br* 1985;67:572–575.
8. Barrett GR, Tomasin JD. Bilateral congenital absence of the anterior cruciate ligament. *Orthopedics* 1988;11:431–434.
9. Johansson E, Aparisi T. Congenital absence of the cruciate ligaments: a case report and review of the literature. *Clin Orthop* 1982;162:108–111.
10. Aichroth PM, Patel DV, Marx CL. Congenital discoid lateral meniscus in children. A follow-up study and evolution of management. *J Bone Joint Surg Br* 1991;73:932–936.
11. Kalamchi A, Dawe RV. Congenital deficiency of the tibia. *J Bone Joint Surg Br* 1985;67:581–584.
12. Spranger J. The epiphyseal dysplasias. *Clin Orthop* 1976;114:46–59.
13. Bradway JK, Klassen RA, Peterson HA. Blount disease: a review of the English literature. *J Pediatr Orthop* 1987;7:472–480.
14. Langenskiold A. Tibia vara. A critical review. *Clin Orthop* 1989;246:195–207.
15. Henderson RC, Kemp J, Hayes PRL. Prevalence of late-onset tibia vara. *J Pediatr Orthop* 1993;13:255–258.
16. Cook SD, Lavernia CJ, Burke SW, et al. A biomechanical analysis of the etiology of tibia vara. *J Pediatr Orthop* 1983;3:449–454.
17. Eckhoff DG, Kramer RC, Alongi CA, et al. Femoral anteversion and arthritis of the knee. *J Pediatr Orthop* 1994;14:608–610.
18. Murphy SB, Simon SR, Kijewski PK. Femoral anteversion. *J Bone Joint Surg Am* 1987;69:1169–1176.
19. Staheli LT. Rotational problems in children. *J Bone Joint Surg Am* 1993;75:939–949.
20. Staheli LT, Corbett M, Wyss C, et al. Lower-extremity rotational problems in children. *J Bone Joint Surg Am* 1985;67:39–47.
21. Salter RB, Best TN. Pathogenesis of progressive valgus deformity following fractures of the proximal metaphyseal region of the tibia in young children. *Instr Course Lect* 1992;41:409–411.
22. Balthazar DA, Pappas AM. Acquired valgus deformity of the tibia in children. *J Pediatr Orthop* 1984;4:538–541.
23. Zionts LE, MacEwen D. Spontaneous improvement of post-traumatic tibia valga. *J Bone Joint Surg Am* 1986;68:680–687.
24. Cooper DE, Warren RF, Warner JJP. The posterior cruciate ligament and posterolateral structures of the knee: anatomy, function, and patterns of injury. *Instr Course Lect* 1991;40:249–268.
25. Curtis BH, Fisher RL. Congenital hyperextension with anterior subluxation of the knee. Surgical treatment and long-term observations. *J Bone Joint Surg Am* 1969;51:255–269.
26. Hubbard DD, Staheli LT, Chew DE, et al. Medial femoral torsion and osteoarthritis. *J Pediatr Orthop* 1988;8:540–542.
27. Yagi T, Sasaki T. Tibial torsion in patients with medial-type osteoarthritic knee. *Clin Orthop* 1986;213:177–182.
28. Hughston JC, Flandry F, Brinker MR, et al. Surgical correction of medial subluxation of the patella. *Am J Sports Med* 1996;24:486–491.
29. Hughston JC, Deese M. Medial subluxation of the patella as a complication of lateral retinacular release. *Am J Sports Med* 1988;16:383–388.
30. Vandermeer RD, Cunningham FK. Arthroscopic treatment of the discoid lateral meniscus: results of long-term follow-up. *Arthroscopy* 1989;5:101–109.
31. Rosenberg TD, Paulos LE, Parker RD, et al. Discoid lateral meniscus: case report of arthroscopic attachment of a symptomatic Wrisberg-ligament type. *Arthroscopy* 1987;3:277–282.
32. Neuschwander DC, Drez D Jr, Finney TP. Lateral meniscal variant with absence of the posterior coronary ligament. *J Bone Joint Surg Am* 1992;74:1186–1190.
33. Howell SM. Arthroscopic roofplasty: a method for correcting an extension deficit caused by roof impingement of an anterior cruciate ligament graft. *Arthroscopy* 1992;8:375–379.
34. Howell SM, Farley TE. A rationale for predicting anterior cruciate graft impingement by the intercondylar roof. A magnetic resonance imaging study. *Am J Sports Med* 1991;19:276–282.
35. McCall RE, Lessenberry HB. Bilateral congenital dislocation of the patella. *J Pediatr Orthop* 1987;7:100–102.
36. Lancourt JE, Cristini JA. Patella alta and patella infera. Their etiologic role in patellar dislocation, chondromalacia, and apophysitis of the tibial tubercle. *J Bone Joint Surg Am* 1975;57:1112–1115.
37. Ogata K. Painful bipartite patella. A new approach to operative treatment. *J Bone Joint Surg Am* 1994;76:573–578.
38. Bourne MH, Bianco AJ Jr. Bipartite patella in the adolescent: results of surgical excision. *J Pediatr Orthop* 1990;10:69–73.
39. Ogden JA, Southwick WO. Osgood-Schlatter's disease and tibial tuberosity development. *Clin Orthop* 1976;116:180–189.
40. Krause BL, Williams JPR, Catterall A, et al. Natural history of Osgood-Schlatter disease. *J Pediatr Orthop* 1990;10:65–68.
41. Kujala UM, Kvist M, Heinonen O. Osgood-Schlatter's disease in adolescent athletes. Retrospective study of incidence and duration. *Am J Sports Med* 1985;13:236–240.
42. Medlar RC, Lyne D. Sinding-Larsen-Johansson disease. Its etiology and natural history. *J Bone Joint Surg Am* 1978;60:1113–1116.
43. Weiner DS, Macnab I. The "fabella syndrome": an update. *J Pediatr Orthop* 1982;2:405–408.
44. Hughston JC, Hergenroeder PT, Courtenay BG. Osteochondritis dissecans of the femoral condyles. *J Bone Joint Surg Am* 1984;66:1340–1348.
45. Terry GC, Flandry F, Van Manen JW, et al. Isolated chondral fractures of the knee. *Clin Orthop* 1988;234:170–177.
46. Hodge JC, Ghelman B. Standard radiologic analysis of the normal and abnormal knee. In: Scott NW, ed. *The knee*. St. Louis: Mosby, 1994:123–128.
47. Hardaker WT, Whipple TL, Bassett FH 3rd. Diagnosis and treatment of the plica syndrome of the knee. *J Bone Joint Surg Am* 1980;62:221–225.
48. Nottage WM, Sprague NF, Auerbach BJ, et al. The medial patellar plica syndrome. *Am J Sports Med* 1983;11:211–214.
49. Metheny JA, Mayor MB. Hoffa disease: chronic impingement of the infrapatellar fat pad. *Am J Knee Surg* 1988;1:134–139.
50. Dinham JM. Popliteal cysts in children. The case against surgery. *J Bone Joint Surg Br* 1975;57:69–71.
51. Curl WW. Popliteal cysts: historical background and current knowledge. *J Am Acad Orthop Surg* 1996;4:129–133.
52. Sabir M, Lyttle D. Pathogenesis of Charcot-Marie-Tooth disease. Gait analysis and electrophysiologic, genetic, histopathologic, and enzyme studies in a kinship. *Clin Orthop* 1984;184:223–235.
53. Conner AN. The treatment of flexion contractures of the knee in poliomyelitis. *J Bone Joint Surg Br* 1990;52:138–144.
54. Asirvatham R, Rooney RJ, Watts HG. Proximal tibial extension medial rotation osteotomy to correct knee flexion contracture and lateral rotation deformity of tibia after polio. *J Pediatr Orthop* 1991;11:646–651.
55. Perry J. Orthopaedic evaluation and treatment of the stroke patient. *Instr Course Lect* 1975;24:26–35.
56. Evans EB. Knee flexion deformity in cerebral palsy. *Instr Course Lect* 1971;20:42–53.
57. Soudry M, Binazzi R, Johanson NA, et al. Total knee arthroplasty in Charcot and Charcot-like joints. *Clin Orthop* 1986;208:199–204.

SECTION II

Function

CHAPTER 5

Mobility of the Knee

John J. O'Connor, Jennifer Feikes, Richie H.S. Gill, and Amy B. Zavatsky

The joints give the skeleton its mobility. The muscles stabilize the skeleton by suppressing joint mobility. This chapter explains how the articular surfaces and the ligaments of the knee interact to control the mobility of the joint. It demonstrates how the ligaments guide the movements of the bones on each other. Chapter 10 describes how the same passive structures interact together and with the muscles to limit mobility and to control stability. It demonstrates how the ligaments restrain the movements of the bones on each other.

In activity, motion occurs under load, combining the mechanisms that control mobility with those that control stability but those mechanisms are most easily understood when they are treated separately. This chapter and Chapter 10 together describe work completed and published by us and others since the publication of the first edition of the book, *Knee Ligaments: Structure, Function, Injury, and Repair,* in 1990. We refer frequently to that book but do not repeat much of what was written there.

MOBILITY

If we were to cut all the soft tissues holding the tibia to the femur and disarticulate the knee, we would give the tibia six degrees of freedom (DOF) relative to the femur, imparting unlimited mobility. It would be free to rotate without restraint about each of three perpendicular axes and to translate along each of those three axes. The passive structures of the joint, the articular surfaces and the ligaments, suppress most of those freedoms, limiting the possible range of movement and the number of DOF within that range. We report first the results of an experimental study of the number of degrees of unresisted freedom (DOUF) exhibited by the human knee within its range of motion, in the process quantifying what has been called the *screw-home mechanism*. We then describe three-dimensional (3-D) and two-dimensional (2-D) mathematical models of the joint that explain and interpret the experimental findings.

EXPERIMENTAL ASSESSMENT

Figure 5.1 shows a simple apparatus, the fixed tibia rig, used to study the mobility of the cadaver knee under minimal load (1). The specimens were fresh frozen at autopsy and thawed just before an experiment. Skin and muscle were removed, but care was taken to leave the capsule and its contents intact. Each specimen retained about 15 cm of the distal femur and of the proximal tibia. The proximal tibia was potted and fixed to the workbench with the tibial plateau approximately horizontal. A Perspex rod was fixed into the femoral shaft; its proximal end lay on a horizontal rod that could be raised and lowered, extending and flexing the knee. The intramedullary rod was free to slide and rotate on the horizontal rod without restraint, apart from friction, so that this apparatus fulfills the criteria for a six-DOF rig (see Chapter 8, "Experimental Methods Used to Evaluate Knee Ligament Function," in first edition), ensuring that the only constraints to motion are those applied by the structures of the specimen joint.

The only load present was the weight of the distal femur and the intramedullary rod, about 10 N (2 lb), partly transmitted across the joint and partly supported on the horizontal rod. This weight was sufficient to keep the intramedullary rod in contact with the horizontal rod during flexion, implying that the passive structures of the knee offered very little resistance to these movements. The experiment therefore examined the kinematics of the joint in the virtually unloaded state: passive motion.

During repeated cycles of flexion and extension, movement of the femur on the tibia was recorded using a magnetic position tracker/digitizer (Isotrack II, Polhemus, Inc., Colchester, VT). Data were analyzed using 3-D kinematic theory (2,3).

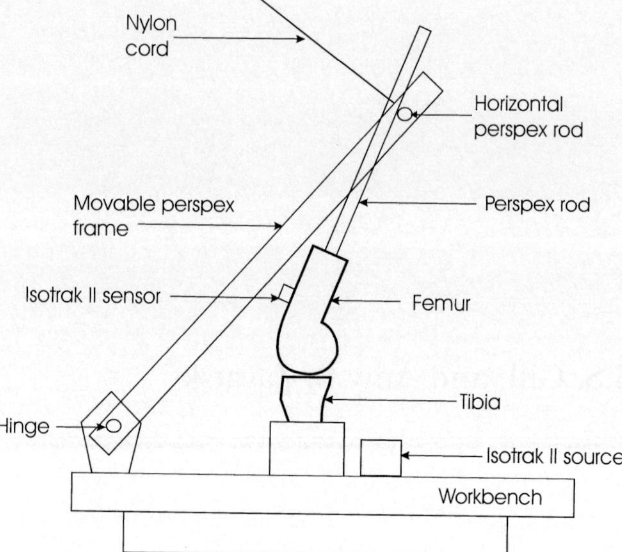

FIGURE 5.1. The fixed tibia rig. The section of distal femur with its intramedullary rod is free to move on the fixed proximal tibia. Flexion and extension of the joint can be controlled by lowering or raising the nylon string attached to the horizontal Perspex rod. The associated movements of the femur on the tibia are recorded with the Isotrack II sensor. (From Wilson DR, Feikes JD, Zavatsky AB, et al. The components of passive knee movement are coupled to flexion angle. *J Biomech* 2000;33:465–473, with permission.)

Motion Path

Figure 5.2 shows that the path of motion exhibited by a single specimen during flexion was repeated in reverse during extension. The graphs show axial rotation and abduction or adduction of the joint and the three components of translation of a single point in the femur (i.e., the most posterior point on the anterior cruciate ligament [ACL] attachment) plotted against flexion angle. The femur followed a unique path of coupled motion relative to the tibia during flexion and extension, with the other five DOF directly related to the flexion angle. The upper curves in the left-hand graph show that the femur rotated externally on the tibia through about 25° over 100° of flexion. This curve is a quantification of the screw-home mechanism, first described by Meyer in 1853 (4). The lower curves show that the femur adducts through about 7° on the tibia from extension to about 40° of flexion and then abducts again. The right-hand graph shows that the chosen point in the femur moves posteriorly and distally during flexion but that the form of the translation curves varies from point to point in the femur. More significant translations, movements of the contact points of the femoral condyles on the tibial plateau, are subsequently described.

Figure 5.3 shows that the mean values (±1 SD) of all five components of movement for 12 intact specimens followed paths similar to those of Figure 5.2 over the flexion range with relatively little scatter.

Figure 5.4 compares the graph of external femoral rotation (±1 SD) for the 12 specimens tested in the fixed tibia

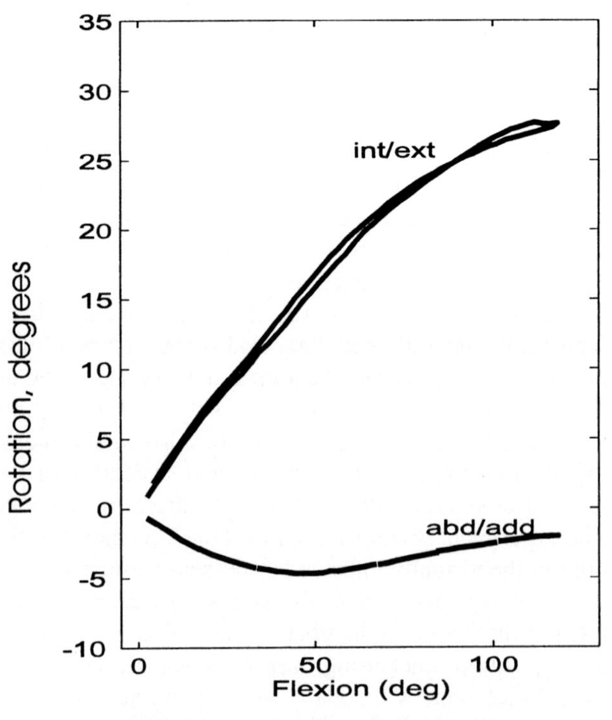

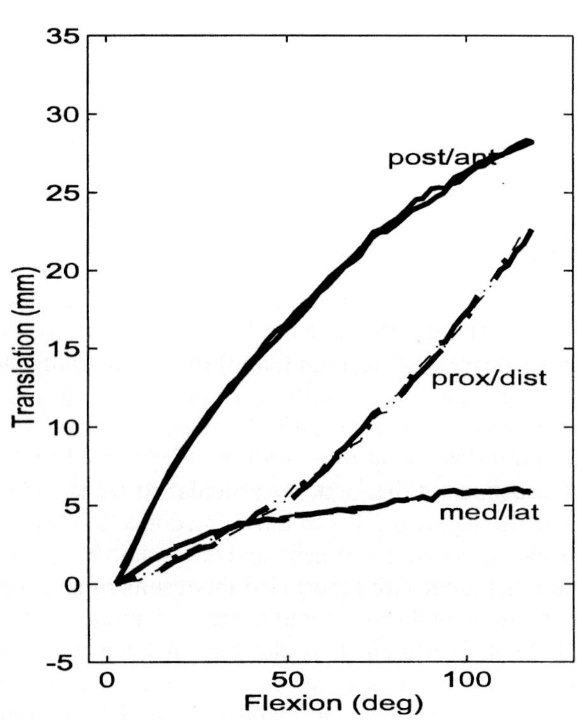

FIGURE 5.2. A: Plots against flexion angle of external (+) and internal femoral rotation, abduction/adduction. **B:** The three components of translation of the most anterior point on the posterior cruciate ligament femoral attachment during a single cycle of flexion and extension of one specimen.

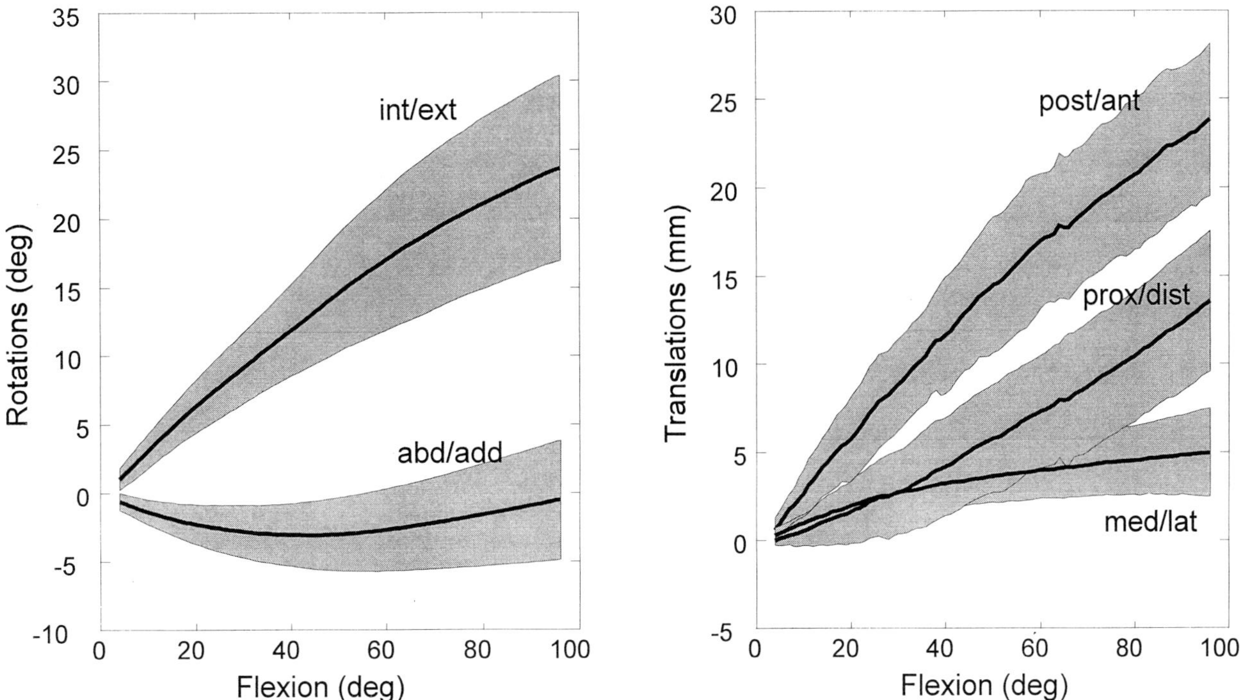

FIGURE 5.3. Rotations and translations plotted against flexion angle. Mean values are given for 12 specimens ± 1 SD. (From Wilson DR, Feikes JD, Zavatsky AB, et al. The components of passive knee movement are coupled to flexion angle. *J Biomech* 2000;33:465–473, with permission.)

rig of Figure 5.1 with the graph of internal tibial rotation for 10 specimens tested in the unloaded state in the flexed-knee stance Oxford rig described in Figure 6.6 (5). The mean values obtained in the two rigs are almost identical; the standard deviations obtained in the flexed knee stance rig are slightly smaller. The comparison demonstrates that external femoral rotation relative to a fixed tibia is the same as internal tibial rotation relative to a fixed femur. The coupling of axial rotation to flexion is independent of the six-DOF rig used for its assessment. The path of unresisted motion is a characteristic of the unloaded human knee rather than an artifact of a particular experiment.

The curves of Figures 5.2 through 5.4 show that all six DOF of motion at the human knee are coupled together. When the value of the flexion angle is chosen, the values of the two other angles of rotation and of the three components

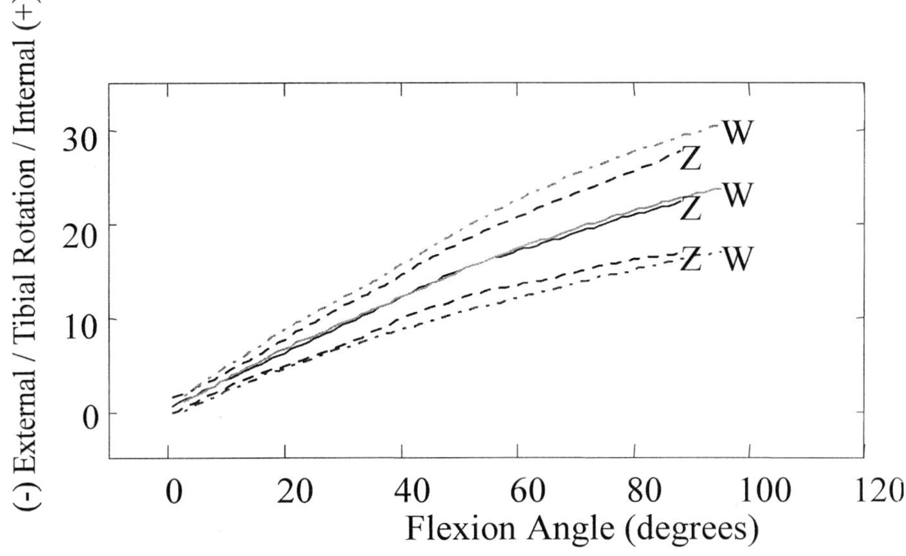

FIGURE 5.4. External or internal rotation of the tibia relative to the femur plotted against flexion angle for 12 specimens tested in the fixed tibia rig *(W)* and 10 specimens tested in the flexed-knee-stance rig *(Z)*. Mean values are given ± 1 SD.

of translation of any point are then fully determined. In other words, the unloaded human knee is a single-DOF system. This implies that the passive structures of the knee suppress five of the six possible DOF by applying five independent constraints to motion of the bones relative to each other. This interpretation is at variance with some recent work; Blankevoort et al. (6) prefer to describe the knee as a two-DOF system, with axial rotation and flexion angle varying independently of each other. They were unable to observe a consistent path of motion in the unloaded knee. Applying successively external and internal tibial torque of 3 Nm, they could twist the knee up to about 40°, defining an "envelope of passive motion" of width varying with flexion angle (7). Bourne et al. (8) and Goodfellow and O'Connor (8a) in similar experiments on the flexed-knee-stance Oxford rig (see Figure 6.6) had previously defined a "range of tibial rotation" varying from zero at full extension to about 30° at 90° flexion.

This study shows that, in the unloaded knee, the internal–external axial rotation can be determined within an average of one degree (the difference between the flexing and extending paths) at a specified flexion angle. Our results for the totally unloaded joint lie within Blankevoort's envelope but closer to their "internal pathway."

Perturbation Tests

With each specimen tested in the fixed tibia rig (Fig. 5.1), the flexing—extending motion was stopped in a number of positions, and manual pressure was applied to move the intramedullary rod in both directions along the horizontal rod until significant resistance to further motion was sensed, at which point the manual pressure was removed. The movements recorded during these perturbation tests were completely recovered, with elastic spring-back, when the manual pressure was removed and motion along the unique path of passive motion was resumed (Fig. 5.5). (A more quantitative description of the movements occurring during perturbation tests and their dependence on load is given in Chapter 10.)

In the perturbation tests, displacement away from the paths defined in Figures 5.2 through 5.4 was resisted, presumably by compression of the articular surfaces and extension of the ligaments and therefore requiring the application of load, whereas motion along the paths was unresisted and presumably did not involve tissue deformation. Removal of the perturbing load brought the specimen back to the position of unresisted motion again, with recovery of the tissue deformation, elastic spring-back. This implies that the unloaded human knee exhibits one degree of *unresisted* freedom (DOUF) and that the five associated constraints to passive motion guide the bones along the path of coupled motion (Figs. 5.2–5.4) without tissue deformation. Because motion along this path is unresisted, it connects a continuum of positions of neutral equilibrium. The knee is unstable with respect to motion along the path; there is no elastic spring-back when it is displaced from

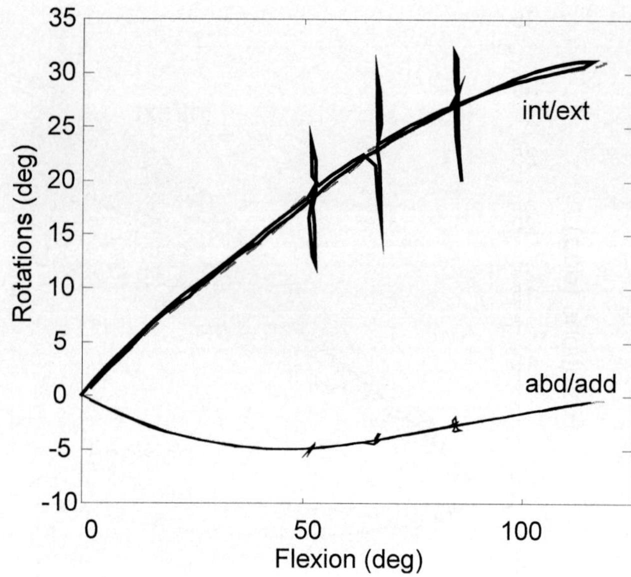

FIGURE 5.5. Perturbations to path of unresisted motion produced in a single specimen at 50°, 65°, and 85° of flexion. (From Wilson DR, Feikes JD, Zavatsky AB, et al. The components of passive knee movement are coupled to flexion angle. *J Biomech* 2000;33:465–473, with permission.)

one point along the path to another. The intervention of forces in other structures (e.g., muscle forces, tension in the posterior capsule near extension) is required if motion along the path is to be resisted. The knee is stable with respect to displacements away from the path of unresisted motion. These displacements are resisted increasingly by forces developed in the passive structures. The displacements occurring during the perturbation tests are a measure of the passive laxity of the joint.

The perturbation tests demonstrated that the path of motion of one bone on the other is readily altered by the application of load to deform the tissues, with different loads producing different alterations to the path. This explains why it is often difficult to reconcile results from different laboratories reporting movement paths under different loading conditions. The path of unresisted passive motion represents the constraints to movement applied by the passive structures of the joint alone. The experiments described by Blankevoort et al. (7), Bourne et al. (8), and Goodfellow and O'Connor (8a) quantify the relation between perturbing load and the associated load-dependent movements. These matters are discussed further in Chapter 10.

Because there is an infinite number of possible loads that could be applied, each eliciting its own movement path, the advantage of studying the unloaded path of motion becomes clear. It provides a unique picture of the mobility of the joint.

Damaged Specimens

Three other specimens did not exhibit the unique paths of coupled motion just described; the flexing path was

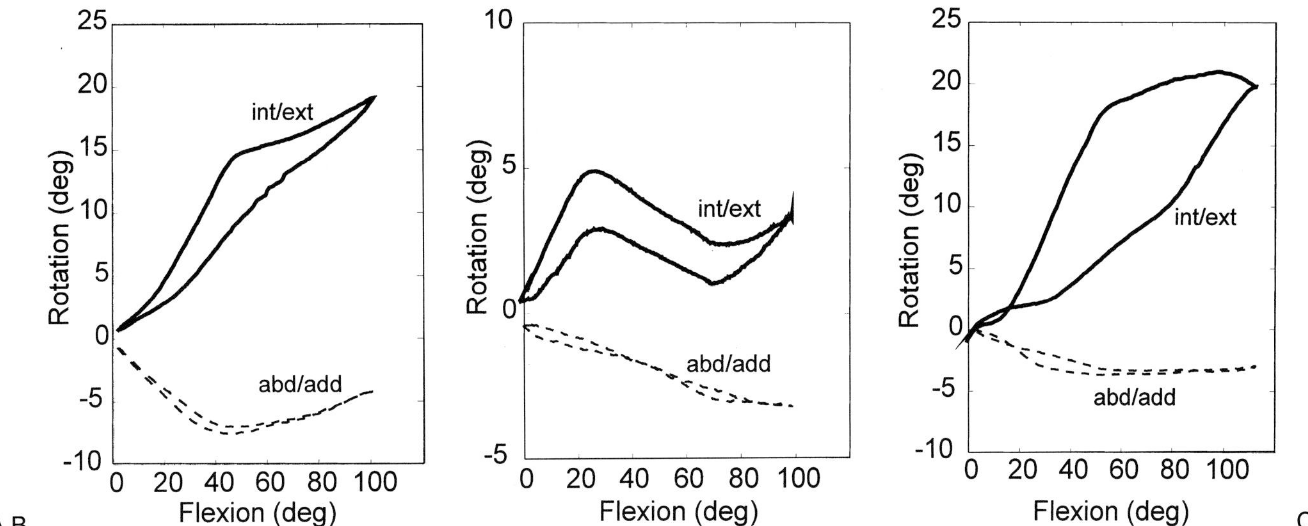

FIGURE 5.6. Three specimens that exhibited different flexing and extending paths. On disarticulation, **(A)** and **(B)** were found to be arthrotic, and **(C)** had a damaged medial collateral ligament.

different from the extending path with distinct hysteresis loops (Fig. 5.6). When these specimens were disarticulated, it was found that two of them exhibited severe osteoarthrotic changes, with erosion of the tibiofemoral articular surfaces, and that the medial collateral ligament of the third specimen had been unwittingly damaged by the scalpel during specimen preparation.

These fortuitous observations confirm the deduction that the articular surfaces and the ligaments act together to constrain the movements of the joint and guide the bones along their path of unresisted passive motion. The constraints to movement are flexible, accounting for the elastic spring-back observed in the perturbation tests.

When the surfaces or the ligaments are damaged, the kinematic behavior of the joint is changed and the number of DOUF is increased.

Helical Axes

There is an alternative way of describing the coupled motion depicted by the graphs of Figures 5.2 through 5.4. As the knee joint flexes, the relative motion of the bones can be described as a pure rotation about a helical axis and as translation along the helical axis (9). Few studies have attempted this description because of poor consistency and reproducibility of results (10). Figure 5.7

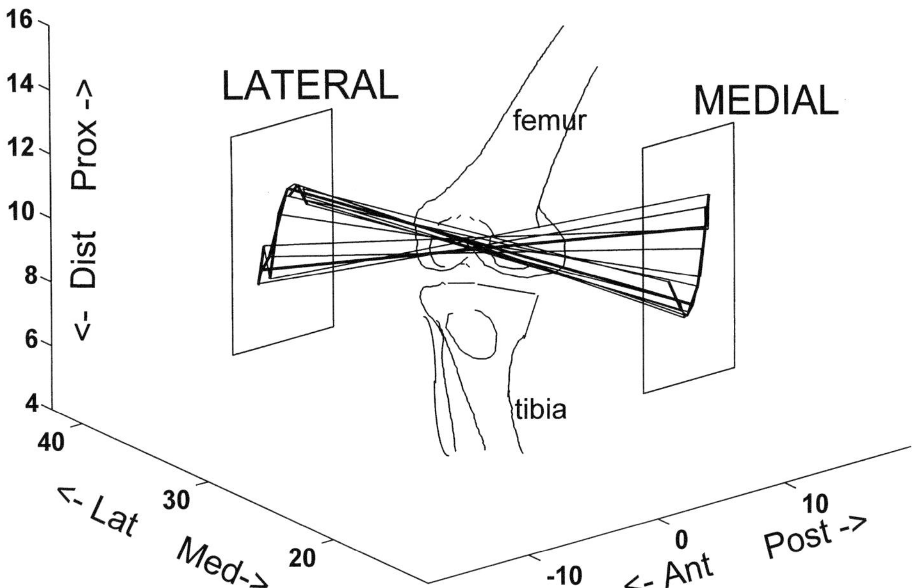

FIGURE 5.7. Finite helical axes of rotation and their tracks on medial and lateral parasagittal planes. (From Wilson DR, Feikes JD, Zavatsky AB, et al. The components of passive knee movement are coupled to flexion angle. *J Biomech* 2000;33:465–473, with permission.)

shows that the helical axis of rotation of the joint at different flexion angles rotates and translates relative to both bones over the flexion range. The positions of the helical axes were calculated from the experiments on the fixed tibia rig using 3-D kinematic theory (9). Similar patterns have been shown by Blankevoort et al. (11), who also found that the axes in the frontal plane were tilted toward the lateral compartment, consistent with the coupling of axial rotation with flexion. Although precise comparison is difficult because of differences in loading conditions in the experiments, they also found a posterior translation of the helical axis of about 8 mm.

Motion of the helical axis relative to the bones demonstrates that the human knee is not a simple hinge with a fixed axis of rotation nor does it move in a single plane. The rotation of the helical axis demonstrates that the coupling between the DOF alters during joint motion, which is also implied by the fact that the curves of Figure 5.1 are not straight. Translation of the helical axis implies that the articular surfaces must roll as well as slide on each other and that the contact point between the femur and the tibia in medial and lateral compartments must translate on the tibial plateau as well as on the femoral condyles.

Contact Point Movement

Another alternative way to describe motion is to track the contact points between femur and tibia in both compartments over the flexion range. The specimens were disarticulated after the tests, and the shapes of the articular surfaces and ligament attachment sites were digitized relative to the positions of reference markers on the bones. Fourth-order polynomial surfaces were then fitted mathematically to each of the articular surfaces. The positions of the bones over the flexion range were reconstructed mathematically from the data collected during the flexion—extension tests, allowing estimation of the point of nearest approach of each femoral condyle to the corresponding tibial plateau.

In the mathematical reconstruction, the modeled surfaces were found not to touch exactly but were apparently separated or interpenetrated because of experimental error.

Table 5.1 includes values of the calculated movement of the medial and lateral contact points in each specimen together with the proximity errors. The proximity error gives a measure of the accuracy with which the positions of the femoral articular surfaces were reconstructed relative to those of the tibia. It represents the accumulation of errors introduced during the measurement of motion of the intact specimens, the digitization of the articular surfaces, the fitting of mathematical surfaces to the digitized data, and the mathematical reconstruction of the motion.

Figure 5.8 shows the movement of the *contact point*, the common normal to the two reconstructed surfaces through their point of nearest approach or maximum interpenetration at more than 100° of flexion.

The proximity error for each specimen for each compartment is included as a pair of error bands. Three of the specimens proved to have proximity errors of more than 5 mm, and their data are not included in the subsequent analysis. Backward movements of the contact point were found in all the remaining nine specimens, averaging 10.4 mm medially (range, 0.7 to 19.6) and 13.4 mm laterally (range, 9.2 to 18.0); the average for both compartments was 11.9 mm.

The difference between medial and lateral contact point movement reflects the coupled external rotation of the femur on the tibia during flexion, reducing the medial movement and increasing the lateral movement from the average. The average medial contact point movement was 12.6% less than the average for both compartments for all

TABLE 5.1. *Calculated posterior movement of medial and lateral tibiofemoral contact point*

Specimen	Medial (mm)	Lateral (mm)	Proximity error (mm)
B	0.7	16.5	3.1
E	6.3	13.1	4.1
F	7.4	18.0	3.9
G	8.8	11.6	3.4
H	9.1	10.2	1.3
I	11.4	9.2	2.3
J	12.4	13.5	2.0
K	18.0	15.2	2.0
L	19.6	12.9	4.2
Mean (n = 9)	10.4	13.4	2.9
SD	5.8	2.9	1.1
SEM	1.7	0.8	0.3
Proximity error > 5 mm			
A	−4.5	9.0	8.7
C	1.9	22.3	6.9
D	3.3	24.6	6.1

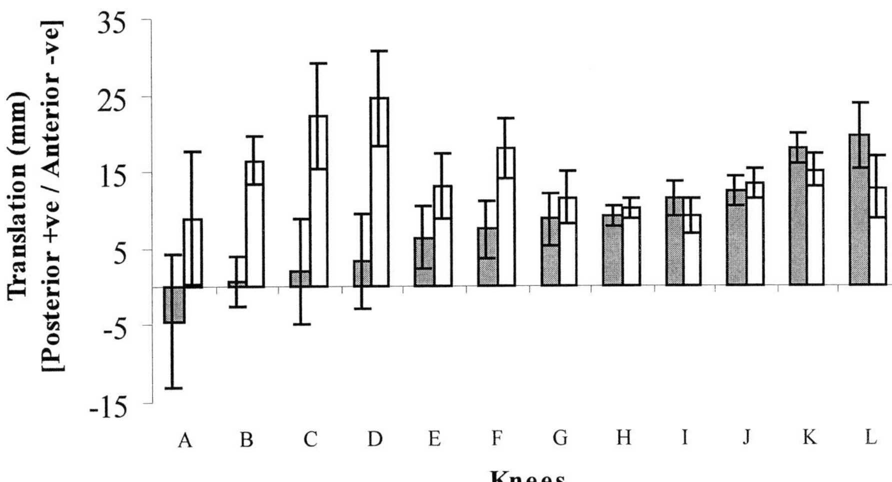

FIGURE 5.8. Contact point movement for 12 specimens in medial and lateral compartments over 100° of flexion. Proximity errors are shown as error bars.

joints, and the average lateral movement was 12.6% more. These proportions are somewhat smaller than the proportion (25%) of external femoral rotation to flexion in the same experiments, but the determination of the bulk movements of the bones is more accurate than the determination of the contact point movements.

We can bring together these various views of passive knee kinematics. Flexion accounts for the average movement of the contact points medially and laterally and for the translation of the helical axis. External rotation of the femur or internal rotation of the tibia reduces medial contact point movement, increases lateral contact point movement from the average, and accounts for the inclination of the helical axis of motion toward the lateral compartment.

Slip Ratio

The movements of the contact points on the tibial plateaus confirm that the femur rolls as well as slides on the tibia during flexion or extension. The methods used to locate the contact points on the tibia were also used to locate them on the femur. Figure 5.9 shows the *slip ratio*, the distance moved by the contact point on the tibia divided by the distance it moved on the femur, for the nine specimens with smaller proximity errors, at various points over the range of flexion.[1] The slip ratio would have the value zero if the contact point remained stationary on the tibia. It would have the value unity for "pure" rolling, with equal contact point movements on the femur and tibia. It did not reach either of these limiting values for medial or lateral compartments, so there was always a combination of continuous rolling and sliding in each compartment. The slip ratio for the medial compartment in the nine specimens tested in the fixed tibia rig remained between 0.2 and 0.4, whereas the values were generally higher in the lateral compartment, between 0.4 and 0.7, indicative of a greater degree of rolling and larger contact point movements in the lateral compartment in most of the specimens (Fig. 5.8).

Iwaki et al. (13) used magnetic resonance imaging (MRI) to study contact point movement. They fitted two circles to sagittal plane images of the femoral condyles and two intersecting straight lines to those of the tibial plateaus. They reported posterior movements of the centers of the femoral circles on the tibia of 8 mm on the medial side and 25 mm on the lateral side. Although the rolling movements on the lateral plateau were described as continuous, increasing steadily with flexion angle, the movements medially were described as discontinuous, with a jump in the position of the medial circle center at about 25° of flexion from an extension position to a flexion position—rock rather than roll. No analysis of experimental error was given.

Our evidence does not support that view. The slip ratios reported in Figure 5.8 remain consistently greater than zero over the flexion range, implying continuous rolling superimposed on sliding. Our analysis involved fitting the surfaces with continuous fourth-order polynomials, a more accurate procedure than the use of discontinuous straight lines or circles.

---

[1]The inverse definition of slip ratio (i.e., femoral contact point movement to tibial contact point movement) was given in Figure 10.14 of the previous edition and in O'Connor et al. (12). The values of slip ratio given there were all greater than unity, and the values given here are all less than unity.

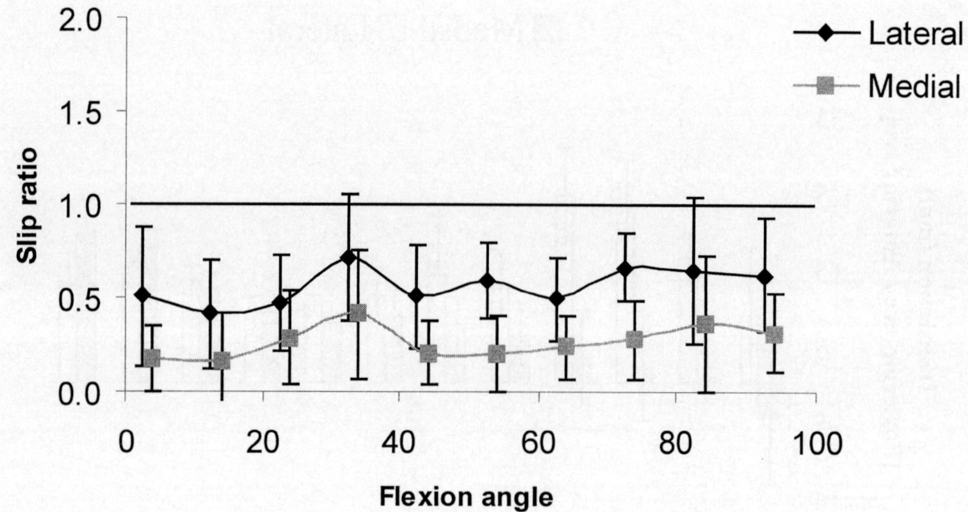

FIGURE 5.9. The slip ratio (i.e., distance moved by the contact point on the tibia divided by the distance moved by the contact point on the femur) is plotted against the flexion angle. Mean values ± 1 SD are given for nine specimens with proximity errors less than 5 mm.

Movements of the Menisci

The menisci are dragged backward and forward to accommodate the contact point movements, as described in 1680 by Borelli (14), in 1987 by Kapandji (15), and in 1991 by Thompson et al. (16) using MRI. Kapandji reported movements of 6 mm for the medial meniscus and 12 mm for the lateral, and Thompson gave values of 5.1 and 11.2 mm, respectively. These values for the lateral side compare reasonably with our value of average contact point movement, but the medial values are smaller than our medial contact point movement. Vedi et al. (17) showed that meniscal movement was slightly increased by weight bearing.

The range of values found in our experiments reflects the inevitable experimental error and could also reflect actual variation from specimen to specimen. The larger range found medially may indicate that inter-specimen variation is found more predominantly in the medial compartment.

Ligament Length Patterns

There has long been interest in the patterns of tightening and slackening exhibited by the ligaments of the knee during flexion and extension, an interest rekindled by the surgical practice of ligament reconstruction. Brantigan and Voshell (18), in their classic 1941 paper, were able to cite 10 references in favor, 10 references against, and 10 references neutral on a range of propositions regarding length-change patterns of a variety of ligament fibers. Development of modern methods of measurement and analysis has provided more, but not complete, unanimity. Although direct *in vivo* methods have been developed by Beynnon and Fleming (19), the range of activities that the subject can perform under local anesthetic is probably limited. Indirect methods using cadaver specimens will continue to be the main source of data until noninvasive imaging techniques become more accurate.

Ligament Architecture

The architecture of ligament fibers or fascicles of fibers is the determining factor. Odensten and Gillquist (20), Arnoczky (21), Friederich et al. (22), and Girgis et al. (23) studied the shapes of the femoral areas of origin and the tibial areas of insertion of the cruciates. Painstaking experiments have been performed by Friederich et al. (22) (Fig. 5.10A, B) and by Mommersteeg et al. (24) (Fig. 5.10C) to trace the tracks of individual fascicles from points within the femoral area of origin to corresponding points within the tibial area of insertion. It is clear from this work that there is a systematic mapping of fascicles from specific points within each area of origin to specific points within the corresponding area of insertion.

Feikes (25) repeated these studies for the cruciates and extended them to the medial collateral ligament (MCL) and the lateral collateral ligament (LCL) (Fig. 5.11). She then developed mathematical formulas that defined the mapping at arbitrary points within the attachments, extrapolating from the known mapping of limited numbers of fibers.

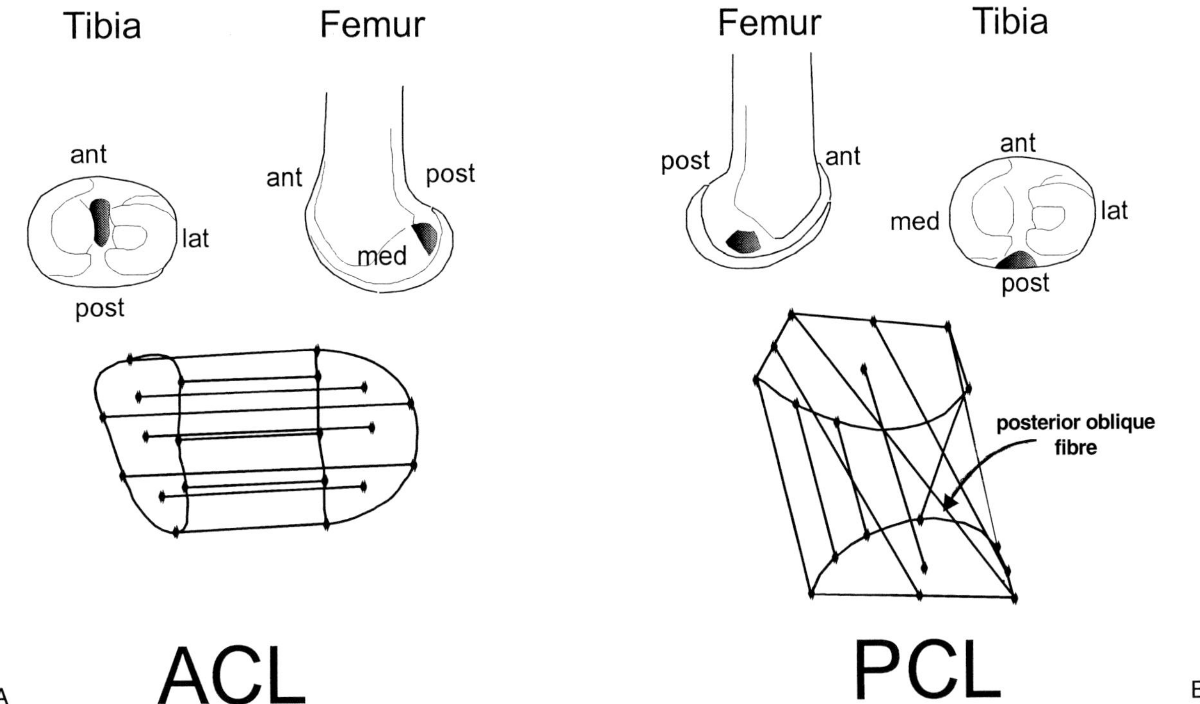

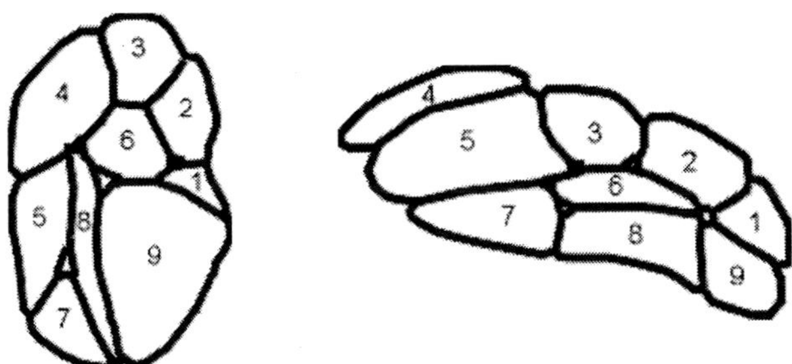

FIGURE 5.10. Fiber mapping of the **(A)** anterior (ACL) and **(B)** posterior cruciate ligaments (PCL) according to Friederich et al. (22) and **(C)** mapping of the ACL according to Mommersteeg et al. (24).(From Friedrich NF, Müller W, O'Brien WR. [Clinical application of biomechanic and functional anatomic finding of the knee joint]. *Orthopade* 1992;21:41–50 and Mommersteeg TJ, Kooloos JG, Blankevoort L, et al. The fibre bundle anatomy of human cruciate ligaments. *J Anat* 1995;187 (Pt2):461–471, with permission.)

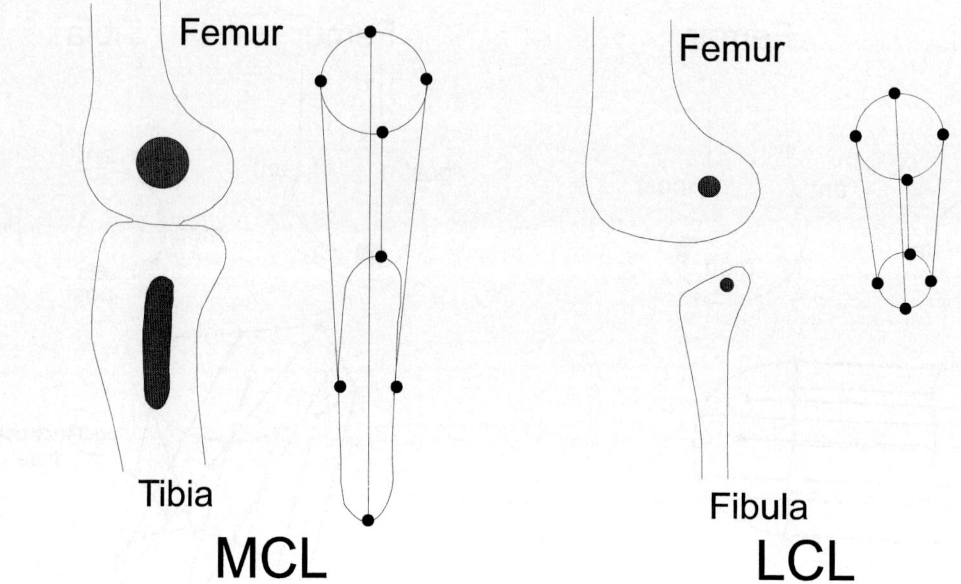

FIGURE 5.11. Mapping of the fibers in the medial (MCL) and lateral collateral ligaments (LCL).

Isometric Ligament Fibers

During flexion and extension, the ligament attachment areas rotate and translate relative to each other, so that the fibers would be expected to slacken or tighten (Fig. 5.12). However, it remains possible that certain fibers could remain isometric. They can rotate about their origins and insertions, following the movements of their attachment areas without stretching or slackening. Knowing the mapping of fibers from one bone to the other (i.e., the position coordinates within the areas of origin and insertion of individual fiber fascicles), the distance between the

points of origin and insertion can be calculated at different positions over the range of passive flexion.

Figure 5.13 shows the positions within the attachment areas of fibers (i.e., physiologic fibers) found to be most nearly isometric in the ACL, posterior cruciate ligament (PCL), and MCL. Similar diagrams for the LCL are not presented because the areas of origin and insertion are so small. Also included in the figure are the positions of digitized points within both areas whose calculated distances apart remained most nearly constant over the range of passive flexion (i.e., combination fibers), as in the technique used by Sidles et al. (26). The combination fibers may also be representative of fiber length patterns determined by measuring movements into and out of the tibia of sutures fixed at different points within the femoral origin area and passing through the tibial insertion area of the ligaments, the technique used by Sapega et al. (27) and Zavras et al. (28).

The figure shows that the femoral origins of the most isometric physiologic fibers were found to be consistent with those of the combination fibers for most specimens. This was not found to be the case for the tibial insertions, especially for the MCL. Table 5.2 shows maximum changes in length, expressed as percentages, for the most isometric fibers, physiologic and combination.

The apparent length changes are well within the errors to be expected from our analysis of proximity error (Table 5.1), and the inconsistencies suggested by some of the data in Figure 5.13 are not surprising. Nonetheless, the percentages of length changes found in all the ligaments in most of the specimens are small (<4%). This justifies the assumption that there are fibers that can remain truly isometric. They could act as constraints to motion and help guide the passive motion of the unloaded

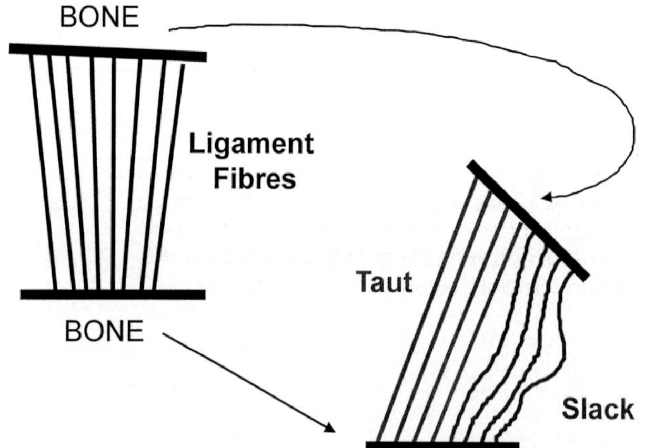

FIGURE 5.12. Ligament fibers or fascicles mapped from the femur to the tibia slacken and tighten as their attachment areas rotate relative to each other during flexion and extension. (From Zavatsky AB, O'Connor JJ, Lu TW. Biomechanical functions of ligaments: implications for ACL reconstruction. *Orthopaedics International Edition* 1996;4:349–357, with permission.)

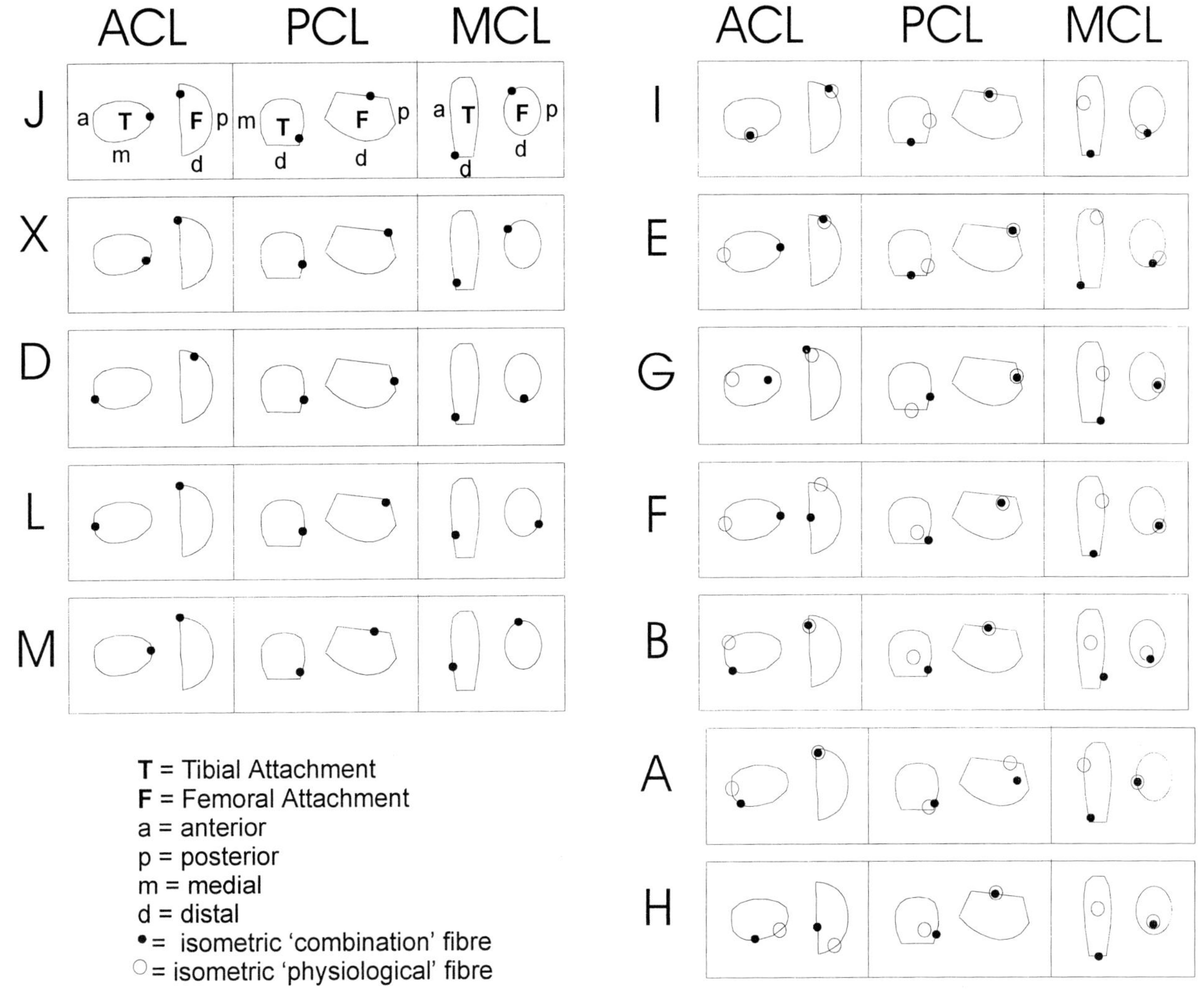

FIGURE 5.13. Positions in femoral and tibial attachments of the four ligaments of physiologic fascicles found to be most isometric in each of 12 specimens. ACL, anterior cruciate ligaments; PCL, posterior cruciate ligaments; MCL, medial collateral ligament.

TABLE 5.2. *Percentage length changes of the most isometric combination fibers in 12 specimens*

Specimen	ACL	PCL	MCL	LCL
J	3.03	14.57	3.95	6.75
D	2.89	6.6	3.74	5.79
L	5.37	7.97	4.68	4.78
M	5.91	18.28	3.21	4.24
X	4.81	8.92	3.72	3.72
I	1.84 (1.93)	3.17 (3.70)	1.46 (1.41)	14.15 (17.23)
E	3.0 (14.82)	1.41 (2.43)	1.2 (1.19)	2.6 (2.86)
G	2.98 (3.31)	2.58 (3.02)	1.67 (2.16)	1.65 (1.73)
F	1.82 (2.63)	1.73 (1.94)	1.4 (1.60)	1.03 (1.42)
B	3.62 (3.43)	4.13 (4.64)	1.67 (1.69)	2.14 (2.22)
A	2.34 (2.39)	6.02 (7.23)	2.53 (3.47)	3.21 (3.92)
H	3.58 (7.33)	2.93 (3.66)	1.2 (1.44)	2.29 (2.49)
Mean	3.43	6.53	2.54	4.36
SD	1.32	5.27	1.26	3.52
Mean (I to H)	2.74 (5.12)	3.14 (3.80)	1.59 (1.85)	3.87 (4.55)
SD (I to H)	0.76 (4.64)	1.56 (1.75)	0.46 (0.78)	4.58 (5.65)

Within parentheses, the most physiologic fibers in seven specimens.
CL, cruciate ligament; A, anterior; L, lateral; M, medial; P, posterior.

joint. They also can be used to explain the coupled motion of the joint observed in our experiments.

Calculation of Ligament Length Patterns

Feikes (25) defined a grid of points on the tibial insertion of each of the ligaments of her experimental specimens. Using the mapping functions described previously, she identified the positions within the corresponding femoral origin of an array of fibers and calculated the distances between the origins and insertions of each fiber within the array. She presented her results in the form of contours of length change (Fig. 5.14).

Figure 5.14 shows contours of length change in the ACL of one specimen, drawn on the tibial attachment of the ligament and expressed as proportions of the lengths of fibers at full extension. The contours define surfaces within the ligament on which all fibers experience the same percentage of length change. There appears to be a surface at the front of the ligament on which fibers remain isometric, whereas all fibers behind that surface slacken as the joint flexes.

The patterns of length change shown in Figure 5.14 were consistent with those found in four of the other six specimens examined and consistent with recent reports in the literature. Sidles et al. (26) showed patterns similar to those of Figure 5.14. Sapega et al. (27) found the anteromedial region of the ACL to be the most isometric and observed slackening followed by lengthening of fibers in the central and posterior regions of the ligament during passive flexion. Blankevoort et al. (29) also found that a posterior bundle shortened and that an anterior bundle remained close to constant length during flexion.

Contours of constant length change are shown in Figure 5.15 for the PCL in the same specimen, with the length change expressed as a proportion of the length at full extension. In the PCL, the isometric surface lies within the body of the ligament. Fibers in front of that surface tighten, and fibers behind it slacken during flexion. This outcome is consistent with Covey's (30) observations that the anterior fibers of the PCL are slack in extension and tighten progressively during flexion, whereas the posterior fibers are tight in extension, slacken, and tighten again during flexion.

The contours of Figures 5.14 and 5.15 show that, in most positions, most fibers in both cruciates in the unloaded joint are slack, with isometry limited to fibers lying along a single surface. These findings explain why the search for isometry is difficult and why many surgeons, observing the ligaments to be slack during surgery, deduce that the ligaments can play no role in guiding the movements of the bones on each other. Strasser (31) is quoted by Pinskerova et al. (32) as stating, "Contrary to the assumption of Zuppinger, the two cruciates cannot remain equally tense because, for example, soon after the beginning of flexion, the whole of the PCL is loose." Not surprisingly, Strasser was unable to observe the isometric surface within the body of the PCL (Fig. 5.15). Unlike Pinskerova et al., we do not regard Strasser's observation as a rebuttal of Zuppinger's assumption (33) that certain ligaments, notably the cruciates, may act as guiding structures, but we consider it to be quite consistent with the results of Figures 5.14 and 5.15. All fibers within a ligament cannot remain isometric during movement, but some can. We demonstrate in Chapter 10 how slack fibers are progressively recruited and stretch when load is applied, allowing the ligaments to develop tension forces and to play their roles as restraining structures, giving the knee its characteristic laxity and stability.

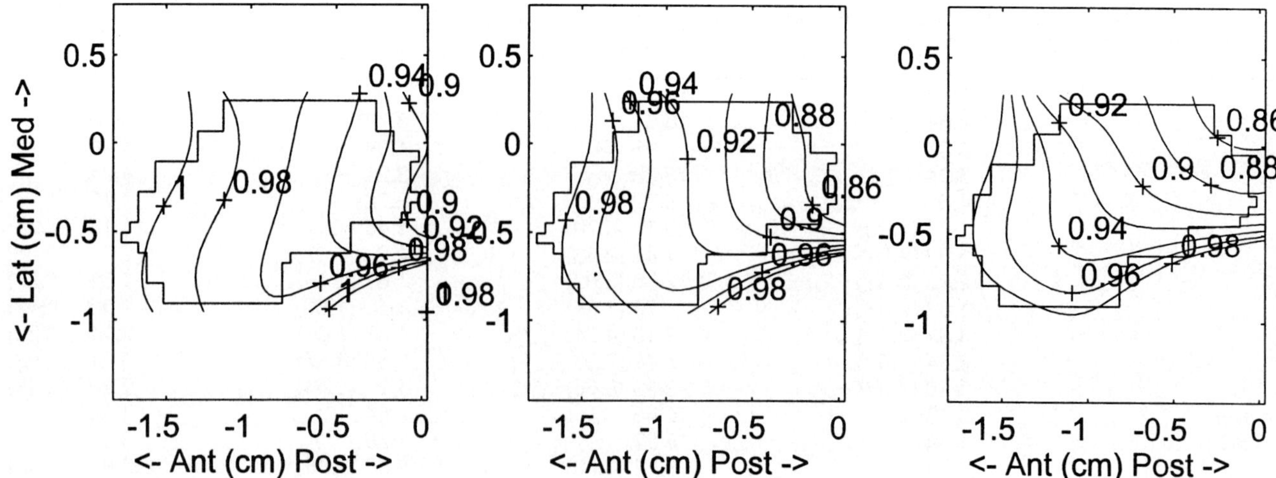

FIGURE 5.14. Outline of the tibial attachment of the anterior cruciate ligament in one specimen showing contours of constant length change at 30°, 60°, and 90° of flexion. Contours are labeled according to fractional length changes with respect to lengths at full extension.

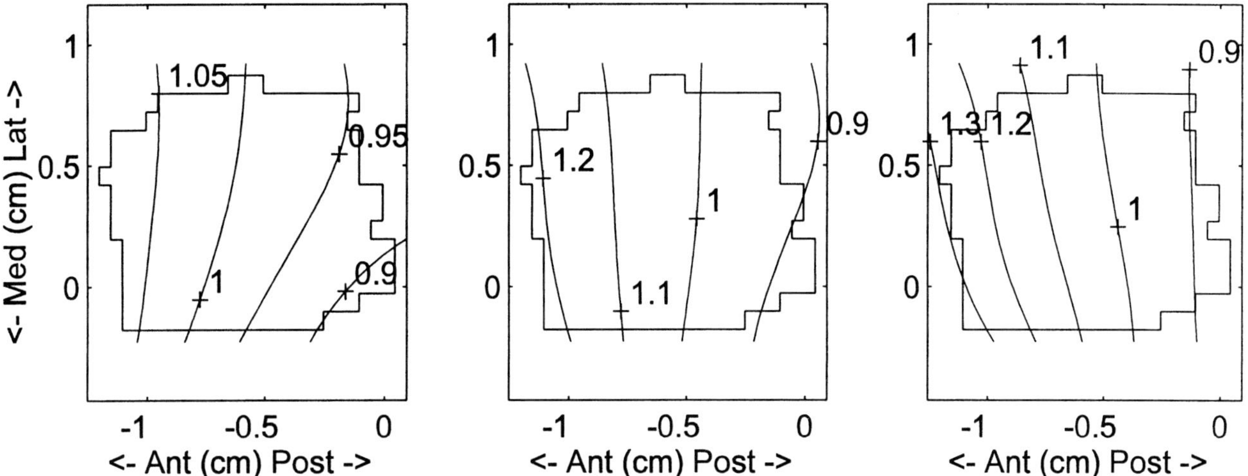

FIGURE 5.15. Outline of the tibial attachment of the posterior cruciate ligament of one specimen at 30°, 60°, and 90° of flexion, showing contours of constant length change relative to fiber lengths at extension. Fibers in front of the contour marked 1.0 are slack in extension and tighten during flexion.

Feikes (25) found that the anterior fibers of the MCL and the LCL remained most nearly isometric. The posterior fibers shortened with flexion. Fiber shortening of up to 20% was found within the range of motion examined. There is very little corroborating evidence in the literature. Warren et al. (34) suggested that anterior and posterior fibers of the MCL experience length changes of less than 2 mm. Blankevoort et al. (29) found that the anterior fibers of the MCL appear to be most isometric, with length changes of about 5%, whereas they found length changes of about 10% in the anterior bundle of the LCL. Rovick et al. (35) found a central fiber of the LCL to shorten by approximately 20%.

THREE-DIMENSIONAL MODEL OF JOINT MOBILITY

There has been speculation for years about the mechanisms that guide the coupled movements of the knee just described. One earlier theory, restated by Blacharski et al. (10), asserts that "the cruciate ligaments have little influence on the kinematics of the knee" and ascribes coupled axial rotation to the different shapes of the articular surfaces in the medial and lateral compartments: "the motion is owing to the geometry of the bones." However, low-friction surfaces spin, like car wheels on ice, and cannot control traction. Such control can only be achieved when the low-friction surfaces are interdigitated, like gear wheels.[2] Ligaments can provide the constraints necessary to control rolling between low-friction articular surfaces. In this section, we describe a mathematical model that demonstrates how the ligaments act together with the articular surfaces to control mobility.

Zuppinger (33) first proposed that the ligaments could act as guiding structures to control the movements of the bones on each other. The article by Pinskerova et al. (32) reproduces his drawings of a four-bar linkage model of the knee, showing how isometric fibers in the two cruciates could control the rolling movements of the femur on the tibia, as exemplified by the data in Figure 5.8. We describe our developments of the four-bar linkage model, but we first outline progress on the development of a 3-D equivalent, which explains the coupling of axial rotation with flexion and the rolling—sliding movements of the bones.

Wilson et al. (36), and Feikes (25) proposed that a parallel spatial mechanism[3] model of the knee could explain coupled passive motion. They suggested five constraints to motion: continuous contact in each of the medial and lateral compartments and isometric fibers in the two cruciate ligaments and in the medial collateral ligament. Five constraints would reduce the six possible DOF at the knee to one. The mathematical problem was then to calculate the path of motion of the bones on each other that would satisfy the constraints that the two pairs of articular surfaces remain continuously in contact and that the three selected ligament fibers remain isometric.[4]

---

[2]The posterior stabilized form of knee replacement uses an interdigitated cam and follower mechanism, with sacrifice of both cruciates to control anteroposterior motion of the bones on each other.

[3]The cockpit simulator used to train pilots is an example of a parallel spatial mechanism. Linear actuators are connected through ball-and-socket joints to two large bodies (i.e., ground and cockpit). Controlled extension and contraction of the actuators move the cockpit in any arbitrary way relative to the ground.

[4]The CD-ROM enclosed with the book contains animations of the three-dimensional and two-dimensional models that can run on a PC in Windows.

This approach to modeling the knee seeks to define the role of the ligaments and articular surfaces in guiding mobility and is quite different from some 3-D models described by Wismans et al. (37), Andriacchi et al. (38), Essenger et al. (39), and Blankevoort et al. (6,40), all of which study motion of the joint under load. These models are unable to predict the fully coupled nature of the motion of the unloaded joint because load is required to hold the knee at any flexion angle and prevent elastic spring-back (37,39,40) and compressive force is required to maintain contact in the model lateral compartment (37,40). Sathasivam and Walker (41) developed finite element models to study load transmission through prosthetic components but without including muscle or ligament simulations. Crowninshield et al. (42) proposed a kinematic model in which they prescribed a certain pattern of coupled motion and then deduced patterns of ligament strain.

Our approach is to assume that the shapes of the articular surfaces and the mapping of isometric fibers joining the bones are known and to calculate the path of coupled motion, the motion of the contact points, and the patterns of fiber slackening and tightening consistent with the ligamentous and articular surface constraints. If the calculated path of motion proves to be reasonably similar to the experimental results described previously, the hypotheses underlying the mathematical model can be advanced as explanations of the experimental results. As discussed in Chapter 10, a model of the kinematics of the unloaded joint can serve as a convenient starting point for the study of its mechanics because it defines the initial lines of action of the intraarticular contact forces and of the ligament and muscle forces at different positions of flexion.

Parameters of the Model

Before a movement path can be calculated, it is necessary to provide the data that specify the shapes of the articular surfaces and their relative location at one position of the joint. The positions of the attachment points on each of the two model bones of each of the three constraining ligament fibers must be specified. These data are the parameters of the model and, between them, imply the specification of the unstretched length of each of the proposed isometric fibers. The resulting movement path depends on the choice of parameters. Specimen-specific models can be generated from parameter data acquired from individual specimens. The calculated movement path can then be compared with the measured movement path of the same specimen.

Surgeons, in performing joint replacements and reconstructing ligaments, impose their own parameters on the joint. Simulation of surgery is therefore possible by studying the effects of parameter variation on the mobility of the model.

Simple Articular Surface Shapes

Wilson et al. (36) and Feikes et al. (43) described a preliminary study in which the surfaces of the femoral condyles were assumed to be spherical and the tibial plateaus were assumed to be planar (Fig. 5.16). The animation of this figure is shown in Image 1 on the enclosed CD-ROM. The radii of the spheres and the positions of spheres and planes on the bones were based on the digitized surface data obtained in the experiments described previously. This model successfully predicts the coupling of external femoral rotation or internal tibial rotation with flexion (Fig. 5.17).

Results of the comparison between specimen movement and the corresponding model varied considerably from model to model. The calculated movements of model D were quite similar to those of the anatomic specimen up to about 100°, although the model exhibited rapid external tibial rotation at higher flexion angles. Model B predicted internal tibial rotation roughly twice the magnitude of the measurement, and both assessments showed that the rotation occurred mainly in the first 40°. Models with nonparallel planar tibial plateaus gave better agreement than those with parallel planes.

All the models predicted internal tibial rotation coupled to the flexion angle. Wilson (44) examined a model with two cruciate ligaments and a lateral collateral ligament and found that the predicted *direction* of the coupled axial rotation was reversed with flexion (i.e., the femur rotated internally, the tibia externally). This finding confirms that it is the MCL rather than the LCL that, together with the cruciates, provides the ligamentous constraints that result in the coupled motions described previously, particularly the coupling of internal tibial rotation with flexion. Kapandji (45) explained coupled internal tibial rotation on the same basis. However, most of the simple surface models (e.g., model B in Fig. 5.17) predicted movements of the contact points on the tibia significantly in excess of the measurements (Fig. 5.8).

Anatomic Surface Shapes

Feikes (25) examined specimen-specific models by fitting the articular surfaces of the experimental specimens with second-, third-, and fourth-order polynomial surfaces (see Color Plate 1, following page 72; the animation of this figure is shown as Image 2 on the CD-ROM). She found that a model with spherical femoral condyles and bi-quadratic, second-order tibial plateaus gave the best match of measured and calculated coupling of axial rotation to flexion (Fig. 5.18A), predicting movements of the contact points (Fig. 5.18B) of similar order to those mea-

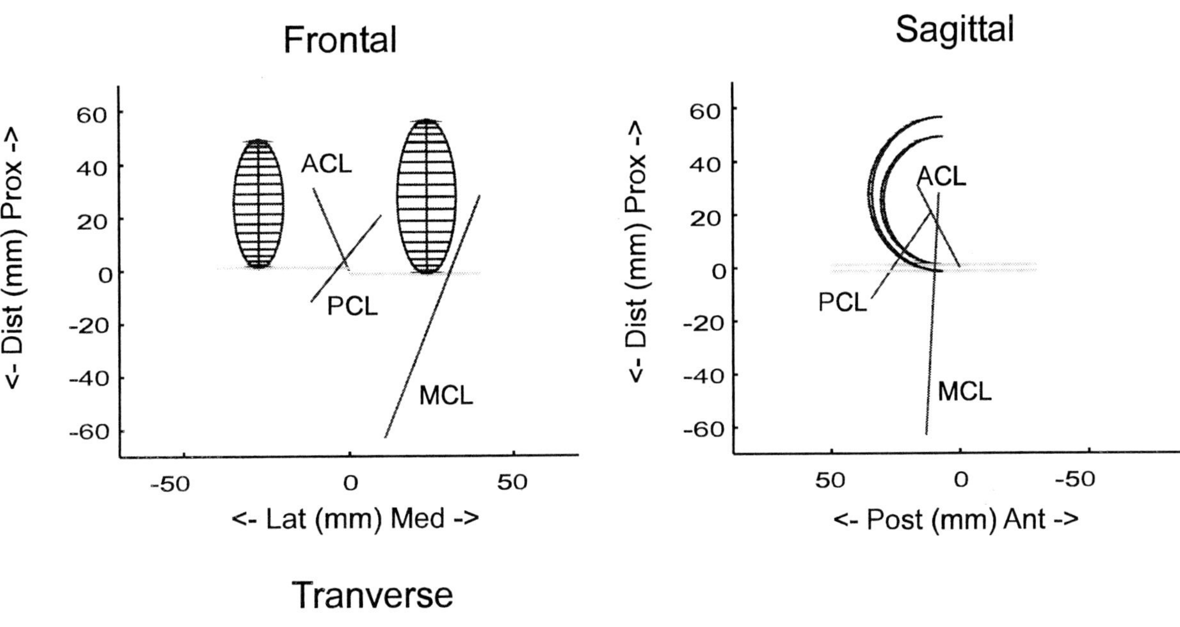

FIGURE 5.16. Parallel spatial mechanism model of the knee with spherical femoral condyles and a flat tibial plateau held together by isometric fibers in the anterior cruciate ligament (ACL), posterior cruciate ligament (PCL), and medial collateral ligament (MCL). (From Wilson DR, Feikes JD, O'Connor JJ. Ligaments and articular contact guide passive knee flexion. *J Biomech* 1998; 31:1127–1136, with permission.

sured experimentally (Fig. 5.8), especially in the lateral compartment. The result for the medial compartment, however, shows forward movement of the contact point in early flexion.

Model Ligament Length Patterns

The basic model uses only the isometric fibers in the ACL, PCL, and MCL. From the digitized data extracted from the specimens, it was possible to locate the attachment areas of the ligaments and to determine their relative motion, as predicted by the model. Using the mapping functions exploited to produce the contours of Figures 5.14 and 5.15, theoretic length-change contours could be calculated (Fig. 5.19).

The model calculations are largely in accord with the experimentally derived curves, although it should be

remembered that the main differences between the two analyses lie in the differences between the actual and the theoretic macroscopic movements of the bones, because the same sources were used for the mapping functions. The calculated patterns of fiber slackening and tightening, based on later descriptions of fiber mapping (Figs. 5.10 and 5.11), are significantly closer to experimental observation than the more speculative patterns described in Chapter 10, "Geometry of the Knee," of the first edition.

Summary of Models of Mobility

The 3-D model of mobility is a purely geometric construct and tells us only how the model bones would move on each other if the two pairs of articular surfaces were to remain continuously in contact and the three identified ligament fibers were to remain isometric over the move-

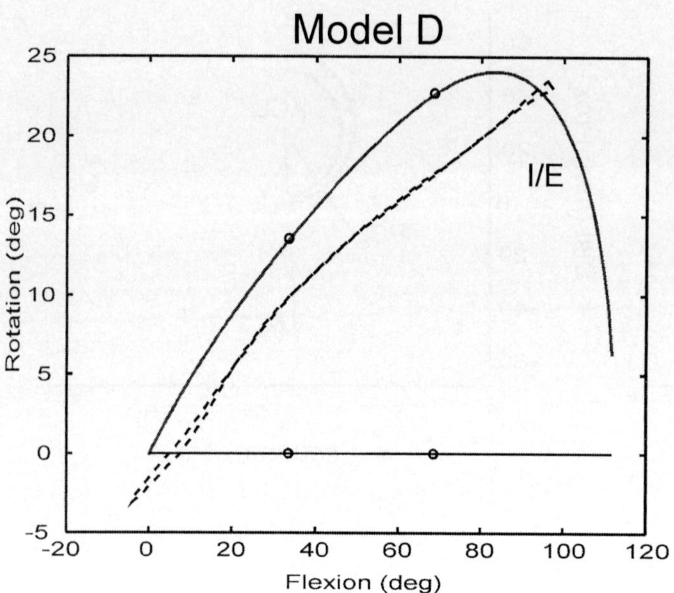

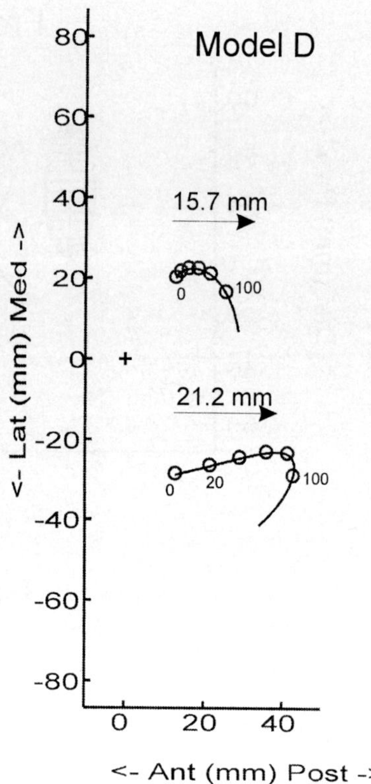

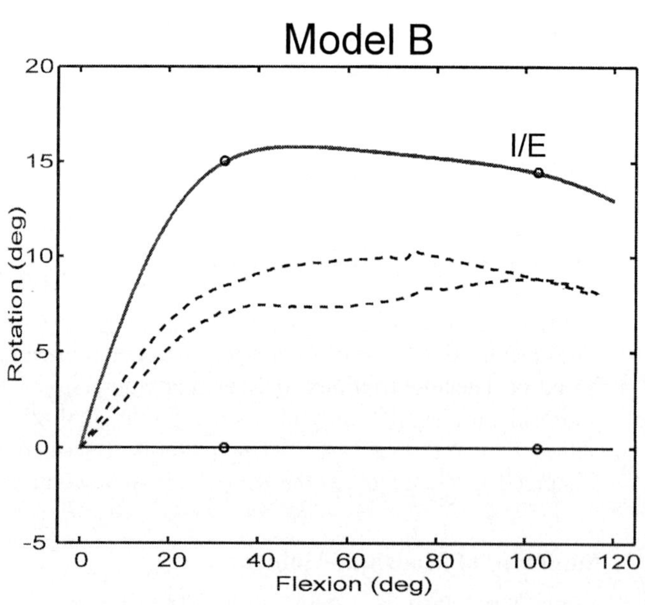

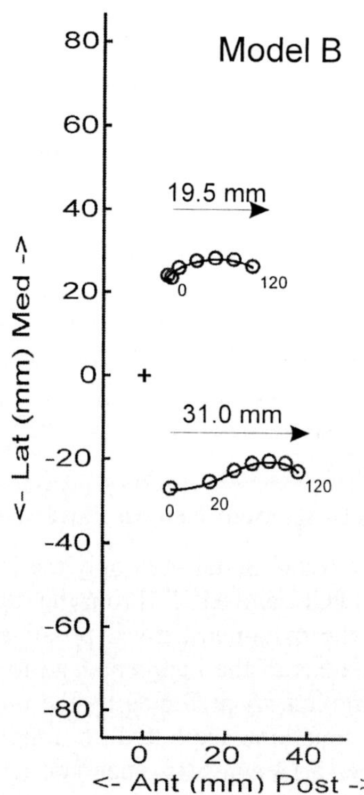

FIGURE 5.17. Calculated *(solid lines)* versus experimental *(dashed lines)* tibial rotation plotted against the flexion angle for two specimen-specific models with spherical femoral condyles and a flat tibial plateau, together with the calculated excursion of contact point in both compartments of the model knees.

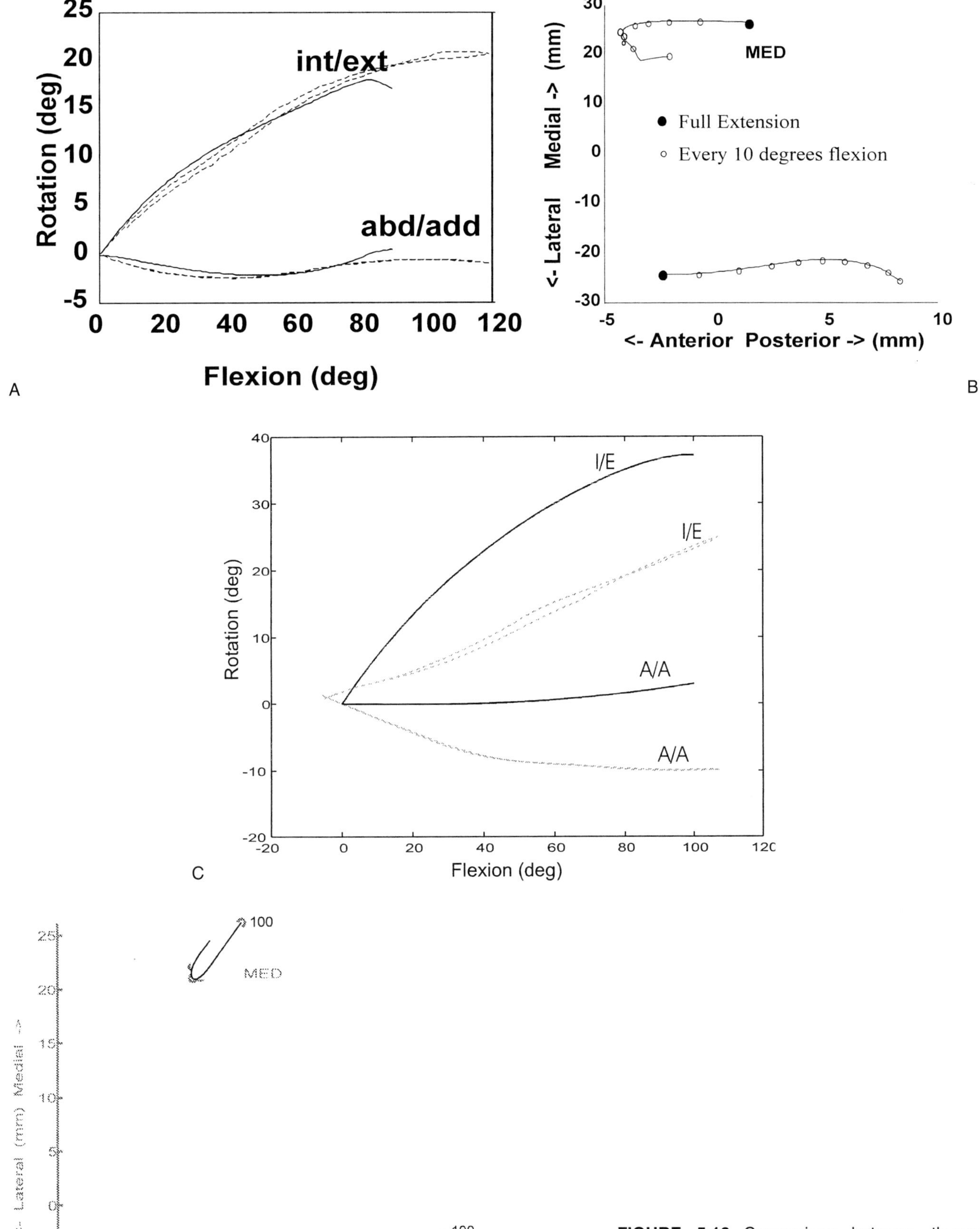

FIGURE 5.18. Comparison between theory *(solid lines)* and experiment *(dashed lines)* for two specimen-specific polycentric surface models. **A, B:** The model ligament fibers connected arbitrarily chosen positions within the attachment areas of the specimen. **C, D:** The model fibers connected the most isometric points detected experimentally.

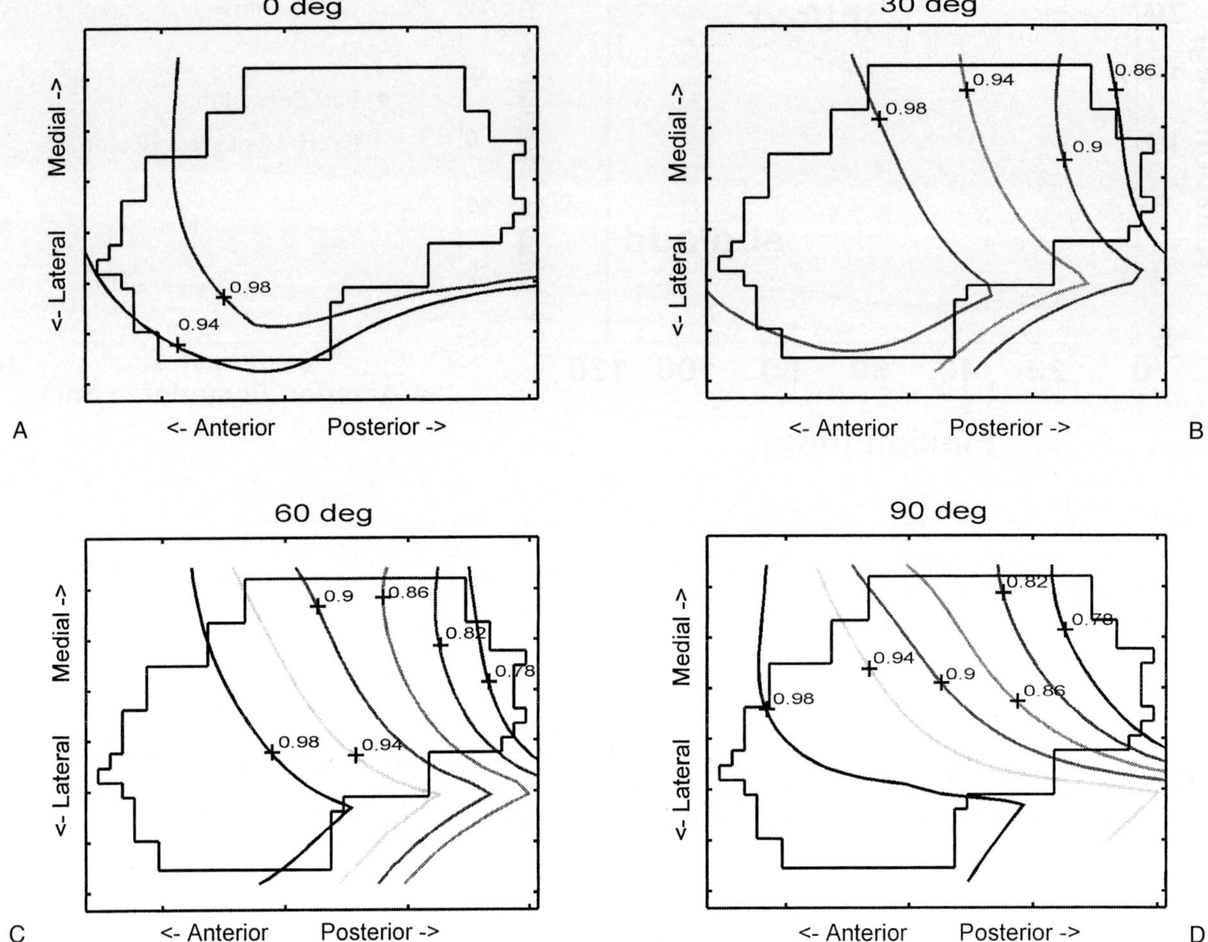

FIGURE 5.19. Contours of constant fiber length of the model anterior cruciate ligament at four positions **(A–D)**. Numbers on the contours give proportions of the reference lengths of the corresponding fiber surfaces.

ment range. There has been no mention of mechanics, of forces or moments, or of stresses or strains. Nonetheless, the model predicts coupled internal tibial rotation with flexion and combined rolling and sliding of the articular surfaces on each other, the main features revealed in the experimental study.

There is reasonable quantitative agreement between experimental and theoretic results. The differences may reflect experimental error as much as the undoubted error in choosing the parameters of the model from the experimental data. Results for different sets of parameters demonstrate that the model is very parameter sensitive. Small differences in the shapes of the articular surfaces or in the geometry of the ligaments of the natural joint could explain the variability in motion detected in the experiments. Equally, changes to the geometry of a joint during arthroplasty or ligament reconstruction must be expected to change its mobility. It may be that a generic model, demonstrating the average behavior of most normal knees, will be the most useful.

The model demonstrates how the combination of surface constraints and ligamentous constraints can work together to define the movement path of the unloaded knee. It represents a series of hypotheses that explain the experimental observations reported previously. By addressing the question of mobility first and explicitly searching for the movement path that allows continuity of contact, the model avoids the difficulty encountered with previous models (6,37) of lift-off of the lateral compartment and the necessity of applying a compressive force merely to maintain contact.

The general agreement between our experimental results and the predictions of the model strengthens our conclusion from the experiments that the unloaded knee joint is a single degree of freedom mechanism and that the two pairs of articular surfaces and the cruciates and MCL provide the constraints needed to reduce six possible DOF to one. The fact that these constraints are flexible explains the laxity of the joint. Rupture of a ligament, increasing the number of DOF from one to two, destabilizes the joint and greatly disrupts function. Combined injuries of more than one ligament are even more damaging. This conclusion justifies attempts at surgical repair and at retention of all the ligaments during joint replacement.

TWO-DIMENSIONAL MODEL OF JOINT MOBILITY

The 3-D model described is still undergoing development. In Chapters 10 and 11, "Geometry of the Knee" and "Mechanics of the Knee," of the first edition, we described the 2-D, four-bar linkage model; and, in Chapter 12, "The Muscle-Stabilized Knee," of the first edition, some of the experimental results used to validate the values of the mechanical variables predicted by the model. We now describe further developments of the four-bar linkage model. Computer-generated colored animations of the model knee in motion can be found in the attached CD-ROM and are easier to interpret than the static diagrams of the printed book. The 2-D model can usefully explain a number of features of the behavior of the knee, and its relevance can be judged from the agreement of model predictions with experimental measurements.

The Four-Bar Linkage Model

Freeman's research (32) revealed that it was Zuppinger (33) who first proposed the four-bar linkage model of the knee. The idea was rediscovered by Kapandji in 1970 (45), Menschik in 1974 (46), and Huson in 1974 (47). It was used by Goodfellow and O'Connor (8a) in 1978 to explain the movements of the meniscal bearings in their proposed knee prosthesis. It was used extensively by Muller to discuss ligament reconstruction (48). We had attributed the idea to Strasser (see Chapter 10, "Geometry of the Knee," in the first edition) but it transpires that he, like many others since then, was dismissive of the idea. However, there is sufficient experimental validation to justify further description of the model that provides insights otherwise difficult to obtain. Leardini et al. (49) proposed a similar four-bar linkage model for the ankle joint.

Figure 5.20 shows a human knee with the lateral femoral condyle removed, revealing the cruciate ligaments. The four-bar linkage comprises the lines *AB* and *CD*, representing isometric fibers within the two cruciates, and the lines *CB* and *AD*, joining the attachments of the isometric fibers to the femur and tibia, respectively. We later discuss the locations of the isometric fibers within the physical ligaments on the basis of the experiments described previously.

During flexion and extension movements, the lines *CB* and *AD* on the two bones rotate relative to each other. To allow these movements, the isometric ligament fibers also have to rotate about their origins on the bones (Fig. 5.21). We have written down the algebraic equations necessary to

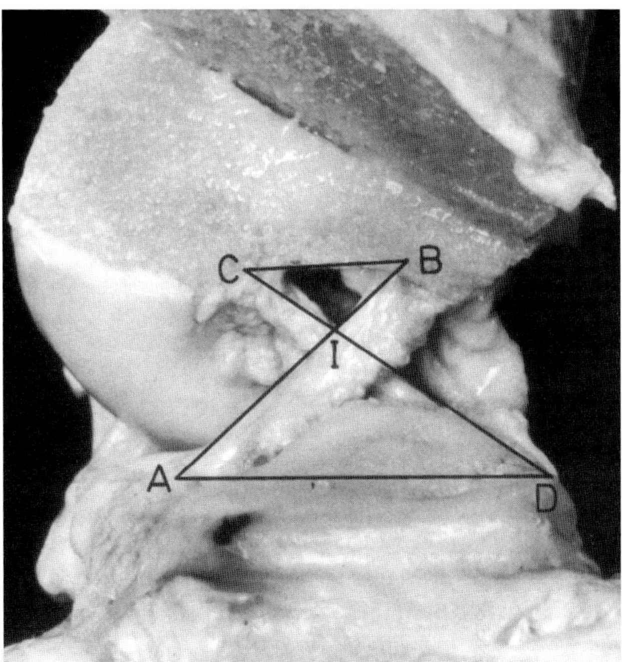

FIGURE 5.20. Section through a human knee with the lateral femoral condyle removed reveals the cruciate ligaments. The four-bar linkage model *(ABCD)* is superimposed. (From O'Connor JJ, Shercliff TL, Biden E, et al. The geometry of the knee in the sagittal plane. *J Engng Med Proc Inst Mech Eng Part H* 1989;203:223–233, with permission.)

calculate the directions of the ligament fibers at any flexion angle (12), and these equations were used to draw Figure 5.21.

Figure 5.21A shows superimposed pictures of the linkage in three positions with the tibia and the tibial link *AD* fixed. The anterior cruciate fiber *AB* rotates about its tibial attachment *A* from AB_1 in extension to AB_3 at 140° flexion, with the femoral origin rotating on a circular path from B_1 to B_3 that is centered at *A*. Figure 5.21B is kinematically identical to Figure 5.21A and shows the linkage in the same three positions but with the femur fixed. The tibial insertions *A* and *D* rotate in circular arcs about their femoral origins, from A_1 and D_1 in extension to A_3 and D_3 at 140°. To achieve 140° of flexion, the isometric fibers have to rotate approximately 100° about their femoral origins and 40° about their tibial insertions. The diagrams demonstrate that they can do this without stretching and remain isometric.

Flexion Axis

An important aspect of the linkage is that its *instant center* (i.e., instantaneous center of zero relative velocity) lies at the point at which the two ligament fibers cross. This is the point about which the bones rotate relative to each other in the sagittal plane during flexion and extension (point *I* in Fig. 5.20). The flexion axis of the model joint passes through the intersection of the isometric fibers, and the instant center is the 2-D equivalent of the helical axis described previously.

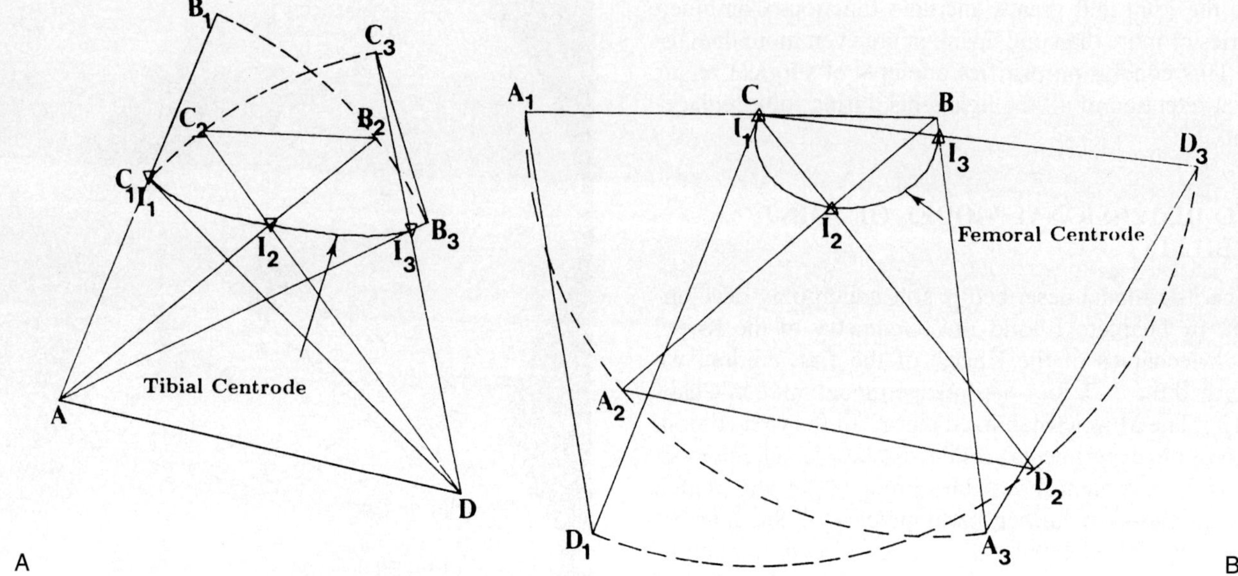

FIGURE 5.21. Superimposed diagrams of the cruciate linkage at extension and at 70° and 140° of flexion with the tibia fixed **(A)** and with the femur fixed **(B)**. (From O'Connor JJ, Shercliff TL, Biden E, et al. The geometry of the knee in the sagittal plane. *J Engng Med Proc Inst Mech Eng Part H* 1989;203:223–233, with permission.)

Because the directions of the two cruciates change during flexion and extension, the instant center, or flexion axis, moves relative to both bones. The curves marked *centrodes* in Figure 5.21 define the successive positions of the flexion axis relative to the tibia (Fig. 5.21A) and relative to the femur (Fig. 5.21B). The shapes of the two centrodes are different, but they are of exactly the same length. The distance along each centrode from the location of the flexion axis in any one position of flexion to its location in any other is also exactly the same. This means that a pair of articular surfaces coinciding with the centrodes would roll without slip on each other (i.e., pure rolling) while allowing the two ligament fibers to remain isometric. The movement of the contact point on each of those surfaces would be identical. Such surfaces would be compatible with the changing geometry of the cruciate mechanism. The shape of the femoral centrode in Figure 5.21B is very similar to that obtained experimentally by Frankel and Burstein (50). Articular surfaces exactly coincident with the two centrodes would roll without sliding on each other. All other possible articular surface pairs would slide as well as roll.

Articular Surface Shapes and Tibiofemoral Joint

The articular surfaces of the human knee lie distal to the intersection of the cruciates (Fig. 5.20) so that these surfaces cannot exhibit pure rolling. Nonetheless, there is an intimate relationship between the geometry of the ligaments and the geometry of the articular surfaces. We have shown (12) that the shapes of possible compatible pairs of articular surfaces have to satisfy the condition that the common normal to both surfaces at their point of

contact has to pass through the flexion axis. If this condition is not satisfied, the articular surfaces would have to separate or interpenetrate during flexion and extension, or the ligaments would have to slacken or stretch.

The common normal theorem implies that there could be a multitude of pairs of articular surfaces, each of which could be compatible with the ligaments. If we specify the shape, for example, of the tibial articular surface, we can use the common normal theorem to calculate the shape of the compatible femoral articular surface. We have shown (12) that the calculated shape of a femoral surface compatible with a concave tibial surface of radius 87.5 mm fits the shape of the natural medial femoral condyle quite well, and the shape compatible with a convex tibial surface of radius 75 mm fits the lateral femoral condyle quite well. For the remainder of this discussion, we treat the tibial plateau as flat, a compromise between the concave medial plateau and the convex lateral plateau of the human knee.

Figure 5.22 shows the 2-D model knee in three positions. Typical parameters needed as input to this model were given in Chapter 10, "Geometry of the Knee," of the first edition. The animation of the figure is shown in Image 3 on the CD-ROM. The tibial plateau is flat and the shape of the compatible femoral condyle was calculated from the common normal theorem. The articular surfaces make contact at the point X, which lies on the perpendicular to the tibial plateau through the flexion axis (I). The contact point moves progressively backward on the tibial plateau during flexion, from X_1 in extension (Fig. 5.22A) through X_2 at 70° flexion to X_3 at 140° flexion, the so-called rollback. The total backward movement

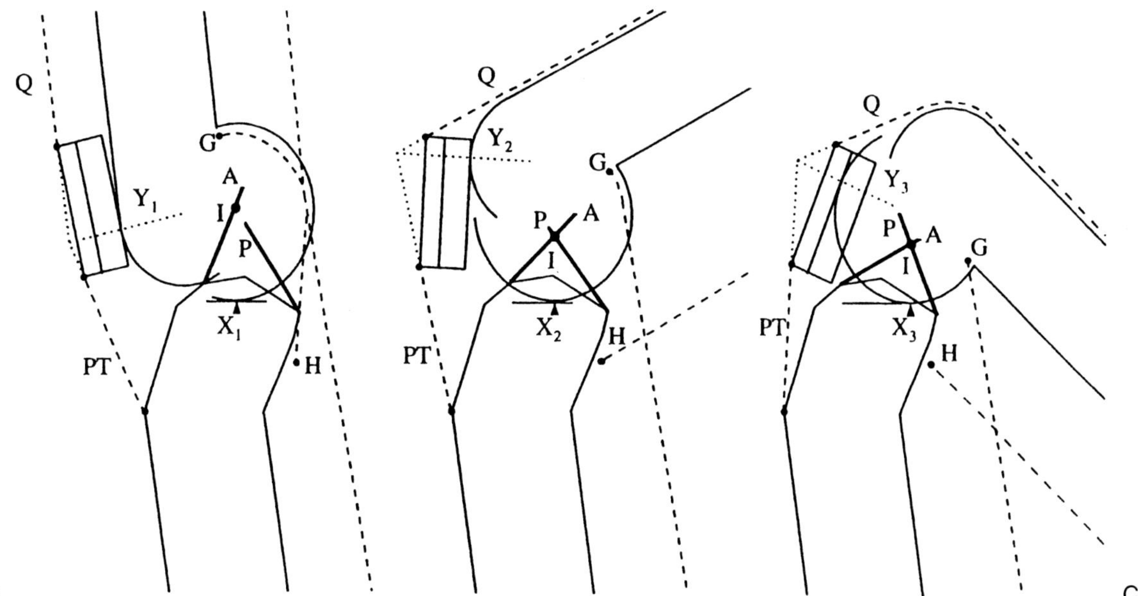

FIGURE 5.22. Two-dimensional model of the knee with the anterior and posterior cruciate ligaments. The tibiofemoral contact point moves from X_1 in extension to X_3 at 140° of flexion. The gastrocnemius arises at point *G* on the femur and inserts into the Achilles tendon (not shown). It wraps around the posterior femoral condyle to about 80° of flexion. The separate heads of hamstrings are amalgamated into one, which inserts on the tibia at point *H*. It wraps around the femoral condyle near extension and lies parallel to the shaft of the femur. The patella is represented as a rectangle connecting the quadriceps *(Q)* and patellar tendons *(PT)*. The quadriceps tendon wraps around the anterior femur in the flexed knee. The line of action of the patellofemoral force lies on the radius of the femoral trochlea perpendicular to the articular surface of the patella and through the intersection of the tendons. Contact on the patella occurs at point Y_1 near its distal pole in extension and at Y_2 near its proximal pole in mid-flexion. Contact passes to Y_3 on the posterior femoral condyles and the medial-lateral patellar facets above about 110° of flexion. (From Lu TW, O'Connor JJ, Taylor SJG, et al. Validation of a lower limb model with *in vivo* femoral forces telemetered from two subjects. *J Biomech* 1998;31:63–69, with permission.)

of the contact point in the model knee is about 12 mm, very similar to the average contact point movement found in the experiments previously described. The calculated value of the contact movement depends on the choices of model parameters (i.e., the lengths of the isometric cruciate ligament fibers and the positions on the model bones of their points of origin and insertion), the chosen shape of the tibial plateau, and its position relative to the insertions of the cruciates.

The diagrams of the model demonstrate that flexion to 140° is possible while the two ligament fibers rotate isometrically about their origins and insertions without stretching or slackening and while the articular surfaces slide and roll on each other without indentation or separation. Mobility of the unloaded joint is therefore possible without tissue deformation, explaining the fact that the human knee exhibits a range of *unresisted* motion, as demonstrated in our experiments and by the 3-D models. To allow the rolling movements in the sagittal plane (and the twisting movements in the transverse plane), the articular surfaces of the tibiofemoral joint have to be incongruous. The menisci, which lie between them, bring the surfaces into effective conformity and spread the trans-

mitted compressive force over a large effective area (51–53).

Muscle Tendons

Figure 5.22 contains lines to represent images of the tendons of the flexor and extensor muscles in the sagittal plane. The hamstrings tendons insert at point H on the posterior proximal tibia and lie parallel to the shaft of the femur, except near extension, where they wrap around the back of the femoral condyles. The directions of the forces that they apply to the tibia therefore vary continuously over the flexion range. The gastrocnemius (G) arises above the posterior femoral condyles and inserts into the Achilles tendon (not shown in the diagrams); it wraps around the posterior femoral condyles even up to 70° of flexion (Fig. 5.22B). Over the flexion range, the direction of the gastrocnemius tendon changes significantly relative to the femur but only a little relative to the tibia. The changing directions of the tendons have important consequences for the loading of ligaments (discussed in detail in Chapter 11, "Mechanics of the Knee," of the first edition).

Patellofemoral Joint

Figure 5.22 differs from the corresponding figure (see Figure 10.31 in first edition) in that it contains a mathematical model of the patella, developed by Gill (54,55). In these diagrams, the trochlear facet of the anterior femur with which the patella makes contact is shown as being separate from the tibial facet of the distal and posterior femoral condyle. This description is based on sections such as in Figure 5.23, which shows the distal femur cut through the sulcus of the trochlea with circles outlining the articular surfaces of the trochlear and tibial facets, showing them to be separate and distinct. The separation is much more distinct in quadrupeds who do not straighten their knees.

In Figure 5.22, the patella is shown with two separate articular surfaces, the more posterior representing the median ridge and more anterior representing the medial and lateral facets of the human bone. The median ridge makes contact with the trochlea over most of the flexion range (Figs. 5.22A, B), and the medial and lateral facets make contact with the femoral condyles in the fully flexed knee (Fig. 5.22C). In the simplest model, the separate articular surfaces of the patella are shown parallel on the basis of sagittal-plane x-ray images.

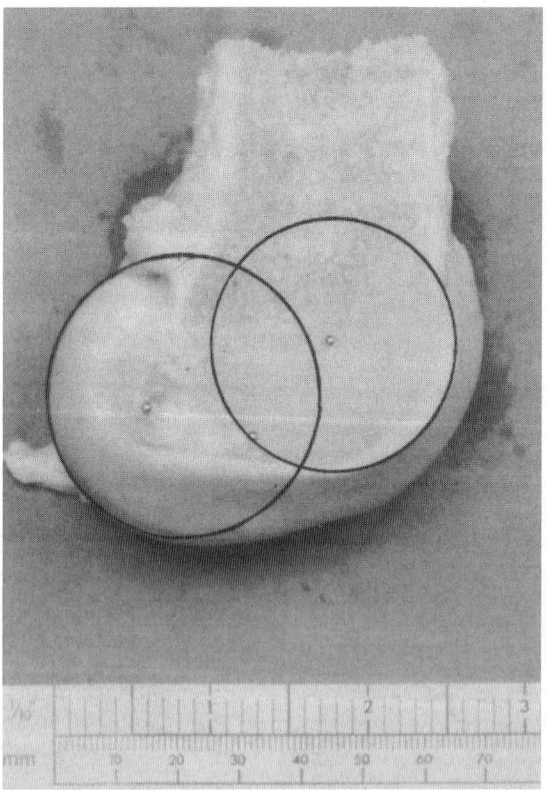

FIGURE 5.23. A section through the sulcus of the femoral trochlea shows that the surface that guides the patella over the femur is distinct and separate from the surface that guides the tibia. Both can be fitted with circular arcs. (From O'Connor JJ, Shercliff TL, Biden E, et al. The geometry of the knee in the sagittal plane. *J Engng Med Proc Inst Mech Eng Part H* 1989;203:223–233, with permission.)

The position of the contact point on the patella is based on the argument from mechanics (the only bit of mechanics used in this chapter) that the lines of action of the three forces acting on the patella—the quadriceps tendon force (QF), the patellar tendon force (PT), and the patellofemoral contact force (PF)—must lie in the same plane and must be concurrent. This assumes that the forces applied to the patella by the retinaculae are small in comparison. This principle was used by Miller et al. (56) to determine the magnitude and line of action of PF over the flexion range in intact cadaver knees and in the same specimens after various replacement arthroplasties (57).

In general, the angle between the line of action of the patellofemoral force and the quadriceps tendon differs from its angle with the patellar tendon. As a result, the forces in the two tendons are not equal, as shown by Maquet (58) and Bishop and Denham (59). The patellofemoral joint is not a frictionless pulley with equal tendon forces, as is sometimes assumed.

Inspection of the line of action of the patellofemoral force in Figure 5.22 shows that the contact point on the patella lies near its distal pole in extension and that it moves proximally during flexion. In the highly flexed knee, it passes onto the medial or lateral facets, which make contact with the condyles; the patella rolls as well as slides on the femur. As a result, the femur flexes through 140° on the tibia, but the patella flexes only 75°. To allow these rolling movements to occur, the articular surfaces of the patellofemoral joint have to be incongruous. Unlike the tibiofemoral joint, there are no menisci available to spread the resulting high-contact stresses that are transmitted through small contact areas. The thick cartilage layer on the posterior surface of the patella may help to increase contact area slightly.

The calculated movement of the contact point on the patella predicted by the model is confirmed by the observations of Goodfellow et al. (60) and Miller et al. (56). The rolling movements of the patella are necessary because, as the knee flexes, the point of intersection of the quadriceps and patellar tendons moves proximally and the line of action of the patellofemoral force has to follow to remain concurrent with that intersection. Figure 5.24 demonstrates that, if the line of action of PF lies proximal to the intersection of the tendons, its moment about the intersection tends to roll the patellar contact point distally toward the intersection. At the same time, the patella has to slide proximally along the trochlea to maintain the length of the patellar tendon constant. If the line of action of PF lies distal to the intersection of the tendons, its moment about the intersection rolls the patellar contact point proximally, again toward that intersection. In the stable position, the three lines of action intersect at the same point.

The model of Figure 5.22 demonstrates that the patellar tendon rotates about its insertion into the tibia. It rotates posteriorly through about 35° during flexion of

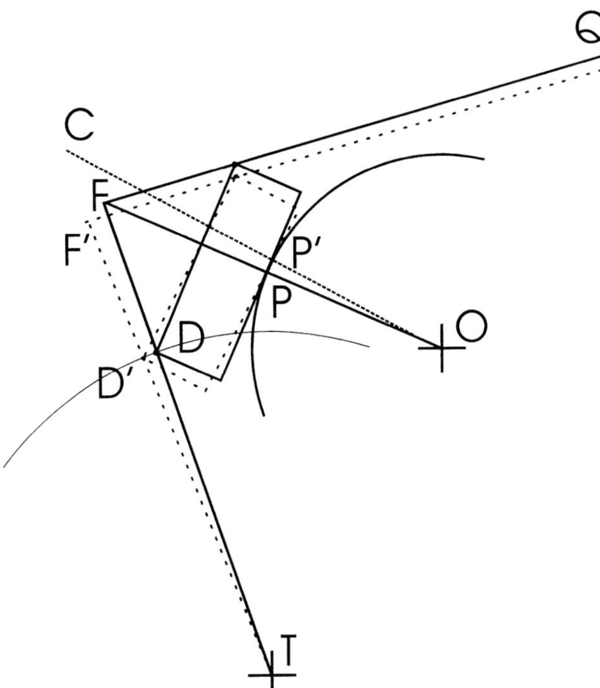

FIGURE 5.24. Model of the patellofemoral joint. The patella makes contact with the trochlea at point *P* on the line joining the center of the trochlea *(O)* to the intersection of the tendons *(F) (solid lines)*. If the patella is moved to the position of the *dashed lines,* the tendon intersection moves to *F'*, but the patellofemoral force on the line *OC* then lies proximal to *F'*. The patellofemoral force applied at *P'* rotates the patella counterclockwise, back toward its equilibrium position, and its distal pole is constrained by the patellar tendon to move from *D'* to *D* along a circle centered at the tibial tubercle *(T)*.

the knee to 140°. The patellar tendon angle (PTA) is now used as a readily measured indicator of tibiofemoral kinematics. It makes it possible to demonstrate the extent to which ACL rupture and reconstruction (61) or various arthroplasties affect the kinematics of the knee. Miller et al. (56) showed that the model of Figure 5.22 gives an estimate of the variation of PTA with a flexion angle that agrees well with their own measurements and those of others. They have also shown that normal PTA can be restored after unicompartmental arthroplasty but is abnormal after ACL-sacrificing, PCL-retaining total-knee replacement (57). We show in Chapter 10 that the anteriorly directed force in the patellar tendon over most of the flexion range has important consequences for the loading of the cruciate ligaments. When flexion reaches about 70° (Fig. 5.22B), the quadriceps tendon begins to wrap around the anterior femur, with an angle of wrap of about 60° in the fully flexed knee (Fig. 5.22C).

Gill and O'Connor (55) have shown that many of the predictions of the patellofemoral model of Figure 5.22 (i.e., patellar mechanism angle, patellar tendon angle, and patellar tendon force) agree well with experimental measurements from various laboratories. The model predicts

slight discontinuities in the values of most variables when the patella makes the transition from trochlear contact to condylar contact. Experiments in which movement of the patella was monitored continuously with an optometric system and the patellofemoral force was measured continuously with a transducer have demonstrated similar discontinuities (62,63).

Ligament Fiber Length Patterns

We have described how the areas of origin and insertion of the ligaments rotate relative to each other during flexion or extension and, as a consequence, most ligament fibers slacken or tighten during these movements. The 2-D model provides further insight into the patterns of ligament fiber strain. We follow the arguments of Chapter 10, "Geometry of the Knee," of the first edition, and use the information on fiber mapping gained in the 1990s and described in the earlier experimental section (Figures 5.10 and 5.11).

Figure 5.25 shows three ligament fibers spanning the knee from femur to tibia and their positions in relation to the isometric fibers of the cruciates (AB and CD). Assuming the femur to be flexing on a fixed tibia and recalling that it rotates in the sagittal plane about a flexion axis passing through the intersection of the cruciates (I), the paths of the femoral origins of the three fibers can be deduced, as shown in the figure.

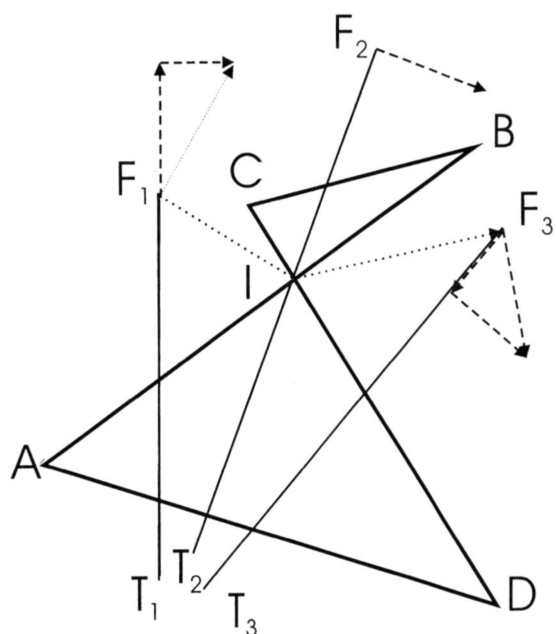

FIGURE 5.25. Fiber F_1T_1 lies in front of the flexion axis through point *I*. With the femur flexing on a fixed tibia, F_1 moves perpendicular to IF_1, with a component of its movement away from its tibial attachment (T_1). The fiber therefore stretches during flexion. Fiber F_2T_2 passes through point *I* and remains isometric during flexion. Fiber F_3T_3 passes behind the flexion axis and slackens during flexion.

The fiber (F_1T_1) passes in front of the flexion axis. The track of its origin (F_1), a circle centered on I, is oblique to the fiber and carries F_1 away from T_1. As a result, fiber F_1T_1 stretches during flexion and slackens during extension. The fiber F_3T_3 passes behind the flexion axis I. The track of its femoral origin F_3 is also a circle centered on I and is oblique to the fiber, but it carries the fiber origin toward its insertion. As a result, the fiber slackens during flexion and tightens during extension. The fiber F_2T_2 passes through the flexion axis; the track of its origin F_2 lies perpendicular to the fiber so that the fiber remains isometric during flexion and extension. The pattern of fiber lengthening and slackening of the ligament as a whole then depends on where within the ligament the isometric fiber lies.

The work of Friederich et al. (22) and Mommersteeg et al. (24) on ligament architecture; the findings of Sidles et al. (26), Fuss (64), Sapega et al. (27), and Covey et al. (30) in searching for isometric fibers within the cruciates; and our own work suggest that, for a 2-D model, the most isometric fibers within the cruciates should be as shown in Figure 5.26. Attachment lines are drawn within the attachment areas for all four ligaments, and the origins and insertions of isometric fibers within the cruciates are shown as heavy dots. The isometric fiber in the ACL lies at the front of the ligament in extension; in the PCL, it lies within the ligament. These assumptions are consistent with the contours of fiber strain shown in Figures 5.14 and 5.15. Based on Friederich's work (22), Zavatsky and O'Connor (65) proposed a proportional mapping for fibers within each model ligament, a fiber arising at a certain proportional distance along the length of the femoral origin line should insert at the same proportion along the length of the tibial insertion line. They also assumed that all fibers in the ACL, MCL, and LCL and the posterior bundle of the PCL are just tight in extension (i.e., the zero-tension reference position), whereas the fibers of the anterior bundle of the PCL were assumed to be just tight at 120° (i.e., the zero-tension reference position). Lu and O'Connor (66) described a computer-graphics representation of such model ligaments, models that could then be animated, as shown on the enclosed CD-ROM.

Figure 5.27 shows the model cruciate ligaments in three positions. The isometric fibers of the two ligaments join the points marked with heavy dots in Figure 5.26.

Length Patterns in the Cruciate Ligaments

The animation of Figure 5.27A is shown as Image 4 on the CD-ROM. The figure shows that the fibers of the model ACL are nearly parallel in extension, but as the femoral attachment line rotates relative to the tibia during flexion, the shape of the ligament changes and fibers that in extension lie at the back of the joint cross the ligament, and their femoral origins lie nearer the front of the joint. The distances between the origin and insertion of each fiber were calculated, and it was found that all but the isometric fibers slacken. Slack fibers are shown buckled. Figure 5.27B shows that the anterior bundle of the PCL tightens with flexion, whereas the posterior bundle tightens and slackens again. Image 5 on the CD-ROM shows the model ACL and PCL with their fibers slackening and tightening systematically.

Figure 5.28A shows the relative lengths during flexion of fibers in the ACL that lie anteriorly, centrally, and posteriorly within the ligament in extension. Length is expressed as a proportion of fiber length at the zero-tension reference position (i.e., in extension). Whereas the most anterior fiber remains isometric, the others slacken initially and then begin to tighten again. They are most slack in the range 50° to 90° of flexion. The calculated length changes reflect the position of fibers relative to the flexion axis of the joint. Slackening occurs as long as the fiber passes behind the flexion axis and retightening

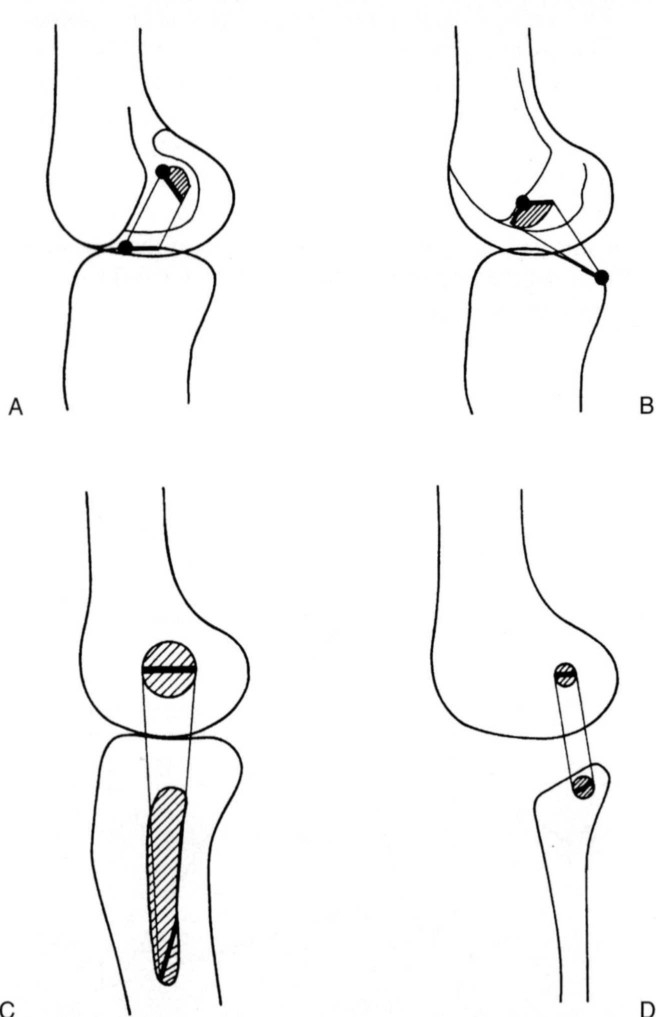

FIGURE 5.26. The knee in extension demonstrates the assumed attachment lines on both bones for each of the four model ligaments **(A–D)**. The assumed isometric fibers in the anterior and posterior cruciate ligaments join the area *(heavy dots)* on the two ligaments. (From Zavatsky AB, O'Connor JJ. A model of human knee ligaments in the sagittal plane. I: response to passive flexion. *J Engng Med Proc Inst Mech Eng Part H* 1992;206:125–134, with permission.)

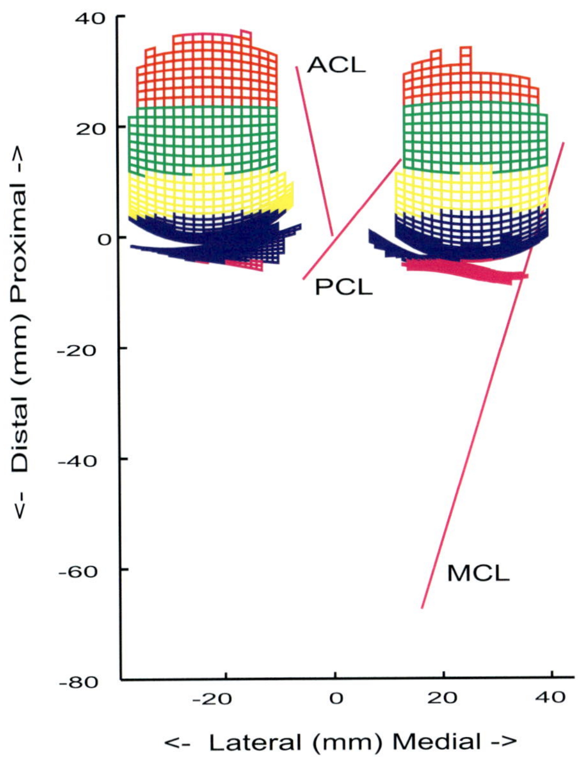

COLOR PLATE 1. Model knee with polynomial femoral and tibial surfaces held together by isometric fibers in the anterior cruciate ligament (ACL), posterior cruciate ligament (PCL), and medial collateral ligament (MCL).

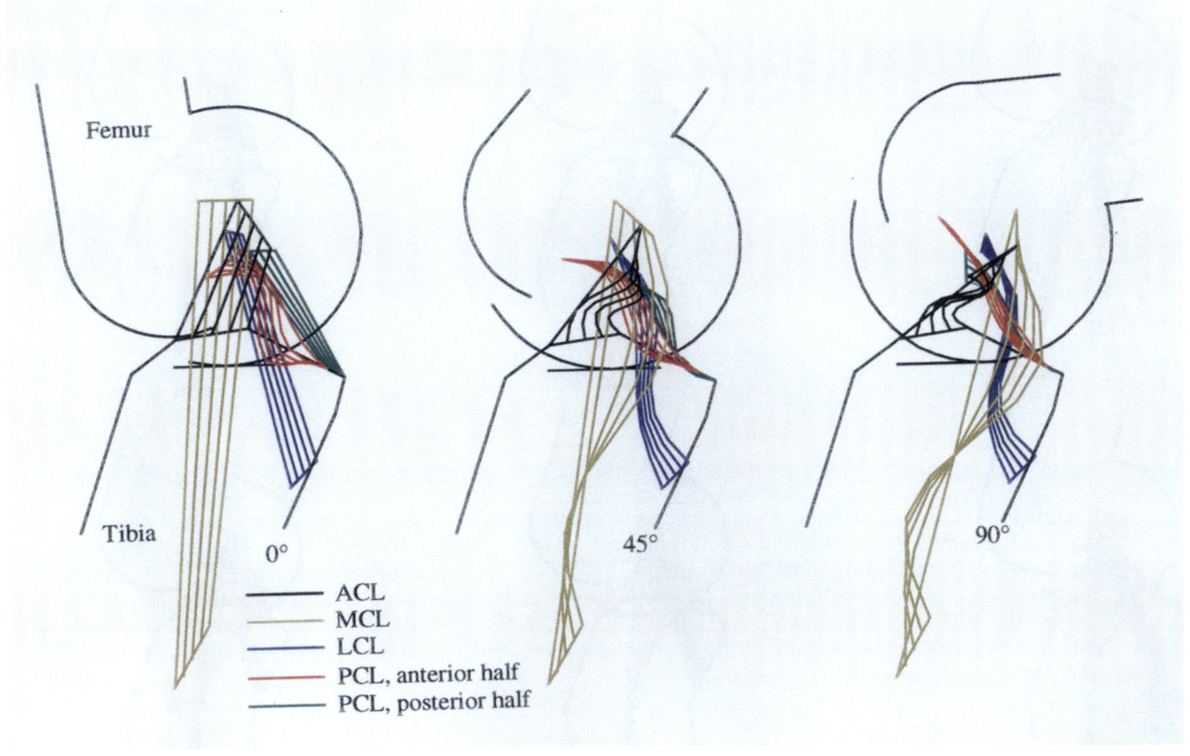

COLOR PLATE 2. Diagrams of the model knee at extension **(A)**, at 45° of flexion **(B)**, and at 90° of flexion **(C)**. The fibers of the anterior cruciate ligament (ACL), medial collateral ligament (MCL), and lateral collateral ligament (LCL) and the posterior fibers of the posterior cruciate ligament (PCL) are tight in extension and slacken during flexion. The anterior fibers of the PCL are slack in extension and tighten during flexion.

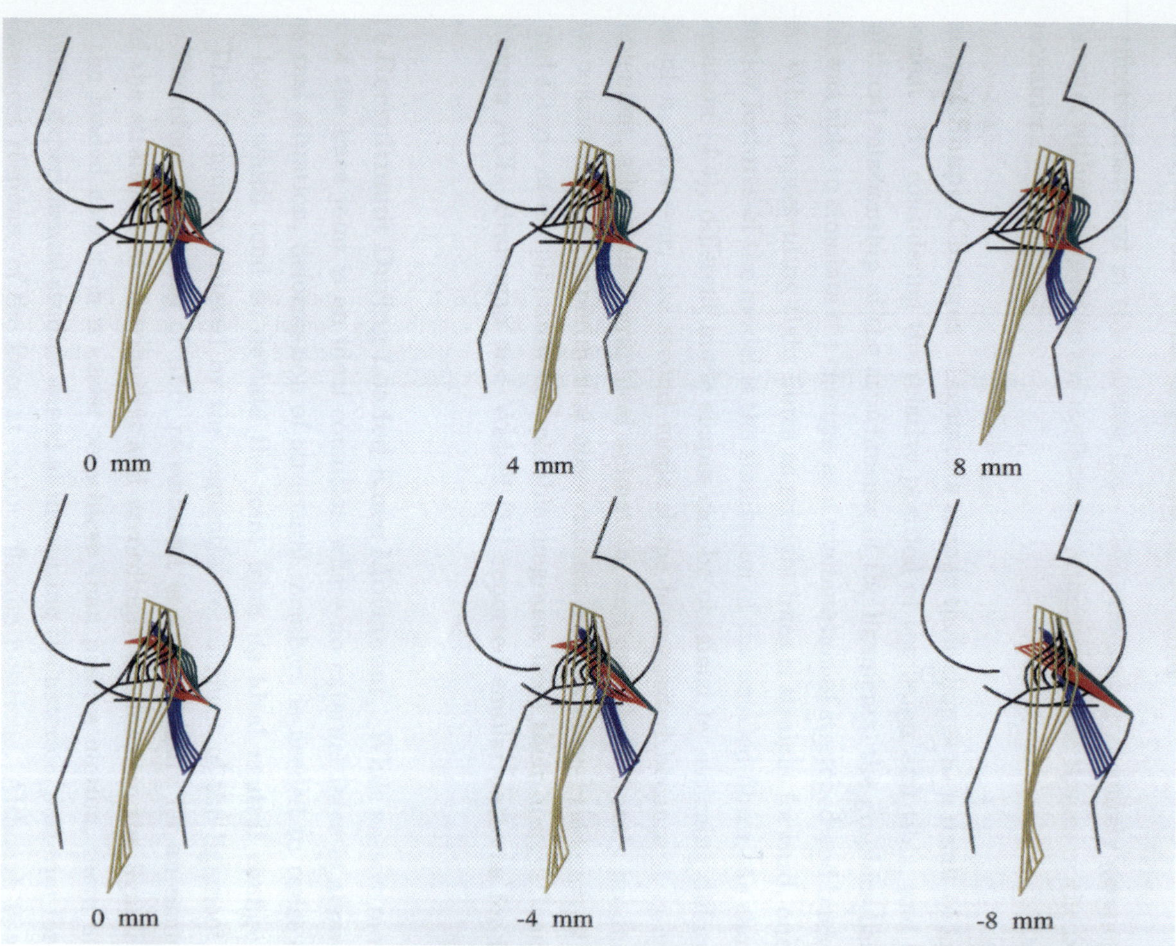

COLOR PLATE 3. Model knee at 25° flexion in the unloaded state (0 mm) and after 4 and 8 mm anterior tibial translation **(top row)** and 4 and 8 mm posterior translation **(bottom row)**. Anterior translation recruits fibers in the anterior cruciate ligament (ACL) and medial collateral ligament (MCL) and slackens the posterior cruciate ligament (PCL) and lateral collateral ligament (LCL). Posterior translation tightens the PCL and LCL and slackens the ACL and MCL. (See also Fig. 10.8.) (From Lu TW. Geometric and mechanical modelling of the human locomotor system. D.Phil. thesis: University of Oxford, 1997, with permission.)

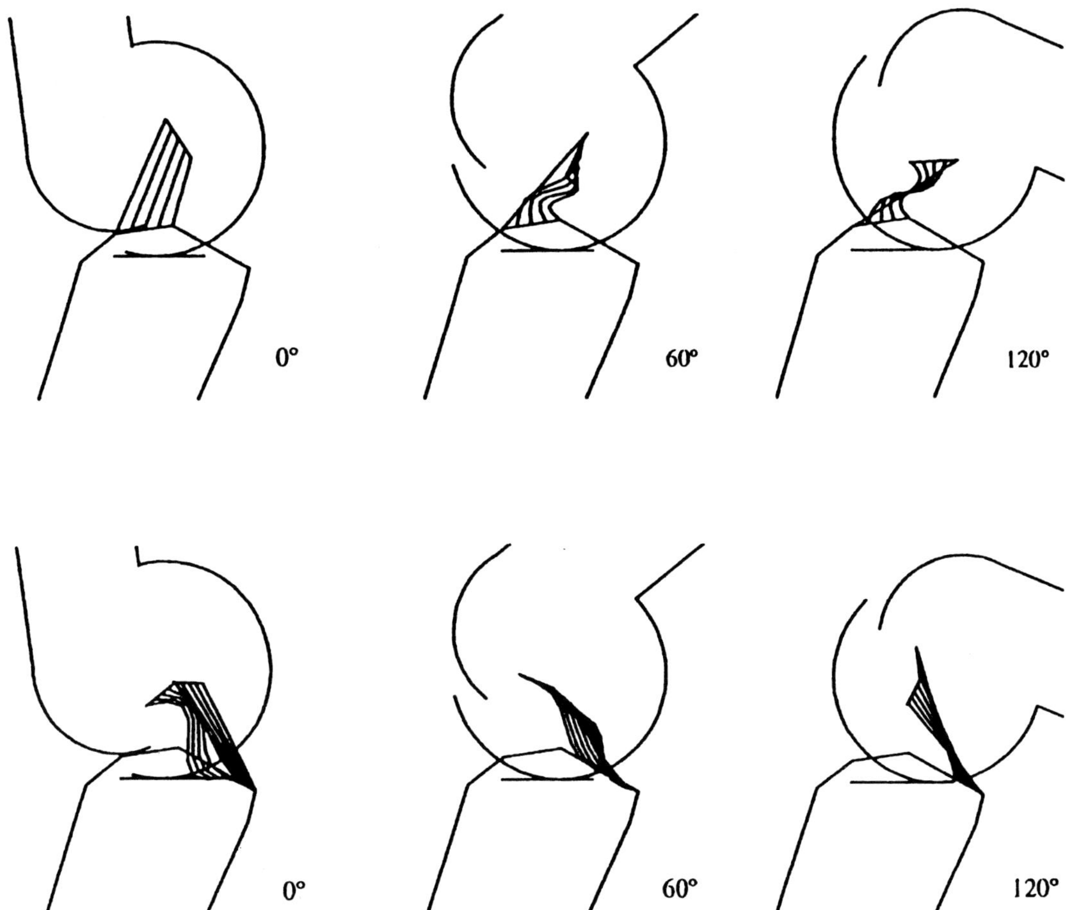

FIGURE 5.27. Models of the anterior cruciate ligament (ACL) and posterior cruciate ligament (PCL) in three positions. All fibers of the ACL and the posterior fibers of the PCL are tight in extension and slacken during flexion. The anterior fibers of the PCL slacken in extension and tighten during flexion. (From Lu TW, O'Connor JJ. Fibre recruitment and shape changes of knee ligaments during motion: as revealed by a computer graphics-based model. *J Engng Med Proc Inst Mech Eng Part H* 1996;210: 71–79, with permission.)

begins when the fiber has crossed over the ligament to lie anterior to the flexion axis.

Figure 5.28B shows length changes for fibers within the anterior bundle of the PCL. All but the isometric fibers tighten continuously with flexion. In contrast (Fig. 5.28C), the posterior bundle of the model PCL behaves much more like the ACL, with slackening followed by retightening.

The shape changes of the cruciates predicted by the model are very similar to those observed by van Dijk et al. (67) who used the Rontgen Stereophotogrammatric Analysis (RSA) technique with stereophotogrammetric x-ray methods to define the length patterns of the cruciates during flexion and extension. The choice of attachment lines for the model cruciates was based on van Dijk's results. The fiber length changes for the ACL are quite similar to those measured by Sapega et al. (27). Amis and Dawkins (68) found similar patterns for the central and posterior fibers of the ACL, but their most anterior fiber showed some initial slackening followed by tightening.

Covey et al. (30) found that the anterior and central fibers of the PCL lengthen by equal amounts and that the posterior longitudinal fibers slacken and then lengthen again. They found the posterior oblique fiber to be the most isometric, as did Friederich et al. (22). The length changes for the model posterior fiber in Figure 5.28C are similar to Covey's, but the length changes for the model anterior fiber are about twice Covey's changes.

Ligament Length Patterns and Collateral Ligaments

Color Plate 2 (following page 72) shows the model joint with all four ligaments; its animation can be found in Image 5 on the CD-ROM. The diagrams of the two cruciates are the same as in Figure 5.27, but diagrams of the collaterals have been superimposed. Comparing the figures at the three positions, it can be seen that the fibers of the lateral collateral ligament, which are all just tight in extension, slacken when the joint begins to flex. The general slackening with flexion occurs because all fibers pass posterior to the flexion axis in all positions of the joint. This outcome is in accordance with the observations of Meister et al. (69), Wang and Walker (70), Rovick et al. (35), and Blankevoort et al. (29).

Although the posterior fibers of the model MCL slacken with flexion, the most anterior fibers remain straight, indicating that they stretch slightly in early flexion before beginning to slacken again. This occurs because the MCL covers the intersection of the cruciates so that the flexion axis of the joint passes through the ligament. The most anterior fibers in the model therefore pass in front of the flexion axis and are expected to stretch during early flexion. Internal tibial rotation would diminish this stretch and further increase the slackening of the LCL. It was this result that prompted the development of the 3-D model described previously, with the two cruciates and the MCL (not the LCL) acting as guides to movement. The shape changes of the MCL during passive flexion suggested by the model are quite similar to those depicted by Muller (48).

Validation of the Model

Although the four-bar linkage model of mobility is 2-D and cannot account for events in the coronal and transverse planes, such as internal tibial rotation, we have been able to cite a significant body of evidence in the literature that can be explained qualitatively and even quantitatively by the model. Lu and O'Connor (52) showed that the predicted variations in direction of the model ligaments and muscle tendons fit well with the measurements of human specimens made by Herzog and Read (71).

Quasi–Three-Dimensional Model of Knee Mobility

Zavatsky and O'Connor (72) proposed a 3-D model of the cruciate ligaments in a model knee in which the movements occurred only in the sagittal plane under the control of the four-bar linkage model. The model areas of origin and insertion were taken to be planar and elliptical, unlike the areas used in the Feikes model (Fig. 5.19), which were based on the digitized shapes of the anatomic attachment areas and the nonplanar geometry of their surfaces. Mapping of fibers from femur to tibia was assumed to be from corresponding points within their elliptical attachment areas such that their coordinates within the ellipses were scaled according to the ratios of their major and minor axes. This was a 3-D analog of the proportional mapping used for the 2-D model (Fig. 5.27A).

Figure 5.29 shows sagittal, coronal, and transverse views of the models' ligaments in extension and at 120° flexion. The shape changes demonstrated by the 2-D model (Fig. 5.27, Color Plate 2 following page 72) are more clearly seen in this quasi–3-D model. To emphasize the

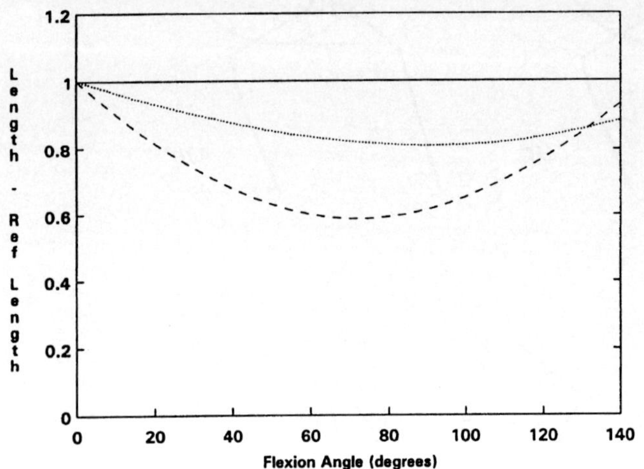

A

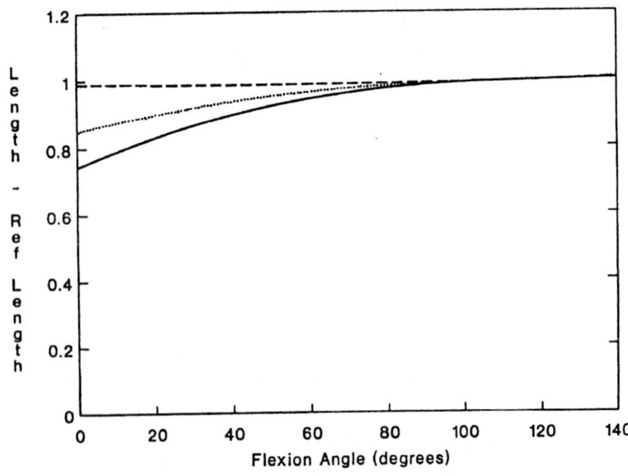

B

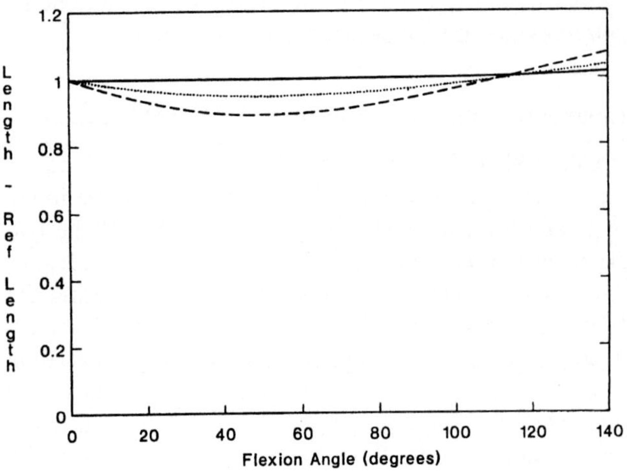

C

FIGURE 5.28. A: Length change patterns with flexion angle of anterior, middle, and posterior fibers of the ACL compared with their lengths in extension. **B:** Anterior, anterocentral, and central fibers of the PCL compared with the lengths in flexion. **C:** Central, posterocentral, and posterior fibers of PCL compared with lengths in extension. (From Zavatsky AB, O'Connor JJ. A model of human knee ligaments in the sagittal plane. I: Response to passive flexion. *J Engng Med Proc Inst Mech Eng Part H* 1992;206:125–134, with permission.)

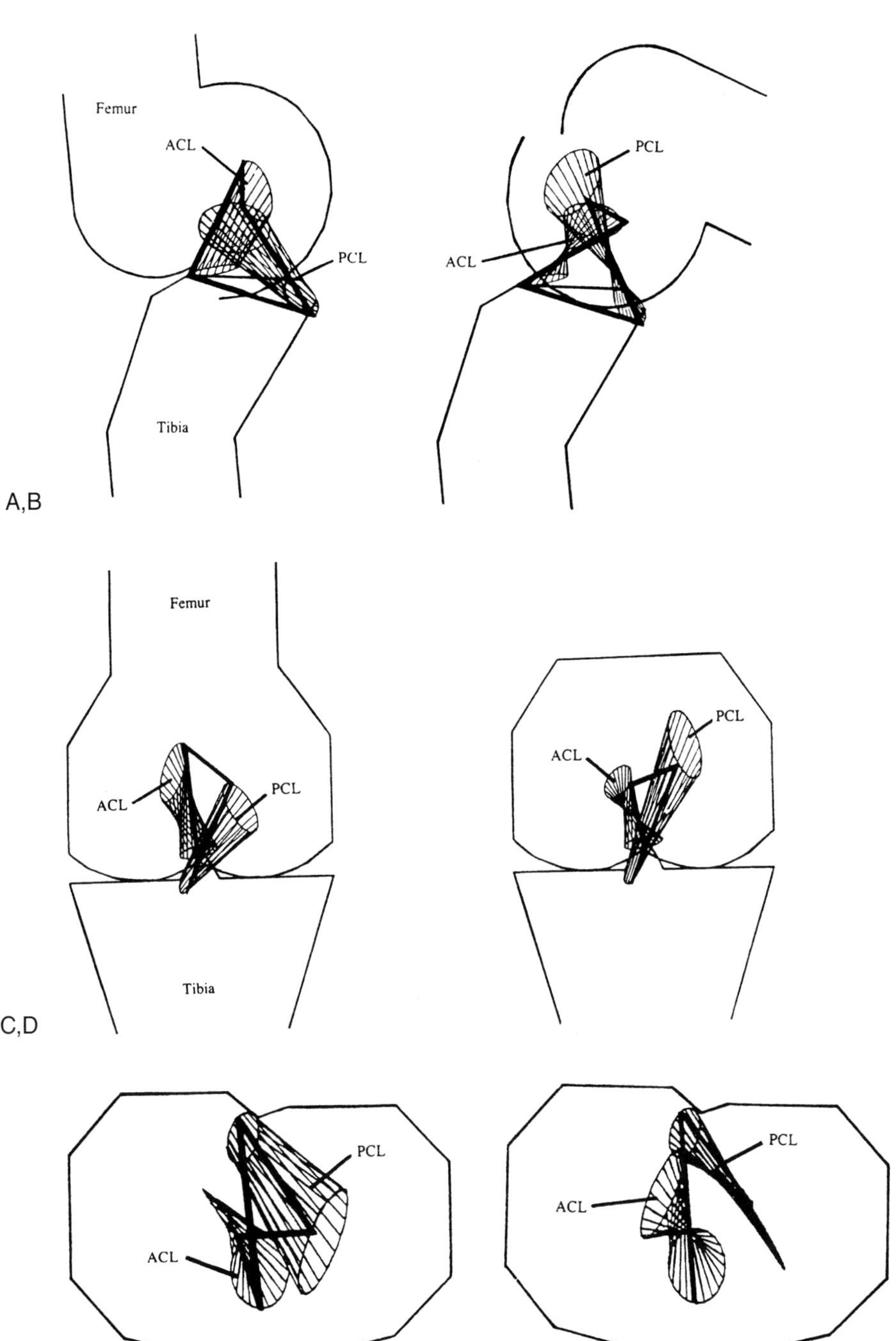

FIGURE 5.29. Model cruciates with elliptical attachment areas in extension **(A, C, E)** and at 90° of flexion **(B, D, F)** in the sagittal plane **(A, B)**, the coronal plane **(C, D)**, and the transverse plane **(E, F)**. The ligaments bend and twist as the joint flexes and extends. The isometric fibers are drawn as *heavy straight lines*. (From Zavatsky AB, O'Connor JJ. Three-dimensional geometric models of human knee ligaments. *J Engng Med Proc Inst Mech Eng Part H* 1994;208: 229–240, with permission.)

shape changes, all fibers are drawn as straight lines connecting their origins and insertions. The ligaments change their shapes because they bend, as reproduced by the purely 2-D model, but also because they twist.

The model assumes that flexion and extension occurs about an axis perpendicular to the sagittal plane but passing through the isometric fibers of the two cruciates. Because the isometric fiber of each cruciate in this model is now inclined to the sagittal plane, the angular velocity vector of the femur relative to the tibia has components perpendicular and parallel to it. The component perpendicular to the isometric fiber causes the ligament to bend in the sagittal plane so that fibers originally anterior and posterior in the ligament in extension cross each other in flexion. The component of the angular velocity vector parallel to the isometric fiber causes the ligament to twist, with the fibers forming a helix-like shape (Fig. 5.30). Van Dijk (73) called this phenomenon *intraligamentary torsion*.

With more than 120° of flexion, the model ACL twists through an angle of about 80°, somewhat more than the measurements reported by van Dijk (73) (Fig. 5.31). The differences can be explained almost entirely by the fact that this model knee does not allow coupled internal tibial rotation, which would reduce the value of the twist calculated by the model.

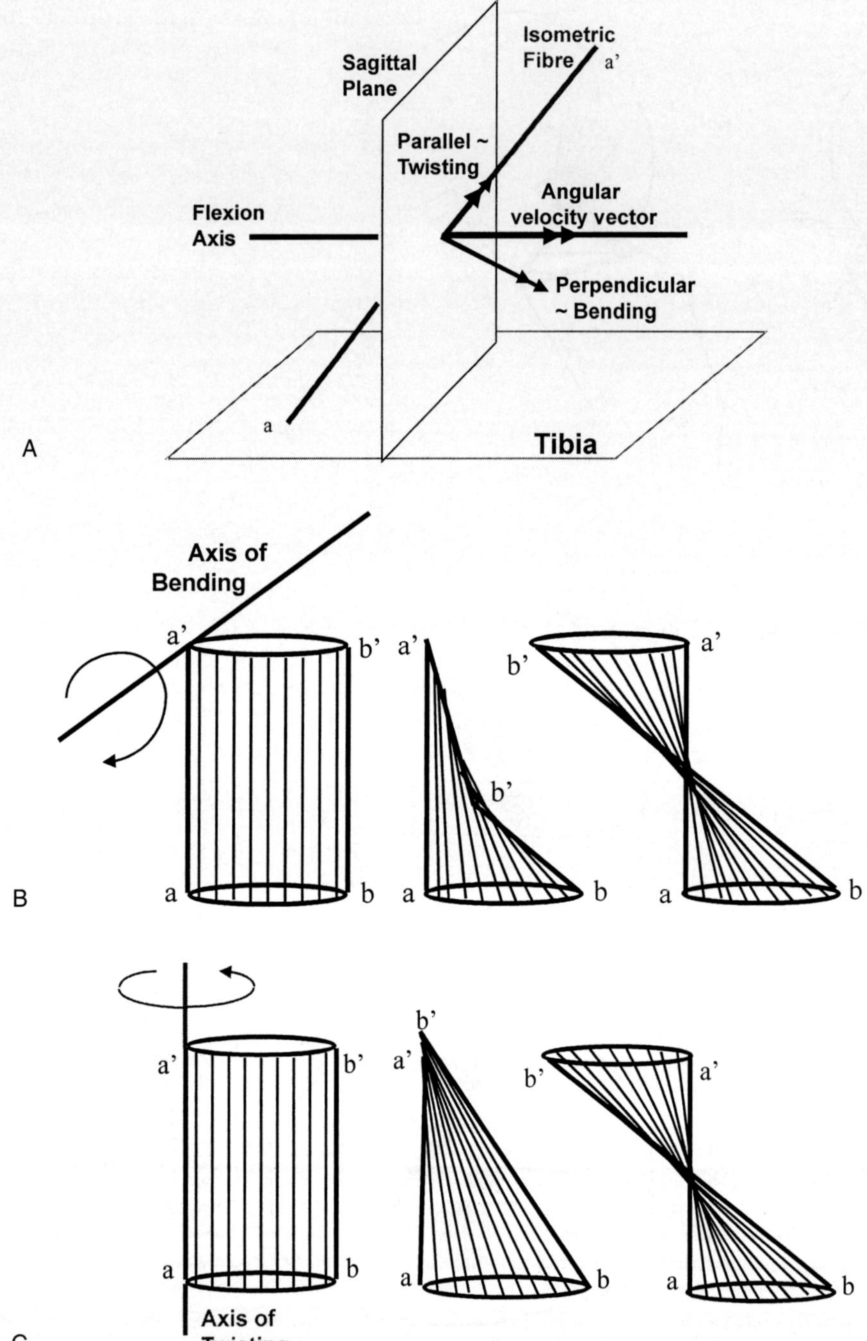

FIGURE 5.30. When the angular velocity vector of the femur relative to the tibia is not perpendicular to the isometric fiber **(A)**, the ligament changes its shape due to bending **(B)** and twisting **(C)**. (From Zavatsky AB, O'Connor JJ, Lu TW. Biomechanical functions of ligaments: implications for ACL reconstructions. *Orthopaedics International Edition* 1996;4:349–357, with permission.)

Figure 5.29 shows that, during flexion and extension movements, the cruciate ligaments bend and unbend as well as twist and untwist and that their fibers cross and uncross in a systematic and repeatable fashion. The calculated shape changes arise because of the relative motion of the ligament attachment areas and are similar to those described by Brantigan and Voschell (18), Friederich et al. (22), Girgis et al. (23), and van Dijk (73). Toutoungi et al. (74) modified the shapes of the ligament attachment areas, eliminating the portions of the ellipses where fibers stretched beyond their reference lengths during passive flexion. The resulting attachment area shapes appear somewhat more anatomic. They also showed that the forces required in the anterior drawer test are very sensitive to the choice of parameters for the model. Clinically, one of the most important considerations must be to position the femoral attachment of a graft ACL as accurately as possible.

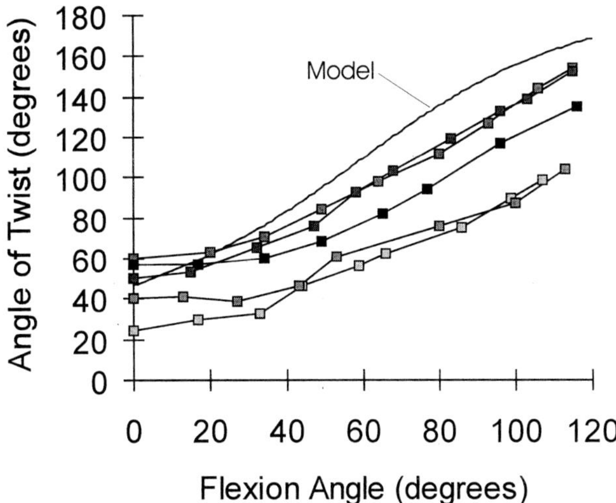

FIGURE 5.31. Twist of the anterior cruciate ligament plotted against the flexion angle. The calculated values from the model exceed the measurements of van Dijk. (From Zavatsky AB, O'Connor JJ. Three-dimensional geometric models of human knee ligaments. *J Engng Med Proc Inst Mech Eng Part H* 1994;208:229–240, with permission.)

DISCUSSION

The experiments described in this chapter demonstrate that the knee joint exhibits a range of unresisted passive motion and that, within that range, the six possible DOF are reduced to one, quantifying in particular the coupling of internal tibial rotation with flexion. The experiments allowed the identification of the constraints to motion, the pairs of articular surfaces in the medial and lateral compartments and isometric fibers in the ACL, PCL, and MCL. Because these constraints are all flexible, the joint exhibits laxity, and only a small force is needed to perturb it from its path of passive motion. The analysis of possible ligament isometry revealed that fibers lying along surfaces near the front of the ACL and MCL and within the bulk of the PCL remained nearly isometric during passive flexion, whereas most other fibers slackened during flexion and tightened again during extension. The PCL was the exception because the anterior fibers were slack in extension but tightened with flexion. These patterns are entirely a consequence of the relative motion of the areas of origin and insertion of the ligaments and the positions within the ligaments of the most isometric fibers. Analysis of the experimental data confirmed that both tibiofemoral compartments exhibit combinations of rolling and sliding.

The 2-D and 3-D models of the knee explain most of the experimentally observed phenomena. The tibia has to rotate internally during flexion to maintain continuous contact in medial and lateral compartments and to avoid stretching of ligament fibers in the ACL, PCL, and MCL. The passive coupled motion of the knee can occur without resistance and without tissue deformation, the articular surfaces rolling and sliding on each other without indentation and the ligament fibers rotating about their origins and insertions without stretching.

The patterns of fiber slackening and tightening revealed by the models agree well with those observed experimentally. Because the mapping functions allow representation of a continuous distribution of fibers within each ligament, rather than a limited number of discrete fibers as in the Mommersteeg model (75), contours of constant fiber strain could be drawn and were found to be similar to those derived from experiment.

The rather complex patterns of slackening and tightening exhibited by the four model ligaments, although developed from simple principles and based on the concept of isometricity of a limited number of fibers, explain why isometric fibers are difficult to observe visually or even by palpation during surgery. Searching for isometric fibers is akin to looking for a needle in a haystack. The concept of isometry is a theoretic ideal that is exhibited by these fibers only when the knee is unloaded, a condition difficult to reproduce experimentally. The analysis of mobility has shown that all fibers within a ligament cannot remain isometric, even within the ideally perfectly unloaded knee. In placing grafts, surgeons should not seek to achieve isometricity of the entire graft, but only of some chosen fibers.

The inferences drawn from the models reveal characteristics that would be difficult to observe experimentally. The direct comparisons between what can be measured and the predictions from the model give a basis for judging the accuracy of model predictions of characteristics that cannot be measured.

Model predictions locate the positions of the contact points and the contact normals and the directions of ligament fibers in the unloaded state. Similarly, the 2-D model defines the directions of the muscle tendons in the unloaded state. This information serves as the common starting point for the analysis of the mechanics of the joint in many different activities (see Chapter 10).

ACKNOWLEDGMENTS

This chapter was based on the insights provided by Mr. John Goodfellow, the surgeon, over many years of happy collaboration. It has benefited from discussions with more recent clinical colleagues, Professor David Murray and Mr. Andrew Price. It summarizes some of the work of a succession of research students—Professor Ed Biden, Dr. David FitzPatrick, Mr. Russell Miller, Professor Jim Collins, Professor David Wilson, Dr. Jennifer Feikes, Dr. David Beard, Dr. Danielle Toutoungi, Professor Tung-Wu Lu, Dr. Ahmed Imran, Dr. Richard Huss, Dr. Alberto Leardini, Dr. Melissa Carson, Dr. Wen Ling Chen, Mr. Paul Oppold, and Mr. Chris Riegger—as well as co-authors Dr. Amy Zavatsky and Dr. Richie Gill. All these contributions are gratefully acknowledged. Our work has been supported with grants from The Arthritis Research Campaign, The Wellcome Trust, The Leverhulme Trust, the EU Commissioners, Biomet Ltd., and De Puy Ltd. The research students have been supported with scholarships and fellowships from the Rhodes Foundation, The Felix Trust, The Thouron Award Scheme (University of Pennsylvania), The Royal College of Surgeons, The Wishbone Trust (British Orthopaedic Association), The Engineering and Physical Sciences Research Council, and The Government of the Republic of China (Taiwan).

REFERENCES

1. Wilson DR, Feikes JD, Zavatsky AB, et al. The components of passive knee movement are coupled to flexion angle. *J Biomech* 2000;33: 465–473.
2. Cole GK, Nigg BM, Ronsky JL, et al. Application of the joint coordinate system to three-dimensional joint attitude and movement representation: a standardization proposal. *J Biomech Eng* 1993;115(4A):344—349.
3. Grood ES, Suntay WJ. A joint coordinate system for the clinical description of three-dimensional motions: application to the knee. *J Biomech Eng* 1983;105:136–144.
4. Meyer H. Die Mechanik des Kniegelinks. *Archiv Anat Physiol* 1853: 497–547.
5. Zavatsky AB. A kinematic-freedom analysis of a flexed-knee-stance testing rig. *J Biomech* 1997;30:277–280.
6. Blankevoort L, Kuiper JH, Huiskes R, et al. Articular contact in a three-dimensional model of the knee. *J Biomech* 1991;24:1019–1031.
7. Blankevoort L, Huiskes R, de Lange A. The envelope of passive knee joint motion. *J Biomech* 1988;21:705–720.
8. Bourne RB, Goodfellow JW, O'Connor JJ. A functional analysis of various knee arthroplasties. *Trans Orthop Res Soc*, Anaheim, 1978:160.
8a. Goodfellow J, O'Connor J. The mechanics of the knee and prosthesis design. *J Bone Joint Surg Br* 1978:60:358–369.
9. Woltring HJ, Huiskes R, de Lange A, et al. Finite centroid and helical axis estimation from noisy landmark measurements in the study of human joint kinematics. *J Biomech* 1985;18:379–389.
10. Blacharski PA, Somerset JH, Murray DG. A three-dimensional study of the kinematics of the human knee. *J Biomech* 1975;8:375–384.
11. Blankevoort L, Huiskes R, de Lange A. Helical axes of passive knee joint motions. *J Biomech* 1990;23:1219–1229.
12. O'Connor JJ, Shercliff TL, Biden E, et al. The geometry of the knee in the sagittal plane. *J Engng Med Proc Inst Mech Eng [H]* 1989;203: 223–233.
13. Iwaki H, Pinskerova V, Freeman MA. Tibiofemoral movement 1: the shapes and relative movements of the femur and tibia in the unloaded cadaver knee. *J Bone Joint Surg Br* 2000;82:1189–1195.
14. Borelli GA. *De motu animalium.* Rome, 1680. English translation: *On the movement of animals.* Berlin: Springer-Verlag, 1989, Maquet PD, translator.
15. Kapandji IA. *The physiology of the joints,* 5th ed. London: Churchill Livingstone, 1987.
16. Thompson WO, Thaete FL, Fu FH, et al. Tibial meniscal dynamics using three-dimensional reconstruction of magnetic resonance images. *Am J Sports Med* 1991;19:210–215, discussion 215–216.
17. Vedi V, Williams A, Tennant SJ, et al. Meniscal movement. An in-vivo study using dynamic MRI. *J Bone Joint Surg Br* 1999;81:37–41.
18. Brantigan OC, Voshell AF. The mechanics of the ligaments and menisci of the knee joint. *J Bone Joint Surg Am* 1941;23:44–66.
19. Beynnon BD, Fleming BC. Anterior cruciate ligament strain in-vivo: a review of previous work. *J Biomech* 1998;31:519–525.
20. Odensten M, Gillquist J. Functional anatomy of the anterior cruciate ligament and a rationale for reconstruction. *J Bone Joint Surg Am* 1985; 67:257–262.
21. Arnoczky SP. Anatomy of the anterior cruciate ligament. *Clin Orthop* 1983;172:19–25.
22. Friederich NF, Muller W, O'Brien WR. [Clinical application of biomechanic and functional anatomical findings of the knee joint]. *Orthopade* 1992;21:41–50.
23. Girgis FG, Marshall JL, Monajem A. The cruciate ligaments of the knee joint. Anatomical, functional and experimental analysis. *Clin Orthop* 1975;106:216–231.
24. Mommersteeg TJ, Kooloos JG, Blankevoort L, et al. The fibre bundle anatomy of human cruciate ligaments. *J Anat* 1995;187[Pt 2]:461–471.
25. Feikes JD. *The mobility and stability of the human knee joint.* [D.Phil. dissertation]. Oxford: University of Oxford, 1999.
26. Sidles JA, Larson RV, Garbini JL, et al. Ligament length relationships in the moving knee. *J Orthop Res* 1988;6:593–610.
27. Sapega AA, Moyer MA, Schneck C, et al. Testing for isometry during reconstruction of the anterior cruciate ligament. *J Bone Joint Surg Am* 1990;72:259–267.
28. Zavras TD, Race A, Bull AM, et al. A comparative study of "isometric" points for anterior cruciate ligament graft attachment. *Knee Surg Sports Traumatol Arthrosc* 2001;9:28–33.
29. Blankevoort L, Huiskes R, de Lange A. Recruitment of knee joint ligaments. *J Biomech Eng* 1991;113:94–103.
30. Covey DC, Sapega AA, Sherman GM, et al. Testing for "isometry" during posterior cruciate ligament reconstruction. *Trans Orthop Res Soc* 1992 :665.
31. Strasser H. *Lehrbuch der Muskel und Gelenkmechanik. III Band: die untere Extremitart.* Berlin: Springer-Verlag, 1917.
32. Pinskerova V, Maquet P, Freeman MAR. Writings on the knee between 1836 and 1917. *J Bone Joint Surg Br* 2000;82:1100–1102.
33. Zuppinger H. Die aktive Flexion in unbelasteten Kniegelenk. In: *Zuricher Habil Schr.* Wiesbaden: Bergmann, 1904:703–763.
34. Warren LA, Marshall JL, Girgis F. The prime static stabilizer of the medical side of the knee. *J Bone Joint Surg Am* 1974;56:665–674.
35. Rovick JS, Reuben JD, Schrager RJ, et al. Relation between knee motion and ligament length patterns. *Clin Orthop* 1991;6:213–220.
36. Wilson DR, Feikes JD, O'Connor JJ. Ligaments and articular contact guide passive knee flexion. *J Biomech* 1998;31:1127–1136.
37. Wismans J, Veldpaus F, Janssen J, et al. A three-dimensional mathematical model of the knee-joint. *J Biomech* 1980;13:677–685.
38. Andriacchi TP, Mikosz RP, Hampton SJ, et al. Model studies of the stiffness characteristics of the human knee joint. *J Biomech* 1983;16:23–29.
39. Essenger JR, Leyvraz PF, Heegard JH, et al. A mathematical model for the evaluation of the behaviour during flexion of condylar-type knee prostheses. *J Biomech* 1989;22:1229–1241.
40. Blankevoort L, Huiskes R. Ligament-bone interaction in a three-dimensional model of the knee. *J Biomech Eng* 1991;113:263–269.
41. Sathasivam S, Walker PS. A computer model with surface friction for the prediction of total knee kinematics. *J Biomech* 1997;30:177–184.
42. Crowninshield RD, Pope MH, Johnson RJ. An analytical model of the knee. *J Biomech* 1976;9:397–405.
43. Feikes JD, O'Connor JJ, Zavatsky AB. A constraint-based approach to modelling the mobility of the human knee joint. *J Biomech* 2002 *(in press)*.
44. Wilson DR. *Three dimensional kinematics of the knee* [D.Phil. dissertation]. Oxford: University of Oxford, 1995.
45. Kapandji IA. *The physiology of the joints.* Edinburgh: Churchill Livingstone; 1970.
46. Menschik A. Mechanik des Kniegelenkes. *Z Orthop* 1974;112:481.
47. Huson A. Biomechanische probleme des kniegelenks. *Orthopade* 1974;3.
48. Muller W. *The knee: form, function and reconstruction.* Berlin: Springer-Verlag, 1983.
49. Leardini A, O'Connor JJ, Catani F, et al. A geometric model of the human ankle joint. *J Biomech* 1999;32:585–591.
50. Frankel VH, Burstein AH. *Orthopaedic biomechanics: the application of engineering to the musculoskeletal system.* Philadelphia: Lea & Febiger, 1970.
51. Seedhom BB, Dowson D, Wright V. The load-bearing function of the menisci: a preliminary study. In: *The knee joint.* Amsterdam: Excerpta Medica, 1974:37–42.
52. Walker PS, Erkman MJ. The role of the menisci in force transmission across the knee. *Clin Orthop* 1975;109:184–192.
53. Shrive NG, O'Connor JJ, Goodfellow JW. Load-bearing in the knee joint. *Clin Orthop* 1978:279–287.
54. Gill HS. The mechanics of heelstrike during level walking [D. Phil. dissertation]. Oxford: University of Oxford, 1996.
55. Gill HS, O'Connor JJ. A bi-articulating two-dimensional computer model of the human patello-femoral joint. *Clin Biomech* 1996;2:81–89.
56. Miller RK, Murray DW, Gill HS, et al. In vitro patellofemoral joint force determined by a non-invasive technique. *Clin Biomech* 1997;12:1–7.
57. Miller RK, Goodfellow JW, Murray DW, et al. In vitro measurement of

patellofemoral force after three types of knee replacement. *J Bone Joint Surg Br* 1998;80:900–906.

58. Maquet PGJ. *Biomechanics of the knee.* Berlin: Springer-Verlag, 1984.

59. Bishop RED, Denham RA. A note on the ratio between tensions in the quadriceps tendon and the infra-patellar ligament. *Eng Med* 1977;6: 53–54.

60. Goodfellow J, Hungerford DS, Zindel M. Patello-femoral joint mechanics and pathology. 1. Functional anatomy of the patello-femoral joint. *J Bone Joint Surg Br* 1976;58:287–290.

61. Beard DJ, Murray DW, Gill HS, et al. Reconstruction does not reduce tibial translation in the cruciate-deficient knee: an in vivo study. *J Bone Joint Surg Br* 2001;83:1098–1103.

62. Oppold PT. *Characterising in vitro patellofemoral kinematics and kinetics* [M.Sc. thesis]. Oxford: University of Oxford, 2000.

63. Price AJ. *Outcome following meniscal bearing unicompartmental arthroplasty of the knee* [D. Phil. dissertation]. Oxford: University of Oxford, 2002.

64. Fuss FK. Anatomy of the cruciate ligaments and their function in extension and flexion of the human knee joint. *Am J Anat* 1989;184:165–176.

65. Zavatsky AB, O'Connor JJ. A model of human knee ligaments in the sagittal plane. Part 1: Response to passive flexion. *Proc Inst Mech Eng [H]* 1992;206:125–134.

66. Lu TW, O'Connor JJ. Fibre recruitment and shape changes of knee ligaments during motion: as revealed by a computer graphics-based model. *J Engng Med Proc Inst Mech Eng [H]* 1996;210:71–79.

67. van Dijk R, Huiskes R, Selvik G. Roentgen stereophotogrammetric methods for the evaluation of the three dimensional kinematic behavior and cruciate ligament length patterns of the human knee. *J Biomech* 1979;12:727–731.

68. Amis AA, Dawkins GPC. Functional anatomy of the anterior cruciate ligament: fibre bundle actions related to ligament replacements and injuries. *J Bone Joint Surg Br* 1991;73:260–267.

69. Meister BR, Michael SP, Moyer RA, et al. Anatomy and kinematics of the lateral collateral ligament of the knee. *Am J Sports Med* 2000;28:869–878.

70. Wang C, Walker PS. The effects of flexion and rotation on the length patterns of the ligaments of the knee. *J Biomech* 1973;6:587–596.

71. Herzog W, Read LJ. Lines of action and moment arms of the major force-carrying structures crossing the human knee joint. *J Anat* 1993; 182[Pt 2]:213–230.

72. Zavatsky AB, O'Connor JJ. Three-dimensional geometric models of human knee ligaments. *J Engng Med Proc Inst Mech Eng [H]* 1994; 208:229–240.

73. van Dijk R. *The behaviour of the cruciate ligaments of the knee.* Nijmegan, Netherlands: Catholic University, 1983.

74. Toutoungi DE, Zavatsky AB, O'Connor JJ. Parameter sensitivity of a mathematical model of the anterior cruciate ligament. *J Engng Med Proc Inst Mech Eng [H]* 1997;211:235–246.

75. Mommersteeg TJ, Huiskes R, Blankevoort L, et al. A global verification study of a quasi-static knee model with multi-bundle ligaments. *J Biomech* 1996;29:1659–1664.

CHAPTER 6

Ligament Cutting Studies

Methodology and Results

Eric C. McCarty, Clemente Ibarra, Peter A. Torzilli, and Russell F. Warren

Normal knee function depends on the perfect balance between mobility and stability. Structural and functional integrity of bones, their articular surfaces, and the soft tissues that surround the joint are crucial for such balance.

Injury to the bony structures of the knee, the articular surfaces, the menisci, and adjacent tendons or muscles commonly results in limitation of mobility. Injury to the ligamentous structures and the joint capsule commonly results in various degrees of instability that can affect the overall function of the knee. Nevertheless, functional stability does not depend on isolated structures.

The role of the ligaments and joint capsule in conferring functional stability to the knee has been recognized and studied by many clinicians. However, most of the knowledge related to the function of the individual ligaments and other structures of the knee was based on subjective clinical observations by the examining physicians. Clinical examination of the knee could reveal the area and mechanisms that produced pain. Historically, limitation of a function was identified by the inability of the patient to perform a specific activity. The cause of that limitation was then identified by the physician who relied on his or her clinical skills. Abnormal motion (decreased or increased motion) was also identified during the clinical examination. This led to the diagnosis of a pathologic process or the identification of an injured structure that was later confirmed during surgery. Development of testing devices that simulated the clinical examination used by the clinician was the first attempt at understanding the functional anatomy of the knee. This has provided a better perspective of how the knee moves and how it is affected by injury.

The *range of motion* or limits of motion of a joint are determined by the different structures that participate in allowing and preventing its movement. The possible motion of one bone with respect to the other, in the three planes and around the three axes (i.e., the degrees of freedom [DOF]), is determined by the configuration of the articular surfaces and by the constraints that the ligaments, capsule, menisci, tendons, and muscles apply on them. For example, when the femur is in a fixed position, the tibia can translate along three axes: anteroposterior or sagittal plane, medial–lateral or coronal plane, and superior–inferior or axial plane. The tibia can also rotate around these axes, conferring three other movements to the tibia relative to the femur. For this reason, the motion of the knee joint is considered to have six DOF. However, the distance that the tibia translates along or around each of these axes under normal conditions varies for each individual plane and axis, and the limits of such a motion are usually determined by the integrity of the different structural components of the joint. The ligaments and capsule play a fundamental role in conferring passive or static stability to the joint, whereas the contraction of the muscles whose tendons insert around the joint, determine the active or dynamic stability to the joint

In the 1940s, Brantigan and Voshell (1) popularized the use of *in vitro* studies in cadaveric knees to identify the role of ligaments and capsule for knee stability when external loads were applied, simulating the clinical procedures used by the physician in the clinical setting. Since their report, numerous studies have addressed the function of ligaments and articular capsule in knee stability. The purpose of this chapter is to describe the methodology used to perform *in vitro* cadaveric knee ligament evaluations and to analyze the results and clinical relevance.

METHODOLOGY

The design of the original knee-testing apparatuses, those used to perform ligament cutting studies to analyze the isolated and combined role of ligaments as knee stabilizers, was first aimed at simulating physical examination procedures used by the clinician to assess knee stability. Although a large amount of information was derived from these studies, it soon became clear that it was crucial to simulate physiologic knee function to obtain more precise information about the individual and combined role of the different structures around the joint. The effect of axial load and the role of muscles and tendons as dynamic stabilizers had to be included if more precise and quantitative information was to be obtained. This led to the design of a second generation of knee-testing apparatuses that allowed greater freedom of motion and included the effect of axial load and muscle function. The advent of electronic transducer technology led to the development of a third generation of studies that used sensors to measure local tissue strains and allowed calculations using computer models. A fourth generation of testing systems is based on the use of robotics technology and finite element computer models. For this reason, the design of the testing apparatuses can be grossly divided in four categories, and although we do not discuss the different designs in separate sections, we try to indicate when and how the transition led to more detailed and complex qualitative and quantitative information.

In 1941, Brantigan and Voshell (1) recognized the controversy regarding the knowledge of the function of the individual ligaments that participated in knee stability. He designed a simple testing apparatus that simulated the examination maneuvers that clinicians used to identify injured collateral ligaments. He was able to determine their role in preventing displacement of the tibia relative to the femur when loads were applied in similar manner as an examiner would place on a patient's knee. The testing apparatus was designed to stabilize the femur (patient's thigh) and allow the examiner to apply a load to the tibia (patient's leg). The medial–lateral load applied to the distal end of the tibia allowed abduction-adduction and internal–external rotation and, in the limits of motion, mediolateral translation (Fig. 6.1).

In 1976, Markolf et al. (2) designed a more sophisticated apparatus with which they could control and measure rotations resulting from applied varus and valgus moments and translations of the tibia relative to the femur when anteroposterior forces were applied with the assistance of force handles attached to the distal tibia (Fig. 6.2). Using this and similar models, Markolf et al. (2), Piziali et al. (3), and Nielsen et al. (4) studied the effects of sectioning isolated ligaments and different combinations of them on the different translations and rotations of the tibia relative to the femur. Their results are subsequently summarized.

The effects of the inherent laxity of the ligaments and capsule were measured in the model described by Wang et al. (5) and Hsieh et al. (6,7). Their findings gave rise to the use of the terms *primary* and *secondary laxity*, which

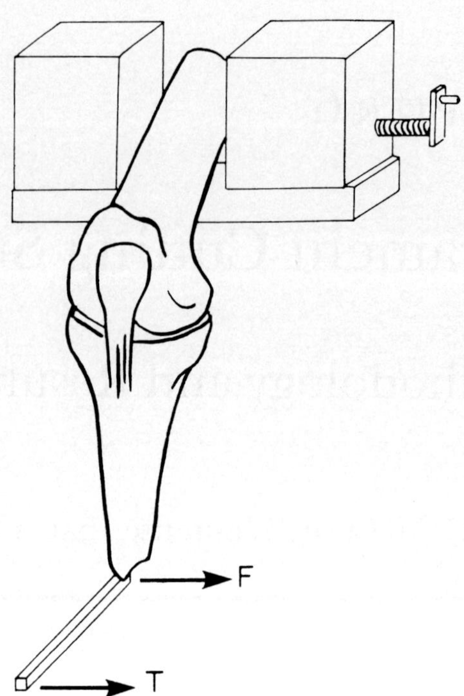

FIGURE 6.1. The test rig used by Brantigan and Voshell (1). The femur was clamped to a rigid base and forces at F or T were applied. Force F acts to abduct or adduct the joint. Force T is intended to produce tibial torsion.

refers to the motion allowed by ligaments and capsule under low loads and high loads, respectively, at the extremes of motion. They also measured the effect of axial joint compression load in relation to its contribution to knee stability and showed that compressive load decreased knee laxity. Markolf et al. (8), Shoemaker et al. (9), Perry et al. (10), and Torzilli et al. (11) described the effect of joint-compressive load and quadriceps muscle force on knee motion in the intact and anterior cruciate ligament (ACL)–sectioned knee.

The information derived from these early studies led to the development of new designs for knee test systems in an attempt to overcome the limitations created by the constrained systems and measuring devices. Kinzel et al. (12,13) and Suntay et al. (14) designed measuring systems that allowed measurement of motion in different planes and axes, regardless of their position in space.

The limitations of overconstrained systems used until then was addressed by Fukubayashi et al. (15), who designed a testing apparatus that allowed four DOF (Fig. 6.3). They measured rotation of the tibia produced by applying anteroposterior loads. By avoiding overconstraint produced by previous testing apparatuses, they allowed near-normal compression between the femur and tibia. The same testing apparatus was also used by Levy et al. (16) to study the role of the medial meniscus as a knee stabilizer. They reported that, in the absence of an

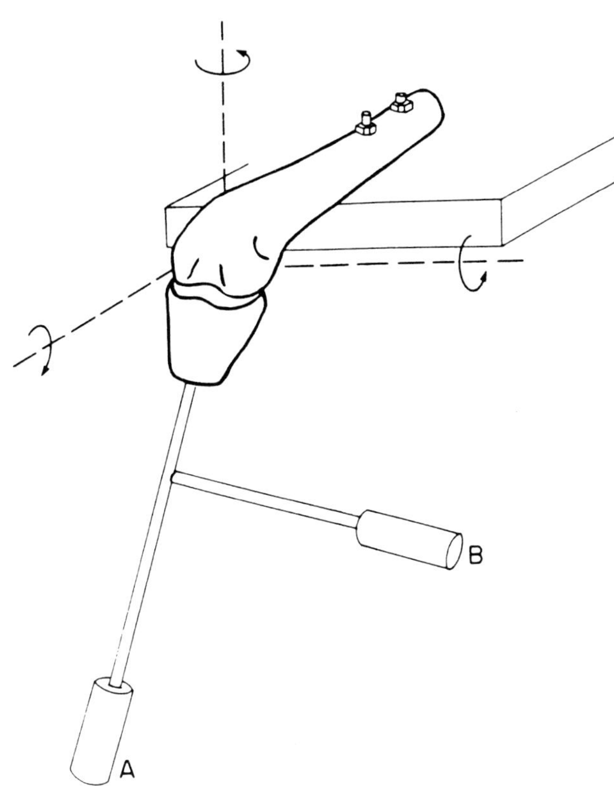

FIGURE 6.2. The test rig used by Markolf et al. (2). The force handles at *A* or *B* can be manipulated to simulate various clinical tests. Forces are well defined in this device, but no muscle action can be simulated.

ACL, the medial meniscus functions as a secondary stabilizer of anterior translation of the tibia relative to the femur. The stabilizing role of the menisci had also been described by Bargar et al. (17) and Shoemaker et al. (9). In later studies, Levy et al. (18), used a five-DOF test system to demonstrate that the lateral meniscus does not contribute significantly to knee stability in the absence of the ACL.

The four-DOF system design suppressed flexion and extension as well as mediolateral translation. Sullivan et al. (19) modified this apparatus, to allow five DOF (Fig. 6.4), and this design was later used by Gollehon et al. (20) and Veltri et al. (21,22) to describe the stabilizing role of the posterolateral structures of the knee. These later studies demonstrated the importance of the posterolateral structures in preventing posterior translation, varus rotation, and external rotation of the tibia, especially after section of the posterior cruciate ligament (PCL). They also showed that when these structures are damaged along with the ACL, internal and external rotation of the tibia increases.

The clinical relevance of these studies was evident from their early stages. However, in 1989, Butler et al. (23) introduced the concept of primary and secondary stabilizers, based on the role that each structure contributes to knee stability and how much it prevents or allows further motion when it is selectively sectioned. When the primary stabilizers are intact, the role of the secondary stabilizer is not as evident as when function of the primary stabilizers is absent. Injury to secondary stabilizers in conjunction with injury to primary stabilizers

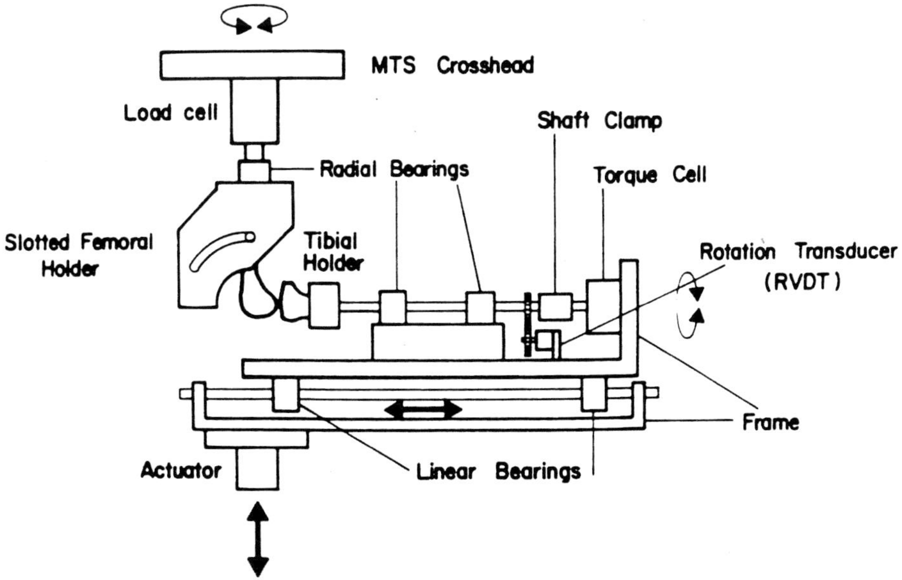

FIGURE 6.3. Schematic representation of a knee-stiffness apparatus mounted on the testing machine by Fukubayashi et al. (15). The radial bearings allow femoral–tibial rotation, and the linear bearings allow sliding and distraction of the joint. Tibial torque is measured by the torque cell when the shaft clamp is tightened, and the rotational transducer measures tibial rotation when the clamp is loosened. The slotted femoral holder provides for a continuously variable position of knee flexion. MTS, Materials Testing System; RVDT, rotary variable differential transformer.

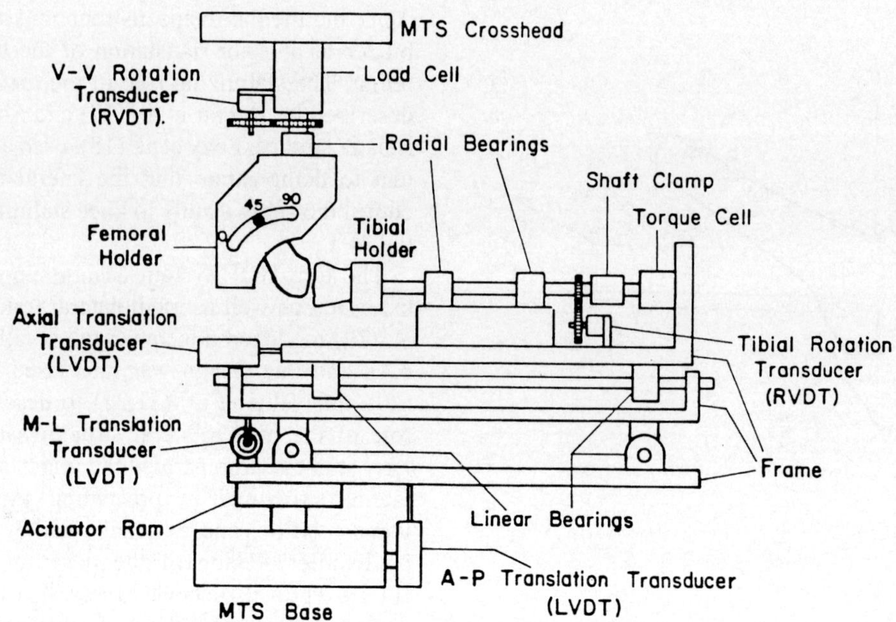

FIGURE 6.4. Diagram represents the five degrees of freedom knee-testing apparatus by Sullivan et al. (19). An anterior and posterior force is applied to the tibia by the actuator ram of the test machine. The resulting anterior, posterior, medial, lateral, and axial displacements (i.e., translations) were measured by the linear variable differential transformers (LVDTs). The resulting varus, valgus, internal, and external tibial rotations were measured by the rotary variable differential transformers (RVDTs). Tests were performed at fixed flexion angles of 0°, 30°, 60°, and 90° of flexion. MTS, Materials Testing System.

can result in more instability than when only the primary stabilizers are injured.

Several selective ligament section studies have concluded that a coupling between anterior force and internal rotation would be expected only when the line of action of the force passes lateral to the axis of tibial internal–external rotation (24). Moreover, looking at the results of most of the studies that until then attempted to analyze the roles of ligaments in knee stability, consensus was reached that each ligament plays a role of primary and secondary stabilizer for different modes of relative motion of the joint. However, the design of the apparatus used in any individual test may show great variability because of the lack of allowance of free motion of the joint.

To complement the information simulating *in vitro* clinical examination techniques, it was necessary to study the function of the stabilizing structures of the knee in activity-simulating conditions. The action of the muscles needed to be considered together with the static stabilizers. *In vivo* studies by Bargar et al. (17) and Markolf et al. (25) demonstrated that the total anteroposterior translation was reduced when muscles were contracted actively. Jurist and Otis (26) found that active contraction of the quadriceps caused anterior and posterior translation, and Daniel et al. (27) demonstrated that anterior translation was limited by active quadriceps contraction with the knee at 90° of flexion with or without ACL function.

In vitro simulation of muscle action was then included in knee ligament testing systems such as the ones used by

Harding et al. (28) and Grood et al. (29) (Fig. 6.5), in which they simulated leg extension. These investigations showed a correlation between early flexion and ACL function. When the ACL was sectioned, there was a greater amount of motion.

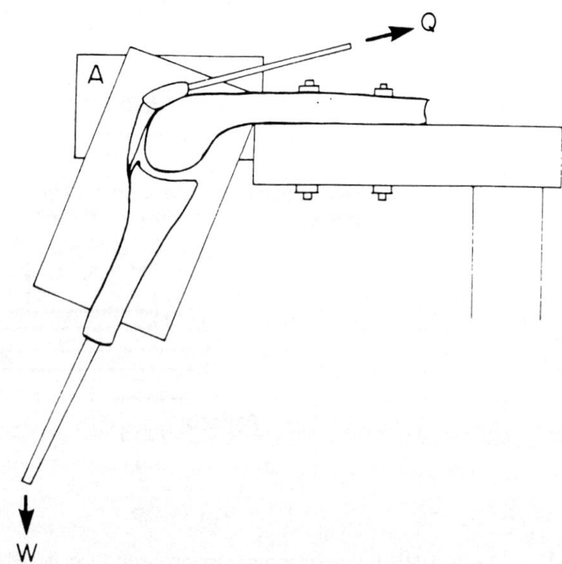

FIGURE 6.5. The testing apparatus is similar to that used by Grood et al. (29). The femur is clamped to a table and a weight *(W)* is applied distal to the joint. The knee is held in equilibrium by a force *(Q)* applied to the end of the quadriceps tendon.

Perry et al. (10) evaluated the stabilizing role of the extensor mechanism by simulating quadriceps function in an *in vitro* testing system, using a tensile load transducer in the quadriceps tendon and a compressive force transducer under the tibial plateau. With this system, they were able to demonstrate the stabilizing effect of muscle forces coupled with axial loading. Torzilli et al. (11) reported a 41% decrease in anteroposterior translation of the knee at 30° of flexion when a joint-compressive load of 444 N was combined with an anteroposterior tibial load of 100 N.

The limitation to these *in vitro* systems resulted from overconstraining knee joint motion. Although they were able to obtain results that were later reproduced using less constraining devices, simulation of lifelike loading still could not be reproduced. Bourne et al. (30) and Biden et al. (31) addressed this problem by using a test apparatus that allowed six DOF, the Oxford rig (Fig. 6.6). In a manner similar to the system used by Perry et al. (10), this apparatus simulated knee loading in a semiflexed position and applied a load to the quadriceps tendon through a load cell. One problem with these systems was that the forces applied to the tendons to simulate muscle function were actually greater than in real life to compensate for greater leverage about the knee available to the applied vertical load (24).

Another approach used by other investigators was the direct measurement of the loads on the individual ligaments with the use of buckle transducers (32–35), strain gages affixed near the ligament insertion sites (36–41), radiographic (5) and kinematic linkage approaches (42), and implantable transducers (43,44) (Fig. 6.7). These systems allowed *in situ* measurement of the loads directly on the ligaments.

A six-DOF apparatus using robotic technology was introduced by Rudy et al. (45). This fully automated, computer-controlled robotics system could apply loads and measure knee motion more precisely. Moreover, by combining these robotics-controlled testing apparatus with the *in situ* measuring devices described previously, the ligaments and other capsular structures could be studied selectively to determine with great precision the role that each one plays in knee stability (46) (Fig. 6.8).

Other investigators have used similar testing designs to evaluate reconstruction of the cruciate ligaments in the presence or absence of damage to medial and lateral capsular structures (47–50). Some studies confirmed the role of capsular structures as secondary restraints to anteroposterior stability of the knee and demonstrated *in vitro* that isolated reconstruction of the cruciate ligaments does not restore stability in cases of combined knee ligament injuries.

It has become evident that each ligament and capsular structure in the knee plays a crucial role in normal knee motion and stability. However, their stabilizing function is supported by neighboring structures, and injury to one

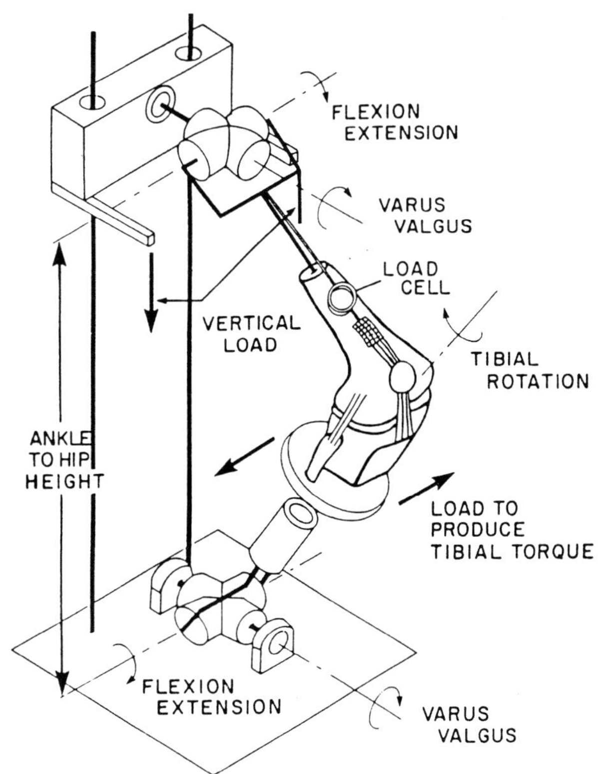

FIGURE 6.6. A: The original Oxford rig. *(Figure continues on next page)*

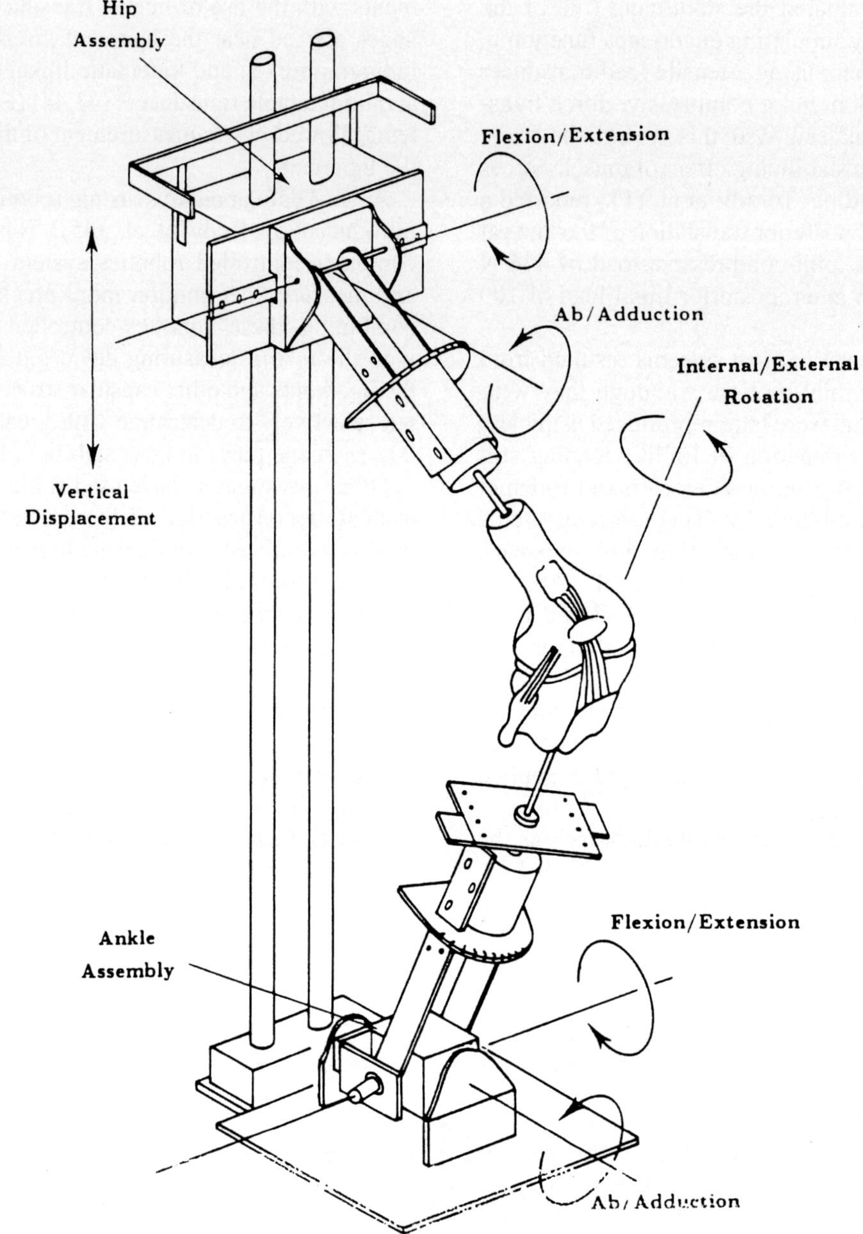

FIGURE 6.6. *Continued.* **B:** The Oxford rig with modification to allow offset of the hip. The Oxford rig allows six degrees of freedom to the knee. The two rotations at the hip and three rotations at the ankle act like a pair of ball-and-socket joints, and the slider allows the height to change as the knee flexes. Simulated muscle action is required for equilibrium except at full extension, in which the load is passed down the tibial axis, producing no flexing or extending moment.

of these structures therefore affects the performance of the others. When addressing an injured knee, the different motions and combinations of them can orient the clinician to the diagnosis, but it must be taken into consideration that the presence of intact secondary restraints and active muscle contraction can obscure the otherwise straightforward identification of the suspected pathology. Moreover, during surgical planning, careful consideration must be given to repairing or reconstructing primary and secondary stabilizers if adequate postoperative perfor-

mance is expected. The evolution of our understanding of knee ligament function is clearly linked to the development of better testing systems that have allowed us to better define the role of each structure in the knee. Advancements in technology have allowed us to replicate the environment and hence have a multiplanar and logical perspective of how the knee moves and functions under different conditions. We have come a long way, but there is even a longer path that we must follow to understand what we once thought of as simple gross anatomy, physi-

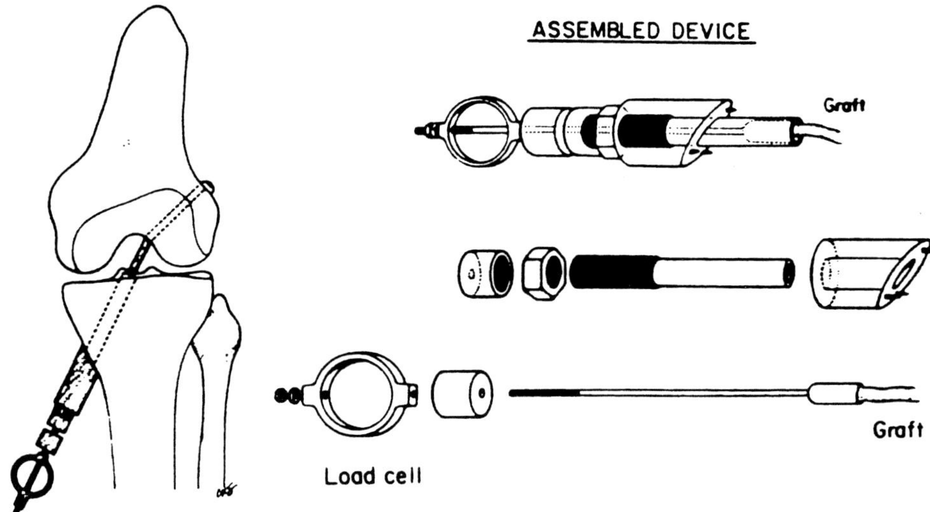

FIGURE 6.7. Schematic drawing of the device used to measure graft tension by Shoemaker et al. (44). The distal bone block of the patellar tendon allograft was cemented to a rod with polymethylmethacrylate (PMMA). The PMMA plug could piston freely in the barrel of the device. Force was measured by a load cell at the distal end of the rod.

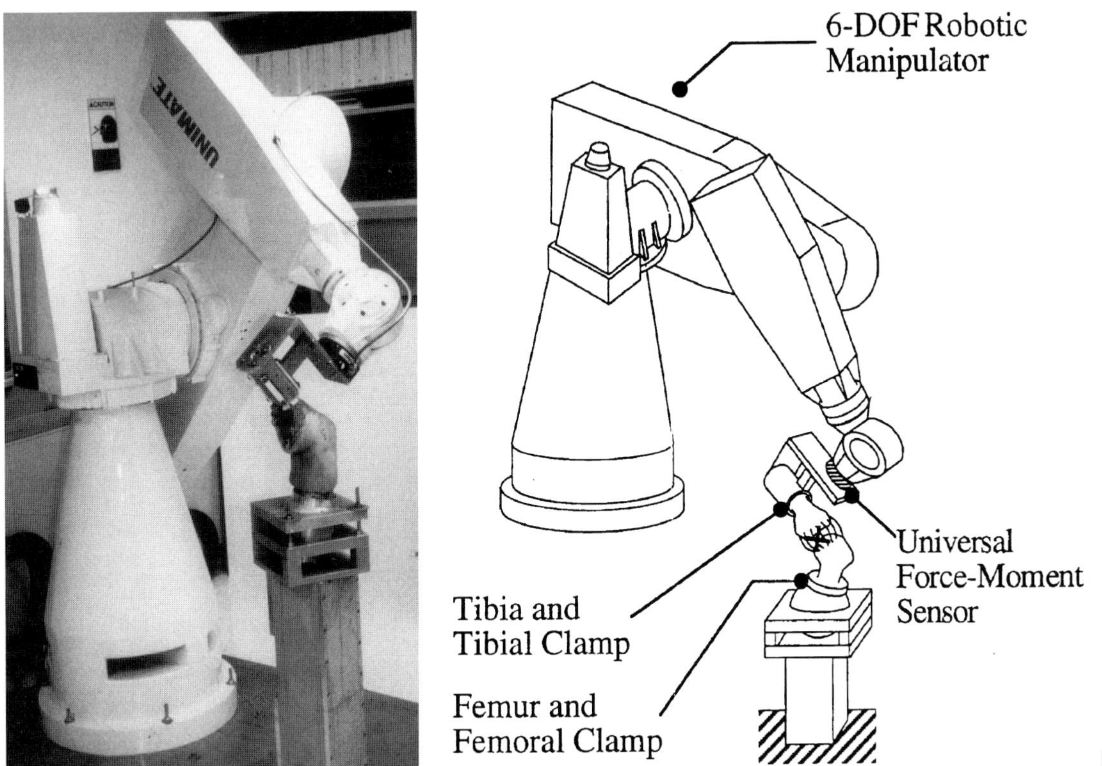

FIGURE 6.8. **A:** The robotic, universal force-moment sensor testing system was used by Fox et al. (46). **B:** The schematic drawing shows the manipulator, universal force-moment sensor, tibial clamp, and femoral clamp. 6-DOF, six degrees of freedom.

ology, and biomechanics. This information will allow us to improve the methods of treatment that we have used to address injuries to the ligaments of the knee.

RESULTS

In this section, we summarize the most relevant results of some selective ligament section studies and highlight their clinical relevance. The concept of ligaments acting as primary and secondary restraints was briefly mentioned earlier. A primary restraint is that structure which accounts for most of the ligamentous force resisting an externally applied force. A secondary restraint provides a smaller contribution. Sectioning a primary restraint typically results in an increase in joint motion. Isolated disruption of a secondary restraint does not result in altering the limits of joint motion, whereas sectioning a secondary restraint in the absence of a primary restraint does alter joint motion. Specific ligaments may be considered in terms of primary and secondary functions. A ligament may function as a primary restraint to motion in one direction and a secondary restraint in another direction. As an illustration, consider the role of the ACL and medial collateral ligament (MCL) in controlling anterior translation. Sectioning the MCL does not result in detectable anterior tibial translation if the primary stabilizer (ACL) is intact. However, if the primary stabilizer has been sectioned, sectioning a secondary restraint, the MCL, results in an increase in anterior translation.

The methods of identifying the primary and secondary stabilizers through selective sectioning of the ligaments were previously discussed. The following section describes the primary and secondary functions of the various structures. The structures are classified as primary, major secondary, or minor secondary restraints.

ANTERIOR CRUCIATE LIGAMENT

Primary function

The ACL has been shown to be the primary structure that limits anterior tibial translation (2,3,6,15,23,48,51,52). The ACL contributes between 80% and 85% of the total resistance to this translation (23,52). With transection of the ACL, a threefold to fourfold increase in laxity has been found (15,48). The ACL is the primary restraint at all angles of knee flexion. Sectioning of this ligament results in greater anterior translation at 30° of flexion than at 90° of flexion (2,3,15,19,23,51–53). Previously, Shoemaker and Daniel reported the testing of ACL-sectioned cadaver knees with the KT-2000 arthrometer (54). They found that sectioning the ACL increased anterior translation from 2.8 mm to 13.0 mm (mean, 6.7 mm) (Fig. 6.9).

Selective cutting studies of the posterolateral and anteromedial bundles of the ACL have found a progressive increase in translation (55,56). These have shown a

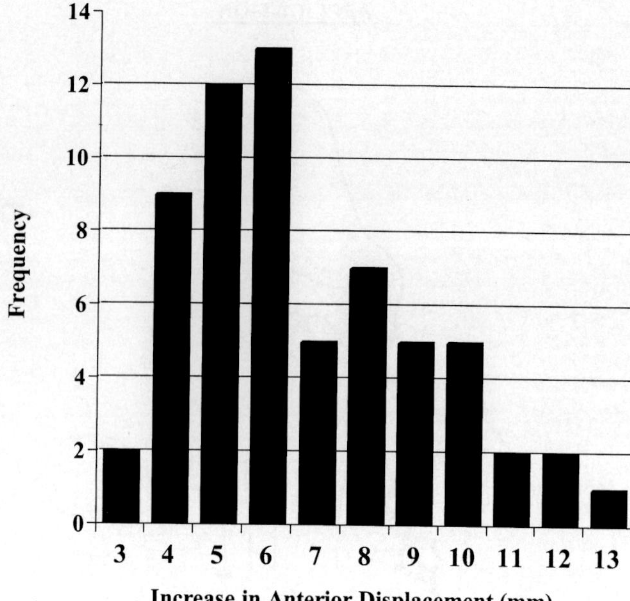

FIGURE 6.9. Effect of anterior cruciate ligament (ACL) section on anterior translation. Anterior translation measurements with the MEDmetric KT-2000 were performed on 65 fresh cadaveric specimens with the ligaments intact and after section of the ACL. The difference between the ligament-intact state and ACL-sectioned state for each specimen is presented (mean, 6.7 ± 2.4 mm [SD]; range, 2.8 to 13.0 mm).

statistically insignificant amount of anterior translation occurs with the sectioning of either bundle. The translation increased with the cutting of at least one half of the other bundle. The amount of translation was not statistically significant until the ACL was completely severed. Hole et al. (55) demonstrated with KT-1000 testing on cadaver knees an average increase of 0.6 mm in translation with severing of the posterolateral bundle. This increased to 3.3 mm with additional cutting of 50% of the anteromedial bundle and an average of 8.0 mm with complete sectioning of both bundles. The nonuniformity of the ACL bundles was demonstrated by Sakane et al. by showing a difference in the distribution of the *in situ* force between the bundles (57). By selectively cutting either bundle, they found the magnitude of force in the posterolateral bundle was more than in the anteromedial bundle in response to anterior tibial loading. This was particularly evident when the knee was near extension. Differences in the direction of the *in situ* force were also present between the bundles at flexion angles from 0° to 60°.

Studies with combined or coupled motion and sectioning of the ACL also have demonstrated the ligament to be the primary restraint to anterior tibial translation (11,15,16,45). Torzilli et al. demonstrated almost a threefold increase in anterior tibial translation with sectioning of the ACL and an externally applied joint compression load combined with a quadriceps force (11). In a model using a six-DOF robotic manipulator, Rudy et al. found that after sectioning the ACL, the anterior translation was 60% greater than when testing with a one-DOF system (45).

Secondary Function

The ACL has a role as a secondary restraint to tibial rotation. Isolated cutting of the ACL has revealed small increases of tibial axial rotation (3° to 4°) with the knee at full extension (2,53). Other studies have demonstrated no or only very small increases of tibial rotation with isolated ACL sectioning (4,20). With combined MCL-ACL sectioning, increases in tibial rotation occurred that were larger than changes from the cutting of these structures individually. This result has also been found for combined posterolateral ligaments and ACL sectioning (22).

From the data available (2,8,22,53,58–60), the ACL appears to function as a major secondary restraint to internal rotation and as a minor secondary restraint to external rotation. The relative contribution of the ACL in restraining rotation is greater in full extension than it is in early (20° to 30°) flexion.

The ACL has some role as a minor secondary restraint to varus-valgus rotation when the knee is in full extension (2,53,61). No significant changes have been observed at 30° to 90° of flexion and isolated sectioning of the ACL (2,53). Markolf et al. identified changes in varus-valgus rotation after combined sectioning of the MCL and ACL that were similar to those of isolated MCL transection (2). Haimes et al. (53), however, had differing results. They observed that a combined MCL plus ACL transection caused a further increase in abduction (i.e., valgus rotation). Combined section of the lateral collateral ligament (LCL) or other posterolateral ligaments and the ACL has been found to cause larger changes than those after isolated LCL transections or posterolateral transections, or both (2,22). Markolf et al. (38), using a load transducer on the ACL in a knee with the posterolateral structures sectioned, found increases in the force on the ACL that was produced with a varus stress. The findings suggest that the ACL provides a small amount of secondary restraint to valgus and varus rotation beyond that from the primary stabilizers of the MCL and LCL (2,38,53,59,61,62).

Clinical Relevance

Findings on clinical examination that best correlate with the sectioning studies of the ACL are demonstrated by the increased anterior tibial translation in a patient with a complete tear of the ACL. Numerous studies have shown this to be most evident at 30° of flexion; this correlates with the position of the Lachman test (2,3,15,19, 23,51–53). Isolated sectioning of the ACL results in decreased anterior stiffness, which is also evident on examination as a soft end point (Fig. 6.10).

Data on sectioning of the anteromedial or posterolateral bundles suggest that isolated rupture of either bundle should not produce significant increased translation on examination (55,56). If there is a clinically detectable increase in translation, functional disruption (i.e., rupture, lengthening) of the remaining bundle has occurred. The authors of the data indicate that, for laxity to be detected, at least 75% of the ACL must be nonfunctional. What is thought to be a partial tear of the ACL as demonstrated by increased translation is in essence almost a complete tear (55,56).

The ACL may also have a role in aligning the knee during the gait cycle, as suggested from the work by Torzilli et al. (11). The ACL was shown to have a significant con-

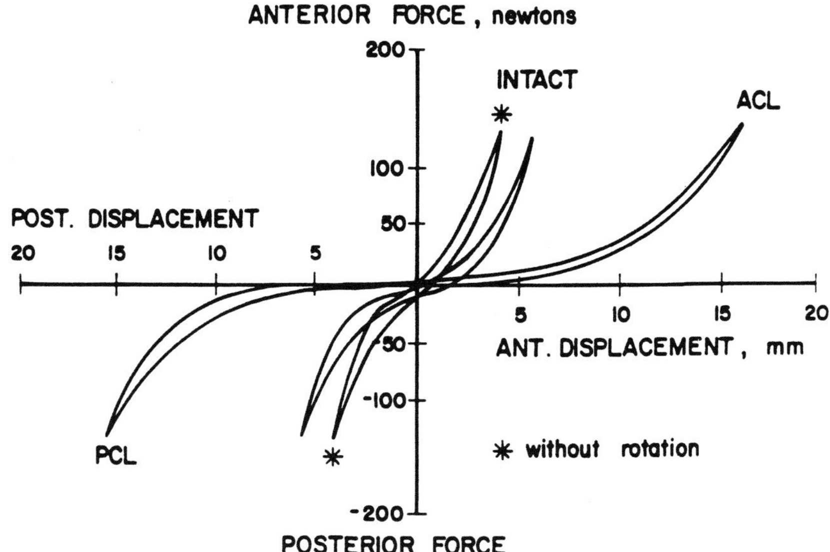

FIGURE 6.10. A typical dynamic recording of anterior–posterior displacement with the knee at 30° of flexion. The displacement increased 30% when the tibia was allowed to rotate freely. Isolated section of the anterior cruciate ligament (ACL) or the posterior cruciate ligament (PCL) produced substantial increases in the measured displacement.

TABLE 6.1. *Primary and secondary restraints to limits of knee motion based on quantitative* in vitro *studies of the anterior cruciate ligament*

Knee motion	Anterior cruciate ligament
Anterior displacement	Primary
Posterior displacement	0
Varus	Minor secondary (full extension)
Valgus	Minor secondary (full extension)
	Major secondary (30° of flexion)
Internal rotation	Major secondary
External rotation	Minor secondary

tribution in restricting coupled anterior translation resulting from a joint-compressive load and a quadriceps force. The investigators state that this may be one component responsible for aligning the tibial plateau surfaces with the femoral condyles during the swing phase and just before heel strike. This would assist in the normal kinematic motion that occurs between the joint surfaces.

The role of the ACL as a secondary restraint may occur in combined injuries of the MCL and ACL. In a biomechanical study using dog knees, Woo et al. (63) found the healing of a transected MCL to be adversely affected when the ACL is concomitantly transected. Their results were consistent with clinical studies in which increased valgus rotation was detected after the conservative management of a combined MCL and ACL injury (64,65) (Table 6.1).

POSTERIOR CRUCIATE LIGAMENT

Primary Function

The PCL is the primary restraint to posterior translation of the tibia. In contrast to the ACL, there is a greater amount of translation at 90° of flexion compared with 30° of flexion (2,3,20,62). The PCL provides approximately 95% of restraint to posterior translation at 90° of flexion (23).The amount of posterior translation in a knee that has undergone transection of the PCL has been shown to be almost three times that of a knee with an intact PCL (15,20). Significantly elevated patellofemoral and medial compartment pressures have been measured after section of the PCL in cadaver knees (66).

In selective cutting of the two bundles of the PCL, Race and Amis found the secondary structures (i.e., arcuate ligament and LCL) to be the primary restraints to posterior translation at extension and the lower angles of knee flexion (67). Their results demonstrated that the anterolateral bundle of the PCL contributed most (50% to 74%) of the primary restraint to posterior translation in the middle range of flexion (40° to 120°). The posteromedial bundle of the PCL contributed more of the primary restraint with further flexion, 57% of the total at 130° knee flexion.

Secondary Function

The PCL acts as a major secondary restraint to external tibial rotation. This is particularly true at 90° of flexion with less of a role as the knee is near full extension (2,3,20,22,62,68). The PCL does not appear to have a role in limiting internal rotation (22). Isolated PCL transection has no effect on external rotation limits (20,68). However, PCL sectioning performed after cutting of the LCL and other posterolateral structures (e.g., popliteus) results in increased primary external rotation (20,22,62, 68). Veltri et al. found that the combined section of the PCL and posterolateral structures resulted in an increase in external rotation at all flexion angles compared with isolated section of the posterolateral structures (22). The greatest increase in external rotation was found at 45° of knee flexion. Gollehon et al. did not find changes with isolated PCL section, but they did report an increase in external rotation with transection of the PCL, LCL, and deep posterior capsule (20). This occurred when the knee was flexed more than 30°. Similar findings were demonstrated by Grood et al. (62) after cutting of the PCL and deep posterior lateral structures. The largest increase in external rotation was seen at 90° of knee flexion, and there were minimal changes evident at 0° and 15° of flexion. These studies differ somewhat, but there is agreement that the PCL functions with some minor secondary restraint to external rotation with the knee extended and with a major secondary restraint to external rotation at 90° of flexion. In addition to an increased amount of external tibial rotation with combined section, Kaneda et al. found that the axis of external tibial rotation changes after isolated section of the PCL (68). There is loss of the posterior tibial translation–external rotation couple. This occurs because the PCL presumably serves as an axis around which the tibia rotates in addition to limiting posterior translation.

Isolated section of the PCL essentially does not affect varus or valgus angulation (2,20,62). However, as Gollehon et al. and others have found, when the LCL and other posterolateral structures are cut, followed by cutting of the PCL, there is an increase in varus rotation (20,22,62). The increases are small at 0° and much larger in flexion near 90°. No increases in valgus rotation has been shown with combined section of the PCL and posterolateral structures. Seering et al. (59) observed a secondary contribution of the PCL to valgus rotation at full extension, more so than the contribution from the ACL. From the results of these studies, it is apparent that the PCL has a role as a minor secondary restraint to varus and valgus rotation.

Clinical Relevance

Physical examination of the knee with a ruptured PCL reveals the greatest increase in posterior translation at

TABLE 6.2. *Primary and secondary restraints to limits of knee motion based on quantitative* in vitro *studies of the posterior cruciate ligament*

Knee motion	Posterior cruciate ligament
Anterior displacement	0
Posterior displacement	Primary
Varus	Minor secondary (full extension)
	Major secondary (30° of flexion)
Valgus	Minor secondary (full extension)
	Major secondary (30° of flexion)
Internal rotation	0
External rotation	Major secondary (90°)
	Minor secondary (full extension)

90°. This is also the position found in the *in vitro* studies to have the greatest increase in translation. This may be caused by the slackening of the medial and lateral extraarticular secondary restraints that occurs with flexion (62). The most sensitive position to clinically detect a rupture of the PCL is flexion at 90° so that these secondary restraints are ineffective in preventing posterior translation of the tibia. This condition should be tested with the tibia in a neutral position to eliminate any coupled motion. With the PCL disruption, there is also decreased posterior stiffness that is evident as a soft end point. An isolated rupture of the PCL does not affect varus laxity or external rotation of the tibia on examination.

The results from studies on the section of the two bundles of the PCL may have clinical implications in the way reconstruction is approached. Race and Amis suggest that for activities in which full flexion is not usually attained, such as walking and running, the anterolateral bundle is the only one that needs to be reconstructed if surgery is indicated (67). However, for activities that require stability in full flexion (e.g., snow boarding), the posteromedial bundle is important as well and a two-bundle PCL reconstruction may be necessary. Many orthopedists may not agree with this assessment, because it has been thought that the posteromedial bundle tightens in extension. Although it has been thought that the anterolateral bundle is tight in flexion and responsible for stability in flexion, few studies have examined this, and only Race and Amis have findings based on selectively cutting the individual bundles. Further work is necessary on the role of the individual bundles (Table 6.2).

MEDIAL STRUCTURES

The medial structures of the knee can be separated into various types of structures. However, for the purpose of this chapter, they are divided into the superficial MCL and the deep medial capsule. The deep medial capsule can be further divided into thirds: the anterior, middle, and posterior aspects. The deep MCL is considered the mid-medial capsule, and the posterior medial corner is the posteromedial capsule. There has been some difficulty in interpreting studies in which the investigators have not used this terminology when assigning their sectioning protocols. Terminology from any studies that depart from these protocols needs to be clarified.

Primary Function

The medial structures, particularly the superficial MCL, act as the primary restraint to limit valgus forces applied at the knee (2,59,61,69). Grood et al. found that the superficial MCL provided 78% of the restraint at 25° of knee flexion compared with 57% at 5° of flexion (61). This may suggest the MCL is more active as a restraint as the knee is flexed. They also found that at 5° of flexion the posteromedial capsule was the most effective secondary restraint. The capsule becomes more relaxed with knee flexion and has a decreased contribution as a secondary restraint. Another study by Haimes et al. found that the posteromedial capsule and posterior oblique ligament acted as secondary restraints in knee extension (53). Seering et al. found a greater contribution of the superficial MCL to restraint of valgus rotation with flexion to 30° (59). Sectioning of the deep MCL resulted only in small increases in valgus rotation.

The medial structures act as primary restraints to internal and external tibial rotation (2,53,59,69–71). Sectioning of the superficial MCL increases the external rotation of the tibia, with the largest increases occurring in the flexed knee (53,69,70). Increased internal rotation has also been observed with section of the superficial MCL (2,59,71). The posteromedial capsule and posterior oblique ligament are important secondary restraints to external tibial rotation, as demonstrated by the increase in external rotation after section of these structures in an MCL-deficient knee (53,69). It is difficult to define the contribution of each medial structure in limiting motion (e.g., rotation) because of differences in the studies in terms of order of section and the angle of flexion the knees were tested in. However, from the information available, it appears that the superficial MCL functions from full extension to full flexion, with a greater contribution at 30° than 0°. The posteromedial capsule has a greater role as the knee approaches extension. The mid-medial capsule acts to limit internal tibial rotation.

Secondary Function

The medial structures act as major secondary restraints to anterior and posterior tibial translation. Several studies have reported no change in anterior or posterior tibial translation when the medial structures were sectioned first (19,53,71). However, when the medial structures were cut after section of the ACL, there was increased translation compared with that of ACL section alone

(19,53). The ability of the MCL to resist anteriorly directed force becomes greater as the knee is flexed (70). Ritchie et al. found the superficial MCL to be the structure responsible for decreased posterior tibial translation in the PCL-sectioned knee (71).

The secondary restraint role of the posteromedial capsule and posterior oblique ligament to external rotation and valgus rotation was mentioned earlier. Valgus rotation increased significantly in the ACL- and MCL-sectioned knee that subsequently underwent posteromedial capsule and posterior oblique transection (53).

Changes in coupled motion occur with ACL- and MCL-transected knees during anterior loading. Haimes et al. found there is no coupled internal rotation in these knees, which contrasted with the coupled internal rotation evident in intact knees and isolated ACL-sectioned knees (53). Fukubayashi et al., however, found coupled internal rotation eliminated in knees with isolated ACL sectioning (15).

Clinical Relevance

Physical examination of the medial structures begins with the superficial MCL, because it contributes most of the restraint to valgus rotation. This is evident particularly at 25° to 30° of knee flexion, whereas in extension, the superficial MCL still has a significant role, but there are other structures that have larger roles as secondary restraints (e.g., posteromedial capsule, PCL). Injury to the superficial MCL is best detected during examination of the knee with application of a valgus stress at 30°. In this position, the superficial MCL has its greatest restraint when the posteromedial capsule and PCL relax. The deep MCL also contributes to valgus rotational testing at 0° and 30°. Valgus loading of the knee with an MCL injury produces 5 to 7 mm of opening medially. This opening is even greater with injury to the secondary restraints. Valgus rotational testing of the knee at full extension is not grossly positive until the secondary restraints, the posteromedial capsule, PCL, and the ACL, are all torn.

Sectioning of the deep MCL only results in small increases in valgus rotation. However, an isolated injury to the deep MCL without an injury to the superficial MCL is unlikely because of the restraint the superficial MCL provides to valgus rotation from full extension to 90°. It is theoretically possible to disrupt the deep MCL without injuring the superficial MCL if the mechanism of injury involves pathologic anterior tibial translation (i.e., concomitant ACL tear). The combination of ACL and deep MCL disruptions would increase the anterior translation limit and be detectable on clinical examination by small changes in valgus stress and internal rotation.

Anterior translation is increased and evident clinically with a combined ACL and superficial MCL injury, as opposed to an isolated ACL tear. This is evident (at 30° and 90°) while doing a Lachman test or an anterior drawer test (53). The anterior drawer test performed with the tibia in external rotation is positive only with a significant medial ligament injury. A patient with a positive anterior drawer result in external rotation may have an intact ACL in view of torn medial structures. Changes in coupled internal rotation are seen in the ACL- or MCL-transected knee. It may be that the restraint to anterior tibial translation provided by the MCL in an intact knee or ACL-deficient knee is more important than previously realized (53).

Combined MCL, posterior oblique ligament, and posteromedial capsule injuries led to findings on examination of large increases in external rotation (best tested at 30° of flexion), internal rotation (especially at 15° of flexion), and valgus rotation (53).

The forces in the ACL increase after disruption of the medial structures. Shapiro et al. demonstrated increased loads in the ACL after section of the MCL (70). This can be important clinically in a patient with an MCL injury and an ACL injury or reconstruction.

When performing a posterior drawer test with internal rotation of the tibia, there is decreased translation in a knee with an intact superficial MCL. The superficial MCL is responsible for the restraint to a posterior drawer performed with the tibia internally rotated compared with a drawer test done in neutral rotation (71) (Table 6.3).

TABLE 6.3. *Primary and secondary restraints to limits of knee motion based on quantitative* in vitro *studies of medial structures*

	Medial structures				
Knee motion	Superficial medial cruciate ligament	Anterior medial capsule	Deep medial cruciate ligament	Posterior medial capsule	Posterior oblique ligament
Anterior displacement	Minor secondary	0	Major secondary	?	?
Posterior displacement	Minor secondary	0	0	0	0
Varus	0	0	0	0	0
Valgus	Primary (full ext. to 90°)	?	Primary (0° to 30°)	Major secondary	Major secondary
Internal rotation	Primary (full ext. to 90°)	?	Primary (0° to 30°)	?	?
External rotation	Primary	?	0	Major secondary	Major secondary

LATERAL STRUCTURES

Similar to the structures on the medial side, the lateral side involves numerous structures that restrain movement. Varus rotation and external tibial rotation are the primary motions restrained by the lateral structures. The role of some of the lateral restraints, such as the popliteus and iliotibial band, are difficult to assess with *in vitro* experiments because they function as dynamic and static stabilizers. The relative contributions of the popliteus have been somewhat defined, but those of the iliotibial band have not been adequately determined. Overall, the lateral structures (i.e., LCL, deep posterior lateral capsule or arcuate ligament, and popliteus tendon) function as a complex. With the exception of the LCL, there is no one structure responsible for most of the restraining force in preventing varus rotation, although the popliteus plays a considerable role.

Primary Function

Several studies have found that the LCL acts as the primary restraint to limit varus rotation (2,3,20,21,61,62). There are, however, some discrepancies in regard to the percentage of restraint provided at different angles of knee flexion. Several studies have reported a small but significant increase in varus rotation (1° to 4°) at all angles of knee flexion (20,21). Markolf et al. found that section of the LCL increased varus rotation 103% at full extension and 30% at 20° and 45° of flexion (2). However, Grood et al. (62) found a relatively constant increase in the amount of varus rotation from 0° to 90° of knee flexion after LCL section. According to these same studies, varus rotation was not significantly altered unless the LCL was cut (2,62). In addition to an increase in varus rotation with section of the LCL, Gollehon et al. reported a small but significant increase at 90° of knee flexion after isolated section of the deep posterior lateral structures composed of the posterior lateral capsule or arcuate ligament and the popliteus tendon (20). They also found a significant increase (5° to 9°) with combined sectioning of these structures and an even greater varus rotation (14° to 19°) with additional section of the PCL (Fig. 6.11). With section of the ACL and LCL, Wroble et al. reported a small (4°) but significant increase in varus rotation occurring maximally at 30° of knee flexion (72).

A consensus finding of these studies was that combined section of the LCL and the deep posterolateral structures led to an increase in varus rotation that was larger than the sum of the increases after individual sectioning. It is evident from these studies that the LCL is the primary restraint to limit a varus rotation but that the posterolateral structures provide considerable restraints as secondary stabilizers.

The lateral structures also play a role as the primary restraints in limiting external rotation of the tibia

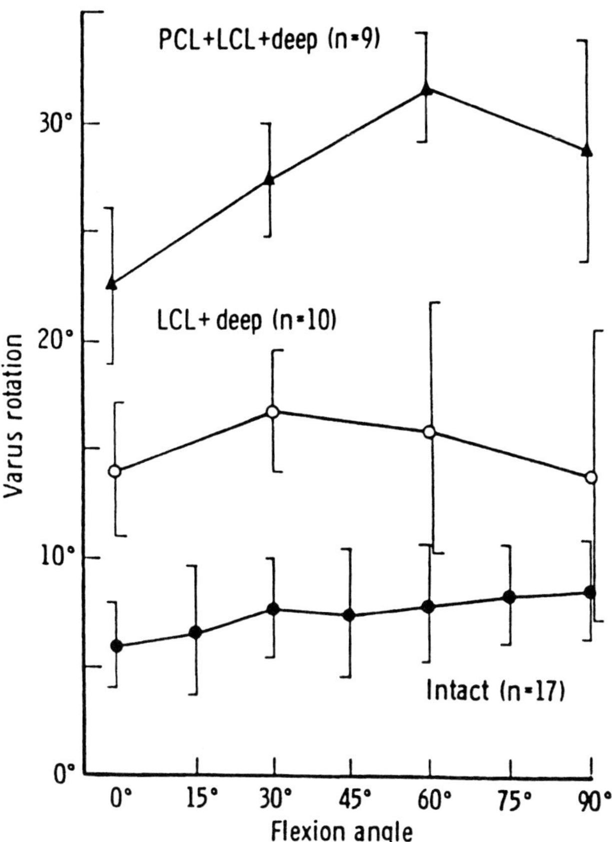

FIGURE 6.11. Primary varus rotations resulting from 10 Nm varus and valgus torque in intact knees and after sectioning. Significant increases in varus rotation were found with combined section of the lateral collateral ligament (LCL) and deep structures and with combined section of the lateral collateral ligament, deep structures, and posterior cruciate ligament (PCL).

(2,20,38,62,68,72,73). Increases in external rotation at all flexion angles have been seen after combined section of the LCL and posterolateral structures (20,38). Markolf et al. found increases in the force in the PCL between 45° and 90° of knee flexion after section of the posterolateral structures (38). Gollehon et al. observed that, when the LCL was left intact and the remaining posterolateral structures were sectioned, the only increase in external rotation was observed at 90° of knee flexion (20). This increase was attributed to the contributions of the popliteus tendon, but the structure was not cut separately to confirm this. Grood et al. observed increases in external rotation after cutting the posterolateral structures. The largest increase was at 30° of knee flexion, which was two times the external rotation at 90° (62). After section of the ACL, Wroble et al. found that cutting the posterolateral structures resulted in small increases in external rotation, but further section of the LCL resulted in a large increase that was evident at all knee flexion angles (72).

A common finding in the previously described studies was that the changes in external rotation limits were small after individual structures were cut, yet the limits increased after combined section of the LCL and other lateral structures, with these numbers exceeding the sum of the component changes. It may be that no individual structure has a role as the primary restraint to external rotation, but that the structures that comprise the posterior lateral corner (i.e., LCL, arcuate ligament, posterior lateral capsule, and popliteus tendon) function in unity to limit external rotation.

Secondary Function

The lateral structures act as secondary restraints to limit anterior and posterior translation. Isolated section of the lateral structures has a minor effect on anterior translation (21,22,72). Section of the ACL and the lateral structures results in increased anterior translation, especially at 30° (21,22). The changes seen with cutting of the lateral structures are small; they act by themselves or in combination to provide minor secondary restraints to anterior translation. The lateral structures have more of a role as a secondary restraint in limiting posterior translation. Some investigators have shown that isolated section of the lateral structures results in increases in posterior translation (21,22). Veltri et al. demonstrated these findings in addition to large increases with additional PCL section and smaller increases with section of the ACL (22). Markolf et al. found that the mean force in the PCL was not affected by sectioning the lateral structures (38).

Gollehon et al. and Grood et al. also demonstrated a role for the lateral structures, but with slightly different findings from those cited earlier (20,62). Gollehon et al. found that isolated cutting of the LCL or posterolateral structures did not change the amount of posterior translation. However, in combination, there were small (3-mm) increases. The changes in posterior translation at 0° and 30° of flexion after combined section of the LCL and posterolateral structures were comparable to increases seen after the PCL was cut. The findings by Grood et al. were similar.

The popliteus plays an important role as a secondary restraint to posterior tibial translation. In PCL-sectioned knees, Harner et al. applied a posterior tibial force and found that adding a 44-N force to the popliteus in a PCL-deficient knee led to a 36% reduction in translation (74). Veltri et al. found increased posterior translation after cutting the popliteus following section of the LCL (21). They also found an increase in translation after section of the popliteofibular ligament. Their results demonstrated maximal posterior translation at 30° after complete posterolateral section. Noyes et al. also found maximal posterior translation at 30° knee flexion after isolated section of the posterolateral structures (75). Other studies have demonstrated the role of the popliteal tendon as a static restraint (2,62,76).

Overall, when the LCL and posterolateral structures are considered individually, they act as minor secondary restraints to posterior translation at full extension. When combined, however, the lateral structures serve as a major secondary restraint from full extension to 30° of knee flexion.

The lateral structures may have a role in the restraint of internal tibial rotation. Section of the anterolateral structures (i.e., iliotibial band and midlateral capsule) and LCL resulted in a significant increase in internal rotation in the flexed knee, greater at 90° than 30° (72). Further increases were found with additional section of the posterolateral structures. Gollehon et al. demonstrated a significant increase in internal rotation only after sectioning of the posterolateral structures in addition to the ACL (20). Lipke et al. similarly found an increase in internal rotation after section of the ACL and posterolateral structures (77). Wascher et al. found small yet significant increases (2.5° to 8°) in internal tibial rotation with complete LCL and posterolateral structure section (76). Small increases in internal rotation were also seen at 60° and 90° knee flexion in a study by Markolf et al. (38).

Clinical Relevance

Disruption of the LCL may result in only a small increase of varus rotation (1° to 4°) and may be difficult to detect clinically, whereas a combined injury to the LCL and posterolateral structures results in large changes (21). Several studies have found that the ideal position to test for an LCL injury is at 30° (21,22,72). With a PCL injury, there is typically significant varus rotation (>10°) that is detected on clinical examination with the knee in full extension. With an isolated LCL injury, there may be a slight varus rotation (<5°) at full extension, but greater degrees of rotation are associated with combination injuries involving the LCL and the posterolateral structures. Data indicate the best position to clinically detect a combined injury of the lateral structures is with the knee at 30° to 45° of flexion (21,22). This is the position in which the greatest increase in primary varus and external tibial rotation and coupled external tibial rotation were seen with combined section. The investigators suggest that if, on physical examination, there is an increase in primary varus and external tibial rotation and coupled external tibial rotation at 30° of knee flexion, but not at 90° of knee flexion, there is a high probability of combined injury to the LCL and posterolateral structures. The same investigators found that combined section of the ACL and posterolateral corner resulted in increases in primary anterior and posterior translation, especially at 30° of knee flexion. They also found an increase in coupled external tibial rotation and primary varus plus internal tibial rotation. Primary external tibial rotation did not differ from intact knees. It was suggested that this con-

TABLE 6.4. *Primary and secondary restraints to limits of knee motion based on quantitative* in vitro *studies of lateral structures*

	Lateral structures		
Knee motion	Lateral cruciate ligament	Deep posterior lateral capsule	Popliteus tendon
Anterior displacement	Minor secondary	Minor secondary	Minor secondary
Posterior displacement[a]	Minor secondary (full ext.)	Minor secondary	Minor secondary
Varus	Primary	Major secondary	Major secondary
Valgus	0	0	0
Internal rotation	Minor secondary	Minor secondary	Minor secondary
External rotation (lateral structures act as complex)	Primary (full ext. to 90°)	Primary (full ext. to 45°)	Primary (90°)

[a]When combined, the lateral structures act as primary restraints to posterior displacement.

tributed to the failure to recognize "posterolateral instability" (i.e., deficiency of the posterolateral structures) in the ACL-ruptured knee with the standard external tibial rotation test performed at 30° of knee flexion. When there is significant posterolateral instability at 90° of knee flexion, a combined injury to the PCL and posterolateral structures is more likely (68).

As reported by Veltri et al., the popliteofibular ligament and the popliteal tendon attachment to the tibia are equal in importance to posterolateral stability of the knee (21). They suggest reconstruction of the LCL and the popliteofibular ligament can suffice in limiting posterior translation, varus rotation, and external tibial rotation. Harner et al. also suggest that restoration of the popliteus muscle function is important when an injury occurs to the popliteus complex (74). They cite its role as an important dynamic stabilizer that helps protect an intact PCL or helps stabilize the knee in the case of a PCL rupture (Table 6.4).

REFERENCES

1. Brantigan OC, Voshell AF. The mechanics of the ligaments and menisci of the knee joint. *J Bone Joint Surg Am* 1941;23:44–66.
2. Markolf KL, Mensch JS, Amstutz HC. Stiffness and laxity of the knee—the contributions of the supporting structures. A quantitative in vitro study. *J Bone Joint Surg Am* 1976;58:583–594.
3. Piziali RL, Seering WP, Nagel DA, Schurman DJ. The function of the primary ligaments of the knee in anterior-posterior and medial-lateral motions. *J Biomech* 1980;13:777–784.
4. Nielsen S, Kromann-Andersen C, Rasmussen O, et al. Instability of cadaver knees after transection of capsule and ligaments. *Acta Orthop Scand* 1984;55:30–44.
5. Wang CJ, Walker PS. Rotatory laxity of the human knee joint. *J Bone Joint Surg Am* 1974;56:161–170.
6. Hsieh HH, Walker PS. Stabilizing mechanisms of the loaded and unloaded knee joint. *J Bone Joint Surg Am* 1976;58:87–93.
7. Hsieh HH, Walker PS. The effect of compressive load of the stability of the knee joint [Proceedings]. *Bull Hosp Joint Dis* 1977;38:10–14.
8. Markolf KL, Bargar WL, Shoemaker SC, Amstutz HC. The role of joint load in knee stability. *J Bone Joint Surg Am* 1981;63:570–585.
9. Shoemaker SC, Markolf KL. The role of the meniscus in the anterior-posterior stability of the loaded anterior cruciate-deficient knee. Effects of partial versus total excision. *J Bone Joint Surg Am* 1986;68:71–79.
10. Perry J, Antonelli D, Ford W. Analysis of knee-joint forces during flexed-knee stance. *J Bone Joint Surg Am* 1975;57:961–967.
11. Torzilli PA, Deng X, Warren RF. The effect of joint-compressive load and quadriceps muscle force on knee motion in the intact and anterior cruciate ligament-sectioned knee. *Am J Sports Med* 1994;22:105–112.
12. Kinzel GL, Hillberry BM, Hall AS Jr, et al. Measurement of the total motion between two body segments. II. Description of application. *J Biomech* 1972;5:283–293.
13. Kinzel GL, Hall AS Jr, Hillberry BM. Measurement of the total motion between two body segments. I. Analytical development. *J Biomech* 1972;5:93–105.
14. Suntay WJ, Grood ES, Hefzy MS, et al. Error analysis of a system for measuring three-dimensional joint motion. *J Biomech Eng* 1983;105:127–135.
15. Fukubayashi T, Torzilli PA, Sherman MF, et al. An in vitro biomechanical evaluation of anterior-posterior motion of the knee. Tibial displacement, rotation, and torque. *J Bone Joint Surg Am* 1982;64:258–264.
16. Levy IM, Torzilli PA, Warren RF. The effect of medial meniscectomy on anterior-posterior motion of the knee. *J Bone Joint Surg Am* 1982;64:883–888.
17. Bargar WL, Moreland JR, Markolf KL, et al. In vivo stability testing of post-meniscectomy knees. *Clin Orthop* 1980:247–252.
18. Levy IM, Torzilli PA, Gould JD, et al. The effect of lateral meniscectomy on motion of the knee. *J Bone Joint Surg Am* 1989;71:401–406.
19. Sullivan D, Levy IM, Sheskier S, et al. Medial restrains to anterior-posterior motion of the knee. *J Bone Joint Surg Am* 1984;66:930–936.
20. Gollehon DL, Torzilli PA, Warren RF. The role of the posterolateral and cruciate ligaments in the stability of the human knee. A biomechanical study. *J Bone Joint Surg Am* 1987;69:233–242.
21. Veltri DM, Deng XH, Torzilli PA, et al. The role of the popliteofibular ligament in stability of the human knee. A biomechanical study. *Am J Sports Med* 1996;24:19–27.
22. Veltri DM, Deng XH, Torzilli PA, et al. The role of the cruciate and posterolateral ligaments in stability of the knee. A biomechanical study. *Am J Sports Med* 1995;23:436–443.
23. Butler DL, Noyes FR, Grood ES. Ligamentous restraints to anterior-posterior drawer in the human knee. A biomechanical study. *J Bone Joint Surg Am* 1980;62:259–270.
24. Biden E, O'Connor J. Experimental methods used to evaluate knee ligament function. In: Daniel DM, Akeson WH, O'Connor JJ, eds. *Knee ligaments: structure, function, injury and repair,* 1st ed. New York: Raven Press, 1990:135–151.
25. Markolf KL, Graff-Radford A, Amstutz HC. In vivo knee stability. A quantitative assessment using an instrumented clinical testing apparatus. *J Bone Joint Surg Am* 1978;60:664–674.
26. Jurist KA, Otis JC. Anteroposterior tibiofemoral displacements during isometric extension efforts. The roles of external load and knee flexion angle. *Am J Sports Med* 1985;13:254–258.
27. Daniel DM, Stone ML, Barnett P, et al. Use of the quadriceps active test to diagnose posterior cruciate-ligament disruption and measure posterior laxity of the knee. *J Bone Joint Surg Am* 1988;70:386–391.
28. Harding ML, Harding L, Goodfellow JW. A preliminary report of a simple rig to aid study of the functional anatomy of the cadaver human knee joint. *J Biomech* 1977;10:517–523.
29. Grood ES, Suntay WJ, Noyes FR, et al. Biomechanics of the knee-extension exercise. Effect of cutting the anterior cruciate ligament. *J Bone Joint Surg Am* 1984;66:725–734.

30. Bourne R, Goodfellow JW, O'Connor JJ. A functional analysis of various knee arthroplasties. In: Orthopaedic Research Society Annual Meeting, Anaheim, 1978:160.
31. Biden E, O'Connor JJ, Goodfellow JW. Tibial rotation in the cadaver knee. In: Society OR, ed. Orthopaedic Research Society Annual Meeting, Atlanta, 1984:30.
32. Lew WD, Lewis JL. The effect of knee-prosthesis geometry on cruciate ligament mechanics during flexion. *J Bone Joint Surg Am* 1982;64:734–739.
33. Lewis JL, Lew WD, Schmidt J. A note on the application and evaluation of the buckle transducer for the knee ligament force measurement. *J Biomech Eng* 1982;104:125–128.
34. Ahmed AM, Burke DL, Duncan NA, et al. Ligament tension pattern in the flexed knee in combined passive anterior translation and axial rotation. *J Orthop Res* 1992;10:854–867.
35. Lewis JL, Lew WD, Hill JA, Hanley P, et al. Knee joint motion and ligament forces before and after ACL reconstruction. *J Biomech Eng* 1989;111:97–106.
36. Arms S, Boyle J, Johnson R, et al. Strain measurement in the medial collateral ligament of the human knee: an autopsy study. *J Biomech* 1983;16:491–496.
37. Markolf KL, Gorek JF, Kabo JM, et al. Direct measurement of resultant forces in the anterior cruciate ligament. An in vitro study performed with a new experimental technique. *J Bone Joint Surg Am* 1990;72:557–567.
38. Markolf KL, Wascher DC, Finerman GA. Direct in vitro measurement of forces in the cruciate ligaments. Part II. The effect of section of the posterolateral structures. *J Bone Joint Surg Am* 1993;75:387–394.
39. Markolf KL, Burchfield DM, Shapiro MM, et al. Combined knee loading states that generate high anterior cruciate ligament forces. *J Orthop Res* 1995;13:930–935.
40. Markolf KL, Willems MJ, Jackson SR, et al. In situ calibration of miniature sensors implanted into the anterior cruciate ligament. Part I. Strain measurements. *J Orthop Res* 1998;16:455–463.
41. Markolf KL, Willems MJ, Jackson SR, et al. In situ calibration of miniature sensors implanted into the anterior cruciate ligament. Part II. Force probe measurements. *J Orthop Res* 1998;16:464–471.
42. Hollis JM, Takai S, Adams DJ, et al. The effects of knee motion and external loading on the length of the anterior cruciate ligament (ACL): a kinematic study. *J Biomech Eng* 1991;113:208–214.
43. Holden JP, Grood ES, Korvick DL, et al. In vivo forces in the anterior cruciate ligament: direct measurements during walking and trotting in a quadruped. *J Biomech* 1994;27:517–526.
44. Shoemaker SC, Adams D, Daniel DM, et al. Quadriceps/anterior cruciate graft interaction. An in vitro study of joint kinematics and anterior cruciate ligament graft tension. *Clin Orthop* 1993;294:379–390.
45. Rudy TW, Livesay GA, Woo SL, et al. A combined robotic/universal force sensor approach to determine in situ forces of knee ligaments. *J Biomech* 1996;29:1357–1360.
46. Fox RJ, Harner CD, Sakane M, et al. Determination of the in situ forces in the human posterior cruciate ligament using robotic technology. A cadaveric study. *Am J Sports Med* 1998;26:395–401.
47. Draganich LF, Vahey JW. An in vitro study of anterior cruciate ligament strain induced by quadriceps and hamstrings forces. *J Orthop Res* 1990;8:57–63.
48. Samuelson M, Draganich LF, Zhou X, et al. The effects of knee reconstruction on combined anterior cruciate ligament and anterolateral capsular deficiencies. *Am J Sports Med* 1996;24:492–497.
49. Draganich LF, Reider B, Ling M, et al. An in vitro study of an intraarticular and extraarticular reconstruction in the anterior cruciate ligament deficient knee. *Am J Sports Med* 1990;18:262–266.
50. Pearsall AT, Pyevich M, Draganich LF, et al. In vitro study of knee stability after posterior cruciate ligament reconstruction. *Clin Orthop* 1996:264–271.
51. Piziali RL, Rastegar J, Nagel DA, et al. The contribution of the cruciate ligaments to the load-displacement characteristics of the human knee joint. *J Biomech Eng* 1980;102:277–283.
52. Takai S, Woo SL, Livesay GA, et al. Determination of the in situ loads on the human anterior cruciate ligament. *J Orthop Res* 1993;11:686–695.
53. Haimes JL, Wroble RR, Grood ES, et al. Role of the medial structures in the intact and anterior cruciate ligament-deficient knee. Limits of motion in the human knee. *Am J Sports Med* 1994;22:402–409.
54. Shoemaker SC, Daniel DM. The limits of knee motion: in vitro studies.
In: Daniel DM, Akeson WH, O'Conner JJ, eds. *Knee ligaments: structure, function, injury, and repair*, 1st ed. New York: Raven Press, 1990:153–161.
55. Hole RL, Lintner DM, Kamaric E, et al. Increased tibial translation after partial sectioning of the anterior cruciate ligament: the posterolateral bundle. *Am J Sport Med* 1996;24:556–560.
56. Lintner DM, Kamaric E, Moseley JB, et al. Partial tears of the anterior cruciate ligament: Are they clinically detectable. *Am J Sports Med* 1995;23:111–118.
57. Sakane M, Fox RJ, Woo SL, et al. In situ forces in the anterior cruciate ligament and its bundles in response to anterior tibial loads. *J Orthop Res* 1997;15:285–293.
58. Shoemaker SC, Markolf KL. Effects of joint load on the stiffness and laxity of ligament-deficient knees. An in vitro study of the anterior cruciate and medial collateral ligaments. *J Bone Joint Surg Am* 1985;67:136–146.
59. Seering WP, Piziali RL, Nagel DA, et al. The function of the primary ligaments of the knee in varus-valgus and axial rotation. *J Biomech* 1980;13:785–794.
60. Ostgaard SE, Helmig P, Nielsen S, et al. Anterolateral instability in the anterior cruciate ligament deficient knee. A cadaver study. *Acta Orthop Scand* 1991;62:4–8.
61. Grood ES, Noyes FR, Butler DL, et al. Ligamentous and capsular restraints preventing straight medial and lateral laxity in intact human cadaver knees. *J Bone Joint Surg Am* 1981;63:1257–1269.
62. Grood ES, Stowers SF, Noyes FR. Limits of movement in the human knee. Effect of sectioning the posterior cruciate ligament and posterolateral structures. *J Bone Joint Surg Am* 1988;70:88–97.
63. Woo SL, Young EP, Ohland KJ, et al. The effects of transection of the anterior cruciate ligament on healing of the medial collateral ligament. A biomechanical study of the knee in dogs. *J Bone Joint Surg Am* 1990;72:382–392.
64. Warren RF, Marshall JL. Injuries of the anterior cruciate and medial collateral ligaments of the knee. A long-term follow-up of 86 cases—Part II. *Clin Orthop* 1978;136:198–211.
65. Fetto JF, Marshall JL. Medial collateral ligament injuries of the knee: a rationale for treatment. *Clin Orthop* 1978;132:206–218.
66. Skyhar MJ, Warren RF, Ortiz GJ, et al. The effects of sectioning of the posterior cruciate ligament and the posterolateral complex on the articular contact pressures within the knee. *J Bone Joint Surg Am* 1993;75:694–699.
67. Race A, Amis AA. Loading of the two bundles of the posterior cruciate ligament: an analysis of bundle function in A-P drawer. *J Biomech* 1996;29:873–879.
68. Kaneda Y, Moriya H, Takahashi K, et al. Experimental study on external tibial rotation of the knee. *Am J Sports Med* 1997;25:796–800.
69. Warren RF, Marshall JL, Girgis F. The primary static stabilizer of the medial side of the knee. *J Bone Joint Surg Am* 1974;56:665–674.
70. Shapiro MS, Markolf KL, Finerman GA, et al. The effect of section of the medial collateral ligament on force generated in the anterior cruciate ligament. *J Bone Joint Surg Am* 1991;73:248–256.
71. Ritchie JR, Bergfeld JA, Kambic H, et al. Isolated sectioning of the medial and posteromedial capsular ligaments in the posterior cruciate ligament-deficient knee: influence on posterior tibial translation. *Am J Sports Med* 1998;26:389–394.
72. Wroble RR, Grood ES, Cummings JS, et al. The role of the lateral extraarticular restraints in the anterior cruciate ligament-deficient knee. *Am J Sports Med* 1993;21:257–262, discussion 263.
73. Nielsen S, Helmig P. Posterior instability of the knee joint. An experimental study. *Arch Orthop Trauma Surg* 1986;105:121–125.
74. Harner CD, Hoher J, Vogrin TM, et al. The effects of a popliteus muscle load on in situ forces in the posterior cruciate ligament and on knee kinematics: a human cadaveric study. *Am J Sports Med* 1998;26:669–673.
75. Noyes FR, Stowers SF, Grood ES, et al. Posterior subluxations of the medial and lateral tibiofemoral compartments. An in vitro ligament sectioning study in cadaveric knees. *Am J Sports Med* 1993;21:407–414.
76. Wascher DC, Grauer JD, Markoff KL. Biceps tendon tenodesis for posterolateral instability of the knee: An in vitro study. *Am J Sports Med* 1993;21:400–406.
77. Lipke JM, Janecki CJ, Nelson CL, et al. The role of incompetence of the anterior cruciate and lateral ligaments in anterolateral and anteromedial instability. *J Bone Joint Surg Am* 1981;63:954–960.

CHAPTER 7

Ligament Mechanics

Structural Behavior and Material Properties of Normal and Injured Ligaments

Nigel G. Shrive, Gail M. Thornton, David A. Hart, and Cyril B. Frank

Ligaments are bands of soft tissue that span from bone to bone across a joint. In conjunction with the muscles, which work across the joint and the surfaces of the bones, ligaments help constrain and control the motion of one bone relative to the other. Typically, there is more than one ligament across a joint, with each ligament usually having the role of being the major passive restraint to a particular distraction of the joint. To constrain that distraction, the ligament becomes subject to tensile load and deformation. For example, in the knee joint (Fig. 7.1), the medial collateral ligament (MCL) has a primary role in resisting valgus moment applied to the joint. Compression develops in the lateral load-bearing compartment to provide the counter-balancing moment to the MCL being stretched and in tension.

Combinations of ligaments can resist other movements. Direct distraction of the knee, for example, would be resisted primarily by the lateral and medial collateral ligaments. The shapes of the bones come into play for other situations. If the femur is twisted about the long axis of the tibia, the femoral condyles rise on the central eminence of the tibia, causing the two bones to separate longitudinally. Direct distraction of the joint is resisted by the two collateral ligaments, so the bone shapes cause relative twist of the bones to be resisted mainly by the same two ligaments. Damage to a ligament can therefore reduce the stability of the joint in respect of more than one relative motion of the bones.

Ligaments must perform their stabilizing roles at different joint angles. The composition of ligaments and the architectural organization of those components are therefore crucial to the ability of the tissues to perform their structural roles. We elucidate the general principles involved in normal ligament function and the factors that affect their behavior. We examine the nature of the loads that ligaments resist, how ligaments are structured, and how they respond to these loads. The growth of ligaments demonstrates the dynamism of these components of the joint organ. Ligaments are shown to be exceptionally well suited to their roles, with an elegant mechanism to resist creep and fatigue. The consequences of ligament injury or reconstruction become comprehensible in the light of normal growth, architecture, and mechanics. We examine how ligaments heal and the processes involved lead to continuing abnormal behavior under load. Attempts at ligament reconstruction inevitably have difficulty in recreating the original structure.

The previous edition of this book offers detailed reviews of certain topics not covered in this chapter. Woo et al. (1) reviewed the experimental techniques for measuring ligament cross-sectional area and strain in addition to the effects of temperature, freezing, maturity, aging, and strain rate on normal ligament structural and mechanical properties. The effects of immobilization and mobilization on normal ligaments (2) and surgically and conservatively treated collateral ligaments injuries (3) were discussed in prior chapters contributed by Woo and colleagues.

LIGAMENT LOADS

During joint motion, ligaments become subject to tensile loads to maintain dynamic equilibrium. Collins and O'Connor (4), for example, demonstrated with a sagittal plane model of the knee that the anterior cruci-

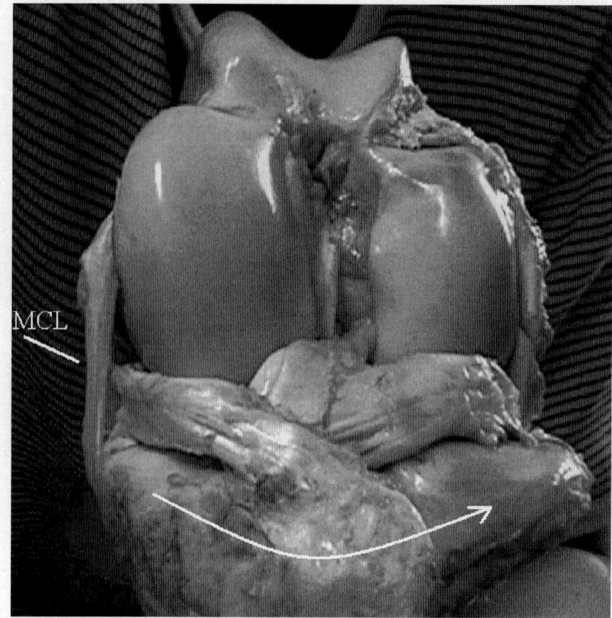

FIGURE 7.1. Frontal view of a bovine knee. A valgus moment *(curved arrow)* is resisted by tension in the medial collateral ligament and compression across the lateral compartment. MCL, medial collateral ligament.

ate ligament (ACL) has to be loaded at certain points of the walking cycle to obtain joint equilibrium. In any repetitive activity such as walking, ground reaction forces repeat step after step, with some natural variation because we do not repeat steps perfectly. Similarly, measurements of the kinematics of limbs show repetition of accelerations and decelerations within a consistent "window" or range. From the ground reaction forces, limb motions and masses, the forces and moments that act at a joint can be estimated. These are repetitive from step to step within a window. Komi et al. (5,6) indicate that muscle—tendon forces repeat in this fashion during walking and running, and Gregor et al. (7) report similar results for cycling. All the previous researchers used buckle transducers, whereas Butler et al. developed techniques involving implantable force and pressure transducers with similar results in tendons and ligaments (8–10). Real-time *in vivo* loads in ligaments have proven elusive and difficult to determine. In an alternate approach, Woo et al. (11–18) used a serial robot to quantify *in situ* load in the ligaments of the knee during *in vitro* passive flexion and extension and when subjecting the knee to motions equivalent to clinical tests. All this work provides the important finding that the magnitude of likely *in vivo* load is a small proportion of ligament structural strength.

This finding is important because we recognize that, *in vivo*, the lines of action of ligament and tendon forces are not altered from step to step. For the resultant forces and moments at a joint to be repeated, those components of the joint that are loaded must be subjected to the same loads from step to step. During repetitive activity, ligaments are subjected to repeated load, and in elastic systems, repetitive loading can lead to failure through fatigue. Fatigue is the phenomenon of increasing damage in the material with increasing numbers of cycles at loads well below those required to cause failure in monotonic loading. The importance of low loads in repetitive activity is that our ligaments are unlikely to fail during normal daily activity with its multiple loadings.

However, ligaments are viscoelastic (19,20), and repeated loads therefore also cause creep (1). Creep is usually defined as the increase in strain over time in a material from the initial elastic strain when the material is subject to constant load (Fig. 7.2). Creep is a viscous response, and viscoelastic materials creep under repetitive loading just as they do under constant load. For viscoelastic materials, there is an interplay between creep and fatigue responses that is receiving increasing recognition in the literature (21,22). Wang et al. recognized that some such interaction must exist in tendons (23,24), and a similar interaction is likely in ligaments. The response of ligaments to load must be considered in light of the need for the tissue to resist fatigue and excessive elongation due to creep. Joints do become looser after activity (25,26), but excessive elongation would lead to instability in the joint.

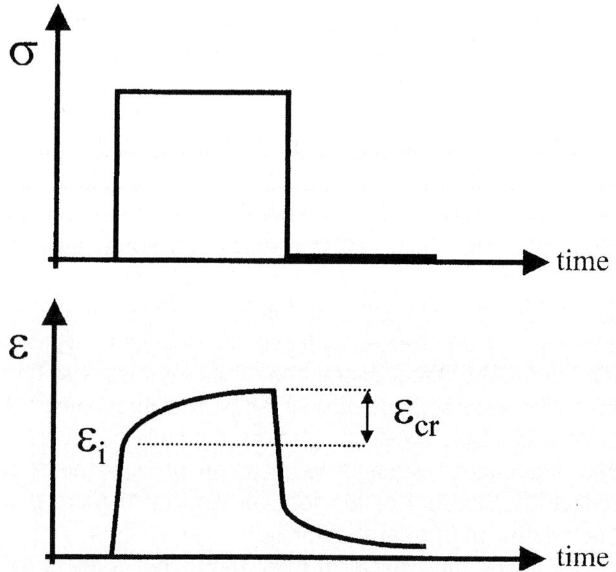

FIGURE 7.2. Schematic of creep test stress input (σ) and strain output (ε), in which ε_i is the initial strain and ε_{cr} is the creep strain.

LIGAMENT CONSTITUENTS AND ARCHITECTURE

Ligaments are bandlike structures that predominantly consist of bundles of collagen fibers. On a local level the bundles appear parallel, but at the tissue level the bundles look interwoven, moving in and out of the plane of the band. Biochemical analysis reveals that ligaments are roughly two-thirds water and one-third solid (27). Most of the solid material is type I collagen. Other collagens—types III, V, VI, XI, and XII—have been identified. Proteoglycans constitute about 1% of the dry weight of a ligament, with decorin being the most prevalent protein. Other proteins such as elastin and fibronectin are also present in small quantities. The functional roles of these various constituents are not fully understood, nor are their interactions with each other and the water in the tissue.

Collagen is a complex protein, essentially a polypeptide chain with a left-handed helical formation. Three such chains aggregate into a tropocollagen molecule with a right-handed helix. The molecules are 340 nm in length and overlap such that there is a characteristic marking, or D-length, of 68 nm in collagen fiber structure. The tropocollagen units aggregate into larger fibrils, which congregate into still larger fibers. The fibers then form the bundles (i.e., fascicles) visible to the naked eye. The formation of collagen provides a characteristic *crimp* when unstretched and viewed under polarized light (Fig. 7.3). The wavelength of the crimp changes as the tissue is stretched and eventually disappears as the molecular structure becomes straight. The D-length also decreases as the fibers are stretched (28,29), suggesting that the collagen straightens and elongates as overall strain is increased. Fibers are thought to be continuous between ligament insertions. There is no direct evidence of such continuity, although fiber ends are difficult to find (30) and ligaments retain their gross structure when the proteoglycans are removed with guanidine (31); they do not collapse into "a pile of spaghetti." Fibers do not connect point to point on insertions directly. Groups of fibers in the form of fascicles can be seen with the naked eye to move in and out of the surface of a ligament. The overall structure therefore is highly complex. The reasons for this complexity have not been delineated, nor has the role of water. Atkinson et al. (32) developed a simple model of part of a fibril as an initial attempt to understand the interaction of the helical structure and water. These investigators suggest that water-saturated matrix within the helix becomes pressurized as the helix begins to straighten (and the radius of the helix decreases). This would make the overall tissue stiffer as load increases. Free water would also be exuded from the pressurized matrix, as observed (33). It is therefore possible that the multiple levels of intertwining of molecules, fibrils, fibers, and fascicles constitute a mechanism to involve a large proportion of water in the tissue in the primary role of tensile load bearing. Other possible causes of fluid exudation on tensile loading include osmotic effects in the highly anisotropic tissue and the straightening of fibers between their ends (34,35).

The crimp pattern observed in a ligament varies with joint position. Different bands of the tissue appear taut at different joint angles. For the MCL in the knee, the posterior band of fibers appears taut when the joint is extended. As the knee is flexed, fibers anterior to this band appear to become taut, while the posterior fibers of the band become slack. This process of recruitment and discharge continues, with the band of apparently taut fibers progressing anteriorly until in full flexion, when the anterior band of fibers of the whole ligament appears taut. The sequential recruitment and discharge of fibers from the taut band is facilitated by the arrangement of the fibers into the femoral insertion and the changing axis of rotation of the femur relative to the tibia (Fig. 7.4).

There are two structural consequences of this shifting band of taut fibers with joint angle. First, the line of action of the force in the ligament changes with joint angle. The apparent line of action of the tension in the tissue lies between different points on the bones meeting at the joint during joint articulation. This presumably provides better stability for the joint throughout its range of motion compared with a single line of action. The second consequence is that the fibers in the ligament are not equally loaded. At any joint angle, some fibers are more tense than others. Neither stress nor strain is evenly distributed over the cross-section of the tissue.

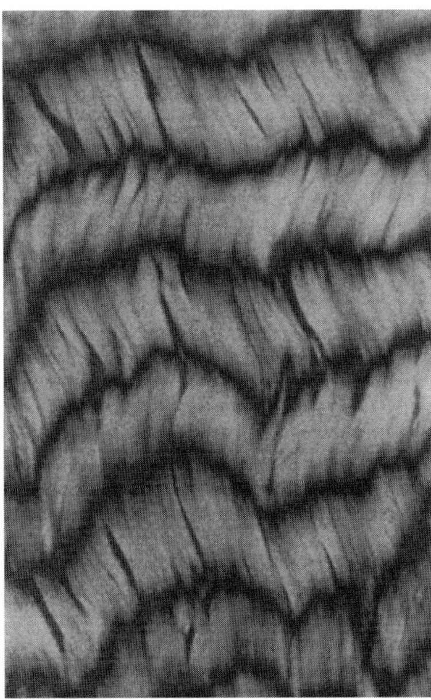

FIGURE 7.3. Photograph of a crimp pattern in a ligament. (Courtesy of J. Matyas, University of Calgary, Alberta, Canada)

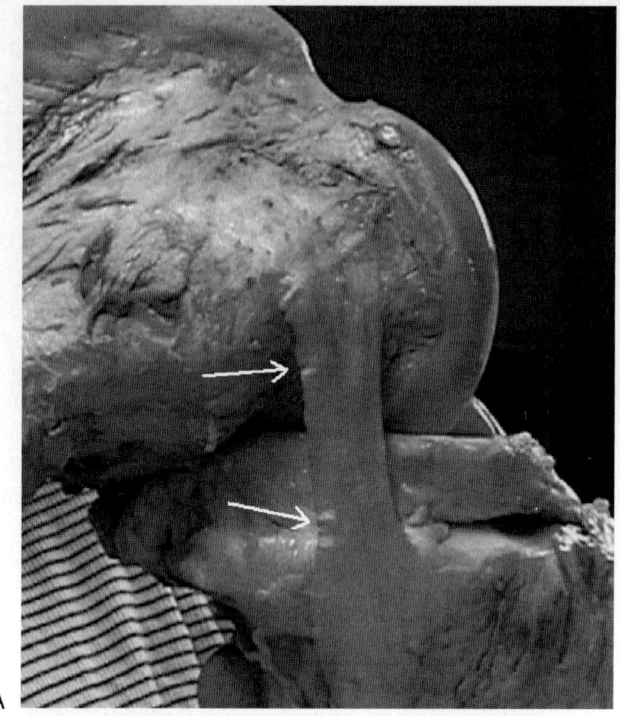

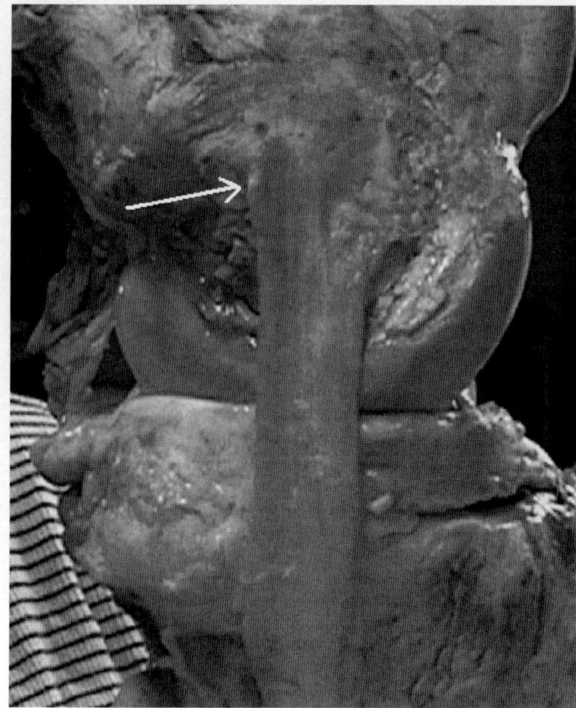

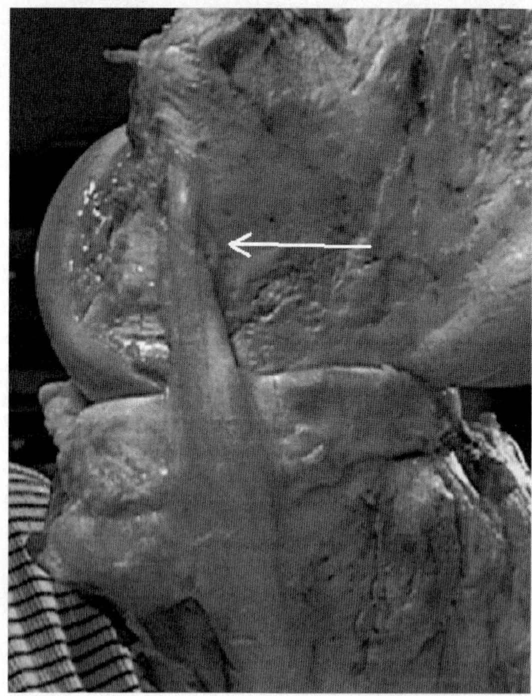

FIGURE 7.4. View of the medial side of a bovine knee. **A:** In full flexion, the anterior fibers of the medial collateral ligament are taut, and the middle and posterior fibers are slack *(arrows)*. **B:** In mid-flexion, the center fibers are straight, and the anterior and posterior fibers are slack *(arrow)*. **C:** In extension, the posterior fibers are taut, and the middle fibers slack, whereas the anterior fibers have rotated in underneath the middle fibers *(arrow)*.

LOAD BEARING BY LIGAMENTS

Traditional thinking is that when a ligament is stretched at a given joint angle, the taut band of fibers picks up the initial load. These fibers are the first to become straight. Other surrounding fibers also stretch, and as the load increases, they also are drawn into load bearing. These fibers must also go through the process of bond straightening (i.e., uncrimping) and chain stretch-ing. The area of stressed fibers increases as more and more fibers are recruited to carry the increasing load. Within the load-bearing area, stress remains unevenly distributed.

As the load-bearing area increases and fibers straighten, the tissue becomes stiffer. There is a nonlinear relationship between load and deformation initially, called the toe region of the load–deformation curve (Fig. 7.5). After all fibers have been recruited and the crimp

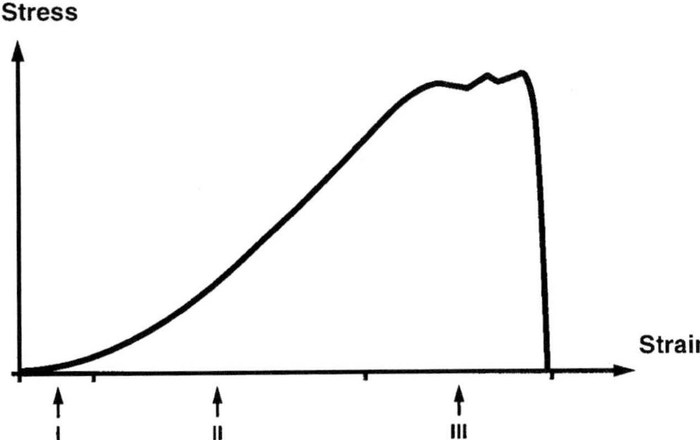

FIGURE 7.5. Schematic stress-strain curve for a ligament. I, toe region; II, linear region; III, failure region. (From Frank CB, Shrive NG. Ligament (2.5). In: Nigg BM, Herzog W, eds. *Biomechanics of the musculoskeletal system,* 2nd ed. New York: John Wiley & Sons, 1999:107–126, with permission.)

removed, there can be no further increase in stiffness, because all fibers are straight, and resistance to further load increments is provided by stretching of the amino acid backbone of the collagen molecules. Viidik (36) used a gradual straining method to relate descriptively the toe region to the straightening out of crimp as fibers are recruited and the linear region to the completion of recruitment and stretching of straightened fibers. Thornton et al. (37) used a rapid monotonic loading method to examine the crimp pattern before and after static creep testing at stresses in the toe and linear regions of the nominal stress-strain curve of the MCL (Fig. 7.6). For the rabbit MCL investigated, the stresses used were 4.1 MPa (toe region), 14 MPa (transition between toe and linear regions), and 28 MPa (linear region). Crimp images captured after creep testing at the linear region stress were consistent with Viidik's (36) description of crimp. However, crimp images captured before creep testing at the linear region stress, on immediate monotonic loading, had more crimp than observed by Viidik (36) using gradual straining. Recruitment occurs, but under monotonic loading the fibers are not completely straight immediately. The water-saturated matrix inside the helical ring may not have time to release all of the bound water under monotonic loading. The structural stiffness is linear because there is insufficient time for any fiber to squeeze out the bound water. The water therefore forces the retention of some crimp under normal dynamic loading, not allowing the fibers to be stretched completely straight. Assuming free water is easily squeezed out of the fiber-reinforced matrix, pressuring the bound water in the matrix within the helix would provide an almost elastic response, because any subsequent water movement would be highly restrained. There would be very little strain-rate dependence of stiffness, as shown by Peterson and Woo (38). However, under the presence of constant

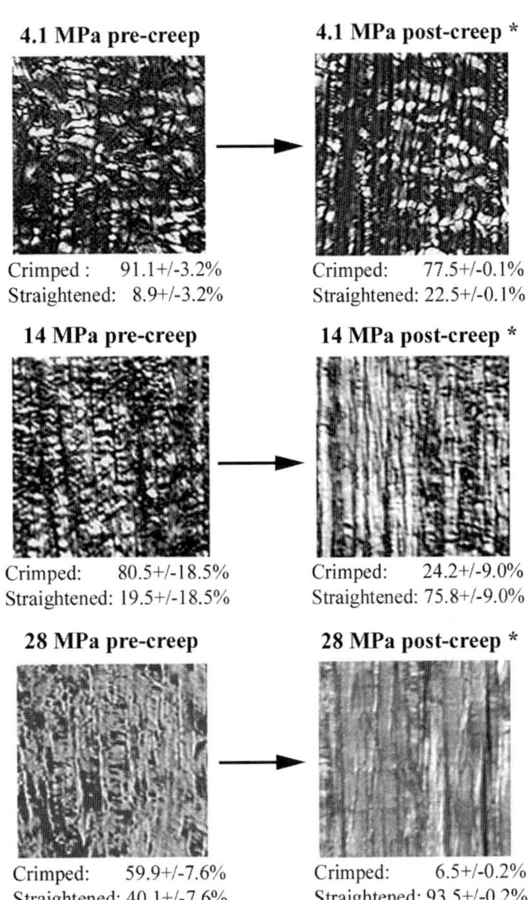

FIGURE 7.6. Crimp images and percent crimped areas of rabbit medial collateral ligaments creep tested at 4.1, 14, and 28 MPa. Image sizes are 280 × 280 µm², and the percent of crimped areas are shown as the mean standard deviation. The *asterisk* indicates the increased area of straightened fibers and decreased area of crimped fibers after creep compared with before creep (*p* < 0.05). (Adapted from Thornton GM, Shrive NG, Frank CB. Ligament creep recruits fibers at low stresses and can lead to modulus-reducing fiber damage at higher creep stresses: a study in a rabbit medial collateral ligament model. *J Orthop Res* 2002;20:967–974, with permission.)

load, there is time for bound water to be exuded so the tissue stretches and the crimp is finally extinguished. A reduction in water content ranging from 4% to 8% occurred during 20 minutes of static creep tests of the rabbit MCL (39), giving the different states shown in Figure 7.7.

The movement of water is one aspect of the time-dependent behavior of ligaments under load. The tissues are viscoelastic, but the microstructural causes of that viscoelasticity are unknown. The 20 minutes of constant high load used to obtain the results seen in Figure 7.6 would be very unusual *in vivo*. *In vivo* loads are usually repetitive in nature, rather than constant, and typically have magnitudes in the toe region of the load-deflection

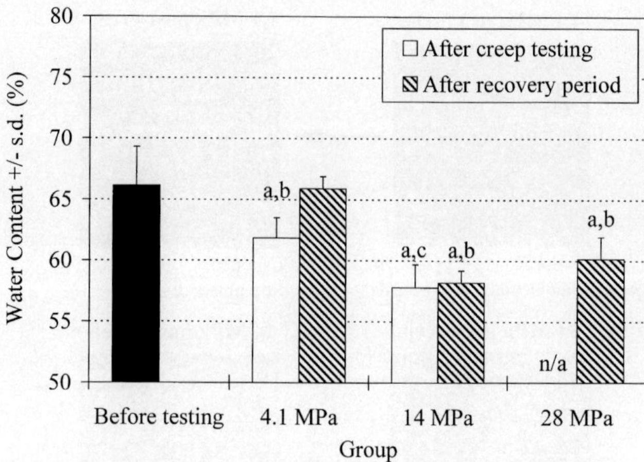

FIGURE 7.7. Water content of rabbit normal medial collateral ligaments before creep testing, after creep testing, and after a recovery period following creep testing. s.d., standard deviation; n/a, not applicable. Significant differences: a = before testing ($p < 0.05$); b = 4.1 MPa after the recovery period ($p < 0.03$); c = 4.1 MPa after creep testing ($p = 0.07$). (Adapted from Thornton GM, Leask GP, Shrive NG, et al. Early medial collateral ligament scars have inferior creep behaviour. *J Orthop Res* 2000;18:238–246, with permission.)

curve (1,8,40,41). Under cyclic loading conditions, the tissue stretches slightly more with each loading cycle. The increments in deformation decrease with each cycle. After a number of cycles, the difference per cycle is so small that many consider a steady state to have been achieved. The static creep strain is similar no matter what the applied average stress in the toe region of the load deformation curve (37). This is a most remarkable response to load. Normally in a structure or material, doubling the stress would double the creep strain. Here, similar creep strains occur over a wide range of stress. This distinctive behavior is achieved through the elegant feature of fiber recruitment. As the taut band at a particular joint angle is loaded and stretches over time, other surrounding fibers are recruited to bear the load, just as occurs with increasing load and deformation in monotonic loading. With an increasing number of fibers resisting the same load, the structure becomes stiffer, limiting the increase in deformation. The stresses carried by the fibers loaded initially reduce over time; the load-bearing area increases, and the peak and average stresses decrease (42).

The limitation of creep is important in normal joint function. Creep increases the length of tissues, and unconstrained creep (i.e., that predicted from stress-relaxation data [43]) would permit length increments that could cause joint instability. Joint laxity does increase with activity (25,26), but joints do not normally become unstable from activity-related increases in laxity.

Variation in the initial levels of crimp in fibers makes strain measurement a difficult task. Surface strains have been measured by various optical means (1,44–49) and individual gauge length strains are measured with an extensometer (50) and differential variable reluctance transducers (DVRTs) (51). Dye lines drawn on a ligament become uneven as the various fascicles stretch differently as load is applied. Extensometer readings vary with the precise locations of contact with the tissue. The DVRT has been used *in vivo* (52) and has revealed that the ACL does "strain" during joint motion. Zero strain is difficult to define in such tests and in general because different fibers are strained in different amounts from the "relaxed" crimp condition as the joint is flexed or extended. Just as stress is distributed unevenly over the cross-section with only some of the cross-sectional area bearing load initially, so is strain unevenly distributed. The average strain over the length of a ligament can be determined from an estimate of the original length of a ligament at zero ligament load and the displacement of the test machine crosshead. However, strain is known to be unevenly distributed over the length of a ligament (53,54). A ligament is longer if its length is measured between the extreme (outer) edges of its insertions than if measured between the inner edges. Because the origin, paths, and ends of fibers are unknown, fiber lengths in a ligament are unknown. Until better techniques are developed, average strain and average stress measures are the closest to real material properties that can be obtained. However, the limitations that both measures are highly unevenly distributed over the cross-section and length of a ligament and depend on joint angle must be recognized.

There is another effect of the fiber recruitment process under repeated load. Reducing the stress on the peak-loaded fibers also increases their fatigue life compared with the situation in which there was no recruitment and no reduction in stress. In the region of the load—the deformation curve, where most *in vivo* loading occurs—ligaments have a sophisticated mechanism for maintaining their function of joint stabilization, which also increases the longevity of the tissue.

From the perspective of structural mechanics, fiber recruitment within creep at toe region stresses means that creep cannot be predicted from load relaxation data at the corresponding deformations. Relaxation is relevant to the group of fibers initially recruited to resist the applied load. Creep at the same initially applied load would involve the same initial group of fibers, but others would become involved in resisting further extension. The benefits of fiber recruitment occur only for loads in the toe region of the monotonic load–deformation relationship (i.e., most *in vivo* loading). After the load reaches levels in the linear portion of that relationship, creep increases with load as expected. Figure 7.6 shows that creep at these load levels involves some fiber straightening and stretching, but there are no more fibers to recruit to increase structural stiffness. The lack of stress reduction on the peak-loaded fibers leaves these fibers prone to fatigue failure under repeated load, or what would be called *creep rupture* under constant load as observed experimentally (37). For viscoelastic materials, therefore, there is interplay between traditional creep and fatigue. These are not independent responses to different loading conditions. Cyclic loading causes creep and fatigue, whereas constant loading can induce time-dependent failure and increased deformation. The growing recognition of this interaction has resulted in some preliminary mathematical models relating the two phenomena (55).

Water is involved in the mechanisms by which a ligament creeps (34). If the water content is increased over the normal *in vivo* level through the use of hypertonic solutions, the creep increases (Fig. 7.8). However, if the water content is reduced from normal, the reduction in creep is less than the previous increase. Water also appears to alter the zero length of ligaments—the length at which the ligament first begins to resist tensile load as it is extended from a no-load position. Increasing water content from normal levels makes the ligament shorter. There is no statistical change in zero position with decreasing water content. If the change in zero length is resisted, forces develop in the tissue with changing water content. The changes with increasing water content may be relevant to inflammation in an injured joint. The increase in water content would tighten the joint. Loading the tissue after changing the water content has the interesting effect after cyclic and static loading of the tissues all being the same length (Fig. 7.9). Whether this finding is fortuitous or a result of a yet to be understood phenomenon remains to be determined.

The postcreep similarity in length with different water contents is just one of many areas for which further understanding is required to obtain full comprehension of how a ligament works. We know there is a reasonable blood supply to the surface of a ligament (56), but the methods by which cells deep within the ligament matrix receive nutrients and dispose of waste is not clear. Introduction of gene therapy vectors, for example, transfects cells only in a small area local to the site of injection (57). If there were rapid movement of fluids, the zone would be expected to be much larger. Nerves are also present in ligaments (58), but their role is not understood. Proprioception has been proposed (59). The mechanism by which the complex architecture is maintained also is not clear. Cells are known to respond to load (60) and may be stimulated to produce the right protein to repair a fatigue fracture, but how the newly produced materials are placed correctly within the organization of the existing extracellular matrix, even in homeostasis, is an enigma. For the full panoply of ligament function to remain effective, it is evident that the fibers must be connected correctly from insertion to insertion. How this is done is unknown. There is evidence that the fibroblasts are fully interconnected

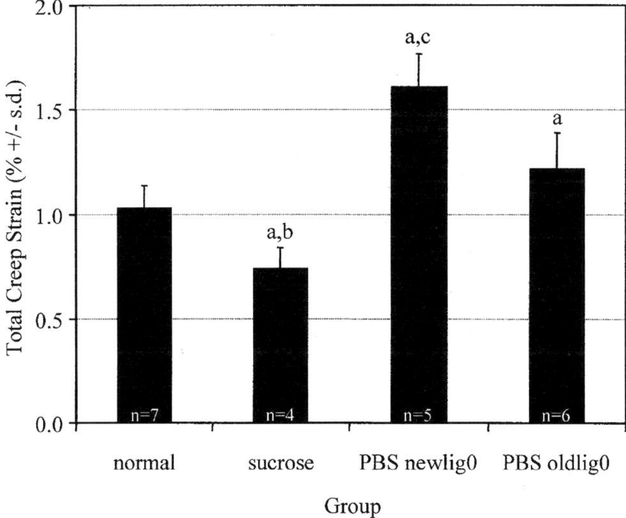

FIGURE 7.8. Total creep strain of normal and soaked rabbit medial collateral ligaments. Soaking ligaments in sucrose significantly reduced water content, and soaking in PBS significantly increased water content from normal values (normal: 67.8 ± 0.5%, sucrose: 52.1 ± 0.8%, PBS newlig0: 73.0 ± 1.6%, PBS oldlig0: 72.1 ± 0.7%). Significant differences: a = normal ($p < 0.02$); b = both PBS groups ($p < 0.0001$); c = PBS oldlig0 ($p = 0.0002$). oldlig0, ligament zero point set before soaking (set to 0 mm at 0.1 N of tension); newlig0, crosshead displacement at 0.1 N of tension after soaking; s.d., standard deviation. (From Thornton GM, Shrive NG, Frank CB. Altering ligament water content affects ligament pre-stress and creep behaviour. *J Orthop Res* 2001;19: 845–851, with permission.)

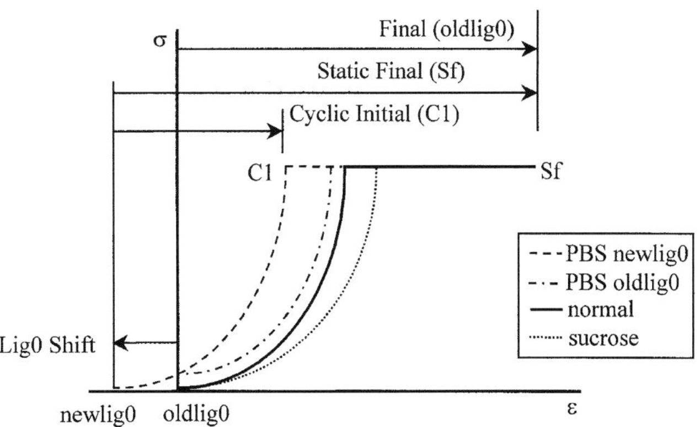

FIGURE 7.9. Creep test point strain of normal and soaked rabbit medial collateral ligaments. Cyclic initial *(C1)* and static final *(Sf)* are measured relative to the creep test start point. Final oldlig0 is measured relative to ligament zero set before soaking. Final oldlig0 values were similar for all groups (normal: 2.65 ± 0.10%, sucrose: 2.61 ± 0.33%, PBS newlig0: 2.77 ± 0.18%, PBS oldlig0 2.77 ± 0.33%). σ, stress; ε, strain; oldlig0, ligament zero point set before soaking (set to 0 mm at 0.1 N of tension); newlig0, crosshead displacement at 0.1 N of tension after soaking; Lig0 Shift, shift in ligament zero as a result of soaking. (From Thornton GM, Shrive NG, Frank CB. Altering ligament water content affects ligament prestress and creep behaviour. *J Orthop Res* 2001; 19:845–851, with permission.)

(61) to form a cellular network in the normal matrix, and the meaning and consequences of this higher-level system should be investigated in more detail.

LIGAMENT GROWTH

Ligaments grow as the skeleton increases in size. Tissue strength increases and peaks around the time the epiphyseal plate closes, with little change thereafter (62,63). The site of failure in strength tests shifts from tibial avulsion in the young to mid-substance tears in the mature person (54,63).

In adult rabbits, there is an almost bimodal distribution of collagen fiber diameters, with smaller fibers interspersed between those of larger diameters (Fig. 7.10). In young animals (3 weeks old), there is a predominance of small fibers (diameters between 48 and 144 nm). By 6 weeks, there has been a rapid increase in size, with an almost gaussian distribution of fiber diameters between 48 and 288 nm. At 14 weeks, the gaussian distribution has stretched on the larger diameter end, with the largest fibers more than 400 nm in diameter. Somewhere between 14 and 52 weeks there are further changes, with increases in the proportions of small (48 to 96 nm) and medium (240 to 340 nm) diameter fibers, giving the distribution seen in Figure 7.10.

The messenger RNA (mRNA) levels for the small, leucine-rich proteoglycans such as biglycan, decorin, fibromodulin, and lumican also change during this period. These proteins are of interest because the leucine-rich core protein contains binding sites for the fibrillar collagens. These four proteins have all been shown to affect fibrillogenesis. It is interesting that the normalized levels of the mRNA for these proteoglycans and collagen type I rise gradually from fetal tissues to week 14. The stimulus for these changes has not been elucidated. By 52 weeks and skeletal maturity, the mRNA level for collagen type I has diminished tremendously; there is probably little need to produce more collagen in the fully developed tissue, rather just enough to maintain the structure. The mRNA

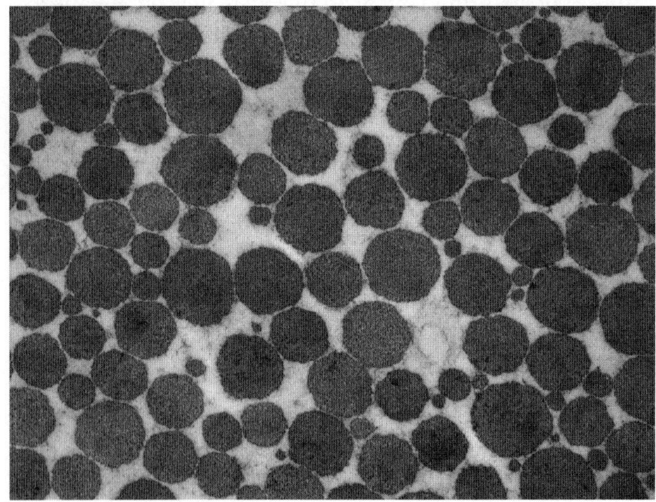

A

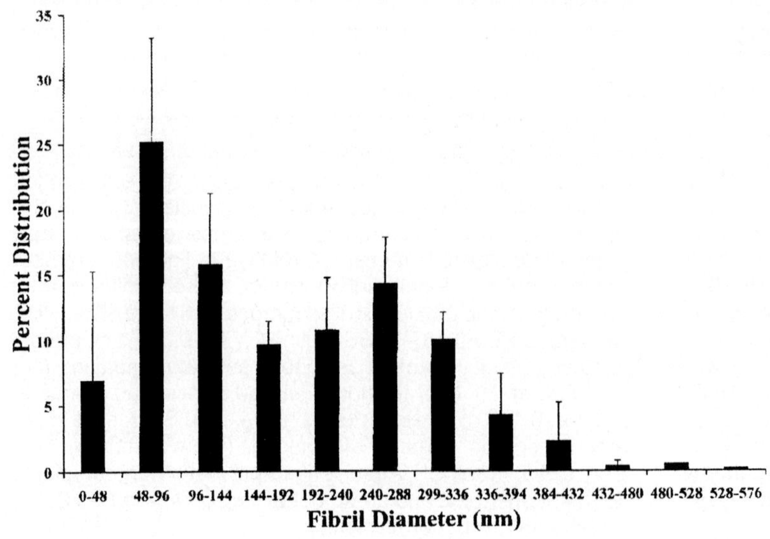

B

FIGURE 7.10. Transmission electron microscopy image **(A)** and fibril diameter distribution **(B)** of the skeletally mature rabbit medial collateral ligament. Notice the bimodal distribution of fibril diameters.

levels for lumican and decorin are maintained, but those for fibromodulin, biglycan, and collagen type I decrease (64). Although it is possible that the mRNA molecules are not translated into actual protein, it is more likely that there are influences other than these molecules in regulating the growth of fibers and maintenance of the extracellular matrix. These proteins are likely to have roles other than regulation of fiber diameter in ligaments. Fiber size is important because it and the quantity of fibers appear essential to tissue strength (65,66). Whether the fibers maintain the same diameter along their length and how cells create and then maintain fiber organization are unknown. Fibers are disrupted during partial or complete failure of a ligament. Such tissue damage leads to a healing response in which there is altered fiber maturation and altered mechanical properties of the ligament tissue.

ABNORMAL LIGAMENT DEVELOPMENT AND MATURATION

The previous discussion focused on normal ligament development and maturation from the mechanical and biologic perspectives. In a number of inherited connective tissue disorders, as well as benign joint hypermobility syndromes, the "normal" ligament laxity parameters of an individual fall outside of the normal range of variability. This finding can be attributed in many instances to alterations in collagen fibril development and matrix assembly in a number of tissues (e.g., skin, ligaments, cardiovascular system components) (reviewed in 67–71). In many of the affected individuals, these changes can be traced to genetic mutations in molecules such as fibrillin-1 or in collagens or their regulatory regions (72,73). In benign joint hypermobility syndromes, the genetic basis has not been identified. Some evidence has implicated collagen regulation (collagen types I and III) (74). However, the finding that the incidence of benign joint hypermobility syndrome is more prevalent in females than males (4:1 to 5:1) has also implicated hormonal factors. Conditions similar to some of those described for humans also have been reported for dogs (75) and other animals. Analysis of these genetic alterations gives rise to the concept that the assembly and maturation of the molecules of the extracellular matrix that lead to the development of collagen fibrils, as well as other structural features of ligaments, are complex processes and do not depend on collagen alone (67,68).

Although these human and animal conditions are rare, they do offer the opportunity for a better understanding of the complexity and basis for the assembly and functioning of ligaments and of the interactions between biology and biomechanics that are required to maintain function within a specific range. Better understanding of the impact of such genetic alterations on function may also be gained from introduction of similar changes in transgenic animals and the assessment of structure–function relationships. Similarly, analysis of matrix assembly during wound healing after disruption of a normal ligament offers the opportunity to investigate development of structure–function relationships in an altered environment without an abnormal genetic influence.

LIGAMENT HEALING

Injury of a ligament is followed by the normal sequence of the body's healing response: inflammation, blood clotting, scar formation, and scar remodeling. These responses overlap but roughly take days, weeks, or months. Each stage of healing involves a complex, coordinated series of cellular events driven and controlled by biochemical and local mechanical factors. All ligaments have a healing response, although in some, particularly the ACL, the healing response frequently may be misdirected. When the ACL is torn, the femoral end has a propensity to heal to the PCL, but the tibial end falls into the space between the femoral condyles and is slowly resorbed. There is no restoration of the ligament, and surgeons have to place a graft in the joint in an attempt to restore the contributions of the ACL to joint function.

When the healing response rejoins the torn ends of a tissue, the original structural architecture is not restored; hence, there is a functional deficit, certainly on a material level. It appears that the initial object of healing is to "fill the gap" created by the injury. Blood collects at the site, and a fibrin-rich clot is formed. Different cells migrate into the clot and begin to perform different tasks—some cleaning up debris and others beginning to produce the proteins needed to create something like the original tissue. Scars in immobilized joints do differentiate into the right sort of tissue with the right sort of organization, albeit very modestly. The load would appear not to be essential to scar formation and initial remodeling, but continued stimulation through loading (from joint motion) appears necessary to generate a scar with sufficient strength to resist the loads applied as the individual gains confidence and greater mobility is attempted. This complementary increase in activity and load, scar strength, and scar remodeling provides additional complexity to the study of healing tissues over those of normal tissues.

Unlike structural properties but similar to material properties (76,77), healing ligaments appear not to recover their ability to resist creep like normal ligaments (Fig. 7.11). This is most probably because the fiber architecture is not restored, and the fibers are not reconnected as before. Within 14 weeks of injury, the water content is almost normal (39), as is the collagen content (78). The orientation of the collagen fibers is more or less back to normal in the longitudinal direction of the ligament, the direction of applied tension (79). However, the distribution in the size of the diameters of the fibers is distinctly abnormal, changing relatively little from 3 to 40 weeks of healing (Fig. 7.12). Two years after injury in the animal

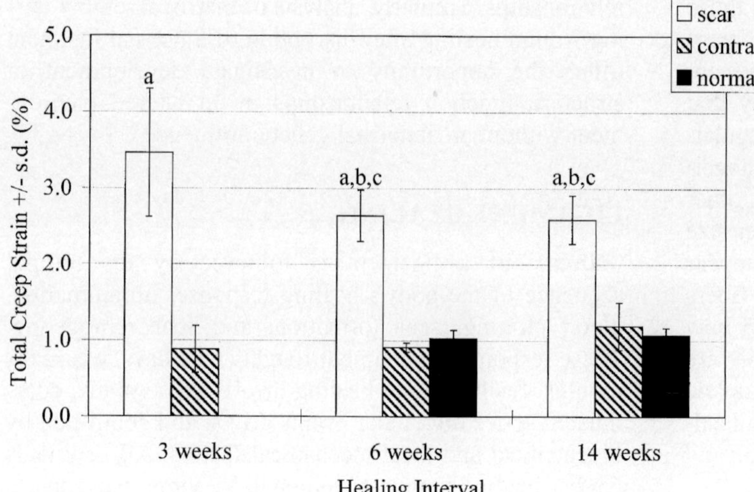

FIGURE 7.11. Total creep strain of rabbit medial collateral ligament gap scars and controls tested at 30% of the ultimate tensile strength of scars. Significant differences: a = contralateral control (contra) ($p < 0.0006$); b = normal ($p < 0.0001$); c = 3-week scar ($p < 0.004$). s.d., standard deviation. (From Thornton GM, Leask GP, Shrive NG, et al. Early medial collateral ligament scars have inferior creep behaviour. *J Orthop Res* 2000;18: 238–246, with permission.)

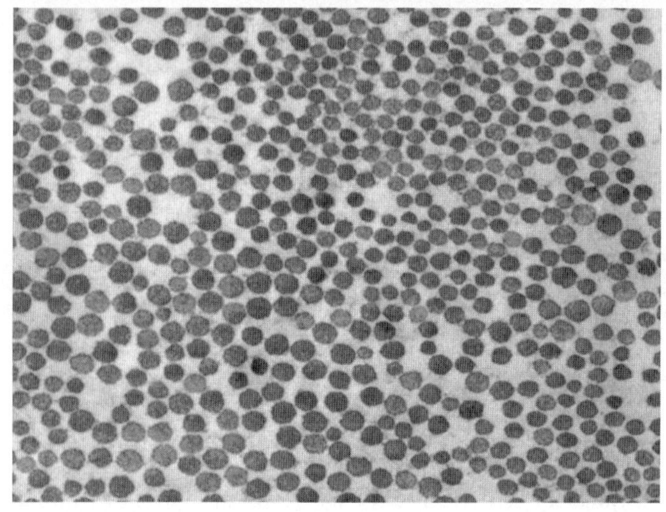

A

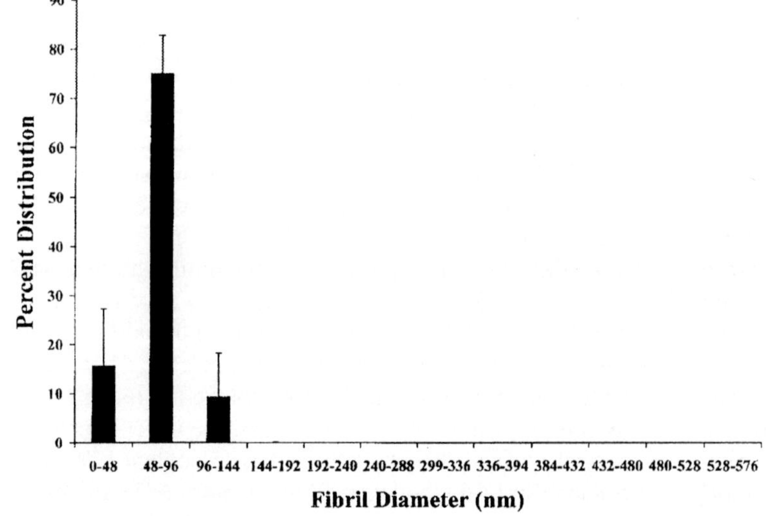

B

FIGURE 7.12. Transmission electron microscopy image **(A)** and fibril diameter distribution **(B)** of the 40-week healing rabbit medial collateral ligament gap scar. Notice the unimodal distribution of fibril diameters.

model used (a surgically created gap in the rabbit MCL), 90% of the fibrils were still small, with some patches of larger fibrils (80).

The mRNA levels and protein synthesis rates for a number of relevant matrix molecules, as well as mRNA levels for other molecules that could potentially influence the synthesis and assembly of collagen fibrils, have been extensively evaluated in the rabbit MCL model in an attempt to understand better how cell activity in a healing ligament differs from normal ligament development and maturation. A series of studies (81–85) indicated that MCL healing in the skeletally mature animal leads to a reproducible pattern of gene expression that differs from normal in a number of aspects. The synthesis rates for the collagen I and III, the major collagens of ligaments, are dramatically altered in the early phases of healing, and the deposition of such altered ratios of these molecules also likely contributes to altered fibril assembly. Although not proven, it is likely that the influence of the inflammatory response during the early phases of healing is a major source of the differences, setting the stage for a pattern of scar maturation. Scar maturation appears programmed to restore some function of the damaged tissue rapidly, but the tissue is altered structurally and mechanically for a prolonged period, if not permanently.

Attempts to remedy partially the altered environment in the healing ligament using gene therapy approaches to influence the expression of molecules believed to be involved in collagen fibril development have been encouraging but only modestly successful (86). The approach used was to curtail the production of the small proteoglycan decorin by the cells. However, the method also affected mRNA levels for other molecules, and a direct cause-and-effect relationship could not be established (87). Decorin is produced in slightly greater quantities than normal early in the healing process, and it is known to influence fibrillogenesis (86). A reduction in decorin production should allow the fibers to aggregate into larger sizes. The strategy was successful locally in cells transfected with the therapy vector, and creep was significantly less than in untreated ligaments. However, the level of *in vivo* scar cell transfection was difficult to control because of delivery limitations and possibly because the cellular organization in a healing ligament is quite different from that in normal tissue (88). Although the approach has merit, current understanding of the associated technical problems means that such techniques are probably a long way from clinical application.

Although it appears technically possible to deal with the problem of small-diameter fibers in ligament scar, there is also much less crosslinking compared with normal tissue (78). It would seem logical to develop a method to stimulate the production of crosslinking proteins while reducing the excess of decorin, collagen type III, and the proteases that can degrade fibrils. The collagen fiber network developed in scar may then resemble more closely that of the original structure. Whether the correct connections would be made in a healed structure, such that recruitment similar to a normal ligament would occur, remains to be seen.

Scar has another feature different from normal tissue: flaws. If flaws are defined as non–load-bearing areas in the tissue (i.e., fat cells, loose collagen, disorganized collagen, blood vessels, and cellular infiltrates), the percentage of a histologic section that is made up of flaw material can be determined, as can the size of the largest flaw (89). After injury, as the scar material remodels, the flaws are slowly removed over time. However, after 14 weeks, the flaw area and the size of the largest flaw remain larger than in normal ligament. In linear elastic fracture mechanics, the critical stress intensity for crack propagation (K_{Ic}) is linearly related to the stress at fracture (σ_c) and the square root of the semi-length of the critical flaw (a_c).

$$K_{Ic} = F\sigma_c\sqrt{\pi a_c}$$

F has to be determined for the particular geometry of the specimen and the flaws. For a single crack in an infinite plate, F = 1; the equation is considered valid if a < 0.4b, in which b is the specimen width. Because the measurement is the area of the largest flaw, the semi-length is some function of the square root of the area. The stress to cause fracture is related to the inverse of the fourth root of the area of the largest flaw. Such a functional relationship appears to exist (Fig. 7.13), but it does not account for the increasing toughness of the scar over the same period as the tissue is remodeled or for the fact that the stress distribution over the cross-section is unlikely to be uniform, especially at the later times of healing when some form of recruitment may have been developed. Nevertheless, there is a clear indication that flaws are a source of weakness and act as stress raisers within the scar matrix. Because stress raisers induce higher creep, particularly if the fiber recruitment mechanism has been restored only in part or not at all, these flaws may also contribute to healing ligaments being unable to resist creep like normal ligaments.

With respect to fatigue, the presence of larger flaws than normal is a major disadvantage, even without the reduced toughness. It is not surprising that scar specimens frequently fail after only a few cycles of cyclic loading, especially in the early stages of healing. K_{Ic} is low, and a_c is large. With healing, K_{Ic} increases, and a_c decreases. More cycles are required to increase the size of flaws until the critical flaw size is reached. A reduction in structural stiffness should occur as the flaws increase in size, because at constant load, the deformation increases as a crack propagates, or at constant deformation, there is a drop in load with increasing crack length. Reductions in structural stiffness are observed before failure in scars (90), typically immediately before failure. In normal ligaments, in which a highly stressed fiber or fiber bundle fails, other less heavily stressed fibers are able to pick up

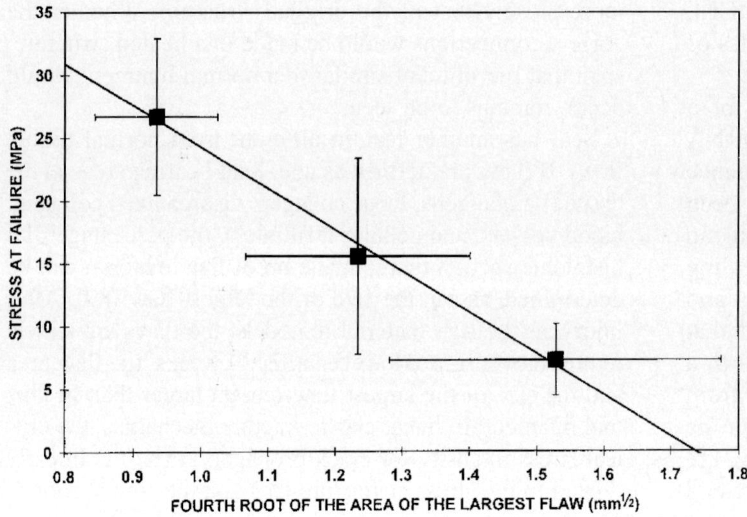

FIGURE 7.13. Stress at failure versus the fourth root of the mean area of the largest flaw of rabbit medial collateral ligament gap scars. Error bars indicate one standard deviation. The maximum likelihood statistical analysis fit shows very strong functional relationship between the variables ($p < 0.001$). (From Shrive N, Chimich D, Marchuk L, et al. Soft-tissue "flaws" are associated with the material properties of the healing rabbit medial collateral ligament. *J Orthop Res* 1995;13:923–929, with permission.)

the load previously carried by the ruptured fibers, and structural stiffness can be restored (37). In this case, crack propagation is not catastrophic for the ligament. *In vivo*; if fatigue or an overload caused failure of a fiber or small group of fibers (as opposed to the whole ligament), the cells presumably would be able to instigate and complete repair if fiber failure occurs within an acceptable, but as yet undefined, extent of damage.

In scar, the growth of flaws may constitute reinjury of developing scar tissue, keeping the cells at a high level of metabolic activity to create sufficient volume of scar to keep stresses sufficiently low to minimize and eventually eliminate crack growth at the increasing levels of stress. Ligament scars are typically much larger in volume than the equivalent material in an uninjured ligament. In the early stages of healing, the scar mass is quite evident, with much larger cross-sectional areas being measured (77,91). As the quality of the scar material for load bearing improves, the cross-sectional area decreases. The delineation between the new ligament and associated fibrous tissue is not clear, and cross-sectional area measures depend on the decision of the person dissecting the preparation about what does or does not constitute part of the healing ligament.

From the perspective of mechanics, all of the extra material generated around the injury site helps keep stresses low to reduce further injury and to restore as much as possible overall stiffness. The stiffness to valgus moment, for example, offered by the whole medial side may be in the same order as the original ligament; isolating the healing "ligament" by removing the additional material in the capsule gives a lower stiffness and does not reflect the response of the whole joint to the injury.

Injury to a ligament does not elicit a healing response in that ligament only. There are changes throughout the joint as stability and load distribution are altered. Healing of the ligament occurs by the production of scar that has an inferior collagen network that may not be connected from insertion to insertion, as in the original tissue. Most of the fiber recruitment mechanism and its distinct benefits appear to be lost, and the ligament does not return to normal after injury, causing compensatory changes in other tissues in the joint.

LIGAMENT RECONSTRUCTION

For injuries to joints in which the level of trauma to a number of structures leaves the joint unstable or when the healing response is known to be inadequate to restore function, orthopedic surgeons have little choice other than to try to reconstruct (replace) the tissues that do not heal. The objective is to provide the patient with a stable joint. The most common ligament requiring reconstruction after complete rupture is the ACL in the knee. The architecture of this ligament is more complex than the normal "straight band of fibrous tissue between two bones" seen for most ligaments. There is a helical twist as the fibers launch posteriorly and proximally off the front of the tibial eminence and swirl round to the medial side of the lateral femoral condyle. In full extension, the posterolateral band of the ACL is taut, whereas in flexion, it is the anteromedial band that becomes tight. As the knee is flexed from full extension, the ligament appears to be subject to torsion about its long axis as well as tension. If the notion that collagen fibers are oriented in directions of maximum principal stress were correct, the helical orientations of the fiber fascicles would support the concept of tension-torsion loading.

Replacing the torn ligament with a piece of tissue with straight fibers (e.g., piece of semitendinosus tendon, middle third of the patellar ligament) cannot restore the complex architecture and its normal function. Knowing this, surgeons are faced with the problem of where to place the graft at each insertion site to obtain the best stability for the joint throughout the range of motion. In the operating room, joint stability is also affected by how tightly the graft is placed; tighter grafts reduce laxity compared with loose grafts. The length of the graft affects its structural stiffness, with longer soft tissues inserted in bone tunnels being much more flexible structurally than shorter ones between bone blocks. The stiffness of the original tissue is unknown, but the surgeon is faced with the difficult challenge to create a graft that can perform like the original structure.

After the surgery is complete, biology takes over. Inflammation in the joint swells the tissue immediately postoperatively, making it prone to creep more than normal. Grafts are susceptible to excessive creep within 2 days of surgery (92). Degradative enzymes are induced and activated and a scarlike tissue begins to form in the scaffold provided by the surgeon within a few weeks. It takes scar months to take over fully, and the graft slowly deteriorates with time because the scar is inferior material compared with normal tissue. Orthotopically placed MCL autografts are slowly taken over by scar and do not have the same properties as normal, even 2 years after surgery (93). In the same model, there was no difference in the laxity of joints 6 months after surgery in which the grafts had been placed tight, loose, or anatomically (94). The effects of the biologic sequelae after surgery are at least as important as the surgery itself. Strategies based on a sound understanding of the postoperative processes need to be developed to control these processes and minimize their negative effects on surgical success and functional outcome.

Clinical evidence suggests that at least 10% to 40% of grafts "stretch out" over time, with the joint tending toward the same level of looseness as before surgery (95–100). This stretching is a scar or tissue remodeling response to creep from repeated loading, with the tissue stretching out from the load and being remodeled to the longer length. The susceptibility of grafts to creep greater than normal is still present 2 years after surgery. Grafts from joints immobilized for 6 weeks after the surgery and then remobilized creep more than grafts from joints allowed freedom of motion after surgery (Fig. 7.14). The reasons for the increased creep are unknown. Some of the problems with scar material have been determined, and methodologies to correct deficiencies are being considered. A multiple molecular, cellular, morphologic, and engineering approach is needed to improve scar and permit healing if the reconstructed tissues are to develop more normal behavior.

Tissue engineering incorporates many of the desired features, and many groups are trying to develop techniques to "grow" an artificial ligament *in vitro* with host cells for later transplantation. However, the effects and control of scar infiltration after implantation must still be considered as part of the overall treatment regimen. An artificial ligament can provide a scaffold, but implanta-

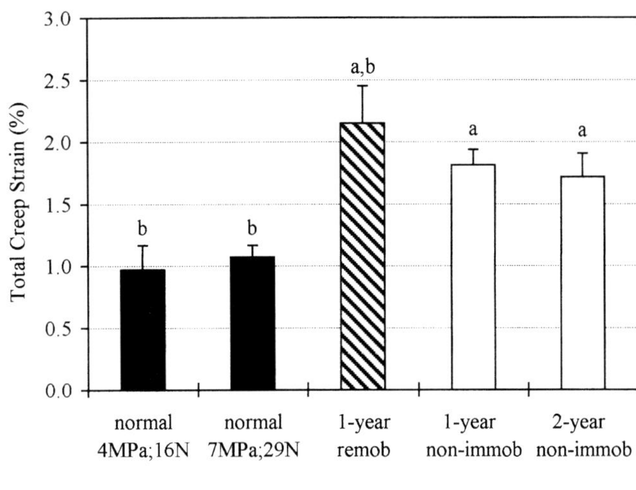

FIGURE 7.14. Total creep strain of rabbit medial collateral ligament (MCL) autografts and normal MCLs. Error bars indicate one standard deviation. Normal MCLs were stress matched (4 MPa) and force matched (29 N) to the MCL autografts. The nonimmobilized (non-immob) group had unrestricted cage activity. The remobilized (remob) group had right hindlimbs immobilized for first 6 weeks after surgery and had unrestricted cage activity for the remainder of the 1-year treatment period. Significant differences: a = normal ($p < 0.0001$) and b = 1-year nonimmobilized autograft ($p < 0.05$). (From Thornton GM, Boorman RS, Shrive NG, et al. Medial collateral ligament autografts have increased creep response for at least two years and early immobilization makes this worse. *J Orthop Res* 2002;20:346–352, with permission.)

tion of such scaffolds may yield a similar end result as current grafts if the postoperative sequelae are not addressed. The problem has many facets and needs a high level of multidisciplinary work in which the effects of one process on another are recognized and the ultimate goal of engineering function is kept in mind.

CONCLUSIONS

Ligaments are complex organs with highly sophisticated architectures. The architecture of each ligament has evolved to optimize the functional role of that ligament. However, there are some common general principles. Fiber recruitment is a mechanism to reduce creep at normal activity loads and thereby constrain the overall laxity that can develop in a joint through repetitive loading (e.g., walking, running); in this way, joint stability is maintained. Fiber recruitment also spreads the repetitious loads over more and more fibers with time, reducing the risk for fatigue failure of those fibers loaded first because the stress on these fibers is reduced over time. There is a nonuniform distribution of stress in a ligament under normal activity loading. This distribution changes with joint angle. At most joint angles, some fibers remain slack under normal loading. Stress measures—the applied load divided by the total cross-sectional area—are only average measures and reflect neither the actual loaded area nor the peak stress. Similarly, strain is nonuniformly distributed along the length and over the cross-section of the tissue. The issue of what constitutes "zero strain" in this milieu remains to be resolved.

Ligaments heal through the formation and remodeling of scar. The rates of healing may differ from tissue to tissue, but scar has distinct deficiencies in the collagen fiber size and interconnections, as well as the presence of flaws that are detrimental to fatigue resistance. Ligament grafts are infiltrated by scar, and therapeutic measures should consider postoperative effects as well as surgical best practice. Because it will be difficult to redevelop the same fiber recruitment regimen as the original, other strategies to provide the engineering function of the original structure need to be considered if a long-term functional outcome is to be achieved. To achieve ligament regeneration will require a transdisciplinary approach with integration of mechanical, biologic, and structural features.

ACKNOWLEDGMENTS

The authors have compounded their views from the work of many students and research fellows. The efforts of these many individuals are gratefully acknowledged. The research was supported by the Medical Research Council of Canada (now the Canadian Institutes of Health Research), The Arthritis Society, the Alberta Heritage Foundation for Medical Research, London Life Ltd., and the McCaig Fund. Nigel G. Shrive is the Killam Memorial Professor, David A. Hart is the Grace Glaum/Calgary Foundation Professor, and Cyril B. Frank is the McCaig Professor. The authors are grateful to all of these organizations for their support.

REFERENCES

1. Woo SLY, Young EP, Kwan MK. Fundamental studies in knee ligament mechanics. In: Daniel DM, Akeson WH, O'Connor JJ, eds. *Knee ligaments: structure, function, injury, and repair.* New York: Raven Press 1990:115–134.
2. Woo SLY, Wang CW, Newton PO, et al. The response of ligaments to stress deprivation and stress enhancement: biomechanical studies. In: Daniel DM, Akeson WH, O'Connor JJ, eds. *Knee ligaments: structure, function, injury, and repair.* New York: Raven Press, 1990: 337–350.
3. Woo SLY, Horibe S, Ohland KJ, et al. The response of ligaments to injury: healing of the collateral ligaments. In: Daniel DM, Akeson WH, O'Connor JJ, eds. *Knee ligaments: structure, function, injury, and repair.* New York: Raven Press, 1990:351–364.
4. Collins JJ, O'Connor JJ. Muscle-ligament interactions at the knee during walking. *Proc Inst Mech Eng [H]* 1991;205:11–18.
5. Komi PV, Salonen M, Jarvinen J. In vivo measurement of Achilles tendon forces in man. *Med Sci Sport Exerc* 1984;16:165–166.
6. Komi PV, Salonen M, Jarvinen M, et al. In vivo registration of Achilles tendon forces in man. I. Methodological development. *Int J Sports Med* 1987;8[Suppl 1]:3–8.
7. Gregor RJ. Komi PV. Jarvinen M. Achilles tendon forces during cycling. *Int J Sports Med* 1987;8[Suppl 1]:9–14.
8. Holden JP, Grood ES, Korvick DL, et al. In vivo forces in the anterior cruciate ligament: direct measurements during walking and trotting in a quadruped. *J Biomech* 1994;27:517–526.
9. Korvick DL, Cummings JF, Grood ES, et al. The use of an implantable force transducer to measure patellar tendon forces in goats. *J Biomech* 1996;29:557–561.
10. Butler DL, Malaviya P, Awad H, et al. A multi-disciplinary approach to analyzing tendon fibrocartilage mechanics, structure and chemistry. In: *Abstracts of the Third World Congress of Biomechanics.* Osaka, Japan: Osaka University, WCB '98 Congress Office, 1998:213.
11. Fujie H, Mabuchi K, Woo SL, et al. The use of robotics technology to study human joint kinematics: a new methodology. *J Biomech Eng* 1993;115:211–217.
12. Takai S, Woo SL, Livesay GA, et al. Determination of the in situ loads on the human anterior cruciate ligament. *J Orthop Res* 1993;11: 686–695.
13. Fujie H, Livesay GA, Woo SL, et al. The use of a universal force-moment sensor to determine in-situ forces in ligaments: a new methodology. *J Biomech Eng* 1995;117:1–7.
14. Livesay GA, Fujie H, Kashiwaguchi S, et al. Determination of the in situ forces and force distribution within the human anterior cruciate ligament. *Ann Biomed Eng* 1995;23:467–474.
15. Rudy TW, Livesay GA, Woo SL, et al. A combined robotic/universal force sensor approach to determine in situ forces of knee ligaments. *J Biomech* 1996;29:1357–1360.
16. Sakane M, Fox RJ, Woo SL, et al. In situ forces in the anterior cruciate ligament and its bundles in response to anterior tibial loads. *J Orthop Res* 1997;15:285–293.
17. Kanamori A, Woo SL, Ma CB, et al. The forces in the anterior cruciate ligament and knee kinematics during a simulated pivot shift test: a human cadaveric study using robotic technology. *Arthroscopy* 2000; 16:633–639.
18. Kanamori A, Sakane M, Zeminski J, et al. In-situ force in the medial and lateral structures of intact and ACL-deficient knees. *J Orthop Sci* 2000;5:567–571.
19. Woo SL, Gomez MA, Akeson WH. The time and history-dependent viscoelastic properties of the canine medial collateral ligament. *J Biomech Eng* 1981;103:293–298.
20. Woo SL. Mechanical properties of tendons and ligaments. I. Quasistatic and nonlinear viscoelastic properties. *Biorheology* 1982;19: 385–396.
21. Perreux D, Joseph E. The effect of frequency on the fatigue performance of filament-wound pipes under biaxial loading: experimental results and damage model. *Compos Sci Technol* 1997;57:353–364.
22. Shenoi RA, Allen HG, Clark SD. Cyclic creep and creep-fatigue interaction in sandwich beams. *J Strain Analysis* 1997;32:1–18.
23. Wang XT, Ker RF. Creep rupture of wallaby tail tendons. *J Exp Biol* 1995;198:831–845.
24. Wang XT, Ker RF, Alexander RM. Fatigue rupture of wallaby tail tendons. *J Exp Biol* 1995;198:847–852.
25. Johannsen HV, Lind T, Jakobsen BW, et al. Exercise-induced knee joint laxity in distance runners. *Br J Sports Med* 1989;23:165–168.
26. Sumen Y, Ochi M, Adachi N, et al. Anterior laxity and MR signals of the knee after exercise. A comparison of 9 normal knees and 6 anterior cruciate ligament reconstructed knees. *Acta Orthop Scand* 1999; 70:256–260.
27. Frank CB, Shrive NG. Ligament (2.5). In: Nigg BM, Herzog W, eds. *Biomechanics of the musculoskeletal system,* 2nd ed. Chichester: Wiley, 1999:107–126.
28. Viidik A, Ekholm R. Light and electron microscopic studies of collagen fibers under strain. *Z Anat Entwicklungsgesch* 1968;127:154–164.
29. Mosler E, Folkhard W, Knorzer E, et al. Stress-induced molecular rearrangement in tendon collagen. *J Mol Biol* 1985;182:589–596.
30. Trotter JA, Kadler KE, Holmes DF. Echinoderm collagen fibrils grow by surface-nucleation-and-propagation from both centers and ends. *J Mol Biol* 2000;300:531–540.
31. Cunningham KD. *The structure-function relationship of the extracellular matrix in the rabbit medial collateral ligament* [M.Sc. thesis]. Calgary: University of Calgary, 1998.
32. Atkinson TS, Haut RC, Altiero NJ. A poroelastic model that predicts some phenomenological responses of ligaments and tendons. *J Biomech Eng* 1997;119:400–405.

33. Hannafin JA, Arnoczky SP. Effect of cyclic and static tensile loading on water content and solute diffusion in canine flexor tendons: an in vitro study. *J Orthop Res* 1994;12:350–356.
34. Thornton GM, Shrive NG, Frank CB. Altering ligament water content affects ligament pre-stress and creep behaviour. *J Orthop Res* 2001;19:845–851.
35. Adeeb S, Shrive N, Frank C, et al. Modeling the behaviour of ligaments: a technical note. Fourth World Congress of Biomechanics. 2002.
36. Viidik A. Simultaneous mechanical and light microscopic studies of collagen fibers. *Z Anat Entwicklungsgesch* 1972;136:204–212.
37. Thornton GM, Shrive NG, Frank CB. Ligament creep recruits fibres at low stresses and can lead to modulus-reducing fibre damage at higher creep stresses: a study in a rabbit medial collateral ligament model. *J Orthop Res* 2002;20:967–974.
38. Peterson RH, Woo SL. A new methodology to determine the mechanical properties of ligaments at high strain rates. *J Biomech Eng* 1986;108:365–367.
39. Thornton GM, Leask GP, Shrive NG, et al. Early medial collateral ligament scars have inferior creep behaviour. *J Orthop Res* 2000;18:238–246.
40. Noyes FR, Butler DL, Grood ES, et al. Biomechanical analysis of human ligament grafts used in knee-ligament repairs and reconstructions. *J Bone Joint Surg Am* 1984;66:344–352.
41. Woo SL, Debski RE, Withrow JD, et al. Biomechanics of knee ligaments. *Am J Sports Med* 1999;27:533–543.
42. Thornton GM, Frank CB, Shrive NG. Ligament creep behaviour can be predicted from stress relaxation by incorporating fibre recruitment. *J Rheol* 2001;45:493–507.
43. Thornton GM, Oliynyk A, Frank CB, et al. Ligament creep cannot be predicted from stress relaxation at low stress: a biomechanical study of the rabbit medial collateral ligament. *J Orthop Res* 1997;15:652–656.
44. Yin FCP, Tompkins WR, Peterson KL, et al. A video dimension analyzer. *IEEE Trans Biomed Eng* 1972;19:376–381.
45. Vito RP. The mechanical properties of soft tissues. I. A mechanical system for bi-axial testing. *J Biomech* 1980;13:947–950.
46. Butler DL, Grood ES, Noyes FR, et al. Effects of structure and strain measurement technique on the material properties of young human tendons and fascia. *J Biomech* 1984;17:579–596.
47. Woo SL, Gomez MA, Inoue M, et al. New experimental procedures to evaluate the biomechanical properties of healing canine medial collateral ligaments. *J Orthop Res* 1987;5:425–432.
48. Amadio PC, Berglund LJ, An KN. Biochemically discrete zones of canine flexor tendon: evaluation of properties with a new photographic method. *J Orthop Res* 1992;10:198–204.
49. Derwin KA, Soslowsky LJ, Green WD, et al. A new optical system for the determination of deformations and strains: calibration characteristics and experimental results. *J Biomech* 1994;27:1277–1285.
50. Shrive NG, Damson E, Frank CB. Technology transfer regarding the measurement of strain on flexible materials with special reference to soft tissues. *Clin Aspects Biomed Exp Mech* 1992;3:121–130.
51. Beynnon BD, Fleming BC. Anterior cruciate ligament strain in-vivo: a review of previous work. *J Biomech* 1998;31:519–525.
52. Beynnon BD, Johnson RJ, Fleming BC, et al. The strain behavior of the anterior cruciate ligament during squatting and active flexion-extension. A comparison of an open and a closed kinetic chain exercise. *Am J Sports Med* 1997;25:823–829.
53. Butler DL, Sheh MY, Stouffer DC, et al. Surface strain variation in human patellar tendon and knee cruciate ligaments. *J Biomech Eng* 1990;112:38–45.
54. Lam TC, Shrive NG, Frank CB. Variations in rupture site and surface strains at failure in the maturing rabbit medial collateral ligament. *J Biomech Eng* 1995;117:455–461.
55. Webster GA. Fracture mechanics in the creep range. *J Strain Analysis* 1994;29:215–223.
56. Arnoczky SP, Matyas JR, Buckwalter JA, et al. Anatomy of the anterior cruciate ligament. In: Jackson DW, Arnoczky SP, Woo SL-Y, et al., eds. *The anterior cruciate ligament: current and future concepts.* New York: Raven Press, 1993:63–73.
57. Nakamura N, Timmermann SA, Hart DA, et al. A comparison of in vivo gene delivery methods for antisense therapy in ligament healing. *Gene Ther* 1998; 5:1455–1461.
58. McDougall JJ, Bray RC, Sharkey KA. Morphological and immuno-histochemical examination of nerves in normal and injured collateral ligaments of rat, rabbit, and human knee joints. *Anat Rec* 1997;248:29–39.
59. Pap G, Machner A, Nebelung W, et al. Detailed analysis of proprioception in normal and ACL-deficient knees. *J Bone Joint Surg Br* 1999;81:764–768.
60. Banes AJ, Tsuzaki M, Yamamoto J, et al. Mechanoreception at the cellular level: the detection, interpretation, and diversity of responses to mechanical signals. *Biochem Cell Biol* 1995;73:349–365.
61. Lo IKY, Chi S, Ivie T, et al. The cellular matrix: a feature of tensile bearing dense soft connective tissues. *Histol Histopathol* 2002;17:523–537.
62. Woo SL, Ohland KJ, Weiss JA. Aging and sex-related changes in the biomechanical properties of the rabbit medial collateral ligament. *Mech Ageing Dev* 1990;56:129–142.
63. Woo SL, Orlando CA, Gomez MA, et al. Tensile properties of the medial collateral ligament as a function of age. *J Orthop Res* 1986;4:133–141.
64. Lo IKY, Leatherbarrow KE, Marchuk LL, et al. Collagen fibrillogenesis in the maturing rabbit medial collateral ligament and patellar tendon. 2002 *(submitted)*.
65. Parry DAD, Barnes GR, Craig AS. A comparison of the size distribution of collagen fibrils in connective tissues as a function of age and a possible relation between fibril size distribution and mechanical properties. *Proc R Soc Lond B Biol Sci* 1978;203:305–321.
66. Parry DAD, Craig AS. Growth and development of collagen fibrils. In: Ruggeri A, Motta PM, eds. *Ultrastructure of the connective tissue matrix.* Boston: Martinus Nijhoff, 1984:34–64.
67. Holbrook KA, Byers PH. Structural abnormalities in the dermal collagen and elastic matrix from the skin of patients with inherited connective tissue disorders. *J Invest Dermatol* 1982;79[Suppl 1]:7s–16s.
68. Holbrook KA, Byers PH. Skin is a window on heritable disorders of connective tissue. *Am J Med Genet* 1989;34:105–121.
69. Grahame R. Joint hypermobility and genetic collagen disorders: are they related? *Arch Dis Child* 1999;80:188–191.
70. Grahame R. Heritable disorders of connective tissue. *Baillieres Best Pract Res Clin Rheumatol* 2000;14:345–361.
71. Giampietro PF, Raggio C, Davis JG. Marfan syndrome: orthopedic and genetic review. *Curr Opin Pediatr* 2002;14:35–41.
72. Smith LT, Schwarze U, Goldstein J, et al. Mutations in the *COL3A1* gene result in the Ehlers-Danlos syndrome type IV and alterations in the size and distribution of the major collagen fibrils of the dermis. *J Invest Dermatol* 1997;108:241–247.
73. Wenstrup RJ, Florer JB, Willing MC, et al. COL5A1 haploinsufficiency is a common molecular mechanism underlying the classical form of EDS. *Am J Hum Genet* 2000;66:1766–1776.
74. Child AH. Joint hypermobility syndrome: inherited disorder of collagen synthesis. *J Rheumatol* 1986;13:239–243.
75. Rodriguez F, Herraez P, Espinosa de los Monteros A, et al. Collagen dysplasia in a litter of Garafiano shepherd dogs. *Zentralbl Veterinarmed A* 1996;43:509–512.
76. Frank C, Woo SL-Y, Amiel D, et al. Medial collateral ligament healing: a multidisciplinary assessment in rabbits. *Am J Sports Med* 1983;11:379–389.
77. Woo SL-Y, Inoue M, McGurk-Burleson E, et al. Treatment of the medial collateral ligament injury. II. Structure and function of canine knees in response to different treatment regimens. *Am J Sports Med* 1987;15:22–29.
78. Frank C, McDonald D, Wilson J, et al. Rabbit medial collateral ligament scar weakness is associated with decreased collagen pyridinoline crosslink density. *J Orthop Res* 1995;13:157–165.
79. Frank C, MacFarlane B, Edwards P, et al. A quantitative analysis of matrix alignment in ligament scars: a comparison of movement versus immobilization in an immature rabbit model. *J Orthop Res* 1991;9:219–227.
80. Frank C, McDonald D, Shrive N. Collagen fibril diameters in the rabbit medial collateral ligament scar: a longer term assessment. *Connect Tissue Res* 1997;36:261–269.
81. Murphy PG, Loitz BJ, Frank CB, et al. Influence of exogenous growth factors on the synthesis and secretion of collagen types I and III by explants of normal and healing rabbit ligaments. *Biochem Cell Biol* 1994;72:403–409.
82. Boykiw R, Sciore P, Reno C, et al. Altered levels of extracellular matrix molecule mRNA in healing rabbit ligaments. *Matrix Biol* 1998;17:371–378.

83. Reno C, Boykiw R, Martinez ML, et al. Temporal alterations in mRNA levels for proteinases and inhibitors and their potential regulators in the healing medial collateral ligament. *Biochem Biophys Res Commun* 1998;252:757–763.

84. Sciore P, Boykiw R, Hart DA. Semiquantitative reverse transcription-polymerase chain reaction analysis of mRNA for growth factors and growth factor receptors from normal and healing rabbit medial collateral ligament tissue. *J Orthop Res* 1998;16:429–437.

85. Hellio Le Graverand MP, Eggerer J, Sciore P, et al. Matrix metalloproteinase-13 expression in rabbit knee joint connective tissues: influence of maturation and response to injury. *Matrix Biol* 2000;19: 431–441.

86. Nakamura N, Hart DA, Boorman RS, et al. Decorin antisense gene therapy improves functional healing of early rabbit ligament scar with enhanced collagen fibrillogenesis in vivo. *J Orthop Res* 2000;18: 517–523.

87. Hart DA, Nakamura N, Marchuk L, et al. Complexity of determining cause and effect in vivo after antisense gene therapy. *Clin Orthop* 2000;379[Suppl]:S242–S251.

88. Lo IKY, Ou Y, Rattner JP, et al. The cellular networks of normal ovine medial collateral and anterior cruciate ligaments are not accurately recapitulated in scar. *J Anat* 2002;200:283–296.

89. Shrive N, Chimich D, Marchuk L, et al. Soft-tissue "flaws" are associated with the material properties of the healing rabbit medial collateral ligament. *J Orthop Res* 1995;13:923–929.

90. Thornton GM, Shrive NG, Frank CB. Reduction in modulus indicates damage in ligaments. *Trans Orthop Res Soc* 2001;26:23.

91. Chimich D, Frank C, Shrive N, et al. The effects of initial end contact on medial collateral ligament healing: a morphological and biomechanical study in a rabbit model. *J Orthop Res* 1991;9:37–47.

92. Boorman RS, Thornton GM, Shrive NG, et al. Ligament grafts become more susceptible to creep within days after surgery: evidence for early enzymatic degradation of a ligament graft in a rabbit model. *Acta Orthop Scand* 2002 *(in press)*.

93. Thornton GM, Boorman RS, Shrive NG, et al. Medial collateral ligament autografts have increased creep response for at least two years and early immobilization makes this worse. *J Orthop Res* 2002;20: 346–352.

94. King GJ, Edwards P, Brant RF, et al. Intraoperative graft tensioning alters viscoelastic but not failure behaviours of rabbit medial collateral ligament autografts. *J Orthop Res* 1995;13:915–922.

95. Daniel DM, Stone ML, Reihl B. Ligament surgery: the evaluation of results. In: Daniel DM, Akeson WH, O'Connor JJ, eds. *Knee ligaments: structure, function, injury, and repair*. New York: Raven Press, 1990:521–534.

96. Howe, JG, Johnson RJ, Kaplan MJ, et al. Anterior cruciate ligament reconstruction using quadriceps patellar tendon graft. Part I. Long-term followup. *Am J Sports Med* 1991;19:447–457.

97. Aglietti P, Buzzi R, D'Andria S, et al. Long-term study of anterior cruciate ligament reconstruction for chronic instability using the central one-third patellar tendon and a lateral extraarticular tenodesis. *Am J Sports Med* 1992;20:38–45.

98. Noyes FR, Barber SD. The effect of a ligament-augmentation device on allograft reconstruction for chronic ruptures of the anterior cruciate ligament. *J Bone Joint Surg Am* 1992;74:960–973.

99. Bach BR Jr, Jones GT, Hager CA, et al. Arthrometric results of arthroscopically assisted anterior cruciate ligament reconstruction using autograft patellar tendon substitution. *Am J Sports Med* 1995;23:179–185.

100. Lerat JL, Moyen B, Mandrino A, et al. Prospective study of postoperative anterior knee laxity after anterior cruciate ligament reconstruction using two different patellar tendon grafts. *Rev Chir Orthop Reparatrice Appar Mot* 1997;83:217–228.

CHAPTER 8

Articular Cartilage and Its Exacting Characteristics

The Benchmark for All Attempts to Achieve Articular Cartilage Regeneration or Repair

Wayne H. Akeson

This chapter provides a capsulized account of structure, composition, and mechanical properties of articular cartilage, which is basic to the understanding of its function. This information is essential for a clear understanding of the therapeutic goals of cartilage restoration by any of the current or future attempts at surgically induced regeneration. Claims are heard occasionally at clinical conferences about full restoration of damaged articular cartilage after surgical intervention. These claims are usually anecdotal, without documentation, and unpublished. Such remarks have tended to confuse thought processes about the underlying biology of the cartilage repair process after injury or surgery. Attempts to achieve hyaline cartilage regeneration in experimental model systems have universally failed, and the anecdotal clinical remarks about hyaline cartilage regeneration must be dismissed as lacking required documentation.

The typical response to cartilage injury in which the subchondral plate is fractured is the formation of fibrocartilage, a scarlike tissue unsuited to the support of compressive loads and shear forces (1,2). If the subchondral plate is not fractured, attempts at healing rely on articular cartilage cells whose response to injury is consistently and completely ineffectual (3).

Given the elegant precision of the morphologic and compositional interdependence of articular cartilage, it is not surprising that attempts at effective regeneration of articular cartilage have frustrated clinicians and basic scientists alike. Mature mammalian cartilage cells have lost the ability to dedifferentiate, a universal property of mammalian cells resulting from evolutionary progress. This circumstance probably is a controlling factor in the limitation of the biologic response of articular cartilage to injury.

Articular cartilage is a unique tissue in many respects, but especially with regard to its structural, metabolic, and functional interactions. Articular cartilage possesses unparalleled biomechanical functional efficiency. This efficiency is derived from design features that are marveled at by physicians and engineers attempting to design artificial substitutes for diseased joints. For example, the articular cartilage lubrication efficiency is an order of magnitude superior to the best bearing surfaces known to modern engineering. Such efficiencies are achieved despite stringent limitations imposed on the tissue, such as the lack of blood supply and a tissue thickness that measures a few millimeters at most. Couple these points with a limited repair capability and the consequent requirement that the tissue survive a lifetime of use, and the question becomes, "How can synovial joints survive as long as they do?" The thrust of this chapter is to describe the morphologic, biochemical, and biophysiologic interactions of the cartilage matrix required to provide insight into the basis of successful long-term survival of cartilage and the requirements for its successful repair or regeneration.

A phenomenologic concept helpful in understanding cartilage function is to consider the air tent, a structure used as a cover for recreational areas such as swimming pools and tennis courts or as a temporary cover for exhibitions (4) (Fig. 8.1). The functional requirements for the air tent are an inflation pump, a fan; an intake tube for the inflation

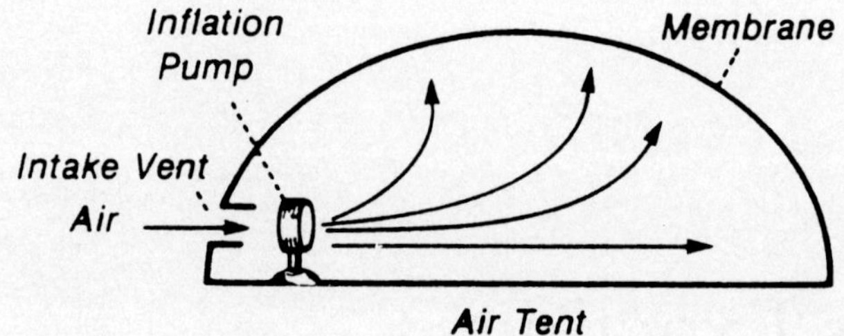

FIGURE 8.1. Articular cartilage is a pressurized structure, conceptually similar to an air tent. The air tent system requires a pump that must be constantly operating to maintain inflation of the tent because of leaks in the fabric. In the case of cartilage, the surface "membrane" is the lamina splendens, consisting of a fine fibrillar network concentrated at the articular surface. The inflation pump mechanism of articular cartilage is served by the proteoglycan molecules, and the inflation medium is an ultrafiltrate of the synovial fluid. In articular cartilage, there is no single intake vent for the inflation medium; rather, the fluid that inflates the structure enters through the same myriad of fine surface pores from which it exits when compressed.

medium; the inflation medium, air; and fabric required to contain the pressurization and to provide the cover. The pump must be working constantly to maintain expansion of the system because of inevitable leaks through the fabric. In the case of cartilage, the surface membrane consists of the fine collagen fibril network concentrated at the articular surface. The inflation pump of cartilage is the proteoglycan molecular structure, and the inflation medium is an ultrafiltrate of synovial fluid. In cartilage, there is no single intake vent for the inflation medium to enter; rather, fluid inflating the tissue enters through a myriad of microscopic pores at the surface, the same pores from which the fluid exits when compressed. These elements are interrelated, and a deficiency in any of them results in failure of the system. In the air tent case, a tear in the fabric for which the pump is not able to compensate results in tent collapse. If the pump fails, the tent gradually collapses as pressurized air leaks through the pores of the fabric.

The fabriclike structure at the cartilage surface, consisting of fine collagen fibrils packed tightly in a matted pattern parallel to the surface, is much different from that seen in the deeper layers, where fibers become thicker, their orientation becomes more vertical, and the spaces between the fibers increase. The surface "fabric" of cartilage has tiny pores that permit fluid and small molecules access to and egress from the tissue but block movement of large molecules. The inflation medium in articular cartilage is fluid, not air. The cartilage fluid is in equilibrium with the synovial fluid, which is essentially an ultrafiltrate of plasma. The fluid in articular cartilage is significantly pressurized. Calculations by Ogston (5) led him to conclude that articular cartilage is inflated to the equivalent of "motor tire pressure." The pump for this pressurized system is not intuitively obvious, but its presence has been established without doubt by modern techniques of rheology and biophysics. The pump for the articular cartilage system is chiefly the proteoglycan subunit (i.e.,

aggrecan) and the proteoglycan aggregate molecule, huge macromolecules locked within the articular cartilage fibrillar matrix by their large size and volume.

In its state of equilibrium, the expansion pressure in the articular cartilage system is in balance with the resisting tension of the collagen fibers, but the balance can be upset by an externally applied load. If the external pressure exceeds the internal pressure, fluid flows outward until a new equilibrium is reached. As the proteoglycan molecules become compressed, their charges become more concentrated. This causes the fluid pressure within the cartilage to be increased until a new equilibrium is reached. The theoretic analysis of the fluid flow patterns and viscoelastic properties under various loading conditions has been studied extensively. This fluid movement is of great interest because it explains the mechanism of several fundamental properties of the articular cartilage system, including lubrication, load bearing, and nutrition.

Chapter 14 describes some of the later attempts to achieve articular cartilage regeneration or repair. The proper evaluation of such attempts must be related to fundamental knowledge of articular cartilage form, composition, and biomechanical characteristics. The collagen matrix of normal articular cartilage, its proteoglycan and proteoglycan aggregate, and the movement of fluid within cartilage with respect to its morphologic, biochemical, and functional features are described in greater detail in the following sections.

COLLAGEN

Morphology of the Collagen Framework

The pattern of collagen fibrils within articular cartilage is well suited to the functional requirements of the tissue. The air tent analogy requires that a pressurized internal medium be constrained from expansion by a membrane. A matted surface layer of collagen fibrils provides this membranelike function.

The collagen pattern in the deeper layers of the cartilage surface is morphologically quite different from the surface pattern. In 1925, Benninghoff (6) described an arcade pattern of articular cartilage collagen organization (Fig. 8.2). This pattern has subsequently been challenged with respect to the precise accuracy of the proposed scheme (7–9), but the concept is at least partially correct and is useful for understanding cartilage function. The surface fibrillar pattern differs from that of fibers in deeper layers (10). The surface collagen fibrils are smaller (30 to 32 nm in diameter) and more closely packed than in the middle and deeper layers. The surface pattern of the collagen framework described has been recognized implicitly for decades by the term *armor plate layer,* referring to the tough, resilient, skinlike cartilage surface (see Color Plate 4, following page 122). The collagen concentration is greatest at the surface, where the small fibrils are compacted tangentially. This arrange-

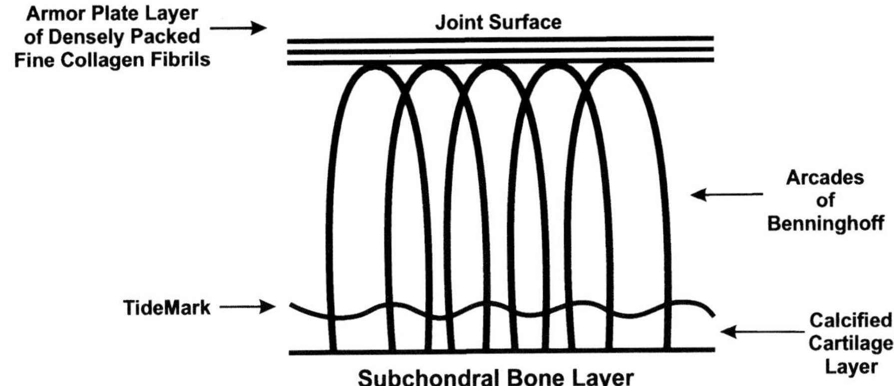

FIGURE 8.2. Benninghoff arcades. In the schematic diagram of the collagen fibril orientation within articular cartilage, the fibrils are tightly packed near the articular surface in a tangential layer that has been called the lamina splendens, or the armor plate layer. Fibrils in the deeper layers become progressively larger as they progress toward the subchondral bone layer. The fibrils are also more widely spaced in the deeper layers of cartilage. Although this is an idealized conception and the fibrils of cartilage are not all ordered so precisely, the concept is still useful in visualizing the fundamental interaction of the fibrils with other constituents of cartilage. The collagen fibrils anchor into the subchondral bone layer after traversing the calcified cartilage, which is demarcated by a change in staining properties called the tidemark line. The anchoring of these fibrils into bone is analogous to the continuation of the ligamentous attachments into bone, called Sharpey's fibers.

ment creates a small pore size, which has been calculated by McCutchen (11) to be about 6 nm. The largest molecule that can traverse a pore of this dimension is hemoglobin. Small ions and glucose, for example, easily traverse these pores, but larger molecules such as most proteins and hyaluronan (hyaluronic acid) do not enter cartilage in significant amounts under normal conditions.

Collagen fibers in the intermediate layers are no longer oriented tangentially to the surface, but rather are directed obliquely or randomly. They are larger than the surface fibrils, with most ranging between 40 and 100 nm. The deepest fibrils are the largest in cartilage. They are disposed perpendicularly relative to the joint surface. They perforate the calcified basal layers of cartilage through the tidemark regions and eventually enter the subchondral bone layer, where they are attached firmly, much as in the case of attachment of Sharpey's fibers of ligament to cortical bone. This feature is crucial for cartilage to be able to resist shearing forces that would otherwise tend to peel cartilage away from the subchondral surface.

It has been well demonstrated clinically that loss of the densely packed collagen mat at the surface of cartilage in weight-bearing regions is the prelude to fibrillation, accelerated wear, and ensuing degenerative arthritis. This seems completely logical, because the coarse, widely spaced fibrils in deeper layers that are oriented principally vertically are poorly suited to constraining the swelling forces generated by the matrix proteoglycans. The term *fibrillation* describes the tendency of these fibrils to be split vertically all the way to their subchondral attachment, much as wood splits along the grain of its fibers. The villus-like strands so exposed collectively resemble a shag rug, and the individual strands are prone to tear off at the base when mechanically loaded and exposed to shear stresses. The armor plate term applies well to the normal surface mat of collagen fibrils, and loss of this layer no longer permits the cartilage to function as a pressurized unit suited to weight bearing.

Evidence supporting the fibril pattern of collagen orientation derives from several types of observation, including routine histology, transmission electron microscopy, scanning electron microscopy, and the demonstration of Hultkrantz lines (12). Hultkrantz lines are typically observed on the surface of cartilage and are analogous to the Langer lines of skin (13). These lines become visible when the surface of cartilage is pricked with a pin. The puncture defects are best demonstrated by coating the cartilage surface with India ink and then wiping it dry. Hultkrantz observed many years ago that the puncture holes appeared as slits rather than round holes. The slits have axes that are generally perpendicular to the principal axis of movement of the joint. Hultkrantz lines are therefore different for each joint of the body. Mechanical tensile tests have confirmed that the Hultkrantz lines indicate the preferred orientation of the collagen fibrils at the surface of the joint resist tensile forces, and Bullough and Goodfellow have shown this characteristic of joint surfaces in experiments illustrated in Color Plate 4 (14). The pattern of matrix and cellular organization of articular cartilage is described in greater detail in a review by Wong and Hunziker (10).

Collagen Chemistry

The molecular structure of collagen has been of considerable interest for more than a century because it is the principal structural protein by mass for all mammals. It constitutes 65% to 80% of the mass by dry weight of such specialized connective tissues as tendons, ligaments, skin, joint capsules, and cartilage. It is the only protein with significant tensile force-resisting properties with the exception of elastin, whose functional role is quite different. Collagen is the key protein in musculoskeletal stability, providing the mechanical properties imparting the "connect" to connective tissue.

The tensile force–resisting properties of cartilage derive from the precise molecular configuration of the collagen macromolecule. This molecule is one of the largest in the body, forming a rodlike structure that is 300 nm in length and 1.5 nm in diameter. These rods are called tropocollagen (15). They are assembled in a three-dimensional array in the extracellular environment, and they are influenced by environmental stresses and additional biologic factors in a way that is not fully understood. The sum of the extracellular influences somehow affects the orientation and size of fibrils that are assembled from the tropocollagen units (15–19). The tropocollagen assembly typically has a quarter-stagger pattern (see Chapter 3).

The α chains are not identical among species or within a single species. Early data on mammalian skin collagen demonstrated two types, α_1 and α_2, in a ratio of 2:1 (15). Miller and Matukas (20) were the first to show that cartilage possesses a collagen different in composition from that in most fibrous connective tissues. This collagen contains a different type of α_2 chain, which they called α_2, type II. The collagen in most cartilages consists of three such identical chains and the abbreviated nomenclature used is $(\alpha_1 [II])_3$, or type II collagen (21).

More than 16 types of collagen have been described in vertebrates. The collagens can be divided into two major classes on the basis of their primary structure and supramolecular assembly: the fibril-forming collagens and the non–fibril-forming collagens. The fibril-forming collagens include types I, II, III, V, and XI (22). Each of these types has a long central triple-helical domain without any interruptions in the Gly-X-Y sequence, where X and Y are amino acids. The rest of the collagens belong to the non–fibril-forming class. Although they vary in size, they share the feature of having imperfections in the Gly-X-Y sequence. Within this class, type IX, XII, and XIV collagens form a subgroup called the fibril-associated collagens with interrupted triple helices (FACITs). They are associated with type I or II collagen fibrils and play a role in the interaction of these fibrils with other matrix components. Although their sizes and primary structures vary, they share several common structural features. Type XVI collagen appears to be a member of this group (23). (A summary of the makeup and distribution of the collagen types currently accepted is provided in several review articles [22–25]). A chart classifying the various collagens is provided in Chapter 3.

The significance of the type II collagen to cartilage is unknown. The principal differences between this collagen and the more common type I found in fibrous connective tissue are in the number of hydroxylysine molecules and the presence of a small number of residues of cysteine. The type II fibrils are thinner near the articular surface and the tangential zone than in the deeper zones, and the collagen concentration is greater at the surface. Evidence is being accumulated that type IX collagen and type XI make critical contributions to the organization and mechanical stability of the type II collagen fibrillar network (Fig. 8.3).

Type IX collagen makes up approximately 10% of the collagen protein in fetal mammalian articular cartilage, but the amount decreases to about 1% in adult tissue. The molecule also is categorized as a proteoglycan because it was originally demonstrated in chicks that there exists a single site for attachment of chondroitin sulfate on the type IX collagen molecule. Type IX is also characterized by the presence of four globular domains in the triple-helix structure (26). In bovine articular cartilage, type IX collagen is found on the surface of type II collagen and appears to be linked covalently to at least one molecule of the type II collagen triple helix (26). From this evidence, it is believed that type IX provides a covalent interface between the surface of type II collagen fibril and the interfibrillar proteoglycan domain. Another theory is that type IX collagen provides interfibrillar linkages between type II fibrils and therefore may enhance the mechanical stability of the fibrillar network.

Type XI collagen makes up about 3% of mature articular cartilage collagen. It has a single globular domain on one end of the triple helix and is located within the type II collagen fibrils (21) (Fig 8.3). Other fibrous collagens found in articular cartilage are type VI and type X; each has a short helix. Type X collagen is found only in hypertrophic zones of growth plates.

Type VI collagen has a globular domain on each end (21). Type VI is unique in that it has no aldehyde crosslink and has arginine–glycine–aspartic acid (RGD) sequences in each α chain, sequences that are important in cell attachment (27). It is known to bind to hyaluronan (28) and to fibronectin (29) and has been identified in the perilacunar matrix surrounding chondrocytes.

The fundamental process of formation of collagen by the chondroblasts and chondrocytes is nearly identical to the process of synthesis by the fibroblast and fibrocyte. The general steps in synthesis are outlined in Chapter 3. The collagen turnover in cartilage proceeds at a rate not unlike that seen in connective tissue of the fibrous type. Because significant collagen synthesis occurs in adult cartilage, it is clear that control processes for spatial orientation of the product, although poorly understood, are of crucial importance.

It is a source of frustration to surgeons and their patients that attempts to achieve cartilage repair, as in surgical arthroplasty, do not successfully regenerate cartilage and seldom produce completely satisfactory clinical results. A major factor contributing to failure of cartilage regeneration is that the collagen fiber architecture of

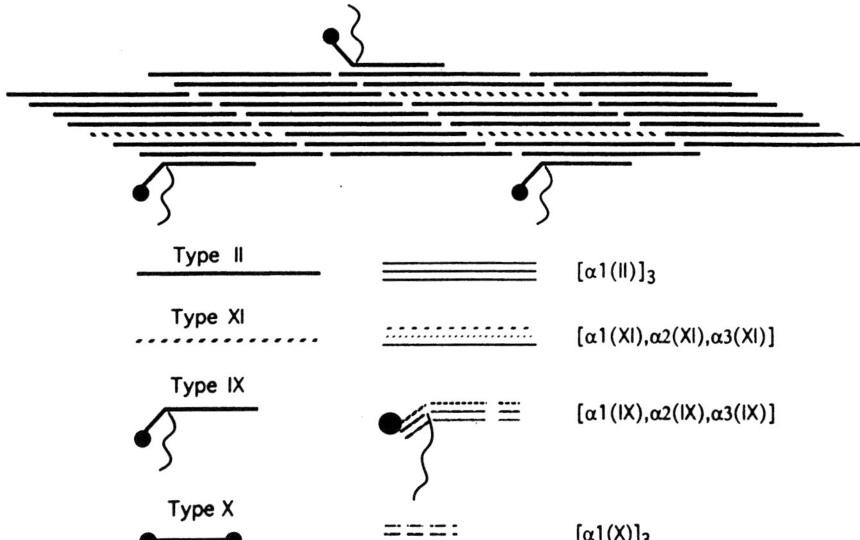

FIGURE 8.3. Collagens of articular cartilage. The assembly of tropocollagen II units into fibers and fibrils in cartilage is controlled in part by the minor collagens. Type IX collagen is a surface molecule that binds to type II and to itself. Its side arms interfere with further growth of the fiber by steric interference with addition of more type II molecules. Type XI collagen is located in the core of the fiber and is thought also to be important in determining ultimate fiber size. Type XI occurs in largest quantities in small fibers. Type X collagen is found in growth plate cartilage, not in articular cartilage. (From Cremer MA, Rosloniec EF, Kang AH. The cartilage collagens: a review of their structure, organization, and role in the pathogenesis of experimental arthritis in animals and in human rheumatic disease. *J Mol Med* 1998;76: 275–288, with permission.)

the arthroplasty repair tissue is disordered throughout the deep layers and lacks the membranelike characteristics so important to the surface layer of articular cartilage. Details of the biology of the cartilage repair process are described later in this chapter.

Collagen Crosslinks

Stabilization of collagen occurs extracellularly after its assembly into the quarter-stagger arrays that make up filaments, fibrils, and fibers. The stabilization and ultimate tensile strength of the fiber structure are thought to result mainly from the development of intramolecular and intermolecular crosslinks. The former occur between α chains of the individual tropocollagen molecule; the latter occur between adjacent tropocollagen molecules. The crosslinks result from enzyme-mediated reactions involving mainly lysine and hydroxylysine. The details of the bifunctional, trifunctional, or quadrafunctional crosslinks so created are beyond the scope of this discussion but are presented briefly in Chapter 3 and are available in detail in several reviews (30–39).

PROTEOGLYCANS OF ARTICULAR CARTILAGE

The proteoglycans of articular cartilage serve as the "pump" of the highly pressurized cartilage system. The characteristics of the proteoglycan molecules that permit this crucial function include their very large size and resulting immobility within the collagen fibril meshwork; their densely concentrated, fixed, negative charges; and the large number of hydroxyl groups. These characteristics collectively serve to attract water and small positively charged ions into the cartilage. This is called the *Donnan osmotic pressure*. The negative charges on the proteoglycan molecules naturally create repulsive forces between each other that are called *chemical expansive stresses*. The sum of the Donnan osmotic pressure and the chemical expansive stress constitutes the cartilage swelling pressure (17). Ogston (5) observed the rough equivalence of the pressure within articular cartilage with "motor tyre pressure!"

The extraordinary size of the proteoglycan aggregate molecules of articular cartilage is achieved by supra-assembly of three types of linear chain molecular species: sulfated glycosaminoglycans, a core protein, and hyaluronan, which is a nonsulfated glycosaminoglycan. The following section briefly describes the chemical structure of the functionally vital proteoglycan and its aggregate and illustrates the manner in which the functional role derives from the chemical structure.

Glycosaminoglycans

Figure 8.4 shows the disaccharide-repeating unit for the glycosaminoglycans of articular cartilage: chon-

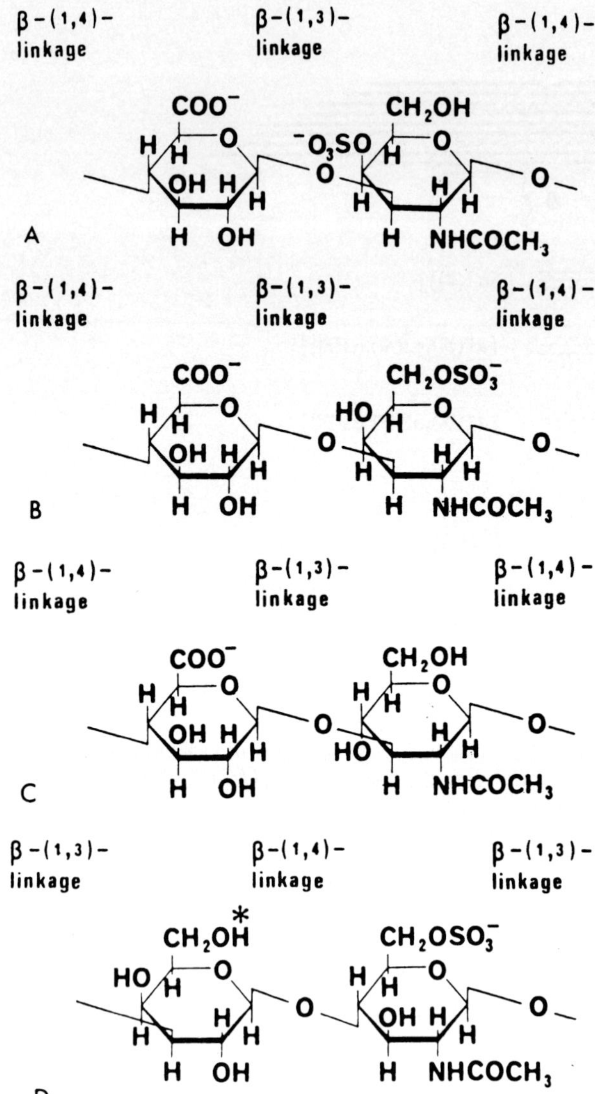

FIGURE 8.4. Disaccharide configuration of the principal glycosaminoglycans of the proteoglycan constituents of articular cartilage. **A:** The molecular configuration of chondroitin-4-sulfate differs from that of chondroitin-6-sulfate only in the location of the sulfate group on the hexosamine molecule. Both contain alternating glucuronic acid and galactosamine sugars. **B:** Chondroitin-6-sulfate. **C:** Hyaluronan is a disaccharide that contains alternating molecules of glucosamine and glucuronic acid but lacks a sulfate group. **D:** Keratan sulfate is a disaccharide that contains galactose rather than a uronic acid moiety. The hexosamine is glucosamine that is sulfated in the C6 position.

droitin-4-sulfate, chondroitin-6-sulfate, hyaluronan, and keratan sulfate. In most of the glycosaminoglycan molecules, hexosamine alternates with another sugar polymerized in a repeating, disaccharide pattern. The predominance of the amine group in this configuration is the reason for the use of *amino* in the term glycosaminoglycan. The common features of the group are obvious at first glance. In particular, the location of the *N*-acety-

lamine group at the number two carbon (C2) of the hexosamine is common to all the disaccharides shown. The hexosamine is galactosamine in three of the four cases; keratan sulfate possesses glucosamine as the alternating hexosamine. All except hyaluronan are sulfated at the C4 or C6 position of the hexosamine. Each disaccharide contains at least three hydroxyl groups. All except keratan sulfate contain uronic acid as the second element of the disaccharide, with a carboxyl terminus at C6. Keratan sulfate possesses galactose rather than uronic acid as the second half of the disaccharide (17).

Aggrecan

The glycosaminoglycans are covalently bound to core protein to form aggrecan in a structure that locates keratan sulfate side arms preferentially close to the linkage region to hyaluronan. The keratan sulfate–rich region of the aggrecan protein polysaccharide is illustrated in Color Plate 5 (following page 122). The keratan sulfate molecules characteristically are of lower molecular weight than the chondroitin sulfate chains. The core protein molecule has three globular domains: G1, G2, and G3. The G1 region is the point of attachment of proteoglycan to hyauronan to create aggregate, G2 is located near the keratan sulfate–rich region, and G3 is located at the opposite terminal end of the core protein (40). Phosphorylation of serine residues occurs adjacent to the chondroitin sulfate–containing peptides of the core protein (41).

Aggregate

The ability of proteoglycan to aggregate further by combining with hyaluronan was originally described by Hardingham and Muir (42), who elaborated on the dissociation and association experiments of Sajdera and Hascall (43) to establish the mechanism of formation of aggregate. Much attention has been given to the degree of aggregate formation in various tissues and in various pathologic conditions (44–48). The ability of the proteoglycan molecule to form aggregates of even greater molecular size amplifies its physiologic functional properties as the "pump" of the articular cartilage system (see Color Plate 5, Fig. 8.5).

Lohmander (49) stated that the molecular mass of aggregate is 100 to 200 million daltons, whereas for a common protein such as insulin, the molecular mass is only 6,000 daltons. Because of its much greater size, the aggregate formed can impose even greater fixation of the proteoglycan molecules, locking them more securely within the interstices of the collagen framework of the tissue and ensuring fixation of the negative charges needed to maintain swelling pressure for expansion of the articular cartilage matrix.

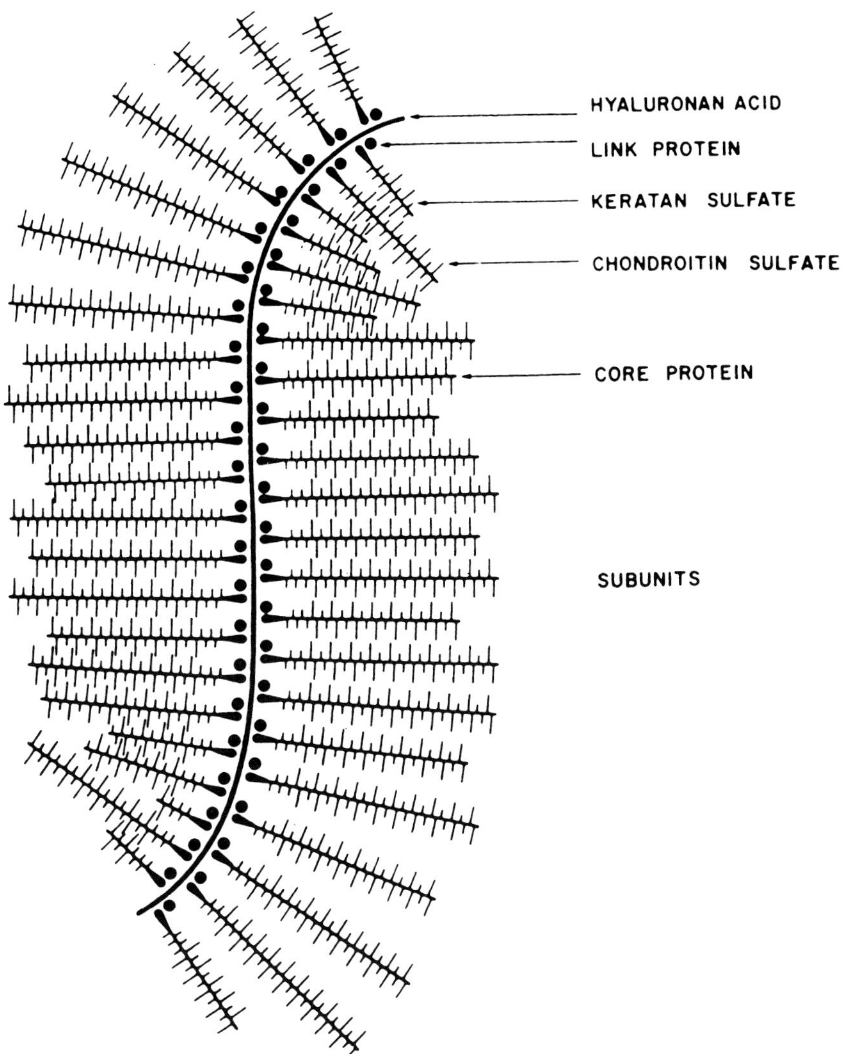

FIGURE 8.5. Aggregate molecule. The aggregate is expanded from the single unit seen in Color Plate 5 (following page 122) to its more fully expanded state in which dozens of aggrecan molecules are linked to the hyaluronan linear chain. The spectacular augmentation in molecular mass from the original glycosaminoglycan mass of approximately 50,000 daltons produces aggrecan with a molecular mass in the millions and an aggregate with a molecular mass of many millions. (From Rosenberg L. Structure of cartilage proteoglycan. In: Simon WH, ed. *The human joint in health and disease.* Philadelphia: University of Pennsylvania Press, 1978, with permission.)

Nature of the Aggregate Linkage

The linkage of proteoglycan subunit, aggrecan, to hyaluronan is noncovalent, in distinction to the covalent linkage of glycosaminoglycans to core protein in aggrecan. The aggregate linkage is facilitated and strengthened by low molecular weight proteins called link proteins (50–54). The linkage can occur without the presence of a link protein, but such proteins have been found in all cartilages examined. The noncovalent linkage of aggrecan and hyaluronan can be dissociated by concentrated solutions of guanidinium hydrochloride, calcium chloride, or magne-

sium chloride (42,43,55–60). The dissociated components can be reassociated by the reduction of the concentration of the dissociative solvents. Under conditions of about 0.5 *M* guanidinium hydrochloride, the three elements—hyaluronan, link protein, and aggrecan—reassociate to form the aggregate again. This process has been the key technique in unraveling the chemical structure of aggrecan and aggregate, in understanding the nature of their association, and in deciphering the role of link proteins. Cartilages from different sources possess differing percentages of aggregation of proteoglycan, but factors controlling this process are not fully understood.

Small Proteoglycans of Articular Cartilage

Small proteoglycan molecules consisting of biglycan, decorin, and fibromodulin represent about 5% of the proteoglycan of articular cartilage. Dermatan sulfate proteoglycans were first observed in articular cartilage by Rosenberg et al. in 1985 (61). The small proteoglycans each consist of a protein core and glycosaminoglycan chain branches. The core protein of the small proteoglycans is only a fourth the length of the core protein of aggrecan and is closely similar in the three molecules. The horseshoe-shaped protein is linked near the open end by a disulfide bond. The glycosaminoglycan side chains are limited in number, consisting of a single chondroitin sulfate–dermatan sulfate side chain in decorin, two such chains in biglycan, and as many as four keratan sulfate side chains in the case of fibromodulin (61–63). Decorin (64) and fibromodulin (65) are located in the superficial zones of articular cartilage in association with collagen fibers. Smaller amounts of decorin are found in deeper cartilage layers (65). Biglycan (65) and decorin (66) are found in the pericellular lacunar regions of chondrocytes.

The small proteoglycans have critical functional roles. Decorin and fibromodulin are associated with collagen fibers. However, decorin inhibits type I and II collagen formation (67–69), and fibromodulin inhibits collagen fibrillogenesis (70). Biglycan and decorin possess properties of competitive binding with transforming growth factor-β (TGF-β), thereby inhibiting the role of this growth factor on repair processes in cartilage (71,72). Because TGF-β is considered the "conductor of the symphony" in connective tissue repair (27), the modulation of its role by biglycan and decorin has great significance in the control of connective tissue repair processes. Decorin and biglycan also bind with other adhesion proteins, including fibronectin (73,74), thrombospondin (75), and type VI collagen (76). Each of these so-called adhesion proteins has the RGD amino acid sequences originally described by Ruoslahti and Pierschbacher (27) as playing key roles in cell adhesion. Decorin or biglycan binding to the adhesion proteins inhibits the cellular attachment of fibroblasts, another key step in the control of connective tissue healing (74). These small proteoglycan roles are most certainly relevant to the questions of limitations of repair potential of articular cartilage. The adhesion proteins—fibronectin, type VI collagen, and thrombospondin—have complex roles in binding to collagen (27,77) and serve to bridge between cells and matrix (27,78), between themselves (79), and to hyaluronan (28). These molecules undoubtedly possess functional roles far greater than quantitative measures of their content in connective tissue matrix suggest, and their functional roles must be understood more completely to provide a comprehensive understanding of normal articular cartilage as well as its repair processes. Facilitation of biologic repair of articular cartilage by surgical procedures may not be made any more feasible by this understanding, given the complexity of the processes involved, but it is unlikely to be achieved without such understanding.

FLUID OF ARTICULAR CARTILAGE

As described in the air tent analogy, the inflation medium of articular cartilage is synovial fluid, which is essentially an ultrafiltrate of plasma plus hyaluronan. The hyaluronan molecules are too large to enter cartilage through its 6-nm diameter surface pores, but most of the remaining ions and molecules of normal synovial fluid, such as water, sodium, potassium, and glucose, are sufficiently small enough to pass through these pores easily (11,80). Movement of fluid into and out of cartilage occurs to some extent by diffusion, but diffusion does not seem adequate itself to provide for cartilage health. The percentage of water in cartilage ranges from more than 60% to nearly 80% (81–83). The water is bound by a variety of weak forces, such as hydrogen bonding to proteoglycan and collagen or simple hydration shell formation, but it is relatively mobile.

Net flow into and out of cartilage is induced by the normal weight-bearing function of synovial joints. Maroudas calculated that, for normal articular cartilage, the sum of swelling pressures is greatly exceeded (10 times) by loading conditions such as walking (84,85). The implications seem to be that cartilage under loading conditions would be compressed rapidly and completely, much as a wet sponge is compressed by weight. However, the rate of fluid movement permitted by the small pore size and the cartilage microarchitecture is sufficiently slow enough that cartilage is compressed only partially, even after loading for hours. The experiments of Linn and Sokoloff illustrate this point well (86–88). These investigators used an apparatus designed to fit into a centrifuge capable of forcing fluid out of cartilage into a receptacle (Fig. 8.6). The cartilage fits into a porous basketlike container into which a plunger rests. The unit is placed into a centrifuge, and the faster the centrifuge revolves, the greater the pressure on the cartilage in the basket. In this way, the effect of varying loads over various periods on the rate of fluid expression from cartilage can be evaluated. These experiments showed that the amount of fluid that can be expressed (about 30%) is extremely small in relation to the total water content. Subsequent experiments by Linn (87) using an animal joint demonstrated the processes of fluid movement in cartilage more directly. The device constructed for this experiment was called an arthrotripsometer (Fig. 8.7). By developing the necessary design criteria, it was possible to vary loading conditions with respect to amplitude of load and to stationary versus cyclic conditions. The joint was immersed in synovial fluid during testing. Deformation versus time is seen to

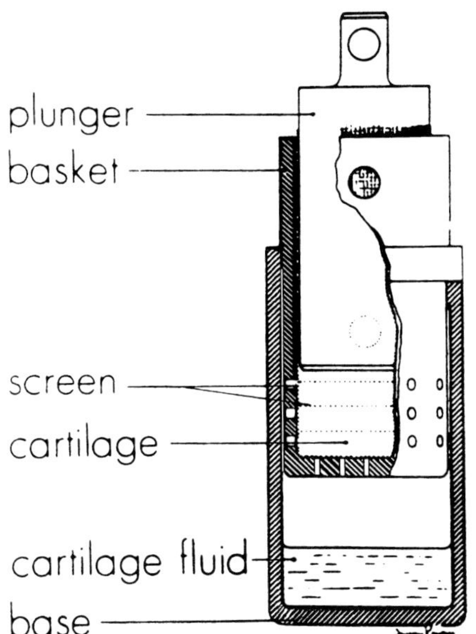

FIGURE 8.6. The device, used by Linn and Sokoloff to express fluid from articular cartilage, consists of a perforated basket within a centrifuge collecting system. A plunger within the basket effectively compresses cartilage at the bottom of the basket when the system is spun in the centrifuge. Time and pressure can be controlled by the duration and speed of the centrifuge operation. This technique permits the amount and composition of cartilage fluid expressed to be analyzed. (From Linn FC, Sokoloff LH. Movement and composition of interstitial fluid of cartilage. *Arthritis Rheum* 1965;8:481, with permission.)

be greater for stationary than for cyclic loads. The explanation for this observation is that, in the cyclic condition, partial recovery occurs because of the effect of swelling pressure in pulling fluid back into cartilage during the phase of the cycle when the cartilage is unloaded. This unparalleled system of load bearing by articular cartilage depends for its effectiveness on functional integrity and detailed interaction of each of the architectural, biomechanical, and biochemical elements within the system. Details of viscoelastic properties of articular cartilage, including Poison's ratio and compressive modulus, are concisely summarized in several reviews (85,89–92).

The fluid movement that occurs during the loading process appears to be important for lubrication of the joint surfaces and for load carriage. On the basis of calculations obtained from complex mathematical models, Mow et al. (89,93) proposed that fluid is expressed out of cartilage in front of the advancing contact surfaces of cartilage. This process provides a fluid film that minimizes cartilage–cartilage contact and therefore minimizes wear. If this analysis is correct, we walk on water.

Cartilage nutrition and metabolism issues are beyond the scope of this chapter. However, it is notable that the cellular population of articular cartilage is sparse and the metabolic domain of a single chondrocyte is huge. Hunziker and associates (10,94,95) calculated the volume of matrix that must be maintained by a single chondrocyte to be 180,000 mμ^3. Given the turnover of matrix components at a level not dissimilar to that of other connective tissues, the miracle of articular cartilage continues to amaze all students of the subject.

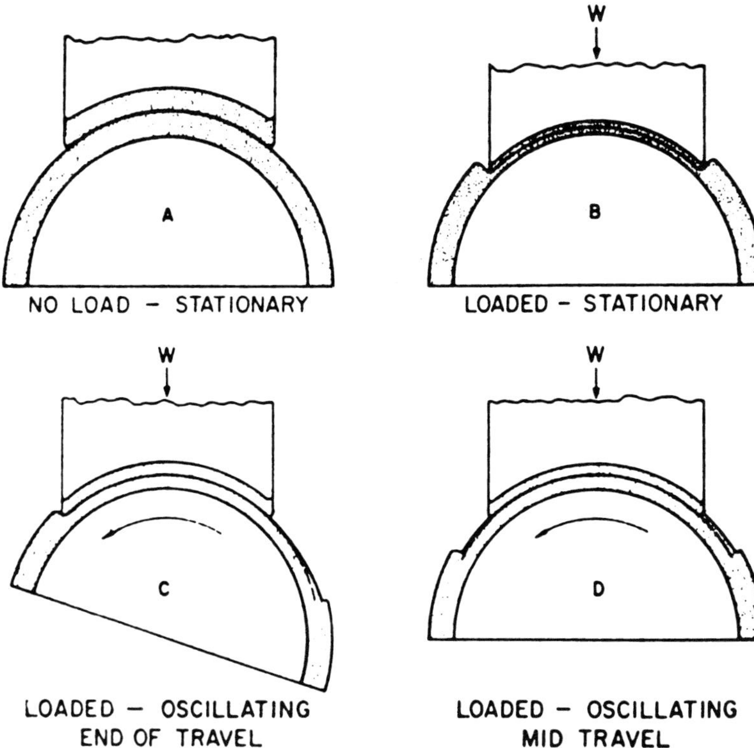

FIGURE 8.7. This figure demonstrates the effect of loading on articular cartilage. A stationary load *(B)* produces significant compression after some time, but when oscillation occurs using the same loading condition, the compressive effect for a given time is considerably less. Because the cartilage is unloaded for a portion of the time, it resorbs some of the fluid that had been expressed. (From Linn FC. Lubrication of animal joints. *J Bone Joint Surg Am* 1967; 49:1079, with permission.)

CARTILAGE HEALING

It is generally agreed that intrinsic healing of cartilage lesions does not occur (1,96–98). There may be a response of the chondrocyte to injury, but the response does not result in cartilage repair. The obvious example is seen in degenerative arthritis (e.g., degenerative joint disease, osteoarthrosis, osteoarthritis) in which chondrocytes often form clones of cells in an attempt to repair damaged surfaces and demonstrate an increased rate of synthesis of matrix components (99–106). However, the synthesized components are not retained within the matrix, and newly synthesized components such as proteoglycans are reduced in concentration despite the increased rate of synthesis. Linear incisions created on articular cartilage surfaces remain indefinitely in reported experimental studies on mammalian joints. Efforts at surgical reconstruction of articular defects therefore have shifted focus to allografts or cartilage autografts developed from cultured cells. These techniques are addressed in Chapter 14.

Historically, most surgical attempts at cartilage healing called on exposure of marrow cells to mount a repair response. This was achieved by subchondral bone resection (e.g., cup arthroplasty) or drilling or abrasion of the subchondral plate (1,3,107–112). When examined histologically a few days after surgery, the response to injury mounted by primitive marrow cells produces an outgrowth of a granulation type tissue (1) (see Color Plate 6, following page 122). This cellular response consists, for the most part, of immature vascular cells, fibroblasts, and macrophages. With time, there is maturation of the surface into fibrocartilage provided that the surface is protected from compressive and shear forces in the early repair stages (see Color Plate 7, following page 122).

The fibrocartilage so formed is remarkably different from hyaline articular cartilage. The fibrocartilage surface is deficient in the precise morphology and composition of normal articular cartilage documented earlier in this chapter. The cells of fibrocartilage vary in shape from place to place in the matrix, occasionally are seen as round cells in a lacunalike structure, but tend more commonly to be spindle shaped (1) (see Color Plates 7–9, following page 122). The fibrous matrix lacks the precise morphology of arcades in the deeper layers and packing of thin, parallel fiber organization at the surface, and it is not anchored securely into the subchondral plate. Strikingly, the proteoglycan content is only a fraction of that of normal articular cartilage (1,113,114). Not surprisingly, this reconstituted surface is not an efficient load-bearing organ. Mechanical tests performed on experimental arthroplasty surfaces show a resistance to compression of only one third of that of normal articular cartilage (2,115–117). As a result, the durability of regenerated arthroplasty surfaces of this type is limited, and the fibrocartilage surface is gradually worn away (1,113,118–120) (see Color Plates 8 and 9, following page 122).

The consequence of the unsatisfactory outcome of the biologic healing response was the relatively rapid abandonment of procedures such as cup arthroplasty of the hip in the late 1960s and early 1970s in favor of total-hip replacement constructs using artificial components. Similarly, arthroscopic débridement of degenerative knee joints using abrasion techniques on exposed bone to stimulate fibrocartilage formation is presently applied principally as a temporizing procedure to defer total-knee replacement.

A related problem encountered surgically is the localized osteochondral defect exemplified by osteochondritis dissecans of the knee or ankle. Frequently, the necrotic fragment with its overlying cartilage is damaged or displaced and is not suitable for replacement and fixation in the cavity from which it originated. In such cases, the surgeon is confronted with a defect of sufficient size to jeopardize long-term survival of the joint because of incongruity of the opposing surfaces. Formerly, this defect was "repaired" by curettage of the cavity and drilling the base of the exposed bone. The expectation was that the cavity would be filled with repair tissue and a new surface would be regenerated. The rationale for this approach was partially derived from small animal experimental studies indicating that drill holes in articular cartilage could heal. The model commonly used in such experiments was the rabbit knee joint in which a 1- to 2-mm drill hole was created, penetrating the subchondral plate. However, the absolute geometry of the larger defects in the human knee—often 2 cm in diameter—respond quite differently from the response seen in the size of defects studied in the small animal models. Experiments performed in large animals represent a more realistic model. The experiments of Convery and Akeson in 1970 (120) on the horse's knee, in which defects of 1.5 to 2.5 cm in diameter were created, demonstrated grossly imperfect healing in all cases (see Color Plate 10, following page 122). Other studies confirmed the limitation of healing of large osteochondral defects (117,121). Such results motivated the search for more realistic solutions to the osteochondritis dissecans lesion in humans such as allografting. Some of the newer surgical approaches to this question are reviewed in Chapter 14.

The implication of the evolving knowledge of normal articular cartilage is the recognition of its phenomenal genius as a biologically engineered construct. It follows that all the evolving surgical attempts at reconstruction are faced with the daunting challenge of the precise requirements of articular cartilage replication. Normal articular cartilage remains the exacting benchmark against which all new therapeutic concepts must be measured. The evolving efforts seeking a biologic solution to repair are exciting, but it is clear that the hurdles remaining are large and the race to the ultimate biologic solution has just begun.

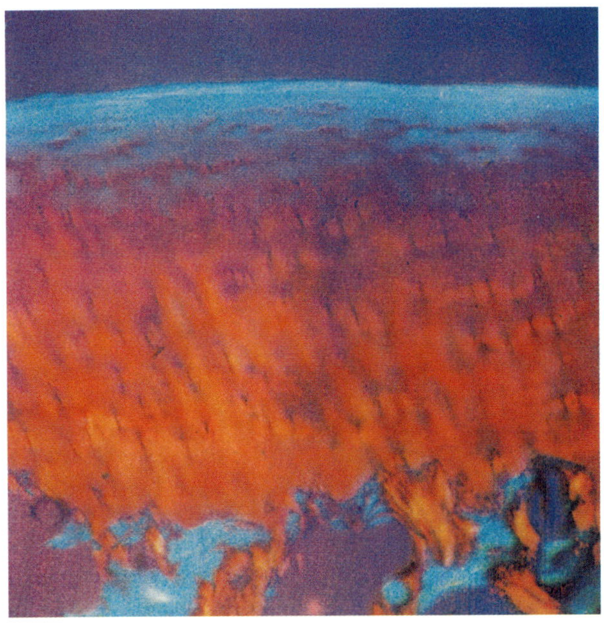

COLOR PLATE 4. This is a ×45 photograph of articular carti-lage under polarized light microscopy. The preferred tangential orientation of the collagen fibrils at the surface creates refractile differences from the deeper layers and is seen on the photograph as a *bright line*. (From Bullough P, Goodfellow J. The significance of the fine structure of articular cartilage. *J Bone Joint Surg Br* 1968;50:852–827, with permission.)

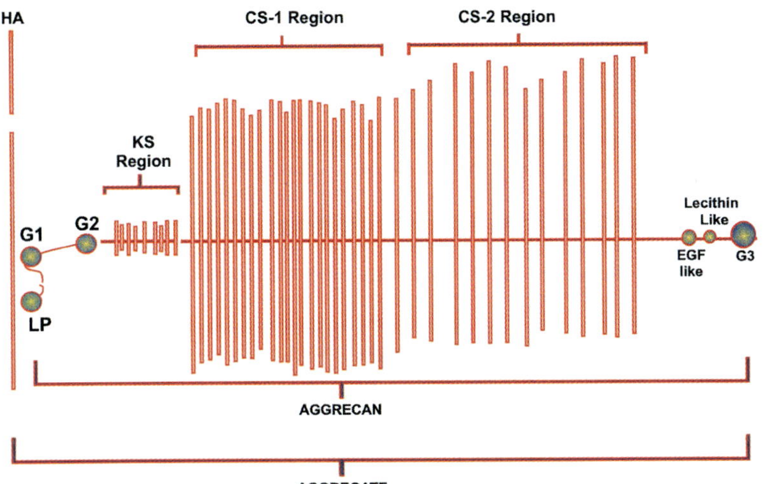

COLOR PLATE 5. Aggregate molecule. The diagram shows the assem-bly of chondroitin sulfate (CS-1 and CS-2, not drawn to scale) and keratan sulfate molecules onto a protein-core linear structure that becomes fixed to hyaluronan by specialized G1 and link protein regions. The various spe-cialized linkage regions are composed of highly specific molecular config-urations. The core protein and its polysaccharide side chains (i.e., aggre-can) attach to hyaluronan to create the aggregate structure. There is typically a high concentration of keratan sulfate with its smaller number of disaccharide units near the attachment site of the core protein to hyaluro-nan. There are usually twice as many molecules in these regions as shown.

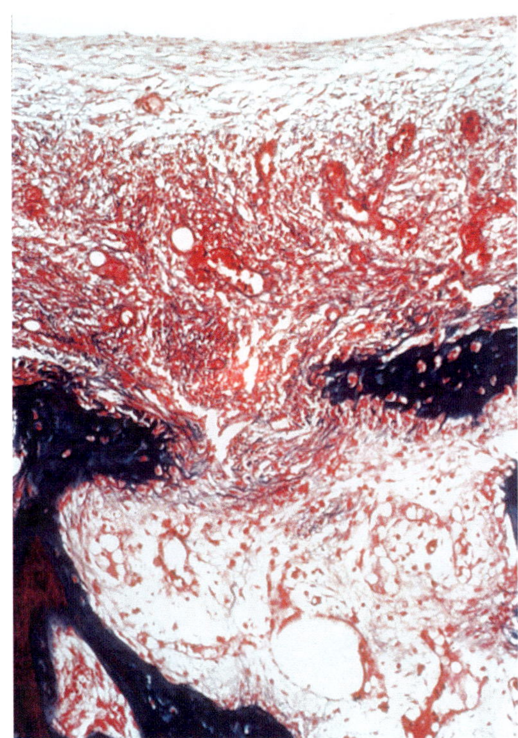

COLOR PLATE 6. Photomicrograph of femur head 10 days after a cup arthroplasty procedure (Masson trichrome stain, original magnification ×80). The hip was denuded of cartilage and sub-chondral bone, and a vitallium cup was placed between the head of the femur and the acetabulum. Grossly and histologically, the tissue at this stage was obviously very soft and highly vascular. The repair tissue has all the characteristics of granula-tion tissue typical of soft tissue repair at other sites. The proliferative response is derived from primitive cellular elements in the subchondral bone marrow.

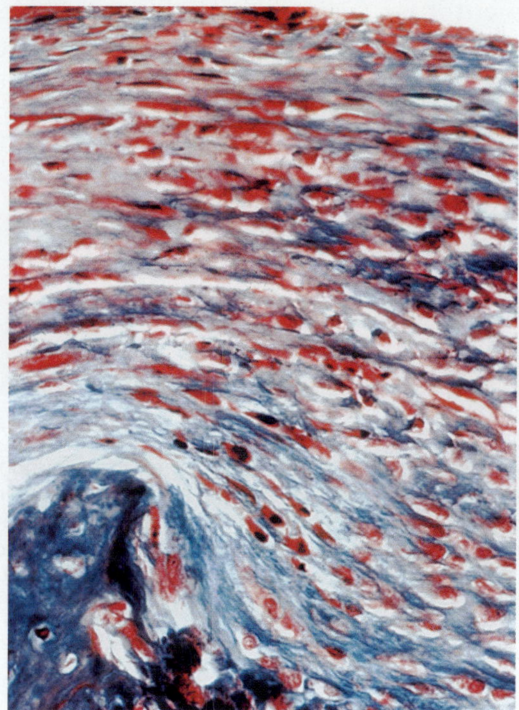

COLOR PLATE 7. Photomicrograph of the canine femur head 1 month after a cup arthroplasty procedure was performed as described in Color Plate 6 (Masson trichrome stain, original magnification ×120). Cellular elements in the non–load-bearing area shown have survived and have undergone metaplasia into fibrocartilage. Notice the coarse nature of the collagen architecture, which has little resemblance to the fibrous architecture of normal articular cartilage. Nothing resembling the architecture of normal hyaline cartilage was seen in this model. Notably, there is only sparse metachromasia. Metachromatic staining indicates glycosaminoglycan or aggrecan molecules in the tissue. This type of repair response is typical of that seen after abrasion arthroplasty or its variants. Such tissue has poor load-bearing characteristics (125).

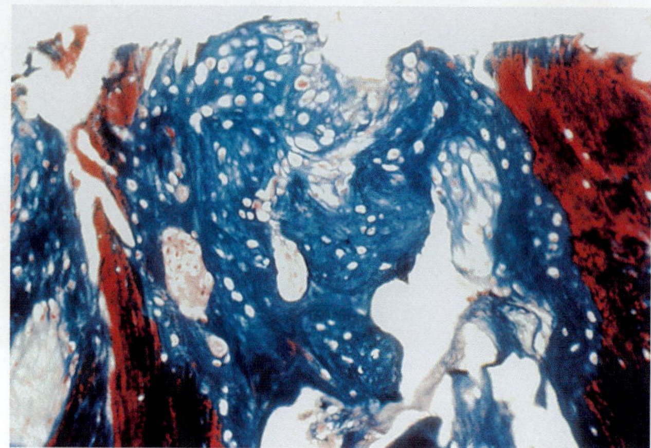

COLOR PLATE 8. Photomicrograph of canine femur head 4 months after a cup arthroplasty procedure was performed, as described in Color Plate 6 (Masson trichrome stain, original magnification ×120). The section is from the superior weight-bearing surface. The repair elements that had grown out from the underlying marrow have been worn away by contact with the opposing surface. Below the surface, between trabecular bone struts, is residual repair tissue. Fibrocartilagelike cells at that site are surrounded by matrix that stains metachromatically. The fiber pattern of the matrix appears random rather than highly ordered. The failure of the repair surface is related to its poor load-bearing characteristics and is predicted by its low proteoglycan content and disordered fiber pattern.

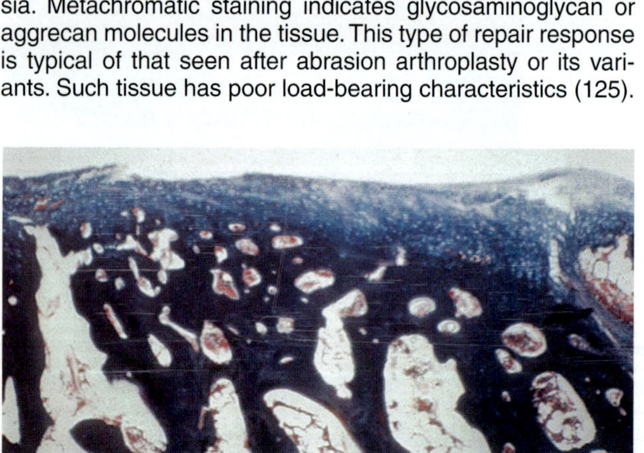

COLOR PLATE 9. Photomicrograph of canine head femur 4 months after a cup arthroplasty procedure was performed, as described in Color Plate 6 (Masson trichrome stain, original magnification ×120). Section is from the inferior non–weight-bearing surface. Fibrocartilaginous cells are seen in lacunae, and metachromasia is evident. However, the surface thickness is irregular, and delamination has occurred through the upper and middle zones of the repair surface. Such tissue does not tolerate even nominal weight bearing over extended periods. Biochemical measures of this surface show hexosamine content to be only one third of normal; hexosamine measures are often used as a rough index of glycosaminoglycan content (1).

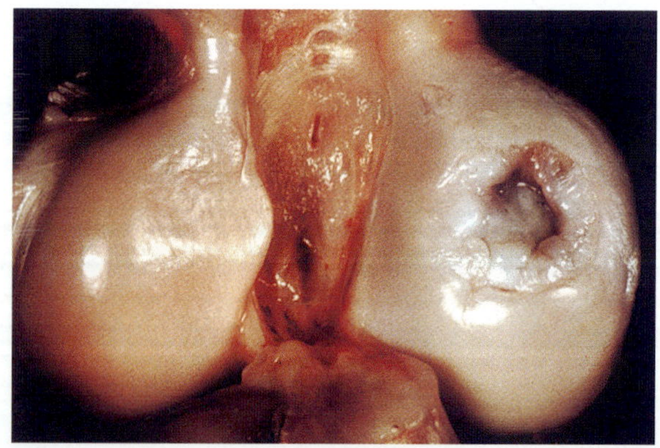

COLOR PLATE 10. Photograph of horse knee 4 months after drilling 4-mm and 2-cm full-thickness defects in the medial femoral condyle. The experiment illustrates the futility of drilling the base of an osteochondritis defect with the expectation of complete repair. Although the 4-mm defect is difficult to see 4 months later (superior and medial to the larger defect), the 2-cm defect has achieved only partial filling. The repair tissue (irregular outline) that does survive is present only at the margin, is fibrocartilaginous, and could not be expected to perform effectively as a functional weight-bearing surface. Therefore, allografting and mosaicplasty techniques are preferred over simple drilling procedures for osteochondritis dissecans lesions when primary healing has failed.

REFERENCES

1. Akeson WH, Miyashita C, Taylor TK, et al. Experimental arthroplasty of the canine hip. Extracellular matrix composition in cup arthroplasty. *J Bone Joint Surg Am* 1969;51:149–164.
2. Coletti JM Jr, Akeson WH, Woo SL. A comparison of the physical behavior of normal articular cartilage and the arthroplasty surface. *J Bone Joint Surg Am* 1972;54:147–160.
3. Mankin H. Current concepts review. The response of articular cartilage to mechanical injury. *J Bone Joint Surg Am* 1982;64:460–466.
4. Akeson W, Amiel D, Gershuni D. Articular cartilage physiology and metabolism. In: Resnick D, ed. *Diagnosis of bone and joint disorders*. Philadelphia: WB Saunders, 1994:23–31.
5. Ogston A. The biological functions of the glycosaminoglycans. In: Balazs E, ed. *Chemistry and molecular biology of the intercellular matrix,* vol 3. London: Academic Press, 1970:1231.
6. Benninghoff A. Form und bau der gelenkknorpel in ihren beziehungen zur funktion. *Z Anat Entwicklungsgesch* 1925;76:43.
7. Weiss C, Rosenberg L, Helfet AJ. An ultrastructural study of normal young adult human articular cartilage. *J Bone Joint Surg Am* 1968;50: 663–674.
8. Clark JM. The organization of collagen in cryofractured rabbit articular cartilage: a scanning electron microscopic study. *J Orthop Res* 1985;3:17–29.
9. Little K, Pimm L, Trueta J. Osteoarthritis of the hip: an electron microscope study. *J Bone Joint Surg Br* 1958;40:123.
10. Wong M, Hunziker E. Articular cartilage biology and mechanics. *Sports Med Arthrosc Rev* 1998;6:4–12.
11. McCutchen C. The frictional properties of animal joints. *Wear* 1962;5:1.
12. Hultkrantz W. Uber die spaltrichtungen der gelenkknorpel. *Verh Anat Ges* 1898;12:248.
13. Langer C. Zur anatomie und physiologie der haut. *Sitzungsb K Acad Wissensch* 1861;45:223.
14. Bullough P, Goodfellow J. The significance of the fine structure of articular cartilage. *J Bone Joint Surg Br* 1968;50:852–857.
15. Piez KA. Characterization of a collagen from codfish skin containing three chromatographically different alpha chains. *Biochemistry* 1965; 4:2590–2596.
16. Mayne R. Preparation and applications of monoclonal antibodies to different collagen types. *Clin Biochem* 1988;21:111–115.
17. Mathews MB. Connective tissue. Macromolecular structure and evolution. *Mol Biol Biochem Biophys* 1975;19:1–318.
18. Eyre DR. The specificity of collagen cross-links as markers of bone and connective tissue degradation. *Acta Orthop Scand Suppl* 1995; 266:166–170.
19. Amiel D, Billings EJ, Akeson W. Ligament structure, chemistry and physiology. In: Daniel DM, Akeson WH, O'Connor JJ, eds. *Knee ligaments: structure, function, injury and repair*. New York: Raven Press, 1990:77–91.
20. Miller EJ, Matukas VJ. Chick cartilage collagen: a new type of alpha 1 chain not present in bone or skin of the species. *Proc Natl Acad Sci U S A* 1969;64:1264–1268.
21. Eyre DR, Wu JJ. Collagen structure and cartilage matrix integrity. *J Rheumatol Suppl* 1995;43:82–85.
22. van der Rest M, Garrone R. Collagen family of proteins. *FASEB J* 1991;5:2814–2823.
23. Pan TC, Zhang RZ, Mattei MG, et al. Cloning and chromosomal location of human alpha 1(XVI) collagen. *Proc Natl Acad Sci U S A* 1992; 89:6565–6569.
24. Cremer MA, Rosloniec EF, Kang AH. The cartilage collagens: a review of their structure, organization, and role in the pathogenesis of experimental arthritis in animals and in human rheumatic disease. *J Mol Med* 1998;76:275–288.
25. Prockop DJ. What holds us together? Why do some of us fall apart? What can we do about it? *Matrix Biol* 1998;16:519–528.
26. van der Rest M, Mayne R. Type IX collagen proteoglycan from cartilage is covalently cross-linked to type II collagen. *J Biol Chem* 1988; 263:1615–1618.
27. Ruoslahti E, Pierschbacher MD. New perspectives in cell adhesion: RGD and integrins. *Science* 1987;238:491–497.
28. McDevitt CA, Marcelino J, Tucker L. Interaction of intact type VI collagen with hyaluronan. *FEBS Lett* 1991;294:167–170.
29. McDevitt D, Francois P, Vaudaux P, et al. Identification of the ligand-binding domain of the surface-located fibrinogen receptor (clumping factor) of *Staphylococcus aureus*. *Mol Microbiol* 1995;16:895–907.
30. Piez KA. Cross-linking of collagen and elastin. *Annu Rev Biochem* 1968;37:547–570.
31. Kang AH, Gross J. Relationship between the intra and intermolecular cross-links of collagen. *Proc Natl Acad Sci U S A* 1970;67:1307–1314.
32. Gallop PM, Blumenfeld OO, Seifter S. Structure and metabolism of connective tissue proteins. *Annu Rev Biochem* 1972;41:617–672.
33. Tanzer ML, Fairweather R, Gallop PM. Isolation of the crosslink, hydroxymerodesmosine, from borohydride-reduced collagen. *Biochim Biophys Acta* 1973;310:130–136.
34. Tanzer MLT, Housley L, Berube R, et al. Structure of two histidine-containing crosslinks from collagen. *J Biol Chem* 1973;248:393–402.
35. Vuorio E, de Crombrugghe B. The family of collagen genes. *Annu Rev Biochem* 1990;59:837–872.
36. Wu JJ, Eyre DR. Cartilage type IX collagen is cross-linked by hydroxypyridinium residues. *Biochem Biophys Res Commun* 1984; 123:1033–1039.
37. Wu JJ, Eyre DR. Identification of hydroxypyridinium cross-linking sites in type II collagen of bovine articular cartilage. *Biochemistry* 1984;23:1850–1857.
38. Wu JJ, Lark MW, Chun LE, et al. Sites of stromelysin cleavage in collagen types II, IX, X, and XI of cartilage. *J Biol Chem* 1991;266: 5625–5628.
39. Wu JJ, Eyre DR. Structural analysis of cross-linking domains in cartilage type XI collagen. Insights on polymeric assembly. *J Biol Chem* 1995;270:18865–18870.
40. Yanagishita M. Function of proteoglycans in the extracellular matrix. *Acta Pathol Jpn* 1993;43:283–293.
41. Anderson RS, Schwartz ER. Phosphorylation of proteoglycans. Identification of phosphorylation sites in chondroitin sulfate-rich region of core protein. *Arthritis Rheum* 1985;28:804–812.
42. Hardingham TE, Muir H. The specific interaction of hyaluronic acid with cartilage proteoglycans. *Biochim Biophys Acta* 1972;279:401–405.
43. Sajdera SW, Hascall VC. Protein-polysaccharide complex from bovine nasal cartilage. A comparison of low and high shear extraction procedures. *J Biol Chem* 1969;244:77–87.
44. Gregory JD. Multiple aggregation factors in cartilage proteoglycan. *Biochem J* 1973;133:383–386.
45. Hascall VC, Sajdera SW. Protein-polysaccharide complex from bovine nasal cartilage. The function of glycoprotein in the formation of aggregates. *J Biol Chem* 1969;244:2384–2396.
46. Hascall VC, Heinegard D. Aggregation of cartilage proteoglycans. II. Oligosaccharide competitors of the proteoglycan-hyaluronic acid interaction. *J Biol Chem* 1974;249:4242–4249.
47. Hascall VC, Heinegard D. Aggregation of cartilage proteoglycans. I. The role of hyaluronic acid. *J Biol Chem* 1974;249:4232–4241.
48. Heinegard D, Hascall VC. Aggregation of cartilage proteoglycans. 3. Characteristics of the proteins isolated from trypsin digests of aggregates. *J Biol Chem* 1974;249:4250–4256.
49. Lohmander S. Proteoglycans of joint cartilage. Structure, function, turnover and role as markers of joint disease. *Baillieres Clin Rheumatol* 1988;2:37–62.
50. Buckwalter JA, Rosenberg LC, Tang LH. The effect of link protein on proteoglycan aggregate structure. An electron microscopic study of the molecular architecture and dimensions of proteoglycan aggregates reassembled from the proteoglycan monomers and link proteins of bovine fetal epiphyseal cartilage. *J Biol Chem* 1984;259: 5361–5363.
51. Fife RS, Myers SL. Evidence for an interaction between canine synovial cell proteoglycans and link proteins. *Biochim Biophys Acta* 1985;843:238–244.
52. Fife RS. Identification of link proteins and a 116,000-Dalton matrix protein in canine meniscus. *Arch Biochem Biophys* 1985;240:682–688.
53. Choi HU, Tang LH, Johnson TL, et al. Proteoglycans from bovine nasal and articular cartilages. Fractionation of the link proteins by wheat germ agglutinin affinity chromatography. *J Biol Chem* 1985;260:13370–13376.
54. Fife RS, Caterson B, Myers SL. Identification of link proteins in canine synovial cell cultures and canine articular cartilage. *J Cell Biol* 1985;100:1050–1055.
55. Rosenberg LC, Pal S, Buckwalter JA. Structural changes related to malignancy in proteoglycans from cartilage neoplasms. *J Med Sci Ala* 1980;17:283–292.
56. Campo RD, Tourtellotte CD. The composition of bovine cartilage and bone. *Biochim Biophys Acta* 1967;141:614–624.
57. Buckwalter JA, Pita JC, Muller FJ, et al. Structural differences

between two populations of articular cartilage proteoglycan aggregates. *J Orthop Res* 1994;12:144–148.

58. Hedlund H, Hedbom E, Heinegard D, et al. Association of the aggrecan keratan sulfate-rich region with collagen in bovine articular cartilage. *J Biol Chem* 1999;274:5777–5781.

59. Roughley PJ, Lee ER. Cartilage proteoglycans: structure and potential functions. *Microsc Res Tech* 1994;28:385–397.

60. Poole AR, Rizkalla G, Ionescu M, et al. Osteoarthritis in the human knee: a dynamic process of cartilage matrix degradation, synthesis and reorganization. *Agents Actions Suppl* 1993;39:3–13.

61. Rosenberg LC, Choi HU, Tang LH, et al. Isolation of dermatan sulfate proteoglycans from mature bovine articular cartilages. *J Biol Chem* 1985;260:6304–6313.

62. Roughley PJ, White RJ. Dermatan sulphate proteoglycans of human articular cartilage. The properties of dermatan sulphate proteoglycans I and II. *Biochem J* 1989;262:823–827.

63. Fisher LW, Termine JD, Young MF. Deduced protein sequence of bone small proteoglycan I (biglycan) shows homology with proteoglycan II (decorin) and several nonconnective tissue proteins in a variety of species. *J Biol Chem* 1989;264:4571–4576.

64. Poole AR, Webber C, Pidoux I, et al. Localization of a dermatan sulfate proteoglycan (DS-PGII) in cartilage and the presence of an immunologically related species in other tissues. *J Histochem Cytochem* 1986;34:619–625.

65. Poole AR, Rosenberg LC, Reiner A, et al. Contents and distributions of the proteoglycans decorin and biglycan in normal and osteoarthritic human articular cartilage. *J Orthop Res* 1996;14:681–689.

66. Roughley PJ, White RJ, Cs-Szabo G, et al. Changes with age in the structure of fibromodulin in human articular cartilage. *Osteoarthritis Cartilage* 1996;4:153–161.

67. Vogel KG, Fisher LW. Comparisons of antibody reactivity and enzyme sensitivity between small proteoglycans from bovine tendon, bone, and cartilage. *J Biol Chem* 1986;261:11334–11340.

68. Vogel KG, Meyers AB. Proteins in the tensile region of adult bovine deep flexor tendon. *Clin Orthop* 1999;(367Suppl):S344–S355.

69. Vogel K, Paulson M, Heinegaard R. Specific inhibition of type I and type II collagen fibrillogenesis by the small proteoglycan of tendon. *Biochem J* 1984;223:587–597.

70. Scott J. Proteoglycan-fibrillar collagen interactions. *Biochem J* 1988;252:313–323.

71. Yamaguchi Y, Mann D, Ruoslahti E. Negative regulation of transforming growth factors by the proteoglycan decorin. *Nature* 1990;346:381–384.

72. Ruoslahti E. Proteoglycans in cell regulation. *J Biol Chem* 1989;264:13369–13372.

73. Winnemoller M, Schmidt G, Kresse H. Influence of decorin on fibroblast adhesion to fibronectin. *Eur J Cell Biol* 1991;54:10–17.

74. Lewandowska K, Choi HU, Rosenberg LC, et al. Fibronectin-mediated adhesion of fibroblasts: inhibition by dermatan sulfate proteoglycan and evidence for a cryptic glycosaminoglycan-binding domain. *J Cell Biol* 1987;105:1443–1454.

75. Winnemoller M, Schon P, Vischer P, et al. Interactions between thrombospondin and the small proteoglycan decorin: interference with cell attachment. *Eur J Cell Biol* 1992;59:47–55.

76. Bidanset DJ, Guidry G, Rosenberg LC, et al. Binding of the proteoglycan decorin to collagen type VI. *J Biol Chem* 1992;267:5250–5256.

77. Watkins SC, Lynch GW, Kane LP, et al. Thrombospondin expression in traumatized skeletal muscle. Correlation of appearance with post-trauma regeneration. *Cell Tissue Res* 1990;261:73–84.

78. Marcelino J, McDevitt CA. Attachment of articular cartilage chondrocytes to the tissue form of type VI collagen. *Biochim Biophys Acta* 1995;1249:180–188.

79. Bornstein P. Diversity of function is inherent in matricellular proteins: an appraisal of thrombospondin 1. *J Cell Biol* 1995;130:503–506.

80. Maroudas A. Transport of solutes through cartilage: permeability to large molecules. *J Anat* 1976;122:335–347.

81. Eichelberger L, Akeson W, Roma M. Biochemical studies of articular cartilage. 1. Normal values. *J Bone Joint Surg* 1958;40:142.

82. Mankin HJ, Thrasher AZ. Water content and binding in normal and osteoarthritic human cartilage. *J Bone Joint Surg Am* 1975;57:76–80.

83. Jaffe FF, Mankin HJ, Weiss C, et al. Water binding in the articular cartilage of rabbits. *J Bone Joint Surg Am* 1974;56:1031–1039.

84. Maroudas A, Bullough P, Swanson SA, et al. The permeability of articular cartilage. *J Bone Joint Surg Br* 1968;50:166–177.

85. Maroudas A. Biophysical chemistry of cartilaginous tissues with special reference to solute and fluid transport. *Biorheology* 1975;12:233–248.

86. Linn F, Sokoloff L. Movement and composition of interstitial fluid of cartilage. *Arthritis Rheum* 1965;8:481.

87. Linn FC. Lubrication of animal joints. I. The arthrotripsometer. *J Bone Joint Surg Am* 1967;49:1079–1098.

88. Linn FC, Radin EL. Lubrication of animal joints. 3. The effect of certain chemical alterations of the cartilage and lubricant. *Arthritis Rheum* 1968;11:674–682.

89. Mow VC, Wang CC, Hung CT. The extracellular matrix, interstitial fluid and ions as a mechanical signal transducer in articular cartilage. *Osteoarthritis Cartilage* 1999;7:41–58.

90. Mow VC, Ateshian GA, Spilker RL. Biomechanics of diarthrodial joints: a review of twenty years of progress. *J Biomech Eng* 1993;115:460–467.

91. Mow VC, Ratcliffe A, Poole AR. Cartilage and diarthrodial joints as paradigms for hierarchical materials and structures. *Biomaterials* 1992;13:67–97.

92. Nordin M, Frankel V. *Basic biomechanics of the musculoskeletal system.* Philadelphia: Lea & Febiger, 1989.

93. Mow VC, Holmes MH, Lai WM. Fluid transport and mechanical properties of articular cartilage: a review. *J Biomech* 1984;17:377–394.

94. Hunziker EB, Herrmann W. In situ localization of cartilage extracellular matrix components by immunoelectron microscopy after cryotechnical tissue processing. *J Histochem Cytochem* 1987;35:647–655.

95. Hunziker EB, Wagner J, Studer D. Vitrified articular cartilage reveals novel ultra-structural features respecting extracellular matrix architecture. *Histochem Cell Biol* 1996;106:375–382.

96. Mankin HJ. The response of articular cartilage to mechanical injury. *J Bone Joint Surg Am* 1982;64:460–466.

97. Hunziker EB. Articular cartilage repair: are the intrinsic biological constraints undermining this process insuperable? *Osteoarthritis Cartilage* 1999;7:15–28.

98. DePalma AF, McKeever CD, Subin DK. Process of repair of articular cartilage demonstrated by histology and autoradiography with tritiated thymidine. *Clin Orthop* 1966;48:229–242.

99. Mankin HJ, Laing PG. Protein and ribonucleic acid synthesis in articular cartilage of osteoarthritic dogs. *Arthritis Rheum* 1967;10:444–450.

100. Mankin HJ, Lippiello L. Biochemical and metabolic abnormalities in articular cartilage from osteo-arthritic human hips. *J Bone Joint Surg Am* 1970;52:424–434.

101. Mankin HJ. The reaction of articular cartilage to injury and osteoarthritis (second of two parts). *N Engl J Med* 1974;291:1335–1340.

102. Mankin HJ. The reaction of articular cartilage to injury and osteoarthritis (first of two parts). *N Engl J Med* 1974;291:1285–1292.

103. Mankin HJ. Biochemical changes in articular cartilage in osteoarthritis. In: *Symposium on osteoarthritis.* St. Louis: Mosby, 1976:1–22.

104. Mankin HJ. Alterations in the structure, chemistry, and metabolism of the articular cartilage in osteoarthritis of the human hip. *Hip* 1982:126–145.

105. Buckwalter J, Mankin H. Articular Cartilage. Part II: Degeneration and osteoarthrosis, repair, regeneration and transplantation. *J Bone Joint Surg* 1997;79:612.

106. Cheung HS, Lynch KL, Johnson RP, et al. In vitro synthesis of tissue-specific type II collagen by healing cartilage. I. Short-term repair of cartilage by mature rabbits. *Arthritis Rheum* 1980;23:211–219.

107. Insall JN. Intra-articular surgery for degenerative arthritis of the knee. A report of the work of the late K. H. Pridie. *J Bone Joint Surg Br* 1967;49:211–228.

108. Insall J. The Pridie debridement operation for osteoarthritis of the knee. *Clin Orthop* 1974;101:61–67.

109. Magnuson P. Technique for debridement of the knee joint for arthritis. *Surg Clin North Am* 1946;24:249.

110. Gomar-Sancho F, Gastaldi Orquin E. Repair of osteochondral defects in articular weightbearing areas in the rabbit's knee. The use of autologous osteochondral and meniscal grafts. *Int Orthop* 1987;11:65–69.

111. Shapiro F, Koide S, Glimcher MJ. Cell origin and differentiation in the repair of full-thickness defects of articular cartilage. *J Bone Joint Surg Am* 1993;75:532–553.

112. Sprague NFD. Arthroscopic debridement for degenerative knee joint disease. *Clin Orthop* 1981;160:118–123.

113. Wei X, Gao J, Messner K. Maturation-dependent repair of untreated osteochondral defects in the rabbit knee joint. *J Biomed Mater Res* 1997;34:63–72.

114. Wei X, Messner K. Maturation-dependent durability of spontaneous cartilage repair in rabbit knee joint. *J Biomed Mater Res* 1999;46:539–548.
115. Nelson BH, Anderson DD, Brand RA, et al. Effect of osteochondral defects on articular cartilage. Contact pressures studied in dog knees. *Acta Orthop Scand* 1988;59:574–579.
116. Wayne JS, Woo SL, Kwan MK. Finite element analyses of repaired articular surfaces. *Proc Inst Mech Eng [H]* 1991;205:155–162.
117. Landells J. The reaction of injured human articular cartilage. *J Bone Joint Surg Br* 1957;39:548.
118. Ghadially FN, Ghadially JA, Oryschak AF, et al. Experimental production of ridges on rabbit articular cartilage: a scanning electron microscope study. *J Anat* 1976;121:119–132.
119. Mitchell N, Shepard N. The resurfacing of adult rabbit articular cartilage by multiple perforations through the subchondral bone. *J Bone Joint Surg Am* 1976;58:230–233.
120. Convery FR, Akeson WH, Keown GH. The repair of large osteochondral defects. An experimental study in horses. *Clin Orthop* 1972;82:253–262.
121. Ghadially JA, Ghadially R, Ghadially FN. Long-term results of deep defects in articular cartilage. A scanning electron microscope study. *Virchows Arch B Cell Pathol* 1977;25:125–136.
122. Rosenberg L. Structure of cartilage proteoglycan. In: Simon WH, ed. *The human joint in health and disease.* Philadelphia: University of Pennsylvania Press, 1978.
123. Linn FC, Sokoloff LH. Movement and composition of interstitial fluid of cartilage. *Arthritis Rheum* 1965;8:481.
124. Linn FC. Lubrication of animal joints. *J Bone Joint Surg Am* 1967;49:1079.
125. Akeson WH, Miyashita C, Taylor T, et al. Experimental arthroplasty of the canine hip: extracelllar matrix composition in cup arthroplasty. Kappa Delta Award Paper. *J Bone Joint Surg* 1969;51A:149–164.

CHAPTER 9

Joint Mechanoreceptors and Knee Function

Tom Hogervorst and Richard A. Brand

Joints are functional units (1,2) consisting of bone, articular surfaces, capsule, ligaments, muscles, aponeuroses, insertions, vascularization, and innervation. With the exception of cartilage, each of these tissues contains neurosensory endings. Ligaments, capsule, and supporting muscle contain nerve endings in the form of mechanoreceptors and free nerve endings.

The study of form and function of the nerve endings can be viewed in three complementary ways (3). The first concerns morphologic classification of the distinctive receptor types (i.e., taxonomy). The second concerns neurophysiologic characterization of the receptors, particularly in relation to taxonomy, including identification of the type of sensory information and the way it is represented in the afferent nerve fiber (e.g., impulse sequence). The third describes the functional significance of the receptors, including signal processing in the central nervous system and its effect on normal movement and alterations with aging, injury, or disease. Light and electron microscopy provide morphologic distinctions, and although newer imaging modalities (e.g., immunohistochemistry) help resolve old issues, new questions arise. New information challenges previous neurophysiologic characterization of the receptors, and definitive clarification of issues will require adaptation of existing technologies or development of new technologies.

The functional significance of receptors (i.e., the information we require clinically) is far less well understood than the morphologic distinctions of the receptors and the physiology of their stimulation. Experiments that can determine the functional significance of knee ligament receptors are difficult to devise. The main reason is the lack of tools to study individual receptors or receptor populations *in vivo*. For example, anterior cruciate ligament (ACL) transection alters knee kinematics (4,5) and most likely induces a change in stimulation and output of the remaining mechanoreceptors of the knee (e.g., mechanoreceptors in intact ligaments and the joint capsule) (6). In view of the large number (7,8) and substantial sensitivity

(9–11) of periarticular receptors, an experimental design explicitly excluding effects from the remaining receptors of the knee is critical to determine the function and significance of loss of ACL receptors alone. This usually means the experiment has to be conducted under artificial conditions in animals, which in itself limits the conclusions for normal human movement. Clearly, we do not have the tools to study the human (central) nervous system during movement. New tools are needed for collecting and interpreting new data. For collecting, new tools to detect *in vivo* neural signals locally, noninvasively, and with rapid response and high spatial resolution are needed. For interpreting, new software and new techniques from computer science and mathematics are needed (12). Despite these difficulties, a body of literature provides substantial information on ligament mechanoreceptors.

Although the presence of joint mechanoreceptors was recognized more than 100 years ago (13–16), most investigators focused on the joint capsule, and not until the 1950s were mechanoreceptors documented in the knee ligaments. Compared with other structures of the knee such as the patellar ligament (17) and posterior joint capsule (9,18), the knee ligaments contain a relatively small number of receptors.

The knowledge of mechanoreceptors in knee ligaments (18–20) resulted in presumptions regarding their function (21–23). Most hypotheses suggested mechanoreceptors served as sensors in reflex arcs influencing motor function in a direct manner. However, only indirect effects of mechanoreceptors in knee ligaments have been convincingly demonstrated (22).

In recent years, the role of mechanoreceptors in the ACL has attracted considerable attention. The relatively high incidence of cruciate ligament injuries, the resulting functional deficits, and the potential for reconstruction explain this interest. However, the neurosensory role of ligaments also relates to questions of cruciate ligament removal or retention in prosthetic knee surgery, particularly with expanding indications for knee arthroplasty in younger persons.

Ascertaining the role of mechanoreceptors in the function of knee ligaments is important for future directions in joint reconstruction. This is true for ligament injuries and prosthetic knee replacement. The functional significance of ligament and other periarticular mechanoreceptors, or lack thereof, determines in part whether future efforts should be directed more toward preservation of the ligament receptors or should remain on purely mechanical and kinematic aspects of joint function.

ANATOMY

Most early investigators of articular neuroanatomy considered ligaments as largely passive joint stabilizers and directed their efforts mainly toward the joint capsule. Although some investigators did recognize the innervation of ligaments, mechanoreceptors in ligaments were not specified (24–27). The first report on knee ligament mechanoreceptors also reflects this view, as Boyd, in 1954, reported ligament mechanoreceptors as an incidental finding when he studied the posterior joint capsule in a cat: "In one case the [capsule] specimen included part of one of the cruciate ligaments, and this contained typical tendon organs of Golgi" (28). Soon after, several reports appeared on mechanoreceptors in the knee ligaments (18,29,30), most of them concerning anatomic studies in the cat. Since the work of Boyd, Skoglund, and others during the 1950s, the cat has become the animal used most for animal experiments. Most researchers assume similarity of the neuroanatomy and neurophysiology of joint receptors in cats and humans, although few have specifically addressed this point (31–33). Only in the last two decades, knee ligament innervation was documented in humans, first with conventional histologic techniques (34) and then with electron microscopy (19) and finally with immunohistochemistry (35).

Anatomic studies suggest a new paradigm for interpreting joint neuroanatomy. In this view, muscle, tendon, ligament, and bone (insertion) are interpreted as one continuous structure, with its components organized "in series." Mechanoreceptors would be predicted at the interfaces between the components where stress is distributed (2,36). This is in agreement with the observation of several anatomic studies that most mechanoreceptors are found near the origin or insertion of ligaments (Tables 9.1, 9.2) and at the muscle–tendon interface (37). The

TABLE 9.1. *Mechanoreceptors in the cat anterior cruciate ligament*

Author, method	Receptor / Receptor types	Total number size (μm)	Location in ligament	Afferent in ligament	fiber (μm)
Boyd (1954), nonserial sections, gold chloride[a]	1 type: Golgi tendon organ	500 × 125	2	Near capsule	12
Skoglund (1956), nonserial sections, gold chloride	1 type: Golgi tendon organ	800 × 300	Not reported	On surface	10–15
Freeman and Wyke (1967), silver and gold chloride, serial sections (insertions not studied?)	2 types: Type III: Golgi-like	100 × 600	"several"	Close to both insertions	14–16
	Type IV: free nerve endings	0.5–1.5	"large numbers"	Mostly superficial	1–5
Sjölander et al. (1989), 20-μm longitudinal serial sections, gold chloride including insertions	4 types: Golgi-like Ruffini Pacini Free nerve endings	Not reported	Not reported	Subsynovial or close to insertions	Not reported
Koch et al. (1995), 70-μm longitudinal serial sections, gold chloride, including insertions	2 types (Freeman and Wyke) Type III: Golgi-like	100 × 600	1–3	Mid-substance	Not reported
	Free nerve endings	Not reported	Not reported	Not reported	Not reported
Gómez-Barrena et al. (1996), (50-μm serial sections, wheat germ agglutinin-horseradish peroxidase of spinal ganglia (retrograde tracer study)	Not applicable	Not applicable	13–52 labeled neurons in spinal ganglia	Not applicable	Not reported
Madey et al. (1997), 20–50-μm longitudinal serial sections, wheat germ agglutinin–horseradish peroxidase (anterograde tracer study)	2 types: Ovoid ending	100	5–17	"Along entire length of ligament"	Not reported
	Large ending	1000–1500	1–3	"In body of each ligament"	Not reported

[a]Insertions not studied.

The posterior joint capsule was studied with observation of ACL receptors as an accidental finding: "In one case the [capsule] specimen included part of one of the cruciate ligaments, and this contained typical tendon organs of Golgi."

TABLE 9.2. *Mechanoreceptors in the human anterior cruciate ligament*

Author, method	Receptor types	Receptor size (µm)	Total number	Location in ligament	Afferent fiber (µm)
Kennedy et al. (1982), silver nitrate, nonserial sections	1 type: Free nerve endings[a]	Not reported	Not reported	Tibial origin or synovia	Not reported
Schultz et al. (1984), gold chloride serial sections	2 types (Freeman and Wyke):				
	Type III: Golgi-like	200 × 75	1–3	On surface	Not reported
	Free nerve endings	Not reported	Not reported	On surface	Not reported
Zimny et al. (1986), 100-µm transverse serial sections, gold chloride	3 types:		"2.5% of total ligament area"	All types: (tibial) insertion and subsynovial	
	Ruffini	Not reported			Not reported
	Pacini	Not reported			Not reported
	Free nerve endings	Not reported			Not reported
Schutte et al. (1987), 100-µm transverse serial sections, gold chloride	4 types:		"1% of total ligament area"	All types: tibial insertion substance or subsynovial	
	2 types of Ruffini	Not reported			Not reported
	Pacini (most frequent)	Not reported			Not reported
	Free nerve endings	Not reported			Not reported
Halata and Haus (1989), electron microscopy	3 types:				
	Ruffini	Not reported	Not reported	Subsynovial	4–6
	Pacini	Not reported	Not reported	Subsynovial	4–8
	Free nerve endings	Not reported	Not reported	Subsynovial	2
Haus and Halata (1990), transverse, glycolmethacrylate, nonserial sections	3 types:				
	Ruffini	=120	9[b]	Interfascicular	3–5
			12[b]	Subsynovial	3–5
	Pacini	=150	5[b]	Subsynovial	Not reported
	Free nerve endings	Not reported	Not reported		Not reported
Amir et al. (1994), 40-µm gold chloride, serial sections	4 types:		3–6% of peri-ligamentous tissue	All types: only in periligamentous tissue	
	2 types of Ruffini	Not reported			Not reported
	Pacini	Not reported			Not reported
	Free nerve endings	Not reported			Not reported
Sparmann et al. (1996) monoclonal antibody	Not reported	Not reported	1–9	Nearest femoral insertion	Not reported
Krauspe et al. (1995), monoclonal antibody, 1 specimen	2 types:				
	Ruffini	60 × 120	15	Subsynovial and near insertions	Not reported
	Free nerve endings	Not reported	Not reported	Not reported	Not reported

[a]Golgi-like receptor reported for posterior cruciate ligament only.
[b]Number of receptors found in a total of 21 anterior cruciate ligament specimens.

conventional distinction between muscle and joint receptors, based on a view of "parallel" organization of joint components, is obsolete in this concept. The same is true for the related discussions of whether joint or muscle receptors are the primary afferents of proprioception (38,39) and whether ligaments contain Golgi tendon organs or Ruffini receptors.

Innervation of the Knee Joint and Its Ligaments

The gross innervation of the human knee has been described in detail (25,26,40,41), but these descriptions do not specify innervation of the knee's ligamentous structures. A detailed description of the variability of human articular nerves is lacking, and most information on innervation of ligaments is still based on animal studies.

Innervation of deeper structures of the knee, such as the joint capsule, menisci, and ligament, is mainly through the posterior, medial, and lateral articular nerves. However, terminal branches from muscle nerves also reach the joint capsule and adjacent structures. Considerable variability exists between species and different nerves. This variability also applies to the innervation of ligaments. Not only is the geography and pattern of nerves variable (40,42,43), but also the number of nerve endings per ligament (17,20,44). In the dog, for example, the posterior articular nerve could not be found in 8 of 18 animals (42), whereas it was reported as the most constant and largest of the articular nerves in the cat (18). Ultimately, these anatomic factors can lead to considerable differences between individuals in the degree of neurologic damage that accompanies a ligament rupture. The precise role of various receptors may vary from individual to individual, and mechanoreceptor loss or failure to adapt from redundant sources may prove more critical in some patients than others.

Medial Aspect of the Knee Joint

The medial side of the knee joint is innervated through four terminal branches of the femoral nerve and the saphenous nerve, itself a branch of the femoral nerve (40,41). After perforating the vastus musculature the femoral nerve sends branches to the ventral side of the joint, the most important of which is the medial femoral cutaneous nerve, ending in the prepatellar plexus. The saphenous nerve divides, most often inside Hunter's canal, in the medial articular nerve, the infrapatellar ramus, and a terminal branch that innervates the medial side of the foot (40). The medial articular nerve innervates the medial joint capsule, the medial meniscus, and the medial collateral ligament (18,42). Innervation of the cruciate ligaments through the medial articular nerve has also been shown in cats and dogs. The infrapatellar ramus innervates the medial and anterolateral skin distal to the patella and the patella ligament. Terminal branches of the nerve to the vastus medialis, also called the medial retinacular nerve, enter the superomedial knee capsule and innervate the medial collateral ligament (40).

Lateral Aspect of the Knee Joint

The common peroneal nerve innervates the anterolateroinferior side of the joint through the lateral articular nerve, branching off at the joint line, and the recurrent peroneal nerve, branching off just distal to the head of the fibula (40). The lateral articular nerve innervates the lateral joint capsule, the lateral meniscus, and the lateral collateral ligament (18,42). The anterolaterosuperior part of the joint is innervated by the superior lateral genicular nerve branching off the sciatic nerve (40) and terminal branches of the nerve to the vastus lateralis muscle (41).

Posterior Aspect of the Knee Joint

The dorsal side of the joint is innervated by the posterior articular nerve that branches off the tibial nerve in the popliteal fossa, the popliteal plexus that receives branches from the obturator nerve, and the posterior articular nerve (25,40,41). The posterior articular nerve innervates the posterior capsule, the posterior horns of the menisci, and the posterior oblique and cruciate ligaments (18). In cats and dogs, it has been shown to contain fibers originating in the popliteus muscle (43,45,46).

The posterior articular nerve is likely not the only nerve innervating human cruciate ligaments. In dogs, microscopic dissection has shown the medial articular nerve innervates medial structures and, through the infrapatellar fat pad, both cruciate ligaments (42). Muscular branches of the obturator nerve were also seen reaching the posterior joint capsule and cruciate ligaments (42).

Similar findings were documented in a neurotracer study in cats (17). After retrograde axonal transport, the tracer was found in lumbar spinal ganglion cells belonging to the posterior articular nerve and to the medial and lateral articular nerves. Quantitative data indicate more than 60% of the innervation of the ACL is through the posterior articular nerve and the remainder through the medial and lateral articular nerves (no distinction was made between medial and lateral articular nerves [17]).

Density of Mechanoreceptors in Knee Ligaments

Neurotracer studies in the cat indicate a total number of 6 to 20 (20) mechanoreceptors or, including afferent free nerve endings, 13 to 52 receptors per ACL (17) (Table 9.1). These numbers probably decrease with age and disease (44,47,48). Quantitative studies in humans are few. Monoclonal antibody stains demonstrated 17 mechanoreceptors in the ACL of a 3-year-old child (35) (Table 9.2). Comparable quantitative studies for other knee structures are lacking, but the innervation of other knee ligaments is presumably comparable to the ACL (Table 9.3). Placed in perspective with the innervation of the entire knee joint (as reflected by total number of nerve fibers), knee ligament mechanoreceptors constitute a small minority (Table 9.4). Most nerve fibers in articular nerves are thin, unmyelinated fibers. In the cat, approximately 87% and 95% of fibers of the posterior and medial articular nerves, respectively, are unmyelinated. Nearly half of the unmyelinated fibers are efferent, forming part of the sympathetic nerve system; the remaining unmyelinated fibers are afferents of the free nerve endings. Myelinated fibers—the afferents of mechanoreceptors—form a small minority. Most mechanoreceptors are located in the posterior joint capsule (9,18), and ligament mechanoreceptors are therefore a minority within the population of joint mechanoreceptors.

Comparable quantitative data are lacking for other ligaments and joints, but available anatomic studies do not indicate principal differences in innervation between the ACL and other knee ligaments. The existence of a small

TABLE 9.3. *Mechanoreceptors in knee structures other than the anterior cruciate ligament*

Author, method	Structure	Description of receptors[a]	Eponyms used
Freeman and Wyke (1967), cat knee, silver, gold chloride, serial sections	Joint capsule	Freeman and Wyke type I, II, IV	Ruffini, Pacini
Halata and Haus (1985), human knee, electron microscopy	Joint capsule	Free nerve endings	
		Small corpuscle without a capsule	Ruffini
		Corpuscle with connective tissue capsule	Ruffini
		Large corpuscle with perineural capsule (resembling Golgi tendon organ)	Ruffini
		Corpuscle with inner cores and perineural capsule	Pacini
O'Connor and McConnaughey (1978), cat knee, gold chloride, nonserial sections	Menisci	Free nerve endings	Not applicable
		"2 Types of mechanoreceptors"	Not reported
Katonis et al. (1991), human knee, gold chloride, nonserial sections	Posterior cruciate ligament	Freeman and Wyke type I, II, IV	Ruffini, Vater-Pacini
		Mainly near bony attachments	
De Avilla et al. (1988), human knee, gold chloride, serial sections	Lateral collateral ligament	Large "spray-shaped" ending	"non-paciniform endings"
		Small ovoid endings	
Andrew (1954), cat, rabbit knee, methylene blue, nonserial sections	Medial collateral ligament	Free nerve endings	
		Variable shape just superficial to ligament and in capsule, thin membrane	Ruffini-type
		Thin "plate" shape, closely applied to bundle of connective tissue	Golgi-type
O'Connor and Gonzales (1979), cat knee, gold chloride, nonserial sections	Medial collateral ligament	Freeman and Wyke type I, II, III, IV	Ruffini, Pacini, Golgi

[a] Terminology of receptor type reported by authors.
Freeman and Wyke = types of nerve ending according to the Freeman and Wyke classification (see Table 9.1).

number of receptors has been used as an argument for assuming they have minor importance. However, there is no *a priori* reason to believe important functions could not be served with small numbers.

TABLE 9.4. *Distribution of fiber types in the joint nerves of the cat knee, disregarding group I fibers*

Nerve	Medial articular nerve	Posterior articular nerve
Total number of fibers	1130	1140
Number of efferent fibers	500	470
Number of afferent fibers	630	670
Percentage group III and IV of afferent fibers	91%	77%

Modified from Grigg P. Nervous system control of joint function. In: Finerman GAM, Noyes FR, eds. *Biology and biomechanics of the traumatized synovial joint: the knee as a model.* Chicago: AAOS Symposium, 1992:275–287.

Morphologic Classification of Mechanoreceptors in Knee Ligaments

Mechanoreceptors were probably first described in the pulp of the fingers, appearing in the thesis of a student of the anatomist Vater in 1741 (49). Considering the optical possibilities of the era, it is not surprising the first observation concerned relatively large mechanoreceptors in an area with a high density of mechanoreceptors. More than a century later, Pacini described the lamellated capsule of this receptor (50). It has since been known as the Pacini or Vater–Pacini receptor. At the end of the 19th century, Rauber described mechanoreceptors around various joints (16), Golgi described the tendon organ, and Ruffini described the subcutaneous receptor of similar appearance (51). Since these early studies, eponyms have been used widely, and the terminology used in discussing mechanoreceptors has varied among investigators. Freeman and Wyke (18) synthesized a variety of previous reports and condensed the varied eponymic terminology into four types (Table 9.5). Many researchers use their terminology.

Interpretation of conventional histology of neurologic structures in ligaments is difficult for three reasons. First, traditional gold and silver chloride stains are nonspecific and stain vascular and other structures containing collagen and elastin (18,19,52); serial sections are essential for proper interpretation; and studies without serial sections are open to question, because what appears to be a mechanoreceptor on one or two sections turns out to be a vascular structure (19,53–55). It can be expected that immunohistochemical techniques will solve these problems in the coming years. Second, there is controversy about classifying individual receptors. Some investigators suggest these are not distinct types but rather a continuum, with types perhaps related to the adaptation of a given receptor to its local conditions (28,29,56). Third, morphologic classification alone does not imply function. It is possible to envision the difficulties in establishing the relationship between a given receptor and function. It would require identification of a single receptor in a living animal; that receptor would then need to be stimulated in a variety of physiologic ways; all afferent, efferent, and end-organ responses would need to be observed; and appropriate morphologic studies of that receptor would be required. These are daunting requirements that have not been met in the literature. Few studies approximate these criteria (57) and much information relating form to function is based on much softer information. Given these and other problems, when inferring function, it is necessary to interpret studies of types and numbers of receptors with considerable caution.

The three difficulties outlined earlier led to controversies that can be summarized in three questions: Is it a receptor? Which one? What does it do? For example, some investigators speak of Golgi tendon organs in the ACL (58,59), others of Golgi-like receptors (18,54,60),

whereas still others have stated there can be no such thing as a Golgi tendon organ in a ligament, preferring the term to be used exclusively for muscle receptors that inhibit muscle contraction (56,61). These investigators consider these mechanoreceptors in the ACL to be a type of Ruffini receptor. The confusion in terms is related to the strong morphologic similarity of Ruffini receptors in dense collagenous tissues (e.g., ligament) and Golgi tendon organs. Based on this similarity, Andrew (29) stated "the form taken by a particular ending depends on the type of tissue in which it is embedded. When applied to the dense connective tissue of a ligament bundle it takes the form of a thin plate on the surface; in diffuse connective tissue it assumes a more cylindrical shape." In 1954, Boyd argued that a continuum might exist for the structure and function of tendon, ligament, and capsule receptors, with both aspects determined by the surrounding tissue (28). Electron microscopy confirms the structure of the Ruffini corpuscle is essentially identical to that of the Golgi tendon organ (56,62). The only important difference is the mechanical bonding of the Golgi tendon organ with muscle fibers at the musculotendinous junction (62,63).

In contrast to morphologic similarity, physiologic similarity, such as the inhibition of motor neurons after activation of Golgi tendon organs, has not been shown for the Golgi-like mechanoreceptors of ligaments. The Golgi tendon organ functions as a force transducer whose major role is providing feedback for reflex regulation (64). The Ruffini receptor functions as a slowly adapting stretch receptor (9). In accordance with the different functions is the difference in diameter of afferent fibers: 18 to 19 μm (group I) for the Golgi tendon organ, which it receives only from intramuscular nerves, and 4 to 6 μm (group II) for the Ruffini receptor in humans, cats, and various other animals. The presence of group I fibers (Table 9.6) in the posterior articular nerve further complicates the matter. However, these fibers apparently originate from muscle spindles in the

TABLE 9.5. *Classification of joint mechanoreceptors*

Receptor type	Morphology	Dimensions average (μm)	Location	Afferent fiber (μm)	Eponyms used by other authors
Type I	Globular or ovoid corpuscle with thin capsule	100 × 40	Joint capsule, periosteum, some in ligaments and tendons	5–8	Ruffini, Golgi-Mazzoni
Type II	Cylindrical or conical corpuscle with thick lamellated capsule	280 × 120	Joint capsule	8–12	Pacini, Krause, Vater-Pacini
Type III	Fusiform corpuscle with thin capsule	600 × 100	Ligaments, tendons	13–17	Golgi, Golgi-Mazzoni
Type IV	Unmyelinated free nerve endings	0.5–1.5	Joint capsule, periosteum ligaments, tendons, blood vessels	0.5–5	Not reported

Modified from Freeman MAR, Wyke B. The innervation of the knee joint. An anatomical and histological study in the cat. *J Anat* 1967;101:505–532.

TABLE 9.6. *Characteristics of fiber types in the joint nerves of the cat knee*

Fiber type	Diameter	Conduction velocity (m/s)	Medial articular nerve	Posterior articular nerve	Receptor type
Efferent fibers					
Group IV	0.2–1.5	0.5–2	500	470	Free nerve endings
Afferent fibers					
Group I	10–20	80–120	0	27[a]	Muscle spindle, Golgi tendon organ
Group II	5–15	35–75	57	150	Ruffini, Pacini
Group III	1–5	5–35	132	85	Free nerve endings
Group IV	0.2–1.5	0.5–2	441	408	Free nerve endings

[a]Group I fibers in the posterior articular nerve originate in the popliteus muscle.
Modified from Langford RA, Schmidt RF. Afferent and efferent axons in the medial and posterior articular nerves of the cat. *Anat Rec* 1983;206:71–78, and Martin JH, Jessel TM. Modality coding in the sensory system. In: Kandell ER, Schwartz JH, Jessel TM, eds. *Principles of Neural Science.* New York: Elsevier, 1992:342–352.

popliteus muscle (42,45,46). Halata modified the ideas mentioned by Andrew (29) and Boyd (28) stating the structure of a Ruffini receptor is modified by the surrounding tissues, but its function is always that of a slowly adapting stretch receptor. In loose connective tissue, they appear as "spray" or branched, complex free nerve endings, similar to the Ruffini receptor of the subcutaneous tissue (56) (Fig. 9.1). In more dense tissue, they seem more organized (Fig. 9.2). In connective tissue with tightly bound parallel collagen fibrils (e.g., ligaments), they merely resemble the Golgi-tendon organ in muscle (Fig. 9.3). This is in accordance with the concept of "in-series" architecture of musculoskeletal tissues in which Golgi tendon organs and Ruffini receptors are considered the same receptor presenting gradual differences depending on the texture of surrounding tissue. Within the collagenous bundles of the ligament can be observed large, fusiform receptors with thick, lamellated capsules (sometimes referred to as Pacini or paciniform receptors) (Fig. 9.4).

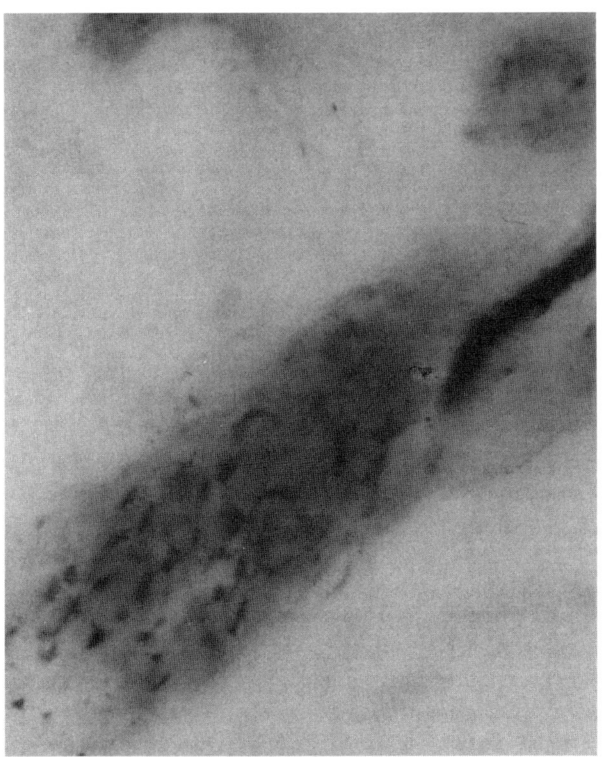

FIGURE 9.1. Light microscopic image of spray ending in loose connective tissue adjacent to the posterior capsule of the cat knee. This is most consistent with a Ruffini ending (Freeman-Wyke type I). All images came from cats and were stained with gold chloride.

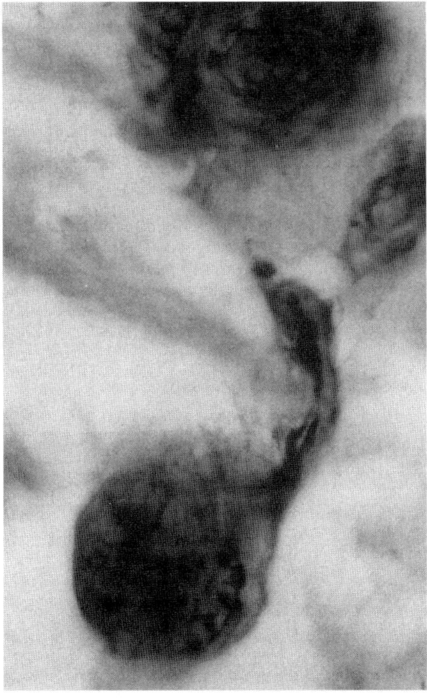

FIGURE 9.2. Light microscopic image of a more organized globular ending with a thin capsule in the subsynovial surface adjacent to the cranial cruciate ligament (analogous to the anterior cruciate ligament in humans). As in Figure 9.1, this most likely represents a Ruffini ending (Freeman-Wyke type I) that has a different morphology because of its environment.

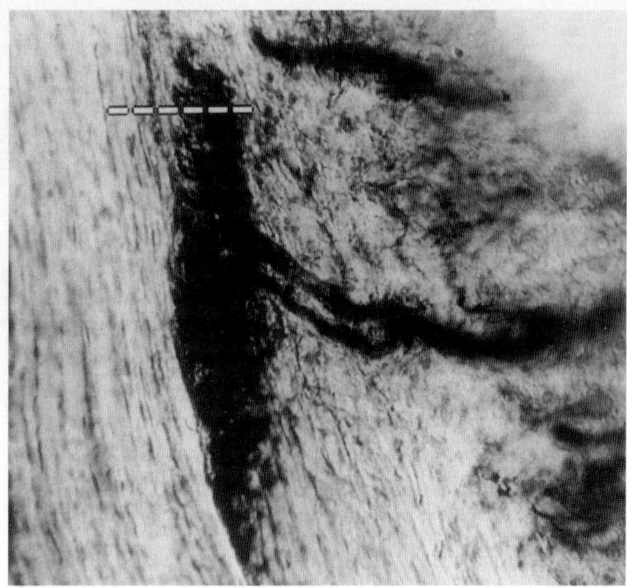

FIGURE 9.3. Light microscopic image of a large fusiform receptor with a thin capsule within the cranial cruciate ligament. This corresponds to a Golgi-like receptor (Freeman-Wyke type III).

Ligament Receptors: Free Nerve Endings and Ruffini Receptors

Nerve endings of intraarticular ligaments are primarily located in the loose connective tissue between the synovium and the ligament, the subsynovial layer (Tables 9.1, 9.2). The synovium (enfolding the cruciate ligaments) consists of an intimal layer facing the joint cavity and a subsynovial layer in direct contact with the ligament. The nerves terminate as free nerve endings or as nerve endings surrounded by an auxiliary structure, the corpuscular nerve endings or mechanoreceptors. The nerve endings are surrounded by a perineurium and consist of unmyelinated or myelinated fibers. Diameter and state of myelinization determine the conduction velocity of the fiber. The fibers originate in nerve cells located in the lumbar dorsal root ganglia.

Ruffini receptors are the most frequently identified mechanoreceptors, with Pacini receptors reported less commonly (Tables 9.1, 9.2). Ruffini receptors are thought to function as stretch receptors (9), whereas Pacini receptors in joints seem to be mainly activated by compression (10,65). A combined study of morphology and physiology of single receptors has been reported for Ruffini receptors in the joint capsule of the cat (57) but not for the Ruffini receptors of ligaments. The Ruffini receptors of the capsule functioned as stretch receptors, and it seems reasonable to infer these receptors function in the knee ligaments as they do in other tissues. The afferent fibers are myelinated and have a diameter of 4 to 6 μm (56). Most Ruffini receptors are located in the posterior joint capsule (9,18).

Ruffini receptors have a variable morphology classified based on electron microscopic images (19,56). The Ruffini receptor of the subsynovial layer of the ACL is ovoid and measures approximately 50 × 500 μm. It is composed of a parent axon that divides into two to six nerve endings to form a spray ending. The nerve endings are enveloped by Schwann cells. The receptor also contains endoneural connective tissue and is enclosed in an incomplete perineural capsule. The endoneural connective tissue consists of collagen fibrils and fibroblasts connected to the surrounding collagen fibrils through gaps in the perineural capsule (19). The nerve endings follow the direction of the local collagen fibrils (66); in ligaments with parallel-oriented fibrils, the nerve endings are aligned along the axis of the ligament, and the perineural capsule is well developed. These Ruffini receptors resemble Golgi tendon organs (56,67). In the posterior joint capsule, the orientation of the nerve endings reflects the different orientations of the collagen fibrils (66).

Pacini receptors are oval and measure approximately 150 × 600 μm. They have a thick, lamellated capsule that consists of 15 to 30 layers of flat perineural cells (Fig.

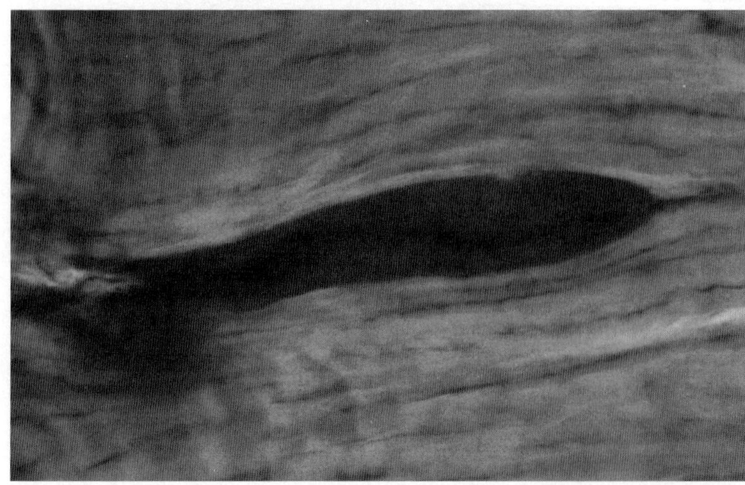

FIGURE 9.4. Light microscopic image of a receptor with a thick, lamellated capsule within the substance of the cranial cruciate ligament. This receptor is most likely a Paciniform variety (Freeman-Wyke type II).

9.3). The single afferent fiber of 4 to 8 μm divides inside the capsule in several branches that then lose their myelin sheath. The nerve terminals are filled with mitochondria and clear vesicles with a diameter of 20 nm. The afferent fibers are myelinated and have a diameter of 4 to 8 μm (19). Free nerve endings are thought to function as nociceptors; they react to noxious influences such as joint inflammation and pain stimuli but also function as high-threshold mechanoreceptors (68,69).

In addition to mechanoreceptors and nociceptors (i.e., afferent sensory innervation), the knee joint also has an important efferent innervation. These unmyelinated fibers of the autonomic nervous system originate in the sympathetic ganglia and are closely associated, functionally and topographically, to the vascularization (70,71). Immuno-histochemistry for a specific sympathetic neuropeptide-Y (NPY) has not shown sympathetic reactivity in the substance of the ACL. Only the subsynovial layer of the surrounding synovium exhibited NPYergic activity (71).

Morphologically, unmyelinated efferent (modulating) and sensory afferent (receptive) fibers cannot be distinguished from each other. Neither is strict functional distinction possible. Neuropeptides such as substance P and gene-related gene product (CGRP) are found in 10% and 33%, respectively, of group III and IV joint afferents. These neuropeptides are capable of causing vasodilatation, plasma extravasation, and angiogenesis (72,73). In response to a stimulus, joint afferents transfer information and can release neuropeptides, the so-called local effector function of joint afferents (74).

Based on these characteristics, afferents and efferents repeatedly have been associated with the mechanisms involved in inflammatory arthritis (75,76). Joint afferents also have been suggested to play a role in the genesis of osteoarthrosis. For example, in a type of mice known to develop degenerative arthritis with aging, the number of knee joint afferents decreased 57% over the average life span. The decrease was particularly apparent in the population of larger neurons, presumably mechanoreceptors. The overall population of afferents decreased 34% over the life span of this mouse (47,77). Loss of knee joint innervation preceded development of osteoarthrosis in the mouse model. Joint mechanoreceptors and free nerve endings may therefore have a modulatory function in tissue homeostasis.

Unlikely Regeneration of Mechanoreceptors in Ligament Grafts

Regeneration of mechanoreceptors has been reported in ACL grafts in humans, sheep, and dogs (59,78,79). The histologic findings of these reports are not, however, convincing, and one such study has been withdrawn (80). Knowledge from healing of nerve lesions and reinnervation of myocutaneous grafts makes regeneration of functional mechanoreceptors in ligament grafts through rein-

nervation of existing mechanoreceptors or axon sprouting rather unlikely.

The cautions that apply to interpretation of histology of mechanoreceptors in normal ligaments also apply to histology of ligament grafts (even more so) because additional factors could cause confusion. First, if regeneration of mechanoreceptors is to be confirmed, examination of the graft material as a control before implantation is needed. Which types of mechanoreceptors are present in the graft before harvest, and what happens to these receptors with remodeling? For example, free nerve endings and Pacini receptors have been described in normal patellar ligament (37). Second, the relation of the neural structures reported with the synovial tissue surrounding the graft should be documented. It may be that the synovium plays a role in vascular (81,82) as well as in neural processes of ligamentization. Regeneration of synovium, including its neural structures, occurs in rheumatoid arthritis in patients and in animal models (83–85). Third, viability and, ideally, function of the mechanoreceptors in the remodeled graft should be verified. Viability can only be verified by using immunohistochemistry. Verification of function is far more difficult and has been attempted with somatosensory-evoked potentials, but it as yet unknown what the value of this method is for this purpose or whether it can distinguish between free nerve endings and mechanoreceptors.

One study used immunohistochemical methods in patients and a rat model (86). In 10 patients, patellar ligament autografts were biopsied 5 to 37 months after surgery. Rats were studied from 2 to 16 weeks after patellar ligament autograft reconstruction. Nerve fibers were identified using protein gene product 9.5, a general neural marker. The viability of the structures was assessed by the expression of growth-associated protein 43/B-50 as a marker for neuronal regeneration. Further characterization of the neural structures was attempted by assessing expression of substance P and calcitonin CGRP. Substance P is thought to be almost exclusively present in small-diameter nociceptive nerve endings, whereas CGRP is present in large proprioceptive and small nociceptive endings (73).

Immunoreactivity for all four neural markers was found in human and rat controls of normal ACL and patellar ligament. Peptide-containing nerves also were seen in the remodeling autografts of rats from 4 to 16 weeks, primarily in the superficial ligament substance near the insertion sites. All biopsies of human patellar ligament autograft (5 to 37 months after surgery) showed signs of the remodeling process being fully completed, with a sinusoidal collagen pattern with fibroblast repopulation. Neuropeptide immunoreactivity, however, was not found in human patellar ligament autografts. The biopsies were taken at identical locations as in the four normal human ACLs (86).

Aune et al. (86) hypothesized expression of sensory neuropeptides in the rat patellar ligament autograft suggested possible involvement of sensory innervation during remodeling of the graft. A modulatory function based on the vascular effects (i.e., vasodilatation, plasma extravasation, and angiogenesis) of the neuropeptides substance P and CGRP can be assumed to contribute to the remodeling of the graft (73). It seems likely in the process of remodeling that vascularization is accompanied by ingrowth of neural structures with a neurosecretory paracrine function. Comparable neurologic findings have been reported in fracture healing (87,88) and the healing of myocutaneous flaps (89,90).

The synovium could take part in the reinnervation of the graft, comparable to the revascularization of the graft that occurs through the synovial sheet. The graft itself has been reported as less vascular (81,91) or avascular in animal (92) and human studies (82).

Only reinnervation with free nerve endings seems possible, however. The synovium of the cat knee joint contains free nerve endings, but only in the form of unmyelinated autonomic fibers near blood vessels. Corpuscular nerve endings occasionally are present at the transition zone to the fibrous layer of the capsule (18,93).

If we consider the scarce reports on ACL mechanoreceptor regeneration in perspective with the large amount of experimental work that has been done on nerve lesions or reinnervation of myocutaneous flaps (review in references 94–96), reinnervation of the ligament grafts with complex nerve endings such as Ruffini receptors is unlikely. In myocutaneous free flaps, reinnervation occurs from the tissue surrounding the graft with mostly unmyelinated fibers (i.e., free nerve endings) that are generally associated with blood vessels. These fibers regenerate along empty neurilemmal sheaths (97).

Most work on nerve or mechanoreceptor regeneration has been done in animal models using crushing, freezing, or transection (with or without suture) of the nerve. During a ligament graft procedure, the mechanoreceptors in the graft are separated from their corresponding nerve cells in the spinal ganglion. This is invariably followed by degeneration of the distal end of the nerve fiber (98). Thick, myelinated fibers have never been shown to form *de novo* complex endings such as mechanoreceptors, but reinnervation of existing mechanoreceptors can occur and depends on viable Schwann cells in the proximal nerve stump and the presence of an end organ distally. It is most likely to succeed if axons are simply crushed or have only a very short (<0.5 cm) gap to cross and is most likely to fail if the gap between nerve stumps is long (>1 cm) and associated with soft tissue damage (96).

In a ligament grafting procedure, concern seems warranted if end organs persist in the graft during the necrosis preceding remodeling. If they do, the only chance for reinnervation appears to be with a nerve suture. However, even in the case of a successful nerve repair, the subsequent organization of the axonal sprouts, particularly their orderly outgrowth to a distal mechanoreceptor, does

not occur in most nerve fibers. With nerve transection and successful suture, only a small proportion of mechanoreceptors is reinnervated, perhaps up to 45% of Golgi tendon organs (99–101) and 25% of muscle spindles (101). If the nerve is cut twice and the interposed segment sutured (i.e., an optimal autograft), both rates are reduced to 10% (101). These mechanoreceptors are mostly abnormal in morphology (98,102,103) and function (99–101,103).

Considering the conditions of graft and native neural tissue during a ligament grafting procedure makes reinnervation of a ligament graft with functional mechanoreceptors unlikely. Nevertheless, reinnervation of a graft with free nerve endings in the subsynovial layer may be part of the ligamentization process. Free nerve endings may play an active role in the remodeling process and possibly in maintaining homeostasis of the graft when remodeling is completed.

NEUROPHYSIOLOGY OF MECHANORECEPTORS

Although mechanoreceptors in joints have been characterized morphologically and physiologically and some of their connections to higher-order neurons have been documented, it is fair to say their functional role, or effect on normal movement, and alterations with aging, injury, or disease remain largely unknown. Most mechanoreceptors in the joint capsule and ligaments of the knee appear to function as limit detectors. Free nerve endings function as nociceptors and as such can contribute to the pathophysiology of arthritis.

When interpreting experimental and clinical work on the function of mechanoreceptors, it should be remembered that neurophysiologic characterization of a single receptor does not necessarily inform us on the role of that receptor in joint function. To understand this role, signal processing in the central nervous system should also be clarified. The effect of mechanoreceptor stimulation on movement or behavior is determined mostly not by a single, a group, or even a type of receptor, but by several groups or types of receptors. For example, proprioception is a compound sense relying on simultaneous activity in a number of mechanoreceptors types: skin, muscle, tendon, and joint mechanoreceptors (104). Another example is the gamma or fusimotor system that influences muscle stiffness; it receives afferent input not only from muscle but also from joint and skin receptors. In other words, redundancy plays an important role (105). Many experiments use nonphysiologic stimulation (e.g., electrical stimulation), and several different receptor populations often are stimulated instead of only the one for which the experiment was intended.

For similar reasons, when interpreting the consequences of the functional loss of mechanoreceptors, such as after a ligament rupture, two considerations apply: the direct effect of loss of ligament receptor output and alterations in output of remaining joint receptors. In the case of the knee joint, altered kinematics after ligament rupture influence output of mechanoreceptors in capsule and remaining ligaments. The latter consideration is supported by an experiment in which the responsiveness of capsule mechanoreceptors in cats was examined before and after ACL transection. Using standardized joint rotations, neural discharge versus joint displacement increased after ACL transection. This was interpreted as reflecting an increase in capsule stress for a given displacement that resulted from altered joint kinematics (6).

The neurophysiologic characterization of joint receptors (i.e., identification of the type of sensory information that is signaled and its representation in the afferent nerve) has been examined in animal experiments with single nerve fiber studies. Nearly all of these experiments have been performed on receptors in the joint capsule, but most investigators assume neurophysiologic characteristics of a given type of receptor are comparable in capsule and ligament. The method used most often is based on the identification of a single afferent fiber of a receptor in the joint nerve. By comparing the action potentials of electrical stimulation of the joint nerve with the action potentials after stimulation by local pressure on the joint capsule, the receptive field and the afferent fiber can be identified. The conduction velocity can be measured, allowing classification of the afferent fiber (i.e., groups I through IV in Table 9.6). Special hairs (i.e., Von Frey hairs) calibrated for micropressure can be used to determine the activation threshold. The response of the receptor to movement of the joint can then be investigated.

The neurophysiology of a mechanoreceptor is partly related to its morphology. The form of the end organ and the properties of the nerve ending's terminal membrane and afferent fiber determine the response to a stimulus. The terminal membrane determines the selectivity and sensitivity of the receptor— the type (pressure, stretch, temperature) and intensity (threshold) of stimulus that activate the receptor (50). The myelinization and diameter of the afferent fiber determine the velocity of impulse conduction to the nerve cell in the dorsal root ganglion. Activation (i.e., depolarization) of a mechanoreceptor is based on deformation of the nerve ending. The deformation opens membrane channels, allowing influx of cations generating a receptor potential. The receptor potential propagates to the first node of Ranvier, where action potentials are produced (105). The end organ modifies the deformation and influences the receptive field (56) and dynamic response or adaptation of a receptor. Adaptation is the decrease in receptor potential in response to a maintained stimulus. A rapidly adapting or phasic receptor responds transiently only at the onset and termination of a stimulus, whereas a slowly adapting or tonic receptor maintains a receptor potential during the complete stimulus period (105).

The few studies that combined morphologic and physiologic studies of single mechanoreceptors demonstrate that Ruffini receptors adapt slowly (tonic) (57) and Pacini receptors adapt rapidly (phasic) (106,107). The lamellated corpuscle of a Pacini receptor dampens the indentation of the terminal membrane and decreases the duration of the receptor potential. Removal of this capsule changes the receptor from rapidly to slowly adapting (108).

Free Nerve Endings as Nociceptors

Free nerve endings in ligament appear to have similar functions as in joint capsules; they have small, spotlike receptive fields (many have multiple receptive fields) and react to noxious stimuli. The stimulus can be mechanical or chemical. A small fraction of the nerve endings responds to normal movement of the joint, but most free nerve endings respond only to movement of the joint when large (noxious) forces are used (68). The spotlike receptive fields of free nerve endings indicate the receptors are not stretch sensors (if they were, they would also react to a stimulus beyond the morphologic limits of the receptor itself). Sensitivity of free nerve endings can be markedly increased by creating a joint inflammation. Free nerve endings that would normally react only to forceful movement then respond to gentle movement of the joint (109). Sensitization of free nerve endings by inflammatory mediators such as prostaglandin E_2 provides the neural substrate for arthritis and arthritic pain (110–112).

Mechanoreceptors of the Knee Joint Capsule as Limit Detectors

Ruffini receptors function as stretch sensors. Stretch of the posterior joint capsule in cats produces a slow-adapting response in the form of a train of action potentials (9). In connective tissue with parallel oriented fibrils (i.e., ligament), the receptors are activated by uniaxial stretching (113). In connective tissue with collagen fibrils oriented at many different orientations, as in the posterior joint capsule, a single receptor can be activated by tissue stretch in many directions (114). Using joint rotations, Ruffini receptors in the joint capsule are stimulated most effectively by movements of the joint to the limit of extension. Receptor output increases when axial rotations are added (115). Receptor output was absent when the joint was not moving and when it was moved at flexion angles in the intermediate range. The Ruffini receptors seem to function as limit detectors. The activation threshold for Ruffini receptors in the joint capsule is low: 250 g/cm extension moment in the cat knee, corresponding to a force of approximately 30 *g* at the ankle (115).

The type of stimulus activating Pacini receptors in joints is not as clear as for Ruffini receptors. Some assume an adequate stimulus activating Pacini receptors is any form of mechanical deformation (49). In the joints of cats, these receptors are stimulated by compression and adapt rapidly. Correspondingly, increased hydrostatic pressure of the joint generates a receptor response, whereas sensitivity to tissue stretch was absent (10).

Ligament mechanoreceptor function is comparable to joint capsule mechanoreceptors, stretch receptors that can signal the limits of knee motion. Mechanoreceptors in the medial collateral ligament produce slow-adapting discharges when steady tension is applied to the ligament (29,116).

Mechanoreceptors in the ACL have been tested using probing, axial traction to a block of bone with the insertion of the ACL (comparable to anterior translation of the tibia in relation to the femur) (117) and with joint rotations (118). In two experiments, only a small number of mechanoreceptors could be identified in each ligament; 15 receptors were identified in 12 cat knees (117) and 26 in 11 cat knees (118). In all animals, substantially larger numbers of mechanoreceptors were found in the posterior joint capsule. Most ACL mechanoreceptors were found near the femoral insertion.

No activity was seen with the knee in the resting position of 30° of flexion. All receptors responded to movement, primarily to extension of the knee. Activity increased markedly when the limits of the range of motion were reached and when internal or external rotation was added, with internal rotation a more potent stimulus than external rotation. A response was also observed in seven of eight receptors tested with flexion up to 60° (118). The output of the ACL mechanoreceptors seems comparable to joint capsule mechanoreceptors; they appear to function as ACL stretch sensors. The ACL is loaded in extension and more so in hyperextension, with a further load increase when internal or external rotation is added. A larger load increase occurs with internal than external rotation (119). However, flexion of the knee unloads the ACL. It is possible to speculate that ACL receptor output with knee flexion results from local compression of the ACL in the femoral notch because of proximal migration of the contact point between the cruciate ligaments (5).

Mechanoreceptor Neurons Connected with Multiple Spinal and Central Nervous System Neurons

After receiving a stimulus from the periphery, the mechanoreceptor neurons project not only to neurons in the central nervous system (through the dorsal column–medial lemniscal system [105]), but also to spinal neurons, such as skeletomotor neurons, interneurons, and fusimotor neurons (120–122). Although these connections have been documented, their precise functional role is not clarified. It is clear, however, that afferent input affords a tremendous opportunity for modulation of the stimulus from the brain to the motoneurons. For example, a dorsal root in the cat carries 15,000 afferent fibers, twice as many as the efferent motor fibers in the ventral root. Between the

afferent dorsal and efferent ventral root fibers, there are more than 300,000 spinal interneurons that integrate peripheral input with descending signals from the brain to control the motoneurons and modulate movement (123). Somatic sensory systems often rely on functionally separate parallel pathways for transmission of complex information to the brain (105). Overlap between these systems exists and can form a basis for compensation of loss of afferent signals after a joint lesion.

FUNCTIONAL ROLE OF JOINT MECHANORECEPTORS

Animal Studies

Determination of the effect of a certain group of mechanoreceptors is difficult because neuromuscular functions typically rely on the input of several different receptor groups (105). This necessitates an experimental design that explicitly isolates the receptor group under study, but such experimental conditions often limit the conclusions permitted for normal movement and behavior.

Lack of Direct Reflex Effect of Joint Mechanoreceptors on Skeletomotor Neurons

Various investigators have proposed joint receptors have a direct reflex effect on skeletomotor neurons of the muscles crossing the knee joint (21,24,124–126). This is the theory of the "protective reflex," a spinal reflex initiated by mechanoreceptors in capsule or ligament, activated by extreme movement of a joint, and leading to contraction of a muscle that antagonizes this movement.

Since the 1950s, several researchers have attempted to document the presence of a direct reflex effect of joint mechanoreceptors on the muscles surrounding the knee (30,116,127–130). Many of the early experiments, however, were confounded by disturbances of muscle or skin receptors. If an influence could be shown, it would often require the use of substantial force, limiting the relation to normal joint function of the experiment.

In perhaps one of the best controlled of these experiments, the influence of joint receptors on skeletomotor neurons was examined by determining the effect of terminal extension of the knee on the (electrically evoked) monosynaptic reflex. A weakly positive feedback was demonstrated after terminal knee extension (i.e., facilitation of quadriceps and inhibition of hamstrings) (131). This effect was much weaker than the effect mediated by muscle afferents. The effect disappeared after cutting of the posterior articular nerve, but it persisted after cutting of the medial articular nerve, demonstrating that it was mediated by the posterior articular nerve only. Although the lateral articular nerve was not examined in this experiment, it is unlikely it mediates a reflex effect of joint receptors on skeletomotor neurons. The lateral articular nerve may contribute a small proportion of the innervation of the cruciate ligaments (but this has not been specifically examined with a neurotracer or immunohistochemistry [17]). In the cat, it does not innervate the posterior joint capsule; it is small and relatively unimportant (17,18) compared with the medial articular nerve, which was not involved in the demonstrated reflex effect.

In view of a putative protective reflex, a reflex that protects from joint damage by contraction of antagonists, it should be noted that the positive feedback found in this experiment does not antagonize terminal knee extension, but enhances it. The reflex effect found has the wrong "sign." A weakly positive feedback was also found in an experiment that used direct stimulation (indentation) of posterior joint capsule mechanoreceptors (120).

Lack of Direct Effect of Anterior Cruciate Ligament Mechanoreceptors on the Electromyogram of Muscles Surrounding the Knee

Traction with a wire loop placed around the ACL has been reported to increase the hamstrings electromyogram (125). Considerable force (130–150 N) was required because low or moderate forces produced no changes. However, when others repeated this experiment with loads up to 125 N (four to five times the body weight of the cats) (132), no quadriceps or hamstring electromyographic effect was observed, although output in the posterior articular nerve was demonstrated. Normal excitability of reflexes was confirmed with tendon taps. To explain the different outcomes, differences in the method of anesthesia were suggested to have induced hyperexcitability in the first experiment (132). Another explanation for the observed hamstring activity may be a flexion (withdrawal) reflex caused by local (noxious) compression of free nerve endings by the wire loop.

Pulling on the ligament with a loop is based on the assumption that no structures other than the intended ligament are stimulated. However, increased discharge patterns in the posterior articular nerve, most likely caused by joint capsule mechanoreceptors, have been documented with as little as 30 µm tibiofemoral motion (133).

Axial traction to a block of bone freed with the tibial insertion of the ACL seems a more appropriate way to isolate mechanical stimulation to the ligament. Using such traction up to 30 N, electromyographic changes were seen in quadriceps and hamstrings of cats and dogs (134). In this experiment, the animals were decerebrated and spinalized by transection of the spinal cord at midthoracic level. Interpretation of these findings is difficult, however, because the latency of the changes seems to have been rather long, with the second and largest peak occurring after 10 to 15 seconds. Moreover, these findings were not verified with a control experiment after posterior articular nerve transection. Based on the available studies, it must be concluded that an effect of ACL mechanoreceptors on the electromyogram of muscles surrounding the knee has not been convincingly demonstrated.

Anterior Cruciate Ligament Receptors Influence Output of Muscle Spindles and Muscle Stiffness through the Fusimotor System

Freeman and Wyke (135) hypothesized ligament receptors influence muscle stiffness (i.e., tone) through reflex effects. Muscle stiffness is defined here as the length change in a muscle–tendon complex for a given force change.

Johansson et al. (122) examined the effects of ligament mechanoreceptor activation on muscle stiffness through the fusimotor system. The ventral root contains alpha (skeletomotor) neurons and gamma (fusimotor) neurons. The efferent fibers innervate striated muscle (extrafusal muscle fibers) and muscle fibers within the muscle spindles (intrafusal fibers), respectively. The muscle spindles are sensitive detectors for the length of a muscle and function in the afferent leg of the stretch reflex. The stretch reflex is essential for the postural muscles and for the execution of voluntary movements. In addition to activation by muscle stretch, the muscle spindles are activated by the fusimotor system. Activation of the fusimotor neurons induces contraction of the intrafusal fibers, stretching the central part that contains the stretch receptor. Contraction of these muscle fibers increases the stretch sensitivity and the basic frequency of the muscle spindles (136). The 1a afferents of the muscle spindles activate skeletomotor neurons that increase the stiffness of the muscle. During muscle contraction (extrafusal fibers), extinction of the 1a output is prevented by simultaneous contraction of the intrafusal fibers through the fusimotor system. This alpha-gamma coactivation allows regulation of muscle stiffness while preserving stretch reflex control, even during movement.

Johansson et al. (122,137) studied fusimotor activity indirectly by monitoring the response of the (1a) afferent nerve fibers of muscle spindles. An alteration in response in most 1a afferent nerve fibers occurred after traction with a wire loop around the cruciate ligaments. Control experiments after posterior articular nerve transection or intraarticular lidocaine administration demonstrated disappearance of the reflex effect (137).

In the experiment of Grigg et al. (131), such a reflex would not have been observed because the 1a fibers in muscle nerves were stimulated, and they do not excite most fusimotor neurons. The influence of ligament afferent nerve fibers on muscle spindle afferent nerve fibers appears convincing, but its functional significance is far from clear. This can be partly explained by the complex input of the fusimotor system with skin, muscle, and joint afferents playing a role (22,138,139).

Johansson et al. (22) suggest the fusimotor system, after integrating complex input, serves as a "final common path" for regulation of muscle stiffness. Although the fusimotor system has a muscle reflex effect, it acts only in an indirect manner. After activation of muscle spindles through the fusimotor system, activation of the skeletomotor neurons occurs through 1a afferent fibers. The indirect route and the low conduction velocity of the fusimotor fibers (15 to 25 m/s) probably preclude a joint protective reflex. We emphasize, however, that an indirect route does not imply the receptors may not be important in daily function and athletic performance.

CLINICAL STUDIES

Neuromuscular changes after knee ligament injury have been studied almost exclusively in the ACL-deficient knee. Rupture or sacrifice of the ACL in humans has been associated with a deficit in proprioception and quadriceps force as well as changes in muscle stiffness and muscle contraction patterns. Neuromuscular changes likely influence functional outcome after a ligament injury, for example, through an effect on dynamic joint laxity. Many reports indicate static laxity, as measured with an arthrometer such as the KT-1000, does not correlate with functional or subjective outcome after ACL injury (140–144), repair (145), or reconstruction (146–149). Dynamic laxity differs from static laxity (150–152) and probably is more important in regard to function and the development of degenerative changes. Dynamic laxity is difficult to measure with sufficient accuracy (153–155), and no studies have specifically addressed the correlation with functional outcome.

The findings of many studies on neuromuscular changes after ACL injury are contradictory. These differences can partly be attributed to differing subject selection criteria and more or less subtle differences in measurement parameters or methods. Individual differences in neuromuscular (compensation) adaptation to a ligament injury may also play a role.

The question can be posed whether the neuromuscular changes are caused by direct loss of mechanoreceptors, altered stimulation of the remaining receptors, or a combination of the two. In clinical research, it is often impossible to make this distinction, although it is clear from the information in preceding sections of this chapter that neuromuscular function is influenced by joint mechanoreceptors and that ligament lesions can influence neuromuscular function.

Given these limitations, it may be more effective for clinical studies to avoid the rigid division of mechanoreceptors in separate groups and to view the substrate of proprioception as one continuous structure of components connected in series. The anatomic basis for this concept has been argued (2,36), and the distribution of mechanoreceptors near the origin or insertion of ligaments and at the muscle–tendon interface appears to support the concept (18,35,37,44,60,118). With the advent of

new methods to study neuromuscular adaptations *in vivo*, we may expect to gain insight into the underlying neural mechanisms and relative contribution of different receptor groups.

Altered Proprioception in Patients with Ligament or Other Lesions of the Knee

Proprioception is the sense of position and movement of the limbs and traditionally has been interpreted using the division between joint and muscle receptors. Several reviews have been based on this idea and have concluded proprioception is a compound sense relying on different receptor populations in skin, muscle, and joints (38,39, 156,157). Muscle mechanoreceptors play a primary role in proprioception (157). It appears large joints may be relying more on proprioceptive input from muscle receptors than small joints (155). Joint mechanoreceptors (of which ligament mechanoreceptors form only a minority) can signal movement, but they are unlikely to play a role in position sense. This conclusion is consistent with the absence of ligament mechanoreceptor output when the knee is not moving (118).

Examiners of knee proprioception use two types of test. Tests ascertaining the threshold to detect passive motion and tests examining the capacity to accurately reposition the limb. The perception of movement is related to the velocity of the movement (156). Normally, a distinction between movement sense and position sense is not possible. However, when a movement is executed with a velocity less than approximately 2° per minute, it is not registered as movement, but as a change in position (158). It is assumed (21,159,160) this makes the test more specific for slowly adapting (joint) mechanoreceptors as opposed to rapidly adapting (joint and muscle) receptors, but this idea is not uncontested (161). Tensing of muscles further increases proprioceptive acuity (162), but currently used tests do not explicitly control for this variable.

For knee ligament injuries, proprioception tests cannot differentiate between ligament and joint capsule mechanoreceptors, and they cannot give conclusive information about the functional significance of ligament mechanoreceptors. Given the complexity of proprioception, neither type of test is ideal.

Proprioceptive acuity decreases with age and osteoarthrosis (163–165). An elastic bandage or taping improves proprioception in persons with a proprioception deficit, possibly through enhanced stimulation of skin receptors (163,166). In persons with unimpaired proprioception the effect is negligible (166).

In ACL-deficient patients, increased (159,167) and unaltered (168,169) thresholds to detection of motion have been reported. Similarly, some investigators (146,167) reported differences with a reposition test in ACL-deficient patients, whereas others could not find important differences (170,171). A substantial correlation of proprioceptive deficits associated with meniscal or chondral lesions also has been reported (172,173). These findings confirm the notion that it is not well known what parameters should be investigated to demonstrate proprioceptive deficits, or what exactly is being tested with current types of examinations. It is likely that some different results of these studies can be explained by differences in patient selection, test method, and specific test devices.

Newer studies suggest potential explanations for reported differences. Several reports document an increased sensitivity in proprioception close to extension (170,174). This is consistent with the finding that capsule and ACL mechanoreceptors primarily respond to terminal extension rather than flexion near extension (31,118). A substantial correlation between proprioception and subjective outcome has been found in ACL-deficient patients (149); after ACL reconstruction, findings confirming (146,149) and contradicting (147) such a correlation have been reported.

Ligament–Muscle Reflex Not Convincingly Demonstrated in Humans

Palmer (24) stated in 1938, "Irritation of the sensory nerve endings of the ligaments through a blow, or a more effective irritant, increased tension, releases protective contraction in a particular group of muscles." Several others (21,124,125) likewise proposed extreme joint movements activate ligament mechanoreceptors, initiating a spinal reflex with contraction of muscles antagonizing the movement (i.e., ligamentomuscular reflex). Such contraction was assumed to take place by direct stimulation of the skeletomotor neurons and prevent ligament and cartilage damage (i.e., a protective reflex). In the case of the ACL, an ACL–hamstring reflex was proposed (175,176).

In clinical studies, convincing demonstration of a ligamentomuscular reflex is mostly impossible because the movement intended to stimulate the ligament receptors also stimulates other receptor groups (6,133), and it is uncertain which receptor population initiates a response. Animal research does not convincingly support a ligament–muscle reflex (131). Regardless of the issue of the origin of neuromuscular alterations, muscle reaction times and contraction sequences after a joint perturbation may differ between ACL-deficient patients and control subjects (144,177). Moreover, subjective and functional results were related to these changes in muscle function. However, the muscular changes found differ considerably between studies. For example, using similar tests with anterior translation of the tibia, one study reported a mean increase of 42 ms for ACL-deficient patients in the fastest hamstring reaction time compared with control subjects (177). In another study, this increase varied from 6 to 14 ms (144), whereas in a third study, no changes were found (178).

Alteration of Muscle Stiffness after Anterior Cruciate Ligament Rupture

Based on the effects of mechanoreceptors on muscle spindles, it would be reasonable to presume such receptors affect muscle stiffness. However, too few clinical studies have addressed this hypothesis to give a clear answer.

Muscle stiffness is defined here as the length change in a muscle–tendon complex for a given force change. Stiffness of a muscle is determined by its viscoelastic properties, which determine the instantaneous stiffness, and by time-related components. After an increase in length, a reduction in the number of actin-myosin crosslinks is seen, reducing its contribution to stiffness. Within 5 ms of reaching a new length, new crosslinks are formed. Muscle stiffness is also reflex mediated, determined by the excitability of the skeletomotor neuron pool. In addition to regulation of the muscle stiffness through the stretch reflex under fusimotor control, higher centers in the central nervous system are also involved. The latency of this reflex-mediated stiffness is approximately 50 ms (179).

Two clinical studies measured muscle stiffness based on the concept of the muscle–tendon complex as a mass spring system with a damping component (180) and found conflicting results in ACL-deficient patients. One study found no difference in hamstring stiffness between injured and uninjured legs (181), whereas another found stiffer hamstrings and less stiff quadriceps in the injured leg (182).

Changes in Neurosensory Feedback as a Central Cause of Quadriceps Force Deficit

ACL deficiency is associated with a quadriceps force deficit that in many patients can only be partially corrected with intensive muscle training. Electrophysiologic evidence indicates a possible neurologic cause for this deficit.

Quadriceps atrophy is a nearly constant finding in ACL deficiency (183–185). Several investigators found the decrease in extensor torque larger than would be expected based on the decrease in quadriceps volume measured by computed tomography (184–188). The hamstring muscles do not show a comparable volume or force deficit (183–185,189). Specific physiotherapy can only partly correct the force deficit (190). A persisting torque difference has been reported after ACL repair (191) or reconstruction using patellar ligament autografts and allografts (190,192–195) and semitendinosus grafts (148,196,197). For example, in a group of 119 patients in which one half had ACL repair with iliotibial band reinforcement and the other half bone–patellar ligament–bone reconstruction, an extensor torque deficit of 9% to 20% compared with the uninjured leg was present at an average of 4 years after reconstruction (191).

Biopsies of quadriceps muscle show minor changes that cannot explain the force deficit (183,185,198). Muscle atrophy is caused primarily by a decrease in the diameter of the muscle fibers. Muscle strength is proportional to the diameter of the muscle fibers, unless the fibers are not fully activated (123). A decrease in activation can be determined by measuring electromyographic activity. Under static conditions, the integrated electromyogram reflects the number of activated muscle fibers and their discharge frequency. Several researchers found a lower integrated electromyogram in the affected leg in operatively (187,199) and conservatively (187,200) treated ACL-deficient patients. However, the electrical efficiency of the muscle (i.e., ratio of integrated electromyogram and work) is not changed for the affected leg (187,199,200). These findings led Elmqvist et al. (200) to propose the strength deficit results from diminished drive of the central nervous system to the quadriceps muscles. A decrease in the activation of quadriceps muscles on a spinal or higher level could be a consequence of an alteration in the afferent signals after ACL rupture. Consequently, a reduction of quadriceps atrophy can be expected when direct electrical stimulation of the muscle is applied. One study confirmed a decrease of quadriceps atrophy, but the investigators did not account for the total work in the two experimental groups (198). The quadriceps force deficit has been reported to be less with direct electrical stimulation compared with volitional muscle exercise (190), but in a study in which torque was monitored during treatment to try to match the absolute muscular tensions in the experimental groups, no difference between the two exercise methods was found (201).

Functional Analysis Shows Neuromuscular Adaptations in Patients with Chronic Anterior Cruciate Ligament Deficiency

Gait analysis in ACL-deficient patients indicates decreased quadriceps activation as a mechanism to reduce anterior tibial translation. This "quadriceps avoidance gait" is seen in approximately two thirds of patients; its prevalence is partly related to the time since injury (202). In the absence of the ACL, quadriceps contraction generates anterior translation of the tibia (4). The finding of reduced quadriceps activation is in agreement with some electromyographic studies (203–205). Alternatively, a decrease in anterior tibial translation can also be affected by an increase in hamstring or gastrocnemius activation (co-contraction), and this has likewise been found in electromyographic studies (206–210). The two mechanisms likely occur simultaneously (203).

For activities that involve knee flexion angles less than 30° (i.e., normal gait), quadriceps avoidance is probably more effective than hamstring co-contraction in preventing anterior tibial translation (211,212), although hamstring co-contraction may also have a stabilizing effect near extension through increasing the joint compressive force (213). In activities that involve knee flexion angles of 40° or more (e.g., jumping, cutting), increased hamstring contraction is effective in preventing anterior tibial translation (211,214–217).

The observed changes do not result from a process that occurs anew with every step. Both adaptations—quadriceps avoidance gait and hamstring co-contraction—precede anterior tibial translation and therefore cannot be the consequence of a reflex mechanism. Functional adaptations appear to be a consequence of a reprogramming of movement strategies that has taken place after an ACL rupture. This can only be attained if the joint receptors that signal the event transfer information to higher centers followed by modification of motor programs—a learning process. Motor programs can be defined as neural networks that govern specific, oft repeated motions. Conversely, reflex-like mechanisms can be excluded based on the time frames involved (218). Another factor that indicates a supraspinal mechanism is the presence of functional adaptations in both limbs of patients with unilateral ACL deficiency (219).

Neuromuscular Adaptations in Anterior Cruciate Ligament Deficiency That Prevent Damage to Secondary Restraints and Stabilize the Knee in Stressful Activities

It is assumed (but not proved) that neuromuscular adaptations are beneficial to ACL-deficient patients. Many patients with lower extremity ligament injury complain of vague symptoms such as the joint feeling unsteady (i.e., giving way). It seems likely at least some aspects of these symptoms are related to mechanoreceptors. It is conceivable that increased anterior tibial translation leads to a feeling of instability in ACL-deficient patients and, in the long term, influences the development of osteoarthrosis. However, direct evidence for either assumption is unavailable. However, several lines of research taken in conjunction do point to a deleterious effect of increased anterior tibial translation and the importance of neuromuscular factors.

ACL transection produces degenerative cartilage changes in the dog, cat, goat, rabbit, and rat (220–224). These changes are not caused by the synovitis after transection of the ligament (225,226). Approximately one half of ACL-deficient patients have radiographic osteoarthritic changes at 10 to 15 years after the initial injury (227,228). In ACL-deficient patients who also had partial meniscectomy, the incidence of radiographic osteoarthrosis was 61% at 20 to 24 years, 71% at 25 to 29 years, and 86% at 30 to 34 years. In patients with partial meniscectomy and an intact ACL, these rates were 40%, 34%, and 50%, respectively, for the same follow-up durations. For the contralateral knee, the rates were below 12% for all groups (229).

Measurement of dynamic laxity during gait is a technical challenge in the ACL-deficient patient (151), and until now, it has only been accomplished in dogs. Increased anterior tibial translation occurs abruptly when the dog lands on the paw and starts to bear weight, and it is maintained throughout stance phase (230,231). The dogs compensate by reducing the limb load and by increasing knee flexion throughout the gait cycle, but they are unable to prevent joint subluxation in stance (230). After 1 and 2 years, dynamic anterior tibial translation was similar to that directly after ACL transection (153). It appears that dogs are not capable of limiting the anterior tibial translation during gait by neuromuscular adaptations. Cats also have stronger knee flexion after ACL transection, but a return to normal flexion range occurs from 3 months after the intervention (dynamic laxity was not measured in this study) (221). Increased anterior tibial translation of the ACL-deficient knee primarily loads the posterior horn of the medial meniscal in cadaver experiments (232) and computer models (214), and it corresponds to the increase in meniscus lesions, mostly medial, seen with time from ACL rupture (233–235).

In dogs, ACL transection leads to slight degenerative cartilage changes at 1 year, but additional deafferentation of the knee joint produces severe degenerative changes within 3 weeks (220,236). Although kinematic studies do not show dogs can effectively limit dynamic laxity, joint sensory input appears to play a role in adapting motor programs so potentially harmful joint positions and loads are prevented, limiting the rate at which an unstable joint degenerates. However, joint sensory input may have a modulatory function in normal tissue homeostasis and can play a role in the development of osteoarthrosis, irrespective of joint instability (47,48).

SUMMARY AND PROPOSALS

We can presume ligament injury has two neurosensory effects: loss of mechanoreceptor signaling from the torn ligament and gain in mechanoreceptor signaling from receptors in the periarticular tissues as a result of instability. Given the fact that functional outcome with a torn ACL does not directly correlate with the amount of laxity, it is possible such lack of correlation relates to variable patient adaptation to loss or gain of signals.

Ligament mechanoreceptors are part of a complex input of several receptor populations that influence muscle stiffness. The fact that several other (potentially redundant) receptor populations have input in this system can be used as an argument for assuming the relatively few receptors in most ligaments may have minor importance in this context and that the loss of receptor input may be compensated for by the remaining receptors of the system. However, the precise role of various receptors may vary from individual to individual, and mechanore-

ceptor loss or failure to adapt from redundant sources may prove more critical in some patients than others.

For the quadriceps, however, specific considerations may be justified. The ACL and quadriceps are mechanical antagonists. Knee extension generates ACL strain, activating mechanoreceptors in the ACL. Quadriceps muscle contraction further increases ACL strain in the extended knee. The ACL is the only structure specifically antagonizing the anterior tibial translation generated by the quadriceps muscle; its mechanoreceptors may be the only mechanoreceptors sensitively and effectively signaling anterior tibial translation. A specific influence of ACL mechanoreceptor output on quadriceps function seems reasonable. In this case, the fact that only a few mechanoreceptors are present need not signify the receptors are unimportant, because they may be the only receptors present with this function. Based on the quadriceps force deficit after ACL rupture, this proposed function may facilitate quadriceps activation when the ACL strain is between certain limits. If we accept a direct reflex influence is not likely, a modulating effect of ACL mechanoreceptor output on motor programs could be proposed in which the quadriceps muscle plays an important role. Traditionally, views on such problems have been based on the notion of direct reflexes, but it may be more realistic to incorporate the notion of a loading *history* instead of a single loading event into any hypothesized function of such receptors.

Based on the neuropeptide expression of afferent free nerve endings, these fibers may play a role, in conjunction with the efferent fibers, in maintaining homeostasis of the ligament (or a remodeled graft). They may play a role in the regulation of blood flow and in the turnover of collagenous tissues. In bone, the primary determinant for control of tissue growth, remodeling, and homeostasis appears to be mechanical factors. In this view, mechanical usage dominates nonmechanical factors (i.e., genes, hormones, cytokines, and calcium). Mechanical factors, especially strain, guide the activities of nonmechanical factors. A primary role of mechanical factors is likewise assumed for soft tissue such as ligament and tendon (237). The precise way in which tissue strain influences mediator mechanisms is unknown. Whether the mechanoreceptor response to the loading history of a ligament also contributes to this is entirely speculative.

For all three functions proposed, potentially testable hypotheses could be formulated. One approach is to design experiments that selectively stimulate or block ligament afferent nerve fibers in combination with a sensitive outcome measure (238). Other approaches can be based on the study of mechanoreceptor function *in vivo*, but this depends on the development of new measurement tools. Whether mechanoreceptors of joint ligaments other than the ACL will have comparable functions seems likely for the first and third function proposed. What seems obvious is the presence of mechanoreceptors and their clear roles in subtle or difficult-to-measure functions. Such subtlety should not be taken as meaning that they do not have important functional or performance implications. As more sensitive measures are developed, it will be possible to study the true roles of these receptors and what must be done to facilitate functional recovery after their loss.

REFERENCES

1. Müller WE. *The knee: form, function and ligament reconstruction.* Berlin: Springer-Verlag, 1983.
2. van der Wal JC. *The organisation of the substrate of proprioception in the elbow region of the rat* [Thesis]. Maastricht, The Netherlands: Rijksuniversiteit Limburg, 1988.
3. Kandel ER, Schwarz SJ, Jessel TM. *Principles of neural science.* New York: Prentice-Hall, 1992.
4. Kaufman KR, Daniel DM, Woo SLY. Joint kinematics in muscle stabilized knees. In: Jackson DW, ed. *The anterior cruciate ligament. Current and future concepts.* New York: Raven Press, 1993;113–130.
5. Müller WE. Kinematics. In: Müller WE, ed. *The knee: form, function and ligament reconstruction.* Berlin: Springer-Verlag, 1983:16–29.
6. Khalsa PS, Grigg P. Responses of mechanoreceptor neurons in the cat knee joint capsule before and after anterior cruciate ligament transection. *J Orthop Res* 1996;14:114–122.
7. Craig AD, Heppelmann B, Schaible HG. The projection of the medial and posterior articular nerves of the cat's knee to the spinal cord. *J Comp Neurol* 1988;276:279–288.
8. Langford RA, Schmidt RF. Afferent and efferent axons in the medial and posterior articular nerves of the cat. *Anat Rec* 1983;206:71–78.
9. Grigg P, Hoffman AH. Properties of Ruffini afferents revealed by stress analysis of isolated sections of cat knee capsule. *J Neurophysiol* 1982;47:41–54.
10. Grigg P, Hoffman AH, Fogarty KE. Properties of Golgi-Mazzoni afferents in cat knee joint capsule, as revealed by mechanical studies of isolated joint capsule. *J Neurophysiol* 1982;47:31–40.
11. Grigg P, Hoffman AH. Stretch-sensitive afferent neurons in cat knee joint capsule: sensitivity to axial and compression stresses and strains. *J Neurophysiol* 1996;75:1871–1877.
12. Dyson FJ. *Imagined worlds* [Jerusalem-Harvard lectures]. Cambridge, MA: Harvard University Press, 1997.
13. Goldscheider A. Untersuchungen über den Muskeln. *Arch Anat Physiol Leipzig* 1889;3:369–502.
14. Krause W. *Die terminalen Körperchen der einfach sensibelen Nerven. Anatomisch physiologische Monographie.* Hanover: , 1870.
15. Krause W. Histologische Notizen. *Zentralbl Med Wiss* 1874;12:211–212.
16. Rauber A. Uber die Vater'schen Körper der Gelenkkapseln. *Zentralbl Med Wiss* 1874;12:305–306.
17. Gomez-Barrena E, Martinez-Moreno E, Munuera L. Segmental sensory innervation of the anterior cruciate ligament and the patellar tendon of the cat's knee. *Acta Orthop Scand* 1996;67:545–552.
18. Freeman MAR, Wyke B. The innervation of the knee joint. An anatomical and histological study in the cat. *J Anat* 1967;101:505–532.
19. Halata Z, Haus J. The ultrastructure of sensory nerve endings in human anterior cruciate ligament. *Anat Embryol* 1989;179:415–421.
20. Madey SM, Cole KJ, Brand RA. Sensory innervation of the cat knee articular capsule and cruciate ligament visualized using anterogradely transported wheat germ agglutinin-horseradish peroxidase. *J Anat* 1997;190:289–297.
21. Barrack RL, Skinner HB. The sensory function of knee ligaments. In: Daniel DM, Akeson WH, O'Connor JJ, eds. *Knee ligaments: structure, function, injury and repair.* New York: Raven Press, 1990:95–114.
22. Johansson H, Sjölander P, Sojka P. Receptors in the knee joint ligaments and their role in the biomechanics of the joint. *Crit Rev Biomed Eng* 1991;18:341–368.
23. Wyke B. The neurology of joints. *Ann R Coll Surg Engl* 1967;41:25–50.
24. Palmer I. On the injuries to the ligaments of the knee joint. A clinical study. *Acta Chir Scand* 1938;81:1–282.
25. Gardner E. The innervation of the knee joint. *Anat Rec* 1948;101:109–130.
26. Jeletsky AG. On the innervation of the capsule and epiphysis of the knee joint. *Vestn Khir* 1931;74–112.
27. Rudinger N. *Die Gelenknerven des menschlichen Korpers.* Erlangen: Ferdinand Enke Verlag, 1857.
28. Boyd IA. The histological structure of the receptors in the knee-joint of the cat correlated with their physiological response. *J Physiol* 1954;124:476–488.
29. Andrew BL. The sensory innervation of the medial ligament of the knee joint. *J Physiol (Lond)* 1954;123:241–250.
30. Skoglund S. Anatomical and physiological studies of the knee joint innervation in the cat. *Acta Physiol Scand* 1956;36:2–101.
31. Grigg P, Greenspan BJ. Response of primate joint afferent neurons to mechanical stimulation of knee joint. *J Neurophysiol* 1977;40:1–8.
32. Hagen-Torn O. Entwicklung und Bau der Synovialmembranen. *Arch Mikr Anat* 1882;21:591–663.
33. Polacek P. Differences in the structure and variability of encapsulated nerve endings in the joints of some species of mammals. *Acta Anat* 1961;47:112–124.
34. Schultz RA, Miller DC, Kerr CS, et al. Mechanoreceptors in human cruciate ligaments. A histological study. *J Bone Joint Surg Am* 1984;66:1072–1076.
35. Krauspe R, Schmitz F, Zoller G, et al. Distribution of neurofilament-positive nerve fibres and sensory endings in the human anterior cruciate ligament. *Arch Orthop Trauma Surg* 1995;114:194–198.
36. Strasmann T, van der Wal JC, Halata Z, et al. Functional topography and ultrastructure of periarticular mechanoreceptors in the lateral elbow region of the rat. *Acta Anat (Basel)* 1990;138:1–14.
37. Stilwell DL. The innervation of tendons and aponeuroses. *Am J Anat* 1957;100:289–311.
38. Matthews PBC. Where does Sherrington's "muscular sense" originate? Muscles, joints, corollary discharges? *Annu Rev Neurosci* 1982;5:189–218.
39. Proske U, Schaible HG, Schmidt RF. Joint receptors and kinaesthesia. *Exp Brain Res* 1988;72:219–224.
40. Horner G, Dellon AL. Innervation of the human knee joint and implications for surgery. *Clin Orthop* 1994;301:221–226.
41. Kennedy JC, Alexander IJ, Hayes KC. Nerve supply of the human knee and its functional importance. *Am J Sports Med* 1982;10:329–335.
42. O'Connor BL, Woodbury P. The primary articular nerves to the dog knee. *J Anat* 1982;134:563–572.
43. O'Connor BL, Seipel J. Anatomical variations of the posterior articular nerve to the cat knee joint. *J Anat* 1983;136:27–34.
44. Sparmann M, Hessel C, Gosztonyi G. Loss of innervation of the anterior cruciate ligament in idiopathic gonarthrosis. *Z Orthop Ihre Grenzgeb* 1996;134:233–237.
45. Burgess PR, Clark FJ. Characteristics of knee joint receptors in the cat. *J Physiol (Lond)* 1969;203:317–335.
46. McIntyre AK, Proske U, Tracey DJ. Afferent fibres from muscle receptors in the posterior nerve of the cat's knee joint. *Exp Brain Res* 1978;33:415–424.
47. Salo PT, Tatton WG. Age-related loss of knee joint afferents in mice. *J Neurosci Res* 1993;35:664–677.
48. Salo PT, Erwin WM. Loss of knee joint innervation precedes the development of degenerative changes in a mouse model of knee osteoarthrosis. *Trans Orthop Res Soc* 1999;24:197
49. Bell J, Bolanowski S, Holmes MH. The structure and function of pacinian corpuscles: a review. *Prog Neurobiol* 1994;42:79–128.
50. Darian-Smith I. The sense of touch: performance and peripheral neural processes. In: Darian-Smith I, ed. *Handbook of physiology,* section 1. *The nervous system,* vol III. *Sensory processes,* part 2. Bethesda, MD: American Physiological Society, 1984;739–788.
51. Ruffini A. *Arch Ital Biol* 1894;21:249.
52. Rivard CH, Yahia LH, Rhalmi S, et al. Immunohistochemical demonstration of sensory nerve fibers and endings in human anterior cruciate ligaments. *Trans Orthop Res Soc* 1993;18:61.
53. De Avila GA, O'Connor BL, Visco DM, et al. The mechanoreceptor innervation of the human fibular collateral ligament. *J Anat* 1989;162:1–7.
54. Koch B, Kurriger G, Brand RA. Characterisation of the neurosensory elements of the feline cranial cruciate ligament. *J Anat* 1995;187:353–359.

55. McLain RF. Mechanoreceptors in human ligaments. *J Bone Joint Surg Br* 1995;77:982.

56. Halata Z. Ruffini corpuscle—a stretch receptor in the connective tissue of the skin and locomotion apparatus. *Prog Brain Res* 1988;74:221–229.

57. Messlinger K, Pawlak M, Steinbach H, et al. A new combination of methods for the localization, identification, and three-dimensional reconstruction of the sensory endings of articular afferents characterized by electrophysiology. *Cell Tissue Res* 1995;281:283–294.

58. Zimny ML, Schutte MJ, Dabezies EJ. Mechanoreceptors in human anterior cruciate ligament. *Anat Rec* 1986;214:204–209.

59. Barrack RL, Lund PJ, Munn BG, et al. Evidence of reinnervation of free patellar tendon autograft used for anterior cruciate ligament reconstruction. *Am J Sports Med* 1997;25:196–202.

60. Sjölander P, Johansson H, Sojka P, et al. Sensory nerve endings in the cat cruciate ligaments: a morphological investigation. *Neurosci Lett* 1989;102:33–38.

61. Grigg P. Nervous system control of joint function. In: Finerman GAM, Noyes FR, eds. *Biology and biomechanics of the traumatized synovial joint: the knee as a model.* Chicago: AAOS Symposium, 1992:275–287.

62. Schoultz TW, Swett JE. The fine structure of the Golgi tendon organ. *J Neurocytol* 1972;1:1–26.

63. Schoultz TW, Swett JE. Ultrastructural organization of the sensory fibers innervating the Golgi tendon organ. *Anat Anz* 1974;179:147–162.

64. Proske U. The Golgi tendon organ. Properties of the receptor and reflex action of impulses arising from tendon organs. *Int Rev Physiol* 1981;25:127–171.

65. Clark FJ. Information signaled by sensory fibers in medial articular nerve. *J Neurophysiol* 1975;38:1464–1478.

66. Halata Z. The ultrastructure of the sensory nerve endings in the articular capsule of the knee joint of the domestic cat (Ruffini corpuscles and Pacinian corpuscles). *J Anat* 1977;124:717–729.

67. Halata Z, Rettig T, Schulze W. The ultrastructure of sensory nerve endings in the human knee joint capsule. *Anat Embryol* 1985;172:265–275.

68. Schaible HG, Schmidt RF. Responses of fine medial articular nerve afferents to passive movements of knee joints. *J Neurophysiol* 1983;49:1118–1126.

69. Schaible HG, Schmidt RF. Effects of an experimental arthritis on the sensory properties of fine articular afferent units. *J Neurophysiol* 1985;54:1109–1122.

70. Samuel EP. The autonomic and somatic innervation of the articular capsule. *Anat Rec* 1952;113:53–70.

71. Schwab W, Bilgicyildirim A, Funk RH. Microtopography of the autonomic nerves in the rat knee: a fluorescence microscopic study. *Anat Rec* 1997;247:109–118.

72. Brain SD, Williams TJ. Substance P regulates the vasodilator activity of calcitonin gene-related peptide. *Nature* 1988;335:73–75.

73. Hokfelt T. Neuropeptides in perspective: the last ten years. *Neuron* 1991;7:867–879.

74. Holzer P. Local effector functions of capsaicin-sensitive sensory nerve endings: involvement of tachykinins, calcitonin gene-related peptide and other neuropeptides. *Neuroscience* 1988;24:739–768.

75. Kidd BL, Mapp PI, Gibson SJ, et al. A neurogenic mechanism for symmetrical arthritis [See comments]. *Lancet* 1989;2:1128–1130.

76. Levine JD, Clark R, Devor M, et al. Intraneuronal substance P contributes to the severity of experimental arthritis. *Science* 1984;226:547–549.

77. Salo PT. Selective loss of knee joint mechanoreceptors in aging mice. *Trans Orthop Res Soc* 1998;23:151.

78. Denti M, Monteleone M, Berardi A, et al. Anterior cruciate ligament mechanoreceptors. Histologic studies on lesions and reconstruction. *Clin Orthop* 1994;308:29–32.

79. Goertzen MJ, Clahsen H, Burrig KF, et al. Sterilisation of canine anterior cruciate ligaments by gamma irradiation in argon. *J Bone Joint Surg Br* 1995;77:205–212.

80. Fulford P. Retraction of a paper [Editorial]. *J Bone Joint Surg Br* 1997;79:705–706.

81. Arnoczky SP. Biology of ACL reconstructions: what happens to the graft? *Instr Course Lect* 1996;45:229–233.

82. Howell SM, Knox KE, Farley TE, et al. Revascularization of a human anterior cruciate ligament graft during the first two years of implantation. *Am J Sports Med* 1995;23:42–49.

83. Goldie I, Wellisch M. The presence of nerves in original and regenerated synovial tissue in patients synovectomised for rheumatoid arthritis. *Acta Orthop Scand* 1969;40:143–152.

84. Bentley G, Kreutner A, Ferguson AB. Synovial regeneration and articular cartilage changes after synovectomy in normal and steroid-treated rabbits. *J Bone Joint Surg Br* 1975;57:454–462.

85. Ranawat CS, Straub LR, Freyberg R, et al. A study of regenerated synovium after synovectomy of the knee in rheumatoid arthritis. *Arthritis Rheum* 1971;14:117–125.

86. Aune AK, Hukkanen M, Madsen JE, et al. Nerve regeneration during patellar tendon autograft remodelling after anterior cruciate ligament reconstruction: an experimental and clinical study. *J Orthop Res* 1996;14:193–199.

87. Hukkanen M, Konttinen YT, Santavirta S, et al. Rapid proliferation of calcitonin gene-related peptide-immunoreactive nerves during healing of rat tibial fracture suggests neural involvement in bone growth and remodelling. *Neuroscience* 1993;54:969–979.

88. Nordsletten L, Madsen JE, Almaas R, et al. The neuronal regulation of fracture healing. Effects of sciatic nerve resection in rat tibia. *Acta Orthop Scand* 1994;65:299–304.

89. Kjartansson J, Dalsgaard CJ. Calcitonin gene-related peptide increases survival of musculocutaneous flap in the rat. *J Pharmacol* 1987;142:355–358.

90. Kostakoglu N, Manek S, Terenghi G, et al. Free sensate secondary skin flaps: an experimental study on patterns of reinnervation and neovascularisation. *Br J Plast Surg* 1994;47:1–9.

91. Jackson DW, Grood ES, Arnoczky SP, et al. Cruciate reconstruction using freeze dried anterior cruciate ligament allograft and a ligament augmentation device (LAD). An experimental study in a goat model. *Am J Sports Med* 1987;15:528–538.

92. Kleiner JB, Amiel D, Harwood FL, et al. Early histologic, metabolic, and vascular assessment of anterior cruciate ligament autografts. *J Orthop Res* 1989;7:235–242.

93. Halata Z, Groth H-P. Innervation of the synovial membrane of the cats joint capsule. *Cell Tissue Res* 1976;169:415–418.

94. Madison RD, Archibald SJ, Krarup C. Peripheral nerve injury. In: Cohen IK, Diegelman RF, Linblad WJ, eds. *Wound healing: biochemical and clinical aspects.* Philadelphia: WB Saunders, 1992.

95. Terenghi G. Peripheral nerve injury and regeneration. *Histol Histopathol* 1995;10:709–718.

96. Hall SM. Regeneration in the peripheral nervous system. *Neuropathol Appl Neurobiol* 1989;15:513–529.

97. Turkof E, Jurecka W, Sikos G, et al. Sensory recovery in myocutaneous, noninnervated free flaps: a morphologic, immunohistochemical, and electron microscopic study. *Plast Reconstr Surg* 1993;92:238–247.

98. Ide C. Degeneration of mouse digital corpuscles. *Am J Anat* 1982;163:59–72.

99. Barker D, Berry RB, Scott JJ. The sensory reinnervation of muscles following immediate and delayed nerve repair in the cat. *Br J Plast Surg* 1990;43:107–111.

100. Collins WF, Mendel LM, Munson JB. On the specificity of sensory reinnervation of cat skeletal muscle. *J Physiol* 1986;375:587–609.

101. Banks RW, Barker D, Brown HG. Sensory reinnervation of muscles following nerve section and suture in cats. *J Hand Surg Br* 1985;10:340–344.

102. Koshima I, Moriguchi T, Soeda S. Reinnervation of denervated pacinian corpuscles: ultrastructural observations in rats following free nerve grafts. *Plast Reconstr Surg* 1993;92:728–735.

103. Quick DC, Rogers SL. Stretch receptors in regenerated rat muscle. *Neuroscience* 1983;10:851–859.

104. Grigg P. Peripheral neural mechanisms in proprioception. *J Sports Rehab* 1994;3:2–17.

105. Martin JH. Coding and Processing of Sensory Information. In: Kandel ER, Schwartz JH, Jessel TM, eds. *Principles of neural science.* New York: Elsevier, 1992:329–340.

106. Gottschaldt K-M, Iggo A, Young DW. Functional characteristics of mechanoreceptors in sinus hair follicles of the cat. *J Physiol (Lond)* 1973;235:287–315.

107. Janig W. Morphology of rapidly and slowly adapting mechanoreceptors in the hairless skin of the cat's hind foot. *Brain Res* 1971;28:217–231.

108. Loewenstein WR, Mendelson M. Components of receptor adaptation in a pacinian corpuscle. *J Physiol (Lond)* 1965;177:377–397.

109. Coggeshall RE, Hong KA, Langford RA, et al. Discharge characteris-

tic of fine medial articular afferents at rest and during passive movement of inflamed knee joints. *Brain Res* 1983;272:185–188.

110. Grubb BD, Birrell GJ, McQueen DS, et al. The role of PGE_2 in the sensitization of mechanoreceptors in normal and inflamed ankle joints of the rat. *Exp Brain Res* 1991;84:383–392.

111. Mapp PI, Kidd BL, Gibson SJ, et al. Substance P, calcitonin gene-related peptide, and C-flanking peptide of neuropeptide Y-immunoreactive fibres are present in normal synovium but depleted in patients with rheumatoid arthritis. *Neuroscience* 1990;37:143–153.

112. Schaible HG, Neugebauer V, Schmidt RF. Osteoarthritis and pain. *Semin Arthritis Rheum* 1989;18:30–34.

113. Grigg P, Hoffman AH. Calibrating joint capsule mechanoreceptors as in vivo soft tissue load cells. *J Biomech* 1989;22:781–785.

114. Grigg P, Hoffman AH. Ruffini mechanoreceptors in isolated joint capsule: responses correlated with strain energy density. *Somatosens Res* 1984;2:149–162.

115. Grigg P. Mechanical factors influencing response of joint afferent neurons from cat knee. *J Neurophysiol* 1975;38:1473–1484.

116. Stener B. Experimental evaluation of the hypothesis of ligamento-muscular protective reflexes. I. A method for adequate stimulation of tension receptors in the medial collateral ligament of the knee joint of the cat, and studies of the innervation of the ligament. *Acta Physiol Scand* 1959;48:5–26.

117. Pope DF, Cole KJ, Brand RA. Properties of anterior cruciate ligament mechanoreceptor afferents. *J Biomech* 1990;23:717.

118. Krauspe R, Schmidt M, Schaible HG. Sensory innervation of the anterior cruciate ligament. An electrophysiological study of the response properties of single identified mechanoreceptors in the cat. *J Bone Joint Surg Am* 1992;74:390–397.

119. Markolf KL, Gorek JF, Kabo JM, et al. Direct measurement of resultant forces in the anterior cruciate ligament. An in vitro study performed with a new experimental technique. *J Bone Joint Surg Am* 1990;72:557–567.

120. Ferrell WRJ, Rosenberg JR, Baxendale RH, et al. Fourier analysis of the relation between the discharge of quadriceps motor units and periodic mechanical stimulation of cat knee joint receptors. *Exp Physiol* 1990;75:739–750.

121. Lundberg A, Malmgren K, Schomburg ED. Role of joint afferents in motor control exemplified by effects on reflex pathways from Ib afferents. *J Physiol (Lond)* 1978;284:327–343.

122. Johansson H, Sjölander P, Sojka P. Activity in receptor afferents from the anterior cruciate ligament evokes reflex effects on fusimotor neurones. *Neurosci Res* 1990;8:54–59.

123. Garrett WE. Skeletal muscle and the knee joint. In: Finerman GAM, Noyes FR, eds. *Biology and biomechanics of the traumatized synovial joint: the knee as a model.* Chicago: AAOS Symposium, 1992: 289–302.

124. Abbott LC, Saunders JB, Dee M, et al. Injuries to the ligaments of the knee joint. *J Bone Joint Surg* 1944;26:503–505.

125. Solomonow M, Baratta R, Zhou BH, et al. The synergistic action of the anterior cruciate ligament and thigh muscles in maintaining joint stability. *Am J Sports Med* 1987;15:207–213.

126. Gardner E. Reflex muscular responses to stimulation of articular nerves in the cat. *Am J Physiology* 1950;161:133–141.

127. Andersson S, Stener B. Experimental evaluation of the hypothesis of ligamento-muscular protective reflexes. II. A study in cat using the medial collateral ligament of the knee joint. *Acta Physiol Scand* 1959; 48[Suppl]:27–49.

128. Cohen LA, Cohen ML. Arthrokinetic reflex of the knee. *Am J Physiol* 1956;184:433–437.

129. Ekholm J, Eklund G, Skoglund S. On the reflex effects from the knee joint of the cat. *Acta Physiol Scand* 1960;50:167–174.

130. Palmer I. Pathophysiology of the medial ligament of the knee joint. *Acta Chir Scand* 1958;115:312–318.

131. Grigg P, Harrigan EP, Fogarty KE. Segmental reflexes mediated by joint afferent neurons in cat knee. *J Neurophysiol* 1978;41:9–14.

132. Pope DF, Cole KJ, Brand RA. Physiologic loading of the anterior cruciate ligament does not activate quadriceps or hamstrings in the anesthetized cat. *Am J Sports Med* 1990;18:595–599.

133. Cole KJ, Daley BJ, Brand RA. The sensitivity of joint afferents to knee translation. *Sportverletz Sportschaden* 1996;10:27–31.

134. Miyatsu M, Atsuta Y, Watakabe M. The physiology of mechanoreceptors in the anterior cruciate ligament. An experimental study in decerebrate-spinalised animals. *J Bone Joint Surg Br* 1993;75:653–657.

135. Freeman MAR, Wyke BD. Articular contributions to limb muscle reflexes. The effects of partial neurectomy of the knee joint on postural reflexes. *Br J Surgery* 1966;53:61–69.

136. Rack PX. Muscle spindles. In: *Handbook of physiology.* Bethesda, MD: American Physiological Society, 1984;

137. Sojka P, Johansson H, Sjölander P, et al. Fusimotor neurones can be reflexly influenced by activity in receptor afferents from the posterior cruciate ligament. *Brain Res* 1989;483:177–183.

138. Johansson H, Sjölander P, Sojka P, et al. Different fusimotor reflexes from the ipsi- and contralateral hind limbs of the cat assessed in the same primary muscle spindle afferents. *J Physiol (Paris)* 1988;83: 281–292.

139. Johansson H, Sjölander P, Sojka P, et al. Effects of electrical and natural stimulation of skin afferents on the gamma-spindle system of the triceps surae muscle. *Neurosci Res* 1989;6:537–555.

140. Buss DD, Min R, Skyhar M, et al. Nonoperative treatment of acute anterior cruciate ligament injuries in a selected group of patients. *Am J Sports Med* 1995;23:160–165.

141. Engstrom B, Gornitzka J, Johansson C, et al. Knee function after anterior cruciate ligament ruptures treated conservatively. *Int Orthop* 1993;17:208–213.

142. Noyes FR, Matthews DS, Mooar PA, et al. The symptomatic anterior cruciate-deficient knee. Part II. The results of rehabilitation, activity modification, and counseling on functional disability. *J Bone Joint Surg Am* 1983;65:163–174.

143. Snyder-Mackler L, Fitzgerald GK, Bartolozzi AR, et al. The relationship between passive joint laxity and functional outcome after anterior cruciate ligament injury. *Am J Sports Med* 1997;25:191–195.

144. Wojtys EM, Huston LJ. Neuromuscular performance in normal and anterior cruciate ligament-deficient lower extremities. *Am J Sports Med* 1994;22:89–104.

145. Sommerlath K, Lysholm J, Gillquist J. The long-term course after treatment of acute anterior cruciate ligament ruptures. A 9 to 16 year follow-up. *Am J Sports Med* 1991;19:156–162.

146. Barrett DS. Proprioception and function after anterior cruciate reconstruction. *J Bone Joint Surg Br* 1991;73:833–837.

147. Harter RA, Osternig LR, Singer KM, et al. Long-term evaluation of knee stability and function following surgical reconstruction for anterior cruciate ligament insufficiency. *Am J Sports Med* 1988;16: 434–443.

148. Kramer J, Nusca D, Fowler P, et al. Knee flexor and extensor strength during concentric and eccentric muscle actions after anterior cruciate ligament reconstruction using the semitendinosus tendon and ligament augmentation device. *Am J Sports Med* 1993;21:285–291.

149. Shiraishi M, Mizuta H, Kubota K, et al. Stabilometric assessment in the anterior cruciate ligament- reconstructed knee. *Clin J Sport Med* 1996;6:32–39.

150. Dyrby CO, Andriacchi TP. Three dimensional measurement of the dynamic envelope of knee motion. *Trans Orthop Res Soc* 1999;24: 934.

151. Hassan SS, Hurwitz DE, Bush-Joseph CA, et al. Dynamic evaluation of knee instability during gait in anterior cruciate ligament deficient patients. *Trans Orthop Res Soc* 1998;23:805.

152. Vergis A, Hindriks M, Gillquist J. Sagittal plane translations of the knee in anterior cruciate deficient subjects and controls. *Med Sci Sports Exerc* 1997;29:1561–1566.

153. Tashman S, Anderst WJ, Schaffler MB, et al. Chronic dynamic instability and osteoarthrosis following ACL loss in dogs. *Trans Orthop Res Soc* 1999;24:457.

154. Andriacchi TP, Alexander EJ, Toney MK, et al. A point cluster method for in vivo motion analysis: applied to a study of knee kinematics. *J Biomech Eng* 1998;120:743–749.

155. Lafortune MA, Cavanagh PR, Sommer HJ, et al. Three-dimensional kinematics of the human knee during walking. *J Biomech* 1992;25: 347–357.

156. Ferrell WR. Articular proprioception and nociception. *Rheumatol Rev* 1992;1:161–167.

157. Martin JH, Jessel TM. Modality coding in the sensory system. In: Kandell ER, Schwartz JH, Jessel TM, eds. *Principles of neural science.* New York: Elsevier, 1992:342–352.

158. Taylor JL, McCloskey DI. Ability to detect angular displacements of the fingers made at an imperceptibly slow speed. *Brain* 1990;113:157–166.

159. Barrack RL, Skinner HB, Buckley SL. Proprioception in the anterior cruciate deficient knee. *Am J Sports Med* 1989;17:1–6.

160. Lephart SM, Pincivero DM, Giraldo JL, et al. The role of proprioception in the management and rehabilitation of athletic injuries. *Am J Sports Med* 1997;25:130–137.

161. Jennings AG. A proprioceptive role for the anterior cruciate ligament: a review of the literature. *J Orthop Rheumatol* 1994;7:3–13.

162. Gandevia SC, McCloskey DI, Burke D. Kinaesthetic signals and muscle contraction. *Trends Neurosci* 1992;15:62–65.

163. Barrett DS, Cobb AG, Bentley G. Joint proprioception in normal, osteoarthritic and replaced knees. *J Bone Joint Surg Br* 1991;73:53–56.

164. Kaplan FS, Nixon JE, Reitz M, et al. Age-related changes in proprioception and sensation of joint position. *Acta Orthop Scand* 1985;56:72–74.

165. Skinner HB, Barrack RL, Cook SD. Age-related decline in proprioception. *Clin Orthop* 1984;184:208–211.

166. Perlau R, Frank C, Fick G. The effect of elastic bandages on human knee proprioception in the uninjured knee. *Am J Sports Med* 1995;23:251–255.

167. Corrigan JP, Cashman WF, Brady MP. Proprioception in the cruciate deficient knee. *J Bone Joint Surg Br* 1992;74:247–250.

168. Klein BP, Blaha JD, Simons W. Anterior cruciate-deficient knees do not have altered proprioception. *Trans Orthop Res Soc* 1992;17:501.

169. Wright SA, Tearse DS, Brand RA, et al. Proprioception in the anteriorly unstable knee. *Iowa Orthop J* 1995;15:156–161.

170. Friden T, Roberts D, Zatterstrom R, et al. Proprioception in the nearly extended knee. Measurements of position and movement in healthy individuals and in symptomatic anterior cruciate ligament injured patients. *Knee Surg Sports Traumatol Arthrosc* 1996;4:217–224.

171. Good L, Beynnon BD, Gottlieb DJ, et al. Joint position sense is not changed after ACL disruption. *Trans Orthop Res Soc* 1995;20:95.

172. Friden T, Roberts D. Proprioceptive deficits after acute knee injury including an ACL rupture is correlated to chondral and meniscal lesions as well as subjective knee function. *Trans Eur Orthop Res Soc* 1997;7:198.

173. Jerosch J, Prymka M. Proprioception of knee joints with a lesion of the medial meniscus. *Unfallchirurgurgie* 1997;100:445–448.

174. Borsa PA, Lephart SM, Irrgang JJ, et al. The effects of joint position and direction of joint motion on proprioceptive sensibility in anterior cruciate ligament-deficient athletes. *Am J Sports Med* 1997;25:336–340.

175. Gruber J, Wolter D, Lierse W. Anterior cruciate ligament reflex (LCA reflex). *Unfallchirurg* 1986;89:551–554.

176. Solomonow M, Baratta R, Zhou BH, et al. Electromyogram coactivation patterns of the elbow antagonist muscles during slow isokinetic movement. *Exp Neurol* 1988;100:470–477.

177. Beard DJ, Kyberd PJ, O'Connor JJ, et al. Reflex hamstring contraction latency in anterior cruciate ligament deficiency. *J Orthop Res* 1994;12:219–228.

178. Jennings AG, Seedhom BB. Proprioception in the knee and reflex hamstring contraction latency. *J Bone Joint Surg Br* 1994;76:491–494.

179. Latash ML, Zatsiorsky VM. Joint stiffness: myth or reality? *Hum Movement Sci* 1993;12:653–692.

180. Hill AV. Production and absorption of work by muscles. *Science* 1960;131:897–903.

181. McNair PJ, Wood GA, Marshall RN. Stiffness of the hamstring muscles and its relationship to function in ACL deficient individuals. *Clin Biomech* 1992;7:131–137.

182. Jennings AG, Seedhom BB. Anterior cruciate ligament injuries and the measurement of muscle stiffness. *J Orthop Rheumatol* 1996;9:143–149.

183. Gerber C, Hoppeler H, Claassen H, et al. The lower extremity musculature in chronic symptomatic instability of the anterior cruciate ligament. *J Bone Joint Surg Am* 1985;67:1034–1043.

184. Kariya Y, Itoh M, Nakamura T, et al. Magnetic resonance imaging and spectroscopy of thigh muscles in cruciate ligament insufficiency. *Acta Orthop Scand* 1989;60:322–325.

185. Lorentzon R, Elmqvist LG, Sjostrom M, et al. Thigh musculature in relation to chronic anterior cruciate ligament tear: muscle size, morphology, and mechanical output before reconstruction. *Am J Sports Med* 1989;17:423–429.

186. Elmqvist LG, Lorentzon R, Johansson C, et al. Knee extensor muscle function before and after reconstruction of anterior cruciate ligament tear. *Scand J Rehabil Med* 1989;21:131–139.

187. Fink C, Hoser C, Benedetto KP, Judmaier W. (Neuro)muscular changes in the knee stabilizing muscles after rupture of the anterior cruciate ligament. *Sportverletz Sportschaden* 1994;8:25–30.

188. Lopresti C, Kirkendall DT, Streete GM. Quadriceps insufficiency following repair of anterior cruciate ligament. *J Orthop Sports Phys Ther* 1988;9:245–249.

189. Friden T, Zatterstrom R, Lindstrand A, et al. Disability in anterior cruciate ligament insufficiency. An analysis of 19 untreated patients. *Acta Orthop Scand* 1990;61:131–135.

190. Snyder-Mackler L, Delitto A, Bailey SL, et al. Strength of the quadriceps femoris muscle and functional recovery after reconstruction of the anterior cruciate ligament. A prospective, randomized clinical trial of electrical stimulation. *J Bone Joint Surg Am* 1995;77:1166–1173.

191. Natri A, Jarvinen M, Latvala K, et al. Isokinetic muscle performance after anterior cruciate ligament surgery. Long-term results and outcome predicting factors after primary surgery and late-phase reconstruction. *Int J Sports Med* 1996;17:223–228.

192. Osteras H, Augestad LB, Tondel S. Isokinetic muscle strength after anterior cruciate ligament reconstruction. *Scand J Med Sci Sports* 1998;8:279–282.

193. Yasuda K, Ohkoshi Y, Tanabe Y, et al. Quantitative evaluation of knee instability and muscle strength after anterior cruciate ligament reconstruction using patellar and quadriceps tendon. *Am J Sports Med* 1992;20:471–475.

194. Tibone JE, Antich TJ. A biomechanical analysis of anterior cruciate ligament reconstruction with the patellar tendon. A two year followup [See comments]. *Am J Sports Med* 1988;16:332–335.

195. Co FH, Skinner HB, Cannon WD. Effect of reconstruction of the anterior cruciate ligament on proprioception of the knee and the heel strike transient. *J Orthop Res* 1993;11:696–704.

196. Maeda A, Shino K, Horibe S, et al. Anterior cruciate ligament reconstruction with multistranded autogenous semitendinosus tendon. *Am J Sports Med* 1996;24:504–509.

197. Rosenberg TD, Pazik TD, Deffner KT. Primary quadrupled semitendinosus ACL reconstruction: a comprehensive 2 year evaluation. *SICOT Congress* 1996;20:177–178.

198. Arvidsson I, Arvidsson H, Eriksson E, et al. Prevention of quadriceps wasting after immobilization: an evaluation of the effect of electrical stimulation. *Orthopedics* 1986;9:1519–1528.

199. Cooper LW, Kadrmas W, Seaber AV, et al. Strength recovery following ACL reconstructive knee surgery: limited by the central nervous system or by muscle. *Trans Orthop Res Soc* 1996;21:777.

200. Elmqvist LG, Lorentzon R, Johansson C, et al. Does a torn anterior cruciate ligament lead to change in the central nervous drive of the knee extensors? *Eur J Appl Physiol* 1988;58:203–207.

201. Lieber RL, Silva PD, Daniel DM. Equal effectiveness of electrical and volitional strength training for quadriceps femoris muscles after anterior cruciate ligament surgery. *J Orthop Res* 1996;14:131–138.

202. Birac D, Andriacchi TP, Bach BR. Time related changes following ACL rupture. *Trans Orthop Res Soc* 1991;16:231.

203. Limbird TJ, Shiavi R, Frazer M, et al. EMG profiles of knee joint musculature during walking: changes induced by anterior cruciate ligament deficiency. *J Orthop Res* 1988;6:630–638.

204. Branch TP, Hunter R, Donath M. Dynamic EMG analysis of anterior cruciate deficient legs with and without bracing during cutting. *Am J Sports Med* 1989;17:35–41.

205. Shiavi R, Zhang LQ, Limbird T, et al. Pattern analysis of electromyographic linear envelopes exhibited by subjects with uninjured and injured knees during free and fast speed walking. *J Orthop Res* 1992;10:226–236.

206. Beard DJ, Soundarapandian RS, O'Connor JJ, et al. Gait and electromyographic changes of anterior cruciate deficient subjects. *Gait Posture* 1996;4:83–88.

207. Kalund S, Sinkjaer T, Arendt-Nielsen L, et al. Altered timing of hamstring muscle action in anterior cruciate ligament deficient patients. *Am J Sports Med* 1990;18:245–248.

208. Lass P, Kaalund S, le Fevre S, et al. Muscle coordination following rupture of the anterior cruciate ligament. Electromyographic studies of 14 patients. *Acta Orthop Scand* 1991;62:9–14.

209. Roberts CS, Rash GS, Honaker JT, et al. Gait adaptations by patients with a deficient anterior cruciate ligament. *Trans Orthop Res Soc* 1998;23:806.

210. Sinkjaer T, Arendt-Nielsen L. Knee stability and muscle coordination in patients with anterior cruciate ligament injuries: an electromyographic approach. *J Electromyogr Kinesiol* 1991;1:209–217.

211. Andriacchi TP. Dynamics of pathological motion: applied to the anterior cruciate deficient knee [Review]. *J Biomech* 1990;23[Suppl 1]:99–105.

212. Mikosz RP, Andriacchi TP, Andersson GBJ. Model analysis of factors influencing the prediction of muscle forces at the knee. *J Orthop Res* 1988;6:205–214.

213. Liu W, Maitland ME. The effect of hamstring muscle compensation for anterior laxity in the ACL-deficient knee during gait. *J Biomech* 1999;33:871–879.

214. Mikosz RP, Wu CD, Andriacchi TP. Model interpretation of functional adaptations in the ACL-deficient patient. In: *Proceedings of the North American Congress on Biomechanics*. Chicago, August 24, 1992. 1992:411–412.

215. More RC, Karras BT, Neiman R, et al. Hamstrings—an anterior cruciate ligament protagonist. An in vitro study. *Am J Sports Med* 1993;21:231–237.

216. O'Connor JJ. Can muscle co-contraction protect knee ligaments after injury or repair? *J Bone Joint Surg Br* 1993;75:41–48.

217. Renstrom P, Arms SW, Stanwyck TS, et al. Strain within the anterior cruciate ligament during hamstring and quadriceps activity. *Am J Sports Med* 1986;14:83–87.

218. Pope MH, Johnson RJ, Brown DW. The role of the musculature in injuries to the medial collateral ligament. *J Bone Joint Surg Am* 1979; 61:398–402.

219. Berchuck M, Andriacchi TP, Bach BR, et al. Gait adaptations by patients who have a deficient anterior cruciate ligament. *J Bone Joint Surg Am* 1990;72:871–877.

220. Brandt KD. Transection of the anterior cruciate ligament in the dog: a model of osteoarthritis. *Semin Arthritis Rheum* 1991;21:22–32.

221. Suter E, Herzog W, Leonard TR, et al. One-year changes in hind limb kinematics, ground reaction forces and knee stability in an experimental model of osteoarthritis. *J Biomech* 1998;31:511–517.

222. Murphy JM, Boynton RE, Kraus K, et al. An experimental model of osteoarthritis in goats. *Trans Orthop Res Soc* 1999;24:435.

223. McBride JT, Rodkey WG, Brooks DE, et al. Early detection of osteoarthritis using technetium 99m MDP imaging, radiographs, histology and gross pathology in an experimental rabbit model. *Orthop Trans* 1991;15:348–349.

224. Williams JM, Felten DL, Peterson RG, et al. Effects of surgically induced instability on rat knee articular cartilage. *J Anat* 1982;134: 103–109.

225. Myers SL, Brandt KD, O'Connor BL, et al. Synovitis and osteoarthritic changes in canine articular cartilage after anterior cruciate ligament transection. Effect of surgical hemostasis. *Arthritis Rheum* 1990;33:1406–1415.

226. Lukoschek M, Boyd RD, Schaffler MB, et al. Comparison of joint degeneration models. Surgical instability and repetitive impulsive loading. *Acta Orthop Scand* 1986;57:349–353.

227. Lohmander LS, Roos H. Knee ligament injury, surgery and osteoarthrosis. Truth or consequences? *Acta Orthop Scand* 1994;65: 605–609.

228. Roos H, Adalberth T, Dahlberg L, et al. Osteoarthritis of the knee after injury to the anterior cruciate ligament or meniscus: the influence of time and age. *Osteoarthritis Cartilage* 1995;3:261–267.

229. Neyret P, Donell ST, Dejour H. Results of partial meniscectomy related to the state of the anterior cruciate ligament. Review at 20 to 35 years. *J Bone Joint Surg Br* 1993;75:36–40.

230. Korvick DL, Pijanowski GJ, Schaeffer DJ. Three-dimensional kinematics of the intact and cranial cruciate ligament-deficient stifle of dogs. *J Biomech* 1994;27:77–87.

231. Tashman S, Kolowich PA, Lock TR, et al. Dynamic knee instability following ACL reconstruction in dogs. *Trans Orthop Res Soc* 1997; 22:97.

232. Shoemaker SC, Markolf KL. The role of the meniscus in the anterior-posterior stability of the loaded anterior cruciate-deficient knee. Effects of partial versus total excision. *J Bone Joint Surg Am* 1986;68:71–79.

233. Irvine GB, Glasgow MM. The natural history of the meniscus in anterior cruciate insufficiency. Arthroscopic analysis. *J Bone Joint Surg Br* 1992;74:403–405.

234. Murrell GAC, Maddali S, Horovitz L, et al. The relationships between time since initial injury and meniscal loss on cartilage damage in ACL insufficient knees. *Trans Orthop Res Soc* 1999;24:293.

235. Cipolla M, Scala A, Gianni E, et al. Different patterns of meniscal tears in acute anterior cruciate ligament (ACL) ruptures and in chronic ACL-deficient knees. Classification, staging and timing of treatment. *Knee Surg Sports Traumatol Arthrosc* 1995;3:130–134.

236. O'Connor BL, Visco DM, Brandt KD, et al. Neurogenic acceleration of osteoarthrosis. The effects of previous neurectomy of the articular nerves on the development of osteoarthrosis after transection of the anterior cruciate ligament in dogs. *J Bone Joint Surg Am* 1992;74:367–376.

237. Frost HM. Changing concepts in skeletal physiology: Wolff's law, the mechanostat and the "Utah paradigm." *Am J Hum Biol* 1998;10: 599–605.

238. Haus J, Halata Z. Innervation of the anterior cruciate ligament. *Int Orthop* 1990;14:293–296.

CHAPTER 10

Stability of the Knee

John J. O'Connor, Amy B. Zavatsky, and Richie H.S. Gill

This chapter explains how the ligaments collaborate with the articular surfaces and with the muscles spanning the knee to control the stability of the joint and to transmit load. The topic is discussed mainly on a theoretical basis, using results obtained from the three-dimensional (3D) and two-dimensional (2D) models of the joint introduced in Chapter 5. For each joint position, these models define the directions of muscle tendon and ligament fibers and of the perpendiculars to the articular surfaces at their points of contact. They therefore provide the lines of action of the forces transmitted by these structures when load is first applied. These lines of action change as tissues deform. A wide variety of external loads can be applied to the joint during different activities, but the geometry of the unloaded joint serves as the common starting point for the analysis of each activity. It is obviously impossible to describe the response to every activity, but those studied here bring out the role of the ligaments in controlling the stability of the joint under load and their contributions to its overall passive and dynamic laxity. Wherever possible, the predictions of the models are compared with experimental results reported from several laboratories, including our own.

Stability

A system in mechanical equilibrium is said to be *stable* when it offers increasing resistance to displacement from its equilibrium position. It is *unstable* when it encounters forces accelerating displacement away from its equilibrium position. It is in *neutral equilibrium* when it encounters no resistance to movement from its equilibrium position.

In Chapter 5, we described the path of unresisted coupled mobility. Any displacement from that path encountered resistance due to tissue deformation so that the knee may be said to be stable with respect to such displacement. We can study the passive stability of the knee by describing how the ligaments and the articular surfaces deform to develop the tensile and compressive forces necessary to resist displacement from the path of unresisted motion. Tissue deformation gives the joint its passive laxity. The passive stability of the joint is compromised when ligaments or articular surfaces are damaged. Various clinical tests have been devised to assess the extent of the damage by exploring the resulting range of unresisted displacement or the increased passive laxity.

The passive structures of knee alone offer no resistance to motion along the path of unresisted mobility, which might therefore be thought of as a succession of positions of neutral equilibrium. We use our muscles mainly to stabilize the skeleton in the presence of gravity and other loads and then to induce and control mobility. Muscle forces stabilize the skeleton by resisting motion along the path of unresisted mobility.

We saw in Figure 5.22 and in Image 3 on the CD-ROM accompanying this book that the muscle tendons are generally inclined to the tibial plateaus so that they apply forces with components parallel to the plateaus. These components cannot be transmitted by the frictionless articular surfaces. The surfaces can transmit only the compressive components of muscle force and external load perpendicular to the tibial plateau. The ligaments are mainly responsible for transmitting the components of muscle force and external load parallel to the plateau. A study of ligament loading inevitably involves consideration of muscle forces and their directions.

In Chapters 11 and 12, "Mechanics of the Knee" and "The Muscle-Stabilized Knee," of the previous edition, *Knee Ligaments,* we analyzed the mechanics of the knee on the assumption that the ligaments do not stretch and the articular surfaces do not indent under load. Despite the simplistic nature of these assumptions, in Chapter 12 of *Knee Ligaments* we showed that estimates from the 2D model of forces in the tendons of the extensor and flexor muscles during simulations of simple sagittal plane activities agreed reasonably well with measurements made in cadaver specimens, although model estimates of cruciate ligament forces were high. In this chapter, we take account of tissue deformation and explain some of our previous results. We analyze passive laxity and passive stability first and then discuss muscle forces.

THREE-DIMENSIONAL MODEL: LIGAMENT FIBER RECRUITMENT IN THE DRAWER TEST

Chapter 5 demonstrated that most ligament fibers in the unloaded joint are slack. However, the ligaments can develop forces progressively to resist movement of the tibia relative to the femur as fibers tighten progressively (1–3). When the positions of the origin and insertion of a fiber are known for the unloaded joint, their increasing separation or approach during increasing tibial translation (drawer) can be calculated.

Figure 10.1 shows how a slack buckled fiber can be straightened back to its unstretched length l_0 by horizontal translation of its tibial insertion from T_1 to T_2 relative to its femoral origin F. Further horizontal translation to T_3 stretches the fiber to length l so that it can now transmit tensile force. The stretch or elongation of the fiber can be calculated from the *geometry* of the triangle FT_2T_3, requiring no knowledge of mechanics. The elongation of the ligament fiber is said to be *geometrically compatible* with the translation T_2T_3 of the tibia relative to the femur. The change in length or elongation l-l_o and the length ratio, length l divided by length l_o, are simple measures of the

strain in the fiber. The force transmitted by the fiber can subsequently be calculated from the elongation if the mechanical properties of the fiber are known. There is extensive literature describing the force–elongation or stress–strain relations for ligaments or ligament fascicles (4,5). A comprehensive review of such studies was given by Woo et al. in Chapter 7, "Fundamental Studies in Knee Ligament Mechanics," in the previous edition of this book.

The geometric relationships between motion of the tibia relative to the femur and the strains in the ligaments were applied to the fibers of the 3D model knee by Feikes et al. (6,7) and to the quasi-3D model by Toutoungi et al. (8). The methodology has been extensively applied to the 2D four-bar linkage model (2, 9–18). Once the geometry of ligament deformation has been established, knowledge of the mechanical properties of ligament fibers allows the calculation of stress distributions throughout the ligaments and, thus, the evaluation of ligament forces. The final step is to relate the tibiofemoral movement induced by tissue deformation to the applied loads (i.e., the analysis of joint laxity). This has been the approach adopted in the papers just cited and forms the basis of this chapter. A similar approach is being applied to the ankle–subtalar complex of joints (19–21).

Fiber Recruitment in the Anterior Cruciate Ligament

Figure 10.2A was derived from the 3D model of the knee (6,22,23), using planar tibial surfaces and spherical femoral surfaces. The figure shows a diagram of the tibial attachment area of the model anterior cruciate ligament (ACL) with contours of fiber length ratio in the unloaded joint (*0 mm*) and when the tibia is translated forward distances of *4 mm* and *8 mm* relative to the femur without axial rotation during anterior drawer. These results are based on a purely geometric analysis. Each contour is labeled with the ratio of current fiber length to its maximum length during passive unloaded flexion.[1] The unloaded contours repeat Figure 5.19. Contours are presented at extension, *25°*, and *90°* flexion. At full extension and no load (*0 mm*), most fibers in the ACL are nearly tight, within 2% of their maximum unloaded lengths (the fibers lying behind the contour labeled *0.98*).

At *90°* and *0 mm* translation, all but the anterior fibers of the unloaded ligament are slack (contours with labels smaller than unity). As the tibia is translated forward, a wave of tension sweeps posteriorly through the ligament. After a translation of *4 mm*, more than half the ligament fibers have tightened (contours with labels >*1.0*) and are transmitting tension force but the remaining fibers at the back of the ligament are still slack. At *90°*, it takes an anterior translation of fully 8 mm to recruit the postero-

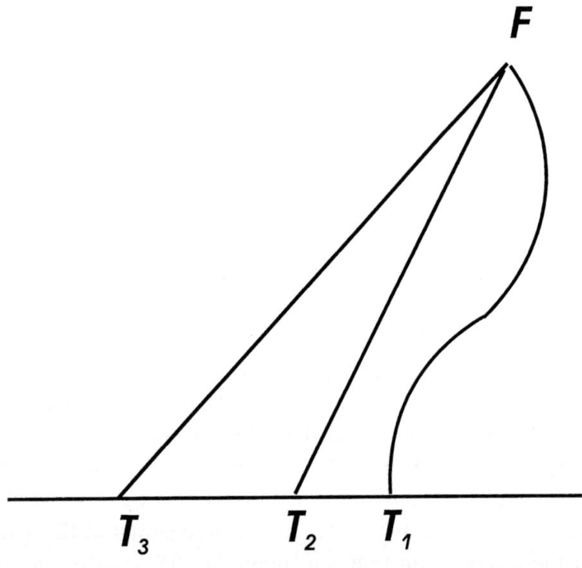

FIGURE 10.1. Fiber recruitment under load. A ligament fiber arising at *F* on the femur, is slack when its tibial insertion is at *T₁*, just tight when movement of the tibia brings it to *T₂*, and stretched at *T₃*. (From Lu TW, O'Connor JJ. Fiber recruitment and shape changes of knee ligaments during motion as revealed by a computer graphics-based model. *J Engng Med Proc Inst Mech Eng* [H] 1996;210:71–79, with permission.)

---

[1]Note that this definition of length ratio is different from that used in Chapter 5 (Fig. 5.14), although the consequences of the differences are slight.

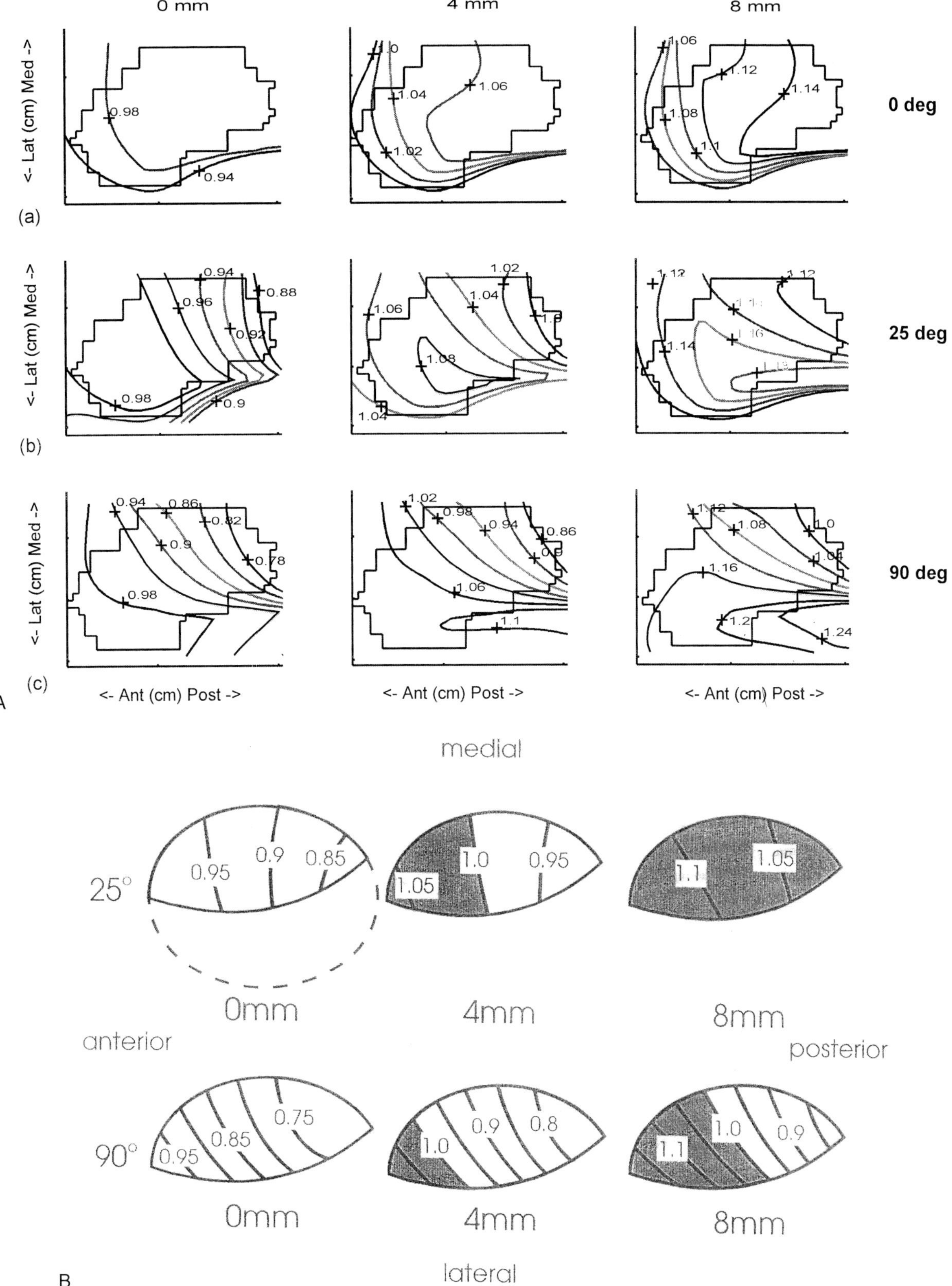

FIGURE 10.2. A: Tibial attachment of the anterior cruciate ligament (ACL) with contours of constant fiber extension ratio in the unloaded state (0 mm) and when the tibia is displaced anteriorly by 4 and 8 mm. At extension (*a*), the posterior fibers tighten more rapidly than the anterior fibers. At 90° flexion (*c*), the antero-lateral fibers tighten first. At 25° (*b*), fibers in the center of the ligament tighten first. (From Feikes JD. The mobility and stability of the human knee joint [D. Phil Thesis]. University of Oxford, 1999, with permission.) **B:** Contours of constant length ratio in the ACL according to the quasi–three-dimensional (3D) model for the unloaded state (0 mm) and after 4 and 8 mm anterior tibial translation. The tibial insertion area is shown as part of an ellipse. (From Toutoungi DE, Zavatsky AB, O'Connor JJ. Parameter sensitivity of a mathematical model of the anterior cruciate ligament. *J Engng Med Proc Inst Mech Eng* [H] 1997;211:235–246, with permission.)

lateral fibers, by which time the anteromedial fibers have stretched by *20%* (contour marked *1.2*). At *25°*, when less slackening occurs passively, a translation of *4 mm* recruits all fibers. In extension, all fibers are more or less tight in the unloaded state (length ratio, *1.0*) and tibial translation results in greater percentage length change of the shorter posterior fibers (contour marked *1.14* after *8 mm* translation) than of the longer anterior fibers (contour marked *1.06*). We will relate these results later to the pattern of partial ligament tears observed at different positions of flexion. In addition, we will discuss magnitudes of anteroposterior translation likely to be encountered in activity and show that an anterior tibial translation of *8 mm* is more than would be expected in activity or during clinical testing of the intact joint.

Figure 10.2B shows patterns of recruitment in the ACL at *25°* and *90°* during anterior tibial translation, according to the quasi-3D model (8). The recruitment pattern of this model is easier to interpret. Waves of tension sweep backward through the model ligament with increasing

tibial translation. Even *8 mm* translation is not sufficient to tighten this model ACL fully at *90°* of flexion.

Fiber Recruitment in the Posterior Cruciate Ligament

Figure 10.3 shows length ratio contours for the posterior cruciate ligament (PCL) during posterior tibial translation, with the isometric band of fibers (lying behind the contour marked *0.98* in extension and within the contour marked *0.98* at *25°* and *90°*) contained within the bulk of the ligament in the unloaded state (*0 mm*). With increasing posterior tibial translation, the more posterior fibers rapidly tighten (contours with labels greater than unity) as a band of tension sweeps backward. Simultaneously, the more anterior fibers tighten as the band of tension moves forward. Load bearing develops from the middle of the ligament. Generally, the strains induced in fibers of the PCL are smaller than those in the ACL for a given distance of tibial translation because the PCL lies more vertically in the sagittal plane over most of the flexion range and is less

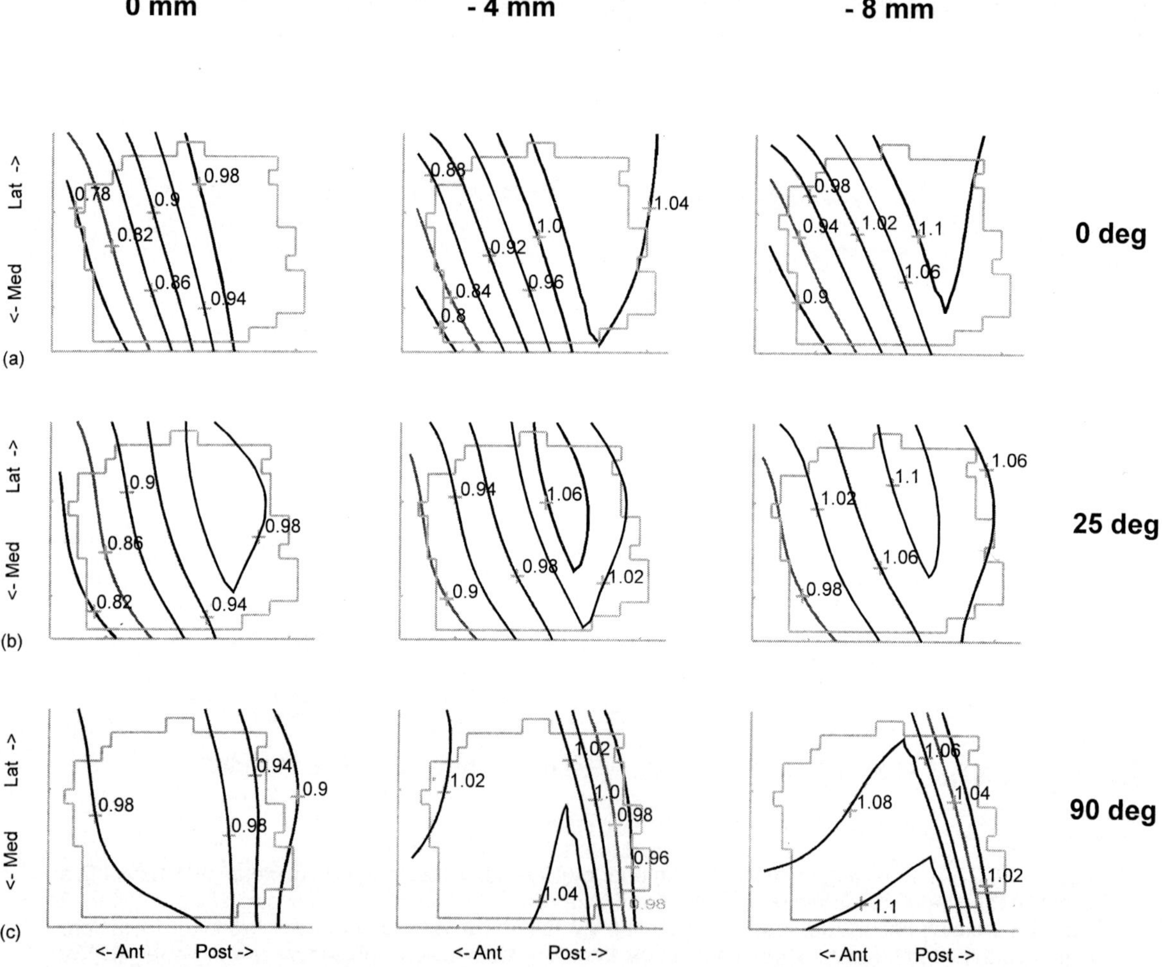

FIGURE 10.3. Tibial attachment of the posterior cruciate ligament (PCL) with contours of constant fiber extension ratio in the unloaded state (0 mm) and when the tibia is displaced posteriorly 4 and 8 mm. (From Feikes JD. The mobility and stability of the human knee joint [D. Phil Thesis]. University of Oxford, 1999, with permission.)

TABLE 10.1. *Maximum and minimum length ratios in each of the four ligaments during anterior and posterior tibial translation*

Ligament	Flexion	4 mm maximum	4 mm minimum	8 mm maximum	8 mm minimum
Anterior tibial translation					
ACL	0	**1.08**	0.98	**1.18**	**1.04**
	25	**1.09**	0.97	**1.21**	**1.10**
	90	**1.11**	0.83	**1.25**	0.96
MCL	0	1.00	0.86	**1.01**	0.86
	25	1.00	0.86	1.00	0.89
	90	**1.01**	0.93	**1.01**	0.94
LCL	0	0.99	0.90	0.97	0.89
	25	0.98	0.90	0.99	0.90
	90	**1.02**	0.96	**1.05**	0.99
Posterior tibial translation					
PCL	0	**1.06**	0.80	**1.13**	0.87
	25	**1.05**	0.88	**1.12**	0.95
	90	**1.05**	0.93	**1.11**	0.98
MCL	0	1.00	0.87	**1.01**	0.88
	25	1.00	0.90	**1.01**	0.91
	90	1.00	0.93	1.00	0.93
LCL	0	**1.02**	0.93	**1.05**	0.96
	25	0.98	0.90	0.98	0.91
	90	0.98	0.92	0.97	0.91

Boldface indicates fiber recruitment.
ACL, anterior cruciate ligament; MCL, medial collateral ligament; LCL, lateral collateral ligament; PCL, posterior cruciate ligament.

efficiently oriented to resisted tibial translation (Images 2 and 3 on the CD-ROM supplied with this book).

Table 10.1 records the largest and smallest length ratios recorded in the four model ligaments for anterior and posterior tibial translations of *4* and *8 mm*. The PCL goes completely slack under anterior drawer and the ACL goes completely slack under posterior drawer. Up to *25%* strain is developed in the ACL at *90°* flexion under *8 mm* anterior drawer, more than the maximum *13%* induced in the PCL at full extension under *8 mm* posterior tibial drawer. In contrast, the maximum strains induced in the collaterals by anteroposterior translations are very small. The strains induced in the medial collateral ligament (MCL) under anteroposterior translation are at most *1%*, whereas the lateral collateral ligament (LCL) develops strains up to *5%* at extension to resist posterior drawer and up to *5%* at *90°* flexion to resist anterior drawer.

Both collaterals can make small contributions in resisting *both* posterior and anterior drawer because most of their fibers are oriented proximodistally and their bulk orientation can be reversed by plus and minus *8 mm* of anteroposterior (A/P) translation. The shifting pattern of fiber recruitment with flexion found in all ligaments reflects the location of fibers that are just taut and ready to bear load. The *8 mm* translation is more than would be exhibited by the intact joint in activity, but these results give an indication of how much tibial translation is necessary to begin to recruit the collaterals when there is cruciate deficiency.

The cruciates are the primary ligamentous stabilizers with respect to anterior or posterior translation, with the collaterals playing only a minor role. This agrees with the conclusions reached in Chapter 9, "The Limits of Knee Motion: *In Vitro* Studies," of the previous edition, based on numerous investigations of sequential cutting of ligaments in cadaver specimens.

Calculation of Applied Drawer Force

Knowing the distribution of strain in each of the ligaments for a given A/P translation and the directions of fibers throughout the strained region, the distribution of stress can be calculated using an appropriate strain–stress relation and, from the stress distribution, we can calculate the total force transmitted by each ligament or portions thereof, in magnitude and direction.

A nonlinear stress–strain relation was assumed, with an initial quadratic relationship to model the unfolding of fiber crimp in the initial toe region up to strains of *3%*, followed by a linear relationship for larger strains (2,4). The values of the Young's Modulus for the linear regions were chosen for the ACL and PCL to match the measurements of Piziali et al. (24) made on cadaver specimens in extension.

Figure 10.4 shows the calculated relationship between A/P load and A/P tibial translation (*solid line*), matched with Piziali's measurements on cadaver specimens (*dashed line*) (24) at full extension. To effect this match, however, it was necessary to assume a large-strain Young's Modulus for the model PCL of *450 Mega Pascals (MPa)*, more than 11 times larger than that assumed for the model ACL, *40 MPa*. The values for fibers of the

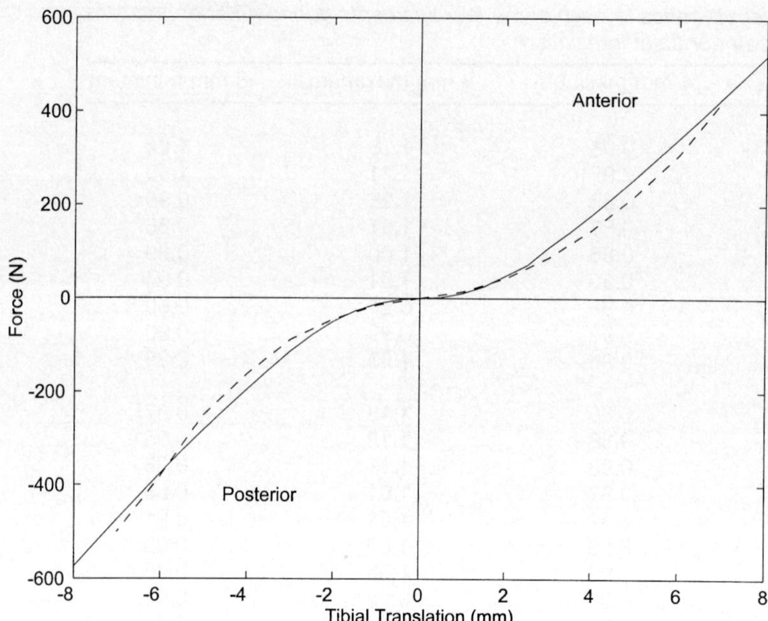

FIGURE 10.4. Drawer force plotted against anteroposterior displacement. Calculated values from model (*solid line*) compared with Piziali's measurements. (From Feikes JD. The mobility and stability of the human knee joint [D. Phil. Thesis]. University of Oxford, 1999, with permission.)

MCL and LCL were *250 MPa*. Although this variation in modulus values seems very large, it spans the range of values reported in the literature.

Modulus Values

The value used for the model ACL modulus is much lower than those reported by Butler et al. (25) (*284 MPa*, anterior subunit; *155 MPa*, posterior subunit), but their reported standard deviations were as large as *100 MPa* and a value of *40 MPa* was found for the posterior subunit of the ligament for one specimen. Our assumed value of *40 MPa* is equivalent to a ligament stiffness of *5,600 N* per unit strain, which is similar to values of *7,136 N* found by Mommersteeg et al. (26), *5,000 N* used by Blankevoort and Huiskes (27), and *7,200 N* used by Andriacchi et al. (28) [as computed by Blankevoort and Huiskes (27)]. There appears to be inconsistency in the experimental results and this topic needs further investigation.

The modulus value chosen for the model PCL is within one standard deviation of the average value reported by Butler et al. (4) (*345 ± 107 MPa*) and within two standard deviations of the average modulus (*248 ± 119 MPa*) reported by Race and Amis (5) for the anterior bundle of the ligament. However, our value was chosen by comparison with the results of Piziali's experiment, carried out on intact cadaver specimens in extension when the posterior capsule would be tight and would contribute to resistance to posterior tibial translation. In the current version of the 3D model, the action of the posterior capsule is not simulated, although our previous experiments (see Fig. 10.14) showed it to contribute to load bearing within about *10°* of full extension. Direct comparison with Piziali's experiment therefore overestimates the PCL modulus.

Anterior Cruciate Ligament Force in the Drawer Test

Figure 10.5A shows that the calculated value of the force in the model ACL during an anterior drawer of *5 mm* decreases steadily from a maximum in extension. This reflects the increasing slackness of most of the ACL ligament fibers with increasing flexion. The calculated value lies between the widely spread experimental estimates of Butler et al. (29) and Vahey and Draganich (30). Toutoungi et al. (8) found that it was possible to fit the results of the quasi-3D model to the results of Butler et al., Vahey and Draganich, or Piziali et al. by appropriate choice of model parameters.

Figure 10.5B shows that the ACL force, expressed as a proportion of the applied drawer force, also diminishes with increasing flexion. The figure confirms the results given by Fitzpatrick and O'Connor (31), Figure 11.8A of the previous edition, Zavatsky and O'Connor (2), and Huss et al. (15) that the value of the ACL force is strongly dependent on tissue deformation. The curve marked *Rigid Model* in Figure 10.5B is based on the assumption that the ACL force is directed along the isometric ACL fiber of the unloaded joint, whereas the other two curves show the effect of ACL elongation. As anterior tibial displacement increases and the ACL stretches, it becomes less steeply inclined to the tibial plateau and more efficient in resisting anterior drawer. Fujie et al. (32) used a force-moment sensor to demonstrate how the direction and line of action of the ACL force changed with increasing applied load. When we assume the ligaments to be inextensible and the articular surfaces to be rigid, we overestimate the values of the ligament forces. This matter will be discussed further below based on the predictions of the 2D model.

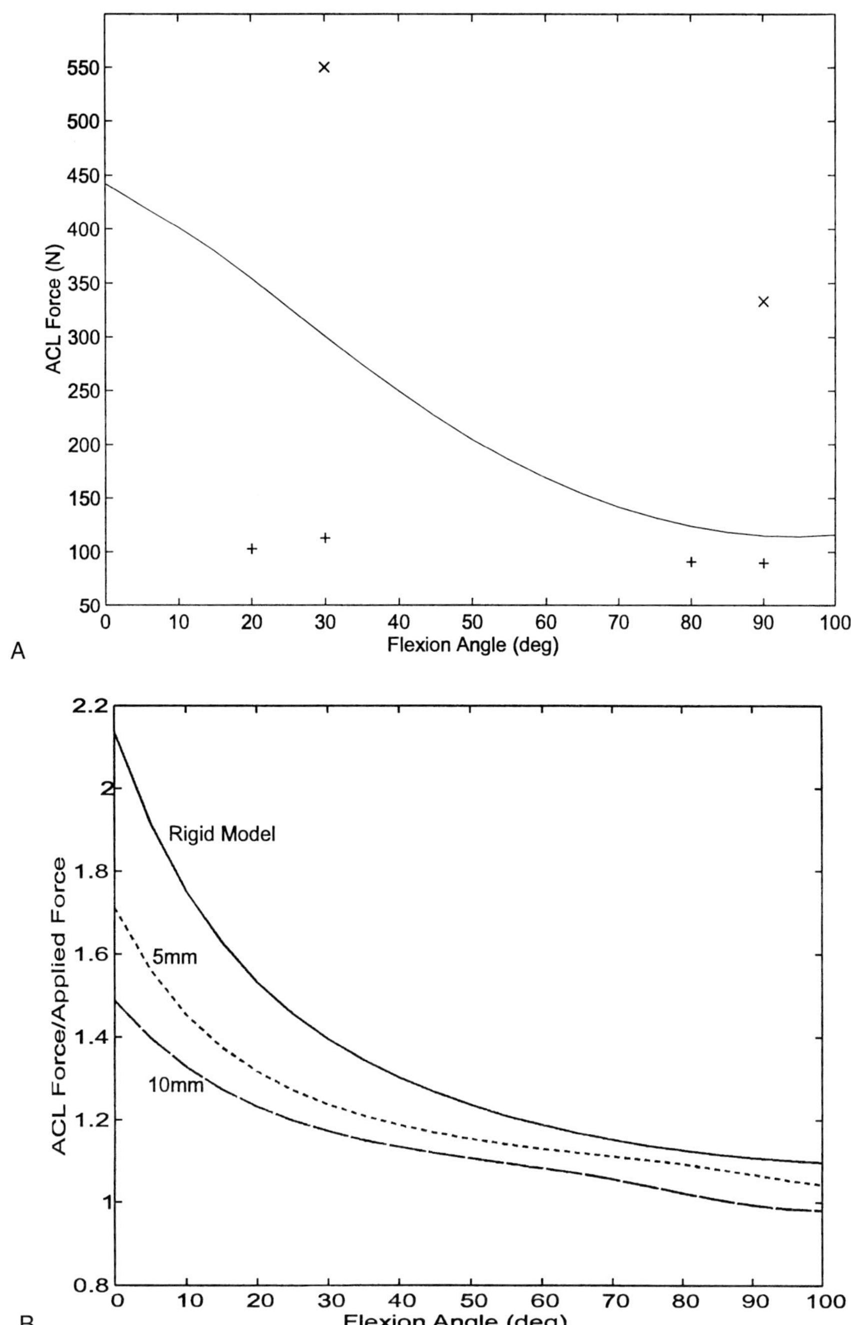

FIGURE 10.5. A: Variation with flexion angle of the anterior cruciate ligament (ACL) force induced by an anterior load of *67 N* applied to the tibia. Solid line curve calculated from model, points marked *x* from Butler et al. (29), points marked + from Vahey and Draganich (30). **B:** ACL force per unit applied drawer force assuming rigid inextensible ligament and articular surfaces and (*lower curves*) assuming 5 and 10 mm anterior tibial displacement. (From Feikes JD. The mobility and stability of the human knee joint [D. Phil. Thesis]. University of Oxford, 1999, with permission.)

The curves in Figure 10.5B are similar in form to those obtained by Lewis et al. (33), using buckle transducers, and by Markolf et al. (34), using a transducer directly transmitting force applied by the ligament through its tibial insertion. However, both these methods gave ligament force values in flexion *less* than the applied drawer force, whereas the model calculation suggests that it is always greater (ligament force divided by applied load greater than unity). The recent study by Chan and Seedhom (35) came to the same conclusion from experiments in which a compressive load, as well as an anterior load, was transmitted across the joint.

Sakane et al. (36), using a robotic manipulator and a universal force–moment sensor, found ACL force values equal to or less than the applied anterior load. They found that the force in the anteromedial bundle was virtually independent of flexion angle, but that in the posterolateral bundle was significantly affected by flexion. This accords with the patterns of fiber recruitment shown in Figure 10.2. Pandy and Shelburne (37) used a 2D knee model with 11 separate fibers representing parts of each of the four ligaments and the posterior capsule but with rigid articular surfaces. They also report ACL forces larger than the applied horizontal force, with small forces in the MCL and in the posterior capsule near extension.

If the horizontal component of the ACL force mainly has to balance the A/P component of the external load, the magnitude of the ACL force would be larger than the applied load (see the discussion of Fig. 10.9 below). If the ACL force is less than the applied drawer force, it must be that the collateral ligaments and the articular surfaces and menisci make much larger contributions to resisting anterior drawer than was previously thought (see Chapter 9, "The Limits of Knee Motion: *In Vitro* Studies," of the previous edition). The strain figures in Table 10.1 suggest that the contribution of the collaterals in resisting A/P tibial translation is very small, as confirmed by the modelling of Pandy and Shelburne. Imran and O'Connor (38) used the 2D cruciate ligament model to examine ligament interactions with convex and concave tibial surfaces, as in the lateral and medial compartments of the human knee. They found that a convex surface gave reduced ACL forces in the drawer test whereas a concave surface gave increased forces. These effects were most marked near extension but diminished in flexion where the two models with curved tibial surfaces gave ACL force values very similar to the model with a flat surface. One might expect that the effects on ACL force of the opposite curvatures of the two tibial plateaus of the knee would balance out. All three 2D models gave ACL values greater than the applied drawer force so that the discrepancy between these results and those of the measurements cannot be due to effects created by the articular surfaces alone.

Joint Laxity

Figure 10.4 shows that the knee offers slowly increasing resistance to A/P translation. The necessary applied force increases slowly from zero but at an increasing rate. Relatively small forces are required to produce the first ±3 mm of A/P translation. Over the flexion range, the joint is initially lax because the bulk of the ligament fibers is initially slack.

Figure 10.6 shows that the calculated total A/P laxity of the model knee at six positions for an applied A/P force of *67 N* compares reasonably with measurements made by Grood and Noyes (39). The model results are divided into anterior (*bottom portion of the bars*) and posterior laxity (*upper portion*). Anterior laxity increases steadily with increasing flexion because of the increasing slackness of the fibers of the ACL in the unloaded state (see Figures 5.14, 5.28A). Posterior laxity is largest in mid-range where most fibers in the unloaded PCL are slack (Fig. 10.3).

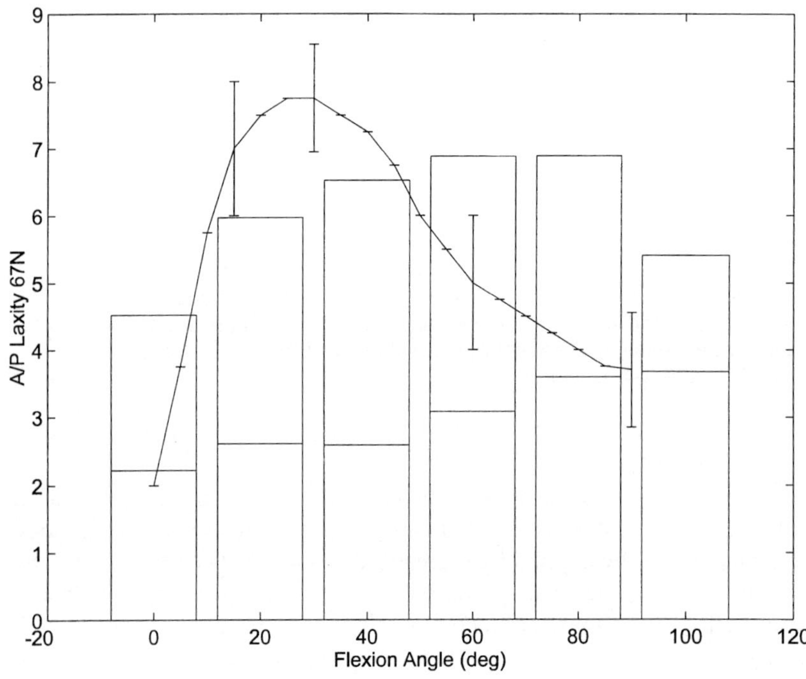

FIGURE 10.6. Calculated anteroposterior laxity (*bar graphs*) at different flexion angles compared with measurements (*solid line curve with error bars*) reported by Grood and Noyes (39). The lower segment of the bar graphs describes anterior laxity, the upper segment posterior laxity. (From Feikes JD. The mobility and stability of the human knee joint [D. Phil. Thesis]. University of Oxford, 1999, with permission.)

Further Development of the Three-Dimensional Model

Development of the 3D model is not yet complete. Its application to the drawer test yields results that accord reasonably with some of the published experimental results but not with others, although the experiments are far from unanimous. An important difficulty lies in the choice of parameters for the model, including the mechanical properties of the ligament fibers. The results of the model calculations can be made to fit the wide range of experimental data available from different laboratories by appropriate choice of parameters, but this is hardly a satisfactory situation. The ideal would be a set of specimen-specific models that fit the range of experimental data obtained in a series of experiments on individual specimens subsequently disarticulated to obtain parameters, as described in Chapter 5. Further development is required, including inclusion of models of the menisci.

The 3D knee model has been incorporated into a muscle–bone model of the lower limb (40,41) so that muscle–ligament interactions can be studied. However, the effects of tissue deformation have not yet been taken into account in that development. Study of the mechanics of the 2D model has revealed how important tissue deformation is in determining the levels of ligament force in activity.

TWO-DIMENSIONAL MODEL OF PASSIVE AND ACTIVE KNEE STABILITY

The 2D four-bar linkage model has been developed extensively in the past 10 years to take account of the deformation both of the ligaments and of the cartilage layers on the articular surfaces.

Passive Stability

Figure 10.7 shows images of the model knee at *20°* and *90°* flexion with its ACL in the unloaded state and after anterior tibial translation of *4 mm* and *8 mm*. Analysis of these figures allows us to determine the strain distribution within the ligament geometrically compatible with translation of the tibia relative to the femur.

In the unloaded state (*0 mm*), all except the isometric fiber at the front of the ligament are slack at both flexion angles. The *8 mm* of anterior drawer is almost sufficient to recruit all ACL fibers at *20°* but not at *90°*. At *90°*, the fibers are more lax in the unloaded state and more anterior

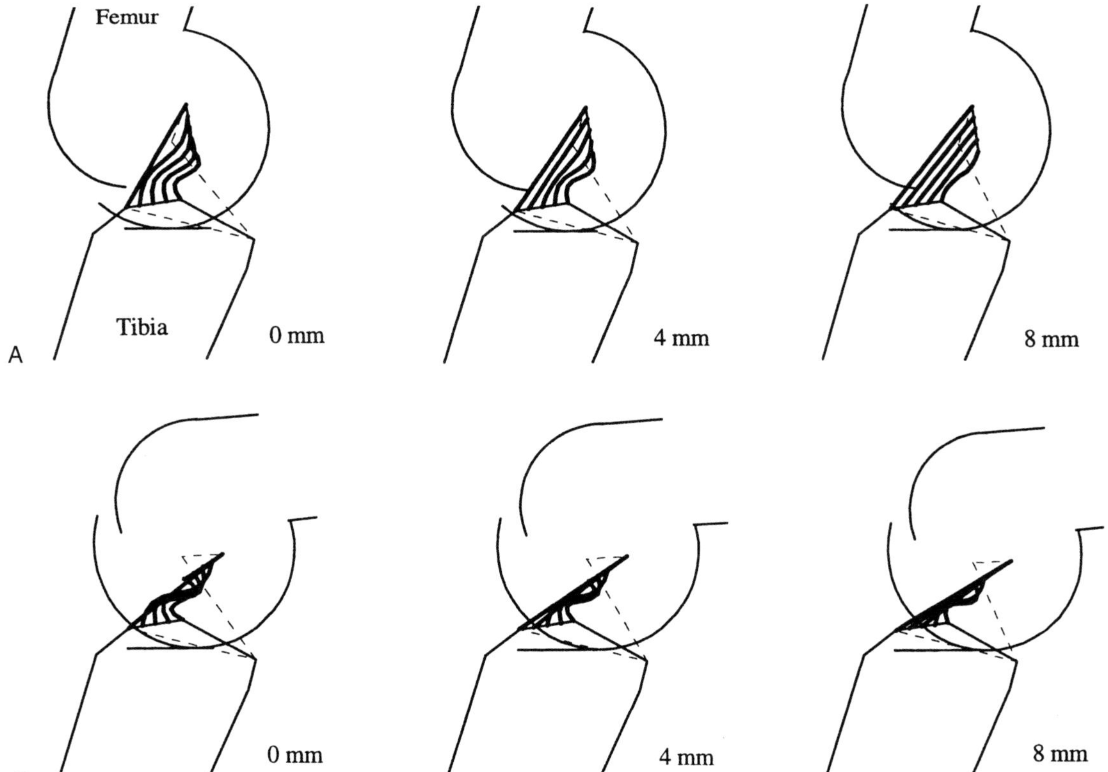

FIGURE 10.7. Recruitment of slack fibers in the anterior cruciate ligament (ACL) during anterior translation of the tibia. At 20° flexion, 8-mm translation tightens more than 80% of the model ligament (**A**) but only 60% at 90° flexion (**B**). (From Lu TW, O'Connor JJ. Fiber recruitment and shape changes of knee ligaments during motion as revealed by a computer graphics-based model. *J Engng Med Proc Inst Mech Eng* [H] 1996;210:71–79, with permission.)

translation is needed to pull them straight and tight. Image 6 on the CD-ROM supplied with this book shows animations of this model during anterior and posterior translation. These images were produced by Lu and O'Connor (14), based on an analysis by Zavatsky and O'Connor (2,9).

The fiber that remains isometric during unloaded motion is stretched during anterior translation and slackens during posterior translation. Fibers that are slack in the unloaded state are progressively stretched with increasing anterior translation and slackened during posterior translation. The effective area of the ligament that can resist anterior translation increases and the ligament gets stiffer with increasing translation. These results are generally consistent with the 3D model (Table 10.1), but the 2D model recruits ACL fibers more slowly.

Figure 10.8 (see also Color Plate 3, following page 72), animated in Image 7 of the CD-ROM accompanying this book, shows similar patterns of fiber recruitment and slackening in all four ligaments during anterior and posterior drawer at *25°* flexion. Fibers in the ACL and MCL tighten and slacken together during anterior and posterior drawer, respectively. Fibers in the PCL and LCL slacken and tighten, respectively, during anterior and posterior drawer. At this flexion angle, a posterior drawer of *8 mm* is sufficient to tighten all PCL and LCL fibers.

Effects of Cartilage Deformation

Huss et al. (15,16) further developed the Zavatsky 2D model by considering the deformation of the cartilage layers covering the bones (Fig. 10.9).

When the tibia is pulled forward a distance δ_x relative to the femur by an horizontal force F_H applied purely parallel to the tibial plateau,[2] the ACL force F_L required to resist the movement is inclined to the tibial plateau and has a component of force F_C perpendicular to the plateau. This force pulls the bones together a distance δ_y and indents the cartilage. The horizontal component of the ligament force, F_H, balances the applied horizontal load.[3]

---

[2]The figure is drawn with the femur pulled backward relative to the tibia.

[3]Both horizontal and vertical components are smaller in magnitude than the ligament force because $F_C = F_L \cdot \sin(\theta)$ and $F_H = F_L \cdot \cos(\theta)$, where θ is the angle between the line of action of the ligament force and the tibial plateau and both the sine and cosine functions are less than unity.

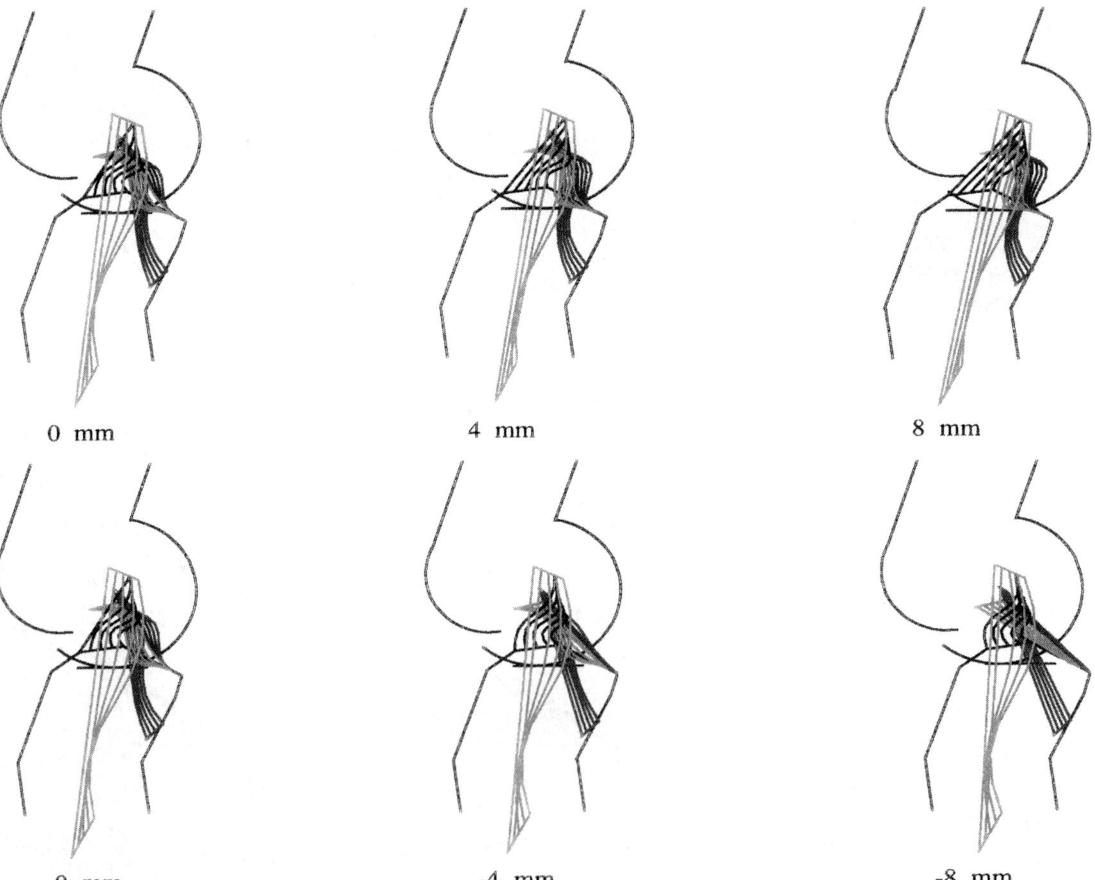

FIGURE 10.8. Model knee at 25° flexion in the unloaded state (0 mm) and after 4 and 8 mm anterior tibial translation (**top row**) and 4 and 8 mm posterior translation (**bottom row**). Anterior translation recruits fibers in the anterior cruciate ligament (ACL) and medial cruciate ligament (MCL) and slackens the posterior cruciate ligament (PCL) and lateral cruciate ligament (LCL). Posterior translation tightens the PCL and LCL and slackens the ACL and MCL. (From Lu TW. Geometric and mechanical modelling of the human locomotor system [D. Phil Thesis]. University of Oxford, 1997, with permission.)

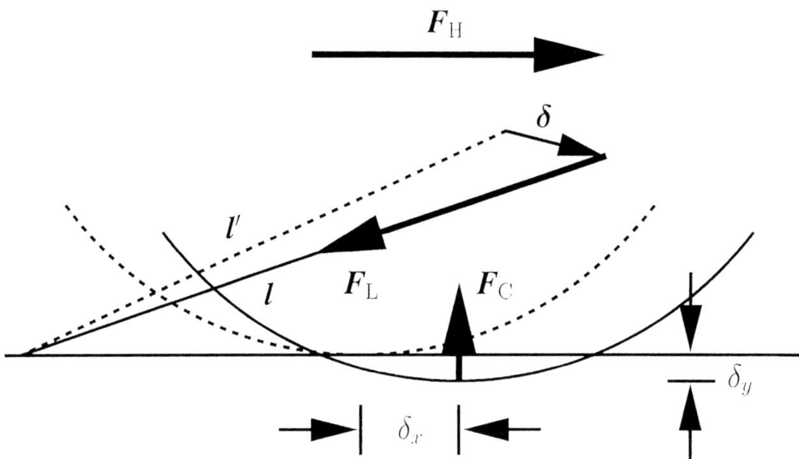

FIGURE 10.9. A horizontal force F_H applied to the femur causes a ligament fiber to stretch from l' to l and cartilage indentation δ_y. The femur moves backward δ_x relative to the tibia. The femoral attachment of the ligament fiber moves δ relative to the tibia, δ_x horizontally and δ_y vertically. (From Huss RA, Holstein H, O'Connor JJ. The effect of cartilage deformation on the laxity of the knee joint. *J Engng Med Proc Inst Mech* [H] 1999;213:19–32, with permission.)

Huss et al. (15) calculated the values of δ_x and δ_y for a specified applied horizontal load F_H. Changes in the direction of ligament forces under increasing load have been observed by Fujie et al. (32). Figure 10.9 suggests that indentation of the cartilage under load could make a significant contribution to this phenomenon.

Figure 10.10 is the 2D model equivalent of the force–tibial translation relation shown in Figure 10.4 from the 3D model and is generally consistent with the 3D model. In addition, it shows that the force required to achieve a specified tibial translation is reduced because of cartilage deformation. Model 1 in the figure was developed by Zavatsky and O'Connor (2), who took account only of the deformation of the ligaments and treated the articular surfaces as rigid. Model 2 was developed by Huss et al. (15). In these calculations, the Young's Modulus values for the anterior and posterior bundles of both ACL and PCL were *200* and *150 MPa,* respectively,

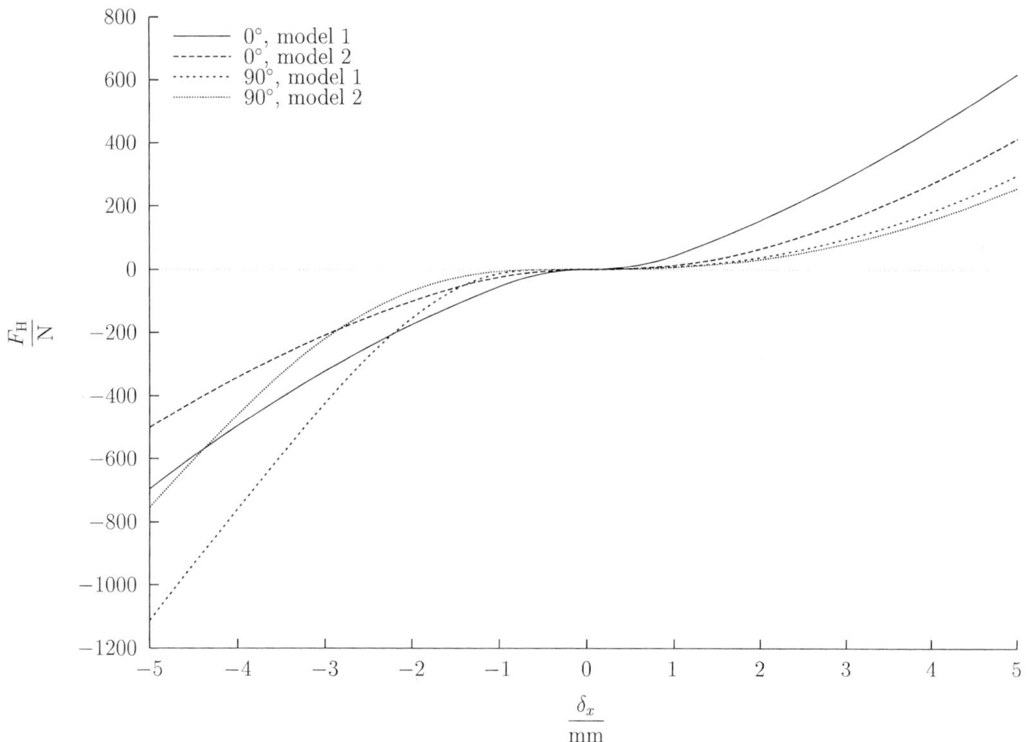

FIGURE 10.10. Applied horizontal force F_H required to produce horizontal displacement of the tibia δ_x at extension and 90° flexion. Model 2 with compressible cartilage requires less force than model 1 with rigid cartilage. The joint is stiffer at extension than at *90°* flexion. (From Huss RA, Holstein H, O'Connor JJ. The effect of cartilage deformation on the laxity of the knee joint. *J Engng Med Proc Inst Mech* [H] 1999;213:19–32, with permission.)

close to the values given by Butler et al. (4) and by Race and Amis (5). The modulus for cartilage was *5.0 MPa*, the value used by Blankevoort et al.(42).

Because of cartilage deformation, the initial laxity of the joint (around $\delta_x = 0$) is increased. In other words, the force required to produce a specified δ_x is reduced. At $\delta_x = 5$ *mm*, force reductions between *35%* at extension and *10%* at 90° flexion were calculated. The magnitude of the effect depends on flexion angle because of the differing inclinations of the ligaments to the horizontal and the differences in initial fiber slackness. Obviously, the main contribution to laxity is the deformability of the ligaments. The contribution of articular surface deformation is relatively small because the compressive contact force (F_C in Fig. 10.9) is equal to the vertical component of the ligament force F_L and therefore smaller than F_L. As we will show, this is not the case when muscle forces are also present and contact forces are much larger than ligament forces.

Deformation of the cartilage layers actually allows the horizontal displacement of the tibia produced by a specified horizontal load to increase.

Figure 10.11A is the 2D model equivalent of Figure 10.6 and shows how the total A/P laxity of the joint for a *67 N* horizontal load is increased over the flexion range because of cartilage deformation; model 1 is the Zavatsky rigid-surface model and model 2 is the Huss model. The separate contributions of anterior and posterior laxity are also included in the figure, showing that anterior laxity makes a somewhat larger contribution to the total. Figure 10.11B shows that the increase in total laxity due to cartilage deformation is largest at extension because of the increased anterior laxity there. In flexion, posterior laxity is the main contributor to the total. The general form of the total laxity curves in Figure 10.11A is similar to that obtained experimentally by Grood and Noyes (39) (Fig. 10.6). The 2D model confirms the result from the 3D model: The contribution of the collateral ligaments to resisting A/P drawer is small.

The calculated total laxity of the joint is maximum at about 20° flexion, as in Grood's experiment, so that a drawer test (the Lachman test) carried out at this position is most sensitive, the application of a given force eliciting the largest displacement. The bulk of the elicited movement is due to ligament deformation, mainly that of the cruciate ligaments; the effects of surface deformation are relatively small. This suggests that a drawer test performed on a patient's knee following a total or unicompartmental knee replacement that allows retention of both cruciates (43,44) can feel quite normal (45) even though the natural articular surfaces have been replaced by surfaces that are more rigid. However, erosion of the natural surfaces by arthrotic lesions can increase the laxity, even in the presence of intact ligaments, with the danger of an erroneous conclusion that increased laxity in these circumstances necessarily implies ligament damage. Most knees with unicompartmental arthrosis have intact cruciates (46). Conversely, the presence of osteophytes can limit A/P laxity and falsely indicate intact ligaments.

Ligament Isometry and Its Role in Guiding Passive Movement

The studies of the drawer test just described throw further light on the concepts of isometry and how the ligaments can be said to *guide* passive movement. As Figures 10.7 and 10.8 suggest, the slightest A/P translation, in response to the slightest load, results in stretching of fibers, which remained isometric during passive movement and the recruitment of others. This points to a further difficulty in detecting such isometric fibers because it is difficult to perform experiments in the completely unloaded state. Fibers that stretch to resist A/P movement induced by external load relax when that load is removed. We saw in Chapter 5 that, during purely passive motion, the contact points of the femur on the tibia move backward during flexion and forward during extension. Figures 10.7 and 10.8 show how the contact points can also be displaced backward and forward during the drawer test, these being examples of the perturbations of Figure 5.5 attributable to tissue deformation. Any deviation from the contact point positions of the unloaded state results in stretching of ligament fibers and indentation of the articular surfaces so that the tissues develop forces tending to resist the deviation. The positions of the bones on each other during passive flexion are therefore those in which all but the isometric fibers are slack and the isometric fibers are just tight. Ligament guidance therefore does not need to rely on complex feedback mechanisms but on the necessity of seeking, for every flexion angle, that position of the bones on each other at which the ligaments and articular surfaces are themselves unloaded when no external loads or muscle forces are applied. This condition of zero tissue strain requires the contact points to be nearer the back of the plateau in flexion and nearer the front on extension.

Sagittal Plane Mechanics: Turning and Nonturning Loads

In Chapter 11, "Mechanics of the Knee," of the previous edition, we considered loads applied in the sagittal plane through the distal tibia or the foot. When the line of action of the load passes through the flexion axis of the knee, it tends to neither extend nor flex the knee so that it can be balanced at the knee by forces in the passive structures, without muscle activity. We therefore called such loads *nonturning loads*. The loads applied during a drawer test at a selected flexion angle are examples of nonturning loads.

When the line of action of a compressive external load passes posterior to the flexion axis, tending to flex the joint, forces are required in the extensor muscles for equilibrium. Compressive loads passing anterior to the flexion axis tending to extend the knee require forces in the flexor muscles for balance. We called these *turning*

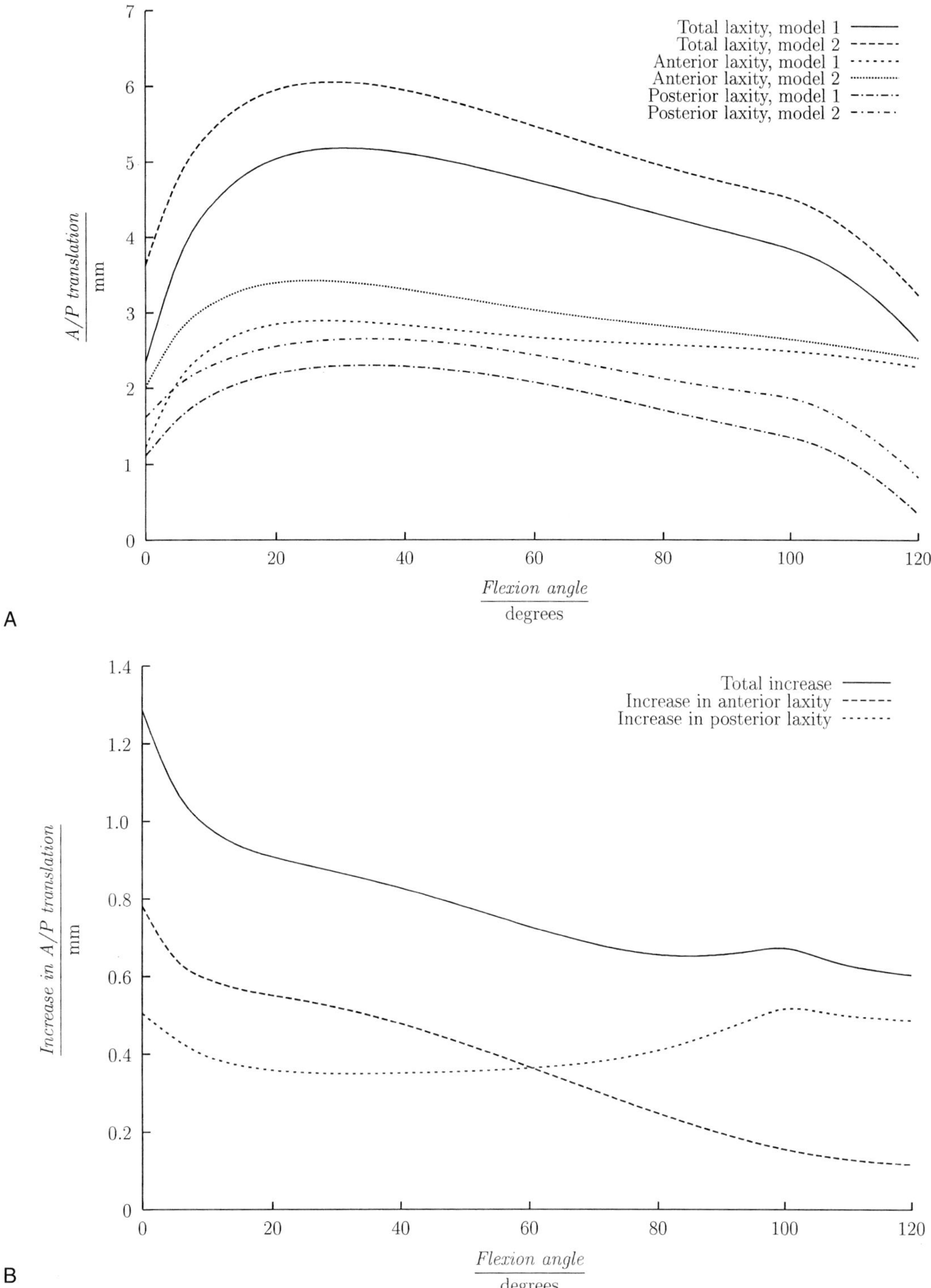

FIGURE 10.11. A: Laxity of the knee over the flexion range under a 67 N horizontal force applied to the tibia, showing the added effects of cartilage deformation and the separate contributions of anterior and posterior laxities. **B:** Increase in total, anterior, and posterior laxities due to cartilage deformation. (From Huss RA, Holstein H, O'Connor JJ. The effect of cartilage deformation on the laxity of the knee joint. *J Engng Med Proc Inst Mech Eng [H]* 1999;213:19–32, with permission.)

loads. The effective lever-arm available to the external load is therefore the perpendicular distance to its line of action from the flexion axis of the joint. Equally, the lever-arm of a muscle tendon is the perpendicular distance from the flexion axis to the tendon.

Leonardo da Vinci (47) in the early 16th century deduced from his anatomic studies that muscle forces are generally larger than external loads because their lever-arms at the joints are shorter. Borelli (48), 170 years later, demonstrated the same result experimentally by hanging weights on the ends of limbs. Muscle force was simulated by weights through wires and pulleys to tendons. Measurements telemetered from instrumented prostheses in living patients triumphantly confirm these early scientific results (49). The geometry of the joint, which determines the lengths of the muscle lever-arms and those of the external loads, fundamentally influences its mechanics. The directions of the muscle tendons fundamentally influence the loading of the ligaments.

Muscle Lever-Arms

The perpendicular distance from the flexion axis to each of the model muscle tendons in Figure 5.23 can be calculated, to give the lengths of the muscle lever-arms about the knee. Because of the changing directions of the tendons during flexion and the associated movements of

the flexion axis, the lever-arm lengths can vary significantly with flexion angle (Fig. 10.12).

Chapter 12, "The Muscle-Stabilized Knee," in the previous edition describes simple experiments on cadaver specimens aimed at validating the lever-arm lengths shown in Figure 10.12. The femur was fixed and weight hung from the distal tibia was balanced by tension force in wires attached to the quadriceps or hamstrings tendons (Figs. 10.13A, B). Experiments were also carried out with the tibia fixed and with tension in the gastrocnemius tendons balancing weight hung from the proximal femur (Fig. 10.13C). These experiments were very similar to those carried out by Borelli in the 17th century (48).

Figures 10.14A–C show plots of the measured muscle force per unit applied load for quadriceps, hamstrings,

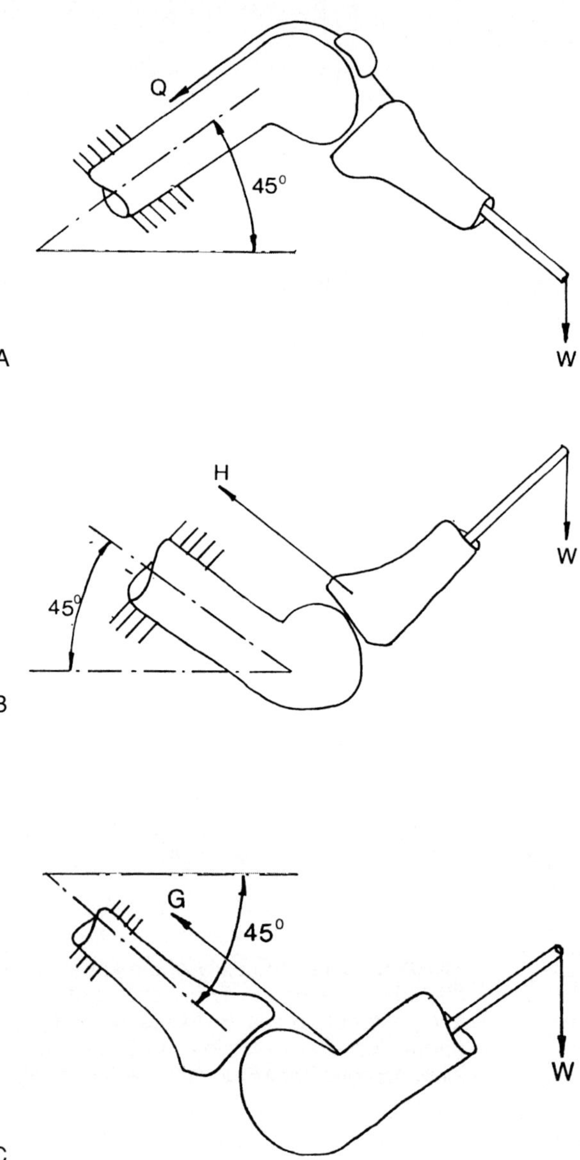

FIGURE 10.13. Experimental configurations for loading the **(A)** quadriceps, **(B)** hamstrings, and **(C)** gastrocnemius tendons.

FIGURE 10.12. Lengths of the lever-arms (moment-arms) of the model patellar tendon, hamstrings, and gastrocnemius tendons plotted against flexion angle. (From O'Connor JJ. Can muscle co-contraction protect knee ligaments after injury or repair? *J Bone Joint Surg Br* 1993;75:41–48, with permission.)

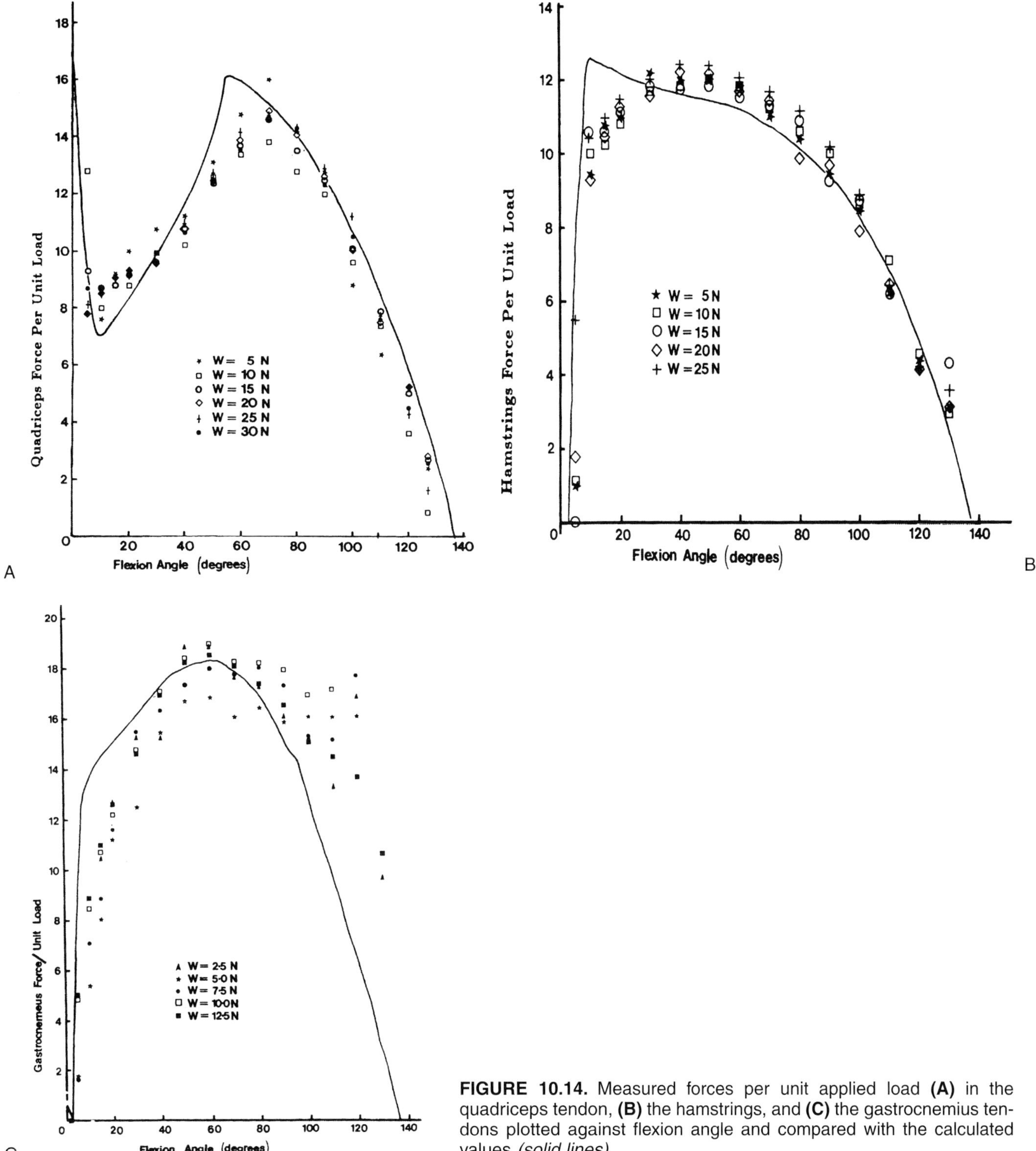

FIGURE 10.14. Measured forces per unit applied load **(A)** in the quadriceps tendon, **(B)** the hamstrings, and **(C)** the gastrocnemius tendons plotted against flexion angle and compared with the calculated values *(solid lines)*.

and gastrocnemius forces, respectively, plotted against flexion angle for a single specimen and compared with calculation of the muscle forces based on the lever-arm lengths of Figure 10.12. A variety of weights were hung from the distal tibia, ranging from 0.5 kg to 3 kg, with corresponding increases in the measured tendon forces. However, when the values of the tendon force were divided by the values of the corresponding applied load, it was found for each muscle that the values of the muscle force per unit load obtained at various loads at a specified flexion angle were about equal, the data collapsing onto single curves when plotted against flexion angle (Fig. 10.14). This implies that, for these simple setups, muscle forces increase *linearly* with increasing applied load, suggesting that the lever-arm lengths do not change much with increasing load and muscle force.

The calculations of muscle force from the model agree reasonably well with the measurements over the flexion range. The model included a simulation of the posterior capsule that limited extension, causing a rapid rise in the value of the quadriceps force and a rapid decrease in the values of the hamstrings and gastrocnemius forces as extension is approached. It is notable that the quadriceps force increased to about 14 times the applied load at about 80° flexion, the hamstrings force to 12 times at about 40°, and the gastrocnemius force to about 18 times at about 50°. It must be emphasized that the experiments were deliberately designed to elicit such large force amplifications by applying the external load perpendicular to the limb at 45° flexion, maximizing its lever-arm length at that position. The results vindicate the conclusions reached by Leonardo and Borelli that muscle forces can be much larger than applied loads because their lever-arms are much shorter. The model included a simulation of the posterior capsule that limited extension, causing a rapid increase in the value of the quadriceps force and a rapid decrease in the values of the hamstrings and gastrocnemius forces as extension is approached.

Note that the quadriceps force peaked at about 70° flexion, not at 45° (where the tibia was horizontal and moment arm of the external load longest, Fig. 10.13A) and where the patellar tendon force would be expected to peak. This is a consequence of the action of the patellofemoral joint and the inequality of the forces in the two tendons. Figure 10.33b of the previous edition shows that the quadriceps force is less than the patellar tendon force between extension and 20° flexion and is larger in the more flexed knee, as suggested by Maquet (50,51) and Bishop and Denham (52). Confirmation of these theoretical results has been obtained in several laboratories.

Imran et al. (53) examined the effects of ligament stretch and cartilage indentation on lever-arm length. They found that deformation-induced backward and forward movements of the tibiofemoral contact points were compensated by associated changes in the directions of the muscle tendons so that deformation-induced changes in the muscle lever-arms were small. Experiments such as those reported in Figures 10.13 and 10.14 are necessarily carried out with small applied loads because of the difficulty of gaining secure attachment to the muscle tendons. Imran et al. (53) concluded that such low-load experiments nonetheless give accurate estimates of the relationships between muscle forces and the larger applied loads typical of activity.

MUSCLE-INDUCED LIGAMENT FORCES

Figure 5.23, animated in Image 3 on the CD-ROM supplied with this book, shows how the models of the muscle tendons rotate relative to the bones during flexion–extension. The tendons are rarely perpendicular to the tibial plateau so that the forces that they apply across the knee pull the tibia either backward or forward relative to the femur. Because the patellar tendon points forward relative to the tibia in extension and backward in flexion (see Figure 5.23), quadriceps action tends to load the ACL near extension and the PCL in flexion. Because the hamstrings point backward relative to the tibia except near extension, they load the PCL over most of the flexion range. The gastrocnemius slopes backward as it spans the gap from femur to tibia at the back of the knee. Its action therefore pulls the tibia forward, loading the ACL. With some muscle tendons pointing forward and others backward, it is possible with appropriately balanced antagonistic action to avoid loading the cruciates at all (54). We shall describe ligament loading by each of the muscle groups separately.

Quadriceps-Induced Ligament Forces

Using the rigid-surface, inextensible ligament model, we studied the leg-lift exercise in Chapter 11, "Mechanics of the Knee," of the previous edition, with the femur held at 45° to the horizontal, and quadriceps force used to raise the tibia under its own weight from the vertical position at 135° flexion, as in Figure 10.13A. The analysis showed that the PCL is loaded from 135° to 85° and the ACL between 85° and extension. At 85°, both cruciates are unloaded because the forward pull of the patellar tendon on the tibia exactly balances the backward push of the external load. Experiments reported in Chapter 12, "The Muscle-Stabilized Knee," of the previous edition found that the calculated values of the ligament forces using the rigid-surface inextensible ligament model were generally very large and, at best, gave upper bounds to the measured values of the ligament forces.

Zavatsky and O'Connor (10,11) studied cruciate ligament loading during isometric quadriceps contraction (Fig. 10.15) using the four-bar linkage model and taking account of ligament extensibility. In this exercise, the extending effect of the quadriceps muscle action, applied

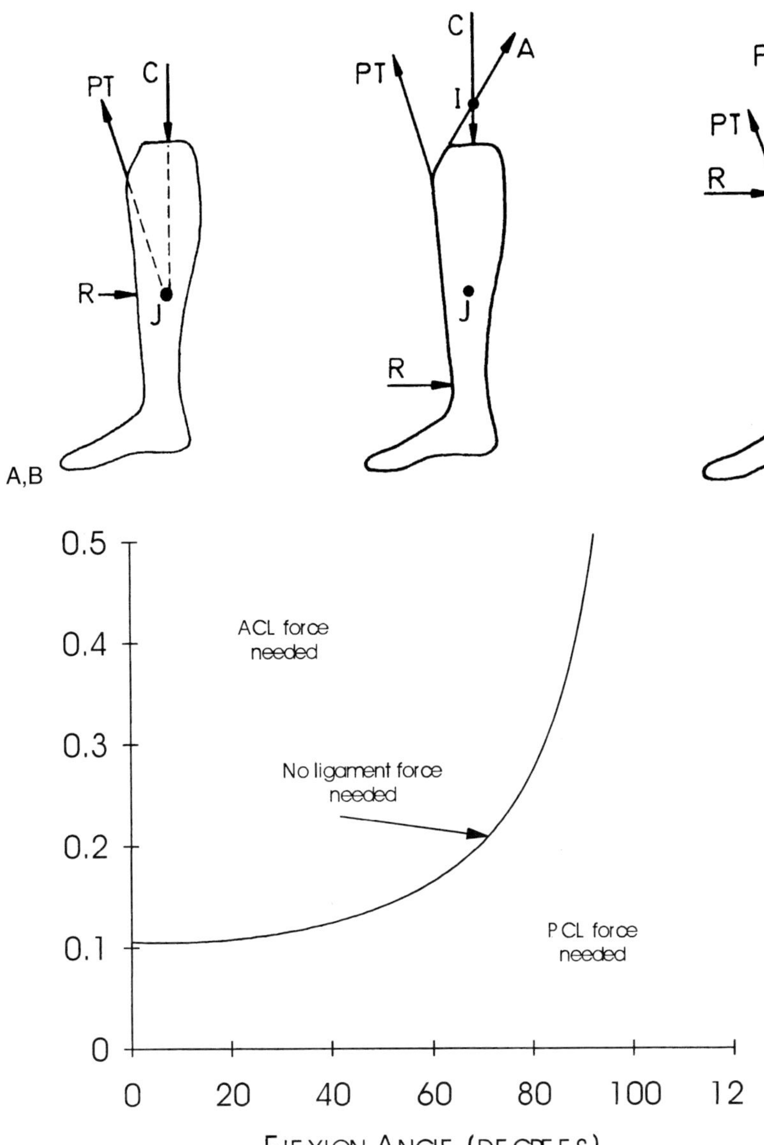

FIGURE 10.15. Isometric quadriceps contraction. Extension is resisted by the force *R*. **A:** When the line of action of *R* passes through the intersection *J* of the lines of the patellar tendon force *PT* and the tibiofemoral contact force *C*, the cruciates are unloaded. **B:** When *R* lies distal to *J*, the anterior cruciate ligament (ACL) is loaded. **C:** When *R* lies proximal to *J*, the posterior cruciate ligament (PCL) is loaded. The curve in **(D)** defines the distance of the resisting force distal to the tibial plateau (in centimeters) at each flexion angle for unloaded cruciates. For placements distal to the values given by the curve, the ACL is loaded. For placements proximal, the PCL is loaded. (From Zavatsky AB, O'Connor JJ. Ligament forces at the knee during isometric quadriceps contractions. *J Engng Med Proc Inst Mech Eng* [H] 1993;207:7–18, with permission.)

to the tibia through the patellar tendon, is balanced by the restraining force *R* applied distally perpendicular to the tibia. In the language of mechanics and using the lever theory, the moment of the patellar tendon force about the flexion axis balances the moment of the restraining force. In this configuration, it is possible to study the effects of increasing quadriceps force at a fixed flexion angle or the effects of increasing flexion with a fixed external lever-arm. A similar configuration is frequently used for rehabilitation after injury to the knee.

Zavatsky and O'Connor showed that the pattern of ligament loading depends not only on the flexion angle but also on the positioning along the tibia of the extension restraint (*R* in Fig. 10.15A). There is a critical restraint position, *J*, at which the moment of the restraining force about the knee is exactly balanced by tension, *PT,* in the patellar tendon while, at the same time, the magnitude of

the horizontal restraining force is equal to the horizontal component of the patellar tendon force. In these circumstances, no action from the cruciates is needed. The position of the tibia on the femur is then exactly that given by the inextensible ligament theory. At each flexion angle, the critical restraining point is the point of intersection of the lines of action of the three forces acting on the leg, the restraining force (*R*), the patellar tendon force (*PT*), and the tibiofemoral contact force (*C*); equilibrium of the leg can be achieved with these three forces alone. Because the direction of the patellar tendon changes with increasing flexion and the relative horizontal component of its force diminishes, the position of the critical restraining point is dependent on flexion angle and moves distally with increasing flexion, as shown in Figure 10.14D. At about 90° flexion, the critical restraining point reaches the ankle.

When the restraint is positioned distal to the critical point, the restraining force has a longer lever-arm and a larger moment about the flexion axis so that a larger patellar tendon force is needed to balance that moment. The horizontal component of the patellar tendon force is now *larger* than the restraining force so that the tibia is pulled forward and force is needed in the ACL to achieve equilibrium in the horizontal direction (Fig. 10.15B). Because of the changing direction of the tendon, the effect depends on flexion angle. The region above the curve in Figure 10.15D defines the conditions of the exercise, the combination of restraint placement and flexion angle, for which the ACL is loaded.

Conversely, when the restraint is placed proximal to the critical point, the horizontal component of the patellar tendon force is now *smaller* than the restraining force so that tension is needed in the PCL to achieve horizontal equilibrium (Fig. 10.15C). At high flexion angles, the patellar tendon is directed backward and its backward pull augments the backward push of the restraining force and augments the requirement for PCL tension. The region below the curve in Figure 10.15D defines the combination of conditions required for PCL loading. Zavatsky and O'Connor (13) described *in vitro* experiments in which restraint placement and flexion angle were varied and the resulting direction of the displacement of the tibia on the femur induced by increasing quadriceps force (anterior or posterior) were found to be in reasonable accord with the predictions of Figure 10.14D and with experimental results published by Jurist and Otis (55), Mandt et al. (56), Howell (57), and Hirokawa et al. (58).

This analysis suggests that the therapist should adjust the conditions of the isometric quadriceps exercise for rehabilitation after ACL or PCL injury. To protect the ACL, a more proximal restraint placement or flexion beyond 90° is required. To protect the PCL, a more distal restraint placement and a straighter leg are required. Zavatsky et al. (11) further discussed the implications of these results for rehabilitation, including also the effects of isometric hamstring contractions.

Effects of Tissue Deformation

The story is not quite as simple as just suggested. As quadriceps force increases, it loads the ligaments and the tibiofemoral articulations. When a ligament is loaded, it stretches and the tibia slips forward or backward relative to the femur, as shown in Figures 10.7 and 10.8 and in Images 6 and 7 on the CD-ROM accompanying this book. The inclination from the tibial plateau of the load-bearing fibers within the ligament diminishes and the ligament becomes more efficient in balancing horizontal load. Increasing muscle force increases the tibiofemoral contact force and the indentation of the cartilage layers. This allows further

tibiofemoral sliding and further changes the inclination of the ligaments. Simultaneously, the directions of the muscle tendons, as they span the joint, change as the tibia slides forward or backward (Fig. 10.8). The relative horizontal component of the muscle tendon force therefore changes and, with it, the demand for ligament force needed to achieve horizontal equilibrium. All of these effects *reduce* the magnitudes of the forces that the ligaments have to carry. We have studied these effects with the 2D sagittal plane model.

Zavatsky used the four-bar linkage model to study the tibial translation induced by quadriceps action over the flexion range, taking account of the extensibility of the ligaments, as in Figures 10.7 and 10.8. The calculation involved incrementing the value of the assumed translation from zero, calculating the consequent ligament force on the basis of its deformation and a nonlinear stress–strain relation, then using two equations of equilibrium in the sagittal plane to calculate the values of the quadriceps and resisting forces. The calculation was repeated with a further increment in the value of the translation until the components of the forces parallel with the tibial plateau balanced.

Huss et al. (16) further extended the model to consider simultaneous indentation of the cartilage. They assumed that both femoral condyles were spherical and used contact theory for a thin layer to relate contact force with indentation. Their analysis involved an additional outer iterative loop with sequential incrementing of the assumed indentation.

The calculated tibial translations, forward (positive) and backward (negative) at different flexion angles, and a restraining load placement *20 cm* below the tibial plateau are plotted against quadriceps force in Figure 10.16. Both models showed that no displacement takes place at a flexion angle of about 70°, consistent with Figure 10.14D. Posterior translation was predicted at higher flexion angles, with loading of the PCL. Anterior translation was predicted with less flexion, the largest occurring at 20°.

The displacements recorded in Figure 10.16A, which accounts for cartilage indentation, are almost double at each flexion angle those of Figure 10.16B, obtained from the extensible-ligament rigid-surface model. This contrasts with the results of Figure 10.11 where only modest increases in passive laxity due to cartilage deformation were observed. The large muscle forces induced in isometric quadriceps contraction are balanced by large compressive contact forces so that the deformation of the cartilage is significantly larger in the dynamic case.

Both models showed that tibial translation grows in a nonlinear manner as quadriceps force increases. There is an initial rapid growth of displacement to about 1 mm with the first 100 N of quadriceps force. Thereafter, displacement grows more slowly and appears to approach limiting asymptotic values for very large quadriceps force. In other words, the bones move rapidly towards

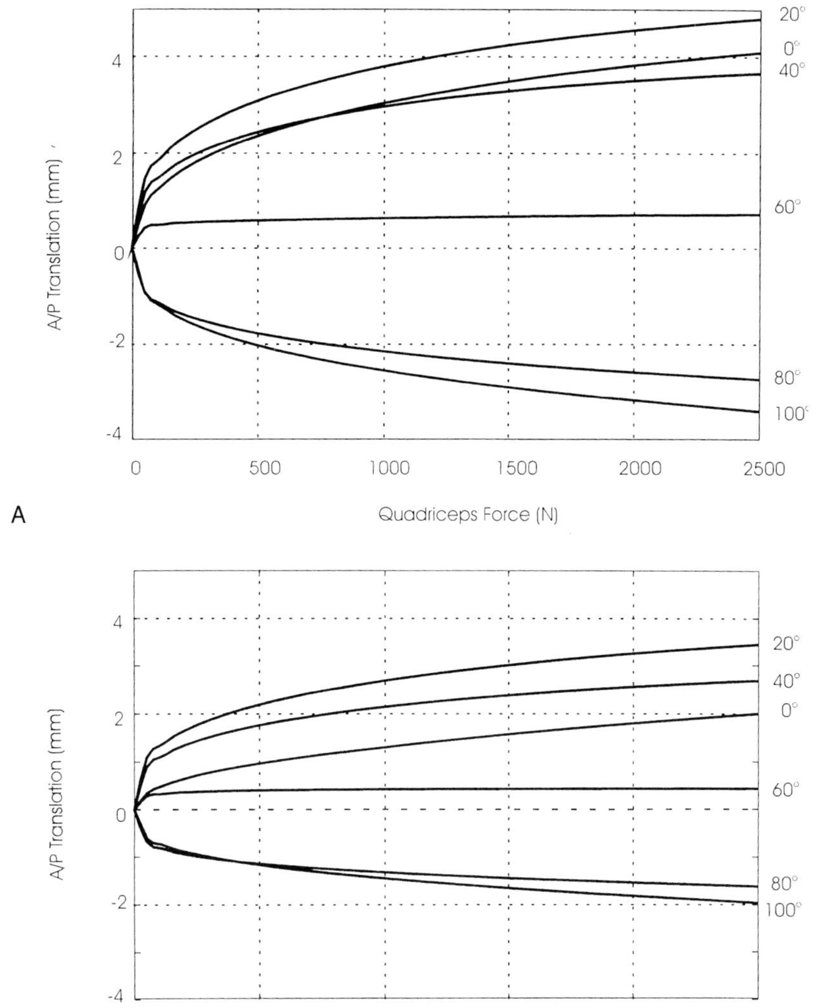

FIGURE 10.16. Anterior (positive) and posterior (negative) tibial displacement induced by increasing quadriceps force against a resistance placed 20 cm distal to the tibial plateau, assuming extensible ligaments and **(A)** compressible articular surfaces, **(B)** assuming rigid articular surfaces. (From Huss RA, Holstein H, O'Connor JJ. A mathematical model of forces in the knee under isometric quadriceps contractions. *Clin Biomech* 2000;15:112–122, with permission.)

positions from which they do not move much further, however large the quadriceps force. Quadriceps forces of *2,500 N* (three times body weight) could not induce anterior translations of more than *5 mm* or posterior translations of more than *4 mm*. The *dynamic laxity* of the joint, the movements due to tissue deformation induced by muscle force, proves to be not much greater than can be induced in the drawer test by an A/P force of only 67 N (Fig. 10.11).

Huss et al. (16) found that their calculations of anterior tibial translation under various values of quadriceps force *underestimated in vivo* measurements by Hirokawa et al. (58), whereas their calculations for *2,500 N* slightly *overestimated* the anterior tibial translation (ATT) reported by Howell (57) for *in vivo* "maximum isometric quadriceps contraction." Their calculations underestimated the measurements of ATT by Kizuki et al. (59) for maximum isometric quadriceps contractions. The values of ATT obtained by Huss et al.

are smaller than those reported by Pandy and Shelburne (37), whose model did not account for cartilage deformation. However, their quadriceps forces (peak value about *6,000 N*) were considerably larger than those considered by Huss et al.

Similar effects were found in the calculated values of the cruciate ligament forces (Fig. 10.17). The ligament forces increase rapidly at first then more slowly with increasing quadriceps force. The ACL force rapidly reaches its asymptotic value, with its largest value of about *130 N* at extension, sensibly reached with a quadriceps force of *1,000 N*. Deformation of the cartilage (Fig. 10.17A) *reduces* ligament force values from those predicted by the rigid-surface theory (Fig. 10.17B). Only the PCL force at high flexion angles fails to exhibit asymptotic behavior because, in these positions, the ligament is most steeply inclined to the tibial plateau and least efficient in resisting posteriorly directed forces.

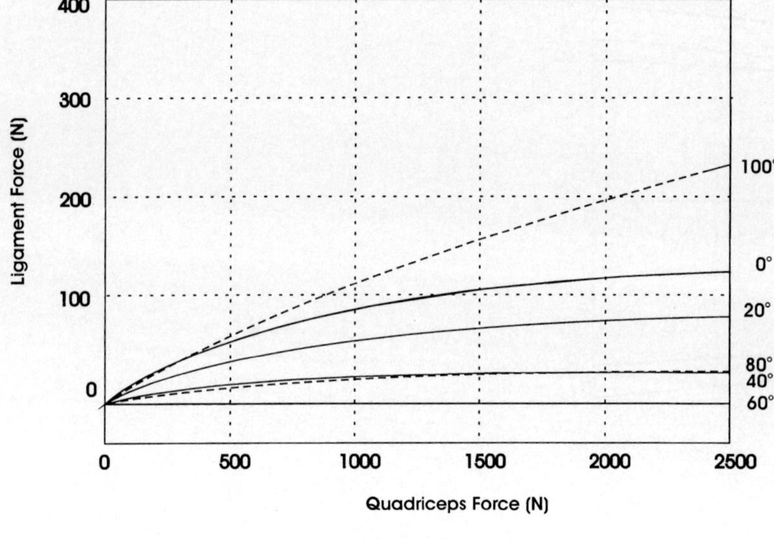

A

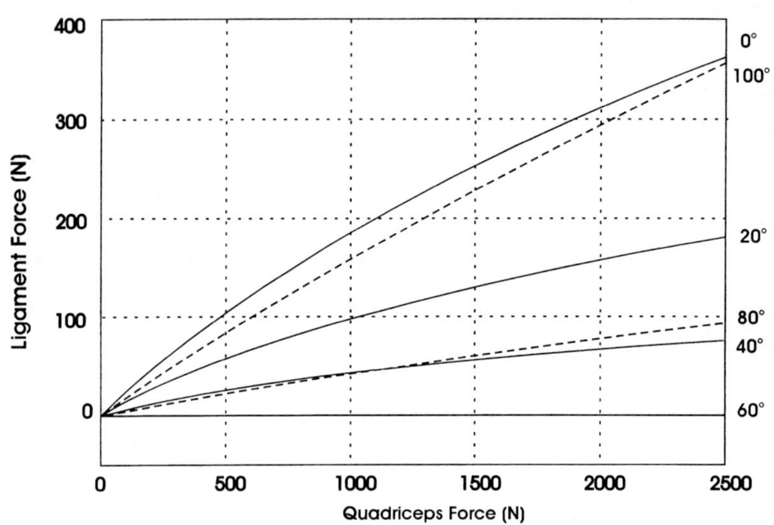

B

FIGURE 10.17. Anterior cruciate ligament (ACL) forces at 0, 20, and 40° and posterior cruciate ligament (PCL) forces (*dashed lines*) at 80 and 100° plotted against quadriceps force for **(A)** compressible and **(B)** incompressible cartilage. (From Huss RA, Holstein H, O'Connor JJ. A mathematical model of forces in the knee under isometric quadriceps contractions. *Clin Biomech* 2000;15:112–122, with permission.)

The ligament forces values calculated by Huss et al. (16) are smaller than those calculated by Pandy and Shelburne (37) whose model did not account for cartilage deformation and whose calculations applied to quadriceps force values up to *6,000 N.*

Zavatsky and O'Connor (10) explained the asymptotic behavior just described. Force in the patellar tendon near extension pulls the tibia forward, stretching the ACL and reducing the inclination of the patellar tendon (Fig. 10.18A). The relative horizontal component of the patellar tendon force is thereby reduced, reducing the demand on the ACL for a further force contribution. Eventually, the tibia can move to a position relative to the femur where further increments in patellar tendon force (δPT, Fig. 10.18B) can be balanced by increments δR in the value of the resisting force without the need for further increases in the ACL force, A. The asymptotic position of the tibia on the femur is akin to that implied by the curve of Figure 10.11D along which the external resisting load is balanced by the patellar tendon force with respect to both moment and horizontal force equilibrium. Tissue deformation results in signif-

icant changes in the geometry of the muscle tendons and in the ligament forces that they induce.

Figure 10.19A, for a quadriceps force of 1,000 N, is equivalent to Figure 10.11D, but considers both ligament and cartilage deformation. For each position of the resisting load below the tibial plateau, there is now a band of flexion angle in which cruciate ligament forces are not required during the isometric quadriceps exercise. Figure 10.19B, which presents the same result for the range of quadriceps force up to 2,500 N and a load placement of 200 mm, shows that the range of flexion over which cruciate ligament force is not required increases with flexion angle. The dashed line in Figure 10.18B defines the solitary flexion angle defined by the rigid surface inextensible ligament model at which cruciate ligament force is not required. Although zero cruciate ligament force is required at *60°* for a restraint placement *20 cm* below the plateau (Fig. 10.17), there is nonetheless a small ATT at this flexion angle (Fig. 10.16).

These diagrams demonstrate that the therapist has to get the initial conditions of the isometric quadriceps exer-

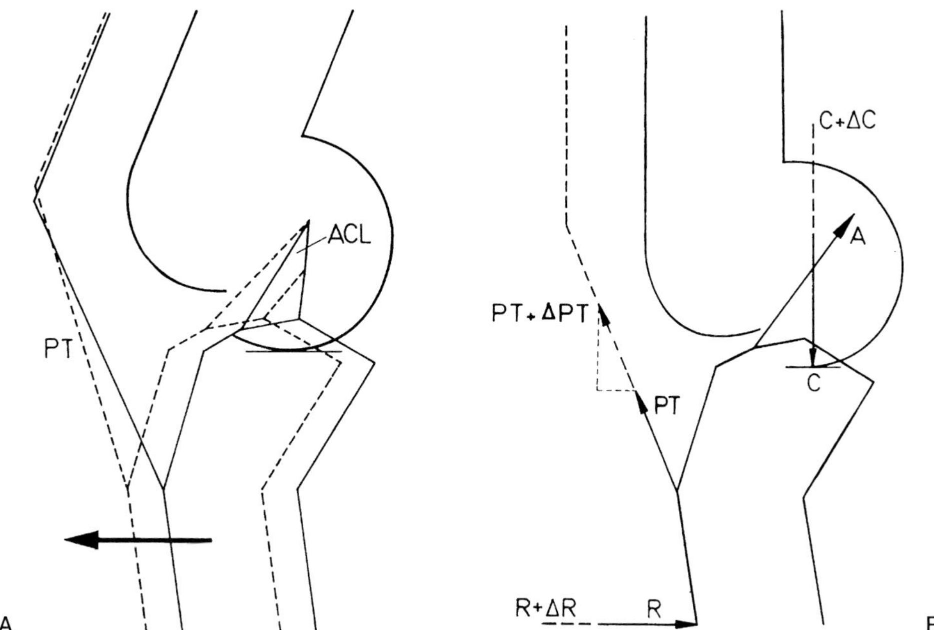

FIGURE 10.18. A: Tissue deformation allows the tibia to slide forward on the femur, reducing the inclination of the patellar tendon to the vertical and reducing the relative horizontal component of the patellar tendon force. **B:** The patellar tendon is now so directed that an increment in the tendon force is completely balanced by increments in the resisting force and tibiofemoral contact force without change in the anterior cruciate ligament (ACL) force. (From Zavatsky AB, O'Connor JJ. Ligament forces at the knee during isometric quadriceps contractions. *J Engng Med Proc Inst Mech Eng* [H] 1993;207:7–18, with permission.)

cise only approximately correct. As the subject increases quadriceps force near but not exactly at the critical conditions of Figure 10.11D, ligament forces can increase and then actually reduce to zero as quadriceps force increases. Near the critical conditions, the subject can be encouraged to apply maximum quadriceps contractions without loading either cruciate severely.

These studies explain how relatively slight structures such as the ACL can survive during even the most intense exercise when muscle forces are very large. The model, of course, does not account for the contribution of the menisci to load bearing. By spreading load over larger surface areas and thereby reducing the levels of contact pressure, the indentation of the cartilage layers may be reduced. The patterns of A/P displacement and ligament force under increasing quadriceps force may lie between the patterns suggested by the rigid surface model (Figs. 10.16B, 10.17B) and the deformable surface model (Figs. 10.16A, 10.17A).

Ligament Forces During Gait

Despite the considerable advances in the clinical use of gait analysis systems, there are surprisingly few estimates of the values of ligament forces encountered during a routine activity such as level walking. Such analysis is not routine, because even the most modern laboratory systems do not use anatomic models of the joints, such as those described in Chapter 5 and above, but content themselves with reporting the values of the resultant

forces and moments transmitted across the joints of the lower limb, without attempting to evaluate muscle, ligament, and contact forces.

The analysis is difficult because there are many more muscles active in the trunk and lower limbs during walking than the number of equations of dynamics available for their evaluation. The locomotor system is *dynamically redundant*. Although this is frustrating to the biomechanic, it is very fortunate for the living subject because it means that there are different strategies available, in terms of which muscles to use, to perform a selected task. When muscles have been injured, or even divided by the surgeon during, for example, a hip replacement, the patient can learn to use alternative muscles to accomplish various tasks. When ligaments are damaged, the patient can learn to use antagonistic muscle action.

Using the methodology of control theory, many schemes have been developed to determine the optimum strategy for the accomplishment of selected tasks (60–64), but an agreed optimization criterion has not yet achieved widespread acceptance (65), and these methods are rarely used in routine clinical gait analysis.

Mikosz et al. (66) developed a stochastic mathematical model of the knee. Although they accounted for the rolling–sliding movements of the articular surfaces on each other, they did not attempt to evaluate ligament forces explicitly. Smidt (67) estimated ligament and muscle tendon directions from serial lateral radiographs and performed an analysis of flexed knee stance. However, he did not calculate the values of the ligament forces but

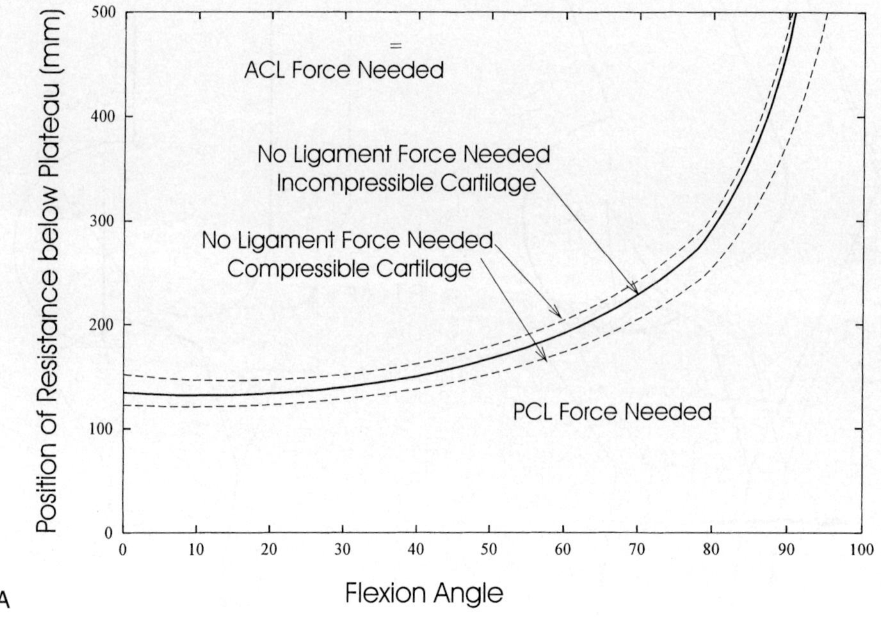

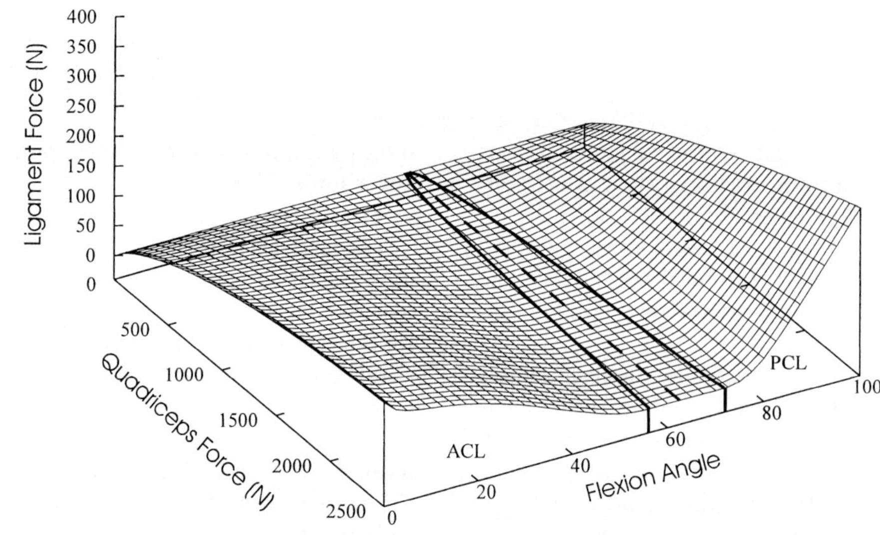

FIGURE 10.19. A: Position of resisting force plotted against flexion angle defining the range within which the resistance can be placed without loading the cruciates. **B:** Plot of cruciate ligament force against quadriceps force and flexion angle when the resistance is placed 20 cm distal to the tibial plateau. (From Huss RA, Holstein H, O'Connor JJ. A mathematical model of forces in the knee under isometric quadriceps contractions. *Clin Biomech* 2000;15:112–122, with permission.)

reported only the values of the shear force transmitted from tibia to femur. Yasuda and Sasaki (68), Balzopolous, Kaufman et al. (69), Nisell et al. (70,71), and Dahlkvist et al. (72) also determined the tibiofemoral shear forces but not the cruciate forces during various exercises.

Morrison (73) provided estimates of ligament forces during gait, using a fixed flexion–axis model of the knee. He based his choice of phasic muscle activity on electromyogram (EMG) data, selecting only a reduced number of agonists, quadriceps, hamstrings, and gastrocnemius, with no abductor–adductor muscles and no antagonists in

his study. His methods were used by Harrington (74) to study normal and pathologic gaits. The estimates of peak cruciate ligament force values during level walking varied in magnitude from 150 to 600 N, the ACL active during most of stance phase and the PCL active in later stance, with larger forces in the PCL. Loading of the MCL during gait was very slight, whereas the LCL force during later stance was thought to rise to about 350 N. Morrison found that cruciate ligament forces were increased during stair rising and descending, the PCL while ascending, and the ACL while descending. However, Andriacchi et al. (75)

found that the absence of a functioning PCL after knee replacement adversely affected stair descent.

Collins and O'Connor (76) used the inextensible ligament rigid surface four-bar linkage model of the knee in a sagittal plane model of the leg. With data from gait analysis, they calculated all the possible combinations of muscle–ligament–contact forces that could be in dynamic equilibrium with the measured external loads. The combinations, including ligament forces, gave very large values of those forces, sometimes exceeding the known measured strength of healthy, young ligaments. They attributed these overestimates to the use of a rigid surface–inextensible ligament model. Wilson et al. (77) showed that estimates of ligament force values were very sensitive to the parameters chosen for the knee model. Force values were largest for those parameters that maximized the inclinations of the ligaments to the tibial plateau.

The smallest values were obtained when ligament elasticity was also taken into account, as demonstrated above.

Lu (40,41) has developed a 3D mathematical model of the lower limb with its muscles and with anatomical models of the hip (a ball and socket joint) and the knee (a parallel spatial mechanism). This model will be the basis for further estimates of ligament force values in activity when it has been developed further to take account of tissue deformation.

Ligament Forces During Isokinetic and Isometric Exercises and Deep Squats

Toutoungi et al.(18) applied a 2D sagittal plane lower limb model with a four-bar linkage knee and extensible ligaments (Fig. 10.20) to analyze data collected in the gait laboratory and to estimate the levels of cruciate ligament

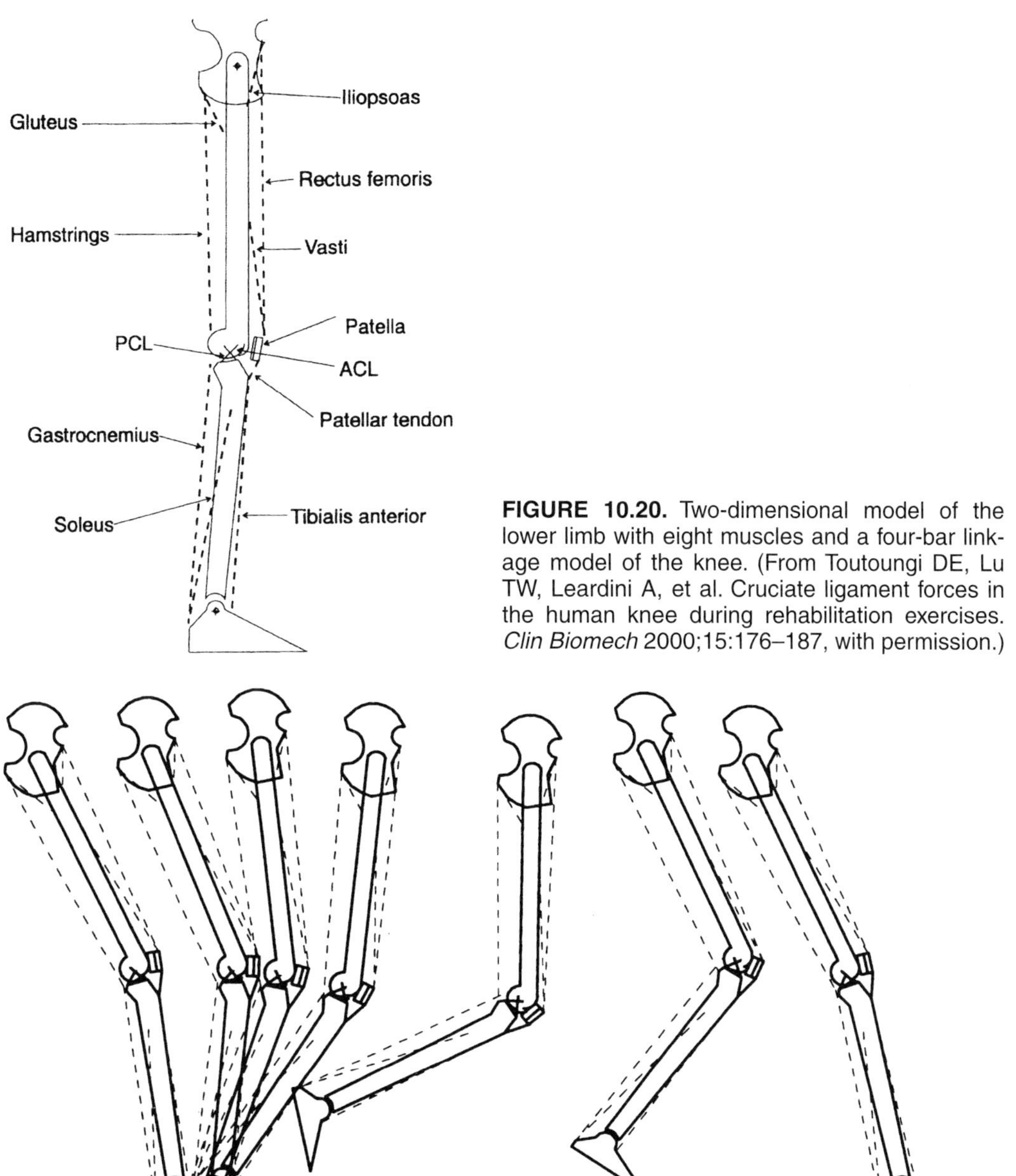

FIGURE 10.20. Two-dimensional model of the lower limb with eight muscles and a four-bar linkage model of the knee. (From Toutoungi DE, Lu TW, Leardini A, et al. Cruciate ligament forces in the human knee during rehabilitation exercises. *Clin Biomech* 2000;15:176–187, with permission.)

force occurring during isokinetic and isometric exercises and deep squats. Optometric data determined the changing shapes of the limb. Force transducer or floor-mounted force-plate data determined the forces applied through the distal leg or floor. EMG from electrodes on the main flexors and extensors indicated which muscles were active at each stage of each exercise. Although the model was 2D, we have found that it reasonably predicted force data telemetered from patients with instrument-implanted hip prostheses during strictly sagittal plane exercises (41). It underestimated forces during gait because it did not account for the actions of the abductors–adductors.

Table 10.2 shows the combinations of forces around the ankle and the knee that were most consistent with the EMG and data that were used for the calculation of ligament forces. The calculations involved the same iterative method to determine the A/P translations occurring during the experiments as described above. During isokinetic and isometric extension involving quadriceps activity, the posterior cruciate was loaded between *100°* and *70°*, whereas the ACL was loaded between *70°* and extension. Isometric and isokinetic flexion involving the hamstrings loaded the PCL over the full range of motion. Squats loaded the ACL from extension to *40°* and the PCL from there to *140°*, both during descent and ascent.

Figure 10.21 shows the calculated values of the ligament forces during the flexion and extension phases of isokinetic exercises carried out by eight young, healthy subjects at three different nominal speeds. Mean values of ligament force together with one standard error of mean (SEM) are plotted against flexion angle. Notice the different scales used to plot ligament forces during flexion and extension. ACL forces peak at about *40°* during extension, but the ACL is not involved during flexion. Much larger peak PCL forces occurred at about 85° during flexion and small PCL forces were found between 100° and 80° during initial extension. The large PCL forces calculated for the flexion exercise arise because, in the flexed knee, the hamstrings are ideally oriented to pull the tibia backward whereas the PCL is much more vertical and inefficient in resisting posterior tibial translation (see the animation in Image 3 on the CD-ROM supplied with this book). The exchange from PCL to ACL forces during extension occurs for the reasons given in the discussion of Figure 10.15D. Ligament force values decreased with increasing exercise speed.

Six of the subjects performed isometric exercises in the isokinetic apparatus. With various fixed angles of flexion, they were invited to pull with maximum force on their extensors and then on their flexors, with suitable resting periods. The patterns of cruciate ligament force calculated from these exercises were broadly similar to those found in the isokinetic exercises, with large PCL forces induced by flexor action in the flexed knee and smaller ACL forces, peaking at about *30°* flexion, induced by extensor action (Fig. 10.22). Again, notice the difference in force scale in the two graphs.

Figure 10.23 shows that only the PCL was seriously involved in three types of deep squat, during both descent and ascent. The heel-off squat (HO) allowed flexion to *140°* whereas heel-on-ground (HG) allowed only *100°* and the one-legged squat (OL) allowed only *85°*. All forces below *40°* flexion were small. The largest ACL forces encountered in these exercises were only *142 N, 0.18* times body weight (BW). Substantial PCL force values were obtained at the depth of the squat. The largest PCL forces were found for HG, with a peak value of *2,704 N, 3.5 BW*.

The largest ACL forces calculated for these *in vivo* exercises are similar in magnitude to those calculated by Zavatsky and O'Connor (10) as described above, taking only ligament elongation into account. Therefore, it is likely that smaller values would be obtained by considering cartilage deformation, as demonstrated by Huss et al. (16) and shown in Figure 10.17. The peak PCL forces calculated during flexor activity and during squats are much larger than those induced by extensor action (Fig. 10.17).

TABLE 10.2. *Combinations of forces at different flexion angles across the ankle, knee, and hip during various exercises*

knee angle	0°		50°		100°		150°
IK/IM extension		TCD-QAC			TCD-QPC		
IK/IM flexion			TCD-HPC				
Squats descent	TGC-QAC-HCD		TGC-QPC-HCD		TSC-QPC-HCD		
Squats ascent	TGC-QAC-HCD		TGC-QPC-HCD		TSC-QPC-HCD		

NOTE: C, contact force; D, direction of contact force; Q, quadriceps; H, hamstrings; G, gastrocnemius; S, soleus; T, tibialis anterior; A, anterior cruciate ligament; P, posterior cruciate ligament. For the squats exercises, the combination of symbols TGC-QPC-HCD means tibialis anterior, gastrocnemius, and tibiotalar contact forces across the ankle and quadriceps, posterior cruciate, and tibiofemoral contact forces at the knee, hamstrings and femoro–acetabular contact forces at the hip with the direction D of the hip contact force determined by the calculation. Forces at the hip were not calculated for the isokinetic or isometric exercises. (From Elsevier Science Ltd., with permission.)

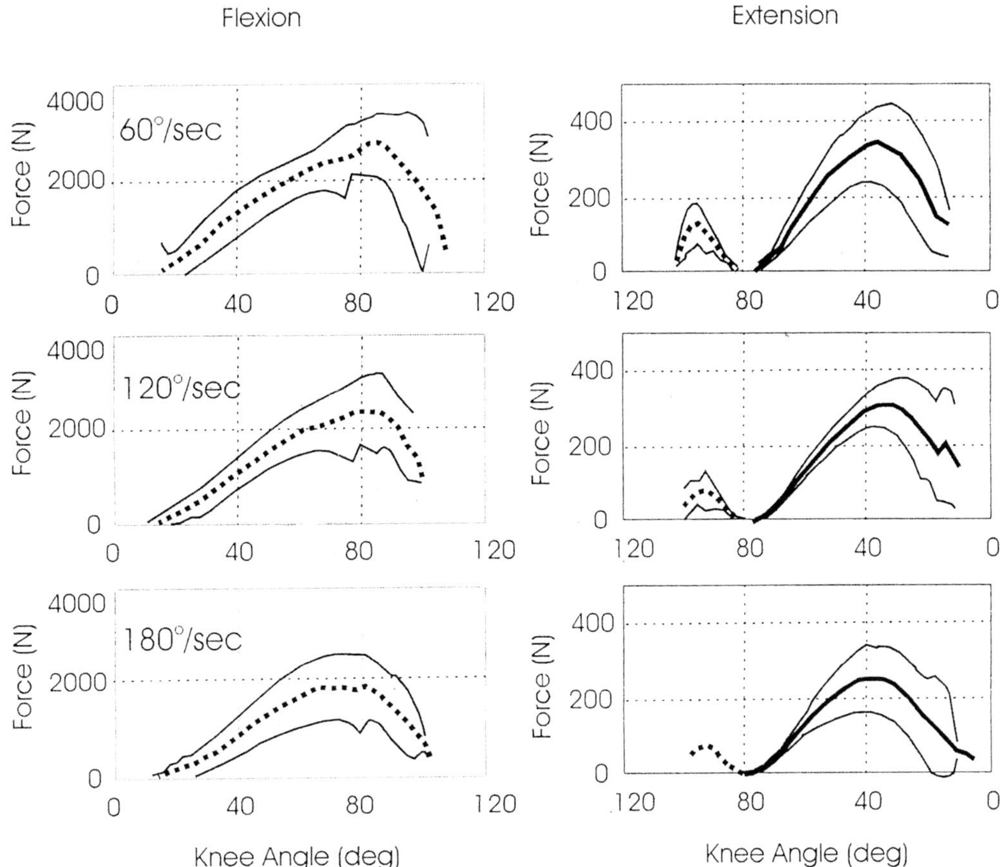

FIGURE 10.21. Calculated values of the cruciate ligament forces at different speeds during isokinetic exercises. *Bold solid lines* are anterior cruciate ligament (ACL) forces, *bold dotted lines* are posterior cruciate ligament (PCL) forces, representing mean values from eight subjects, *light solid lines* give ±1 SEM. (From Toutoungi DE, Lu TW, Leardini A, et al. Cruciate ligament forces in the human knee during rehabilitation exercises. *Clin Biomech* 2000;15:176–187, with permission.)

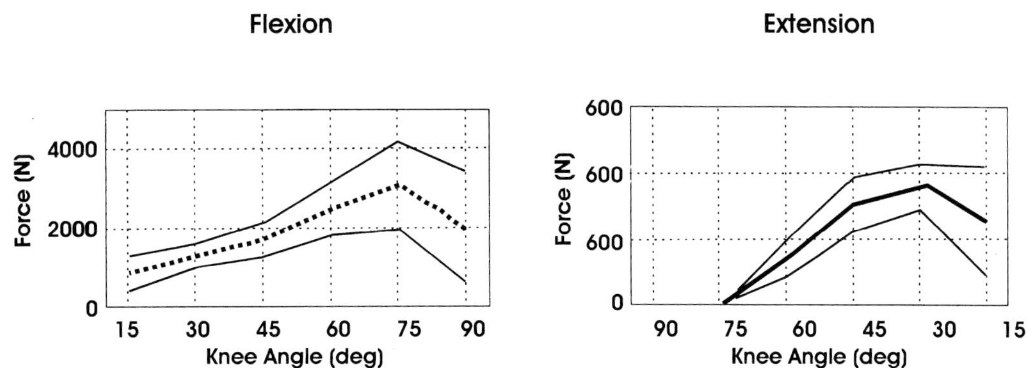

FIGURE 10.22. Cruciate ligament forces during isometric exercises. *Bold lines* show mean values from six subjects; *light solid lines* show ±1 SEM; *solid bold line* indicates anterior cruciate ligament (ACL) force; and *dotted bold line* indicates posterior cruciate ligament (PCL) force. (From Toutoungi DE, Lu TW, Leardini A, et al. Cruciate ligament forces in the human knee during rehabilitation exercises. *Clin Biomech* 2000;15:176–187, with permission.)

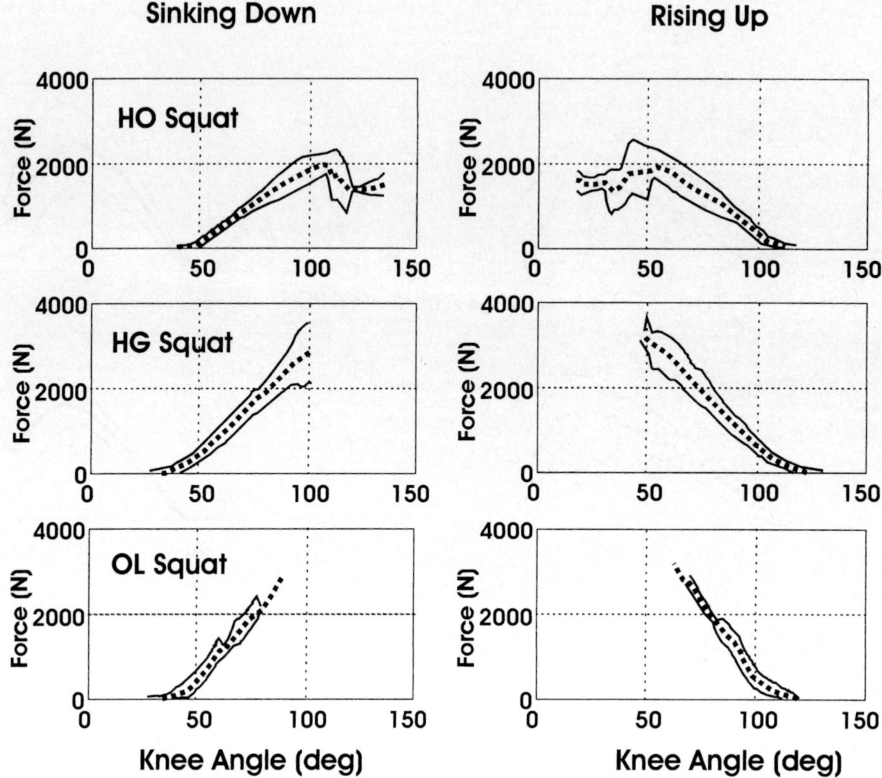

FIGURE 10.23. Cruciate ligament forces (±1 SEM) for heel-off, heel-on-ground, and one-legged squats. Mean values for eight subjects. (From Toutoungi DE, Lu TW, Leardini A, et al. Cruciate ligament forces in the human knee during rehabilitation exercises. *Clin Biomech* 2000;15:176–187, with permission.)

The direct backward pull of the hamstrings on the flexed knee is a potent loader of the PCL.

The peak ACL values found in these calculations are still a small fraction of the ultimate tensile strength of the ACL of the young healthy adult (78), but the peak PCL values are almost *85%* of its reported strength (5). Our PCL values are undoubtedly too large, because cartilage deformation was not accounted for in the calculations. Nonetheless, our values are consistent with the values of tibiofemoral shear forces estimated by other investigators.

For instance, the posterior shear force values reported by Dahlkvist et al. (72) during deep squats (*3.66 BW*) were actually larger than the peak PCL force values calculated by our method (*3.5 BW*). Although the values of the peak anterior shear force reported by Nisell et al. (70) (*0.9 BW*) and by Baltzopolous (*0.9 BW*) for isokinetic extension are higher than our peak ACL forces, their knee moment values are also higher. The peak posterior shear forces reported by Kaufman et al. (69) during isokinetic extension are much higher (*1.7 BW*) than our peak PCL forces (*0.1 BW*), whereas their peak posterior shear forces during isokinetic flexion (*1.7 BW*) are reasonably consistent with our PCL force values.

Toutoungi et al. (18) discussed the safety or otherwise of these exercises during rehabilitation after ACL or PCL repair. They concluded that squats are a safe exercise after ACL reconstruction, once early healing is com-

pleted, whereas they should be limited to about *50°* flexion after PCL reconstruction. Exercises involving very high PCL forces should be avoided after reconstruction of that ligament.

Antagonistic Muscle Action and Ligament Protection

O'Connor (54) (see Chapter 11, "Mechanics of the Knee," in the previous edition) used the inextensible ligament rigid surface 2D model to demonstrate that, over most of the flexion range, some of the flexors and extensors pull the tibia backward, whereas others pull the tibia forward. Their relative contributions vary with flexion angle because of their changing directions. They should therefore, between them, be able to develop appropriate levels of force to balance not only the moment of the external loads but also the component of the external load parallel to the tibial plateau. The flexors and extensors should be able to compensate completely for ligament force while keeping the contact points between the bones near their unloaded positions (i.e., without excessive subluxation). They should be able to protect healthy or healing ligaments and to compensate for ruptured ligaments. Whether it is possible to teach patients to apply the appropriate levels of muscle force is not a question that can be answered in terms of engineering mechanics. Compensation was not possible near extension because all three muscles pull the tibia forward in those positions (see Figure 5.23).

Imran and O'Connor (17) have reexamined quadriceps–hamstrings interactions using the extensible ligament 2D model. They examined the isometric quadriceps exercise as discussed earlier (Fig. 10.15) and considered two cases: (a) the ACL was ruptured or incapable of bearing load and (b) the ACL was intact or reconstructed and capable of bearing load. Calculations were carried out for placement of the resisting force *30 cm* below the tibial plateau (Fig. 10.15). At this placement, ACL force would be expected from extension up to about *85°* flexion in an intact knee under isometric quadriceps contraction.

Figure 10.24 shows the values of quadricep, hamstring, and tibiofemoral contact force expected in the ACL-deficient knee, plotted against flexion angle. The solid lines assume that there is no ATT. The dashed and dotted lines show force values with varying levels of ATT. Force values are expressed as multipliers of the value of the resisting force.

The force levels per unit resisting force are not strongly influenced by tissue deformation and ATT in the flexed knee where relatively small values of the hamstrings force can balance relatively large values of quadriceps force. However, as the knee is extended, tissue deformation plays an important role. Without tissue deformation, all forces become impossibly large near *20°* flexion. This remains true for an ATT of 2 mm, but an ATT of *3 mm* makes compensation for loss of an ACL possible near extension and larger ATTs reduce the required force levels considerably. Near extension, an ATT of *6 mm* reduces the required quadriceps force to less than 10 times the resisting force and the required hamstrings force to less than 6 times. There are corresponding reductions in the value of the tibiofemoral contact force. However, note that the contact force levels are generally very high near

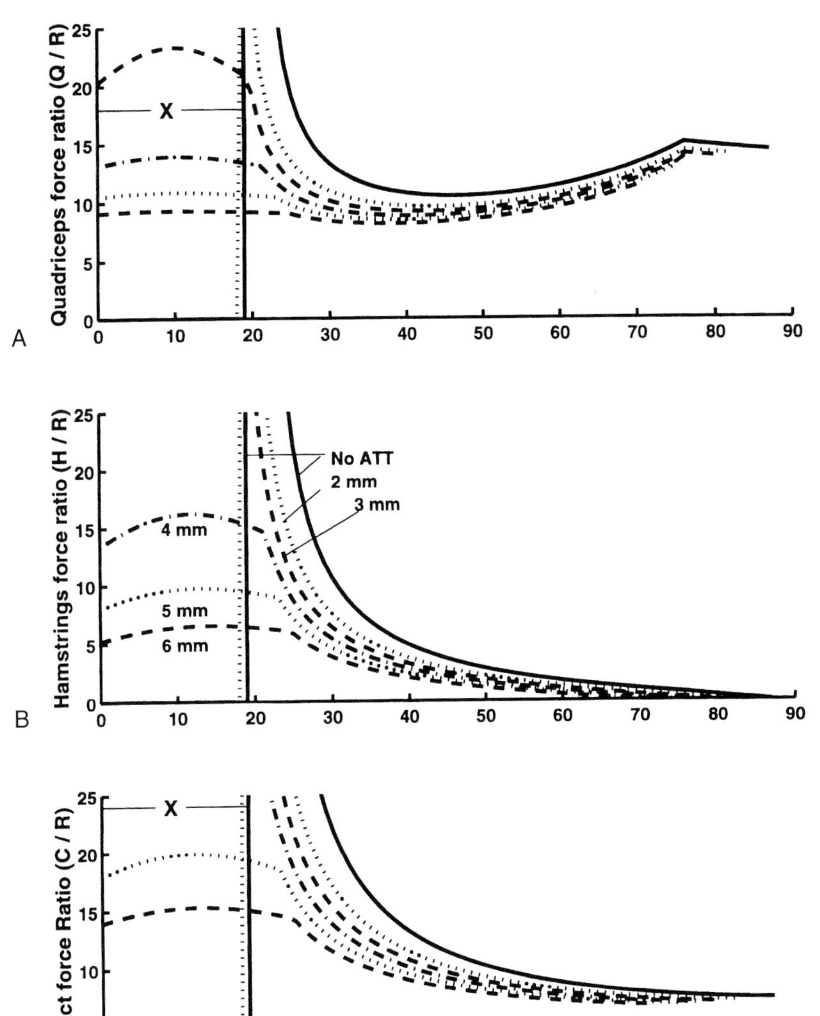

FIGURE 10.24. Quadriceps **(A)**, hamstrings **(B)**, and tibiofemoral contact forces in **(C)** the anterior cruciate ligament (ACL)–deficient knee plotted against flexion angle for various anterior tibial translations during quadriceps isometric exercises against a resistance placed 30 mm distal to the tibia plateau. Antagonistic quadriceps–hamstrings action cannot compensate for an absent ACL in the flexion range marked *X* unless the tibia translates anteriorly. (From Imran A, O'Connor JJ. Control of knee stability after ACL injury or repair: interaction between hamstrings contraction and tibial translation. *Clin Biomech* 1998;13:153–162, with permission.)

extension because they balance the upward pulls of both extensors and flexors.

The effect of ATT is to redirect the directions of the muscle tendons so that equilibrium in the A/P direction can be achieved, with the anteriorly directed component of the patellar tendon force relatively reduced and the posteriorly directed component of the hamstrings force increased. These levels of ATT are not unphysiologic. Howell (57) has reported ATT of the order of *8 mm* in ACL-intact knees during "manual maximum A/P laxity tests." However, they are larger than would be expected in the intact model joint even under quadriceps forces as large as *2,500 N*, three times BW (Fig. 10.17). Therefore, it seems possible for the ACL-deficient patient to use antagonistic muscle action over the full range of flexion and therefore stabilize the knee but at the expense of increased anterior tibial translation. This, combined with the increased values of the tibiofemoral contact force, may have deleterious effects on the menisci. Whether a patient can learn to tune muscle tension so precisely is another matter.

Figures 10.25 and 10.26 refer to the ACL-intact or -reconstructed knee. Figure 10.25 shows how, at *45°* flexion, ligament, quadriceps, and contact forces all grow with increasing levels of resisting force.[4] Curves are plotted for four levels of hamstrings force from zero to *375 N* in Figure 10.25A and for zero and *375 N* hamstrings force in Figures 10.25B and 10.25C. Note that quadriceps force reaches values greater than *2,500 N*.

Figure 10.25A shows how ACL force diminishes for these modest increases in hamstrings force at a selected value of resisting force. For small resisting forces, less than *100 N*, increasing hamstrings force can eventually unload the ACL and load the PCL, as the directions of the muscle tendons change due to tissue deformation. Figure 10.25B shows that the required levels of quadriceps force

---

[4]Here, we are regarding resisting forces as independently applied and the quadriceps force as the reaction to it, whereas the opposite is the reality. However, the relations between the forces remain the same. The resisting force can readily be measured. It is directly related to the torque measured in an isokinetic machine.

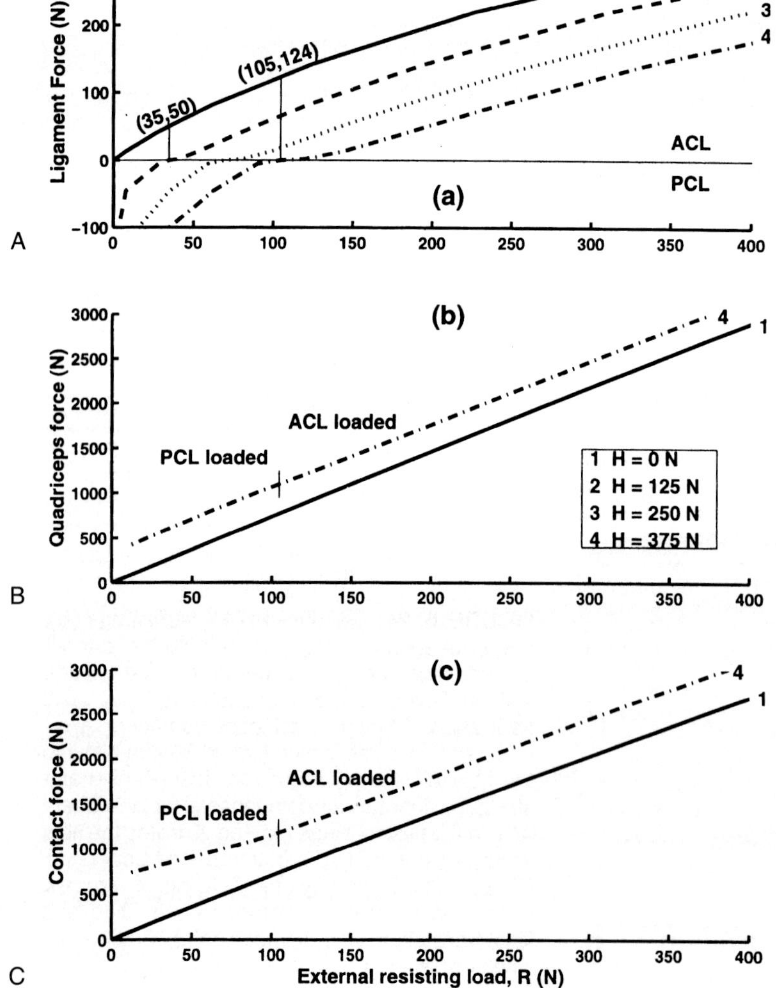

FIGURE 10.25. Cruciate ligament **(A)**, quadriceps **(B)**, and tibiofemoral contact forces **(C)** during isometric quadriceps exercise at 45° flexion, plotted against value of resisting force. The *solid* and *chain-dotted curves* in **(B)** and **(C)** give quadriceps and contact force values in the presence of zero and 375 N hamstring force, respectively. (From Imran A, O'Connor JJ. Control of knee stability after ACL injury or repair: interaction between hamstrings contraction and tibial translation. *Clin Biomech* 1998;13: 153–162, with permission.)

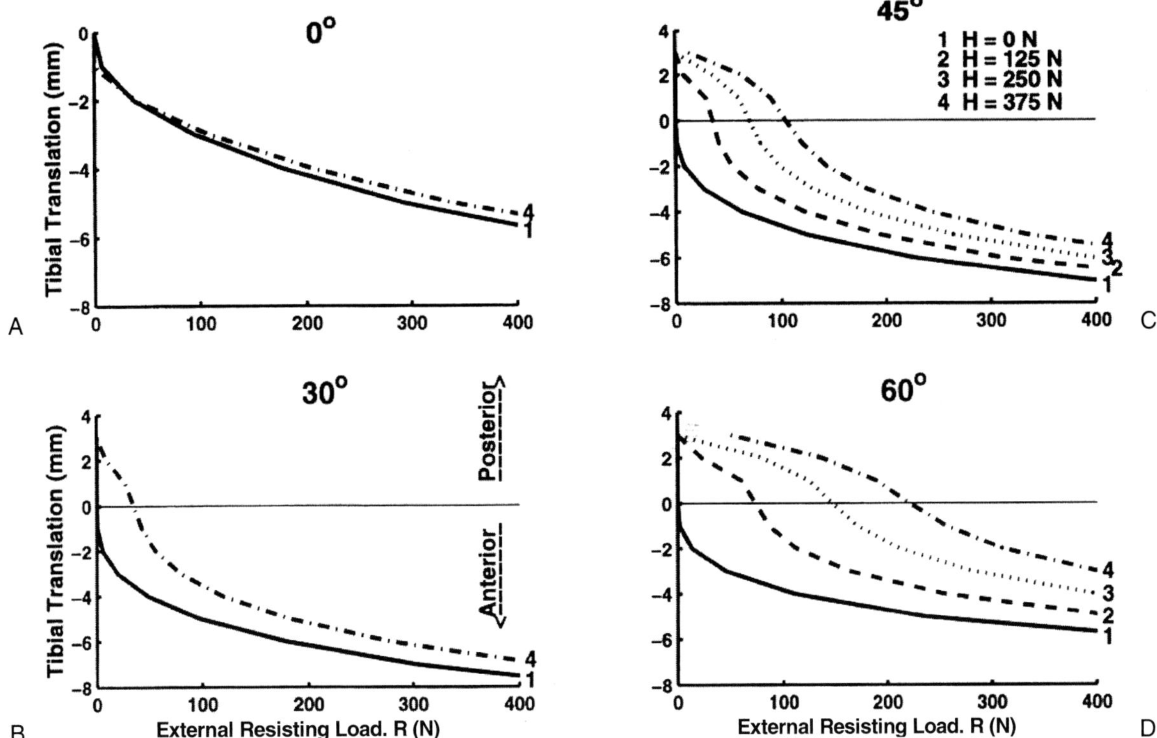

FIGURE 10.26. Tibial translation (positive posterior, negative anterior) produced by combined quadriceps–hamstrings action plotted against the value of the resisting force at four flexion angles. At each flexion angle, different combinations of forces unload the ligaments and produce zero tibial translation. (From Imran A, O'Connor JJ. Control of knee stability after ACL injury or repair: interaction between hamstrings contraction and tibial translation. *Clin Biomech* 1998;13:153–162, with permission.)

are little affected by levels of hamstrings force necessary to make significant differences to the ligaments. At *45°* flexion, small quadriceps forces load the PCL and larger quadriceps forces load the ACL. These levels of hamstrings force have only modest effects on the values of the tibiofemoral contact force (Fig. 10.26C).

Figure 10.26 shows how tibial translation increases with increasing resisting force, responding to increased quadriceps force, but it is significantly moderated by the intervention of antagonistic hamstring action. Hamstrings are relatively ineffective at extension because of their near-perpendicular orientation relative to the tibial plateau and only slight alteration in the value of ATT are produced. The flexed knee gives hamstrings better advantage and only *375 N* of hamstrings force can reverse the direction of tibial translation. At *60°* flexion, posterior tibial translation is produced by hamstrings forces of only 375 N and the ACL is fully protected even when quadriceps is pulling with a force of about *2,000 N (2.5 BW)*. At 45°, the same hamstring pull protects the ACL up to a resisting force of about *100 N*, a quadriceps force of about *1,000 N*. That is what deformable body mechanics predicts. Methods of teaching patients to exploit their muscle activity appropriately need to be developed.

This analysis suggests that the cost in terms of the increased levels of quadriceps force needed to compen-

sate for the antagonistic hamstring activity is small. Conversely, Berchuk et al. (79) suggest that ACL-deficient patients adapt their gait to minimize use of quadriceps. Beynnon et al. (80) measured ACL strain *in vivo* during leg-lift exercises and found that antagonistic hamstrings action protected the ACL at *30°* flexion and above but not at *15°* when the quadriceps were obviously active, confirming the predictions of the theory. Beard et al. (81) examined the gait and EMG of ACL-deficient subjects and found that they exhibited no decrease in quadriceps' EMG duration but they did show increased hamstrings' EMG duration into midstance and a significant increase in knee flexion at heel-strike and before toe-off. They concluded that the patients walked with a crouched gait and avoided extension to orient the hamstrings appropriately and thus compensate for ACL deficiency during quadriceps activity. Several *in vitro* studies have confirmed the protective action of hamstrings, except near extension (82–86). The current analysis suggests that the required levels of hamstrings force are small, of the same order as the ACL forces in the intact knee (Fig. 10.17).

The 2D model used for the analysis does not allow for tibial rotation. However, Des Jardins et al. (87) showed that axial rotation is much reduced in the presence of simultaneous quadriceps and hamstrings activity. The analysis does not consider cartilage deformation. This would not be expected to have much influence on the values of the quadriceps force (53) but may further reduce the predicted values of hamstring force needed to compensate for ACL deficiency.

INITIATION AND PROGRESSION OF ANTERIOR CRUCIATE LIGAMENT INJURY

Despite the large volume of published work devoted to the ACL, there is a surprisingly small amount of literature describing the mechanisms of injury and of partial tears. Noyes et al.(88) found that fully one third of patients could not describe the displacement or rotation of the knee at the time of injury. From those identified, there was no common joint position at which ACL disruption occurred. Partial tears are difficult to detect using laxity tests (89,90). Detailed arthroscopic assessment (91) or instrumented arthrometry (92) is required for their diagnosis. Aune et al. (93) applied high-speed anterior tibial translations to human knee specimens but they were interested in the anterior force level required to cause injury and the effect of quadriceps load rather than the mechanisms of initiation and progression of injury. There has been no theoretical analysis using mathematical models of the progression of the ACL from intact to fully ruptured.

Zavatsky and Wright (94) have recently used the 2D extensible ligament model to study the effects of increasing anterior tibial translation on strain within the ACL. They used a maximum critical strain criterion to identify the point of fiber rupture, based on the work of Butler et al. (4,25). They studied several possibilities: the critical strain was the same across the ACL with values of *10%*, *15%*, or *20%*; the critical strain was *20%* for the anterior half of the ligament and *15%* for the posterior half; the critical strain decreased linearly from *20%* for the most anterior fiber to *15%* for the most posterior. They calculated strains in five representative fibers (anterior, midanterior, central, midposterior, and posterior) over the flexion range from extension to *140°* for ATT between zero and *15 mm*.

Figure 10.27 shows that the ATT required for rupture of each of the five representative fibers according to each of the five criteria outlined above varies significantly with flexion angle. At low flexion angles ($< 20°$), the posterior fibers failed before the anterior. The tear started posteriorly and progressed anteriorly (Fig. 10.28A). At higher flexion angles, the tear started anteriorly and progressed posteriorly (Fig. 10.28B). Near extension, all fibers are nearly tight in the unloaded state; the posterior fibers are shorter and build up strain more rapidly than do the longer anterior fibers. Early failure of the posterior fibers is even more marked when they are assumed to have a lower critical strain to rupture (compare Fig. 10.27A with Fig. 10.27C). In the flexed knee, the posterior fibers are initially slack and require up to *5 mm* ATT before they begin to take up load. Thus, very large ATTs are required for full rupture so that partial tears are more likely in this flexion range.

The flexion angle at which the transition from posterior initiation to anterior initiation happened depended on the critical strain criterion adopted. For uniform critical strains between *10%* and *20%*, the transition flexion angle lay between *5°* and *15°* (Figs. 10.27A–C). For the other two criteria, it was about *20°* (Figs. 10.27D, E). Near the transition angles, all fibers failed at approximately the same ATT. At other flexion angles, fibers failed progressively over a much wider range of ATTs. The smallest and largest ATTs at fiber failure corresponded to the *10%* and *20%* uniform critical strain criteria, respectively (Figs. 10.27A, C). At flexion angles between *40°* and *120°*, more than *15 mm* ATT was required to create a full thickness rupture.

These values of failure ATT may seem high, but we estimate from the typical load–deformation graph in the article by Aune et al. (93) that a failure ATT of about *25 mm* was necessary in their experiments.

Locations of partial tears within the ACL have been reported but without correlation with flexion angle at the time of injury. Noyes et al. (88,95) found many more anterior tears, as did McDaniel (96) and Farquharson–Roberts and Osborne (97). In contrast, Sandberg and Balkfors (98) saw more tears that are partial posteriorly. The present model cannot explain the proximal–distal localization of tears along the ligament nor does it model bone evulsion.

The model suggests that a partial tear of the posterior half of the ACL would be difficult to detect clinically because above *30°* flexion, the applied anterior force supported by the intact and torn ligament are almost the same up to first-fiber rupture. Anterior tears should be easier to detect because the anterior component of force in the intact ligament is greater than that of the torn ligament.

A 3D model is required to investigate the effects of axial rotation under load. Markolf et al. (99) found that internal tibial torque combined with an anteriorly directed load applied to the tibia generated increased strain in the ACL at full extension and in hyperextension. We will now describe some experimental work on tibial rotation under load carried out as a preliminary to this stage of our model development.

TIBIAL ROTATION

The *6-df* flexed knee stance rig (100), Figure 6.6A,B, is an ideal system for studying the laxity of the joint under load, particularly when stabilized by the tension in the quadriceps tendon. Similar rigs have been used by Des Jardins et al. (87) to study effects of antagonistic quadriceps–hamstrings action, by Shoemaker et al. (101) to study quadriceps–ACL graft interactions, and by Ezzet et al. (102) to study extensor mechanics after total knee replacement.

Figure 10.29 shows that internal tibial rotation for 10 knee specimens in the flexed knee stance rig increases

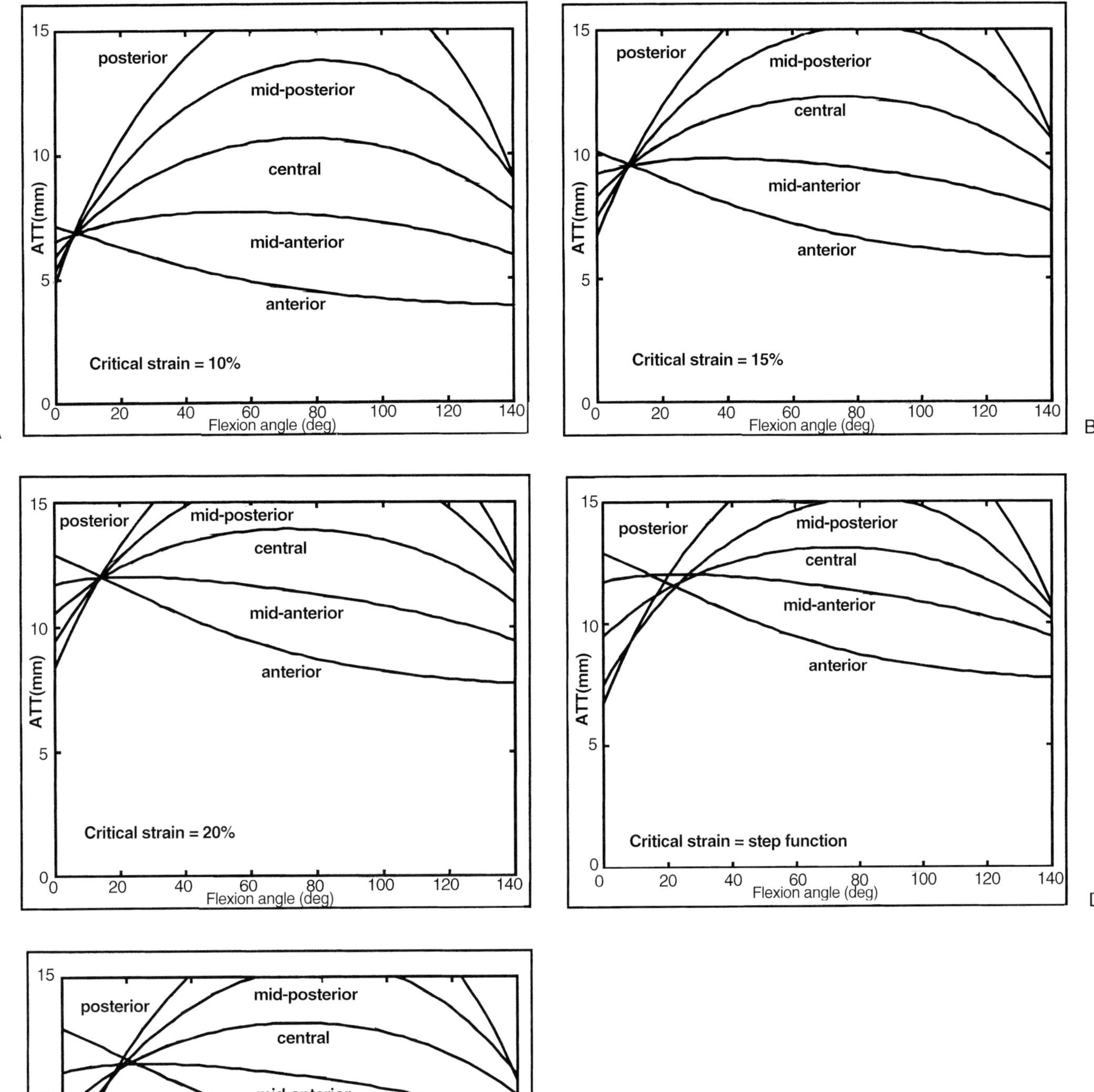

FIGURE 10.27. Anterior tibial translation (ATT) required at different flexion angles to initiate failure in different parts of the anterior cruciate ligament (ACL) according to five different failure criteria. Uniform critical strains of 10%, 15%, and 20% give the results of **A–C. D:** The critical strain was assumed to change discontinuously from 20% in the anterior fibers to 15% in the posterior fibers. **E:** The critical strain varied linearly from 20% for the most anterior fiber to 15% for the most posterior. (From Zavatsky AB, Wright HJ. Injury initiation and progression in the anterior cruciate ligament. *Clin Biomech* 2001;16:47–53, with permission.)

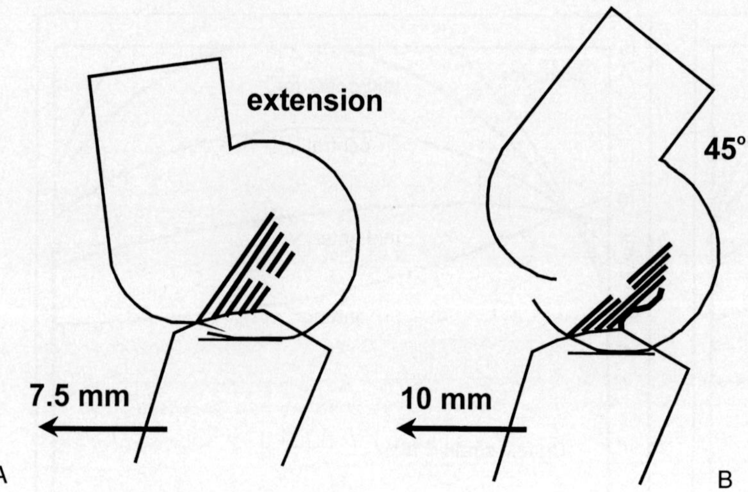

FIGURE 10.28. Models of initial posterior rupture **(A)** and initial anterior rupture **(B)**. (From Zavatsky AB, Wright HJ. Injury initiation and progression in the anterior cruciate ligament. *Clin Biomech* 2001; 16:47–53, with permission.)

steadily with flexion angle in the unloaded state but that it occurs over the first *40°* of flexion when the knee is subjected to vertical load on the hip–ankle axis and stabilized by quadriceps force. The graphs for the unloaded knee are the same as those in Figure 5.4 and therefore the same as those in Figure 5.3 for specimens tested in the fixed tibia rig. The concentration of rotation near extension in the presence of quadriceps force may be the reason why the phenomenon is called "terminal rotation" because the clinical test is probably carried out in the presence of at least passive forces in the extensor mechanism. It should be emphasized that in the flexed knee stance rig, quadriceps force grows rapidly with increasing flexion, rising from zero in full extension to about 12 times the applied vertical load at *120°* flexion (see Fig. 12.5 of the previous edition) so that the stabilizing effects of quadriceps force are more effective in the flexed specimen in this experiment. The quadriceps dependent results in Figure 10.29 are similar to those reported by Rovick et al. (103).

Blankevoort et al. (104) described the "envelopes of passive motion," the increase in external and internal rotation when the otherwise unloaded knee was taken over the range of flexion first with an applied externally rotating torque and then an internally rotating torque. Goodfellow and O'Connor (105) had obtained similar results in the first version of our flexed knee stance rig but they described the phenomenon as the range of tibial rotation. Bourne et al.(106) reported the range of tibial rotation measured in the same rig before and after knee replacement. Goodfellow and O'Connor (107) reported the range of tibial rotation measured clinically in patients after knee replacement. These are all measures of the torsional laxity of the joint, reflecting the deformation of the ligaments and articular surfaces in response to applied torque.

Figure 10.30, in the format used by Blankevoort et al. (104), shows that there is a family of paths of tibial rotation for various values of external and internal torque

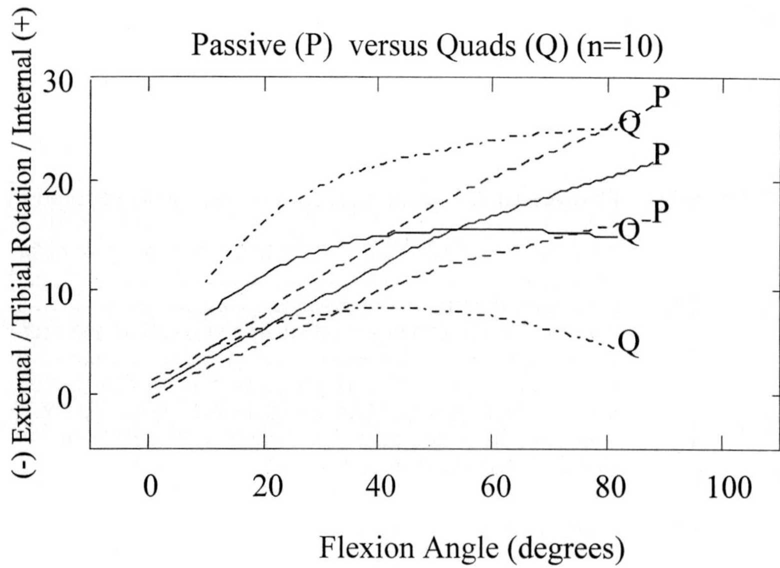

FIGURE 10.29. Internal tibial rotation plotted against flexion angle for unloaded specimens (*P*) and quadricep-loaded specimens (*Q*).

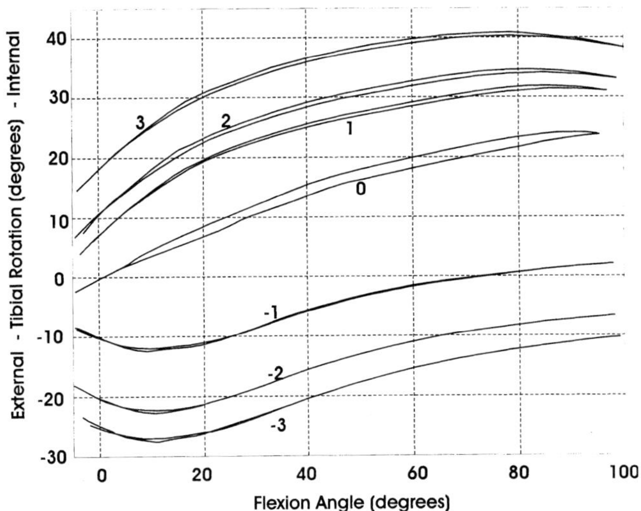

FIGURE 10.30. Tibial rotation plotted against flexion angle for a single specimen in the unloaded state (curve marked 0) and when internal (curves with positive numbers) and external (negative numbers) torques of 1, 2, and 3 Nm were applied to the tibia.

applied to the tibia. (This work soon will be submitted for publication.) Torques as small as ±0.5 Nm produce definite stable envelopes surrounding the path of unresisted motion exhibited by the unloaded joint. The envelopes for torques of ±0.5 Nm, ±1 Nm, and ±2 Nm all fit within the envelopes for ±3 Nm, the values of torque used by Blankevoort et al. (104).

This family of curves reflects increasing resistance to perturbation from the path of unresisted motion, resistance exerted by tension in the ligaments and compression of the articular surfaces and menisci. Figure 10.31

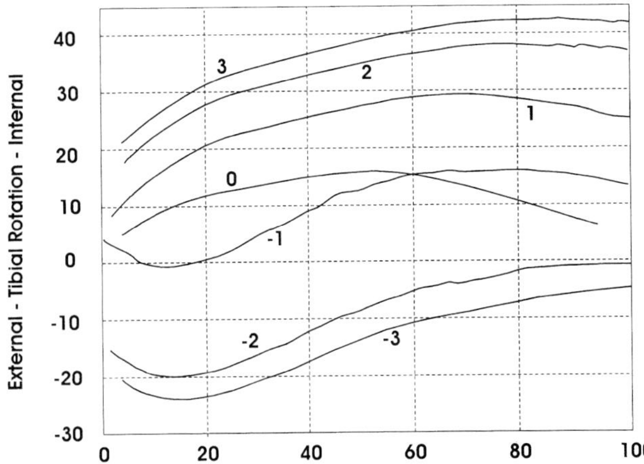

FIGURE 10.31. Tibial rotation under a vertical load of 40 N and associated quadriceps force with internal (curves marked with positive numbers) and external (negative numbers) tibial torques and zero tibial torque (curve marked zero).

shows that these paths are further modified by the presence of quadriceps force. Rovick et al. (103) showed similar effects of internal and external torques.

Figures 10.29 and 10.30 show how the unique path of unresisted motion displayed by the unloaded knee, as described in Figures 5.2–5.4, is profoundly altered by load and tissue deformation. Further alteration would be expected in the presence of medial or lateral hamstrings or gastrocnemius forces, as demonstrated by Des Jardin's work (87). Each such path will result in a pattern of contact point movement different from those shown in Figures 5.8 and 5.9. The path of unresisted passive motion is a more unequivocal characteristic of a knee than the wide variety of paths that can be elicited by a variety of loads.

CONCLUSION

The work described in this chapter and Chapter 5 leads us to conclude that the knee joint exhibits unresisted mobility because its articular surfaces can roll and slide on each other, without indentation, and its ligaments can rotate about their origins and insertions on the bones, without stretching. Unresisted mobility can be accomplished without tissue deformation. Conversely, the knee joint exhibits stability because its articular surfaces indent to develop the compressive contact forces and its ligaments stretch to develop the tensile forces—both necessary to resist displacement from the path of unresisted mobility. In activity, both these phenomena occur simultaneously, the surfaces indenting as well as sliding and rolling, the ligaments stretching as well as rotating. The dynamic laxity of the joint is different from the passive laxity because of the large muscle forces and large balancing contact forces. Muscle forces in activity determine the pattern of ligament loading but they can be tuned to protect ligaments when they are injured or reconstructed.

This chapter and Chapter 5 illustrate the insights that can be gained when mathematic modeling work is used to interpret the results of experimental work and to amplify the deductions that can be drawn from experiments. Mathematic models can be used to evaluate quantities that are difficult—if not impossible—to measure. The models are validated by comparison with the values of quantities that can be measured. The validation of our 3D models in this way has been found to be imperfect and needs further work; but, in surveying the literature, we have found significant differences in the results of published experimental work. Many of the predictions of the 2D model agree well with experiment, but choice of model parameters is critical. The sequential approach, study of mobility followed by study of stability, was shown to be advantageous. However, further effort is needed before we reach a full understanding of the mechanisms that control the mobility and the stability of the knee and of other joints.

ACKNOWLEDGMENTS

This chapter was based on the insights provided by Mr. John Goodfellow, the surgeon, over many years of happy collaboration. It has benefited from discussions with more recent clinical colleagues, Prof. David Murray and Mr. Andrew Price. It summarizes some of the work of a succession of research students: Prof. Ed Biden, Dr. David FitzPatrick, Mr. Russell Miller, Prof. Jim Collins, Prof. David Wilson, Dr. Jennifer Feikes, Dr. David Beard, Dr. Danielle Toutoungi, Prof. Tung-Wu Lu, Dr. Ahmed Imran, Dr. Richard Huss, Dr. Alberto Leardini, Dr. Melissa Carson, Dr. Wen Ling Chen, Mr. Paul Oppold, and Mr. Chris Riegger, as well as coauthors Dr. Amy Zavatsky and Dr. Richie Gill. All these contributions are gratefully acknowledged.

Our work has been supported with grants from the Arthritis Research Campaign, Wellcome Trust, Leverhulme Trust, EU Commissioners, Biomet, and De Puy. The research students have been supported with scholarships and fellowships from the Rhodes Foundation, Felix Trust, Thouron Award Scheme (University of Pennsylvania), Royal College of Surgeons, Wishbone Trust (British Orthopaedic Association), Engineering and Physical Sciences Research Council, and Government of the Republic of China (Taiwan).

REFERENCES

1. Blankevoort L, Huiskes R, de Lange A. Recruitment of knee joint ligaments. *J Biomech Eng* 1991;113:94–103.
2. Zavatsky AB, O'Connor JJ. A model of human knee ligaments in the sagittal plane, II: fibre recruitment under load. *Proc Inst Mech Eng [H]* 1992;206:135–145.
3. Mommersteeg TJ, Huiskes R, Blankevoort L, et al. A global verification study of a quasi-static knee model with multi-bundle ligaments. *J Biomech* 1996;29:1659–1664.
4. Butler DL, Kay MD, Stouffer DC. Comparison of material properties in fascicle-bone units from human patellar tendon and knee ligaments. *J Biomech* 1986;19:425–432.
5. Race A, Amis AA. The mechanical properties of the two bundles of the human posterior cruciate ligament. *J Biomech* 1994;27:13–24.
6. Feikes JD. *The mobility and stability of the human knee joint* [D. Phil thesis]. University of Oxford; 1999.
7. Feikes JD, Zavatsky AB, O'Connor JJ. A three-dimensional model of knee stability. In: Prendergast PJ, Lee TC, Carr AJ, eds. *Proceeding of 12th Conference of the European Society of Biomechanics.* Dublin: Royal Academy of Medicine in Ireland; 2000:359.
8. Toutoungi DE, Zavatsky AB, O'Connor JJ. Parameter sensitivity of a mathematical model of the anterior cruciate ligament. *J Engng Med Proc Inst Mech Eng [H]* 1997;211:235–246.
9. Zavatsky AB, O'Connor JJ. A model of human knee ligaments in the sagittal plane, I: response to passive flexion. *J Engng Med Proc Inst Mech Eng [H]* 1992;206:125–134.
10. Zavatsky AB, O'Connor JJ. Ligament forces at the knee during isometric quadriceps contractions. *J Engng Med Proc Inst Mech Eng [H]* 1993;207:7–18.
11. Zavatsky AB, Beard DJ, O'Connor JJ. Cruciate ligament loading during isometric muscle contractions. A theoretical basis for rehabilitation. *Am J Sports Med* 1994;22:418–423.
12. Zavatsky AB, O'Connor JJ. Three-dimensional geometric models of human knee ligaments. *J Engng Med Proc Mech Eng [H]* 1994;208:229–240.
13. Zavatsky AB, O'Connor JJ. Anteroposterior tibial translation during simulated isometric quadriceps contractions. *Knee* 1995;2:85–91.
14. Lu TW, O'Connor JJ. Fibre recruitment and shape changes of knee ligaments during motion: as revealed by a computer graphics-based model. *J Engng Med Proc Inst Mech Eng [H]* 1996;210:71–79.
15. Huss RA, Holstein H, O'Connor JJ. The effect of cartilage deformation on the laxity of the knee joint. *J Engng Med Proc Inst Mech Eng [H]* 1999;213:19–32.
16. Huss RA, Holstein H, O'Connor JJ. A mathematical model of forces in the knee under isometric quadriceps contractions. *Clin Biomech* 2000;15:112–122.
17. Imran A, O'Connor JJ. Control of knee stability after ACL injury or repair: interaction between hamstrings contraction and tibial translation. *Clin Biomech* 1998;13:153–162.
18. Toutoungi DE, Lu TW, Leardini A, et al. Cruciate ligament forces in the human knee during rehabilitation exercises. *Clin Biomech* 2000;15:176–187.
19. Leardini A, O'Connor JJ, Catani F, et al. A geometric model of the human ankle joint. *J Biomech* 1999;32:585–591.
20. Stagni R, Leardini A, Cappozzo A, et al. Effects of hip joint centre mislocation on gait analysis results. *J Biomech* 2000;33:1479–1487.
21. Corazza F, O'Connor JJ, Leardini A, et al. Ligament fibre recruitment and forces for the anterior drawer test at the human ankle joint. *J Biomech* 2002 (in press).
22. Wilson DR, Feikes JD, O'Connor JJ. Ligaments and articular contact guide passive knee flexion. *J Biomech* 1998;31:1127–1136.
23. Feikes JD, O'Connor JJ, Zavatsky AB. A constraint-based approach to modelling the mobility of the human knee joint. *J Biomech* 2002 (in press).
24. Piziali RL, Rastegar JC, Nagel DA. Measurement of the non-linear coupled stiffness characteristics of the human knee. *J Biomech* 1977;10:45–51.
25. Butler DL, Guan Y, Kay MD, et al. Location-dependent variations in the material properties of the anterior cruciate ligament. *J Biomech* 1992;25:511–518.
26. Mommersteeg TJ, Blankevoort L, Huiskes R, et al. The effect of variable relative insertion orientation of human knee bone-ligament-bone complexes on the tensile stiffness. *J Biomech* 1995;28:745–752.
27. Blankevoort L, Huiskes R. Ligament-bone interaction in a three-dimensional model of the knee. *J Biomech Eng* 1991;113:263–269.
28. Andriacchi TP, Mikosz RP, Hampton SJ, et al. Model studies of the stiffness characteristics of the human knee joint. *J Biomech* 1983;16:23–29.
29. Butler DL, Noyes FR, Grood ES. Ligamentous restraints to anterior-posterior drawer in the human knee. *J Bone Joint Surg Am* 1980;62:259–270.
30. Vahey JW, Draganich LF. Tensions in the anterior and posterior cruciate ligaments of the knee during passive loading: predicting ligament loads from in situ measurements. *J Orthop Res* 1991;9:529–538.
31. FitzPatrick DP, O'Connor JJ. Theoretical modelling of the knee applied to the anterior drawer test. *Proceedings of IMechE Conference on the changing role of engineering in orthopaedics,* 1989, paper C384/033, pp 79–83 (Mechanical Engineering Publications, London).
32. Fujie H, Livesay GA, Woo SL, et al. The use of a universal force-moment sensor to determine in-situ forces in ligaments: a new methodology. *J Biomech Eng* 1995;117:1–7.
33. Lewis JL, Lew WD, Schmidt J. A note of the application and evaluation of the buckle transducer for knee ligament force measurement. *Trans ASME - J Biomech Eng* 1982;111:125–128.
34. Markolf KL, Gorek JF, Kabc JM, et al. Direct measurement of resultant forces in the anterior cruciate ligament—an in vivo study with a new experimental technique. *J Bone Joint Surg Am* 1990;72:557–567.
35. Chan SC, Seedhom BB. Equivalent geometry of the knee and the prediction of tensions along the cruciates: an experimental study. *J Biomech* 1999;32:35–48.
36. Sakane M, Fox RJ, Woo SL, et al. In situ forces in the anterior cruciate ligament and its bundles in response to anterior tibial loads. *J Orthop Res* 1997;15:285–293.
37. Pandy MG, Shelburne KB. Theoretical analysis of ligament and extensor-mechanism function in the ACL-deficient knee. *Clin Biomech* 1998;13:98–111.
38. Imran A, O'Connor JJ. Theoretical estimates of cruciate ligament forces: effects of tibial surface geometry and ligament orientations. *J Engng Med Proc Inst Mech Eng [H]* 1997;211:425–439.
39. Grood ES, Noyes FR. Diagnosis of knee ligament injuries: biomechanical precepts. In: Feagin JA Jr, ed. *The crucial ligaments: diagnosis and treatment of ligamentous injuries about the knee.* New York: Churchill Livingstone; 1988:245–285.

40. Lu T-W. *Geometric and mechanical modeling of the human locomotor system* [D. Phil thesis]. Oxford University; 1997.

41. Lu T-W, O'Connor JJ, Taylor SJG, et al. Comparison of telemetered femoral forces with model calculations. In: *Proceedings of the european society of biomechanics.* Toulouse: J Biomech, 1998:47.

42. Blankevoort L, Kuiper JH, Huiskes R, et al. Articular contact in a three-dimensional model of the knee. *J Biomech* 1991;24:1019–1031.

43. Stiehl JB, Komistek RD, Cloutier JM, et al. The cruciate ligaments in total knee arthroplasty: a kinematic analysis of 2 total knee arthroplasties. *J Arthroplasty* 2000;15:545–550.

44. Murray DW, Goodfellow JW, O'Connor JJ. The Oxford medial unicompartmental arthroplasty: a ten-year survival study. *J Bone Joint Surg Br* 1998;80:983–989.

45. White SH, O'Connor JJ, Goodfellow JW. Sagittal plane laxity following knee arthroplasty. *J Bone Joint Surg Br* 1991;73:268–270.

46. White SH, Ludkowski PF, Goodfellow JW. Anteromedial osteoarthritis of the knee. *J Bone Joint Surg Br* 1991;73:582–586.

47. da Vinci L. *Leonardo on the human body.* O'Malley CD, Saunders JBdCM, ed. New York: Dover Publications, 1983;192.

48. Borelli GA. *De motu animalium.* Rome, 1680.

49. Bergmann G, Graichen F, Rohlmann A, et al. Hip joint forces during load carrying. *Clin Orthop* 1997:190–201.

50. Maquet P. Advancement of the tibial tuberosity. *Clin Orthop* 1969;115:225–230.

51. Maquet PGJ. *Biomechanics of the knee.* Berlin: Springer-Verlag, 1984.

52. Bishop RED, Denham RA. A note on the ratio between tensions in the quadriceps tendon and the infra-patellar ligament. *Eng Med* 1977;6:53–54.

53. Imran A, Huss RA, Holstein H, et al. The variation in the orientations and moment arms of the knee extensor and flexor muscle tendons with increasing muscle force: a mathematical analysis. *Proc Inst Mech Eng [H]* 2000;214:277–286.

54. O'Connor JJ. Can muscle co-contraction protect knee ligaments after injury or repair? *J Bone Joint Surg Br* 1993;75:41–48.

55. Jurist KA, Otis JC. Anteroposterior tibiofemoral displacement during isometric extension exercises. *Am J Sports Med* 1985;13:254–258.

56. Mandt PR, Daniel DM, Biden E, et al. Tibial translation with quadriceps force: an in vitro study of the effect of load placement, flexion angle and ACL sectioning. *Trans Orthop Res Soc* 1987;33:243.

57. Howell SM. Anterior tibial translation during a maximum quadriceps contraction: is it clinically significant? *Am J Sports Med* 1990;18:573–578.

58. Hirokawa S, Solomonow M, Lu Y, et al. Anterior-posterior and rotational displacement of the tibia elicited by quadriceps contraction. *Am J Sports Med* 1992;20:299–306.

59. Kizuki S, Shirakura K, Kimura M, et al. Dynamic analysis of anterior tibial translation during isokinetic quadriceps femoris muscle concentric contraction exercise. *Knee* 1996;2:151–155.

60. MacConaill MA. The ergonomic aspects of articulated mechanics. In: Evans FG, ed. *Studies of the anatomy and function of bones and joints.* New York: Springer, 1967:69–80.

61. Seireg A, Arvikar RJ. A mathematical model for evaluation of forces in lower extremities of the musculoskeletal system. *J Biomech* 1973;6:313–326.

62. Pedotti A, Krishnan VV, Stark L. Optimization of muscle force sequencing in human locomotion. *Math Biosci* 1978;38:57–76.

63. Crowninshield RD, Brand RA. A physiologically based criterion of muscle force prediction in locomotion. *J Biomech* 1981;14:793–801.

64. Patriarco AG, Mann RW, Simon SR, et al. An evaluation of the approaches of optimization models in the prediction of muscle forces during human gait. *J Biomech* 1981;14:513–525.

65. Collins JJ. The redundant nature of locomotor optimization laws. *J Biomech* 1995;28:251–267.

66. Mikosz RP, Andriacchi TP, Andersson GB. Model analysis of factors influencing the prediction of muscle forces at the knee. *J Orthop Res* 1988;6:205–214.

67. Smidt GL. Biomechanical analysis of knee flexion and extension. *J Biomech* 1973;6:79–82.

68. Yasuda K, Sasaki T. Exercise after anterior cruciate ligament reconstruction: the force exerted on the tibia by separate isometric contractions of the quadriceps and hamstrings. *Clin Orthop* 1987;220:275–283.

69. Kaufman K, An KN, Litchey W, et al. Dynamic joint forces during knee isokinetic exercise. *Am J Sports Med* 1991;19:305–316.

70. Nisell R, Ericson M, Nemeth G, et al. Tibio-femoral joint forces during isometric knee extension. *Am J Sports Med* 1989;17:49–54.

71. Nisell R, Nemeth G, Ohlsen H. Joint forces in extension of the knee: analysis of a mechanical model. *Acta Orthop Scand* 1986;57:41–46.

72. Dahlkvist N, Mayo P, Seedhom B. Forces during squatting and rising from a deep squat. *Eng Med* 1982;11:69–76.

73. Morrison JB. The mechanics of the knee joint in relation to normal walking. *J Biomech* 1970;3:51–61.

74. Harrington IJ. A bioengineering analysis of force actions at the knee in normal and pathological gait. *Biomed Eng* 1976:167–172.

75. Andriacchi TP, Galante JO, Fermier RW. The influence of total knee-replacement design on walking and stair-climbing. *J Bone Joint Surg Am* 1982;64:1328–1335.

76. Collins JJ, O'Connor JJ. Muscle-ligament interactions at the knee during walking. *Proc Inst Mech Eng [H]* 1991;205:11–18.

77. Wilson DR, Zavatsky AB, O'Connor JJ. Cruciate ligament forces at the knee in gait: parameter sensitivity and effects of ligament elasticity. In: *International Society of Biomechanics XIVth Congress.* Paris, 1993:1466–1467.

78. Noyes FR, Butler DL, Grood ES, et al. Biomechanical analysis of human ligament grafts used in knee-ligament repairs and reconstructions. *J Bone Joint Surg Am* 1984;66:344–352.

79. Berchuck M, Andriacchi TP, Bach BR, et al. Gait adaptations by patients who have a deficient anterior cruciate ligament. *J Bone Joint Surg Am* 1990;72:871–877.

80. Beynnon BD, Fleming BC, Johnson RJ, et al. Anterior cruciate ligament strain behavior during rehabilitation exercises in vivo. *Am J Sports Med* 1995;23:24–34.

81. Beard DJ, Soundarapandian RS, O'Connor JJ, et al. Gait and electromyographic analysis of anterior cruciate ligament deficient subjects. *J Gait Post* 1996;4:83–88.

82. Durselen L, Claes L, Kiefer H. The influence of muscle forces and external loads on cruciate ligament strain. *Am J Sports Med* 1995;23:129–136.

83. More RC, Karras BT, Neiman R, et al. Hamstrings—an anterior cruciate ligament protagonist: an in vitro study. *Am J Sports Med* 1993;21:231–237.

84. Hirokawa S, Solomonow M, Luo Z, et al. Muscular co-contraction and control of knee stability. *J Elect Kinesiol* 1991;1:199–208.

85. Draganich LF, Vahey JW. An in vitro study of anterior cruciate ligament strain induced by quadriceps and hamstrings forces. *J Orthop Res* 1990;8:57–63.

86. Renstrom P, Arms SW, Stanwyck TS, et al. Strain within the anterior cruciate ligament during hamstring and quadriceps activity. *Am J Sports Med* 1986;14:83–87.

87. Des Jardins JD, MacWilliams BA, Wilson DR, et al. The in vitro assessment of knee joint kinematics under physiologic loading. In: *Trans Orthop Res Soc.* San Francisco; 1997:260.

88. Noyes FR, Bassett RW, Grood ES, et al. Arthroscopy in acute traumatic hemarthrosis of the knee. Incidence of anterior cruciate tears and other injuries. *J Bone Joint Surg Am* 1980;62:687–695, 757.

89. Hole RL, Lintner DM, Kamaric E, et al. Increased tibial translation after partial sectioning of the anterior cruciate ligament: the posterolateral bundle. *Am J Sports Med* 1996;24:556–560.

90. Lintner DM, Kamaric E, Moseley JB, et al. Partial tears of the anterior cruciate ligament: Are they clinically detectable? *Am J Sports Med* 1995;23:111–118.

91. Duri ZAA, Aichroth PM. Partial anterior cruciate ligament ears: evaluation and a clinical review. *Knee* 1995;2:131–138.

92. Rijke AM, Perrin DH, Goitz HT, et al. Instrumented arthrometry for diagnosing partial versus complete anterior cruciate ligament tears. *Am J Sports Med* 1994;22:294–298.

93. Aune AK, Cawley PW, Ekeland A. Quadriceps muscle contraction protects the anterior cruciate ligament during anterior tibial translation. *Am J Sports Med* 1997;25:187–190.

94. Zavatsky AB, Wright HJ. Injury initiation and progression in the anterior cruciate ligament. *Clin Biomech* 2001;16:47–53.

95. Noyes FR, Mooar LA, Moorman CT III, et al. Partial tears of the anterior cruciate ligament. Progression to complete ligament deficiency. *J Bone Joint Surg Br* 1989;71:825–833.

96. McDaniel WJ. Isolated partial tear of the anterior cruciate ligament. *Clin Orthop* 1976:209–212.

97. Farquharson–Roberts MA, Osborne AH. Partial rupture of the anterior cruciate ligament of the knee. *J Bone Joint Surg Br* 1983;65:32–34.

98. Sandberg R, Balkfors B. Partial rupture of the anterior cruciate ligament: natural course. *Clin Orthop* 1987:176–178.

99. Markolf KL, Burchfield DM, Shapiro MM, et al. Combined knee loading states that generate high anterior cruciate ligament forces. *J Orthop Res* 1995;13:930–935.

100. Zavatsky AB. A kinematic-freedom analysis of a flexed-knee-stance testing rig. *J Biomech* 1997;30:277–280.

101. Shoemaker SC, Adams D, Daniel DM, et al. Quadriceps/anterior cruciate graft interaction. An in vitro study of joint kinematics and anterior cruciate ligament graft tension. *Clin Orthop* 1993:379–390.

102. Ezzet KA, Hershey AL, D'Lima DD, et al. Patellar tracking in total knee arthroplasty: inset versus onset design. *J Arthroplasty* 2001;16:838–843.

103. Rovick JS, Reuben JD, Schrager RJ, et al. Relation between knee motion and ligament length patterns. *Clin Biomech* 1991;6:213–220.

104. Blankevoort L, Huiskes R, de Lange A. The envelope of passive knee joint motion. *J Biomech* 1988;21:705–720.

105. Goodfellow J, O'Connor J. The mechanics of the knee and prosthesis design. *J Bone Joint Surg Br* 1978;60:358–369.

106. Bourne RB, Goodfellow JW, O'Connor JJ. A functional analysis of various knee arthroplasties. In: *Trans Orthop Res Soc.* Anaheim 1978:160.

107. Goodfellow JW, O'Connor JJ. Clinical results of the Oxford knee: surface arthroplasty of the tibiofemoral joint with a meniscal bearing prosthesis. *Clin Orthop* 1986:21–42.

CHAPTER 11

Ligament Injury and Repair

Monti Khatod, Wayne H. Akeson, and David Amiel

LIGAMENT INJURY

Clinical

Ligamentous injuries of the knee joint are among the most common ligament injuries encountered by orthopedists (1). The anterior cruciate ligament (ACL) and medial collateral ligament (MCL) are major ligaments contributing to the stability and normal functioning of the knee joint (2–5). Injuries of various degrees occur to these ligaments during exercise, sports, and nonspecific trauma (6,7). Injuries to these ligaments can be clinically classified, as described by Rockwood et al. (8), into three degrees. A first-degree sprain involves a tear of a minimum number of fibers (microtears) or less than one third of the ligament. There is minimal hemorrhage and swelling, localized tenderness, and no clinical instability or laxity. Second-degree sprains involve a tear of more ligamentous fibers (one third to two thirds of the ligament) with a greater loss of function, localized tenderness, and an effusion, but there is no laxity or noticeable instability. Third-degree injuries have greater disruption (greater than two thirds of the ligament), more tenderness, and demonstrable laxity of the knee joint. Laxity of the knee joint can be evaluated clinically on a 0 to 3+ scale or a grade 1 to 3 scale. Gradation is dependent on the distance of translation of the joint reflecting injury severity in the ligament.

It is well known that the ACL mounts a poor to negligible repair response to injury (9–13), whereas the MCL heals readily without even the need for surgical repair in most cases (11–14). The most frequently cited exception is in the case of the so-called terrible triad injury (12) where reconstruction of the ACL is required to prevent lax healing of the MCL (15,16). Reconstruction with autograft tissue, either medial hamstring or patellar tendon (bone–tendon–bone) grafts, has become the treatment of choice for disabling instability due to ACL deficiency. Allograft replacement and prosthetic replacement have been universally abandoned (17,18).

Multiple structural factors influence knee ligament injury and repair: (a) location of the injury within the ligament determines the type of reparative cell, osteoblast versus fibroblast; (b) the size of the injury in the collateral ligament potentially affects the mechanical strength of the repair scar; (c) the blood supply to each ligament affects its nutrition (Urban [19] has also postulated that variation of oxygen tension in ligaments during healing may be an important modulator of successful repair); and (d) the location of the ligament, intrasynovial versus extrasynovial, may play a role in its ability to mount a repair process.

Morphology Issues in Knee Ligament Repair

To understand the healing response of the ligament to injury, one must examine the structural factors involved in the injured ligament. Location of the injury within the ligament is one such factor. Sherman and Bonamo (20) found that proximal stump tears (those injuries involving the proximal 20% of the ligament) accounted for more than 80% of ACL tears. Midsubstance or "mop end" tears accounted for another 10% of all tears, and avulsion injuries accounted for less than 5% of ACL injuries. Lyon et al. (21) found that the only exception to poor ACL healing is seen in avulsion injuries of the ligament from its attachment to bone. The repair response in the avulsion injuries is mounted by the bone cells, not by the cells of the ACL. The cells of the ACL do not mount an effective repair response. The ACL will occasionally drop down after injury and become affixed to the PCL (22), but in this altered location it is not functionally adequate in the athletically inclined patient. The location of injury within the ligament substance of the MCL does not seem to alter its ability to undergo functional repair, but, as mentioned earlier, if the injury occurs in combination with ACL tears, the MCL will tend to heal with laxity unless the ACL is first reconstructed (15).

The size of the injury was also found to be of importance in the eventual mechanical strength of healing in the collateral ligament. Loitz–Ramage et al. (23) created an 8-mm gap injury compared with a 4-mm Z-plasty injury in the MCL of a rabbit knee. Mechanical testing at 40, 78, and 104 weeks showed the scar material properties in both injury models remained markedly inferior to normal, and gap injuries showed significantly inferior structural properties at all intervals. These results suggest that a large initial gap between ligament ends in the extraarticular space predispose scars to long-term structural weakness. Still, clinical studies have generally found no benefit of suture versus closed management of the MCL (see Chapter 21A).

To allow us to understand structural issues of intrinsic healing mechanisms in knee ligament healing, a surgical model was developed to explore the role of surgical repair methods in repair of the ACL (24). Initial attempts to repair a complete laceration of the ACL were carried out on rabbits with complete midsubstance lacerations, using a technique described by Marshall et al. (25) (Fig.

11.1A). Six weeks after surgery, none of the repaired ligaments showed evidence of healing. All specimens were in the process of resorption, and a large gap spanned by suture was uniformly evident. A second group was operated on in a similar manner, except the sutures were placed before lacerating the ACL in an attempt to decrease the interstump gap. The same resorptive process and lack of healing response were observed in all animals 6 weeks after surgery.

To limit stump retraction and ensure accurate approximation of the lacerated portions of the ACL, a Z-plasty repair was attempted (Fig. 11.1B). Six weeks later, no evidence of healing was observed. Failure of this technique was again related to the retraction of lacerated ACL stumps, followed by resorption of the exposed ligament ends.

Partial transection of the ACL has been attempted previously in animal models. O'Donoghue et al. (27) described poor results, and Arnoczsky et al. (28) noted a vascular proliferation in the area of the injury but detected no evidence of bridging in a gap injury.

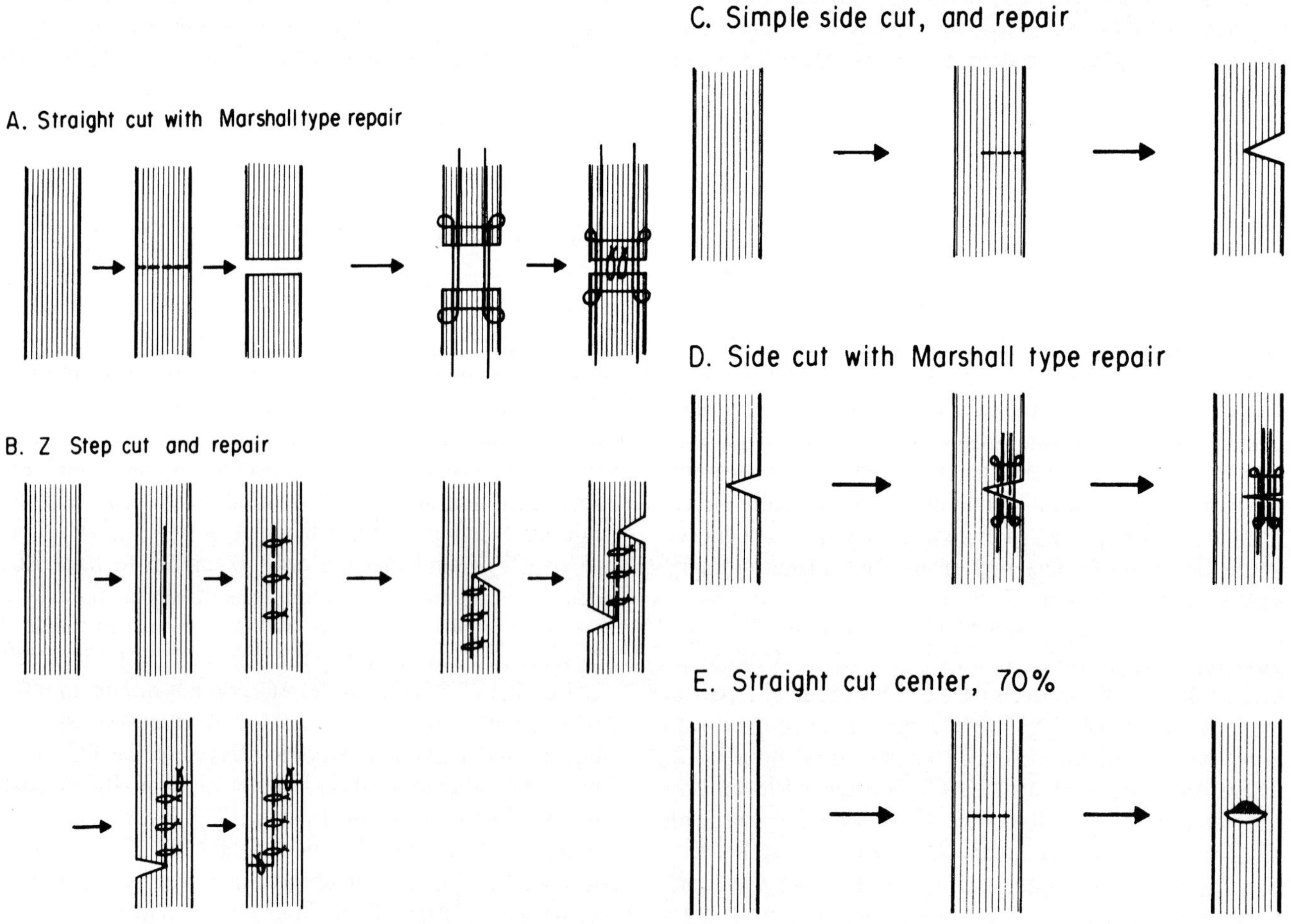

FIGURE 11.1. Surgical models for evaluation of anterior cruciate ligament healing. **A, B:** Complete laceration models. **C–E:** Partial laceration models. (From Amiel D, Kleiner JB. Biochemistry of tendon and ligament. In: Nimni M, Olsen B, eds. *Collagen: biotechnology.* Vol. 3. Cleveland, OH: CRC Press, 1988, with permission.)

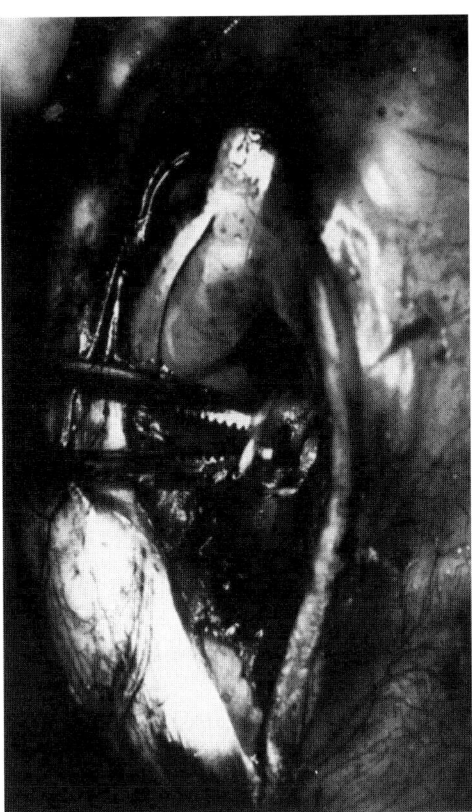

FIGURE 11.2. Midsubstance partial laceration in rabbit anterior cruciate ligament.

Arnoczsky et al. concluded that the inability to heal might be related to the fact that the "anteromedial band" of the ACL, a portion of the ACL that is taut throughout the normal range of motion, had been lacerated

To obviate this problem, our laboratory (Fig. 11.1C) transected the posterolateral portion of the ACL. An immediate retraction of the incised portion of the ligament was noted. In all animals, no evidence of gap reduction was shown. A modified Marshall procedure was then attempted to hold the edges of the partially transected ACL together (Fig. 11.1D). Six weeks after this operation, none of the animals revealed evidence of ACL wound healing. It became obvious that a stent of uncut tissue on one side of the laceration was insufficient to control retraction of the cut ends of the ligament. To circumvent this problem, a model was developed where only the midportion of the ligament was transected (Fig. 11.1E). This model minimally disturbs the biomechanical stability of the ligament by retaining lateral and medial ligament continuity. Thus, the lacerated ends stay in close proximity to each other during the postlaceration recovery period (Fig. 11.2).

The surface area of the ligament exposed to joint fluid is also limited in this model to the site of the perforation into the ligament by a 2-mm-wide, razor-thin, square-edged Beaver blade. Access to the area of injury by potentially harmful enzymes contained in the synovial fluid is thereby restricted. The model largely, although not totally, eliminates two mechanisms proposed to be responsible for failure of ACL healing: (a) destabilizing biomechanical forces at the injury site and (b) enzymatic degradation of ligament substance along with inhibition of fibroblast activity by synovial fluid. Using the surgical ACL laceration model described herein, we have observed a partial healing response in a small percentage (5%) of ACLs tested in a reproducible fashion (Fig. 11.3).

Another morphologic reason postulated for the difference in healing responses between the ACL and the MCL

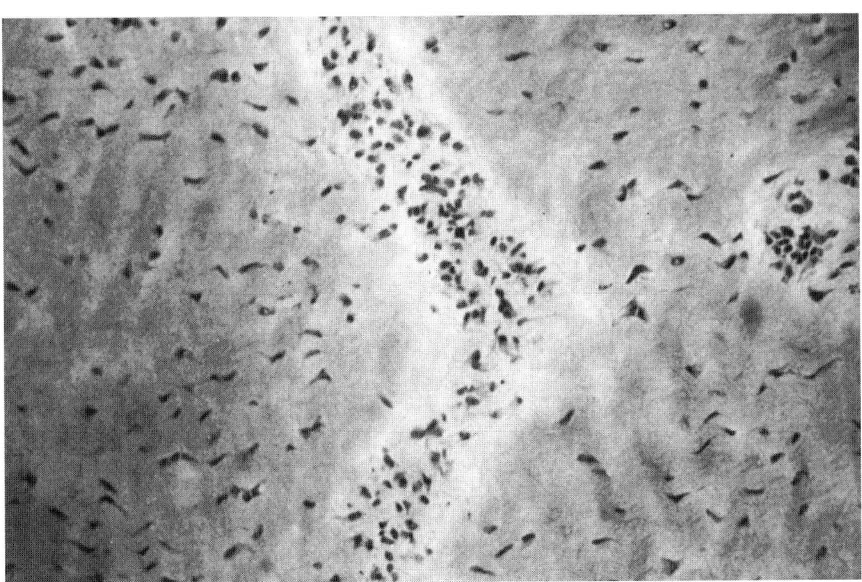

FIGURE 11.3. Laceration site, 12 weeks after surgery (hematoxylin and eosin, ×50). (From Amiel D, Kleiner JB. Biochemistry of tendon and ligament. In: Nimni M, Olsen B, eds. *Collagen: biotechnology.* Vol. 3. Cleveland, OH: CRC Press, 1988, with permission.)

is their differences in blood supply. The MCL has a rich blood supply, which it derives from the inferior medial geniculate artery and from its osseous attachments (29). The blood supply to the ACL is described as poor (28–30). A paraligamentous network of vessels courses through the synovial membrane. These vessels enter the ligament transversely and anastamose freely with endoligamentous vessels. The core of the midportion of the cruciate ligament is less well vascularized than the proximal and distal cores.

Of the many morphologic factors important in ligament healing—mechanical forces, blood supply, and local environment—it is the local environment that has often been used as an explanation for the poor healing capacity of the cruciate ligaments (27). The cruciate ligaments reside in a unique environment. Both ligaments are intracapsular, and both are enveloped by a synovial membrane, effectively making them extrasynovial. The synovial membrane is only a few cells thick and separates the cruciates from the synovial fluid that bathes the other intracapsular knee joint structures. During ACL injury, the synovial membrane is usually torn, exposing the frayed ligament ends to the synovial fluid and to a host of potentially destructive enzymes released by the breakdown of hemarthrosis fluid in the injured joint. This local environment has been referred to as the "hostile" environment of the synovial joint space.

Synovial fluid, formed from an ultrafiltrate of blood (31), has been shown to adversely affect ligament fibroblasts and to stimulate them (32–34). Andrish and Holmes (32) demonstrated that ACL fibroblast proliferation was diminished *in vitro* when exposed to synovial fluid. Synovial fluid has also been shown to be a physiologically important nutrient delivery pathway for the ACL (35). Nickerson et al. (33,34) found that bovine synovial fluid stimulates proliferation of rabbit ACL and MCL cells. Maximum stimulation occurred at 20% concentration with diminishing stimulation at higher concentrations; however, even high concentrations were not inhibitory.

Our laboratory studied the role of synovial fluid in providing nutrition to rabbit knee ligaments and menisci, *in vivo*, by intraarticular injection of titrated proline (a collagen precursor) (35). Measurements of [³H]-hyp incorporation showed that all knee structures tested utilized synovial fluid–derived proline. The cruciate ligaments demonstrated the highest uptake of [3H]-hyp (Fig. 11.4). Control ligaments and menisci showed no detectable isotopes. These findings indicate that intraarticular structures can derive nutrition from a synovial fluid source.

Rapid degeneration of the ACL occurs after acute rupture. Warren (36) described this phenomenon clinically wherein ruptured ACL ligament substance could completely disappear six weeks after injury. These findings were confirmed by Kohn (37), who noted either complete disappearance or only a remnant of the ACL in patients who underwent arthroscopy.

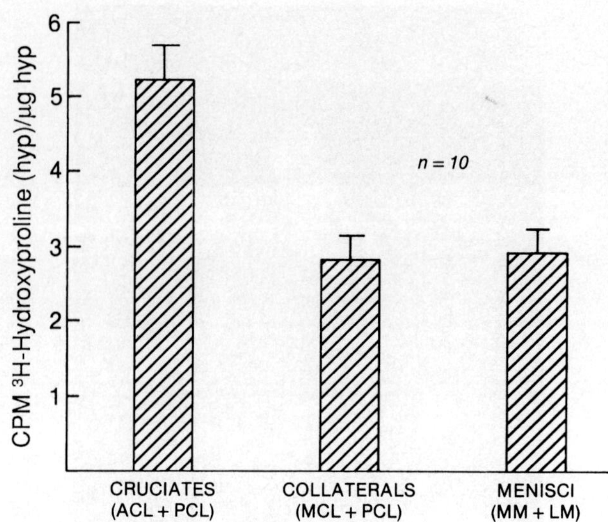

FIGURE 11.4. Nutrient uptake of the various periarticular connective tissue structures. (From Amiel D, Abel MF, Kleiner JB, et al. Synovial fluid nutrient delivery in the diarthrial joint: an analysis of rabbit knee ligaments. *J Orthop Res* 1986;4:90–95, with permission.)

To test the hypothesis that ligament resorption after ACL injury represents a cellular response of intrinsic ligamentous cells to degrade their extracellular matrix, a rabbit model of ACL injury was created by our laboratory with the development of an *in vitro* assay for collagenase activity (38). A collagenase assay was used because collagen represents the major structural protein of the cruciate ligament. The left ACL was transected off its tibial insertion, whereas the right knee served as a sham-operated control. The ACL and menisci were harvested 10 days after surgery, placed in tissue culture, and assayed for collagenase 3 days later. Results demonstrated a relatively large increase (82%) in injured ACL collagenase content compared with control ACLs (Fig. 11.5). This was consistent with the average net loss of 34% in total collagen mass from the injured ACLs.

In addition, the transected ACLs were swollen and retracted (Fig. 11.6). The free transected ligament ends displayed a relative hypocellularity and loss of collagen matrix organization, histologically confirming the observation that, once ruptured, the free ends of the ACL undergo rapid degeneration (28,36,37) (Fig. 11.7). The transected ACL tissue itself may be responsible for this degenerative process. Cells within the ACL may respond to injury by degrading their collagenous matrix.

Collagenase release has been documented from other articular structures such as synovium (39,40) and articular cartilage (41,42). These structures synthesize and release a latent form of collagenase. The data from our experiment indicate that the ACL and menisci secrete only active enzymes, which may be detrimental to intraarticular structures (43). The ACL may be a privileged intraarticular structure, because it possesses a syn-

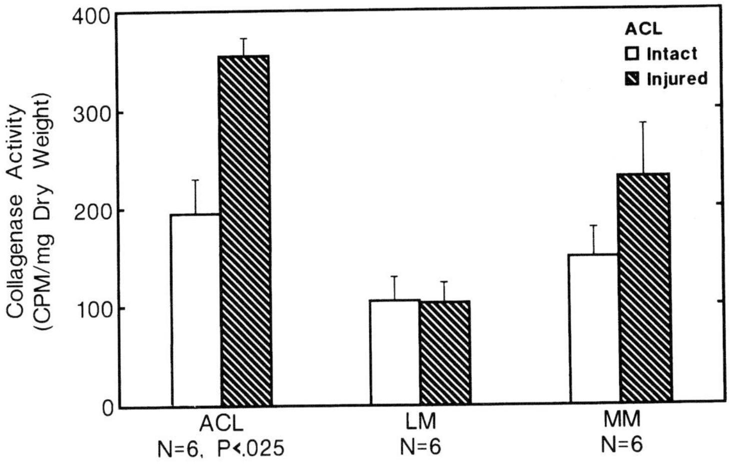

FIGURE 11.5. Collagenase activity. Note significant increase in collagenase activity in injured anterior cruciate ligaments. No differences were noted in menisci. (From Amiel D, Ishizue KK, Harwood FL, et al. Injury of the ACL: the role of collagenase in ligament degeneration. *J Orthop Res* 1989;7:486–493, with permission.)

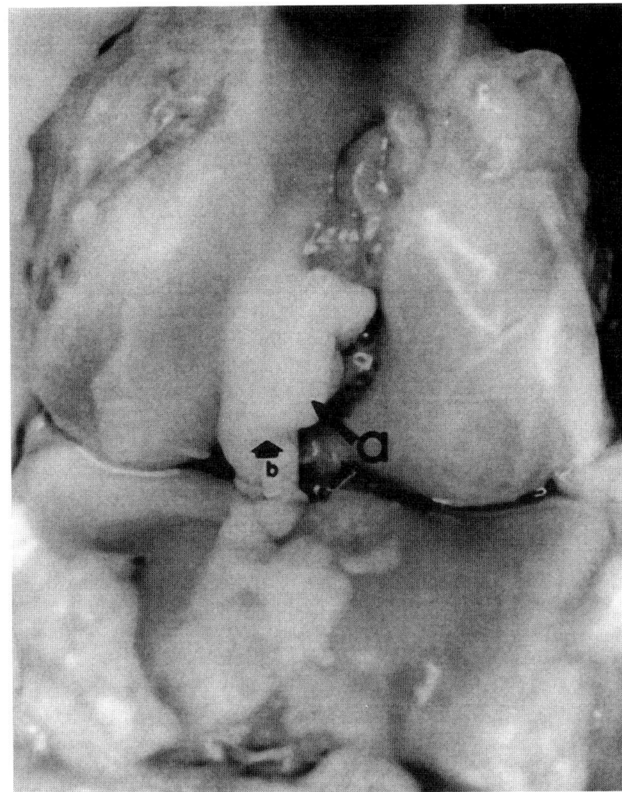

FIGURE 11.6. Gross morphology showing transected anterior cruciate ligament. Note swollen (*a*) and retracted (*b*) appearance. (From Amiel D, Ishizue KK, Harwood FL, et al. Injury of the ACL: the role of collagenase in ligament degeneration. *J Orthop Res* 1989;7:486–493, with permission.)

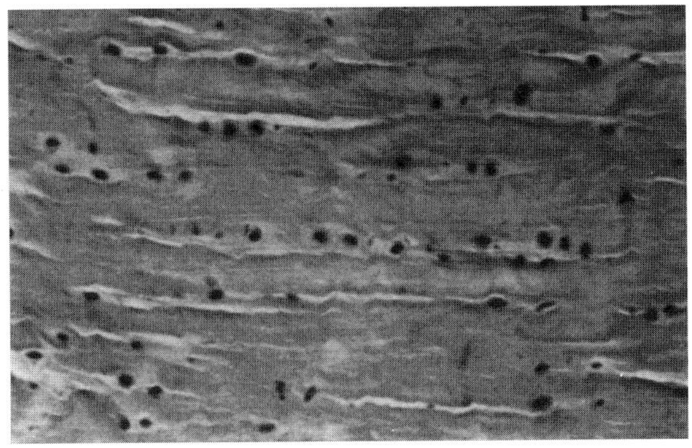
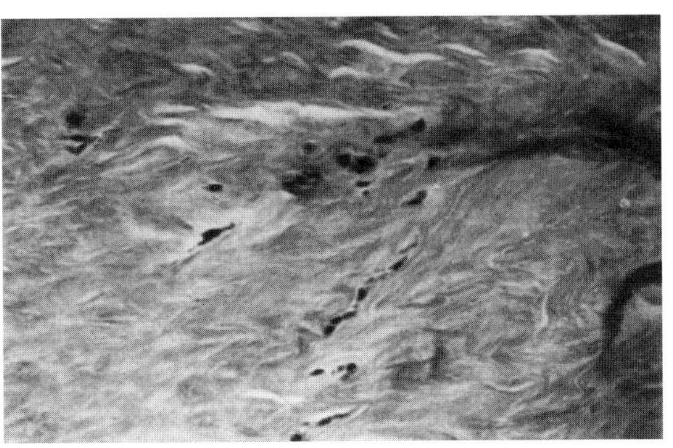

FIGURE 11.7. Microscopic evaluation (final magnification, ×30). **A:** Anterior cruciate ligament (ACL) in region of bony attachment (normal cellular organization). **B:** ACL near transected end of ligament. Note loss of cellularity and loss of organization. (From Amiel D, Ishizue KK, Harwood FL, et al. Injury of the ACL: the role of collagenase in ligament degeneration. *J Orthop Res* 1989;7:486–493, with permission.)

ovial covering that allows it to be protected from the intraarticular environment. With acute rupture of the ACL and resultant synovial injury, this protective barrier may be lost. Subsequent exposure of ligament substance to the intraarticular environment may produce changes in the ligament and may explain, in part, the poor results reported with attempts to primarily repair the ACL.

Cellular–Biologic ACL-MCL Differences

Cellular and biologic processes need to be discussed to understand the responses to ligament injury. The cellular differences in the ACL versus the MCL include differences in phenotype, cellular alignment, proliferation, migration, adhesion to substrates, responses to mechanical forces, and signaling. Nagineni et al. (44) studied knee ligament histology and found that MCL cells exhib-

ited a typical fibroblastic morphology. The cells were elongated and spindle-shaped. ACL cells, however, were slightly larger and more ovoid in shape. Lyon et al. (21), in our laboratory, reported that ACL cells had a more fibrocartilage characteristic.

Cellular cytoplasmic processes were found to be different. The MCL fibroblast has long cytoplasmic processes extending outward into the surrounding matrix. In striking contrast, the ACL cells are devoid of any long cytoplasmic processes, and the cell membrane and the adjacent collagen fibrils are separated by an amorphous matrix (21). When these cells were stained for fibronectin, both cell types showed intense staining in the area of the cell membrane. The major difference was that the fibronectin stain followed the MCL processes far out into the matrix. Because the ACL cells lack the long processes, they did not have the same staining pattern

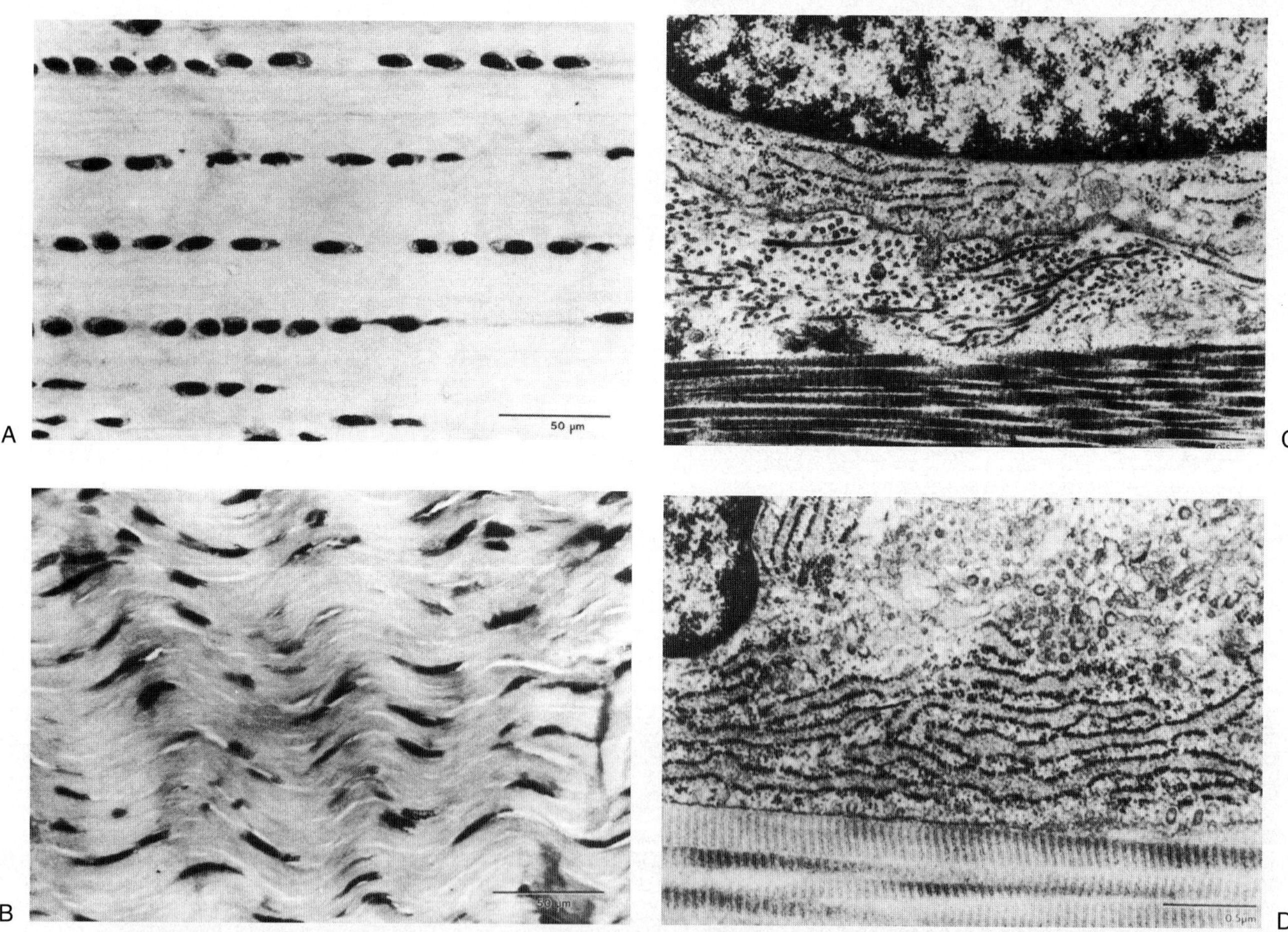

FIGURE 11.8. A: Longitudinal section from the deep midportion of the rabbit anterior cruciate ligament (ACL). The cells are strung out like pearls on a string and lack long cellular processes [hematoxylin and eosin (H&E), ×100]. **B:** Photomicrograph of longitudinal section from the deep midportion of a rabbit medial collateral ligament (MCL). The cells are spindle-shaped with long cytoplasmic processes extending distances many times the length of the cell body (H&E, ×100). **C:** High-power transmission electron microscopy (TEM) of rabbit ACL reveals an amorphous matrix separating the cell membrane and the adjacent collagen fibrils. The mature collagen fibrils are not closely approximated by the cell membrane. **D:** High-power TEM of rabbit MCL shows a fibroblast whose cell membrane is in close proximity to the mature collagen fibrils adjacent to it. (From O'Donoghue DH, Frank GR, Jeter GL, et al. Repair and reconstruction of the anterior cruciate ligament in dogs: factors influencing long-term results. *J Bone Joint Surg Am* 1971;53:710–718, with permission.)

(21) (Fig. 11.8). Burridge and Chrzanowska–Wodnicka (45) found more bundles of microfilaments (representing stress fibers) in the ACL than in the MCL. The results supported the conclusion that the ACL cells are able to form more stable adhesion plaques than the MCL cells.

Lyon et al. (21) further revealed cellular alignment differences. The deep portion of the central one third of the MCL had compact collagen fiber bundles oriented along the longitudinal axis of the ligament. Spindle-shaped MCL fibroblasts were interspersed throughout the collagen fiber bundles. Transillumination of the MCL using polarized light demonstrated a high-amplitude, low-frequency crimp pattern of the collagen fibers, which parallels that of adjacent fiber bundles. MCL fibroblasts were oriented at angles corresponding to the angle of collagen fiber crimp (Fig. 11.9A). The deep portion of the central third of the ACL also had compact, parallel collagen fiber bundles ori-

ented along the long axis of the ligament. However, the fiber bundles were separated by narrow spaces containing ovoid cells arranged in columns like pearls on a string. The crimp pattern for the ACL collagen fiber bundles demonstrated a low-amplitude, high-frequency pattern (Fig. 11.9B). Furthermore, the cells within the narrow spaces did not conform to the crimp pattern of the adjacent fibers. In a recent study, the anteromedial bundle of human ACLs distinguished three different zones along the length of the ligament. These zones were characterized by fusiform, ovoid, and spheroid cell shapes. Fusiform and ovoid cells occupied the proximal quarter of the anteromedial bundle of the ACL and were found to express the α–smooth muscle actin isoform. In the spheroid zone, which constitutes the distal three fourths of the ACL, only a portion of cells expressed the α–smooth muscle actin isoform (46). These cellular alignment differences may represent a spectrum

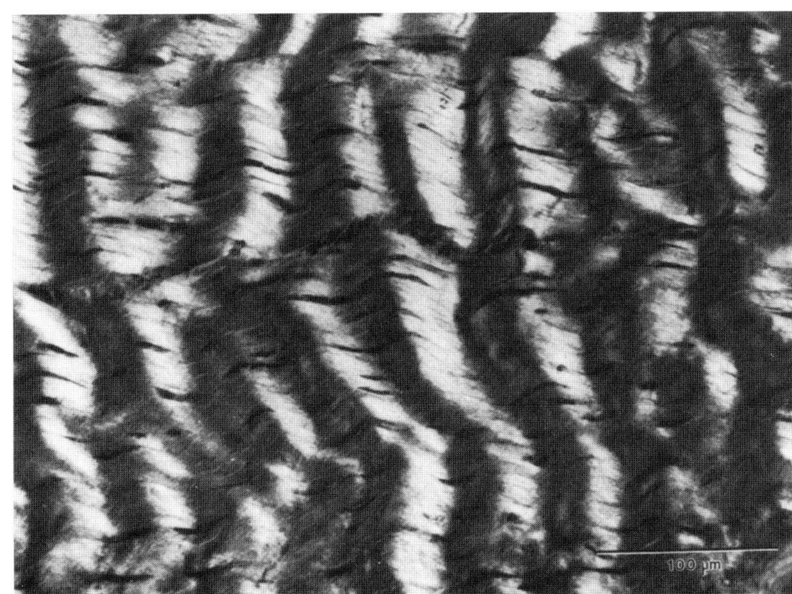

A

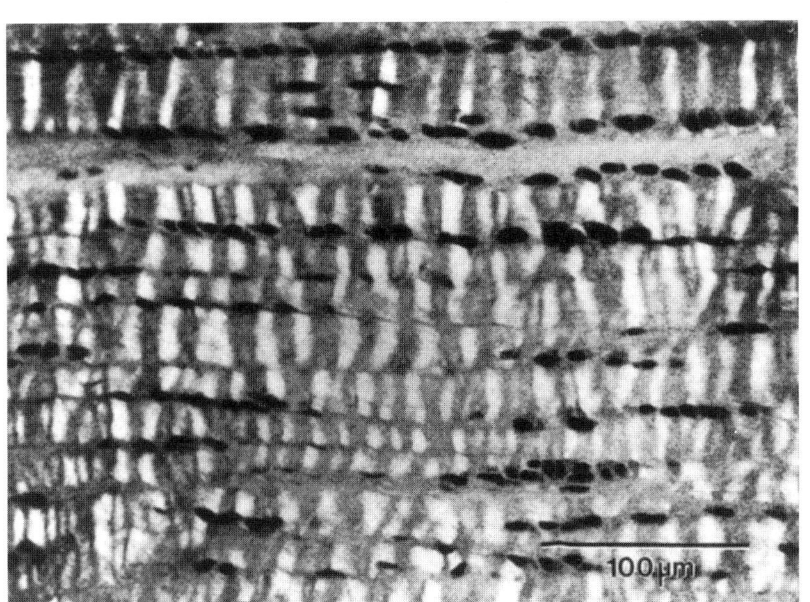

B

FIGURE 11.9. **A:** Polarized light photomicrograph of the midportion of the medial collateral ligament showing the sharp waveforms roughly parallel to each other across the section. The cell bodies and processes closely follow the waveform configuration (hematoxylin and eosin [H&E], ×50). (From Sherman MF, Bonamo JR. Primary repair of the anterior cruciate ligament. *Clin Sports Med* 1988;7:739–750, with permission.) **B:** Polarized light appearance of the rabbit anterior cruciate ligament shows lack of register of waveforms of adjacent bundles. Cells are not tightly adherent to matrix. They do not deform in register with the waveforms of the matrix (H&E, ×50).

among ligamentous cells with the classic fibroblast–fibrocyte at one end and the chondroblast–chrondrocyte at the other end (46). But, in general, the MCL histologically appears to favor the fibroblast–fibrocyte phenotype, whereas the ACL cell tends to favor a fibrocartilage phenotype (21).

Proliferative differences between ACL and MCL cells have been well demonstrated. The outgrowth of cells from ACL explants was slower than that from MCL explants and slower in closing *in vitro* confluent culture streak wounds (44). Growth curves of ACL and MCL cultures at both passage numbers two and six showed a significantly slower rate of proliferation of ACL cells than MCL cells (Fig. 11.10) (47–49). DNA synthesis measured in terms of tritiated thymidine incorporation of both log phase and confluent cultures, supports the conclusion that differential proliferation rates of these cells exist in culture (44). Furthermore, an *in vitro* wound created in a confluent layer of ACL and MCL cells, revealed that 48 hours after injury, the cell-free zones created in ACL cultures were occupied partially by single cells in a nonconfluent fashion. In contrast, the wounded zone in the MCL cultures was almost completely covered by cells (44) (Fig. 11.11). These results demonstrate a lower proliferation and migration potential of ACL cells in comparison with MCL cells in response to injury.

Another factor important in the migration of ligament fibroblasts is the expression of fibronectin (50). The ACL and PCL each contain twice the amount of fibronectin found in either MCL or patellar tendon. The cellular–biologic characteristics of phenotype, cellular alignment and crimp pattern, proliferation, and migration reveal differences in the intrinsic properties of the normal ACL versus MCL cells. These different intrinsic properties between the cells of these ligaments have been proposed as important factors in their differential repair mechanisms.

LIGAMENT REPAIR

General Healing Process

Andriacchi et al. (51) and Arnoczsky (52) described four phases of healing in the injured ligament. According to their description, phase I occurs within the first 72 hours after injury, and encompasses the acute inflammatory response. This phase has two distinct components important for understanding potential therapeutic control approaches to stimulate or to reduce scar proliferation. Hematoma formation is the first element with its associated platelet aggregation and degranulation. The platelet release of growth factors stimulates the second element, the trafficking of white cells into the area of injury (see Chapter 12). Phase II lasts over the next 6 weeks and is associated with a marked proliferation of both cellular and extracellular components. This phase involves the inward migrating monocyte transformation into macrophages, which in turn stimulate fibroplasia. Remodeling in the Andriacchi–Arnoczsky conceptual framework involves two phases. Phase III occurs from 6 weeks to several months and involves the initial remodeling of the early scar. Finally, in phase IV, the final remod-

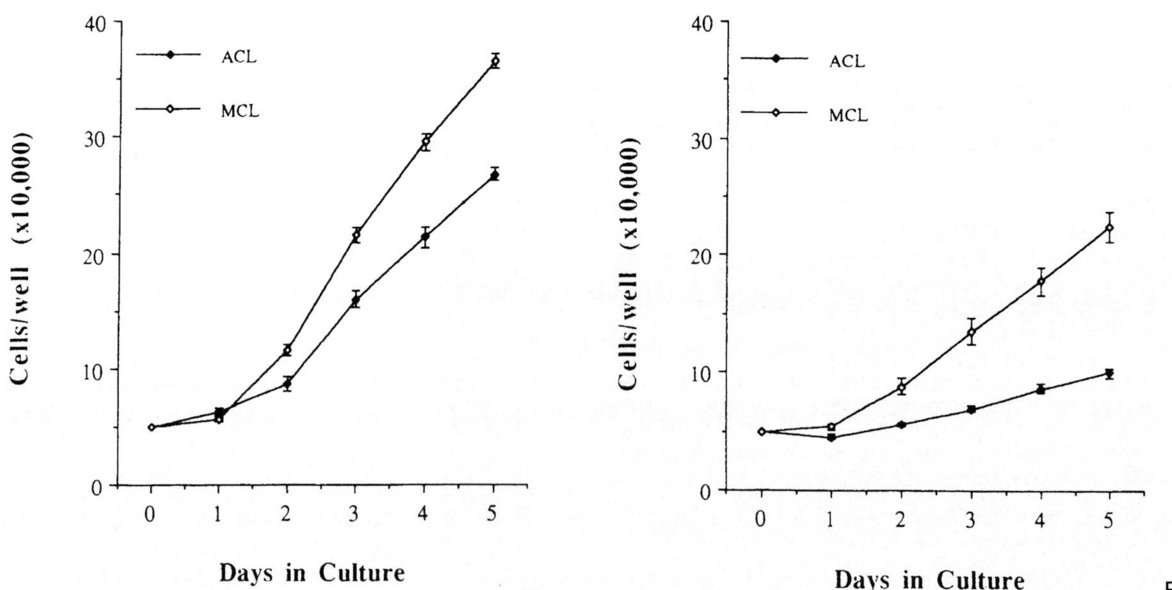

FIGURE 11.10. Growth curves of anterior cruciate ligament (ACL) and medial collateral ligament (MCL) at passages two (**A**) and six (**B**). Results are means ± SEM of duplicate samples of six batches of cultures derived from ACL and MCL tissues of six rabbits. (From Nagineni CN, Amiel D, Green MH, et al. Characterization of the intrinsic properties of the anterior cruciate and medial collateral ligament cells: an *in vitro* cell culture study. *J Orthop Res* 1992;10:465–475, with permission.)

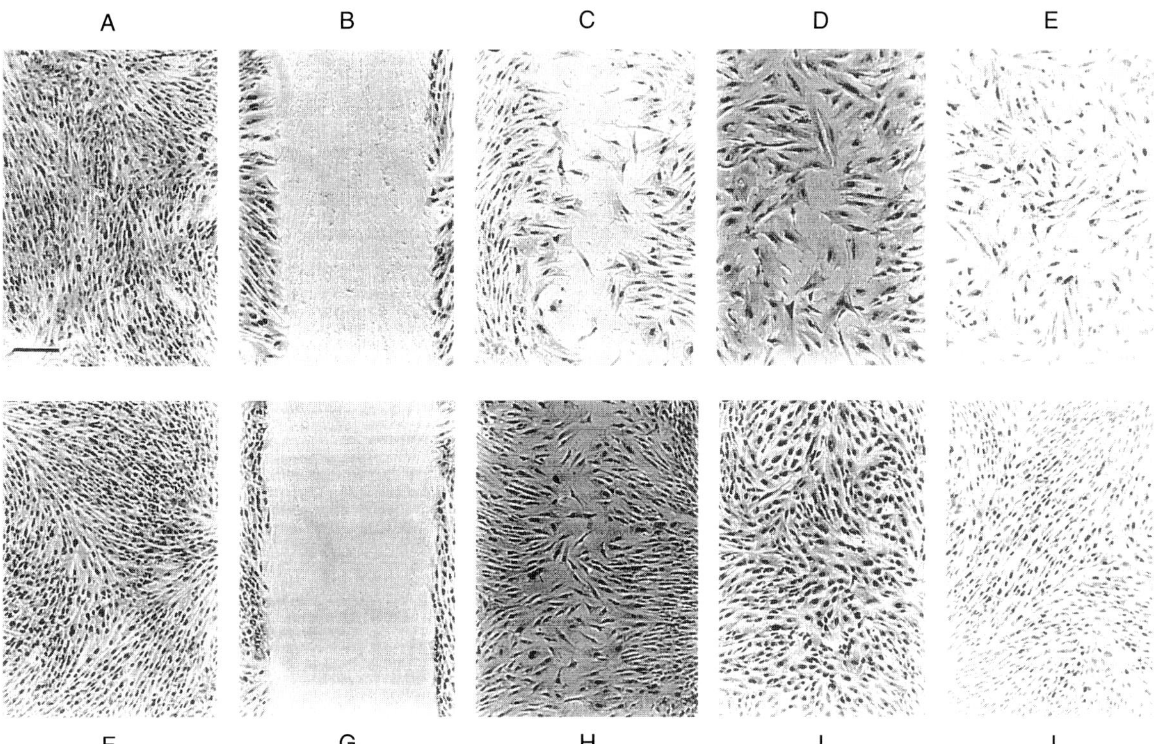

FIGURE 11.11. Representative pictures of anterior cruciate ligament (ACL) and medial collateral ligament (MCL) cultures subjected to *in vitro* wounding and allowed subsequent healing. **A–E:** ACL cultures. **F–J:** MCL cultures. **A, F:** Control cultures. **B, G:** Immediately after wounding. **C, H:** Twenty-four hours after wounding. **D, I:** Forty-eight hours after wounding. **E, J:** Seventy-two hours after wounding. Bar in **(A)** represents 200 μm. All pictures are at the same magnification. (From Nagineni CN, Amiel D, Green MH, et al. Characterization of the intrinsic properties of the anterior cruciate and medial collateral ligament cells: an *in vitro* cell culture study. *J Orthop Res* 1992;10:465–475, with permission.)

eling of the area of injury occurs with maturation of the repair tissue, which can continue for years. Neurath et al. (53) reviewed these phases in human ACL injuries and found that in phase I, erythrocytes, lymphocytes, and mononuclear macrophages were common. In the extracellular matrix, fibrinous exudate and cell debris was observed predominantly near the ruptured area. At the end of this phase, Day 3, a marked proliferation of fibroblasts occurred with a markedly enhanced expression of type III procollagen in the pericellular area. Phase II revealed proliferation of fibroblasts in the stumps of the ruptured ACL. This proliferation was even more pronounced than in phase I. However, the cellular ultrastructure of these cells was increasingly distorted. More fibroblasts became necrotic with increasing time from injury. Surprisingly, there were only a few myofibroblasts in the ligament stumps during this phase. Phase III revealed increasing variance from patient to patient. Overall, there was a slight reduction in the number of altered fibroblasts compared with phase II, but these differences were not significant. The repair tissue in the stumps of the ACL never approached normal ligament characteristics and no adequate tissue remodeling occurred.

The MCL is found to have a distinctly different repair process. Frank et al. (14) reviewed the healing of the MCL in rabbits. Grossly, all ligaments in this experiment "healed" by bridging their gap injury with "scar tissue." Scar tissue is defined as *the new connective tissue that replaces tissue that has been injured* (54). The MCL defect was filled by vascular inflammatory tissue by 10 days as seen by histology. In the "scar zone" itself, the preponderance of inflammatory cells then subsided and active fibroblasts then dominated most fields by 3 weeks. Between 3 and 6 weeks, there was a decrease in fibroblast numbers and size, and some evidence of longitudinal (along the long axis of the ligament) alignment of their nuclei. At 14 weeks, continued remodeling had occurred, with improving realignment and a further decrease in cell numbers. Between 14 and 40 weeks, few changes were noted. Cells remained larger and more numerous than those seen in normal MCLs (Fig. 11.12).

Schreck et al. (55,56) performed a comparison of ACL and MCL ligament healing in the rabbit model. The histology of the wounded MCL revealed a rapidly proliferative, increasingly cellular repair site with time. This was consistent with observations by other investigators (20,54). On the first day after injury, the wound gap

FIGURE 11.12. Representative sections of scar tissue taken from midsubstance areas of healing medial collateral ligaments at different intervals. Progressive changes in cell numbers, size (metabolic activity), distribution, and orientation are noted as stages of inflammation, proliferation, and remodeling take place (hematoxylin and eosin, ×30). (From Frank C, Woo SL-Y, Amiel D, et al. Medial collateral ligament healing: a multidisciplinary assessment in rabbits. *Am J Sports Med* 1983;11:379–389, with permission.)

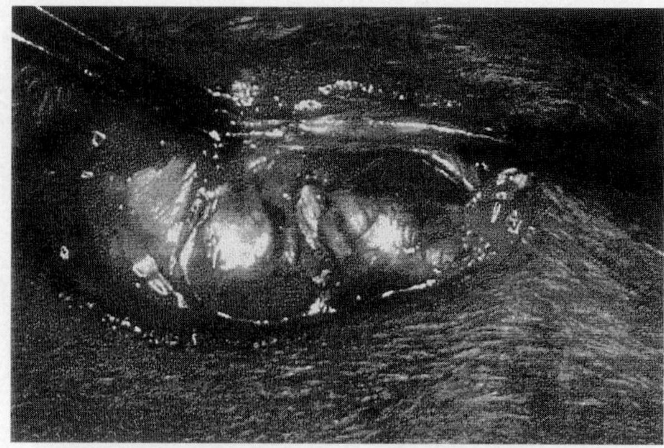

Ruptured Ligament

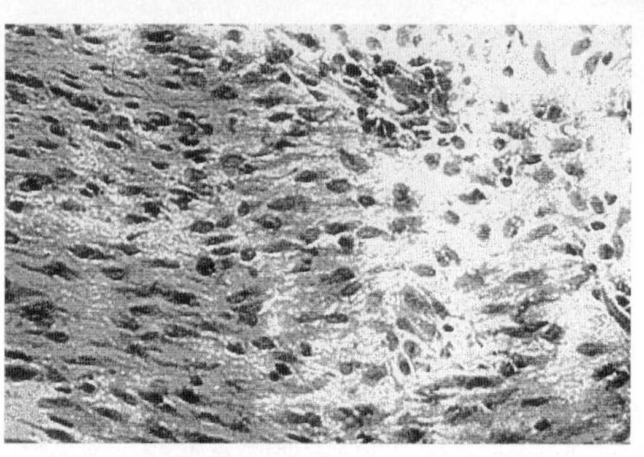

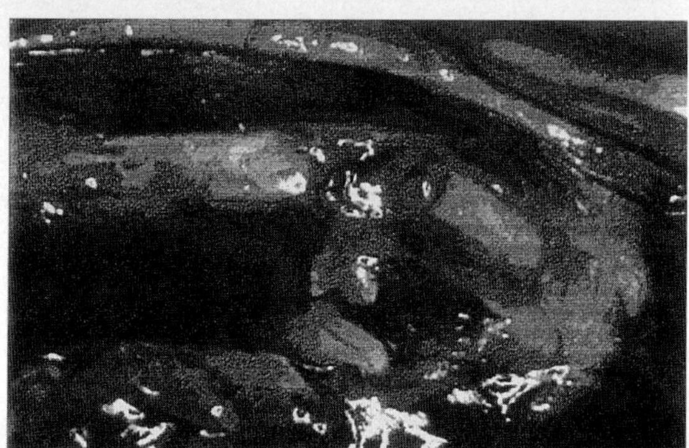

3 weeks

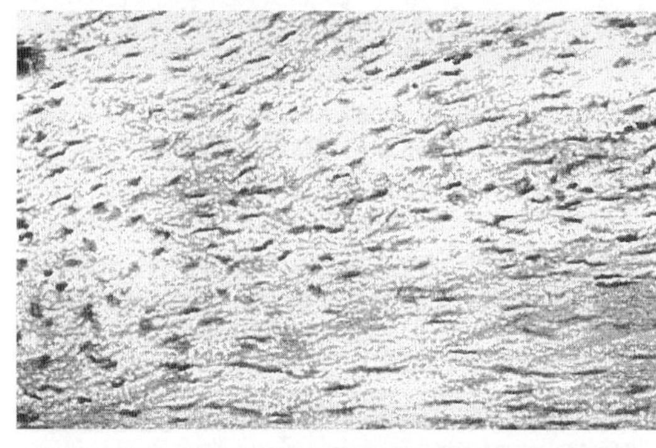

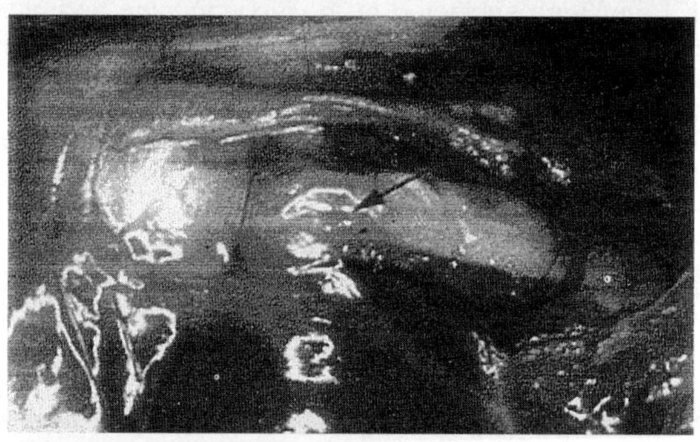

14 weeks

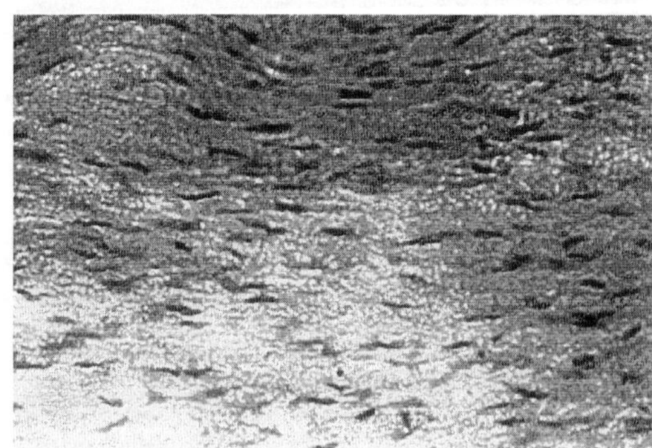

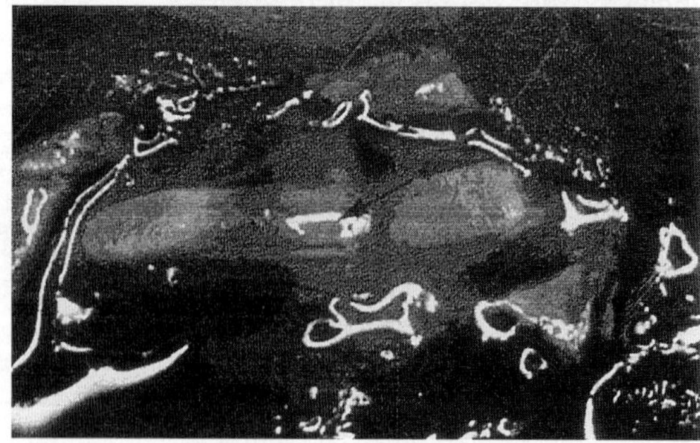

40 weeks

appeared to be relatively acellular, but a larger number of inflammatory cells appeared in the wound as early as 3 days after injury. By 7 days, all of the specimens demonstrated a disorganized, hypercellular repair site with an increased number of inflammatory cells and fibroblasts with plump nuclei. Ingrowth of capillaries was prominent at the margins of the wound. This neovascularity tapered off gradually with increasing distance from the wound. In the specimens collected on Day 10, the transition between the wound and the adjacent MCL tissue became less clear. This was caused by the fibroblasts and vessels, which appeared to be streaming into the injury site from the adjacent tissue. In contrast, the ACL did not mount an effective repair response. No similar neovascularization or evidence of cellular proliferation appeared in any of the specimens. Several sections taken on Day 10 actually appeared relatively hypocellular near the edge of the wound. In these sections, nuclei of fibroblasts nearest the edge of the wound demonstrated less distinct staining, possibly representing cellular lysis. Inflammatory cells were only sparsely interspersed at the margins of the wound. Witkowski et al. (57), in Sung's group, demonstrated reduced migration of ACL and MCL cells under inflammatory conditions induced by tumor necrosis factor-α. (TNF-α), C5a, or lipopolysaccharide *in vitro*. The ACL cells were inhibited to a greater degree than the MCL cells by a factor of between 1.2- to 3.4-fold.

These studies confirm the ACL's inability to mount an effective repair process while the MCL undergoes the appropriate phases of ligament healing. Aside from the cellular invasion of inflammatory cells followed by fibroblasts, the ligament was also shown to undergo neovascularization. Bray et al. (58) performed studies on the healing MCL using microspheres and ink–gelatin perfusion techniques. The normal rabbit MCL is relatively hypovascular, highly organized, and oriented in a longitudinal fashion. The healing MCL scar becomes twice as vascular early on, but returns to near normal values by 40 weeks. The scar vascular channels also appear less organized, but do show some remodeling with time. These experiments revealed that MCL injury is a potent stimulus for increasing blood flow, most pronounced at 3 weeks, remaining elevated at 6 weeks, and slightly elevated at 17 weeks.

Maturation of Extracellular Matrix During the Healing Process

As the MCL heals, the biochemical and biomechanical properties of the healing scar tissue are altered from normal values (20). Biochemically, the water content of the injury site is significantly elevated at 10 days and at 3 weeks. By 6 weeks, however, it returns to normal values. The glycosaminoglycan (GAG) content, a measurement of the proteoglycan content in the matrix, also increases significantly. This increase occurs early and remains ele-

vated at all postinjury intervals. There was a trend toward normal, but the GAG content remained elevated at 40 weeks. The collagen content is found to be normal at 10 days but drops significantly by 3 weeks. A subsequent return toward normal values is seen, but never completely attained. Collagen typing also shows an altered ratio of type III to type I collagen. Type III collagen, an immature form of collagen, is found to be significantly increased in the ligament scar at all time intervals. DNA content, as well, is significantly elevated at all intervals except 40 weeks where the content is slightly, but not significantly, elevated. Type III collagen is thought to be of particular use in the early repair process because of its ability to form rapid cross-links that stabilize the repair site (59). In the Sherman study (20), the authors concluded that despite the apparent healing of the MCL, a continuous remodeling of the ligament, primarily at the site of injury, was still occurring even at one year after injury.

Structural alterations of the healing ligament include changes in the cross-sectional area of the midsubstance of the ligament scar tissue. This is significantly increased over normal values at all time intervals. The increased diameter is greatest by 3 weeks, corresponding to the increased water content, and then undergoes a gradual decrease from 3 to 14 weeks. The diameter then remains stable through 40 weeks. Ligament scar laxity was significantly increased at 3 weeks. The laxity decreased slightly by 6 weeks and was not significantly different from normal values at 14 weeks. This decrease in laxity is presumably caused by contraction of the scar by myofibrils. At 40 weeks, however, a significant amount of laxity is once again detected in the healed MCL. Another mechanical property, load at ligament failure, was significantly lower for all experimental ligaments compared with their contralateral shams. These experiments reveal that the injured MCL will heal without primary repair, but that the resultant ligament scar will have altered biochemical and biomechanical properties. The remodeling that occurs appears to favor a return of the biochemical properties such as water content, GAG content, and collagen content at the expense of biomechanical measurements such as ligament laxity and load at failure. Although further remodeling may occur to create functional recovery of the MCL, studies have not shown a similar biologic recovery of the ligament scar. The ACL mounts neither a functional nor a biologic recovery. The factors involved in the various stages of ligament and tissue recovery are currently under intense investigation.

Cell Receptors Involved in Healing

After tissue injury, inflammatory cells become established in the wound, and tissue fibrocytes are activated into fibroblasts and stimulated to migrate. Fibronectin, collagen fragments, and various growth factors are some of the many substances involved in this activation process, which occurs through integrins and other cell membrane receptors (56). The integrins are a ubiquitous family of cell surface proteins that mediate many essential cellular functions, including adhesion, migration, proliferation, and elaboration of the extracellular matrix (60) (Fig. 11.13 and Table 11.1). The adhesive interactions of cells with other cells and with the extracellular matrix play a fundamental role in the organization of cell motility, and the healing process. The adhesion characteristics of ligament fibroblasts depend on the expression of cell surface molecules and their interaction with the extracellular matrix. Fibronectin molecules are dimeric glycoproteins, which consist of two similar 250-kD disulfide bond subunits. Although many receptors mediating

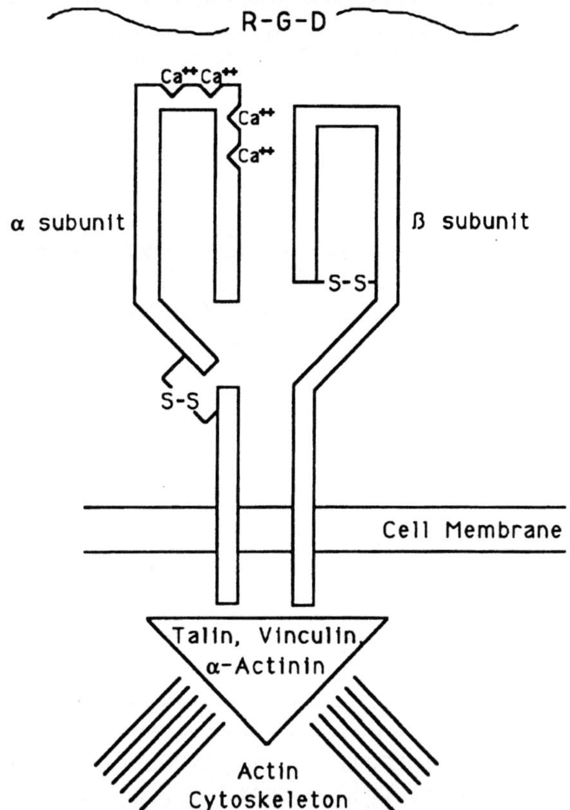

FIGURE 11.13. Integrin structure. This schematic representation of a typical integrin demonstrates the large globular extracellular region, the single short membrane-spanning domain, and the carboxy-terminal cytoplasmic domain of each subunit. The extracellular ligand-binding domain of a particular integrin is created by an association of the amino-terminal domains of both α and β chains (61). Ligand recognition by these binding pockets uses specific amino acid sequences within the ligand peptide; the best described is the tripeptide sequence arginine-glycine-aspartic acid (R-G-D). This sequence is involved in binding a variety of ligands, including fibronectin, fibrinogen, thrombospondin, vitronectin, laminin, and type I collagen (62). The cytoplasmic domains of the integrin are physically linked to the actin-containing cytoskeleton, probably through intermediary cytoplasmic proteins, including talin, vinculin, and α-actinin (63–65).

TABLE 11.1. *Integrin heterodimers and their ligands*

β Chain	α Chain	Ligand
β1	α1	laminin, collagen
	α2	laminin, collagen, fibronectin
	α3	laminin, collagen, fibronectin
	α4	fibronectin (CSI-1), VCAM
	α5	fibronectin (RGD)
	α6	laminin
	α7	laminin
β2	αL	ICAM
	αM	C3bi, fibrinogen
	αX	C3bi ?
β3	αIIb	vitronectin, VWF, fibrinogen, TSP, fibronectin, laminin
	αv	vitronectin, fibrinogen, VWF, fibronectin, TSP, OP, laminin

VCAM, vascular cell adhesion molecule; ICAM, intercellular adhesion molecule; TSP, thrombospondin; VWF, von Willebrand factor; OP, osteogenic protein.

the effects of the extracellular matrix components on ligament cell function remain poorly defined, it is known that fibronectin allows ligament cells to adhere through its RGD sequence to the VLA-5 integrin (α-5β-1) (47).

Under suitable conditions, a given integrin can bind to elements outside of the cell and at the same time bind to cytoskeletal components inside the cell, and thereby form a mechanical link (56). Thus, integrins play a crucial role in cell migration, and fibronectin plays a crucial role in fibroblast cell migration. Through its multiple specific adhesive domains, fibronectin attaches simultaneously to collagen or fibrin and its cell surface receptors to permit fibroblastic migration through connective tissue or blood clots (66). Gesink et al. (67) first demonstrated the presence of β-1, α-1, and α-5 integrins on the tissue fibroblasts of both normal ACL and MCL cells of rabbit and human ligaments.

Integrins have been found to be responsible for cellular adhesion and therefore play an important role in cellular migration. Cellular migration is a crucial component of wound healing models. Sung et al. (47,48) reported that the adhesion strength of ACL fibroblasts versus MCL fibroblasts is not random, but has a well-defined functional relationship with the fibronectin concentration and the seeding time. The seeding time is defined as the time cells are allowed to adhere to a coated culture dish. Through micromanipulation techniques, ACL cells were found to have a stronger dependence on fibronectin concentration for short seeding times than for long seeding times. MCL cells revealed a dependence on seeding time for all concentrations of fibronectin. For all seeding times studied and all fibronectin concentrations used, the MCL cells had higher adhesion strength than ACL cells (47). Tenascin, laminin, and fibronectin were sparsely distributed in normal ACL, but strongly expressed in ruptured ligaments (68). Nagineni et al. (44) concluded that the capacity of any cell to migrate on a substratum is generally inversely proportional to its number of focal adhesions. Ruoslahti et al. (69), however, found that while seemingly strong cellular adhesions limit cellular motility, so does no adhesion. The latter is analogous to trying to run on a frictionless surface. Moderate or "appropriate" adhesion permits and promotes cellular motility. The role of cytoskeletal proteins, paxillin and tensin, in adhesion were studied by Zamir and colleagues (70). Adhesions were shown to be of two types: focal contacts and fibrillar adhesions. Focal contacts were located at the cell periphery with high concentrations of paxillin, vinculin, and the α-v β-3 integrin. Fibrillar adhesions were noted to be elongated, beaded structures with high content of tensin and α-5, β-1 integrins. These authors propose a dynamic model in which transitions of the two forms of adhesions are operative in producing cell motility (70). Integrins have also been found to effect proliferation of fibroblastic cells that likely represent the combined effects of migration and division (56).

Regulation of the extracellular matrix composition mediated by integrins has also been described. The actin–integrin–fibronectin complex is crucial in tissue remodeling by providing for the transduction of biomechanical signals for the cellular machinery to modulate the phenotypes of the fibroblasts (71). Conversely, integrins also allow the cytoskeleton of the cell to exert mechanical forces on the surrounding extracellular matrix (56). Integrins thereby appear to play a central role in the construction of extracellular matrix. In tissue culture, fibroblasts first produce the soluble building blocks of the extracellular matrix, including procollagens and fibronectin dimers, and then assemble these soluble precursors into an insoluble three-dimensional structure (56).

Integrin display has been studied in the injured MCL and ACL tissue. Integrin display increases in the wounded MCL but not the wounded ACL. Between 3 and 7 days, the wounded MCL demonstrates a striking increase in staining for the α-1, α-5, and α-v subunits on the fibroblasts. In marked contrast, the ACL, which does not mount an effective repair response, demonstrated no comparable alteration of integrin expression from baseline levels (55).

Another factor involved in adhesion and consequently cellular migration is laminin. Laminin, a matrix glycoprotein found in the basement membrane, surrounds the exterior of the ligaments. Laminin is a large complex of three very long polypeptide chains arranged in the shape of a cross and held together by disulfide bonds. It consists of a number of functional domains. Adhesion strength assays, using micromanipulation techniques, showed higher forces for the adhesion of fibroblasts from the ACL to laminin than for fibroblasts from the MCL, even after normalization (48). Laminin and fibronectin both play roles in the adhesion and migration of ligamentous

cells. Fibronectin may also play a role in the fibroblast's regulation of extracellular matrix. The fibroblasts must have appropriate adhesion to the extracellular matrix in order to migrate effectively. Both ACL and MCL fibroblast adhesion depends on cytoskeletal assembly, but differ in many ways. In particular, the actin filament capping protein, tropomodulin, delivered exogenously, increases MCL adhesion, but decreases ACL adhesion (72). In addition, signaling differences between the two ligament cell types have been described (73,74), and differences in adhesion to type I and type III collagen have been noted (75) (see Chapter 12). Multiple factors play a role in the adhesion strength of fibroblast to the extracellular matrix including seeding time and concentration of fibronectin or laminin. Mechanical factors are obviously important (76), but the variable, or variables, responsible for the ACL cells' lack of proliferation, both division and migration, and the MCL's more rapid proliferation have yet to be conclusively defined.

Growth Factors Involved in Healing

Understanding the phases of ligament healing uncovers the rapidly expanding field of factors involved in the healing process. Initially, the ligament injury results in localized bleeding and clot formation. The resultant inflammatory phase brings with it not only cells, but also growth factors that are being found to be crucial in wound healing models (77,78). These factors act in an autocrine, paracrine, and endocrine fashion with multiple manifestations dependent on their location and concentration. The overall function of growth factors, as described by McGrath (79), is to undergo receptor-mediated second messenger regulation of gene transcription. This will result in an alteration of cellular function. For ligamentous tissue in repair, proliferation, migration, and matrix synthesis are the most important parameters under investigation.

After injury, the platelets migrate to the wound site, form a clot, and hemostasis is obtained. Platelets secrete peptides such as platelet-derived growth factor (PDGF), transforming growth factor-β (TGF-β), and other factors. PDGF and TGF-β play important roles in the initiation of repair processes after injury. These factors are chemotactic for inflammatory cells and appear to regulate proliferation and differentiation of fibroblasts (78,80–83). Inflammatory cells at the wound site then release other peptides such as basic fibroblast growth factor (bFGF) and epidermal growth factor (EGF).

PDGF has been shown to affect fibroblast cellular proliferation. In thymidine uptake studies, it was shown to increase ACL proliferation equal to that of MCL cells (84). However, other studies claim that PDGF has no effect on cellular proliferation (85) or only increases cellular outgrowth in MCL cells but not in ACL cells (86). Batten et al. (87) showed that if PDGF was administered within 24 hours of injury, the MCL showed an increase in biomechanical strength, otherwise PDGF had no effect on MCL strength. DesRosiers et al. (88) found that PDGF had its maximal effect on stimulating ACL fibroblast proliferation but had no effect on collagen synthesis and only a small increase in proteoglycan synthesis. Hannafin et al. (89), using recombinant human PDGF to stimulate canine fibroblast motility observed accelerated migration of both intrarticular (ACL and PCL) and extraarticular (MCL and LCL) fibroblasts. Proliferation of the intraarticular fibroblasts was slower than the extraarticular fibroblasts, amplifying previous studies restricted to ACL and MCL cells.

TGF-β has been shown to have a multitude of effects as well. Many investigators have shown TGF-β to have a stimulatory effect on proliferation of both ACL and MCL cells in a dose-dependent manner (84,85,88,90). These studies show that TGF-β, in particular TGF-β₁, a subtype of the TGF-β family, has inhibitory effects on thymidine uptake at high concentration (90). TGF-β₁ has also been shown to increase collagen synthesis in MCL tissue (91), as well as collagen and proteoglycan synthesis in ACL cells (88). Cell adhesion receptors were also found to be regulated by TGF-β₁ with the concomitant regulation of integrins that share a common β-1 subunit (92). This may play an important role in regulation of migration by TGF-β₁ on fibroblasts.

Fibroblast growth factor (FGF) has been shown to have its greatest effects on cellular proliferation. Schmidt et al. (84) found that bFGF caused an approximate eightfold increase in thymidine uptake in MCL and ACL cells. The results concluded that with the administration of bFGF, the ACL cells were proliferating at a rate equivalent to MCL cells. Lee et al. (86), however, did not find an increase in cellular proliferation in MCL or ACL cells using a cellular outgrowth model, supplemented with bFGF. When evaluating the healing MCL scar ligament cells, bFGF had no effect on collagen synthesis (91). However, bFGF receptors were increased in the healing MCL scar ligament cells (58).

EGF had a potent eightfold increase in thymidine uptake in both MCL and ACL cells (84). This was confirmed by DesRosiers et al. (88), who found that the ACL cells had an increase in proliferation as well as an increase in proteoglycan synthesis when exposed to EGF; however, a decrease in collagen synthesis was noted. And, once again, EGF receptors were up-regulated in the healing MCL scar ligament (58).

Other growth factors have been analyzed as well. Insulin has been shown by one investigator to increase cell proliferation and proteoglycan synthesis (88), whereas another investigator has found no increase in cell outgrowth cultures for either ACL or MCL cells (86). Insulin-like growth factor (IGF) has also been evaluated with respect to ligamentous cells. In one study, IGF was found to cause ACL cells to proliferate as rapidly as MCL cells using thymidine uptake assays (84). Another investigator found that IGF type I increased ACL proliferation as well as increasing collagen and proteoglycan synthesis (88). Murphy et al. (91), however, in studying healing MCL scar ligament, found that IGF type I had no effect on collagen synthesis whereas type II had a positive effect on the synthesis of collagen (91).

Studies have not limited themselves to analyzing the effects of only one growth factor. In an attempt to find synergistic effects between growth factors that utilize different messengers at different times in the cell cycle, studies have been performed using a combination of growth factors. Lee et al. (86) combined bFGF, insulin, TGF-β₁, and platelet-derived growth factor-B (PDGF-B). This combination resulted in a threefold increase in cell outgrowth of MCL cells *in vitro*, and a 10- to 20-fold increase in cell outgrowth of ACL cells. Even with the remarkable increase in cellular outgrowth of ACL cells, the MCL cells were still found to outgrow the ACL cells. Berry et al. (93) presented a combination of TGF-β₁, PDGF-BB, bFGF, and insulin, which caused a threefold increase at three days and 16-fold increase at six days of cell outgrowth by MCL cells. The same mixture of growth factors had a twofold increase at three days and at six days of cell outgrowth in ACL cells. The investigator then added hyaluronic acid, a proteoglycan that has long been implicated in remodeling the extracellular matrix to aid in cell locomotion (94). The MCL cells showed a 50-fold increase in cellular outgrowth and the ACL cells had a sixfold increase at three days and a 15-fold increase at six days in cellular outgrowth. This study concluded that hyaluronic acid would be a good carrier for growth factors. The mechanism by which growth factors affect proliferation, migration, and extracellular matrix synthesis is under active investigation (73). Focal adhesion kinase (FAK) is a nonreceptor protein–tyrosine kinase downstream signaling molecule that indirectly localizes to sites of integrin-receptor clustering through interactions with paxillin and talin (integrin-associated proteins) (95). FAK associates with activated PDGF and EGF receptor signaling complexes and is an important receptor–proximal link between growth factor receptor and integrin signaling pathways. The activation of downstream signaling pathways by integrins is obviously an area deserving considerable focus of interest.

CONCLUSION AND FUTURE DIRECTIONS

Knee ligament injury remains one of the most common injuries encountered by orthopedists (1). Structural factors such as laxity, location of tear, size of gap in injury, and the local environment of injury as well as biologic factors such as proliferation, migration, and extracellular matrix synthesis are important in the healing of the knee ligament. Recently, growth factors, integrins, and other molecular factors have been discovered to also play crucial roles in ligament healing. The injured knee ligament has multiple variables influencing its repair, however, the relative importance of one variable over another is not yet understood. It has been well described that the MCL is capable of producing a functional ligament scar even without primary surgical repair (11–14) whereas the ACL is incapable of a functional repair even with the isolation of biomechanical factors (9–13). What is the explanation for this enigma? Multiple differences have been discovered between the MCL and ACL cells. The healing MCL and the healing ACL display even greater differences, any of which could play a role in their contrasting repair response. Environmental factors, especially differences in the intraarticular versus extraarticular environments are undoubtedly important in the healing differences between these ligament types as are differences in vascularity. It is likely that a combination of the observed differences between these ligaments accounts for their vastly different response to injury.

Directions for the future of ligament healing lie in the field of molecular biology. Sung et al. (73) and others (74,89,95) are analyzing the signal pathways involved in ligament cell adhesion and signaling pathways. Further investigation into the mechanism of the healing processes between the ACL and MCL described in this chapter may elucidate a pattern with which a conclusion of repair response differences will be better understood. Tissue engineering is another field of increasing interest. The manufacturing of tissue or aids that will enhance the inherent repair capabilities of the healing ligament is a field of rapid growth. Yannas (96) proposes the introduction of new ACL grafts composed of cells and matrix that will function superior to autografts or synthetic fiber grafts. The cells used in tissue engineering experiments can also be enhanced through molecular biology means.

Manipulation of the genetic machinery of cells is becoming an ever-more-important means of elucidating pathways of molecular and cellular biochemistry. In addition, gene therapy is a potentially powerful tool for enhancing fibroblast regeneration, migration, and extracellular matrix synthesis. This process may offer "customized" cells that when placed into a biologic scaffold, will enhance the reparative efforts of the healing ligament (97). Our laboratory and those of others (98–100) are investigating novel techniques in genetic transfection to enhance the efficiency of gene transfer and eliminate the negative side effects of viral transfection. Goomer et al. (100) have been able to show a transfection rate of greater than 70% efficiency when utilizing a receptor/liposome-mediated transfection system. This is an outstanding improvement over the previous 15% efficiency rate published by investigators (98,99). With the improvement of transfection techniques, the delivery of factors involved in ligament healing will be made available. Growth factors, as described, have a multitude of potentially beneficial effects in the healing ligament. Their delivery into the genetic machinery of the healing fibroblast may have a

profound influence on the ability of the ligament to heal effectively.

Further investigation in the fields of ligament repair using cellular and environmental factors continues, and the task of producing a healed ACL ligament, which is biochemically and biomechanically equivalent to the original ligament, is a common goal.

REFERENCES

1. Fetto JF, Marshall JL. The natural history and diagnosis of anterior cruciate ligament insufficiency. *Clin Orthop* 1978;132:206–218.
2. Kennedy JC, Fowler PJ. Medial and anterior instability of the knee: an anatomic and clinical study using stress machines. *J Bone Joint Surg Am* 1971;53:1257–1270.
3. Kennedy JC, Weinberg HW, Wilson AS. The anatomy and function of the anterior cruciate ligament, as determined by clinical and morphological studies. *J Bone Joint Surg Am* 1974;56:223–235.
4. Norwood LA, Cross MJ. Anterior cruciate ligament: functional anatomy of its bundles in rotatory instabilities. *Am J Sports Med* 1979; 7:23–26.
5. Odensten M, Gillquist J. Functional anatomy of the anterior cruciate ligament and a rationale for reconstruction. *J Bone Joint Surg Am* 1985;67:257–262.
6. Balkfors B. The course of knee ligament injuries. *Acta Orthop Scand (suppl)* 1982;198:1– 99.
7. O'Donoghue DH, Frank GR, Jeter GL, et al. Repair and reconstruction of the anterior cruciate ligament in dogs: factors influencing long-term results *J Bone Joint Surg Am*1971;53:710–718.
8. Scuderi GR, Scott WN, Insall JN. Injuries of the knee. In: Rockwood CA Jr, Green DP, Bucholz RW, Heckman JD, eds. *Fractures in adults.* 4th ed. New York: Lippincott-Raven, 1996.
9. Arnold JA, Coker TP, Heaton LM, et al. Natural history of anterior cruciate tears. *Am J Sports Med* 1979;7:305–313.
10. Cabaud JE, Rodkey WG, Feagin JA. Experimental studies of acute anterior cruciate ligament injury and repair. *Am J Sports Med* 1979; 7:18–22.
11. Clayton ML, Miles JS, Abdulla M. Experimental investigations of ligamentous healing. *Clin Orthop* 1968;61:146–153.
12. O'Donoghue DH. An analysis of end results of surgical treatment of major injuries to the ligaments of the knee. *J Bone Joint Surg Am* 1955;37:1–13.
13. Wiig ME, Amiel D, Vandeberg J, et al. The early effect of high molecular weight hyaluronan (hyaluronic acid) on anterior cruciate ligament healing: an experimental study in rabbits. *J Orthop Res* 1990;8: 425–434.
14. Frank C, Woo SL-Y, Amiel D, et al. Medial collateral ligament healing: a multidisciplinary assessment in rabbits. *Am J Sports Med* 1983; 11:379–389.
15. Woo SL, Young EP, Ohland KJ, et al. The effects of transection of the anterior cruciate ligament on healing of the medial collateral ligament: a biomechanical study of the knee in dogs. *J Bone Joint Surg Am* 1990;72:382–392.
16. Anderson DR, Weiss JA, Takai S, et al. Healing of the medial collateral ligament following a triad injury: biomechanical and histological study of the knee in rabbits. *J Orthop Res* 1992;10:485–495.
17. Jackson DW, Corsetti J, Simon TM. Biologic incorporation of allograft anterior cruciate ligament replacements. *Clin Orthop* 1996;324: 126–133.
18. Rivard CH. Studies on the anterior cruciate ligaments: a 10-year experience review. *Nippon Seikeigeka Gakkai Zasshi* 1989;63:687–691.
19. Femor B, Urban J, Murray D, et al. Proliferation and collagen synthesis of human anterior cruciate ligament cells *in vitro*: effects of ascorbate-2-phosphate, dexamethasone and oxygen tension. *Cell Biol Int* 1998;22:635–640.
20. Sherman MF, Bonamo JR. Primary repair of the anterior cruciate ligament. *Clin Sports Med* 1988;7:739–750.
21. Lyon RM, Akeson WH, Amiel D, et al. Ultrastructural differences between the cells of the medial collateral and the anterior cruciate ligaments. *Clin Orthop* 1991;272:279–286.
22. Lo IK, de Naat GH, Valk JW, et al. The gross morphology of torn

human anterior cruciate ligaments in unstable knees. *Arthroscopy* 1999;15:301–306.

23. Loitz-Ramage BJ, Frank CB, Shrive NG. Injury size affects long-term strength of the rabbit medial collateral ligament. *Clin Orthop* 1997;337:272–280.

24. Kleiner JB, Roux RD, Amiel D, et al. Primary healing of the ACL. *Trans Orthop Res Soc* 1986;11:131.

25. Marshall JL, Rubin RM, Wang JB, et al. The anterior cruciate ligament: the diagnosis and treatment of its injuries and their serious prognostic implication. *Orthop Rev* 1978;7:35–46.

26. Amiel D, Kleiner JB. Biochemistry of tendon and ligament. In: Nimni M, Olsen B, eds. *Collagen: biotechnology.* Vol. 3. Cleveland, OH: CRC Press, 1988:223–250.

27. O'Donoghue DH, Rockwood CA Jr, Frank GR, et al. Repair of the ACL in dogs. *J Bone Joint Surg Am* 1966;48:503–519.

28. Arnoczsky SP, Rubin RM, Marshall JL. Microvasculature of the cruciate ligaments and its response to injury. *J Bone Joint Surg Am* 1979; 61:1221–1229.

29. Alm A, Stromberg B. Vascular anatomy of the patellar and cruciate ligaments. A microangiographic and histologic investigation in the dog. *Acta Chir Scand* 1974;445(suppl):25–35.

30. Wallace CD, Amiel D. Vascular assessment of the periarticular ligaments of the rabbit knee. *J Orthop Res* 1991;9:787–791.

31. Ropes MW, Bennett GA, Bauer W. The origin and nature of normal synovial fluid. *J Clin Inves* 1939;18:351–372.

32. Andrish J, Holmes R. Effects of synovial fluid on fibroblasts in tissue culture. *Clin Orthop* 1979;138:279–283.

33. Nickerson DA, Joshi R, Williams S, et al. Synovial fluid stimulates proliferation of rabbit ligament. *Clin Orthop* 1992;274:294–299.

34. Nickerson DA, Joshi R, Williams S, et al. Synovial fluid stimulates the proliferation of rabbit ligament fibroblasts in vitro. *Clin Orthop* 1992; 274:294–299.

35. Amiel D, Abel MF, Kleiner JB, et al. Synovial fluid nutrient delivery in the diarthrial joint: an analysis of rabbit knee ligaments. *J Orthop Res* 1986;4:90–95.

36. Warren RF. Primary repair of the ACL. *Clin Orthop* 1983;172:65–70.

37. Kohn D. Arthroscopy in acute injuries of anterior cruciate-deficient knees: fresh and old intraarticular lesions. *Arthroscopy* 1986;2:98–102.

38. Amiel D, Ishizue KK, Harwood FL, et al. Injury of the ACL: the role of collagenase in ligament degeneration. *J Orthop Res* 1989;7:486–493.

39. Cheung HS, Halverson PB, McCarty DJ. Release of collagenase, neutral protease, and prostaglandins from cultured mammalian synovial cells by hydroxyapatite and calcium pyrophosphate dihydrate crystals. *Arthritis Rheum* 1981;24:1338–1344.

40. Werb Z, Reynolds JJ. Stimulation of endocytosis of the secretion of collagenase and neutral proteinase from rabbit synovial fibroblasts. *J Exp Med* 1974;140:1482–1497.

41. Ehrlich MG, Mankin HJ, Jones H, et al. Collagenase and collagenase inhibitors in osteoarthritic and normal cartilage. *J Clin Invest* 1977; 59:226–233.

42. Ridge SC, Oransky AL, Kerwar SS. Induction of the synthesis of latent collagenase and latent neutral protease in chondrocytes by a factor synthesized by activated macrophages. *Arthritis Rheum* 1980;23: 448–454.

43. Lindy S, Turto H, Sorsa T, et al. Increased collagenase activity in human rheumatoid meniscus. *Scand J Rheum* 1986;15:237–242.

44. Nagineni CN, Amiel D, Green MH, et al. Characterization of the intrinsic properties of the anterior cruciate and medial collateral ligament cells: an in vitro cell culture study. *J Orthop Res* 1992;10: 465–475.

45. Burridge K, Chrzanowska–Wodnicka M. Focal adhesions, contractility, and signaling. *Annual Review of Cell and Developmental Biology* 1996;12:463–518.

46. Murray MM, Spector M. Fibroblast distribution in the anteromedial bundle of the human anterior cruciate ligament: the presence of alpha-smooth muscle actin positive cells. *J Orthop Res* 1999;17:18–27.

47. Sung PK-L, Kwan MK, Maldanado F, et al. Adhesion strength of human ligament fibroblasts. *J Biomech Eng* 1994;116:237–242.

48. Sung PK-L, Steele LL, Whittermore D, et al. Adhesiveness of human ligament fibroblasts to laminin. *J Orthop Res* 1995;13:166–173.

49. Hannafin JA, Attia ET, Warren RF, et al. Characterization of chemotactic migration and growth kinetics of canine knee ligament fibroblasts. *J Orthop Res* 1999;17:398–404.

50. Amiel D, Foulk RA, Harwood FL, et al. Quantitative assessment by competitive ELISA of fibronectin (Fn) in tendons and ligaments, *Matrix* 1989;9:421–427.

51. Andriacchi T, Sabiston P, DeHaven K. Ligament: injury and repair. In: Woo SL-Y, Buckwater JA, eds. *Injury and repair of the musculoskeletal soft tissues.* Chicago: American Academy of Orthopedic Surgeons, 1988.

52. Arnoczsky SP. Physiologic principles of ligament injuries and healing. In: Scott NA, ed. *Ligament and extensor mechanism injuries of the knee: diagnosis and treatment.* St. Louis: CV Mosby, 1991;67–81.

53. Neurath MF, Printz H, Stofft E. Cellular ultrastructure of the ruptured anterior cruciate ligament. *Acta Orthop Scand* 1994;651:71–76.

54. Jack EA. Experimental rupture of the medial collateral ligament of the knee. *J Bone Joint Surg Br* 1950;32:396–402.

55. Schreck PJ, Kitabayashi LR, Amiel D, et al. Integrin display increases in the wounded rabbit medial collateral ligament but not the wounded anterior cruciate ligament. *J Orthop Res* 1995;13:174–183.

56. Schreck PJ, Amiel D, Woods VL Jr, et al. The role of integrin adhesion receptors in anterior cruciate ligament physiology. In: Jackson DW, ed. *The anterior cruciate ligament: current and future concepts.* New York: Raven Press, 1993:423–430.

57. Witkowski J, Yang L, Wood DJ, et al. Migration and healing of ligament cells under inflammatory conditions. *J Orthop Res* 1997;15:269–277.

58. Bray RC, Butterwick DJ, Doschak MR, et al. Coloured microsphere assessment of blood flow to knee ligaments in adult rabbits: effects of injury. *J Orthop Res* 1996;14:618–625.

59. Liu SH, Yang RS, al-Shaikh R, et al. Collagen in tendon, ligament, and bone healing: a current review. *Clin Orthop* 1995; 318:265–278.

60. Ruoslahti E. Integrins. *J Clin Invest* 1991;87:1–5.

61. Hynes RO. Integrins: a family of cell surface receptors. *Cell* 1987;48: 549–554.

62. Ruoslahti E. Fibronectin and its receptors. *Annu Rev Biochem* 1988; 57:375–413.

63. Burridge K, Fath K, Kelly T, et al. Focal adhesions: transmembrane junctions between the extracellular matrix and the cytoskeleton. *Annu Rev Cell Biol* 1988;4:487–525.

64. Horwitz A, Duggan K, Buck C, et al. Interaction of plasma membrane fibronectin receptor with talin—a transmembrane linkage. *Nature* 1986;320:531–533.

65. Otey CA, Pavalko FM, Burridge K. An interaction between α-actinin and the $\beta1$ integrin subunit in vitro. *J Cell Biol* 1990;111:721–729.

66. Humphries MJ, Obara M, Olden K, et al. Role of fibronectin in adhesion, migration, and metastasis. *Cancer Invest* 1989;7:373–393.

67. Gesink DS, Pacheco HO, Kuiper SD, et al. Immunohistochemical localization of beta-1 integrins in anterior cruciate and medial collateral ligaments of human and rabbit. *J Orthop Res* 1992;10:596–599.

68. Neurath M. Expression von tenacin, laminin und fibronectin nach traumatisher vorderer Kreuzbandruptur. *Z Orthop Ihre Grenzgeb* 1993;131:168–172.

69. Ruoslahti E, Giancotti FG. Integrins and tumor cell dissemination, *Cancer Cells* 1989;1:119–126.

70. Zamir E, Katz M. Posen Y, et al. Dynamics and segregation of cell-matrix adhesions in cultured fibroblasts. *Nature Cell Biol* 2000;2: 191–196

71. Unemori EN, Werb Z. Reorganization of the polymerized actin: a possible trigger for induction of procollagenase in fibroblasts cultured in and on collagen gels. *J Cell Biol* 1986;103:1021–1031.

72. Sung KL, Yang L, Whittemore DE, et al. The differential adhesion forces of anterior cruciate and medial collateral ligament fibroblasts: effects of tropomodulin, talin, vinculin, and alpha-actin. *Proc Natl Acad Sci U S A* 1996;93:9182–9187.

73. Sung PK-L, Whittemore DE, Yang L, et al. Signal pathways and ligament cell adhesiveness. *J Orthop Res* 1996;14:729–735.

74. Hung CT, Allen FD, Pollack SR, et al. Intracellular calcium response of ACL and MCL ligament fibroblasts to fluid-induced shear stress. *Cell Signal* 1997;8:587–594.

75. Yang L, Tsai CM, Hsieh AH, et al. Adhesion strength differential of human ligament fibroblasts to collagen types I and III. *J Orthop Res* 1999; 17:755–762.

76. Derosiers EA, Methot S, Yahia L, et al. Responses des fibroblastes ligamentaires a la stimulation mecanique. *Ann Chir* 1995;49:768–774.

77. Mustoe TA, Pierce GF, Thomason A, et al. Accelerated healing of incisional wounds in rats induced by transforming growth factor-β. *Science* 1987;237:1333–1336.

78. Deuel TF, Senior M, Huang JS, et al. Chemotaxis of monocytes and

neutrophils to platelet derived growth factor. *J Clin Invest* 1982;169:1046–1049.

79. McGrath MH. Peptide growth factors and wound healing. *Clin Plas Surg* 1990;17:421–432.

80. Roberts AB, Anzano MA, Lamb LC, et al. New class of transforming growth factors potentiated by epidermal growth factor: isolation from non-neoplastic tissues. *Proc Natl Acad Sci U S A* 1981;78:5339–5343.

81. Roberts AB, Sporn MB, Assoian RK, et al. Transforming growth factor type β: rapid induction of fibrosis and angiogenesis in vivo and stimulation of collagen formation in vitro. *Proc Natl Acad Sci U S A* 1986;83:4167–4171.

82. Seppa H, Grotendorst G, Seppa S, et al. Platelet-derived growth factor is chemotactic for fibroblasts. *J Cell Biol* 1982;92:584–588.

83. Sporn MB, Roberts AB, Wakefield LM, et al. Transforming growth factor β: biological function and chemical structure. *Science* 1986;233:532–534.

84. Schmidt CC, Georgescu HI, Kwoh CK, et al. Effect of growth factors on the proliferation of fibroblasts from the medial collateral and anterior cruciate ligaments. *J Orthop Res* 1995;13:184–190.

85. Spindler KP, Imro AK, Mayes CE, et al. Patellar tendon and anterior cruciate ligament have different mitogenic responses to platelet-derived growth factor and transforming growth factor β. *J Orthop Res* 1996;14:542–546.

86. Lee J, Green MH, Amiel D. Synergistic effect of growth factors on cell outgrowth from explants of rabbit anterior cruciate and medial collateral ligaments. *J Orthop Res* 1995;13:435–441.

87. Batten ML, Hansen JC, Dahners LE. Influence of dosage and timing of application of platelet-derived growth factor on early healing of the rat medial collateral ligament. *J Orthop Res* 1996;14:736–741.

88. DesRosiers EA, Yahia LH, Rivard CH. Proliferative and matrix synthesis response of canine anterior cruciate ligament fibroblasts submitted to combined growth factors. *J Orthop Res* 1996;14:200–208.

89. Hannafin JA, Attia ET, Warren RF, et al. Characterization of chemotactic migration and growth kinetics of canine knee ligament fibroblasts. *J Orthop Res* 1999; 17:398–404.

90. Amiel D, Nagineni CN, Choi SH, et al. Intrinsic properties of ACL and MCL cells and their responses to growth factors. *Med Sci Sports Exerc* 1995;6:844–851.

91. Murphy PG, Barbara JL, Frank CB, et al. Influence of exogenous growth factors on the synthesis and secretion of collagen types I and III by explants of normal and healing rabbit ligaments. *Biochem Cell Biol* 1994;72:403–409.

92. Gove PB ed. *Webster's Third New International Dictionary*. Springfield, MA:G & C Merriam, 1976.

93. Berry SM, Green MH, Amiel D. Hyaluronan: a potential carrier for growth factors for the healing of ligamentous tissues. Presented at: Fourth Annual Meeting of the Wound Healing Society, May 18–21, 1994; San Francisco, CA.

94. Turley EA. Hyaluronan and cell locomotion. *Cancer Metast Rev* 1991;11(suppl 1):21–30.

95. Sieg DJ, Hauck CR, Illic D, et al.. FAK integrates growth-factor and integrin signals to promote cell migration. *Nature Cell Biol* 2000;2:249–256.

96. Yannas IV. Application of ECM analogs in surgery. *J Cell Biochem* 1994;56:188–191.

97. Mann MJ, Morishita R, Gibbons GH, et al. DNA transfer into vascular smooth muscle using fusigenic Sendai virus (HVJ)-liposomes. *Mol Cell Biochem* 1997;172:3–12.

98. Fortunati E, Bout A, Zanta MA, et al. In vitro and in vivo gene transfer to pulmonary cells mediated by cationic liposomes. *Biochim Biophys Acta* 1996;1306:55–62.

99. Brant WO, Goomer RS, Amiel D. Assessment of liposome-mediated transfectional efficacy of aged human chondroprogenitor cells. Abstract at the Western Student Medical Research Forum at the American Medical Association Education and Research Foundation, Feb 5–8, 1997; Carmel, CA.

100. Goomer RS, Coutts RD, Maris T, et al. High efficiency gene transfer into perichondrium derived cells using a novel receptor/liposome mediated transfection system. Presented at: 44th Annual Orthopaedic Research Society Meeting, Mar 16–19, 1998; New Orleans, LA.

CHAPTER 12

Cell Adhesion and the Signaling Biology of Ligament Healing

K-L. Paul Sung, Wayne H. Akeson, and Adam H. Hsieh

Knowledge of the basic intrinsic properties of fibroblasts from the anterior cruciate ligament (ACL) and medial collateral ligament (MCL) and their molecular responses to injury conditions are essential for understanding the healing processes of ligaments and the problems associated with healing and ligament remodeling. It is well documented that following a traumatic knee injury in adults, the MCL heals much more effectively than the ACL, usually without surgical repair. In general, the injured adult human ACL does not have a functional healing response. These complicated natural differences between the ACL and MCL can be appreciated by using cellular and molecular approaches in studying their intrinsic properties. Injuries to the MCL generally follow a classical healing response that can be divided into three overlapping phases: inflammation, cellular proliferation, and matrix synthesis and remodeling (1–5). Because of its extraarticular location and vascular bed environment, the ACL is incapable of forming intermediate scar tissue and lacks an initial inflammatory response, resulting in poor tissue repair (6,7). The ACL is surrounded by a thin layer of synovial tissue within an intraarticular environment (*extrasynovial structure*), which, when ruptured due to injury, causes the ACL to be exposed to synovial fluid containing inflammatory cells and their mediators, hemorrhagic breakdown products, hyaluronan, and proteolytic enzymes (8). Although the ACL has an active vascular response after injury (9,10), the lack of spontaneous healing has led to the support of the primary repair of ACL injuries. This deficiency in healing capacity of the ACL has been a topic of great interest in orthopedic research for decades (10–12).

Although much is known about the anatomic differences between the ACL and MCL, such as vascularity, superficial layers, innervation, matrix composition, biomechanical loading, and gross morphology, much less is known about the intrinsic cellular differences that may account for their different functional healing responses (13–17). The cells of the ACL are arranged in columns and are rounded, resembling cells of fibrocartilage, whereas the cells of the MCL are spindle-shaped fibroblastlike cells that rest directly on a collagen matrix. Collagen molecules secreted locally by fibroblasts are embedded in the matrix and have a high turnover rate. They form the intermolecular cross-links, which give the ligament its tensile strength characteristics. The proper alignment of fibroblasts within its surrounding extracellular matrix (ECM) and their interaction with matrix molecules like collagen (structural protein) and fibronectin (adhesive protein) reflect the ligament's physical properties. Experiments have shown a greater migratory ability of MCL fibroblasts compared with ACL fibroblasts (16,18) as well as greater proliferation (19). Growth factors have also been shown to affect ACL and MCL fibroblast proliferation differently (20). We have determined that a number of additional intrinsic differences exist between ACL and MCL fibroblasts in regard to their adhesiveness to fibronectin and laminin, signal pathway processes, and gene expression under mechanical loading. This chapter presents the experimental design and research conducted to determine the cellular behavior of the ACL and MCL and their gene activities under biochemical and mechanical stimuli to help us understand the mechanisms involved in ligament repair processes after injury.

ADHESIVENESS OF LIGAMENT FIBROBLASTS BY MICROPIPETTE ASPIRATION OF SINGLE CELLS

Cellular adhesion and migration are fundamental biologic processes in health and disease. Cell attachment and detachment are of considerable importance in development, growth, differentiation, immune response, wound healing, and the functioning of multicellular organisms under physiologic conditions. In an injured ligament,

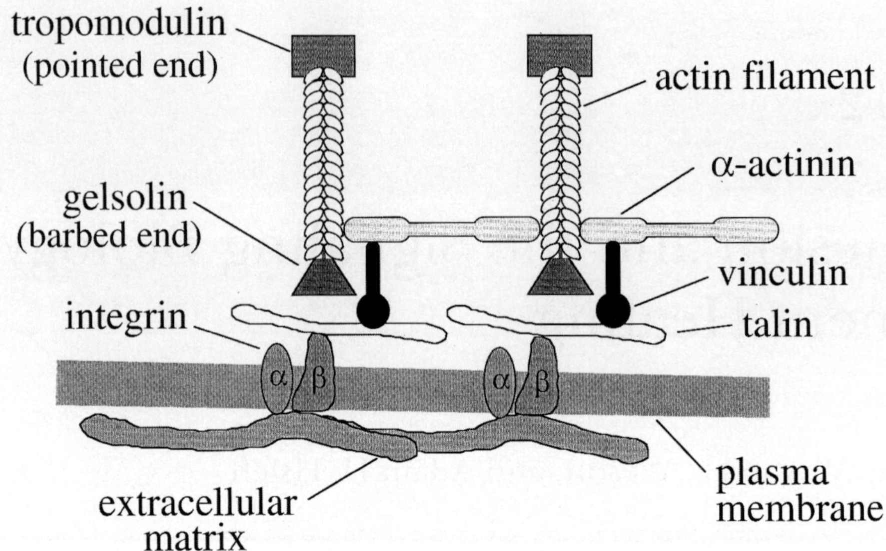

FIGURE 12.1. Schematic drawing of cytoskeleton–integrin–extracellular matrix complex. Tropomodulin, located at the pointed end of actin filament, gelsolin, located at the barbed end of actin filament, and the bridging proteins (talin, vinculin, and α-actinin), located between actin filaments and integrins, are shown.

fibroblasts embedded in the amorphous healing tissue matrix of ligaments have been found to migrate into a damaged site. We look at cell adhesion as a fundamental part of cell migration, and these two cellular events must be delicately balanced for functional wound repairing and tissue remodeling. Adhesion also plays an important role in many pathologic states (e.g., inflammation, thrombus formation, tumor metastasis, artificial organ development, etc.). This chapter will determine individual cell adhesion strengths using a micropipette–micromanipulation system after cells were treated with or without signal pathway–inhibiting agents. Determining cell adhesion and signal pathway and understanding such mechanisms may have implications in many physiologic systems in addition to the ligament healing process.

Experiments also determined the adhesion strength through integrin–cytoskeleton complexes, which transduce mechanical and chemical signals into the cytoplasm and the nucleus. The integrin–cytoskeleton complex has been described by other investigators (16,21–24). Detailed linkages among integrins, stress fibers, and actin-binding proteins (e.g., talin, vinculin, α-actinin) have been described in Luna and Hitt (23). The lengths of actin fibers can be regulated by tropomodulin at the pointed ends of actin filaments, and by the gelsolin family at the barbed end (Fig. 12.1) (25).

METHODS AND RESULTS

Cell Preparation and Adhesion Force Assay

Cell Isolation

Human ligament fibroblasts were obtained from ACL and MCL explants from five subjects (one woman and four men, 30–52 years old). Fibroblasts were freshly harvested at autopsy (within 24 hours) as described previously (19) and showed no difference in viability between subjects. Details of the cell culture management are given in recent articles from this laboratory (26–28).

Micropipette Chamber Preparation

Details of the micropipette chamber and its preparation are also given in recent articles (26–28) (Fig. 12.2).

Adhesion Strength of Human Ligament Fibroblasts to Fibronectin

A direct measurement of the adhesion between ACL or MCL fibroblasts to fibronectin (FN) through the very late antigen-5 (VLA-5) receptor ($\alpha_5\beta_1$) was achieved (Fig. 12.3). We found that the adhesion strength is not random, but has well-defined functional relationships with the FN concentration and the time allowed for the cell to establish attachment (Fig. 12.4). The adhesion strength (i.e., force required to detach) of ACL fibroblasts showed a stronger dependence on FN concentration (1, 2, and 5 µg/mL) for a short period of seeding time (15 to 30 minutes) than for a long period (40 to 75 minutes). For MCL fibroblasts, the effect of the seeding time on adhesion strength was apparent for all concentrations. For all the seeding times studied and FN concentrations used, MCL fibroblasts had higher adhesion strengths than ACL fibroblasts in RPMI medium. These results can be reversed under Dulbecco's modified Eagle's (DME) medium (29). The adhesion strength of the ACL and MCL fibroblasts was normalized to cell adhesion area. The MCL fibroblasts showed an increase in normalized force after 45 minutes, however,

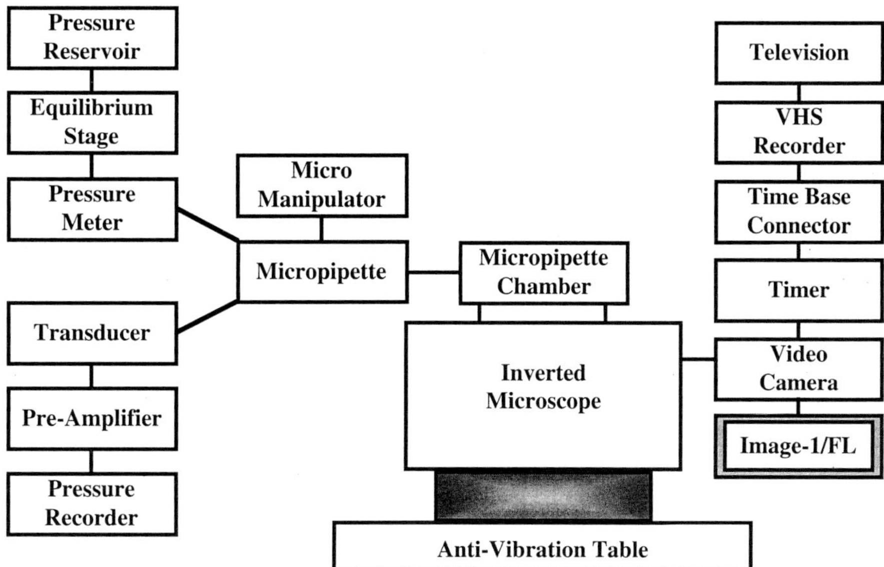

FIGURE 12.2. Schematic drawing of micropipette and micromanipulator system for single-cell adhesion study. The system is composed of four parts: (i) pressure regulator system to provided accurate pressure (fraction of millimeter hydraulic pressure) applied to single cells; (ii) pressure recording system to provided time-based recording of small pressure; (iii) micropipette and micromanipulator system linked to inverted microscope to study single cell under high magnification; and (iv) video recording system, which allows us to dynamically record all experiment events and can be linked to a computer for image analysis.

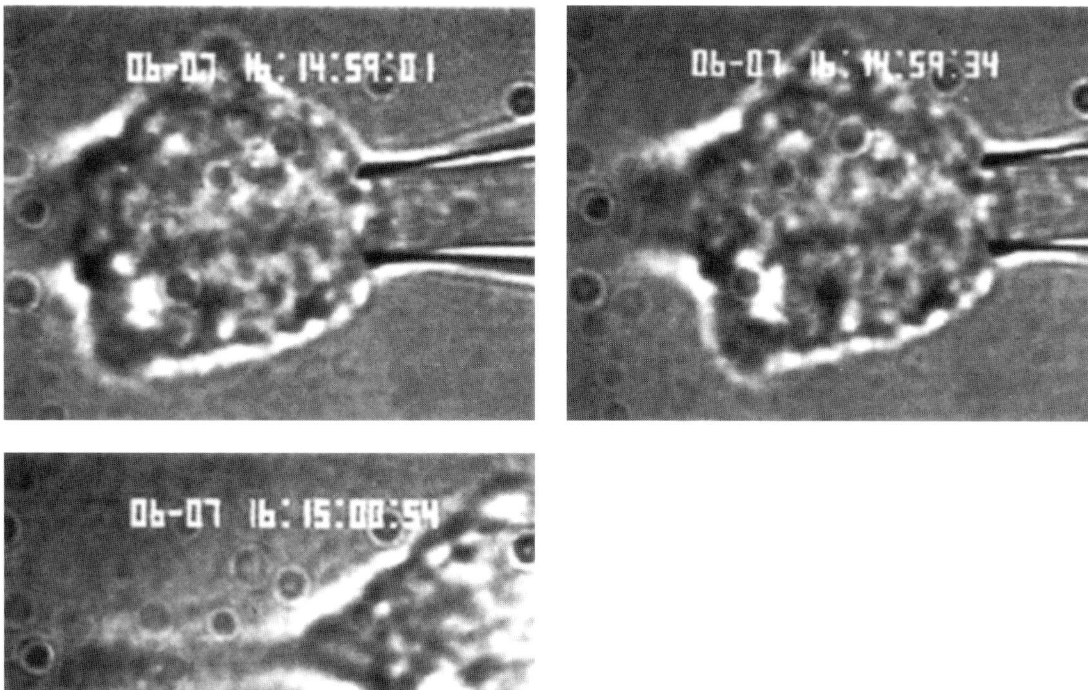

FIGURE 12.3. Sequential pictures showing cell adhesion force measurement by separating a human anterior cruciate ligament (ACL) fibroblast from a coverglass precoated with fibronectin (5 µg/mL) using a micropipette (tip radius, ~2.5 µm).

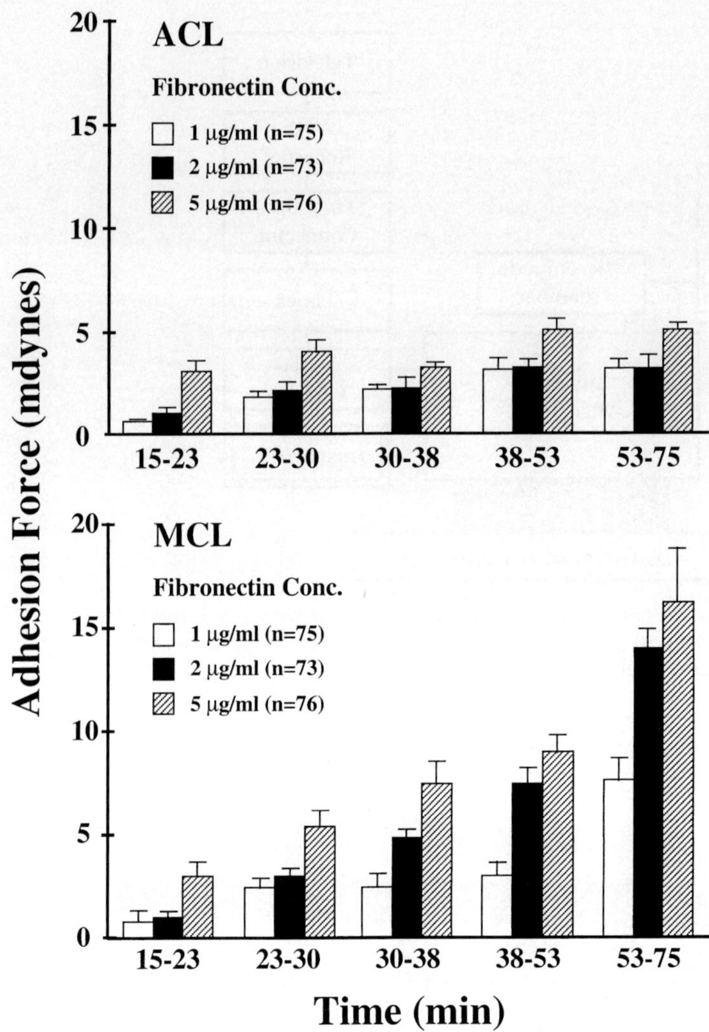

FIGURE 12.4. Adhesion forces of anterior cruciate ligament (ACL) and medial collateral ligament (MCL) fibroblasts to fibronectin (FN). Measurements were taken at variable FN concentrations and seeding times.

the ACL fibroblasts showed no change in normalized adhesion force throughout the time course of the experiment (Fig. 12.5).

Adhesiveness of Human Ligament Fibroblasts to Laminin

This session focused on the intrinsic differences between ACL and MCL fibroblasts with regard to their adhesion properties to laminin, one of the major adhesive macromolecules that make up the extracellular matrix. The adhesion strength of ACL fibroblasts to laminin varied from 0.59 to 3.8 times greater than from MCL fibroblasts ($p < 0.0001$), depending on the laminin concentration (Table 12.1). ACL fibroblasts also exhibited a laminin concentration dependent increase in adhesion strength up to 30 µg/mL where the laminin receptors were thought to be saturated. MCL fibroblasts did not show a laminin concentration-dependent increase in adhesion strength except between 5 and 10 µg/mL laminin (Table 12.1). There was no significant difference in adhesion area between ACL and MCL fibrob-

lasts except after 45 minutes at a laminin concentration of 40 µg/mL ($p < 0.05$). Adhesion strength (normalized by adhesion area) had no correlation to seeding time ($r^2 < 0.15$) for both ACL and MCL fibroblasts (results not shown). Taking into account all times, however, normalized adhesion strength for ACL fibroblasts was approximately two to three times higher and significantly different ($p < 0.0001$) than MCL fibroblasts (20 to 80 µg/mL laminin). Although ACL and MCL fibroblasts behaved similarly in their adhesion to laminin in many ways, it can be concluded from this study that the ACL fibroblasts adhere much stronger to laminin when compared with MCL fibroblasts.

Signal Pathway Studies

Cyclic Adenosine Monophosphate Pathway

Pertussis toxin (Calbiochem, San Diego, CA) made by the bacterium that causes whooping cough, was used as a potent inhibitor of the inhibitory G protein (Gi-protein). Pertussis toxin works by maintaining high levels of cyclic

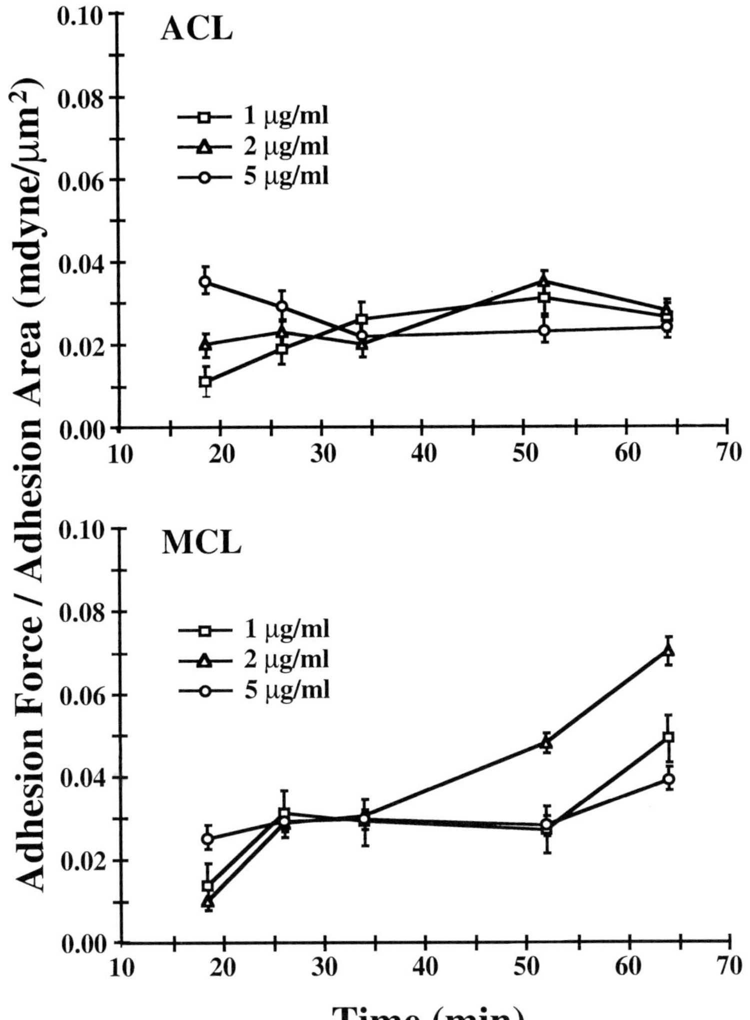

FIGURE 12.5. Adhesion force normalized to apparent adhesion area. Comparison between anterior cruciate ligament (ACL) and medial collateral ligament (MCL) fibroblasts for the three different concentrations of fibronectin (FN). The normalized force for MCL cells increased after 50 minutes compared with other periods, whereas the normalized force for ACL cells stayed constant for each time. This cell behavior difference between ACL and MCL fibroblasts after interaction with FN could be due to their intrinsic characteristics.

adenosine monophosphate (cAMP) by adenosine diphosphate (ADP)–ribosylating the α-subunit (Giα) of the Gi-protein complex (30). KT5720 (Calbiochem) was used as a selective and potent inhibitor of PKA (protein kinase A) (31,32). KT5823 (Calbiochem) was used to selectively inhibit PKG (protein kinase G) (7).

Ca²⁺/Phospholipid Pathway

Neomycin (Calbiochem), a common antibiotic that binds to inositol phospholipids and inhibits their metabolism, synthesis, and degradation, was used as an inhibitor of PLC (phospholipase C) (33,34). Polymyxin B (Cal-

TABLE 12.1. Adhesion force (mean ± SEM) of ligament fibroblasts to laminin-coated surface

Laminin concentration[a] (µg/mL)	Adhesion force (mdyne)		Mean ratio of ACL/MCL
	ACL fibroblast	MCL fibroblast	
5	0.57 ± 0.0027	0.96 ± 0.0099	0.59
10	5.83 ± 0.17	4.59 ± 0.036	1.27
20	7.07 ± 0.059	3.06 ± 0.026	2.31
30	14.58 ± 0.081	6.35 ± 0.040	2.30
40	14.05 ± 0.079	3.68 ± 0.035	3.82
80	15.37 ± 0.079	6.38 ± 0.055	2.41

ACL, anterior cruciate ligament; MCL, medial collateral ligament.
[a]For each concentration, laminin was layered onto a coat of poly-D-lysine (2 µg/mL).

biochem) was used as a selective inhibitor of PKC (protein kinase C) (35–38). Chlorpromazine (Calbiochem), a calmodulin antagonist, was used to inhibit the calmodulin stimulation of cyclic nucleotide phosphodiesterase (39). Individual signal pathway–inhibiting drugs were added directly from a concentrated stock to the cell suspension according to the following working concentrations determined from inhibitory concentrations in the literature (7, 30–39): pertussis toxin (10 nM), KT5720 (50 nM), KT5823 (0.2 μM), neomycin (1 mg/mL), polymyxin B (10 μM), and chlorpromazine (10 μM). Cells were incubated at 37°C with the inhibiting agents for up to 60 minutes (up to 3 hours for neomycin) before loading them into the micropipette chamber. Incubation times were based on signal pathway and protein activation times found in the literature (7, 30–42). Controls (without agents) were run simultaneously with each agent treatment.

Chemical Perturbation

The effects of IP$_3$ (inositol 1,4,5-triphosphate) in its signal pathway were mimicked by the addition of pharmacologic agents to healthy cells affecting intracellular free calcium concentration ([Ca^{2+}]$_i$) The calcium ionophore, A23187 (Molecular Probes, Eugene, OR), was used to increase [Ca^{2+}]$_i$ by causing Ca^{2+} to move into the cytosol from the extracellular medium (43). BAPTA (Molecular Probes), an intracellular calcium chelator, was used to mimic an inhibition of the IP$_3$ pathway and decrease the available intracellular free calcium (44). A23187 was added directly to the cell suspension (at a working concentration of 10 nM) and incubated at 37°C (5% CO$_2$) for 30 minutes before seeding the micropipette chamber. Conversely, BAPTA was loaded into the cells using its acetoxymethyl (AM) ester, BAPTA-AM, according to the following protocol. Stock BAPTA within dimethyl sulfoxide (DMSO; Sigma, St. Louis, MO) at 10 mM concentration was stored in prealiquoted portions at −20°C. When ready

for use, the BAPTA was transferred into a nonionic detergent (mixture of 3:1 ratio by weight DMSO and low-toxicity dispersion agent Pluronic F-127; Molecular Probes) to facilitate cell loading. BAPTA was then added to the cell suspension (at a working concentration of 25 μM) and incubated at 37°C (5% CO$_2$) for 60 minutes before seeding the micropipette chamber. A23187 and BAPTA working concentrations and incubation times were based on literature findings (43,44).

Fluorescent Microscopy

Video microscopy and a quantitative fluorescence system were used to measure fluctuations in [Ca^{2+}]$_i$ of ACL and MCL fibroblasts seeded onto a monolayer of FN for 60 minutes. Details of the technique are presented in recent articles from this laboratory (45–47).

Signal Pathway Dependence in Ligament Fibroblast Adhesion

The influence of signal pathways involved in the adhesion of ACL and MCL fibroblasts to fibronectin was investigated. Specific emphasis was made on the cAMP and Ca^{2+}/phospholipid pathways to determine the signaling mediated by integrin receptors during cell binding and spreading on a fibronectin-coated glass surface. Individual cell adhesion strengths were determined after treating cells with signal pathway–inhibiting agents. MCL fibroblast adhesion was significantly reduced by Gi-protein, PKA, PKC, PKG, PLC, and calmodulin-inhibiting agents, suggesting a crucial role of cAMP and Ca^{2+}/phospholipid signaling in MCL fibroblast integrin-mediated adhesion. Conversely, ACL fibroblast adhesion was only reduced by a PKC-inhibiting agent and increased by PKA, PKG, and calmodulin-inhibiting agents, suggesting only a partial role of Ca^{2+}/phospholipid signaling in ACL fibroblast integrin-mediated adhesion (Tables 12.2 and 12.3).

TABLE 12.2. *Adhesion force (mean ± SEM) of ligament fibroblasts to 5 μg/mL fibronectin-coated surface under the influence of cAMP pathway-inhibiting agents*

cAMP pathway-inhibiting agents	Adhesion force (mdyne)	
	ACL fibroblast	MCL fibroblast
Control	12.08 ± 1.00	7.80 ± 0.07
Pertussis toxin[a]	12.30 ± 1.05	5.50 ± 0.60[d]
KT5720[b]	16.00 ± 2.05[d]	5.50 ± 0.95[d]
KT5823[c]	15.00 ± 2.00[d]	4.75 ± 0.90[d]

ACL, anterior cruciate ligament; MCL, medial collateral ligament; cAMP, cyclic adenosine monophosphate.
[a]Inhibitory G protein (G$_1$ protein) inhibitor.
[b]Protein kinase A inhibitor.
[c]Protein kinase G inhibitor.
[d]Significant difference with respect to control ($p < 0.05$).

TABLE 12.3. *Adhesion force (mean ± SEM) of ligament fibroblasts to 5 µg/mL fibronectin-coated surface under the influence of Ca^{2+}/phospholipid pathway–inhibiting agents*

Ca²⁺/phospholipid pathway–inhibiting agents	Adhesion force (mdyne)	
	ACL fibroblast	MCL fibroblast
Control	12.02 ± 2.11	7.70 ± 0.09
Neomycin[a]	10.95 ± 2.33	5.95 ± 0.10[d]
Polymyxin B[b]	7.20 ± 0.15[d]	4.97 ± 0.05[d]
Chlorpromazine[c]	14.00 ± 2.40[d]	5.05 ± 0.01[d]

ACL, anterior cruciate ligament; MCL, medial collateral ligament.
[a]Phospholipase C inhibitor.
[b]Protein kinase C inhibitor.
[c]Calmodulin antagonist.
[d]Significant difference with respect to control ($p < 0.05$).

Based on additional parallel studies on the role of intracellular calcium in integrin-mediated adhesion, MCL fibroblast adhesion was calcium-dependent, whereas ACL fibroblast adhesion was less sensitive to calcium fluctuations throughout the 60-minute time course of adhesion experiments. Both ACL and MCL fibroblasts had reduced adhesion on incubating cells with BAPTA, a calcium chelator. Likewise, both ACL and MCL fibroblasts showed a significant increase in adhesion with increased calcium after incubation with A23187, a calcium ionophore (Fig. 12.6). For both BAPTA and A23187 treatments, MCL fibroblast adhesion was more affected by calcium fluctuations than ACL fibroblast adhesion.

Microfilament- and Microtubule-Disrupting Agents and Treatment Studies

Actin-Filament–Disrupting Agent

Actin-filament–disrupting agent, cytochalasin D (CD) (48), and the microtubule disrupting agent, colchicine (CC) (49), were obtained from Sigma. CD and CC were used at final concentrations of 0.5 and 0.1 µM, respectively, sufficient to inhibit cytoskeletal assembly within the time course of our experiments. Experimental details are described in recent articles (48). This treatment is intended to elucidate the effects of actin-filament– and microtubule-disrupting agents before and after the formation of stress fibers and adhesion plaques during cell

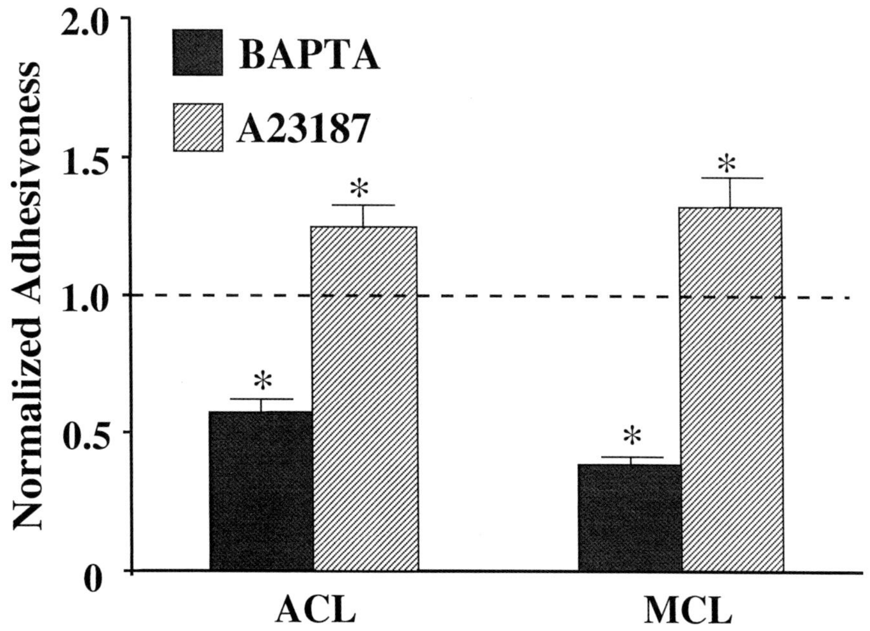

FIGURE 12.6. Effect of intracellular free calcium on the adhesion of anterior cruciate ligament (ACL) and medial collateral ligament (MCL) fibroblasts to 5 µg/mL fibronectin. The calcium ionophore A23187 was used to increase the intracellular calcium, and the calcium chelator BAPTA was used to decrease the available intracellular free calcium. Values equal force ± SEM normalized to a control (*dotted line*). *Asterisk* represents significant difference with respect to control ($p < 0.05$).

attachment and spreading. Control experiments were conducted without any agent.

Electroporation Technique

Electroporation (50) was used to deliver tropomodulin (Tmod) (25 and 50 µg/mL) and monoclonal antibodies (mAbs) against Tmod (mAb Tmod-204, 25 and 50 µg/mL), talin (200 and 385 µg/mL), vinculin (30 and 100 µg/mL), and α-actinin (50 and 100 µg/mL) into fibroblasts. The mAbs against talin, vinculin, and α-actinin were anti-human antibodies from mouse ascites fluid (Sigma) and mAbs to Tmod and albumin (control mAb) were rabbit antihuman mAbs. Antibody concentrations were chosen based on reports in the literature (51–56). Electroporation was accomplished by using a T820 electroporation system (BTX, San Diego, CA) with a setting (1 pulse, 99 µsec pulse length, 300 V) that yields 90% cell viability (trypan blue exclusion). Control cells were electroporated with nonspecific albumin (50 µg/mL, control for Tmod) or anti-albumin antibody (150 µg/mL, control for mAbs). A negative control in the absence of protein or antibody was used to monitor the nonspecific effects of the treatment. The cells were used 2 to 3 hours after electroporation, allowing time for the cells to recover and for the exogenous proteins or mAbs to bind.

Effect of Cytoskeleton Integrity on Ligament Fibroblast Adhesion Strength

This study focused on using fibroblasts to demonstrate that cellular adhesion to FN involving integrins requires an intact cytoskeleton, especially the integrity of actin filaments, microtubules, actin-filament pointed-end capping protein (tropomodulin), and actin-filament/integrin bridging proteins (talin, vinculin, and α-actinin). ACL and MCL cell adhesions were affected differently after delivering exogenous tropomodulin and its antibody intracellularly. Monoclonal antibody antitropomodulin (50 µg/mL) significantly reduced MCL cell adhesion by 19% ($p < 0.002$), but had no effect on ACL cell adhesion (Table 12.4). Less-concentrated antitropomodulin (25 µg/mL) was unable to affect either ACL or MCL cell adhesion (Table 12.4). ACL cells electroporated with tropomodulin had a decrease in adhesion strength of 30% with respect to controls (25 and 50 µg/mL tropomodulin), whereas MCL cells showed a 79% increase in adhesion at the higher tropomodulin concentration of 50 µg/mL (Table 12.5). Prevention of actin filament bundle (stress fiber) formation using cytochalasin D (5×10^{-7} M) significantly reduced ACL and MCL fibroblast adhesion strength by 80% to 90%. However, after allowing fibroblast attachment to FN and the formation of stress fibers, cytochalasin D treatment was only able to significantly reduce the adhesion strength by approximately 30%. ACL and MCL fibroblast adhesion strength was significantly reduced by 20% and 29%, respectively, after incubating cells with 10^{-7} M colchicine (a microtubule disrupting agent) before cell attachment to FN. After fibroblasts were allowed to attach to FN, colchicine had a slightly smaller effect on MCL cells (23% reduction in adhesion strength), but had no effect on ACL cell adhesion (Fig. 12.7). The mAbs against talin, vinculin, and α-actinin were introduced intracellularly to bind to the bridging proteins that link the actin filaments to FN receptor molecules (integrins) within

TABLE 12.4. *Adhesion force (mean ± SEM) of ligament fibroblasts to 5 µg/mL fibronectin-coated surface normalized to control under the influence of antibodies against actin-associated proteins*

Antibody	Concentration (µg/mL)	Normalized adhesion force	
		ACL fibroblast	MCL fibroblast
Tmod	25	0.92 ± 0.06	1.01 ± 0.08
	50	0.89 ± 0.09	0.81 ± 0.06[a]
Talin	200	0.90 ± 0.07	0.69 ± 0.07[a]
	385	0.71 ± 0.10[a]	0.80 ± 0.07[a]
Vinculin	30	0.54 ± 0.01[a]	0.89 ± 0.04
	100	0.52 ± 0.05[a]	0.80 ± 0.08[a]
α-actinin	50	0.65 ± 0.02[a]	0.98 ± 0.11
	100	0.64 ± 0.03[a]	0.62 ± 0.04[a]

ACL, anterior cruciate ligament; MCL, medial collateral ligament; Tmod, tropomodulin.
Antialbumin at 150 µg/mL was used in the control group.
[a]Significant difference with respect to control ($p < 0.05$).

TABLE 12.5. *Adhesion force (mean ± SEM) of ligament fibroblasts to 5 µg/mL fibronectin-coated surface under the influence of tropomodulin*

	Adhesion force (mdyne)	
Treatment	ACL fibroblast	MCL fibroblast
Tmod (25 µg/mL)	12.08 ± 1.00	7.80 ± 0.07
Tmod (50 µg/mL)	12.30 ± 1.05	5.50 ± 0.60[a]

ACL, anterior cruciate ligament; MCL, medial collateral ligament; Tmod, tropomodulin.
[a]Significant difference with respect to control ($p < 0.05$).

the plasma membrane. Adhesion strength of ACL fibroblasts was significantly reduced by antitalin (29% reduction), antivinculin (48% reduction), and anti–α-actinin (36% reduction), whereas MCL fibroblast adhesion was only significantly reduced by antitalin (20% reduction) (Table 12.4).

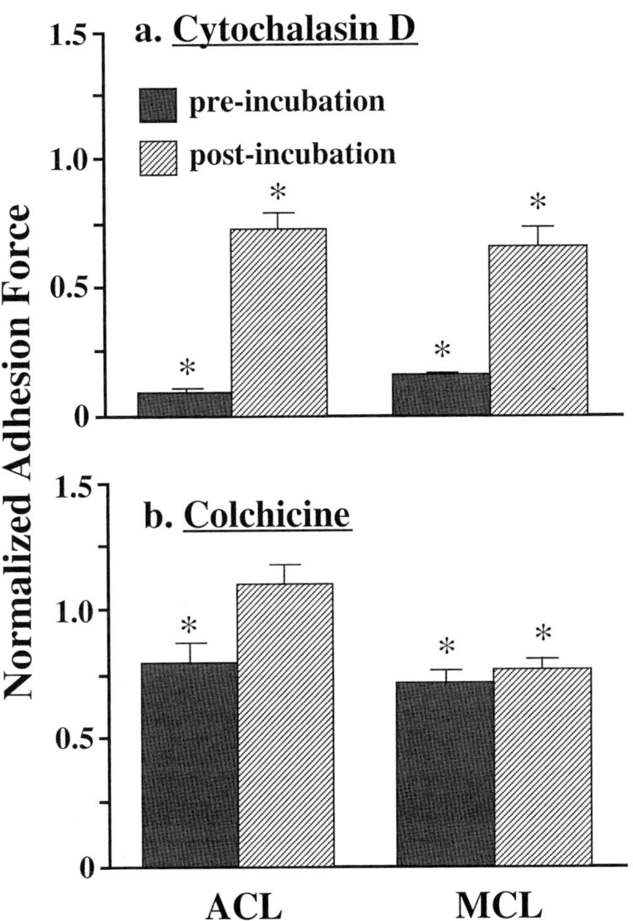

FIGURE 12.7. Effect of cytochalasin D (0.5 µM) and colchicine (0.1 µM) on the adhesion of anterior cruciate ligament (ACL) and medial collateral ligament (MCL) fibroblasts to a fibronectin-coated (5 µg/mL) surface. Cytochalasin D is an actin-filament–disrupting agent, whereas colchicine is a microtubule-disrupting agent. Values equal force ± SEM normalized to a control without reagent treatment. *Asterisk* represents significant difference with respect to control ($p < 0.05$).

INFLUENCES OF MECHANICAL STRETCH ON LIGAMENT FIBROBLASTS

Mechanical forces have long been recognized as one of the factors that govern behavior in biologic tissues. Original studies that examined the effects of mechanical forces were based on hypotheses generated from macroscopic observations of the responses of particular tissues to external physical stimuli (57). As such, most of the earlier investigations focused on bone in their experiments because this was the most intuitively obvious tissue that was dependent on mechanical forces. With the progression of studies in this area, scientists began to realize the role that mechanical stimuli had in all living tissue, and, thus, the scope of these investigations broadened to a variety of tissues including blood vessels, muscle, heart, kidney, lungs, and ligaments. Once thought of as being passive structures, knee ligament tissue was soon recognized as being capable of responding to mechanical stimuli and that tissue function may be dependent on these mechanical factors (58–64).

On the modulation of structural characteristics during remodeling and repair of knee ligament tissue by mechanical forces, several studies used animal models to study the shielding of stresses from ligaments by immobilization of joints and subsequently analyzing the structure and properties of ligament tissue over a period of time (65–71). Although these studies were able to use elegant systems to study the response of ligament tissue to stretch, the influences of mechanical strains, or lack thereof, on the fibroblasts themselves could not be determined directly. In addition, strains imposed on the tissue were not well characterized and could not be controlled. While these experiments reveal the pathologic effects of removing mechanical stimulation to ligament tissue, they do not show how the tissue responds to mechanical strain. More recently, deformable substrates have become widely used as means to apply mechanical strains to cell monolayers *in vitro* (72–75). Although earlier studies using this technique applied strains that were not well characterized, apparatuses have been designed to apply static homogeneous well-defined strains over the entire substrate (76); thus, all cells in the monolayer were subjected to the same magnitudes and directions of strain. Further evolution of these devices brought the ability to apply customized dynamic strains to the deformable substrate using either mechanical or pneumatic means (77,78). Such advances have allowed the study of the role of mechanical stresses on cells in a much more carefully controlled environment.

Although deformable substrates have been used extensively to apply mechanical strains to cell monolayers in other cell types, their use in ligament fibroblast studies has been very limited. Aside from our group, the only other reported investigation applying mechanical strains to knee ligament fibroblasts was by Bhargava and Hannafin (79). In their flow cytometric studies performed on ACL and MCL fibroblast monolayers, they demonstrated that integrin receptors on the surface of cell membranes were differentially expressed during mechanical strain application depending on the protein coating of the elastomer substrate.

METHODS AND RESULTS

Cyclic Strain and Northern Blot of Type I and III Collagen Genes

This section concentrates on the expression of genes encoding the extracellular matrix proteins type I collagen and type III collagen for two different amplitudes of strain at various time points during a continuous dynamic strain regimen (80). Type I collagen is the predominant protein of ligament tissue, making up approximately 90% of the dry weight, and type III collagen is also present in ligaments but has been found to be more involved in healing and remodeling processes (81,82). Because there is still a lack of information on how ligament tissue strengthens and remodels, this study serves as a first step toward determining the mechanisms that may be involved in strain-mediated events in knee ligaments and could provide insight into the basis of the healing differential between the ACL and MCL.

Cyclic Strain

Cells were trypsinized and seeded into type I collagen–coated 6-well BioFlex plates (Flexcell International, McKeesport, PA), which possess elastomer membrane bottoms. These BioFlex plates were specially designed for use in dynamic mechanical strain application in the Flexercell Strain Unit (Flexcell International). Using computer-controlled vacuum pressure, flex plates were deformed to apply precalibrated strains to the elastomer membranes by pulling the membranes over a lubricated polymer platen. Such a setup allows strains over most of the membrane area to be equibiaxial. Following a 24-hour serum-starvation period, cell monolayers were strained using a sinusoidal strain profile at 1 Hz (60 cycles/min) with 5% and 7.5% strain amplitudes for 0.5, 1, 2, 4, 16, and 24 hours. Unstrained controls consisted of cell monolayers cultured simultaneously in identical Flex plates under the same conditions, but not subjected to substrate deformation. All conditions were performed in triplicate for each cell type (n = 3) using cells from a different patient for each repetition. Relative changes in the levels of messenger RNA (mRNA) were assessed by Northern blot analysis. After autoradiography, intensity of bands was quantified by National Institutes of Health (NIH) (Bethesda, MD) Image software. Intensities of types I and III collagens were normalized with the housekeeping gene *GAPDH* to account for loading differences, and

then normalized with respect to unstretched controls to obtain a percent change relative to control.

Type I and III Collagen Gene Expression Under Cyclic Strain

For 5% strain magnitudes, type I collagen mRNA levels increased for ACL fibroblasts at 2 and 24 hours, whereas only the 24-hour group was statistically significant. Conversely, MCL fibroblasts exhibited statistically significant decreases in type I collagen mRNA for the 24-hour stimulation period (Fig. 12.8). Type III collagen showed similar trends for ACL and different trends for MCL fibroblasts. MCL fibroblasts demonstrated increases in expression of type III collagen mRNA that were statistically significant in both 2- and 24-hour time groups compared with controls; however, statistically significant increases in ACL fibroblasts were seen only at 24 hours (Fig. 12.9). These increases in ACL fibroblasts were much more modest compared with MCL fibroblasts.

For 7.5% strain amplitudes, type I collagen mRNA levels increased to statistically significant levels at 24 hours for ACL fibroblasts, whereas for MCL fibroblasts, there was no significant change in type I collagen expression for 2 or 24 hours compared with control (Fig. 12.10). Type III collagen did not change significantly for ACL fibroblasts, but MCL fibroblasts exhibited increases that were statistically significant for 2 and 24 hours (Fig. 12.11).

The results that were found indicate very different profiles of expression for genes encoding types I and III collagens between ACL and MCL fibroblasts. Whereas dynamic mechanical strains resulted in increases in mRNA levels of type I collagen in ACL fibroblasts, there was a decrease in type I collagen mRNA in MCL fibroblasts. Type III collagen mRNA levels, on the other hand, increased to a greater extent in MCL fibroblasts than in ACL fibroblasts.

Previous studies using rabbit MCL (65,83) found that all ligaments require the bridging of scar tissue, which is predominantly composed of type III collagen, for adequate healing. We can infer that the initial expression of type III collagen is crucial to this process and that the overexpression of type I collagen may not be as useful during the early stages of ligament healing. In addition, the influence of tension on ligament healing has also been studied. One report (84) demonstrated the enhanced formation of scar tissue when rabbit MCL wound sites were subjected to constant tension. Tension is believed to act as an environmental cue for reparative callus formation (85). These phenomena suggest that early mobilization of ligament repairs would serve to aid in the formation of bridging scar tissue and promote healing in ligaments. Because the MCL exhibits increased type III collagen expression, the ability of the ligament to heal adequately,

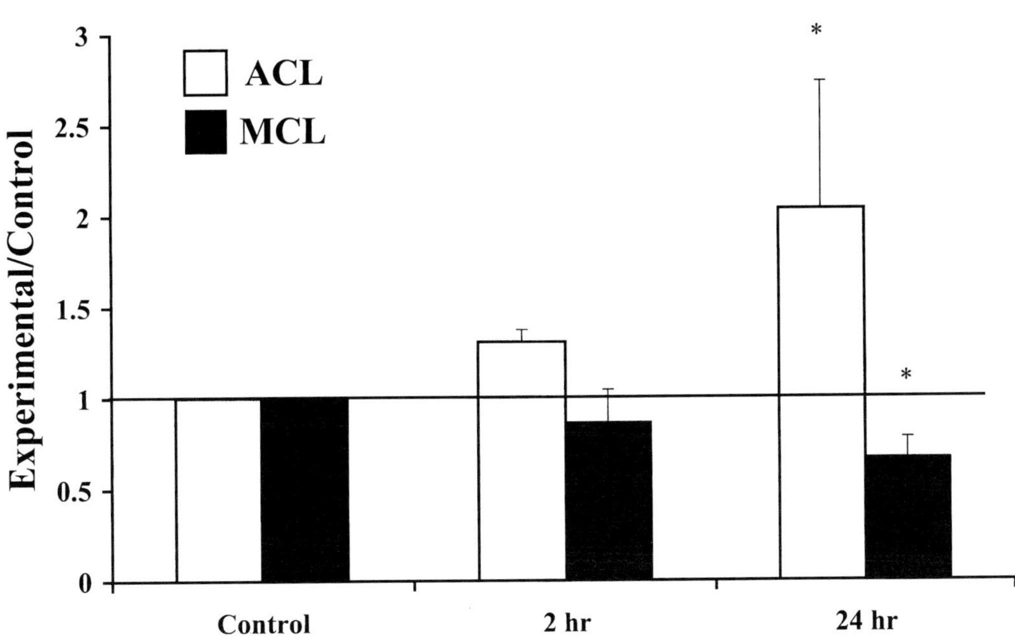

FIGURE 12.8. Expression of type I collagen in anterior cruciate ligament (ACL) and medial collateral ligament (MCL) fibroblast monolayers subjected to 5% strains at a frequency of 1 Hz. Quantification of Northern blot analysis was performed by measurement of band intensities. Values represent intensities of type I collagen bands normalized by their respective GAPDH bands. Each sample was then normalized with control. *Asterisk* represents statistically significant differences ($p < 0.05$; n = 3) of individual time groups compared with control samples. Error bars represent SEM.

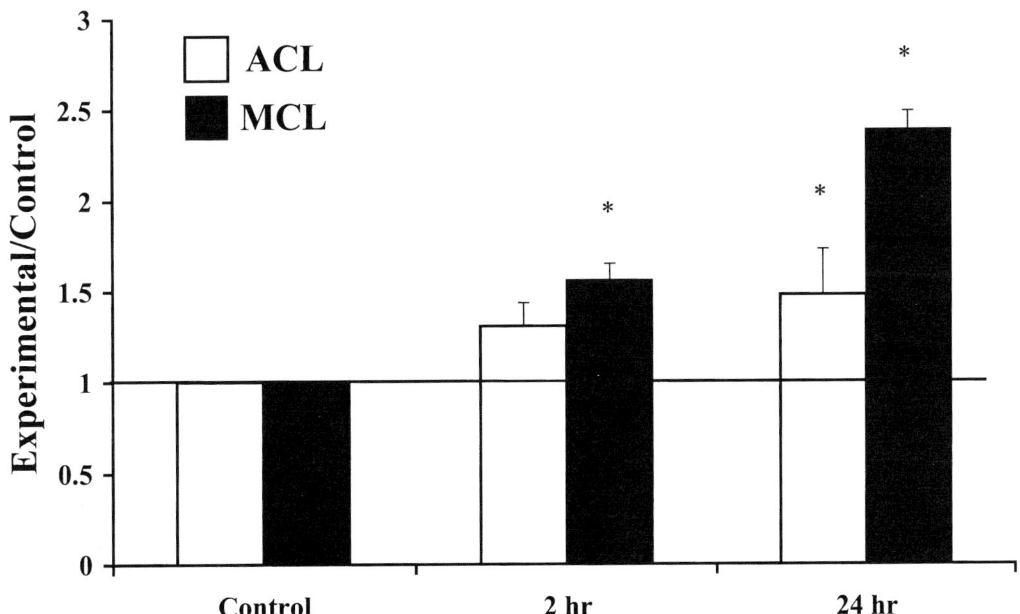

FIGURE 12.9. Expression of type III collagen in anterior cruciate ligament (ACL) and medial collateral ligament (MCL) fibroblast monolayers subjected to 5% strains at a frequency of 1 Hz. Quantification of Northern blot analysis was performed by measurement of band intensities. Values represent intensities of type III collagen bands normalized by their respective GAPDH bands. Each sample was then normalized with control. *Asterisk* represents statistically significant differences ($p < 0.05$; n = 3) of individual time groups compared with control samples. Error bars represent SEM.

Type I Collagen - 7.5% Strains

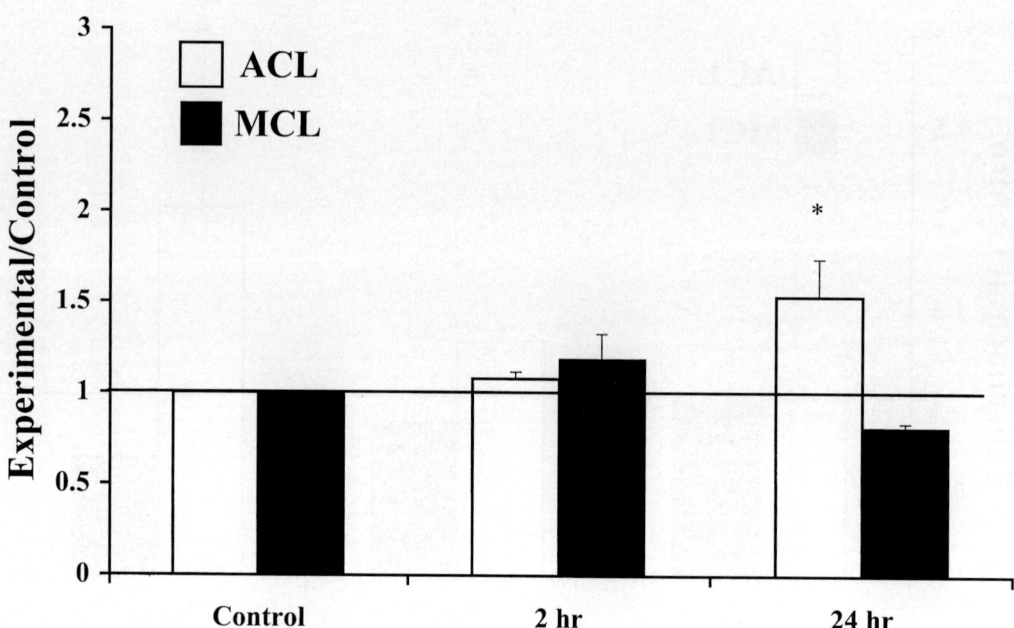

FIGURE 12.10. Expression of type I collagen in anterior cruciate ligament (ACL) and medial collateral ligament (MCL) fibroblast monolayers subjected to 7.5% strains at a frequency of 1 Hz. Quantification of Northern blot analysis was performed by measurement of band intensities. Values represent intensities of type I collagen bands normalized by their respective GAPDH bands. Each sample was then normalized with control. *Asterisk* represents statistically significant differences ($p < 0.05$; n = 3) of individual time groups compared with control samples. Error bars represent SEM.

Type III Collagen - 7.5% Strains

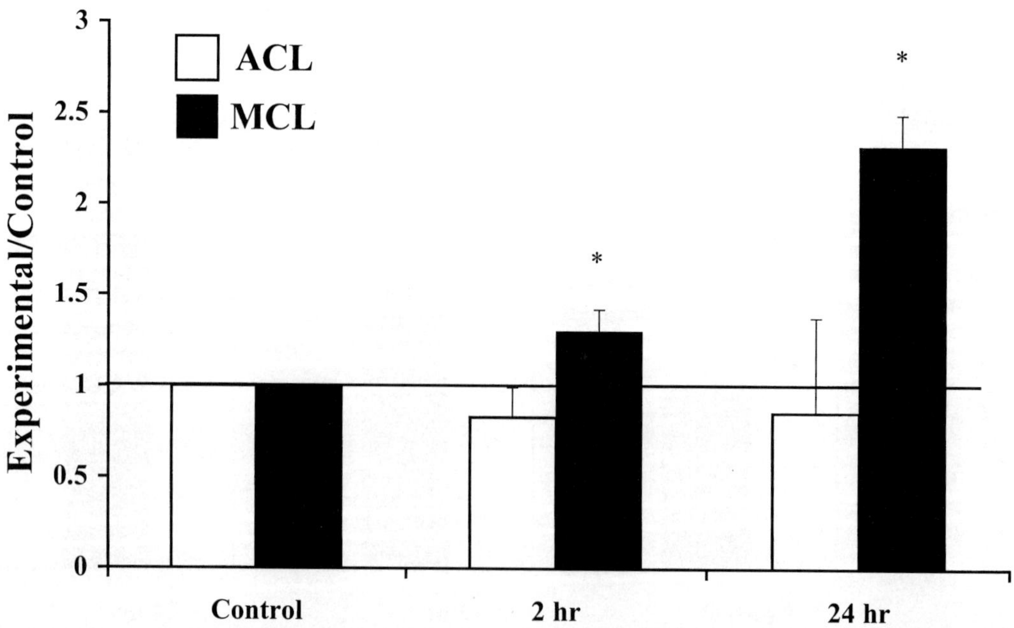

FIGURE 12.11. Expression of type III collagen in anterior cruciate ligament (ACL) and medial collateral ligament (MCL) fibroblast monolayers subjected to 7.5% strains at a frequency of 1 Hz. Quantification of Northern blot analysis was performed by measurement of band intensities. Values represent intensities of type III collagen bands normalized by their respective GAPDH bands. Each sample was then normalized with control. *Asterisk* represents statistically significant differences ($p < 0.05$; n = 3) of individual time groups compared with control samples. Error bars represent SEM.

albeit slowly, after injury and repair does not appear to be too surprising.

DISCUSSION

This chapter describes experiments performed to investigate the intrinsic differences that exist between ACL and MCL fibroblasts that can aid the understanding of the ACL and MCL healing differential. The following cell properties were studied: (a) the adhesion strength of ligament fibroblasts to fibronectin and laminin, (b) the signal pathway dependence of ligament fibroblast adhesion, (c) the effects of cytoskeletal integrity on ligament fibroblast adhesion, and (d) the effects of mechanical stimuli on ligament fibroblasts. The large amount of data and results generated from these properties are discussed in the following five sections.

Adhesion Strength of Human Ligament Fibroblasts to Fibronectin

This study revealed an additional intrinsic difference between ACL and MCL fibroblasts and showed that intrinsic differences in cellular adhesion can be determined by using the micropipette technique. Greater adhesion to FN seen in MCL fibroblasts compared with ACL fibroblasts may account for the normal migration of fibroblasts into the ligament rupture site during granulation tissue formation of ligament healing. Results indicated that cell adhesiveness depends on matrix concentration and fibroblast seeding time.

We also found that the intracellular free calcium levels in MCL fibroblasts change during cell adhesion processes. From our previous study (86), the fluorescence calcium imaging experiments revealed interesting results concerning the change in intracellular calcium upon cell binding to FN. The results indicated that after approximately 12 minutes of seeding to an FN-coated glass surface, the ACL free intracellular calcium level of ~70 nM stayed constant up to the 60-minute seeding time. However, the cytosolic free calcium in MCL fibroblasts showed a 2.2-fold increase from approximately 22 minutes (~44 nM free calcium) to 43 minutes (~97 nM free calcium) after initial seeding. Therefore, the increase in MCL adhesion force may be due to an increase in intracellular calcium shown to occur after 45 minutes in MCL fibroblasts but not ACL fibroblasts.

Adhesiveness of Human Ligament Fibroblasts to Laminin

The results from animal studies have shown that there were no laminin receptors ($\alpha_6\beta_1$ integrin) on fibroblasts from the MCL and a relatively small number of receptors on fibroblasts from the ACL. The absence of a significant increase in adhesion force with increasing concentration,

adhesion strength, and adhesion area over the time course of the experiment for fibroblasts from the MCL indicates that the adhesion forces we were characterizing were nonspecific. This may relate directly with the notion that there were very few or no laminin receptors on fibroblasts from the MCL in humans. Because of the location of laminin in relation to the ACL and MCL *in vivo*, fibroblasts may not express as many laminin receptors (or any, as is the case for fibroblasts from the medial collateral ligament) as, for example, fibronectin receptors. This could be due to cellular adaptation to the environment (fibronectin molecules were in local contact with the ligaments and laminin molecules were located outside leaflet of the synovial sheath. The functional significance of adhesive property differences remains unclear, but the physiologic incongruities, which create these differences, need further study.

This study may prove useful in understanding ACL and MCL fibroblast adhesion to the basal lamina within the extracellular matrix and add insight into the natural healing process of the ACL and MCL. This study revealed an additional intrinsic difference between ACL and MCL fibroblast.

Signal Pathway Dependence in Ligament Fibroblast Adhesion

The regulation of cell signal pathways and the cellular response to the matrices were important for a number of tissue remodeling and healing events, including cell adhesion, migration, and proliferation. In the present study, we have shown that the signal pathway regulation of ACL cells is dramatically different to MCL cells in response to FN–integrin interaction during cell adhesion. In particular, (a) adhesion behavior of ACL and MCL fibroblasts was significantly different for all inhibiting agents except polymyxin B, which inhibits PKC. PKC has been shown previously to reduce focal adhesion to a FN surface and to markedly reduce stress fiber formation in fibroblasts (87); (b) ACL fibroblast adhesion was significantly increased by PKA, PKG, and calmodulin inhibiting agents while MCL fibroblast adhesion was reduced by PLC, PKA, PKC, PKG, Gi-protein and calmodulin inhibiting agents; and (c) both ACL and MCL fibroblast adhesion was dependent on sufficient intracellular calcium levels, but MCL cells were more dependent on intracellular calcium for normal adhesion than were ACL cells.

It is well understood that during tissue remodeling, which involves cell adhesion and migration, cells not only change their shape, but also redistribute their cytoskeletal proteins by way of polymerization, phosphorylation, and assemblage of cytoskeletal molecules. All these processes require cell communication with the ECM to direct its activities. These activities include triggering signal receptors and activating signal transduction pathways that convert the integrin receptor and ECM binding event into a cascade of intracellular signals and final protein phosphorylation.

Effect of Cytoskeleton Integrity on Ligament Fibroblast Adhesion Strength

Our studies have shown that the cytoskeletal proteins have striking effects on ACL and MCL cell adhesion and on the formation of stress fibers during cell spreading. A disruption in the cytoskeleton–integrin bridging proteins resulted in significantly reduced adhesion. The reduction in adhesion is most likely due to the reduced formation of stress fibers and cell attachment area seen in fibroblasts introduced with mAbs against talin, vinculin, and α-actinin.

By disrupting the assembly of actin filaments with CD, adhesion force can be drastically decreased by 80% to 90% when ACL and MCL cells were preincubated with the agent before cell attachment. A previous study strongly suggested the involvement of the cytoskeleton in the regulation of integrin-mediated cell adhesion after it was found that CD abolished chimeric receptor adhesion to immobilized fibrinogen (88). Therefore, the reduction in adhesion force observed in our experiments may be caused by a loss of adhesion function of the β_1-integrin receptor for FN. It is possible that this loss in function could stem from a conformational change in the integrin receptor brought on by the disruption in the association between the actin filaments of the cytoskeleton and the integrin receptor. Another possibility is that actin filaments were anchored to the integrin receptor by bridging proteins. The assembly of many actin filaments into stress fibers requires that the barbed ends of the actin filaments be anchored to the integrin receptors. This condensed area of integrin receptors and stress fibers is built up to form a functional adhesion plaque. Any disruption in stress fiber assembly will disrupt adhesion plaque formation. Microtubule assembly also appears to be an important factor in fibroblast adhesion to the FN molecule, but not as essential as actin filament assembly. This mechanism, however, is not completely understood yet.

The role of Tmod in ACL and MCL fibroblast adhesion is less clear. It is assumed that the capping of actin filaments at the pointed end (nonpreferred end of polymerization) with Tmod serves in accelerating the polymerization of actin filaments at the barbed end near the focal contacts. This allows for greater bundling of actin filaments into stress fibers, which, in turn, results in greater adhesion. Fibroblasts from the ACL, on the other hand, showed a much different effect of Tmod on adhesion behavior compared with that of MCL fibroblasts. This finding is consistent with past findings about the contrasting intrinsic properties between ACL and MCL fibroblasts in regards to their adhesion and migration

behavior (19,27,89) and also is consistent with new findings on intracellular differences.

We conclude that the cytoskeletal integrity contributes to the adhesiveness of ligament cells and that the loss of the integrity of their cytoskeletal apparatus leads to a reduction of their adhesion strength. In addition, integrins were able to transduce signals through cytoskeleton from the extracellular matrix to the cytoplasm and to the nucleus of the cell. Therefore, the cytoskeleton plays a particularly important role in ligament cells, which is the constant involvement in the remodeling process, requiring the translation of adhesion force and changes in the extracellular environment into internal biochemical signals which leads to the formation and remodeling of the ligament. The integrity of actin filament bundles plays an essential role in cellular adhesion based on our findings.

Effects of Mechanical Stimuli on Ligament Cell Gene Expression

The observation that type III collagen expression is deficient in ACL fibroblast monolayers at short time periods (2 hours) for 5% strains and especially under higher strains of 7.5% implies that unless carefully treated, the ACL may not provide enough of a response in type III collagen expression to form an adequate bridging scar tissue after injury. It is possible that at the injury site, instead of the normal progression of formation of scar tissue followed by remodeling of the scar, there were greater numbers of type I collagen molecules that were not being incorporated into the extracellular matrix, leading to a deficiency in ACL healing response.

The results of this study motivate the need for further in-depth studies on mechanisms that regulate mechanically induced changes in gene expression in ligament fibroblasts. The finding that type III collagen expression is augmented in MCL fibroblasts and deficient in ACL fibroblasts with mechanical strain supports the possibility that the ACL does not heal after injury because of inadequate scar formation.

SUMMARY

These studies represent only a portion of the potential avenues of research in the area of knee ligament healing. An understanding of the intrinsic characteristics of ligament fibroblasts is the first crucial step for the future development of methods both to compensate for dysfunctional healing responses and to accelerate existing healing processes in ligament tissue after injury. In addition to determining these cellular and molecular characteristics, efforts must be made to delve into the mechanisms that regulate these events. This next step will elucidate the signal pathways and the molecules involved so that, through the use of mechanical and biochemical stimuli, cellular processes can be orchestrated by scientists to direct healing processes toward a positive direction.

ACKNOWLEDGMENTS

The authors would like to thank John Kim for his technical assistance. This work was supported by NIH AR 14918 and OREF 59212A.

REFERENCES

1. Akeson WH, Woo SLY, Amiel D, et al. The biology ligaments. In: Hunter LY, Funk FJ, eds. *Rehabilitation of the injured knee*. St. Louis: CV Mosby, 1984;93–148.
2. Frogameni AD, Jackson DW, Simon TM. Collagen remodeling in ACL reconstruction (goat model). In: Jackson DW, Arnoczky SP, Frank CB, Woo SLY, Simon TM, eds. *The anterior cruciate ligament: current and future concepts*. New York: Raven Press, 1993;219–226.
3. McDevitt CA, Marcelino J. Adhesion macromolecules of the ligament: the molecular glues in wound healing. In: Jackson DW, Arnoczky SP, Frank CB, Woo SLY, Simon TM, eds. *The anterior cruciate ligament: current and future concepts*. New York: Raven Press, 1993:179–188.
4. Murphy PG, Frank CB, Hart DA. The cell biology of ligaments and ligament healing. In: Jackson DW, Arnoczky SP, Frank CB, Woo SLY, Simon TM, eds. *The anterior cruciate ligament: current and future concepts*. New York: Raven Press, 1993;165–177.
5. Woo SLY, Horibe S, Ohland KJ, et al. The response of ligaments to injury: healing of the collateral ligaments. In: Daniel D, Akeson W, O'Connor J, eds. *Knee ligaments: structure, function, injury, and repair*. New York: Raven Press, 1990:351–364.
6. Jackson DW. ACL reconstruction and substitutes (biologic). In: Jackson DW, Arnoczky SP, Frank CB, Woo SLY, Simon TM, eds. *The anterior cruciate ligament: current and future concepts*. New York: Raven Press, 1993:237.
7. Kase H, Iwahashi K, Nakanishi S, et al. K-252 compounds: novel and potent inhibitors or protein kinase C and cyclic nucleotide-dependent protein kinases. *Biochem Biophys Res Comm* 1987;142:436–440.
8. Barlow Y, Willoughby J. Pathophysiology of soft tissue repair. *Br Med Bull* 1992;48:698–711.
9. Arnoczky SP. Physiologic principles of ligament injuries and healing. In: Scott, WN, ed. *Ligament and extensor mechanism injuries of the knee: diagnosis and treatment*. St. Louis: CV Mosby, 1991:67–81.
10. O'Donoghue DH, Rockwood CA Jr. Repair of the anterior cruciate ligament in dogs. *J Bone Joint Surg Am* 1966;48:503–519.
11. Hefti FL, Kress I, Fasel J, et al. Healing of the transected anterior cruciate ligament in the rabbit. *J Bone Joint Surg Am* 1991;73:373–383.
12. O'Donoghue DH. An analysis of end results of surgical treatment of major injuries to the ligaments of the knee. *J Bone Joint Surg Am* 1955;37:1–13.
13. Amiel D, Billings E Jr, Akeson WH. Ligament structure, chemistry, and physiology. In: Daniel D, Akeson W, O'Connor J, eds. *Knee ligaments: structure, function, injury, and repair*. New York: Raven Press, 1990: 77–91.
14. Bray RC, Frank CB, Miniaci A. Structure and function of diathrodial joints. In: McGinty JB, ed. *Operative arthroscopy*. New York, Raven Press, 1991:79–123.
15. Sung KLP, Kwan M, Maldonado F, et al. Deformation, adhesion patterning and adhesion strength of ligament fibroblasts. *Proc Ann Fall Meeting Biomed Engin Soc* 1992;1:17.
16. Witkowski J, Yang L, Wood DJ, et al. Migration and healing of ligament cells under inflammatory conditions. *J Orthop Res* 1997;15:269–277.
17. Mow VC, Hayes WC. *Basic orthopaedic biomechanics*. New York: Raven Press, 1991.
18. Geiger MH, Green MH, Monosov A, et al. An *in vitro* assay of anterior cruciate ligament (ACL) and medial collateral ligament (MCL) cell migration. *Connective Tiss Res* 1994;30:215–224.
19. Nagineni CN, Amiel D, Green MH, et al. Characterization of the intrinsic properties of the anterior cruciate and medial collateral ligament cells: an *in vitro* cell culture study. *J Orthop Res* 1992;10:465–475.
20. Schmidt CC, Georgescu HI, Kwoh CK, et al. Effect of growth factors on the proliferation of fibroblasts from the medial collateral and anterior cruciate ligaments. *J Orthop Res* 1995;13:184–190.
21. Holzmann B, McIntyre BW, Weissman IL. Identification of a murine Peyer's patch-specific lymphocyte homing receptor as an integrin molecule with an alpha chain homologous to human VLA-4 alpha. *Cell* 1989; 56:37–46.
22. Hynes RO. Integrins: a family of cell surface receptors. *Cell* 1987;48: 549–554.
23. Luna EJ, Hitt AL. Cytoskeleton-plasma membrane interactions. *Science* 1992;258:955–964.
24. Ruoslahti E. Fibronectin and its receptor. *Ann Rev Biochem* 1988;57: 375–413.
25. Sung KLP, Yang L, Whittemore DE, et al. The differential adhesion forces of anterior cruciate and medial collateral ligament fibroblasts: effects of tropomodulin, talin, vinculin, and α-actinin. *Proc Natl Acad Sci U S A* 1996;93:9182–9187.
26. Kato G, Wakabayashi K. Effect of polylysine-bound laminin on human retinoblastoma cell lines. *In Vitro Cell and Develop Biol* 1988;24: 274–280.
27. Sung KLP, Kwan MK, Akeson WH. Adhesion strength of human ligament fibroblasts. *J Biomech Engin* 1994;116:237–242.
28. Sung KLP, Sung LA, Crimmins M, et al. Determination of junction avidity of cytolytic T-cell and target cell. *Science* 1986;234:1405–1408.
29. Yang L, Tsai CMH, Kwon SY, et al. Ligament cell adhesiveness and repairing in vitro under inflammatory conditions. *Cells Materials* 1998;8:183–197.
30. Pirotton S, Erneux C, Boeynaems JM. Dual role of GTP-binding proteins in the control of endothelial prostacyclin. *Biochem Biophys Res Comm* 1987;47:1113–1120.
31. Guidry C. Fibroblast contraction of collagen gels requires activation of protein kinase C. *J Cell Physiol* 1993;15:358–367.
32. Irie K, Tokuda H, Hagiwara N, et al. Structure-activity relationship in the induction of Epstein–Barr virus by teleocidin derivatives. *Int J Cancer* 1985;36:485–488.
33. McDonald LJ, Mamrack MD. Phosphoinositide hydrolysis by phospholipase C modulated by multivalent cations La(3+), Al(3+), neomycin, polyamines, and melittin. *J Lipid Med Cell Signal* 1995;11:81–91.
34. Vassbotn FS, Östman A, Siegbahn A, et al. Neomycin is a platelet-derived growth factor (PDGF) antagonist that allows discrimination of PDGF α- and B-receptor signals in cells expressing both receptor types. *J Biol Chem* 1992;267:15635–15641.
35. Pugazhenthi S, Mantha SV, Khandelwal RL. Inhibitory effect of H-7, H-8, and polymyxin B on liver protein kinase C-induced phosphorylation of endogenous substrates. *Biochem Int* 1990;20:941–948.
36. Qi DF, Schatzman RC, Mazzei GJ, et al. Polyamines inhibit phospholipid-sensitive and calmodulin-sensitive Ca^{2+}-dependent protein kinases. *Biochem J* 1983;213:281–288.
37. Raynor RL, Zheng B, Kuo JF. Membrane interactions of amphiphilic polypeptides mastoparan, melittin, polymyxin B, and cardiotoxin: differential inhibition of protein kinase C and Ca^{2+}/calmodulin-dependent protein kinase II and synaptosomal membrane Na, K-ATPase, and Na pump and differentiation of HL60 cells. *J Biol Chem* 1991;266:2753–2758.
38. Schachtele C, Seifert R, Osswald H. Stimulus-dependent inhibition of platelet aggregation by the protein kinase C inhibitors polymyxin B, H-7 and staurosporine. *Biochem Biophys Res Comm* 1988;151:542–547.
39. Marshak DR, Lukas TJ, Watterson DM. Drug-protein interactions: binding of chlorpromazine to calmodulin, calmodulin fragments, and related calcium binding proteins. *Biochemistry* 1985;24:144–150.
40. Bokoch GM, Katada T, Northup JK, et al. Identification of the predominant substrate for ADP-ribosylation by islet activating protein. *J Biol Chem* 1983;258:2072–2075.
41. Molski TF, Naccache PH, Marsh ML, et al. Pertussis toxin inhibits the rise in the intracellular concentration of free calcium that is induced by chemotactic factors in rabbit neutrophils: possible role of the "G proteins" in calcium mobilization. *Biochem Biophys Res Comm* 1984;124:644–650.
42. Wyatt TA, Pryzwansky KB. KT5823 activates human neutrophils and fails to inhibit cGMP-dependent protein kinase phosphorylation of vimentin. *Res Comm Chem Path Pharm* 1991;74:3–14.
43. Takasu N, Yamada T, Shimizu Y, et al. Generation of hydrogen peroxide in cultured porcine thyroid cells: synergistic regulation by cytoplasmic free calcium and protein kinase C. *J Endocrin* 1989;120:503–508.
44. Tsien RY, Pozzan T, Rink TJ. Calcium homeostasis in intact lymphocytes: cytoplasmic free calcium monitored with a new, intracellularly trapped fluorescent indicator. *J Cell Biol* 1982;94:325–334.

45. Tsien RY, Harootunian RT. Practical design criteria for a dynamic ratio imaging system. *Cell Calcium* 1990;11:93–109.

46. Tsien RY, Pozzan T. Measurement of cytosolic free Ca^{2+} with quin2. *Methods Enzymol* 1989;172:230–262.

47. Tsien RY. New calcium indicators and buffers with high selectivity against magnesium and protons: design, synthesis, and properties of prototype structures. *Biochemistry* 1980;19:2396–2404.

48. Wodnicka M, Pierzchalska M, Bereiter–Hahn J, et al. Comparative study on effects of cytochalasins B and D on F-actin content in different cell lines and different culture conditions. *Folia Histochem Cytobiol* 1992;30:107–111.

49. Salmon ED, McKeel M, Hays T. Rapid rate of tubulin dissociation from microtubules in the mitotic spindle in vivo measured by blocking polymerization with colchicine. *J Cell Biol* 1984;99:1066–1075.

50. Chakrabarti R, Wylie DE, Schuster SM. Transfer of monoclonal antibodies into mammalian cells by electroporation. *J Biol Chem* 1989;264:15494–15500.

51. Kreis TE, Birchmeier W. Microinjection of fluorescently labeled proteins into living cells with emphasis on cytoskeletal proteins. *Int Rev Cytol* 1982;75:209–227.

52. Lee SW, Wulfkuhle JD, Otto JJ. Vinculin binding site mapped on talin with an anti-idiotypic antibody. *J Biol Chem* 1992;267:16355–16358.

53. Mueller SC, Kelly T, Dai MZ, et al. Dynamic cytoskeleton-integrin associations induced by cell binding to immobilized fibronectin. *J Cell Biol* 1989;109:3455–3464.

54. Nuckolls GH, Romer LH, Burridge K. Microinjection of antibodies against talin inhibits the spreading and migration of fibroblasts. *J Cell Sci* 1992;102:753–762.

55. Pavalko FM, Schneider G, Burridge K, et al. Immunodetection of alpha-actinin in focal adhesions is limited by antibody inaccessibility. *Exp Cell Res* 1995;217:534–540.

56. Samuelsson SJ, Luther PW, Pumplin DW, et al. Structures linking microfilament bundles to the membrane at focal contacts. *J Cell Biol* 1993;122:485–496.

57. Wolff J. *Das Gesetz Der Transformation Der Knochen.* Berlin: Hirschwald, 1892.

58. Adams A. Effect of exercise upon ligament strength. *Res Quarterly* 1966;37:163–167.

59. Klein KK. A continuation study of specific progressive resistive exercises for increasing medial lateral collateral ligament stability: an isometric concept. *J Assoc Phys Mental Rehab* 1966;20:196–198.

60. Zuckerman J, Stull GA. Effects of exercise on knee ligament separation force in rats. *J Appl Physiol* 1969;26:716–719.

61. Meyers EJ. Effect of selected exercise variables on ligament stability and flexibility of the knee. *Res Quarterly* 1971;42:411–422.

62. Noyes FR, Torvik PJ, Hyde WB, et al. Biomechanics of ligament failure, II: an analysis of immobilization, exercise, and reconditioning effects in primates. *J Bone Joint Surg Am* 1974;56:1406–1418.

63. Noyes FR. Functional properties of knee ligaments and alterations induced by immobilization: a correlative biomechanical and histological study in primates. *Clin Orthop Rel Res* 1977;59:210–242.

64. Tipton CM, Matthes RD, Maynard JA, et al. The influence of physical activity on ligaments and tendons. *Med Sci Sports* 1975;7:165–175.

65. Frank C, Woo SL, Amiel D, et al. Medial collateral ligament healing: a. multidisciplinary assessment in rabbits. *Am J Sports Med* 1983;11:379–389.

66. Woo SL, Gomez MA, Sites TJ, et al. The biomechanical and morphological changes in the medial collateral ligament of the rabbit after immobilization and remobilization. *J Bone Joint Surg Am* 1987;69:1200–1211.

67. Newton PO, Woo SL, Kitabayashi LR, et al. Ultrastructural changes in knee ligaments following immobilization. *Matrix* 1990;10:314–319.

68. Newton P, Woo S, MacKenna D, et al. Immobilization of the knee joint alters the mechanical and ultrastructural properties of the rabbit anterior cruciate ligament. *J Orthop Res* 1995;13:191–200.

69. Bray RC, Shrive NG, Frank CB, et al. The early effects of joint immobilization on medial collateral ligament healing in an ACL-deficient knee: a gross anatomic and biomechanical investigation in the adult rabbit model. *J Orthop Res* 1992;10:157–166.

70. AbiEzzi SS, Gesink DS, Schreck PJ, et al. Increased expression of the beta 1, alpha 5, and alpha v integrin adhesion receptor subunits occurs coincident with remodeling of stress-deprived rabbit anterior cruciate and medial collateral ligaments. *J Orthop Res* 1995;13:594–601.

71. AbiEzzi SS, Foulk RA, Harwood FL, et al. Decrease in fibronectin occurs coincident with the increased expression of its integrin receptor alpha5beta1 in stress-deprived ligaments. *Iowa Orthop J* 1997;17:102–109.

72. Birukov KG, Shirinsky VP, Stepanova OV, et al. Stretch affects phenotype and proliferation of vascular smooth muscle cells. *Mol Cell Biochem* 1995;144:131–139.

73. Harter LV, Hruska KA, Duncan RL. Human osteoblast-like cells respond to mechanical strain with increased bone matrix protein production independent of hormonal regulation. *Endocrinology* 1995;136:528–535.

74. Sun YQ, McLeod KJ, Rubin CT. Mechanically induced periosteal bone formation is paralleled by the up-regulation of collagen type one mRNA in osteocytes as measured by in situ reverse transcript-polymerase chain reaction. *Calc Tiss Int* 1995;57:456–462.

75. Yasuda T, Kondo S, Homma T, et al. Regulation of extracellular matrix by mechanical stress in rat glomerular mesangial cells. *J Clin Invest* 1996;98:1991–2000.

76. Lee AA, Delhaas T, Waldman LK, et al. An equibiaxial strain system for cultured cells. *Amer J Physiol* 1996;271:C1400–1408.

77. Sotoudeh M, Jalali S, Usami S, et al. A strain device imposing dynamic and uniform equi-biaxial strain to cultured cells. *Ann Biomed Eng* 1998;26:181–189.

78. Gilbert JA, Weinhold PS, Banes AJ, et al. Strain profiles for circular cell culture plates containing flexible surfaces employed to mechanically deform cells in vitro. *J Biomech* 1994;27:1169–1177.

79. Bhargava MM, Hannafin JA. Effect of cyclic strain on integrin expression by ligament fibroblasts. *Ann Biomed Eng* 1997;25:S77.

80. Hsieh A, Tsai CMH, Ma QJ, et al. Time-dependent increases in type III collagen gene expression in MCL fibroblasts under cyclic strains. *J Orthop Res* 2000;18:220–227.

81. Arnoczky SP. Anatomy of the anterior cruciate ligament. *Clin Orthop Rel Res* 1983;11:19–25.

82. Dodds JA, Arnoczky SP. Anatomy of the anterior cruciate ligament: a blueprint for repair and reconstruction. *Arthroscopy* 1994;10:132–139.

83. Frank C, Schachar N, Dittrich D. Natural history of healing in the repaired medial collateral ligament. *J Orthop Res* 1983;1:179–188.

84. Gomez MA, Woo SL, Amiel D, et al. The effects of increased tension on healing medial collateral ligaments. *Am J Sports Med* 1991;19:347–354.

85. Mass DP, Tuel RJ, Labarbera M, et al. Effects of constant mechanical tension on the healing of rabbit flexor tendons. *Clin Orthop Rel Res* 1993;79:301–306.

86. Sung KLP, Whittemore DE, Yang L, et al. Signal pathways and ligament cell adhesiveness. *J Orthop Res* 1996;14:729–735.

87. Woods A, Couchman JR. Protein kinase C involvement in focal adhesion formation. *J Cell Sci* 1992;101:277–290.

88. Peter K, O'Toole TE. Modulation of cell adhesion by changes in alpha L beta 2 (LFA-1, CD11a/CD18) cytoplasmic domain/cytoskeleton interaction. *J Exp Med* 1995;181:315–326.

89. Sung KLP, Steele LL, Whittemore D, et al. Adhesiveness of human ligament fibroblasts to laminin. *J Orthop Res* 1995;13:166–273.

CHAPTER 13

Arthrofibrosis

The Mechanism of Proliferative Scar Production and Potential Therapeutic Remedies to Modulate the Healing Response

Wayne H. Akeson

Traditional therapy for prevention of arthrofibrosis follows well-recognized principles of careful tissue handling during surgery, avoidance of excessive bleeding and hematoma formation, judicious use of drains, and active early mobilization of affected joints after surgery. In spite of these measures, an unacceptable number of arthrofibrotic complications continue to be observed. The purpose of this chapter is to review the biologic processes leading to proliferative scar formation that apply to the postoperative or postinjury knee and to outline potential pharmacologic interventions on the near horizon.

Injury invokes a vigorous healing response in soft tissue as it does in bone. The needs of individual survival undoubtedly required such an evolutionary response as a survival mechanism. Inevitably, the control mechanisms of the healing response will not infrequently extend beyond the range of the ideal. When the response to soft tissue injury is excessively exuberant, complications are encountered such as keloid formation, peritoneal adhesion, intestinal stricture, tendon adhesion, epidural fibrosis, and arthrofibrosis with attendant joint contractures, to name just a few. An important case in point is the loss of range of motion that occurs occasionally after knee injuries or knee surgery in spite of seemingly appropriate initial management and subsequent rehabilitation. It follows that an understanding of the healing process is necessary to explore potential therapeutic remedies to minimize these complications.

OVERVIEW OF NORMAL WOUND HEALING

The healing of soft tissues is a continuum of five general phases (1) (Table 13.1).

- *Hemorrhage* and formation of a blood clot followed by platelet degranulation
- *Leukocyte* trafficking into the wound
- *Inflammation*, during which neutrophils phagocytose bacteria and debris and degranulate, releasing proteolytic enzymes, and the monocytic cells become transformed into macrophages
- *Repair*, during which macrophages stimulate fibroblast proliferation and the resulting extracellular matrix synthesis
- *Remodeling* of the initial scar

Initial bleeding is followed promptly by platelet aggregation and degranulation and vasoconstriction of neighboring vessels. Extravasation of blood proteins, including fibronectin, vitronectin, and fibrinogen, occurs with the initial hemorrhage. Fibrin formation and clotting ensue. An inflammatory process occurs next, triggered by growth factors and cytokines initiating a cascade of events starting with activation of selectins and cell adhesion molecules (CAMs), which modulate the initial leukocyte trafficking across the endothelium of postcapillary venules. Platelets will have released transforming growth factor-β (TGF-β) and tumor necrosis factor-α (TNF-α), among other factors, immediately after wound-

TABLE 13.1. *Wound healing stages*

Step 1: Hemorrhage	Platelets degranulate releasing
	   TGF β
	   TNF α
	   Other cytokines
	Blood proteins are spilled
	   Fibrinogen
	   Vitronectin
	   Fibronectin
	Blood clot forms

Step 2: Leukocyte trafficking	Selectins > leukocyte rolling +Chemoattractants +Cell adhesion molecules ↓ Leukocyte–endothelial cell adhesion cascade ↓ Transmigration of leukocytes into the wound
Step 3: Inflammation	Neutrophils enter the wound in the first few hours, sterilize the wound by phagocytosis of bacteria and release of oxygen radicals, and degranulate releasing proteolytic enzymes. Monocytes enter the wound at about 18 h. They proliferate rapidly and are transformed into macrophages. Macrophages phagocytose cellular, bacterial, and matrix debris.
Step 4: Repair	Macrophages stimulate fibroblasts > fibroplasia and neovascularization > granulation tissue. Further collagen synthesis produces mature matrix.
Step 5: Remodeling	Fibroblasts, haphazard collagen fiber deposition is remodeled by an iterative process of resorption and synthesis. The process is guided by cellular mechanoreceptors that respond to stresses applied to the tissue.

TGF, transforming growth factor; TNF, tumor necrosis factor.

ing, causing leukocyte margination, or "rolling." This results in slowing of the passage of leukocytes through the venule, which allows the leukocytes to monitor the environment for chemoattractants. The CAMs and chemoattractants are programmed in a sequential manner to form a leukocyte–endothelial cell adhesion cascade (2–5). Chemoattractants bind to serpentine receptors on the leukocytes, which then activate G proteins that signal up-regulation of integrins on the leukocyte cell surface. The arrested cells subsequently undergo transmigration between the endothelial cells under the influence of the adhesion proteins plus PECAM-1 (platelet endothelial cell adhesion molecule-1), chemoattractant gradients aided by chemoattractant–proteoglycan binding (6–8), and chemotaxins in the wound environment. After entry into the wound, these cells are free to react with matrix proteins and to stimulate mitogenesis and additional chemotaxis through autocrine and paracrine functions.

The sequence of leukocyte classes recruited into the wound environment is observed to include neutrophils in the first few hours followed by monocytes at 18 hours and T cells and macrophages at 36 to 48 hours. Sequential changes in the adhesion molecule system are presumably the mechanism of selection and control of specific leukocyte transendothelial migration. Notably, there are clear differences in adhesion requirements for particular types of inflammation (2,9). The polymorphonuclear leukocytes that initially populate the wound sterilize the wound by phagocytosis and the release of oxygen radicals. They bind to complement fragments on bacterial

surfaces. Neutrophils are quickly followed by lymphocytes and monocytes. Between Days 3 and 4, monocytes proliferate rapidly. The infiltrating cells release a plethora of cytokines, growth factors, and chemokines that collectively orchestrate the local cellular response, which includes the transformation of monocytes into macrophages. The macrophages phagocytose cellular, bacterial, and matrix debris. Macrophages assume a crucial role in further modulating the healing process by stimulating the proliferation of reparative cells, including fibroblast, epithelial, and capillary endothelial cells (10). This step is followed by the synthesis of complex components that form the extracellular matrix. The breadth of activities of TGF-β have given it the appellation "the conductor of the symphony" with regard to the healing process (11). Initially the extracellular matrix is high in proteoglycan content, which soon gives way to increased collagen synthesis and scar formation. The initial scar presents as a random display of collagen fibers in what is commonly referred to as a "haystack pattern" (12). The final chronic remodeling phase occurs over many months. Mechanical factors, particularly tensile stresses, are perceived by adhesion receptors and mechanoreceptors of the fibroblasts, and the matrix is gradually remodeled by an iterative process of matrix resorption and new matrix synthesis. In this complex process the collagen molecules become aggregated by intra- and intermolecular cross-links modulated in part by other matrix components such as the minor collagens and the small proteoglycans described in previous chapters (12).

Definitive candidates for postsurgical scar control have recently emerged following an explosion of progress in understanding and prevention of a variety of chronic fibrotic conditions of the skin, lung, heart, liver, kidney, and vasculature. Extensive studies on the processes of leukocyte trafficking in wounds have broadened the understanding of the underlying processes at work in the early wound. These concepts have been clarified and phenomenologically synthesized by Butcher (13) and others (3,14,15). Progress in this field now provides an exciting opportunity to approach the problem of control of fibrosis with a plethora of potentially important scar-neutralizing agents. This discussion will focus on some of the new concepts that are of interest as potential therapeutic approaches to the problem of arthrofibrosis and related problems of interest to the orthopedic surgeon.

Fetal Healing

Fetal healing—the healing that occurs in the early fetus without scar—was observed in 1971 by Burrington (16) in the fetal lamb. Subsequently, it was noted that the effect is not seen uniformly during development. Fetal healing is dependent on stage of gestation and on wound characteristics (17). Incisional scarless healing is most evident in the early fetal gestation periods, generally through midgestation. Later in gestation, the healing of incisional wounds tends with time gradually to resemble the healing of adult wounds. In mice, for example, fetal wounds heal without scar at gestational (gd) day 14, but at gd 18, heal with scar (mouse term = 20 days) (18). Excisional wounds heal without scar in the very early fetus, but lose that capacity sooner than in the case of the incisional wound healing with respect to time of gestation (17).

Fetal healing occurs in a unique extracellular matrix environment. Key conditions include a high concentration of high molecular weight (HMW) hyaluronan (18–24) and very low levels of TGF-β-1 and -2 (25,26). Other differences are gradually being reported such as the presence of low levels of hyaluronidase (23,26), increased amounts of tenacin (27), and differences in content of the CD44 HA receptor noted to be four times the level in the fetal wound compared with the adult wound (24).

If the early fetal environment could be reproduced therapeutically, excessive scar formation could potentially be prevented in strategic sites after surgery. Indeed, several investigators have provided evidence that conditions that partially mimic the environment of fetal connective tissue matrix can, in fact, result in modified healing in certain animal models that demonstrate reduced scar formation, with more orderly collagen patterning, and with tensile strength of postoperative incisional wounds equivalent to that of normal adult wounds (18,20,26–28). Potential applications of fetal healing concepts in orthopedic surgery include the modulation of scar formation after tenolysis performed to correct tendon adhesions, prevention of arthrofibrosis, and

prevention of epidural adhesions, to name just a few examples. And strikingly, a new branch of surgery is on the doorstep in which the possibility of correcting certain fetal deformities *in utero* is becoming a reality (28).

Whitby and Ferguson were the first to show that TGF-β-1 was missing in the connective tissue matrix of the early fetus (25,26). They demonstrated that blockade of TGF-β-1 and -2 activity encouraged scarless healing in the skin of adult animal models (27). The effective agents they used to inhibit TGF-β-1 and -2 included mannose-6-phosphate and decorin and antibodies against TGF-β-1 and -2.

A profusion of reports in recent years have described additional differences between the fetal and adult wound. An abbreviated listing of relevant observations includes the following:

Adult wound fluids have a higher concentration of hyaluronidase than fetal wound fluids (23).

Fetal healing response to injury can be converted toward the adult form of healing by the injection of TGF-β in the Institute of Cancer Research (ICR) mouse fetus (29).

Hyaluronan injected repeatedly into sponge implants in mice (every 3 days) over 1 and 2 weeks altered the adult healing so that it resembled fetal healing in respect to the histologic amount and character of collagen fibers. Injection of hyaluronidase into the sponges reversed that effect (30).

Fetal articular cartilage heals, whereas adult cartilage does not (31) (a possible focus of importance in the field of cartilage healing research).

The fetal immune response differs—the cellular infiltrate is mainly a small number of macrophages, with few polymorphonuclear leukocytes (32,33).

Fetal cytokine profile differences exist (33).

Fetal fibroblasts have different collagen gel contraction ability (34,35).

Metalloproteinases differ between fetal and adult wounds (36).

COL1A1 gene expression is absent in fetal fibroblasts but is up-regulated by the addition of TGF-β (37).

Type V collagen α1(V)/α2(V) chains differ in fetal and adult sheep sponges, type I collagen cross-links increase during gestational development as scar formation begins to appear (38).

Interleukin-8 (IL-8) is absent in fetal fibroblasts (39).

HA inhibits fetal platelet aggregation and impairs the release of platelet-derived growth factor-AB (PDGF-AB) (40).

There is more rapid up-regulation of integrins (α2, α3,α5,α6 and β, β4, and β6) in the fetal wound and more rapid reepithelialization by keratinocytes (41).

This necessarily sketchy account of the recent literature suggests the breadth of interest in the fetal healing phenomenon. It is not yet possible to synthesize all these findings meaningfully, but many, if not all, may be derivative of the two central observations in the fetal wound:

the high concentration of HA and the low concentration of TGF-β-1 and -2 that inhibit inflammation.

Hyaluronan

Hyaluronan is a ubiquitous component of the extracellular matrix (ECM) and occurs transiently in both the cell nucleus and cytoplasm. It promotes cell motility, adhesion, and proliferation and has an important role in morphogenesis, wound repair, and tumor metastasis (42,43). Cell motility is central to the effect of each of these processes. HA is actively synthesized during wound healing and is an important substrate for leukocyte migration during inflammation (24,42,44–47). Disturbance of regulation of these processes has been alleged to be responsible for errors in morphogenesis, aberrant repair, exaggerated inflammatory responses, and tumorigenesis. HA binding, ligand specificity, and stimulation of signal pathways can be modulated by soluble forms of the receptors, by alternatively spliced cell surface isoforms, and by glycosylation variants of the receptors (42).

Scarless healing has been noted in the sheep embryo up through the 130th day of gestation, when high levels of HA are found. After 130 days, HA was observed to decline to a trough (21). In an adult rat model it was possible to inhibit scar formation in skin wounds by treating the wound with a HA–protein–collagen form of HA (48). In this experiment, the treated wounds had more organized collagen fibers, less TGF-β-1 and -2 and increased TGF-β-3 (an inhibitor of TGF-β-1 and -2). An *in vitro* model has also been studied in which HA concentration was varied in fibroblast cell culture (49). In this experiment, streak "wounds" were created in confluent fibroblast cultures under the influence of exogenous HA (5 mg/mL). These wounds closed more rapidly than untreated wounds. Studies on incisional wound healing in fetal limb organ cultures to which exogenous HA was added with each change of media, showed results similar to the scarless healing seen in other models mimicking fetal healing. Repair site collagen fibers in the treatment group had the typical "basket weave" pattern of normal dermal collagen in contrast to the less well-organized collagen in the control groups (30).

Crucial to the work in the proposed project is the discovery of the bimodal action of HA in the ECM with respect to reaction of HA with various receptors. A collection of inflammatory genes is induced in macrophages by HA oligosaccharides, but not by native HMW HA (50). HMW HA is antiangiogenic, whereas oligosaccharide degradation products of HA actively stimulate endothelial cell proliferation and migration and induce angiogenesis *in vivo* (51).

Clearly, it is the HMW form of HA, which is the requisite molecular form of HA in the fetal scarless healing environment. A fascinating complement to this requirement is the observation that low hyaluronidase levels exist in the fetal connective tissue matrix (23). A potential mechanism for control of this process has been found by the discovery that anti-CD44 monoclonal antibody (mAb), which blocks the fibroblast cell receptor for low molecular weight (LMW) HA binding, also inhibits the LMW HA induced release of IL-12 by elicited macrophages (52). Furthermore, native HMW HA has a dose-dependent inhibitory effect on induced gene expression by HA oligosaccharides (53). Three cell surface receptors that are important for the cell interaction with HA of the matrix have been identified: CD44, RHAMM (receptor for HA-mediated motility—the HA motogenic receptor), and ICAM-1 (42). As with other adhesion receptors, binding of the cell through the HA-mediated receptors triggers signal transduction events. These events are central to the control of cytoskeletal structure and cell trafficking.

Also central to arthrofibrosis research is the recent discovery that TGF-β is involved in RHAMM message regulation (54). This finding presents an interesting juxtaposition of a counter-mechanism between TGF-β and HA. The half-life of RHAMM messenger RNA (mRNA) has been shown to be increased threefold in cells treated with TGF-β (55). Possibly, by blocking TGF-β, RHAMM synthesis may be inhibited—a step that could thereby inhibit leukocyte trafficking into the area of concern (50).

The author's laboratory reported in the 1970s that a single injection of HA inhibited contracture formation about 50% in an experimental animal model (56). More recently, we have shown the efficacy in reducing epidural scar after surgery with topical HA in a standard rat model (57). The observation that HA injection into arthritic joints may be beneficial symptomatically is likely a result of its antiinflammatory action. That action would also hold promise as a neutralizing agent against the inflammatory response that occurs after knee joint manipulation and in the management of complications of knee joint contracture occurring after surgery.

TGF-β

The production of scar through the stimulation of collagen synthesis by CTGF (connective tissue growth factor) in the injured tissue is believed to be coordinated by TGF-β. TGF-β has been called the "conductor of the symphony" of the healing response by Grotendorst (11). TGF-β stimulates connective tissue cell growth, stimulates extracellular matrix synthesis, and modulates the immune response. It acts on fibroblasts and smooth muscle cells. It increases mRNA for CTGF. CTGF is chemotactic and mitogenic for connective tissue cells and stimulates extracellular matrix production. TGF-β exists in tissue in a latent form, bound by LAP (latency associated peptide), LTBP (latent TGF-β-binding protein), decorin, and biglycan (58). Recombinant LAP is a potent inhibitor of TGF-β *in vivo* and *in vitro* (59). TGF-β exists in several isoforms, including β-1, -2, and -3. Neutralization of

TGF-β1 and -2 or the addition of TGF-β-3 reduces scarring in several models (27). Different fibroblasts react differently to TGF-β, emphasizing the fact that all fibroblasts are not the same (60). Work in our laboratory characterizing differences between ligaments of the knee has clearly shown that ligaments that heal well (medial collateral ligaments) have fibroblastic characteristics quite different from ligaments that fail to heal (anterior cruciate ligaments) (61–64).

TGF-β is overproduced in fibrotic lesions and is a key factor in the pathogenesis of organ fibrogenesis (9,27, 65,66). Fibrosis resembles normal wound healing, but fails to terminate, leading to replacement of normal tissue with scar. Most fibrotic reactions (lung, heart, vascular system, kidney, liver, skin, brain, gastrointestinal tract, synovial joints) appear secondary to trauma, infection, or inflammation. Studies using immunohistochemical techniques have demonstrated that TGF-β is overproduced in areas of chronic fibrosis. The reason for the continued scar proliferation is not always clear, but it is possible that some fibroblasts become permanently altered and do not respond appropriately to the usual regulatory controls (60). Both TGF-β-3 and decorin, which inhibits the actions of TGF-β-1 and -2, may represent a local regulatory control elements (27,59,67). The exaggerated behavior of TGF-β in the fibrotic syndromes has been termed "The Dark Side of TGF-β" in an article by Border et al. (3) and termed "The Good, the Bad and the Ugly" by Wahl (68). A hemarthrosis after trauma, surgery, or manipulation will inevitably contain platelets that release cytokines into the joint. These cytokines, including TGF-β, provoke an inflammatory response that can result in arthrofibrosis and joint contracture. The use of neutralizing agents against TGF-β holds promise for minimizing this troublesome complication of knee injuries. Controlled clinical studies on their use should be forthcoming in the near future.

Decorin

Decorin is a powerful molecule with wide-ranging regulatory effects. Decorin is characterized as a member of the class of small proteoglycan molecules. It contains a protein core with leucine-rich motifs and a single side chain of dermatan–chondroitin sulfate.

It is ubiquitously distributed in the extracellular matrix of mammals. It binds to fibrillar collagens, including minor collagens, influencing kinetics of fibril formation and final diameter of fibrils (69,70). It has profound effects on matrix assembly and cellular growth including cytostatic effects on transformed cells with diverse histogenic backgrounds (71). It influences embryogenesis, inflammation, wound healing, and neoplastic growth (71–75). Decorin antagonistically regulates the action of TGF-β (76). It binds TGF-β-1, co-localizing in many tissues (77,78). Decorin inhibits some actions of TGF-β and its synthesis is stimulated by TGF-β, suggesting that it

provides a negative feedback control for TGF-β activity (77–79). The bound form may serve as a tissue reservoir of TGF-β in a manner similar to the binding interaction between TGF-β and LAP or β-glycan (80). Release of TGF-β from its bound form with decorin is regulated by proteases including MMP-2,3 and 7 (81). Decorin also reacts with HA (82) and has been reputed to possess close similarities to the CD44 family (83).

Decorin also interacts with other growth factors. TNF-α has the ability to transcriptionally inhibit decorin gene expression in growth-arrested cells and may be a key modulator of decorin (84). Decorin is proposed as a novel ligand for EGF and, in this role, may regulate cell growth in tissue remodeling and cancer (71). Decorin activates the EGF receptor triggering a signaling cascade, which leads to phosphorylation of mitogen-activated protein (MAP) kinase, induction of p21, and growth suppression. IL-1 and IL-4 inhibit decorin expression (85,86). Overexpression of v-src selectively abolishes the expression of decorin (87). Because of its interaction with growth factors, decorin expression can substantially alter the cellular response to injury (88).

Decorin synthesis has been inhibited by antisense nucleotides in ligament healing studies using gene delivery methods and this has been proposed as a technique to accelerate scar production (89). However, most potential pharmacologic applications of decorin have addressed application as a TGF-β inhibitor for decreasing inflammation and scar production and for increasing the tissue immune response (72,75). Decorin's scar-inhibitory activity has been proposed for treatment of inflammatory kidney diseases (90), pulmonary fibrosis (91), tuberculosis (92), and diabetic vascular disease (93) are among just a few of the proposed applications.

The exciting breadth of antifibrotic agents becoming available for research studies on fibrosis inhibition can be illustrated by the following examples of neutralizing agents to consider (Table 13.2):

Other antagonists to TGF-β: Blocking peptides to TGF-β-1 and -2, LAP (latency-associated peptide), TGF-β-3 (which neutralizes isoforms 1 and 2), decorin, mannose-6-phosphate, TGF-β antisense nucleotides, nonviral gene therapy, soluble receptors to TGF-β-1 and -2 and peptidomimetics that react with and block the TGF-β receptors.

Other classes of antifibrotics: These include the interferons, relaxin, certain peptidomimetics such as RGD peptides or fibronectin (FN) fragments against integrins, certain glycomimetics, mAbs against selectins, lysyl oxidase inhibitors of collagen cross-linking, collagen prolyl hydroxylase inhibitors, to name just some of the potential candidates. Recently, anti-cd44 antibody has been shown to induce cultured fibroblast detachment from substratum and morphologic change compatible with apoptosis (94).

TABLE 13.2. *Potential clinically useful antifibrotics*

Antifibrotics blocking TGF-β
  Antibodies to TGF-β 1 and 2
  Soluble receptors to TGF-β 1 and 2
  Peptidomimetics against the TGF-β receptor
  TGF-β antisense nucleotides
  TGF-β 3
  Recombinant LAP
  M-6-P
  Antibodies to the M-6-P receptor on LAP
  Decorin, biclycan
  α₂-macrroblobulin (in serum)
Other antifibrotics
  Interferons
  Relaxin
  RGD peptides or peptidomimetids
  Fibronectin fragments
  mAms against selectins
  Lysyl oxidase inhibitors of collagen crosslinking
  Collagen prolyl hydroxylase K inhibitors

TGF, transforming growth factor; LAP, latency-associated peptide; M-6-P, mannose-6-phosphate; mAbs, monoclonal antibodies.

The systematic application of fetal healing concepts to minimize scarring in the knee joint has not yet been applied systematically. The time is ripe for such studies aimed at minimizing proliferative scar after knee ligament repair or after knee manipulation. Hyaluronan and decorin are powerful agents for the control of the inflammatory process. Hyaluronan, at one time thought to be simply a tissue lubricant, is strongly antiinflammatory in its HMW form, whereas in its degraded oligomeric form it has powerful inflammatory effects. Among the several functional properties of the ubiquitous small proteoglycan, decorin, is the inhibition of the inflammatory response by binding TGF-β. The door is open for focused scholarly pursuit of these opportunities to potentially minimize arthrofibrosis and other problems of exuberant scar proliferation following injuries to the knee joint.

REFERENCES

1. Schall T, Bacon K. Chemokines, leukocyte trafficking and inflammation. *Curr Opin Immunol* 1994;6:865–873.
2. vonAndrian U, Chambers J, McEvoy L, et al. Two-step model of leukocyte-endothelial cell interaction in inflammation. *Proc Nat Acad Sci U S A* 1991;88:7538–7542.
3. Border W, Noble N, Yamamoto T, et al. Antagonists to TGF-beta: treatment of glomerulonephritis and prevention of glomerulosclerosis. *Kidney Int* 1992;41:566–570.
4. Pober J, Cotran R. The role of endothelial cells in inflammation. *Transplantation* 1990;50:537–544.
5. Smith C. Endothelial adhesion molecules and their role in inflammation. *Can J Physiol Pharmacol* 1993;71:76–87.
6. Muller W, Weigl S, Deng X, et al. PECAM-1 is required for transendothelial migration of leukocytes. *J Exp Med* 1993;178:449–460.
7. Webb L, Ehrengruber M, Clark-Lewis I, et al. Binding to heparan sulfate or heparin enhances neutrophil responses to interleukin 8. *Proc Natl Acad Sci U S A* 1993;90:7158–7162.
8. Witt D, Lander A. Differential binding of chemokines to glycosaminoglycan subpopulations. *Curr Biol* 1994;4:394–400.
9. Weyrich A, Ma X, Lefer D, et al. In vivo neutralization of P-selectin protects feline heart and endothelium in myocardial ischemia and reperfusion injury. *J Clin Invest* 1993;91:2610–2629.
10. Hernandez-Pando R, Orozco H, Arriaga K, et al. Analysis of the local kinetics and localization of interleukin-1 alpha, tumour necrosis factor-alpha and transforming growth factor-beta, during the course of experimental pulmonary tuberculosis. *Immunology* 1997;90:607–617.
11. Grotendorst GR. IBC Int Conf on therapeutic advances in fibrosis. 1996, Washington, DC.
12. Akeson WH, Amiel D, Mechanic GL, et al. Collagen cross-linking alterations in joint contractures: changes in the reducible cross-links in periarticular connective tissue collagen after nine weeks of immobilization. *Connect Tissue Res* 1997;5:15–19.
13. Butcher E. Leukocyte-endothelial cell recognition: three (or more) steps to specificity and diversity. *Cell* 1991;67:1033–1036.
14. Collins T. Adhesion molecules in leukocyte emigration. *Sci Am Sci Med* 1995:28–37.
15. Schall T, Bacon K. Chemokines, leukocyte trafficking and inflammation. *Curr Opin Immunol* 1994;6:865–873.
16. Burrington J. Wound healing in the fetal lamb. *J Pediatr Surg* 1991;6:523–528.
17. Cass DL, Bullard KM, Sylvester KG, et al. Wound size and gestational age modulate scar formation in fetal wound repair. *J Pediatr Surg* 1997;32:411–415.
18. Ioncono J, Ehrlich H, Keefer K, et al. Hyaluronan induces scarless repair in mouse limb organ culture. *J Pediatr Surg* 1998;33:546–547.
19. DePalma R, Krummel T, Durham L, et al. Characterization and quantitation of wound matrix in the fetal rabbit. *Matrix* 1999;9:224–231.
20. Cabrera R, Siebert J, Eidelman Y, et al. The in vivo effect of hyaluronan associated protein-collagen complex on wound repair. *Biochem Mol Biol Int* 1995;37:151–158.
21. Freund R, Siebert J, Carera R, et al. Serial quantitation of hyaluronan and sulfated glycosaminoglycans in fetal sheep skin. *Bioch Mol Biol Int* 1993;29:773–783.
22. Shepard S, Becker H, Hartman L. Using hyaluronic acid to create a fetal-like environment in vitro. *Ann Plast Surg* 1996;36:65–69.
23. West DC, Shaw DM, Lorenz P, et al. Fibrotic healing of adult and late gestation fetal wounds correlates with increased hyaluronidase activity and removal of hyaluronan. *Int J Biochem Cell Biol* 1997;29:201–210.
24. Alaish S, Yager D, Diegelmann R, et al. Biology of fetal wound healing: hyaluronate receptor expression in fetal fibroblasts. *J Pediatr Surg* 194;29:1040–1043.
25. Whitby DJ, Ferguson MW. The extracellular matrix of lip wounds in fetal neonatal and adult mice. *Development* 1991;12:651–668.
26. Whitby DJ, Ferguson MW. Immunohistochemical localization of growth factors in fetal wound healing. *Devel Biol* 1991;147:207–215.
27. Shah M, Foreman D, Ferguson M. Neutralisation of TGF-beta 1 and TGF-beta 2 or exogenous addition of TGF-beta 3 to cutaneous rat wounds reduces scarring. *J Cell Sci* 1995;108:985–1002.
28. Adzick NS, Lonaker MT. *Fetal wound healing.* New York: Elsevier, 1991.
29. Stelnicki EJ, Bullard KM, Harrison MR, et al. A new in vivo model for the study of fetal wound healing. *Ann Plast Surg* 1997;39:374–380.
30. Ioncono J, Krummel T, Keefer K, et al. Repeated additions of hyaluronan alters granulation tissue deposition in sponge implants in mice. *Wound Repair Regen* 1998;6:442–448.
31. Namba RS, Meuli M, Sullivan KM, et al. Spontaneous repair of superficial defects in articular cartilage in a fetal lamb model. *J Bone Joint Surg Am* 1998;80:4–10.
32. Mackool RJ, Gittes GK, Longaker MT. Scarless healing: the fetal wound. *Clin Plast Surg* 1998;25:357–365.
33. Cowin AJ, Brosnan MP, Holmes TM, et al. Endogenous inflammatory response to dermal wound healing in the fetal and adult mouse. *Dev Dyn* 1998;212:385–393.
34. Coleman C, Tuan TL, Buckley S, et al. Contractility, transforming growth factor-beta, and plasmin in fetal skin fibroblasts: role in scarless wound healing. *Pediatr Res* 1998;43:403–409.
35. Irwin CR, Myrillas T, Smyth M, et al. Regulation of fibroblast-induced collagen gel contraction by interleukin-1beta. *J Oral Pathol Med* 1998;27:255–259.
36. Bullard KM, Cass DL, Banda MJ, Adzick NS. Transforming gowth factor beta-1 decreases interstitial collagenase in healing human fetal skin. *J Pediatr Surg* 1997;32:1023–1027.

37. Gallivan K, Alman BA, Moriarty KP, et al. Differential collagen1 gene expression in fetal fibroblasts. *J Pediatr Surg* 1997;32: 1033–1036.

38. Lovvorn HN III, Cheung DT, Nimni ME, et al. Relative distribution and crosslinking of collagen distinguish fetal from adult sheep wound repair. *J Pediatr Surg* 1998;34:218–223.

39. Liechty KW, Crombleholme TM, Cass DL, et al. Diminished interleukin-8 (IL-8) production in the fetal wound healing response. *J Surg Res* 1998;77:80–84.

40. Olutoye OO, Barone EJ, Yager DR, et al. Hyaluronic acid inhibits fetal platelet function: implications in scarless healing. *J Pediatr Surg* 1997; 32:1037–1040.

41. Cass DL, Bullard KM, Sylvester KG, et al. Epidermal integrin expression is upregulated rapidly in human fetal wound repair. *J Pediatr Surg* 1998; 33:312–316.

42. Entwistle J, Hall CL, Turley EA. HA receptors: regulators of signaling to the cytoskeleton. *J Cell Biochem* 1998;61:569–577.

43. Naot D, Sionov RV, Ish-Shalom D. CD44: structure, function, and association with the malignant process. *Adv Cancer Res* 1997;71:241–319.

44. Asari A, Morita M, Sekiguchi T, et al.. Hyaluronan, CD44 and fibronectin in rabbit corneal epithelial wound healing. *Jpn J Ophthalmol* 1996;40:18–25.

45. Rudzki Z, Jothy S. CD44 and the adhesion of neoplastic cells. *Mol Pathol* 1997;50:57–71.

46. Shyjan AM, Heldin P, Butcher EC, et al. Functional cloning of the cDNA for a human hyaluronan synthase. *J Biol Chem* 1996;271:23395–23399.

47. Wang C, Entwistle J, Hou G, et al. The characterization of a human RHAMM cDNA: conservation of the hyaluronan-binding domains. *Gene* 1996;174:299–306.

48. Greco RM, Iocono JA, Ehrlich HP. Hyaluronic acid stimulates human fibroblast proliferation within a collagen matrix. *J Cell Physiol* 1998; 177:465–473.

49. Shepard S, Becker H, Hartmann JX. Using hyaluronic acid to create a fetal-like environment in vitro. *Ann Plast Surg* 1996;36:65–69.

50. McKee CM, Penno MB, Bowman M, et al. Hyaluronan (HA) fragments induce chemokine gene expression in alveolar macrophages: the role of HA size and CD44. *J Clin Invest* 1996;98:2403–2413.

51. Lees VC, Fan TP, West DC. Angiogenesis in a delayed revascularization model is accelerated by angiogenic oligosaccharides of hyaluronan. *Lab Invest* 1995;73:259–266.

52. Hodge-Dufour J, Noble PW, Horton MR, et al. Induction of IL-12 and chemokines by hyaluronan requires adhesion-dependent priming of resident but not elicited macrophages. *J Immunol* 1997;159:2492–2500.

53. Deed R, Rooney P, Kumar P, et al. Early-response gene signaling is induced by angiogenic oligosaccharides of hyaluronan in endothelial cells: inhibition by nonangiogenic, high-molecular-weight hyaluronan. *Int J Cancer* 1997;71:251–256.

54. Hall C, Laange L, Prober D, et al. pp60 (c-src) is required for cell locomotion regulated by the hyaluronan receptor RHAMM. *Oncogene* 1996;13:2213–2224.

55. Amara FM, Entwistle J, Kuschak TI, et al. Transforming growth factor-beta1 stimulates multiple protein interactions at a unique cis-element in the 3′-untranslated region of the hyaluronan receptor RHAMM mRNA. *J Biol Chem* 1996;271:15279–15284.

56. Amiel D, Frey C, Woo SL, et al. Value of hyaluronic acid in the prevention of contracture formation. *Clin Orthop Related Res* 1985;196: 306–311.

57. Waters SN, Massie JB, Amiel D, et al. *A role for anti-fibrotics in the prevention of epidural fibrosis. Proceedings of the Orthopedic Research Soc 0071,* Orlando, FL, Mar 12–15, 2000.

58. Tamaki K, Okuda S, Miyazono K, et al. Matrix-associated latent TGF-beta with latent TGF-beta binding protein in the progressive process in adriamycin-induced nephropathy. *Lab Invest* 1995;73:81–89.

59. Bottinger EP, Factor VM, Tsang ML, et al. The recombinant proregion of transforming growth factor beta1 (latency-associated peptide) inhibits active transforming growth factor beta1 in transgenic mice. *Proc Natl Acad Sci U S A* 1996;93:5877–5882.

60. Davidson J. Cell biology of tissue repair and fibrosis. In: IBC Int Conf on Therapeutic Advances in Fibrosis. Martin G, ed. Washington DC: InformaLife Sciences Group, 1996.

61. Nagineni CN, Amiel D, Green MH, et al. Characterization of the intrinsic properties of the anterior cruciate and medial collateral ligament cells: an in vitro cell culture study. *J Orthop Res* 1992;10:465–475.

62. Schreck PJ, Kitabayashi LR, Amiel D, et al. Integrin display increases in the wounded rabbit medial collateral ligament but not the wounded anterior cruciate ligament. *J Orthop Res* 1995;13:174–183.

63. Geiger MH, Green MH, Monosov A, et al. An in vitro assay of anterior cruciate ligament (ACL) and medial collateral ligament (MCL) cell migration. *Conn Tiss Res* 1994;30:215–224.

64. Amiel D, Kuiper SD, Wallace CD, et al. Age-related properties of medial collateral ligament and anterior cruciate ligament: a morphologic and collagen maturation study in the rabbit. *J Gerontol* 1991; 46:B159–B165.

65. Albelda S, Smith C, Ward P. Adhesion molecules and inflammation injury. *FASEB* 1994;8:504–512.

66. Kavanaugh A, Heudebert G, Cush J, et al. Cost evaluation of novel therapeutics in rheumatoid arthritis (CENTRA). *Sem Arthritis Rheum* 1995;25:1–12.

67. Shah M, Whitby D, Ferguson M. Fetal wound healing and scarless surgery. In: Jackson D, Sommerlad B, eds. *Recent advances in plastic surgery,* vol. 5. Edinburgh: Churchill Livingstone, 1996.

68. Wahl SM. Transforming growth factor beta: the good, the bad, and the ugly. *J Exp Med* 1994;180:1587–1590.

69. Weber IT, Harrison RW, Iozzo RV. Model structure of decorin and implications for collagen fibrillogenesis. *J Biol Chem* 1996;271: 31767–31770.

70. Kresse H, Liszio C, Schonherr E, et al. Critical role of glutamate in a central leucine-rich repeat of decorin for interaction with type I collagen. *J Biol Chem* 1997;272:18404–18410.

71. Iozzo RV, Moscatello DK, McQuillan DJ, et al. Decorin is a biological ligand for the epidermal growth factor receptor. *J Biol Chem* 1999;274: 4489–4492.

72. Munz C, Naumann U, Grimmel C, et al. TGF-beta-independent induction of immunogenicity by decorin gene transfer in human malignant glioma cells. *Eur J Immunol* 1999;29:1032–1040.

73. Olsson U, Bondjers G, Camejo G. Fatty acids modulate the composition of extracellular matrix in cultured human arterial smooth muscle cells by altering the expression of genes for proteoglycan core proteins. *Diabetes* 1999;48:616–622.

74. Okamoto O, Fujiwara S, Abe M, et al. Dermatopontin interacts with transforming growth factor beta and enhances its biological activity. *Biochem J* 1999;337:537–541.

75. Stander M, Naumann U, Dumitrescu L, et al. Decorin gene transfer-mediated suppression of TGF-beta synthesis abrogates experimental malignant glioma growth in vivo. *Gene Ther* 1998;5:1187–1194.

76. Khanna A, Li B, Li P, et al. Transforming growth factor-beta 1: regulation with a TGF-beta 1 antisense oligomer. *Kidney Int Suppl* 1996;53: S2-S6.

77. Redington AE, Roche WR, Holgate ST, et al. Co-localization of immunoreactive transforming growth factor-beta 1 and decorin in bronchial biopsies from asthmatic and normal subjects. *J Pathol* 1998; 186:410–415.

78. Schonherr E, Broszat M, Brandan E, et al. Decorin core protein fragment Leu155-Val260 interacts with TGF-beta but does not compete for decorin binding to type I collagen. *Arch Biochem Biophys* 1998;355: 241–248.

79. Asakura S, Kato H, Fujino S, et al. Role of transforming growth factor-beta1 and decorin in development of central fibrosis in pulmonary adenocarcinoma. *Hum Pathol* 1999;30:195–198.

80. Mogyorosi A, Ziyadeh FN. Increased decorin mRNA in diabetic mouse kidney and in mesangial and tubular cells cultured in high glucose. *Am J Physiol* 1998;275:F827-F832.

81. Imai K, Hiramatsu A, Fukushima D, et al. Degradation of decorin by matrix metalloproteinases: identification of the cleavage sites, kinetic analyses and transforming growth factor-beta1 release. *Biochem J* 1997;322:809–814.

82. Roughley PJ, White RJ, Mort JS. Presence of pro-forms of decorin and biglycan in human articular cartilage. *Biochem J* 1996;318:779–784.

83. Ehnis T, Dieterich W, Bauer M, et al. A chondroitin/dermatan sulfate form of CD44 is a receptor for collagen XIV (undulin). *Exp Cell Res* 1996;229:388–397.

84. Mauviel A, Santra M, Chen YQ, et al. Transcriptional regulation of decorin gene expression. Induction by quiescence and repression by tumor necrosis factor-alpha. *J Biol Chem* 1995;270:11692–11700.

85. Kuroda K, Shinkai H. Decorin and glycosaminoglycan synthesis in skin fibroblasts from patients with systemic sclerosis. *Arch Dermatol Res* 1997;289:481–485.

86. Demoor-Fossard M, Redini F, Boittin M, et al. Expression of decorin

and biglycan by rabbit articular chondrocytes: effects of cytokines and phenotypic modulation. *Biochim Biophys Acta* 1998;1398:179–191.

87. Kolettas E, Rosenberger RF. Suppression of decorin expression and partial induction of anchorage-independent growth by the v-src oncogene in human fibroblasts. *Eur J Biochem* 1998;254:266–274.

88. Brown CT, Nugent MA, Lau FW, et al. Characterization of proteoglycans synthesized by cultured corneal fibroblasts in response to transforming growth factor-beta and fetal calf serum. *J Biol Chem* 1999;274:7111–7119.

89. Nakamura N, Timmermann SA, Hart DA, et al. A comparison of in vivo gene delivery methods for antisense therapy in ligament healing. *Gene Ther* 1998;5:1455–1461.

90. Peters H, Noble NA, Border WA. Transforming growth factor-beta in human glomerular injury. *Curr Opin Nephrol Hypertens* 1997;6:389–393.

91. Giri SN, Hyde DM, Braun RK, et al. Antifibrotic effect of decorin in a bleomycin hamster model of lung fibrosis. *Biochem Pharmacol* 1997;54:1205–1216.

92. Hirsch CS, Ellner JJ, Blinkhorn R, et al. In vitro restoration of T cell responses in tuberculosis and augmentation of monocyte effector function against Mycobacterium tuberculosis by natural inhibitors of transforming growth factor beta. *Proc Natl Acad Sci U S A* 1997;94: 3926–3931.

93. Yokoyama H, Deckert T. Central role of TGF-beta in the pathogenesis of diabetic nephropathy and macrovascular complications: a hypothesis. *Diabet Med* 1996;13:313–320.

94. Henke C, Bitterman P, Roongta U, et al. Induction of fibroblast apoptosis by anti-CD44 antibody: implications for the treatment of fibroproliferative lung disease. *Am J Pathol* 1996;149:1639–1650.

CHAPTER 14

Cartilage Therapies

Chondrocyte Transplantation, Osteochondral Allografts, and Autografts

Constance R. Chu

Articular cartilage is a connective tissue organ with remarkable mechanical properties. It possesses a unique functional structure that allows for near frictionless multiplanar motion. Adult articular cartilage also possesses a limited capacity to heal (1). Once destroyed, its highly ordered matrix and cellular architecture are not readily restored by mature chondrocytes. Thus, the treatment of symptomatic, full-thickness articular cartilage defects is a clinical and scientific challenge.

Loss of articular cartilage can occur in many ways. Patients with inflammatory arthritis generally sustain cartilage damage in multiple joints. Tricompartmental disease is frequently present when the knee is affected. Similarly, patients with genetic factors predisposing them to the development of degenerative arthritis and those with idiopathic primary osteoarthritis often present with tricompartmental findings. The surgical options discussed in this chapter are not intended for the treatment of knees with generalized arthritis. Rather, they represent biologic treatment options for the repair of focal chondral and osteochondral lesions of the knee.

To make useful comparisons between several treatment options, it is necessary to establish standard criteria for documenting the initial cartilage lesion and for assessing outcome following the selected procedure. To date, clinical series on articular cartilage treatments have not used uniform evaluation standards. Before considering treatment options, it is important to assess and define the extent of injury.

The foundation for modern classification of articular cartilage damage was laid by Outerbridge (2) in 1961 when he described four grades of chondromalacia patella.

Outerbridge grade I consisted of cartilage softening and swelling; grade II represented fragmentation and fissuring of less than 0.5 inch; grade III defects had clefts and fissures in an area greater than 0.5 inch; and grade IV lesions had exposed subchondral bone. In 1976, Insall et al. (3) classified chondromalacia patella into similar grades with minor differences: grade II was differentiated from grade III not by size of the lesion but by the depth of the fissures. Insall's grade II consisted of deep clefts extending to the subchondral bone, whereas grade III had fibrillation giving a "crab meat" appearance.

In 1988, Bauer and Jackson (4) described a six-grade system based on appearance of the lesion. Grades I through IV describe relatively fresh lesions without significant degenerative changes. Grade I is linear; grade II, stellate; grade III, a flap tear; and grade IV, a crater. Grade V (fibrillation) and grade VI (degrading) with exposed subchondral bone represent early degenerative joint disease.

A comprehensive evaluation was proposed by Noyes and Stabler (5) in 1989. This system used a scoring system based on the magnitude of articular cartilage damage and the size of the lesion. Location and appearance of the lesion were also documented. Three grades of lesions were described and subdivided into subtypes A and B. The A subtypes represented less involvement than B subtypes. Grade I lesions were closed lesions with gross pathology confined to cartilage softening. Grade II lesions were characterized by disruption of the articular surface and grade I lesions represented any surface with exposed bone.

Despite the need for wide use of a comprehensive evaluation system, no consensus exists concerning which system to use. Perhaps the most widely used grading system continues to be a modified Outerbridge system (6). Under this system, grade I consists of softening and swelling of the cartilage; grade II lesions consist of partial-thickness fibrillation; grade III defects consist of lesions with clefts down to subchondral bone; and grade IV defects consist of exposed subchondral bone. The treatment options discussed in this chapter are for these types of focal grade III and grade IV articular cartilage lesions with full-thickness involvement greater than 1 cm^2 in any of the three compartments of the knee.

The prevalence of chondral defects in the symptomatic knee is high. In a retrospective review of 31,516 knee arthroscopies, Curl and colleagues (6) determined that modified Outerbridge grade III lesions were present in 41% of the knees and grade IV lesions in 19.2%. Grade III lesions were most commonly found in the patella and the medial femoral condyle and were the most common lesions in patients older than 30 years. Grade IV lesions were seen in 20% of arthroscopies with 72% found in patients older than 40 years. The medial femoral condyle was the most common location for single grade IV defects. Another study determined that the incidence of chondral injuries in knees with acute hemarthrosis was 20% (7). Untreated, focal chondral injuries are thought to progress to degenerative arthritis in most patients. Lesions greater than 1 to 2 cm^2 often become symptomatic long before the onset of osteoarthritic changes. Traumatic and degenerative lesions of articular cartilage are a frequent cause of disability.

Recent advances in chondrocyte transplantation techniques, autograft mosaicplasty and renewed interest in allograft transplantation have increased the number of treatment options for patients with symptomatic focal chondral defects (8). These procedures, along with more traditional treatments, including marrow-based techniques, such as microfracture, subchondral drilling, and abrasion arthroplasty, will be the principal topics reviewed in this chapter.

MARROW STIMULATION TECHNIQUES

When confronted at arthroscopy with a chondral defect, surgeons will frequently treat the lesions with interventions ranging from debridement of fibrillated cartilage and unstable chondral flaps to stimulation of a marrow-based repair response through microfracture, subchondral drilling, and abrasion arthroplasty. Relief of pain and mechanical symptoms of catching have been observed following arthroscopic debridement. Marrow-based techniques consisting of systematic violation of the subchondral bone plate to access reparative cells from the bone marrow are reported to provide varying degrees of success. It has been difficult to separate the treatment effect of the marrow stimulation from that of arthroscopy alone.

In 1959, Pridie (9) described generating a fibrocartilaginous repair tissue to damaged femoral condyles following joint debridement and drilling of the cartilage defect with a ¼-inch drill. Forty-six of 62 knees treated in this fashion were reported to be a success (10,11). The poor results were largely attributed to patellofemoral malfunction associated with patellectomy. Because all patients in this series underwent thorough open joint debridement to include osteophyte resection when necessary, it is unclear whether the clinical successes occurred because of the debridement alone.

Richards and Lonergen (12) separated 43 patients into 2 groups, with 22 patients undergoing arthroscopic joint debridement alone and 21 patients undergoing arthroscopic joint debridement combined with the Pridie procedure. All of these patients also underwent concomitant meniscal debridement. Overall, 80% of patients undergoing the Pridie procedure at average follow-up of 25 months and 81% of patients undergoing debridement alone at average follow-up of 40 months had satisfactory results. Unfortunately, the study did not carefully segregate patients on the basis of degree of degenerative arthritis present. Thus, patients with worse disease (grades III and IV chondromalacia) tended to undergo the Pridie procedure, thereby confounding the results.

Using a rabbit model, Mitchell and Shepard (13) demonstrated in 1976 that subchondral drilling could stimulate the repair of large chondral defects. The reparative cells appeared to originate from the bone marrow. Histologic studies showed that the repair tissue emanated from the drill holes to gradually cover areas of exposed subchondral bone. Although the repair tissue was cartilaginous in appearance, the tissue could not withstand the mechanical stresses within the joint and degenerated by one year. These findings were reconfirmed by Shapiro and colleagues (14) in 1993. These investigators used tritiated thymidine injections to show that the repair tissue originated from the primitive mesenchymal cells of the marrow.

Johnson (15) built on the principles of subchondral drilling to access marrow mesenchymal cells by abrading the superficial layer of subchondral bone using a motorized burr to expose interosseous vessels. This technique became known as *abrasion arthroplasty*. Protected weight bearing was instituted for 4 to 6 weeks after the procedure. He biopsied the resulting repair tissue. It was found to be fibrocartilage containing predominantly type I collagen. Only one of eight biopsies contained any of the type II collagen that is characteristic of hyaline cartilage.

Bert and Maschka (16) reported on 59 patients at a minimum of 5 years after abrasion arthroplasty and arthroplastic debridement. These patients had severe unicompartmental degenerative arthritis with Ahlback's grade 2 radiographic changes (complete loss of joint space). Half of these patients exhibited joint space widening on radiographs obtained following abrasion arthroplasty. Nevertheless, there was no correlation between radiographic joint-space widening and clinical results. Fifteen of these patients, including several with radiographic evidence of joint-space widening, underwent total knee replacement. At the time of total knee replacement, several of these patients were found to have residual regenerative fibrocartilage. Meanwhile, 20% of patients with persistent joint space collapse continued to maintain satisfactory clinical results.

Reporting on a similar patient population, Rand (17) compared 131 knees with grades III and IV chondromalacia and radiographic joint space collapse treated with arthroscopic debridement to 28 knees with similar abnormalities treated by arthroscopic debridement and abrasion arthroplasty. Whereas 50% of the patients with abrasion arthroplasty knees failed and underwent total knee replacement at an average of 3 years following the procedure, 67% of the patients in the simple debridement group reported satisfactory results through 5-year follow-up. On the basis of these results, Rand concluded that arthroscopic debridement alone was preferable to abrasion arthroplasty in the management of grades III and IV chondromalacia of the knee.

Although reports following subchondral drilling and abrasion arthroplasty do not appear to demonstrate a positive treatment effect specific to the marrow stimulation procedure, Blevins et al. (18) and Steadman et al. (19) have reported encouraging results through microfracture. The microfracture technique differs from subchondral drilling or abrasion in that motorized instruments are not used to expose the bone marrow. Rather, an arthroscopic awl is used to penetrate the subchondral bone at approximately 3- to 4-mm intervals. In theory, this technique allows preservation of the subchondral bone plate and reduces the potential for tissue damage through thermal necrosis. A comprehensive rehabilitation program, including immediate postoperative continuous passive motion (CPM), protected weight bearing for 6 to 8 weeks, and early progressive strength training, is used (20). These factors, combined with a tendency toward use of microfracture in patients with focal chondral defects and no radiographic changes, may account for the improved results over what has been reported for subchondral drilling and abrasion arthroplasty.

AUTOGENOUS CHONDROCYTE TRANSPLANTATION

Transplantation of autologous chondrocytes can take place within bioresorbable matrices or as a cell suspension contained within the chondral defect by a periosteal patch. Currently, only the latter technique has been approved by the Food and Drug Administration (FDA) for use in the United States.

The technique of autologous chondrocyte transplantation (ACT) was first reported by Grande et al. (21) in 1989 as an animal study using a rabbit model. The authors performed a series of three experiments using 3-mm, full-thickness defects placed in the patellae of adult New Zealand white rabbits. In the primary experimental group, autologous chondrocytes were enzymatically liberated from the removed patellar cartilage and expanded *in vitro*. The passaged chondrocytes were then injected into the defect under an autogenous flap of periosteum sutured over the defect. Control knees either had no treatment or received the periosteal patch without cells. Animals were killed 6 weeks after chondrocyte transplantation. On average, the repair tissue was found to fill 82.4% of the 3-mm defects, which were injected with approximately 1 million autologous chondrocytes. Ungrafted defects had 16.5% fill, whereas defects treated with periosteum alone had 18.8% fill when evaluated by the same criteria. Autoradiography revealed the presence of approximately 8% labeled cells within grafted defects, suggesting that implanted cells participated in the repair process.

Petersen, one of the investigators in the study, subsequently applied the technique to patients in his native Sweden. The findings were published by Brittberg et al. (22) in 1994 in the *New England Journal of Medicine*. This study ignited tremendous worldwide interest in chondrocyte transplantation for the repair of articular cartilage defects.

The initial publication reported on short-term results in 23 patients who ranged in age from 14 to 48 years. All of the patients were treated for symptomatic cartilage defects ranging in size from 1.6 to 6.5 cm². Thirteen patients had traumatic defects to the femoral condyles, three patients suffered from osteochondritis dissecans, six patients had debilitating chondromalacia patella, and one patient had a traumatic chondral defect to the patella.

Articular cartilage biopsies were obtained arthroscopically from the upper medial trochlear rim of the affected knee. Chondrocytes were extracted from the cartilage through enzymatic digestion. These chondrocytes were expanded in cell culture to approximately 10 times the original number and reimplanted as a cell suspension of 2.6 to 5 million cells.

Implantation was performed through arthrotomy approximately 2 to 3 weeks after chondrocyte harvest. The chondral lesion was debrided to surrounding normal cartilage and underlying bone (Fig. 14.1). Care was taken to avoid violation of the subchondral bone. A periosteal patch slightly larger than the chondral defect was obtained from the ipsilateral proximal medial tibia and sutured to the rim of the defect (Figs. 14.2A, B). Cultured autologous chondrocytes were then injected under the patch (Fig. 14.2C). Patients were non–weight bearing initially, but were permitted to perform range of motion exercises by 2 to 3 days after surgery. Weightbearing was gradually introduced during the first 8 weeks.

Patients in this initial study were evaluated every 8 to 12 weeks. Arthroscopic evaluation was performed at 3

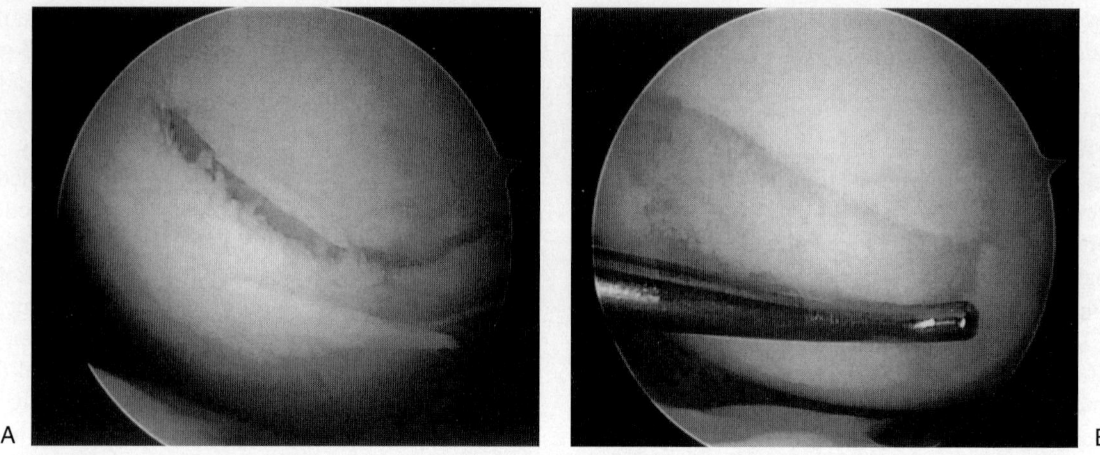

FIGURE 14.1. Full-thickness chondral defect. **A:** Unstable chondral flap found at arthroscopy. **B:** Debridement of the flap reveals a grade IV lesion with exposure of subchondral bone.

months and again at 12 to 46 months after the procedure. Full-thickness biopsies were obtained from the central area of the repair at the second arthroscopy in 15 patients. Eleven of 15 biopsies were reported to be hyaline cartilage by histologic examination with 5 of the biopsies positive for the presence of type II collagen by immunohistochemistry. The six histologic failures consisting of fibrous repairs were all in the patella. At 2-year follow-up, clinical evaluation revealed that 14 of 16 patients with femoral condylar transplants received good to excellent ratings. Only two of seven patients receiving patellar grafts had similar clinical results. On the basis of these findings, the authors concluded that the procedure could be used with reasonable expectations for success in the treatment of femoral condylar lesions. They suggested that the poor results in the patella may be due to mal-

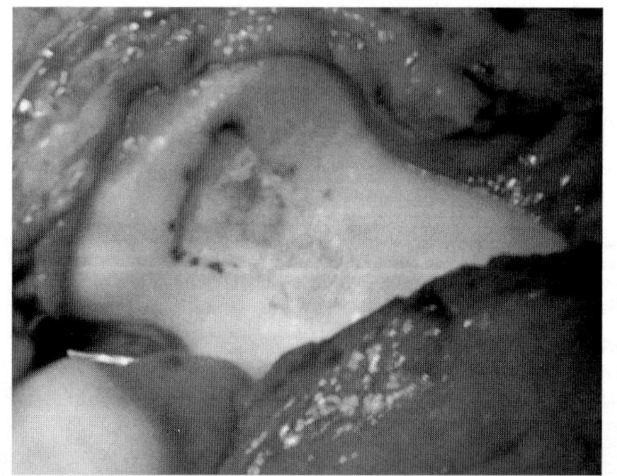

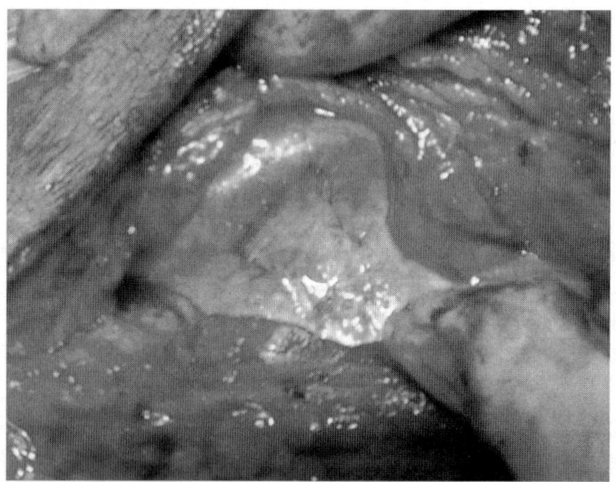

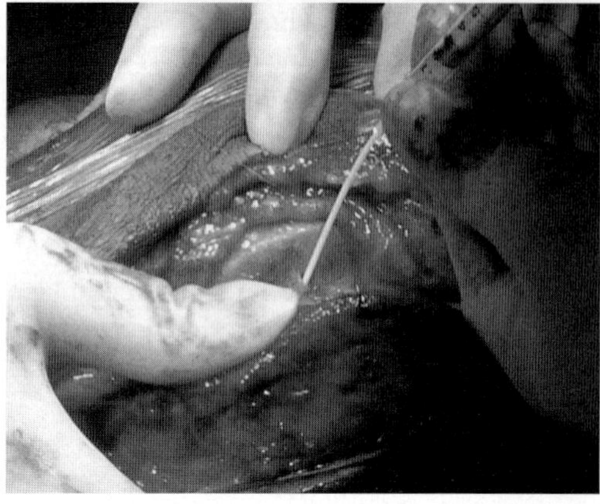

FIGURE 14.2. Autologous chondrocyte implantation. **A:** Large, full-thickness defect to the trochlea after debridement of damaged cartilage. A previous marrow stimulation procedure had failed. A medial intralesional osteophyte is present. **B:** Trochlear defect after suture of an autologous periosteal patch to the rim of the defect. **C:** Injection of autologous chondrocytes underneath the periosteal patch into the chondral defect.

tracking. Thus, results in the patella could be improved by concomitant correction of patellar maltracking at the time of chondrocyte implantation.

Subsequent reports on the first 100 consecutive patients treated in Sweden with 2 to 9 years of follow-up have demonstrated encouraging clinical results (8). The average follow-up was 3 years and 11 months. Ninety-two percent of isolated femoral condylar repairs were rated good to excellent. Among condylar lesions that required anterior cruciate ligament reconstruction, 75% achieved similar clinical ratings. According to this report (8), 80% of biopsies performed at second arthroscopy were consistent with a hyaline cartilage repair. The hyaline repairs were firm to probing while fibrous repairs were softer.

Animal studies using a canine model demonstrated hyaline repairs at 6 months, which rapidly deteriorated by 1-year follow-up. Breinan and colleagues (23) evaluated 44 defects in 14 dogs separated into three treatment groups. Group I lesions received autologous chondrocyte transplantation under a periosteal flap sutured to the surrounding cartilage. Group II lesions received the sutured periosteal flap alone without cells. Group III lesions were left empty. At the end of 12 and 18 months, no difference between any of the treatment groups could be detected by histologic evaluation. Repairs were generally inadequate with only 36% to 76% fill. Hyaline cartilage was present in only 10% to 23% of the repair area. Autologous chondrocyte implantation was associated with the least fill. Repair fill and quality declined between 12 and 18 months. In addition, suturing of the periosteum to the adjacent cartilage appeared to disrupt the normal cartilage. Increased proteoglycan depletion and more chondrocyte cloning was seen surrounding lesions that received sutured periosteum (groups I and II). In contrast to the 1989 rabbit study (21) that reported on the repair tissue at an early time point of 6 weeks, this longer term canine study failed to demonstrate a long-term treatment effect from autologous chondrocyte transplantation.

Although clinical results approaching 10 years appear to be more positive than what would be expected from experiments in the dog, patients require careful monitoring during the 2-year healing process (8). Difficulties that may be encountered after ACT include repair tissue and periosteal delamination. The delamination can be classified as marginal, partial, or complete on the basis of the amount of separation from the adjacent host articular cartilage and the underlying subchondral bone. There is frequently antecedent trauma. Marginal or partial delamination can be treated by arthroscopic debridement. Small cartilage defects uncovered by debridement of delaminated tissue can be managed by microfracture. Larger defects have been addressed with revision chondrocyte transplantation. When complete delamination of the repair tissue is present, the grafting procedure has failed and revision surgery through repeated ACT or another cartilage resurfacing procedure is indicated.

Problems can also occur with periosteal overgrowth. Hypertrophy of the periosteal graft is reported to occur about 10% to 15% of the time. Patients who were progressing well during the first 3 to 6 months will suddenly complain of pain and catching. A new effusion may be present. Patients with these complaints should undergo arthroscopy. Several patterns of periosteal flap abnormalities have been noted. Superficial fibrillation is most frequently encountered. Overgrowth of the periosteal patch over the surrounding cartilage is also common. The periosteum sometimes completely delaminates from the underlying cartilage repair, which remains intact. Occasionally, a mound of periosteum-derived tissue forms at one end of the repair. Areas of hypertrophic or delaminated periosteum are readily debrided at arthroscopy.

ACT is currently approved by the FDA for the treatment of chondral defects to the distal femur. The biologic processes of cartilage regeneration through ACT are not well understood. Questions remain concerning whether the repair tissue arises primarily from the transplanted cells, the periosteal graft, or intraarticular tissues. Long-term durability of the repair tissue has not been consistently demonstrated in animal studies (23,24). Nevertheless, patient satisfaction with the procedure has been reported to be greater than 92% at medium-term follow-up of 2 to 9 years. Individual patients appear to undergo continued improvement over a 3-year period. The procedure has been shown to be cost-effective when evaluated against other relatively costly treatments for chronic diseases (25). Whether ACT, or a derivative of the current technique, proves to deliver a durable repair tissue or not, it remains one of the first FDA-approved medical treatments based on laboratory-manipulated cells. It is currently the most sophisticated cell-based treatment for articular cartilage repair available for general use.

ARTICULAR CARTILAGE TRANSPLANTATION

A major obstacle to successful articular cartilage regeneration through cell-based therapies centers on coercing the correct cells into the appropriate three-dimensional location for replicating the cellular and matrical architecture of adult articular cartilage (26). Interest in transplanting the intact articular cartilage organ is not new. Articular cartilage transplantation concepts and techniques differ mainly in regards to whether the tissue is obtained from another site within the same patient (autograft) or from a cadaveric donor (allograft). Among allograft treatments, differences may be found in the use of refrigerated (fresh) or cryopreserved (frozen) osteochondral grafts.

AUTOGENOUS TRANSPLANTS

Use of autogenous osteochondral grafts have been sporadically reported in the literature (27–30). The advantages of using the patient's own tissues involve less risk for disease transmission and less risk for graft failure due to immunologic reactions or to failure of subchondral bone incorporation. Bone-to-bone healing between autogenous graft and host bone should occur through a standard fracture-healing mechanism. Concerns over donor site morbidity center around two issues: (a) Are there truly areas where articular cartilage can be spared? and (b) What damage to the joint may arise from either the insult of graft harvesting or from the presence of the resulting osteochondral defect?

Osteochondral mosaicplasty of focal chondral defects to the knee represents a method aimed at minimizing concerns over donor site morbidity through harvesting small-diameter osteochondral plugs (27,28,31,32). These grafts measuring 2.7 to 4.5 mm in diameter are obtained from the supracondylar ridges or the intercondylar notch of the affected knee. Harvested grafts consist of the articular surface along with approximately 10 mm of underlying bone. These plugs are then press-fit into similarly sized recipient holes within the previously prepared lesion site.

Mosaicplasty techniques were introduced in 1992 by Hangody and colleagues. Small plugs of intact articular cartilage are anchored in their new location by press-fit of the underlying bone. This bone rapidly unites with the recipient bone bed and provides a stable platform for the cartilage. The exposed bone provides a conduit for marrow-based repair cells to form a bridging fibrocartilage between the transplanted articular cartilages. Effort is made to preserve the viability of the chondrocytes within the transplanted articular cartilage through gentle harvest and implantation techniques. The resulting surface appears to function well in short-term follow-up.

Using a modified Hospital for Special Surgery Knee Score (HSSKS), Hangody and colleagues reported on 57 patients with more than 3 years of follow-up. Patients were evaluated by clinical examination and plain radiographs. Some patients underwent computed tomography, magnetic resonance imaging studies, arteriography, and ultrasound evaluations. Using the modified Hospital for Special Surgery (HSS) knee scoring system, 91% of the patients achieved a good or excellent result.

This technique has been used by the originators and others to treat a variety of chondral defects, including traumatic osteochondral defects and osteochondritis dissecans (31). The ideal defect is smaller than 2 cm and has a discrete margin surrounded by normal appearing articular cartilage. Patients should not have thin, chondromalacic cartilage that is less than 3-mm thick or synovitis, marginal osteophytes, or similar indicators of osteoarthritis that have reached a progressive stage. Additionally, patients with inflammatory arthritis are not candidates for the procedure.

The procedure can be performed arthroscopically, through arthroscopic assist, mini-arthrotomy, or formal arthrotomy. Approach choice is frequently dependent on size and location of the lesion as well as surgeon preference and experience. Currently, patellar lesions are approached by standard medial parapatellar arthrotomy with eversion of the patella. Small lesions (< 1.5 cm) to the medial femoral condyle can be treated arthroscopically.

Although the short- to medium-term results are encouraging, only longer term follow-up can determine the ultimate fate of the composite repair tissue. Biopsies of the treated regions and the donor sites generally reveal survival of the transplanted articular cartilage with intervening areas of fibrocartilage (27).

The strength of the fibrocartilaginous grout may or may not be sufficient to prevent debonding and degeneration of the repair over time. Nevertheless, the procedure appears effective in short- to medium-term relief of pain and disability arising from full-thickness focal chondral defects.

OSTEOARTICULAR ALLOGRAFTS

Articular cartilage allograft transplantation has a long history. In the last century, Lexer (33) performed two transplants on November 3, 1907. One was what he termed a "half-joint transplant." The second was a whole-joint transplant. The first case was a 38-year-old man who needed a new left proximal tibia after resection of a myeloid sarcoma. Lexer transplanted a right proximal tibia salvaged from an elderly man undergoing amputation for peripheral vascular disease. The right-to-left mismatch apparently did not adversely affect the outcome. The graft incorporated and the man was able to exercise, stand, and walk. Approximately 1.5 years later, the man requested an amputation for religious reasons. On retrieval, the specimen had complete union with the diaphysis and the joint cartilage was well maintained.

The second case consisted of a femoral and tibial epiphyseal transplantation performed in a 19-year-old woman who developed a right-angle synostosis of the left knee as a result of osteomyelitis. Again, the fresh donor tissue was obtained from the amputated limb of an elderly man. Her native patella continued to limit motion and was removed. At this operation, Lexer noted that the transplanted epiphyses had healed to host bone and that the articular surfaces looked normal. He followed her progress over the next 16 years during which she maintained painless weight bearing and sufficient joint motion to go up and down stairs. Notably, she was captured during the Great War in the Russian drive on East Prussia and had to march for days at a time. During these forced marches, the knee that did not require surgery swelled painfully, forcing the patient to rely on her transplanted knee.

Lexer reported a 50% success rate using articular cartilage allografts to resurface knees, fingers, and elbows in 23 joints (33). Five of 14 transplanted knees failed, all due to infection. All five infected knees were in patients who received transplants as treatment for ankylosis resulting from osteomyelitis. Three of the five failed knees had recurrent infection with tuberculosis. Foci of encapsulated pus were present at the time of joint transplantation in the other two failed knees. In this report, Lexer stated that fresh transplants were superior to fresh cadaver transplants mainly because of a high infection rate following cadaver transplants. Notably, the cadaver knees were apparently harvested in the morgue, not under aseptic conditions. Failures not due to infection were most frequently attributed to collapse of the subchondral bone followed by degeneration of the articular surface.

Although Lexer used fresh tissues, time constraints associated with storage and transport of fresh allografts may limit their utility (34–36). Frozen allografts have mostly been used for large joint reconstruction following tumor surgery. Mankin and colleagues reported early results following use of large cryopreserved allografts with largely positive clinical results. In this series of 150 allograft implantations, 91 had 2 or more years of follow-up. Of these patients, 70% of the patients had good to excellent functional results. The authors noted that transplantations that did not involve a joint had better results. In a later study, analysis of the joint surfaces revealed that 75% of the grafts exhibited subchondral fractures indicative of cartilage destruction. At retrieval through autopsy or revision, the articular surfaces were acellular (36). The articular cartilage of frozen osteochondral allografts appear to undergo degenerative changes within 5 to 8 years.

Cryopreservation of intact articular cartilage has been shown to kill articular chondrocytes in all but the most superficial layers (37). Although the biomechanical properties may be preserved in the short term (38), viable chondrocytes are necessary for maintenance of the functional structure under long-term *in vivo* mechanical demands.

Renewed interest in the fresh osteochondral allograft has ensued in part due to the failure of frozen grafts to retain chondrocyte viability and in part due to the strong interest in articular cartilage repair generated by chondrocyte transplantation, mosaicplasty and tissue engineering. The use of fresh osteochondral allografts for the treatment of chondral defects has been reported on by at least three centers with consistent clinical results.

Clinical Series

Gross et al. (39) and McDermott et al. (40) have used small fragment osteochondral allografts for the treatment of traumatic injuries since 1972. In a survivorship analysis performed on 92 knees in 91 patients (of a series of 99 knees in 98 patients), Beaver et al. (41) reported a 75% success rate at 5 years, 64% at 10 years, and 63% at 14 years. Failure in this report was defined as either need for reoperation or persistence of preoperative symptoms. The

authors described a higher failure rate in bipolar grafts when compared with unipolar grafts. A more recent report with average follow-up of 7.5 years (range, 1–22 years) showed a 95% success rate at 5 years, 71% at 10 years, and 66% success at 20 years (42). The overall success rate was 85%.

Results from Chu et al. (26) and Meyers and colleagues (43) are quite similar. With a minimum of 2-year follow-up, Meyers et al. reported a 77.5% success rate using a fresh, osteochondral shell allograft to resurface 40 damaged knees. At 5 to 10 years after receiving a fresh osteochondral shell allograft, Chu et al. (26) reported on 55 knees with an overall success rate of 76%. Success in this series was defined as a good to excellent clinical result based on a modified D'Aubigne and Postel rating scheme. Knees treated with unipolar transplants had an 84% success rate while bipolar replacements were successful 50% of the time.

A 1986 report by Garrett (44) on treatment of unipolar femoral condylar defects in 24 patients showed no failures at short-term follow-up of 1 to 4 years. Only 1 of 24 grafts did not have radiographic evidence of bony union within 6 to 12 weeks. This graft eventually healed by 12 months. Eleven of the 24 patients had a second operation. Seven of these second surgeries were for removal of hardware and four were arthroscopic examinations at 1 to 2 years to determine clearance for full activity. The grafts appeared healthy in all 11 cases; fraying was limited to the periphery in all but two cases and there were no signs of graft collapse. Longer follow-up of this series of patients would provide additional information concerning the longevity of unipolar fresh osteochondral allografts.

Graft Retrieval and Storage

Fresh cadaver knees are harvested in accordance with the guidelines of the American Association of Tissue Banks. Grafts are procured in operating rooms under aseptic conditions within 24 hours after death. The knees are placed in sterile physiologic solutions and refrigerated at 4°C. Ghazavi et al. (42) and Garrett (44) advocated transplantation of the allograft tissue within 12 to 24 hours after graft procurement. The donors in the series from these authors were younger than the age of 30 years.

Patients in the series reported at different time intervals by Chu et al. (26) received their transplants 3 to 7 days after donor death. The waiting period permitted more complete testing of the donor tissue for evidence of infectious agents. It also exploited the differing biologic and metabolic properties of bone and cartilage to create a safer osteochondral allograft. Analysis of retrieved human grafts have confirmed animal study data indicating that chondrocytes can survive for several days to weeks within intact articular cartilage maintained at 4°C (34,45,46). In contrast, bone and hematologic cells do not survive longer than 48 hours after death even when refrigerated at 4°C (47). Within the 3- to 7-day window, the articular cartilage maintains its viability and is transplanted alive. At the same time, the more infectious and more immunogenic bone and marrow cells die and can then be removed by pulsatile lavage. This leaves an acellular subchondral bone to serve as a scaffold for the ingrowth of host bone. This treatment protocol serves to minimize risks for immune reactions and disease transmission without demonstrable compromise to articular cartilage viability (26).

Surgical Technique

All transplantation procedures were accomplished by arthrotomy. Garrett operated only on isolated femoral condylar lesions between 1.2 and 2.75 cm in diameter. He converted the defects into cylindrical shapes 8 to 10 mm deep using specially designed instruments. An identically sized plug was then obtained from the donor and press-fit into position. Internal fixation using Kirschner wires was used as needed. In the series reported at different time intervals by Meyers, Convery, and Chu, focal unipolar lesions of the femoral condyles were similarly treated by press-fit of an identically sized shell allograft of 5- to 10-mm thick obtained from an orthotopic location (Fig. 14.3). Most lesions in this series were converted to a trapezoidal shape. Biodegradable pins were used to supplement fixation when necessary.

Larger lesions in the series of Meyers, Convery, and Chu frequently required fixation using bone screws. In cases where the patella, trochlea, or entire medial or lateral compartment were resurfaced, allografts were secured using extraarticular screws. Similarly, in the treatment of posttraumatic knee defects, Gross implanted small-fragment allografts to reconstruct deficient condyles and tibial plateaus. For lesions of this size, two partially threaded cancellous screws were routinely used to fix the graft to the host bone. Patients in this series often required a realignment osteotomy to correct malalignment and to unload the transplanted cartilage.

Rehabilitation

Protected weight bearing is instituted until there is radiographic evidence of bone incorporation. Smaller condylar lesions may incorporate within 6 weeks, whereas larger transplants may take 1 to 2 years to heal. Patients are non–weight bearing for a minimum of 6 weeks. Early motion is initiated through immediate use of continuous passive motion machines. Active and active assisted range of motion along with isometric strengthening exercises are permitted. Resistive exercises are not

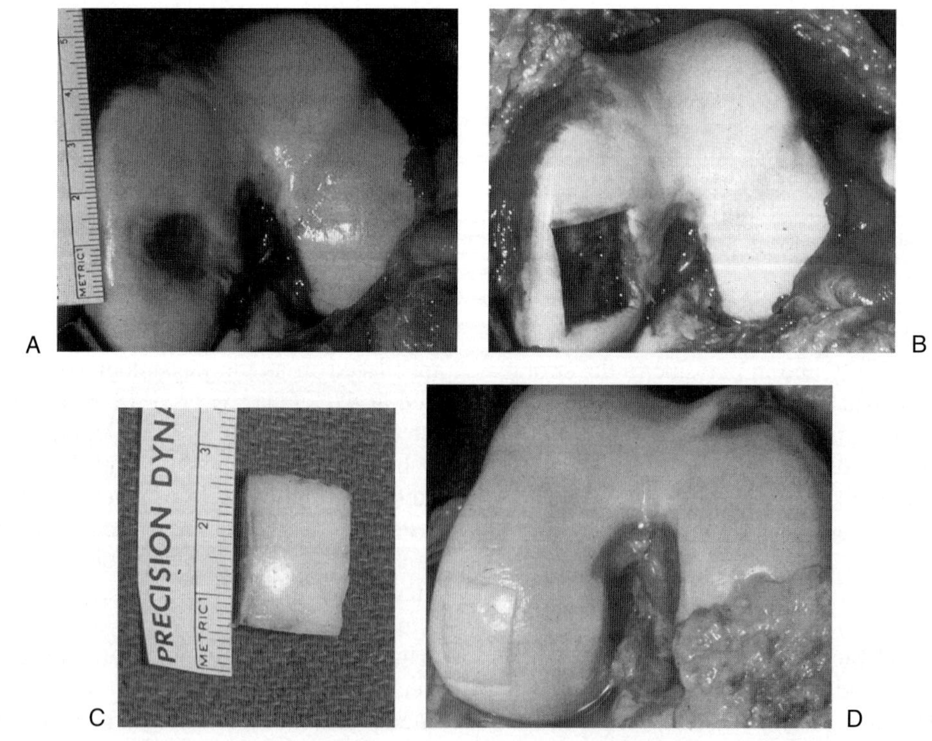

FIGURE 14.3. Osteochondral allograft. **A:** Large ulcerative lesion to the medial femoral condyle. **B:** Same defect as **(A)** after removal of damaged cartilage and "squaring-off" the lesion. **C:** An osteochondral allograft harvested from the orthotopic location in the medial femoral condyle of a size-matched donor. **D:** The graft has been "press-fit" into the defect.

permitted until the graft is healed. Patients with larger grafts or concomitant osteotomies or ligament reconstructions may require supplemental bracing for 1 to 2 years. Gross and colleagues routinely placed patients in ischial bearing braces for a full year to assist with prolonged, protected weight bearing.

Analysis of Failures

Bipolar grafts and grafts in older patients had a greater tendency toward failure (26,48). In an analysis of failures among 108 patients, Oakeshotte et al. (48) reported that the average age of those with successful grafts was 37.8 years, whereas the average age of patients with failed grafts was 57. Most failed grafts had some radiographic evidence of subchondral pathology. Subchondral collapse, fracture, or sclerosis were most frequently seen (49). Firm fixation with use of pins and screws as needed and proper size-matching of the grafts are important in achieving optimum results. Other reasons for failure included progression of osteoarthritic changes in other compartments, failure to correct instability or malalignment at the time of allografting, or systemic illnesses such as multiple sclerosis or lupus, which adversely affected healing or rehabilitation.

The procedure is considered to be bone-sparing. In posttraumatic defects with bone loss, the allograft serves to improve available bone stock. Conversion to total knee replacement or to unicondylar knee replacement is usually straightforward.

Immunology

The high success rate with fresh osteochondral allografts reported in clinical series from three separate institutions suggests that rejection of these grafts in most patients may be clinically insignificant. No effort was made in any of these institutions to match donor to recipient by histocompatibility antigens. Immunosuppressive agents were not used. The rationale behind the clinical success of these grafts centers around the insulating effect of the dense, cartilage matrix. In theory, this dense, avascular matrix serves to shield membrane-associated histocompatibility antigens present on viable chondrocytes from cellular and humoral immune responses.

The immune response to the transplanted bone and marrow cells may be transient because those cells do not survive and persist in the transplanted tissue. For grafts transplanted within 12 to 24 hours after harvest, donor bone and marrow cell necrosis can be expected to occur within the first 24 to 48 hours, quite possibly accompanied by some type of host immune response to foreign antigens. The protocol originating in San Diego serves to minimize transfer of bone and marrow cells by delaying the time of transplant for several days to allow for extra-

corporeal cell death. These dead cells are then flushed away with pulsatile lavage prior to graft implantation.

Animal studies and human case reports exist, however, that indicate that there may be a host immune response to osteocartilaginous transplants (50–54). Some patients form cytotoxic antibodies after receipt of musculoskeletal transplants (55). Allograft bone and tissues incorporate slower than autogenous transplants. In some instances, persistent effusions or even bone resorption were associated to graft failure. These cases all suggest the presence of host immune factors that may ultimately compromise graft longevity. Further study in this area may lead to improved patient and donor selection criteria. Control of potential immune responses may also lead to more predictable clinical outcomes.

Transmission of Disease

The transfer of organs, tissues, and cells between individuals always carries the risk for disease transmission. The risk for transmitting blood-borne pathogens is proportional to the amount of hematologic cells and fluids that are transferred (56,57). Musculoskeletal connective tissues generally carry lower risk than solid organs such as kidney, heart, or lung (58). Bones and tendons that have a blood supply are frequently transplanted dead following cryopreservation. Viruses and bacteria, however are quite capable of surviving extended periods of cold storage.

The primary means for minimizing disease transmission is through careful screening of donors and testing of donor tissue for evidence of microbial contamination or infection with known pathogens such as human immune deficiency virus (HIV 1, 2, and other strains as they become known), hepatitis B (HBV), and hepatitis C (HCV). In 1996, Schreiber et al. (56) reported the risk for transmitting HIV, HBV, and HCV by transfusion of blood from donors who passed all routine screening tests to be as follows: HIV, 1 in 493,000; HBV, 1 in 63,000; and HCV, 1 in 103,000. Osteochondral grafts from donors who test negative for known infectious agents should carry no additional risk for disease transmission above that of blood transfusion. In theory, the risk is likely to be substantially less than that of blood transfusion.

A 1995, a report by Tomford (58) estimated the use of musculoskeletal allografts of bone, tendon, and cartilage to be approximately 150,000 transplants annually in the United States. There have been only two reported cases of HIV transmission from musculoskeletal transplants. The first case occurred in 1984 when a young woman developed acquired immunodeficiency syndrome (AIDS) after receiving a frozen femoral head allograft during spine arthrodesis to treat idiopathic scoliosis. The femoral head came from an untested donor with lymphadenopathy and risk factors now widely recognized as associated with

HIV infection. Using current screening tests, tissues from this donor would be rejected.

Since 1985, donors of blood, organs, tissues, and semen have been routinely screened for HIV-1 antibody. In 1987, an elderly woman, with no risk factors aside from receiving a femoral head during her hip replacement in 1985, tested positive for HIV. The donor was a young man with no known risk factors whose serum tested negative for HIV-1 antibody using the technology of the time (59). Reexamination of the tissues in 1991 revealed that the donor was infected with HIV-1. Of 48 identified recipients of tissues from this donor, 41 were tested for HIV-1 antibody. All four recipients of organs (liver, heart, and kidneys) and three of four recipients of unprocessed, fresh frozen musculoskeletal tissues were infected with HIV. All 25 identified recipients of processed bone tested negative. The bone was processed by removal of blood and bone marrow through high-pressure washes and treatment with ethanol followed by lyophilization. The individual receiving unprocessed frozen bone who tested negative had a proximal femur allograft as part a revision total hip replacement. Unlike the other transplanted fresh frozen bone allografts from the donor, the medullary canal of this proximal femur had been extensively reamed before implantation. The reaming likely removed most of the marrow and blood cells. Heat generated from reaming and cement polymerization may have then killed any remaining HIV infected cells.

HIV appears to be most efficiently transmitted through cells containing the CD4 surface receptor. Cells from the hematopoietic system are CD4-containing cells. Chondrocytes do not have the CD4 receptor. However, there is one report in which HIV DNA was detected in the articular cartilage of individuals with HIV infection (60). Transmission of hepatitis infection are also strongly associated with transfer of blood and blood products or with transplantation of viable, blood-containing organs. There are only a handful of reports in the literature implicating musculoskeletal allografts in the transmission of hepatitis. The transmission of viral disease has not been reported following cartilage transplantation (58). Removal of blood and bone marrow from fresh osteochondral allografts probably removes a large portion of the potential viral load. The San Diego protocol involving delayed transfer of osteochondral grafts for 3 to 7 days to allow for death of the more potentially infectious marrow and bone cells also provides additional time to obtain more comprehensive testing of donor tissues for infectious agents.

It is important to discuss with patients the risks of disease transmission when transplanting fresh, osteochondral allografts. Informed consent must be obtained before surgery. When compared with the risks of cancer, heart disease, or accidental death, the risk for disease transmission through musculoskeletal tissue transplantation is quite small; however, fresh osteochondral allografts can transmit disease. To minimize the risks of disease transmission, surgeons should ensure grafts are obtained from suppliers adhering to current standards for tissue banking as specified by the American Association of Tissue Banks and the FDA.

SUMMARY

Just a few years ago, few treatment options were available for the treatment of focal chondral defects of the knee. Although much research and development remains to be performed before clinically proven and widely applicable treatments become available, there is widespread optimism that solutions to the problem of articular cartilage regeneration exist. Consistent treatment algorithms reflecting current thinking have been established at several institutions.

REFERENCES

1. Mankin HJ. The response of articular cartilage to mechanical injury. *J Bone Joint Surg Am* 1982;64:460–466.
2. Outerbridge RE. The etiology of chondromalacia patellae. *J Bone Joint Surg Am* 1961;4:752–757.
3. Insall J, Falvo KA, Wise DW. Chondromalacia patellae: a prospective study. *J Bone Joint Surg Am* 1976;58L:1–8.
4. Bauer M, Jackson RW. Chondral lesions of the femoral condyles: a system of arthroscopic classification. *Arthroscopy* 1988;4:97–102.
5. Noyes FR, Stabler CL. A system for grading articular cartilage lesions at arthroscopy. *Am J Sports Med* 1989;17:505–513.
6. Curl WW, Krome J, Gordon ES, et al. Cartilage injuries: a review of 31,516 knee arthroscopies. *Arthroscopy* 1997;13:456–460.
7. Noyes FR, Bassett RW, Grood ES, et al. Arthroscopy in acute traumatic hemarthrosis of the knee: incidence of anterior cruciate tears and other injuries. *J Bone Joint Surg Am* 1980;62:687–695, 757.
8. Minas T, Nehrer S. Current concepts in the treatment of articular cartilage defects. *Orthopedics* 1997;20:525–538.
9. Pridie A. The method of resurfacing osteoarthritic knee joints. *J Bone Joint Surg* 1959;41:618.
10. Insall JN. Intra-articular surgery for degenerative arthritis of the knee: a report of the work of the late K. H. Pridie. *J Bone Joint Surg Br* 1967;49:211–228.
11. Insall J. The Pridie debridement operation for osteoarthritis of the knee. *Clin Orthop* 1974;101:61–67.
12. Richards R, Lonergen R. Arthroscopic surgery for relief of pain in the osteoarthritic knee. *Orthopedics* 1984;7:1705.
13. Mitchell N, Shepard N. The resurfacing of adult rabbit articular cartilage by multiple perforations through the subchondral bone. *J Bone Joint Surg Am* 1976;58:230–233.
14. Shapiro F, Koide S, Glimcher MJ. Cell origin and differentiation in the repair of full-thickness defects of articular cartilage. *J Bone Joint Surg Am* 1993;75:532–553.
15. Johnson LL. Arthroscopic abrasion arthroplasty historical and pathologic perspective: present status. *Arthroscopy* 1986;2:54–69.
16. Bert J, Maschka K. The arthroscopic treatment of unicompartmental gonarthrosis: a five year follow-up study with abrasion arthroplasty plus arthroscopic debridement and arthroscopic debridement alone. *Arthroscopy* 1989;5:25–32.
17. Rand J. Role of arthroscopy in osteoarthritis of the knee. *Arthroscopy* 1991;7:358.
18. Blevins FT, Steadman JR, Rodrigo JJ, et al. Treatment of articular cartilage defects in athletes: an analysis of functional outcome and lesion appearance (see comments). *Orthopedics* 1998; 21:7:761–767; discussion 767–768.
19. Steadman JR, Rodkey WG, Briggs KK, et al. (The microfracture technic in the management of complete cartilage defects in the knee joint). *Orthopade* 1999;28:26–32.
20. Rodrigo J, et al. Improvement of full-thickness chondral defect healing in the human knee after debridement and microfracture using continuous passive motion. *Am J Knee Surg* 1994;7:109–116.

21. Grande DA, Pitman MI, Peterson L, et al. The repair of experimentally produced defects in rabbit articular cartilage by autologous chondrocyte transplantation. *J Orthop Res* 1989;7:208–218.
22. Brittberg M, Lindahl A, Nilsson A, et al. Treatment of deep cartilage defects in the knee with autologous chondrocyte transplantation (see comments). *N Engl J Med* 1994;331:889–895.
23. Breinan HA, Minas T, Hsu HP, et al. Effect of cultured autologous chondrocytes on repair of chondral defects in a canine model. *J Bone Joint Surg Am* 1997;79:1439–1451.
24. Brittberg M, Nilsson A, Lindahl A, et al. Rabbit articular cartilage defects treated with autologous cultured chondrocytes. *Clin Orthop* 1996;326:270–283.
25. Minas T. Chondrocyte implantation in the repair of chondral lesions of the knee: economics and quality of life. *Am J Orthop* 1998;27:739–744.
26. Chu CR, Convery FR, Akeson WH, et al. Articular cartilage transplantation: clinical results in the knee. *Clin Orthop* 1999;360:159–168.
27. Hangody L, Kish G, Karpati Z, et al. Arthroscopic autogenous osteochondral mosaicplasty for the treatment of femoral condylar articular defects: a preliminary report. *Knee Surg Sports Traumatol Arthrosc* 1997;5:262–267.
28. Hangody L, Kish G, Karpati Z, et al. Mosaicplasty for the treatment of articular cartilage defects: application in clinical practice (see comments). *Orthopedics* 1998;21:751–756.
29. Outerbridge HK, Outerbridge AR, Outerbridge RE, et al. The use of lateral patellar autologous grafts for the repair of large osteochondral defects in the knee. *Acta Orthop Belg* 1999;65(suppl 1):129–135.
30. Yamashita F, Sakakida K, Suzu F, et al. The transplantation of an autogeneic osteochondral fragment for osteochondritis dissecans of the knee. *Clin Orthop* 1985;201:43–50.
31. Berlet GC, Mascia A, Miniaci A. Treatment of unstable osteochondritis dissecans lesions of the knee using autogenous osteochondral grafts (mosaicplasty). *Arthroscopy* 1999;15:312–316.
32. Kish G, Modis L, Hangody L. Osteochondral mosaicplasty for the treatment of focal chondral and osteochondral lesions of the knee and talus in the athlete: rationale, indications, techniques, and results. *Clin Sports Med* 1999;18:45–66, vi.
33. Lexer E. The classic: joint transplantation. *Clin Orthop Rel Res* 1985;197:4–10.
34. Amiel D, Harwood FL, Hoover JA, et al. A histologicand biochemical assessment of the cartilage matrix obtained from in vitro storage of osteochondral allografts. *Connect Tissue Res* 1989;23:89–99.
35. Malinin TI, Martinez OV, Brown MD. Banking of massive osteoarticular and intercalary bone allografts: 12 years' experience. *Clin Orthop* 1985;197:44–57.
36. Sammarco VJ, Gorab R, Miller R, et al. Human articular cartilage storage in cell culture medium: guidelines for storage of fresh osteochondral allografts. *Orthopedics* 1997;20:497–500.
37. Ohlendorf C, Tomford WW, Mankin HJ. Chondrocyte survival in cryopreserved osteochondral articular cartilage. *J Orthop Res* 1996;14:413–416.
38. Kiefer GN, Sundby K, McAllister D, et al. The effect of cryopreservation on the biomechanical behavior of bovine articular cartilage. *J Orthop Res* 1989;7:494–501.
39. Gross AE, Silverstein FA, Falk J, et al. The allotransplantation of partial joints in the treatment of osteoarthritis of the knee. *Clin Orthop* 1975;108:7–14.
40. McDermott AG, Langer F, Pritzker KP, et al. Fresh small-fragment osteochondral allografts: long-term follow-up study on first 100 cases. *Clin Orthop* 1985;197:96–102.
41. Beaver RJ, Mahomed M, Backstein D, et al. Fresh osteochondral allografts for post-traumatic defects in the knee: a survivorship analysis. *J Bone Joint Surg Br* 1992;74:105–110.
42. Ghazavi MT, Pritzker KP, Davis AM, et al. Fresh osteochondral allografts for post-traumatic osteochondral defects of the knee. *J Bone Joint Surg Br* 1997;79:1008–1013.
43. Convery FR, Meyers MH, Akeson WH. Fresh osteochondral allografting of the femoral condyle. *Clin Orthop* 1991;273:139–145.
44. Garrett JC. Treatment of osteochondral defects of the distal femur with fresh osteochondral allografts: a preliminary report. *Arthroscopy* 1986;2:222–226.
45. Convery FR, Akeson WH, Amiel D, et al. Long-term survival of chondrocytes in an osteochondral articular cartilage allograft. A case report. *J Bone Joint Surg Am* 1996;78:1082–1088.
46. Kwan MK, Wayne JS, Woo SL, et al. Histologicand biomechanical assessment of articular cartilage from stored osteochondral shell allografts. *J Orthop Res* 1989;7:637–644.
47. Rodrigo JJ, Thompson E, Travis C. Deep-freezing versus 4 degrees preservation of avascular osteocartilaginous shell allografts in rats. *Clin Orthop* 1987;218:268–275.
48. Oakeshott RD, Faine I, Pritzker KP, et al. A clinical and histologic analysis of failed fresh osteochondral allografts. *Clin Orthop* 1988;233:283–294.
49. Kandel RA, Gross AE, Ganel A, et al. Histopathology of failed osteoarticular shell allografts. *Clin Orthop* 1985;197:103–110.
50. Langer F, Czitrom A, Pritzker KP, et al. The immunogenicity of fresh and frozen allogeneic bone. *J Bone Joint Surg Am* 1975;57:216–220.
51. Stevenson S, Dannucci DA, Sharkey NA, et al. The fate of articular cartilage after transplantation of fresh and cryopreserved tissue-antigen-matched and mismatched osteochondral allografts in dogs. *J Bone Joint Surg Am* 1989;71:1297–1307.
52. Stevenson S. The immune response to osteochondral allografts in dogs. *J Bone Joint Surg Am* 1987;69:573–582.
53. Rodrigo JJ, Heiden E, Hegyes M, et al. Immune response inhibition by irrigating subchondral bone with cytotoxic agents. *Clin Orthop* 1996;326:96–106.
54. Rodrigo JJ, et al. Inhibition of the immune response to experimental fresh osteoarticular allografts. *Clin Orthop* 1989;243:235–253.
55. Strong DM, Friedlaender GE, Tomford WW, et al. Immunologic responses in human recipients of osseous and osteochondral allografts. *Clin Orthop* 1996;326:107–114.
56. Schreiber GB, Busch MP, Kleinman SH, et al. The risk of transfusion-transmitted viral infections. *N Eng J Med* 1996;334:1685–1690.
57. Williams AE, Thomson RA, Schreiber GB, et al. Estimates of infectious disease risk factors in US blood donors. Retrovirus Epidemiology Donor Study (see comments). *JAMA* 1997;277:967–972.
58. Tomford WW. Transmission of disease through transplantation of musculoskeletal allografts. *J Bone Joint Surg Am* 1995;77:1742–1754.
59. Simonds RJ, Holmberg SD, Hurwitz RL, et al. Transmission of human immunodeficiency virus type 1 from a seronegative organ and tissue donor (see comments). *N Eng J Med* 1992;326:726–732.
60. Campbell DG, Li P, Oakeshott RD. HIV infection of human cartilage. *J Bone Joint Surg Br* 1996;78:22–25.

CHAPTER 15

Meniscus Injury and Repair

Albert M-H. Tsai and Robert A. Pedowitz

HISTORICAL REVIEW

The first reported meniscal repair was performed on November 16, 1883 by Thomas Annandale (1) at the University of Edinburgh. His patient was a 30-year-old miner, who 10 months before presentation, had suffered a torn anterior horn of the medial meniscus. Two months after suture repair of the meniscus, the patient was dismissed cured.

Despite Annandale's success with this new procedure, the prevailing sentiment of the time was that total meniscectomy was the standard of care. Sutton (2) in 1897 believed that the menisci merely represented the "functionless vestigial remains of leg muscle origins." Sir Robert Jones (3) in 1909 reported on his experience on more than 500 knee arthrotomies. He stated that "stitching the cartilage should be an obsolete operation. If the cartilage is only slightly mobile and the history characteristic, it should be removed forthwith." Gibson (4) in 1931 reported that after total meniscectomy in dogs, there was regeneration of the meniscus, which he thought, if anything, was superior to the original. Smillie (5) observed the same thing in human meniscectomy patients and therefore concluded that "if it be accepted that the meniscus performs any function, that function can best be performed by the most perfect replica of the original. The most perfect replica possible follows total meniscectomy."

It was not until King's classic article (6) in 1936 that some evidence emerged that perhaps total meniscectomy was not a completely benign procedure. In his article, *The Function of Semilunar Cartilages*, King performed varying degrees of partial or total meniscectomies in dogs and then examined their articular cartilage for degenerative changes. What he found was that the amount of cartilage degeneration was proportional to the amount of meniscus removed, and he concluded that "the semilunar menisci

serve to protect the articular hyaline cartilages, and probably operative excision should be limited to removal of the mobile portion."

Fairbank (7) reviewed pre- and postoperative radiographs in patients up to 14 years after meniscectomy and consistently observed changes including osteophyte formation, joint space narrowing, and flattening of the femoral condyle. He suggested that these changes were caused by loss of the weight-bearing function of the meniscus, and concluded correctly that meniscectomy was not entirely benign.

In 1975, Cox et al. (8) demonstrated in the canine knee that the amount of articular cartilage degeneration was related to the amount of meniscus excised. Jackson (9) conducted a radiographic study using the unoperated knee as a control and confirmed that there were more degenerative changes in postmeniscectomy knees. Since then, many investigators (7–27) have observed the detrimental effects of meniscectomy on the knee joint, some reporting the relative risk of radiographic arthritis after meniscectomy being up to 14 times greater (24).

Since it was determined that meniscectomy was undesirable, the question arose whether meniscus tears could heal or be repaired. Another of King's classic articles from 1936 reports on the healing of meniscus tears in dogs (28). He observed first that there was only a very limited, peripheral blood supply to the meniscus. He then created a variety of meniscus tears and observed that tears isolated to the meniscus did not heal, but if the tears were extended the to the synovium, they could heal with fibrous tissue. Nearly 100 years after Annandale's article, Heatley (29) and DeHaven (30,31) reported on their experience with meniscus repairs, Heatley in rabbits and DeHaven in an early clinical series. They both demonstrated that meniscus healing could take place if the peripheral rim was excised and the inner fragment was sutured directly to the synovial margin.

ANATOMY AND BIOMECHANICS

The menisci are crescent-shaped fibrocartilaginous structures (Fig. 15.1) that act to increase joint congruity by forming a concavity on the tibial plateaus to articulate with the femoral condyles. The medial meniscus covers 51% to 74% of the medial tibial plateau, while the lateral meniscus covers 75% to 93% of the lateral tibial plateau (32). Both menisci have firm bony attachments at the anterior and posterior horns to help resist the hoop stresses that occur with axial loading of the joint. Despite these attachment sites, the menisci are mobile during flexion, with approximately 5 mm of excursion medially and 11 mm laterally (33,34). The medial meniscus peripherally is firmly attached to the medial collateral ligament (MCL), whereas the lateral meniscus has no strong ties to the lateral collateral ligament, accounting in part for its increased mobility.

Mechanically, the meniscus is best understood by examining the organization of its collagen fibrils. Older light microscopic anatomical studies (35–38) have demonstrated an "arcade-like" orientation of the collagen fibrils, mainly running in a radial direction in the internal circumference and in a circular direction in the external circumference. Newer scanning electron microscopic studies (39), however, have found three distinct layers. The tibial and femoral surfaces of the meniscus are covered by a meshwork of delicate thin fibrils. Beneath this superficial network, there is one lamellar layer each at the tibial and femoral surfaces, with radially oriented fibrils peripherally at the anterior and posterior horns. Elsewhere in this layer, the fibrils intersect at various angles. The chief portion of the collagenous fibrils runs in the central main part and is arranged in a circular fashion in all segments of the meniscus (Fig. 15.2).

This longitudinal collagen fiber arrangement makes the meniscus much stiffer in the circumferential direction. During axial loading of the knee joint, the radial component of the force on the knee tends to extrude the meniscus towards the periphery of the joint. The tensile stiffness of the circumferential collagen bundles, together with the strong bony attachments of the anterior and posterior horns, act to resist this extrusive force. This tensile stress that develops is often referred to as hoop stress.

Biomechanical studies have suggested that one of the most important roles of the meniscus is as a load-bearing member of the knee (7,8,10–12,14,15,23,25). Meniscectomy has been shown to alter the pattern and distribution of load transmission across the knee joint. Kurosawa et al. (40) studied the physical properties of cadaver knee joints that were loaded with up to 1,500 N both before and after performing meniscectomies. In the intact joint, the femoral condyles contact both menisci and the exposed cartilage is relatively spared. After removal of both menisci, the contact area was reduced by a third to a half and became concentrated into two small round areas on the tibial plateaus. The average stresses, being load divided by contact area, consequently increased by two to three times. Baratz et al. (11) performed similar measurements in cadaver knees using pressure sensitive film.

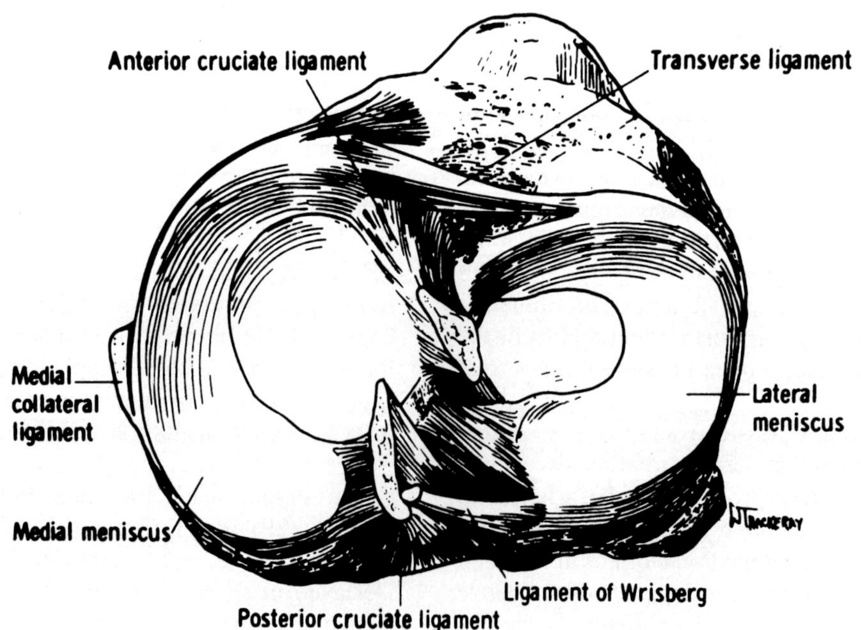

FIGURE 15.1. Drawing of the human tibial plateau, showing the attachments of the menisci and cruciate ligaments. (From Warren RF, Arnoczky SP, Wickiewicz TL. Anatomy of the knee. In: Nicholas JA, Hershman EB, eds. *The lower extremity and spine in sports medicine.* St. Louis: CV Mosby, 1986: 657–694, with permission.)

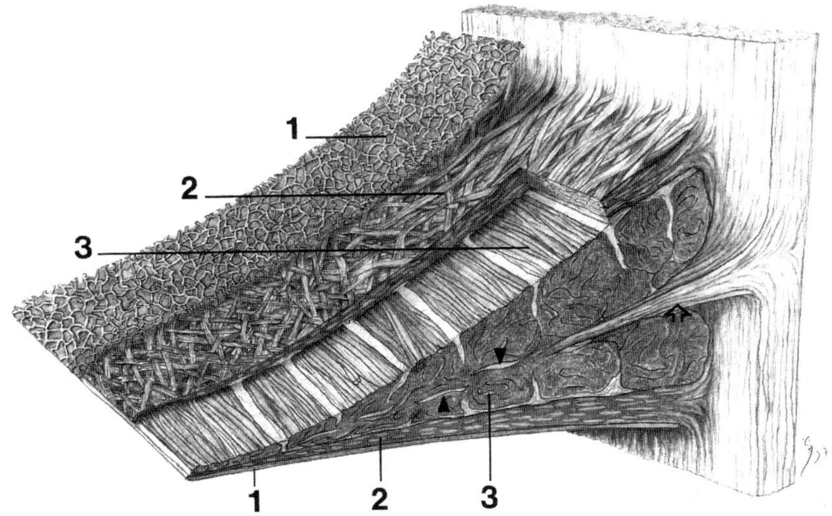

FIGURE 15.2. Scanning electron microscopy reveals three distinct layers in the meniscus cross-section. 1, superficial; 2, middle; 3, deep layer. (From Petersen W, Tillmann B. Collagenous fibril texture of the human knee joint menisci. *Anat Embryol* 1998;197:323, with permission.)

After partial meniscectomy, contact areas decreased approximately 10%, and peak local contact stresses increased approximately 65%. After total meniscectomy, contact areas decreased approximately 75%, and peak contact stresses increased approximately 235%.

The vascular supply to the medial and lateral menisci originates predominantly from the medial and lateral genicular arteries (41). Branches from these vessels give rise to a perimeniscal capillary plexus that supplies the peripheral border of the meniscus at its attachments to the synovial joint capsule. India ink injection studies have demonstrated that the degree of peripheral vascular penetration is 10% to 25% of the width of the meniscus (Fig. 15.3). A small portion of vascular synovial tissue also is

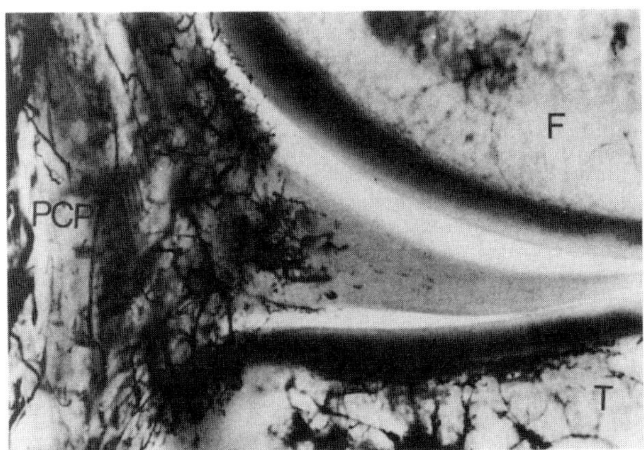

FIGURE 15.3. Frontal section of the medial compartment of the knee after vascular injection and tissue clearing. F, femur; T, tibia; PCF, peripheral capsular fibers. (From Arnoczky SP, Warren RF. Microvasculature of the human meniscus. *Am J Sports Med* 1982;10:90–95, with permission.)

present throughout the peripheral attachment of the menisci on both the femoral and tibial articular surfaces. This synovial fringe extends for a short distance over the articular surfaces of the menisci and does not contribute vessels to the meniscus itself, but does contribute greatly to the healing response of the meniscus.

MENISCAL HEALING

When considering meniscus tears for potential repair, lesions are often classified by their location with regard to the peripheral blood supply. The so-called RED–RED tear has a functional blood supply on both the capsular and meniscal sides of the lesion. A tear in this location, which is usually within 3 mm of the synovial margin, obviously has the best prognosis for healing. A RED—WHITE tear occurs within the transitional area between 3 and 5 mm from the synovial margin where there is an active peripheral blood supply, but the central inner surface of the tear is in the avascular zone. Theoretically, these tears should have enough vascularity to heal. Finally, a WHITE–WHITE tear occurs in the completely avascular zone of the meniscus more than 5 mm from the synovial margin, and these tears are unlikely to heal on their own (28,42,43).

There are two general pathways through which meniscal healing occurs. The extrinsic pathway is activated following injury within the peripheral vascular zone of the meniscus. A fibrin clot is formed, which acts as a scaffold for proliferation of vessels from the perimeniscal capillary plexus. Undifferentiated mesenchymal cells are attracted from the outside, and fill the lesion with a fibrovascular scar tissue (28,42,44). The second pathway is intrinsic to the meniscal chondrocytes and involves unlocking the inherent capacity of meniscal chondrocytes to heal, even in the avascular white zone. Webber et al. (45,46) and Arnoczky et al. (44) have both shown in animal studies that these cells can proliferate and synthesize matrix, without a blood supply, if they are provided with the proper working environment. Work is still under way to precisely define the requisite ingredients to nurture this intrinsic meniscal healing.

Meniscal repair has generally been limited to the peripheral vascular area of the meniscus, but a significant number of lesions occur in the central avascular zone. Experimental and clinical observations have shown that these lesions are incapable of healing and therefore provided the rationale for partial meniscectomy (28,42,43). However, in an effort to extend meniscal repair into these avascular zones, certain techniques have been proposed to provide vascularity to the WHITE–WHITE tears, thereby improving the potential for healing. In addition, these techniques are used in RED–WHITE tears to optimize the healing environment.

Early reports of meniscal repairs used excision of the peripheral white rim to suture the central avascular portion directly to the well-vascularized synovial rim (30,47). This effectively converted a WHITE–WHITE tear into a RED–WHITE tear, with improved healing potential. However, excision of the peripheral rim pulls the residual meniscus outward and deforms the shape, leading to a decrease in the width and cross-sectional area of the meniscus. This leads to a delay in meniscal contact with the femoral condyle until higher joint loads are reached, and performs no better long term than a partial meniscectomy (47).

Arnoczky et al. (42) demonstrated in dogs that healing would occur after complete transection of the meniscus, as long as the laceration was extended into the peripheral attachment of the meniscus. The defect healed with fibrovascular scar tissue and was covered by a vascular pannus extending from the synovial fringe (Fig. 15.4). Longitudinal lesions within the avascular region of the meniscus never healed. However, if they were connected to the peripheral synovial tissues by a vascular access channel, all the lesions healed with fibrovascular scar by 10 weeks. The vascular access channel connects the avascular meniscal lesion to the peripheral vasculature. Unfortunately, creation of an adequately sized vascular access channel cuts across the circumferential orientation of the collagen fibers and adversely affects the biomechanical functioning of the meniscus.

In an effort to minimize damage to the collagen architecture of the meniscus while still taking advantage of the ability of the peripheral vasculature to migrate along access corridors, the technique of trephination was suggested (48). This entails using a needle to create holes through the peripheral meniscal rim, producing a series of bleeding puncture sites. This allows influx of a vascular response with relatively minimal damage to the colla-

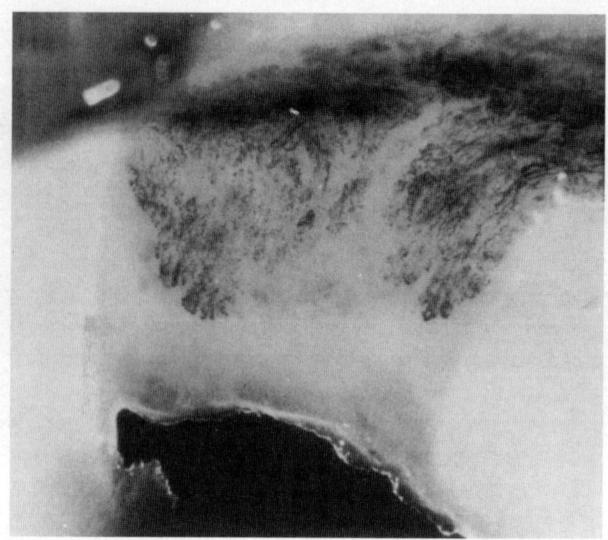

FIGURE 15.4. Healing radial tear in the medial meniscus of a dog 6 weeks after injury. The synovial fringe produces a vascular pannus over the surface of the repair. (From Arnoczky SP, Warren RF. Microvasculature of the human meniscus. *Am J Sports Med* 1982;10:90–95, with permission.)

gen architecture of the meniscus. A number of studies in both animal and human models suggest enhanced healing with trephination (48,49).

In the normal repair process of a peripheral meniscus tear, the vascular synovial fringe often extends over the femoral and tibial surfaces of the meniscus. Because this response is often extensive, it was theorized that stimulation of the synovial fringe could accentuate this response and help extend it into avascular or marginally vascularized tears (47,50–53). One of the most widely accepted methods of inducing neovascularization is synovial abrasion, where a rasp is used to abrade the synovial fringe on the superior and inferior surfaces of the peripheral white rim. Henning et al. (47) reported a 22% failure rate in meniscal repair without synovial abrasion compared with a failure rate of 9% using abrasion technique.

Several studies (44,50,54–57) have shown that when meniscal chondrocytes are exposed to some of the growth factors normally found in a blood clot, such as platelet-derived growth factor and fibronectin, the cells demonstrate an increase in proliferation and matrix synthesis. The clot itself acts as a scaffold for repair. A fibrin clot is formed by stirring 50 to 60 mL of whole blood in a glass container until a clot precipitates. The clot is capable of holding sutures placed through its substance. Arnoczky et al. (44) demonstrated in dogs that avascular meniscal defects healed when they were filled with fibrin clot. By providing the factors necessary for repair as well as a scaffold for the repair process, the fibrin clot was able to induce and support a healing response in the avascular portion of the meniscus. Henning et al. (55) reported a 41% failure rate in isolated repairs without fibrin clot, versus 8% with the clot. So, it may be that the absence of a hematoma and its associated factors, and not the absence of a blood supply per se, limits healing in the avascular portion of the meniscus.

A corollary of the fibrin clot technique is the use of synthetic fibrin glue that is formed by combining various factors in the normal clotting cascade. The adhesive property of fibrin glue is superior to that of natural fibrin clot, but it lacks the biologically active factors normally found in fibrin clot. The technique is described by Ishimura et al. (58–60) in recent clinical studies. Two solutions are simultaneously injected into a meniscus tear, which is then reduced and held in place for 1 to 2 minutes. In one study, only 4 of 61 tears required supplemental suturing after fixation with fibrin glue, and the overall failure rate was 10% (60).

Another repair enhancement technique that has been investigated is the use of synovial grafts (61–63). The high vascularity of synovial tissue makes it an attractive potential substrate for the repair process, and in some animal studies, enhanced healing has been demonstrated. However, the clinical use of this technique in humans has not been examined. Laser energy to oppose tissue and stimulate repair has also been reported in various experimental models (64–66), but to date none of these studies conclusively demonstrates an ability to weld or repair meniscal tears. More work is needed before widespread clinical use.

MENISCAL REPAIR IN THE CRUCIATE-UNSTABLE KNEE

The anterior cruciate ligament (ACL)–deficient knee is subjected to repeated instability episodes resulting in recurrent trauma to the menisci and articular surfaces (67–71) and progressive degenerative arthritis (69–73). In patients with an acute ACL injury, the incidence of meniscal tears has been reported as approximately 65%, with nearly equal numbers of lateral and medial meniscal tears (74–76). In the chronic ACL-deficient knee, meniscus tears are found in as many as 98% of patients (70,76–78). The ratio of medial-to-lateral meniscal tears is nearly 3:1 (79), most likely related to the observation that the medial meniscus is a significant restraint to anterior tibial translation after ACL disruption (80). In contrast, it has been noted that lateral meniscectomy after ACL sectioning failed to cause a significant increase in anterior tibial translation (81).

Preservation of the meniscus is associated with a decreased incidence of osteoarthritis and therefore, meniscal repair is the preferred treatment (82,83). Healing of repaired meniscal tears has been reported in 50% to 98% of cases (51,71,76,82-91). There are multiple factors responsible for the variability of meniscal repair success. The most significant factor for long-term success, however, is the status of the ACL (50,52,76,82,86,87,89,90,92,93). DeHaven (94) found a 30% recurrent tear rate in ACL-deficient knees but only an 8% recurrent tear rate when the meniscus was repaired in conjunction with an ACL reconstruction. Hanks et al. (87) reported a 13% failure rate of meniscal repair when performed in ACL-deficient knees compared with an 8% failure rate in stable knees. Keene et al. (71) reported an 8% incidence of failed meniscal repair at an average follow-up of 40 months, and all of these failures occurred in unstable knees. Morgan et al. (90) reported a 16% failure rate of meniscal repair, all of which occurred in ACL-deficient knees. Many authors have confirmed these findings. In addition, lateral meniscal repairs have been found to have a higher healing rate than medial meniscal repairs, both in stable and ACL-reconstructed knees (95,96). This again is likely related to the greater mobility of the lateral meniscus compared with the medial meniscus.

It has also been shown that a meniscal repair performed simultaneously with an ACL reconstruction is especially likely to heal (95,97). The reasons for this higher healing rate may be a combination of factors. Meniscal tears that occur in conjunction with an acute ACL injury afford healthier repair tissue and are less likely to show histologic evidence of degeneration when compared with meniscal tears without an ACL injury. In addition, the significant hemarthrosis that develops after ACL reconstruction bathes the tear site in growth factors that have been shown to stimulate healing (44,50,54–57), and the additional stability as well as postoperative protection following ACL reconstruction may protect the repair site more than in an isolated meniscus repair. Cannon and Vittori (95) found that the healing success rate for isolated meniscal repairs in stable knees is 50% compared with a 93% healing rate in repairs performed simultaneously with ACL reconstruction. Tenuta and Arciero (97) confirmed these findings in their study, finding a 90% healing rate of meniscal repairs performed with ACL reconstruction and a 57% healing rate of meniscal repairs performed in cruciate-stable knees.

The timing of meniscal repair may affect the success rate. Some authors (95,97) have found that acute repairs less than 8 weeks old were more successful in healing than chronic tears. However, other studies (52) have not demonstrated a significant effect of repair timing on healing rates. Similarly, some studies show that patient age may be a factor in meniscal healing, whereas others report no significant relationship to the healing rate (55,95,97).

The treatment of meniscus tears in the posterior cruciate ligament (PCL)–deficient knee remains controversial. Clinical studies have documented an increased incidence of degenerative changes in PCL-deficient knees with or without meniscal pathology (98). In isolated PCL-deficient knees, meniscal tears should be repaired if the tear is amenable. Isolated PCL reconstruction with meniscus repair is more controversial, because PCL reconstruction is unlikely to play the protective role that is afforded by ACL reconstruction. However, in patients with PCL and posterolateral ligament complex instability, meniscus repair and concurrent ligament reconstruction should be undertaken, because nonsurgical treatment with this combination of injuries is associated with a poor outcome (98).

MENISCUS REPAIR TECHNIQUES

Certain principles are common to all successful meniscal repair techniques. The nature and location of the tear must be thoroughly understood using arthroscopic examination. All unstable tissue must be debrided from the meniscal rim and capsule, and the surfaces of the tear must be freshened with a rasp or curette to optimize vascularity on the capsular side of the repair. Finally, as many sutures or alternative fixation devices as are needed to make the tear secure and anatomic should be placed.

The first open meniscal repair was performed by Annandale (1) in 1883, but these techniques were refined in the late 1970s by DeHaven and others (30). These open approaches allowed the neurovascular structures to be identified and protected, and there was direct visualization of the tear that allowed for freshening up of the tear surfaces and good stable suture fixation. However, only tears that were within 2 mm of the meniscosynovial junction were accessible, and extensive dissection which could damage the medial or lateral collateral ligaments was needed to reach tears not restricted to the anterior or posterior thirds of the meniscus.

Ikeuchi (99) performed the first arthroscopic meniscal repair in Tokyo in 1969, but it was Henning (47,100) who popularized the technique in the United States in the 1980s. The most important advantage of arthroscopic versus open repair is that it allows repair of meniscal lesions that are not strictly peripheral, and which are in areas of questionable vascularity or even in the central avascular zone. It may be important therefore, to combine arthroscopic repair with one or more of the healing-enhancement techniques such as synovial abrasion (47,50–53), vascular access channels (42), or fibrin clot insertion (44,50,54–57). Two basic types of arthroscopic repair have evolved, the "inside-out" technique pioneered by Henning (47,100) and others, and the "outside-in" technique developed by Warren (101) and others.

Meniscal repair using the inside-out technique is currently the most commonly performed technique for meniscal repair (102). After confirming the reparability of a tear, the meniscus repair bed is properly prepared using a rasp or arthroscopic shaver to abrade the perimeniscal synovial fringe to stimulate a vascular healing response. Further enhancement of the healing response may be achieved by the use of a fibrin clot (44,50,54–57). A separate posteromedial or posterolateral skin incision is then made (103, 104). The purpose of the approach is to develop the interval down to the level of the capsule to place a retractor for visualization of the suture needles while protecting the posterior neurovascular structures. The suture needles are advanced through either a single- or double-lumen cannula system, advanced across the tear and through the capsule, and collected out through the accessory incision. After all sutures have been passed, they are pulled taut and the meniscus is probed and inspected to verify a stable and anatomic reduction. The sutures are then tied over the joint capsule (Fig. 15.5).

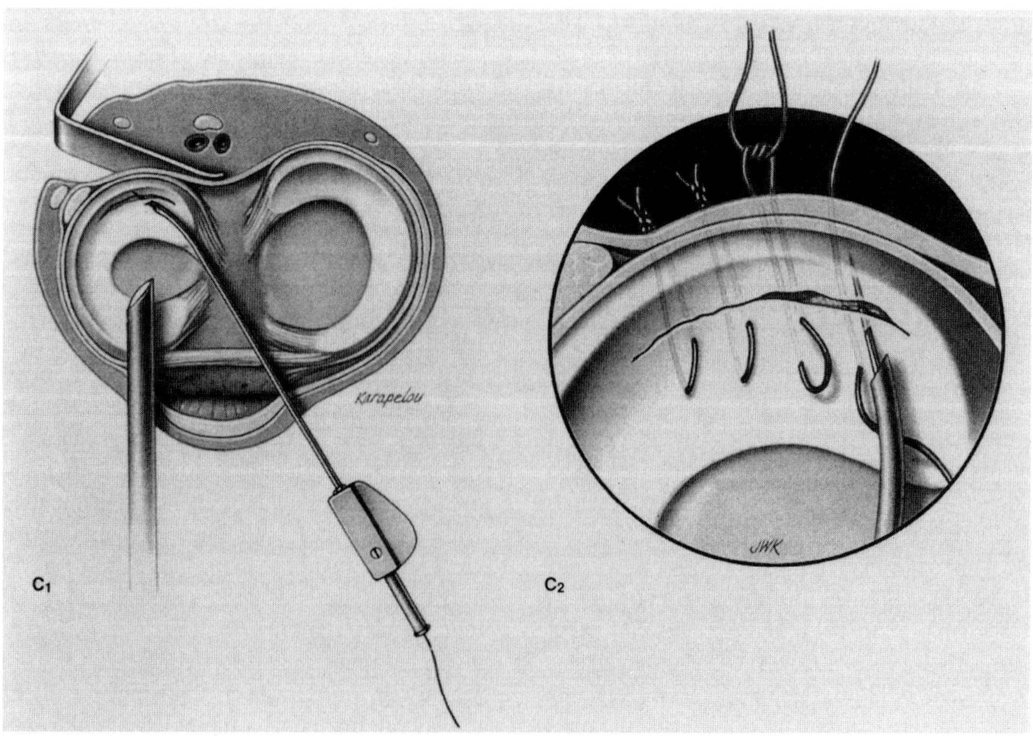

FIGURE 15.5. Inside-out meniscal repair. (From Miller MD. Atlas of meniscal repair. *Op Tech Orthop* 1995;5:70–71, with permission.)

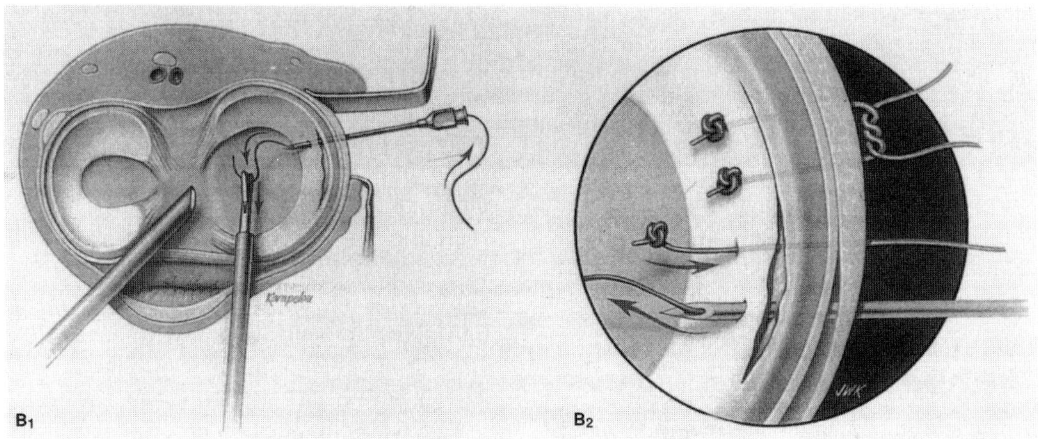

FIGURE 15.6. Outside-in meniscal repair. (From Miller MD. Atlas of meniscal repair. *Op Tech Orthop* 1995;5:70–71, with permission.)

The outside-in technique involves passage of spinal needles across the tear from outside into the joint (105). Suture is passed through the needle and brought out through an anterior portal, a knot is tied in the suture, and the knot is then pulled back into the joint to lie against the meniscus and maintain it in a reduced position. The free ends of adjacent sutures are then tied subcutaneously (Fig. 15.6). This technique allows safe passage of the needles based on anatomic landmarks; for example, laterally the needle entry site is anterior to the biceps tendon to avoid the peroneal nerve. It also minimizes the chance that the surgeon or assistant will suffer a needle stick, which is a potential danger with the inside-out technique.

The all-inside repair technique was developed by Morgan (106) and Mulhollan (107) as a means to access posterior horn tears arthroscopically. A 70° arthroscope is advanced into the posterior compartment through the intercondylar notch and operative instrumentation is placed through either a posteromedial or posterolateral portal. The sutures are placed across the tear and then tied intraarticularly (Fig. 15.7).

There is some controversy regarding the type of suture that should be used in meniscal repair. Advocates of absorbable suture material believe that nonabsorbable sutures may scuff the articular cartilage and that the meniscal puckering that occurs after suture placement might cause permanent deformation (108). Advocates of nonabsorbable suture believe that absorbable suture material degrades too rapidly to accommodate the slow meniscal healing process (109–111).

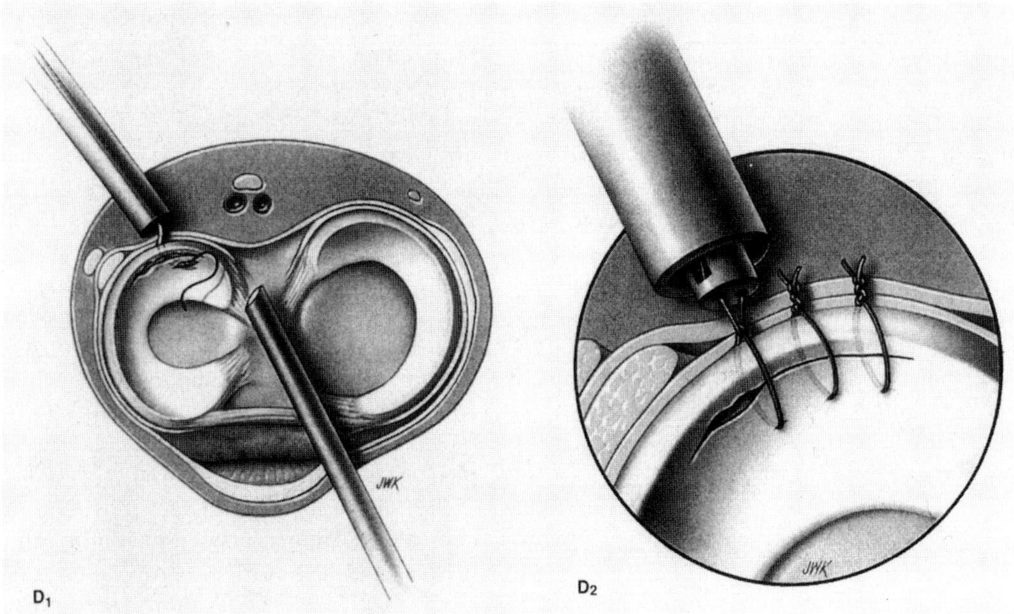

FIGURE 15.7. All-inside meniscal repair. (From Miller MD. Atlas of meniscal repair. *Op Tech Orthop* 1995;5:70–71, with permission.)

Newer techniques and instrumentation for meniscal repair are under investigation. There has been a rapid increase in the options available for all-inside meniscal repair using various bioabsorbable arrows, darts, screws, and staples. Short-term studies have been published reporting surgical techniques and comparisons to suture fixation (112–115). However, additional long-term studies are needed to accurately assess meniscal healing rates using these newer instrumentation techniques.

POSTOPERATIVE REHABILITATION AFTER MENISCAL REPAIR

Postoperative rehabilitation following meniscal repair is a controversial area of discussion. In the past, some authors found that re-tears occurred in patients who returned to sports activities before 6 months after repair, which led to recommendations that weight bearing be restricted for 6 weeks with the knee in 45° flexion, with running allowed at 3 months, but no sports until 6 months had passed (116). The length of immobilization varied from 2 weeks (117,118), 3 to 4 weeks (90), and up to 6 weeks (51,104). However, canine studies have demonstrated that full-thickness meniscal incisions in the vascularized portion of the medial meniscus show a significantly greater collagen percentage in animals that underwent an immediate mobilization protocol when compared with those that were cast-immobilized (119). Extrapolating these results to human patients is difficult, but many authors now advocate immediate range of motion following meniscal repair (86,120). Some authors have become even more aggressive, allowing "accelerated" programs that permit unlimited weight bearing, full motion, and no restrictions on pivoting sports. Many studies comparing these accelerated programs with more standard rehabilitation protocols fail to show any statistical difference in repair failures (85,121,122).

During the initial stages of rehabilitation, goals should be to achieve full weight bearing and full range of motion. Functional training is then designed to improve strength, endurance, power, and coordination. Activities such as deep squatting, which may unduly load the meniscus and jeopardize the repair, should be avoided in the early stages. In addition, twisting and pivoting motions should be limited for 4 to 6 months in stable repairs, and perhaps longer in complex or radial tears. The multiple factors involved in healing rates of meniscus tears are still not completely understood. No long-term studies in an animal or human model exist to strongly support any specific rehabilitation protocol. Therefore, clinical experience is invaluable.

MENISCAL ALLOGRAFT TRANSPLANTATION

Despite advances in meniscal repair techniques and healing enhancement techniques, there remains a group of patients who have undergone previous meniscectomy or require total or near-total meniscectomy for irreparable tears. These patients are at risk for the development of progressive degenerative osteoarthritis. Studies with synthetic meniscal prostheses (123–127) have been discouraging and have therefore prompted the investigation into meniscal allograft transplantation. The first attempts at such allografts were massive proximal tibial osteochondral allografts transplanted for the treatment of tumors (128). This led to the first isolated meniscal allograft transplantation performed by Milachowski et al. (129) in 1984. Since then, a number of clinical and experimental studies have been reported in the literature (130,131).

Several techniques to process and preserve meniscal allografts have been used, each with specific advantages and disadvantages. Some processes are used to maintain donor cell viability, whereas others emphasize storage, reduction of disease transmission, and reduction of graft antigenicity.

Some investigators believe that transplanting viable donor fibrochondrocytes maintains the extracellular matrix and the mechanical integrity of the transplanted tissue. This belief has led to techniques designed to preserve the donor cells. The simplest technique is to transplant fresh meniscal tissue; however, this method is impractical for many reasons. The graft must be transplanted quickly to maintain cell viability, so there is little or no opportunity to match the graft size to the host. Also, the risk of disease transmission is high, because there may not be time for serologic testing of the donor, and secondary methods of graft sterilization cannot be used because they would destroy the cells.

Cryopreservation is another technique designed to maintain donor fibrochondrocytes in suspended animation while allowing storage of the graft for a limited time. The technique involves placing the tissue in preservation medium and then gradually freezing the graft. Cell viability after cryopreservation has ranged from 10% to 40% (132,133). Serologic testing can then be performed, reducing the risk of disease transmission. In addition, the graft can be appropriately size-matched to a host, and surgery can be scheduled electively. Disadvantages include the expense and technical difficulty of freezing and thawing the graft correctly, and secondary sterilization techniques that affect cell viability cannot be used, increasing the risk of disease transmission in the donor with false-negative serologic tests. Finally, it is unclear whether efforts to maintain donor cell viability are worthwhile, because donor cells have been shown to be entirely replaced by host cells in as little as 4 weeks after transplantation in a goat model (134).

Freezing musculoskeletal allografts destroys donor cells and denatures histocompatibility antigens, making the material less likely to provoke an immune response (135). Freezing of allografts preserves the collagen framework of the graft, but may affect graft incorporation adversely and may lead to graft shrinkage (129). However, the technique is simple and inexpensive. Freeze-drying is much like fresh-freezing, but the dehydration of the graft allows for indefinite storage, the major advantage of this technique. The technique has disadvantages: The graft is brittle and handling of the graft before rehydration may damage collagen fibers, thus altering the biomechanical properties of the graft (136).

Several animal studies have been done to evaluate the feasibility and long-term viability of meniscal allograft transplantation. In a canine model using cryopreserved allografts, Arnoczky (137) demonstrated that there was healing to the capsule by 6 months, with a normal cell population. Other authors have used a variety of animal models and a variety of graft preservation techniques and have demonstrated healing of the allograft and no problems with rejection (133,137–139).

Jackson et al. (133) transplanted fresh and 30-day cryopreserved allografts in a goat model and examined the menisci at 6 months. Grossly the menisci appeared healthy, but Jackson et al. found that water content was increased 12% to 24% and uronic acid was decreased up to 56%, suggesting degeneration of the meniscal tissue. Although this was only a single time point and no upward or downward trend could be established, they hypothesized that if the biochemical parameters did not return to a more normal level, the meniscus might eventually break down.

Several authors have suggested that allograft transplantation may offer some protection to the articular cartilage of the knee following meniscectomy (137,140–142). Cummins et al. (140) demonstrated that fewer degenerative changes occurred in the articular cartilage of rabbits receiving a meniscal transplantation when compared with control animals that underwent meniscectomy. Paletta et al. (142) showed in cadaver human knees that the decrease in contact area and increase in contact pressure after meniscectomy could be partially relieved by implantation of a meniscal allograft. After total meniscectomy, contact area decreased 45% to 50% and contact pressure increased 235% to 335%. Allograft replacement increased the contact area 42% to 65% and decreased the pressure 55% to 65% when compared with total meniscectomy. They attributed the fact that the numbers did not return completely to normal to imperfect size-matching and possibly suboptimal fixation of the anterior and posterior horn attachment sites.

The surgical indications for transplantation are still not well defined. Factors that must be considered include patient age, knee stability, alignment, and the degree of articular cartilage wear. Most authors reserve meniscal transplantation for the patient with pain and discomfort associated with early osteoarthrosis of the involved compartment, before severe bony architectural changes including ostephytes have developed (143). One might also consider an allograft in the young athlete who has undergone a previous meniscectomy, who has relatively few symptoms, and who is active in a high-risk sport. Recommending the procedure in a young, meniscectomized patient with no symptoms is difficult to justify at this time, but this may be the group that stands to benefit the most should meniscal transplantation prove to be effective in protecting hyaline cartilage.

Clinical results of allograft meniscal transplantation have been difficult to interpret, because most series are small, with limited follow-up (129,144–146). The Meniscus Transplant Study Group met in 1995 and presented their pooled data from a 5-year period (146). From 110 clinicians, 625 allografts were implanted into 591 patients. Their results demonstrated an 89% overall survival rate. Other reports have demonstrated capsular healing of meniscal allografts and viable active fibrochondrocytes in the grafts. Long-term follow-up and additional biomechanical and biochemical evaluations are needed to evaluate the ability of transplanted menisci to protect the hyaline cartilage of the knee.

MENISCAL REPLACEMENT

Stone et al. (147) performed subtotal resection of canine menisci with immediate autologous reimplantation. This represented an idealized model of allografting, because the tissue was fresh, autogenous, and perfectly sized. However, gross healing was achieved in only 50% of the cases and the authors concluded that if an autogenous replant could not reliably heal, success with allografts is unlikely. Efforts were therefore directed at regrowing the meniscus. The belief that meniscal fibrochondrocytes can migrate, divide, and make appropriate extracellular matrix was supported by the work of Webber et al. (45,46), Smillie (5), and others.

Stone et al. (148) designed collagen-based scaffolds by reconstituting enzymatically purified collagen from bovine Achilles tendons (Fig. 15.8). *In vitro* experiments were performed to determine whether the templates were toxic to meniscal fibrochondrocytes, whether the cells

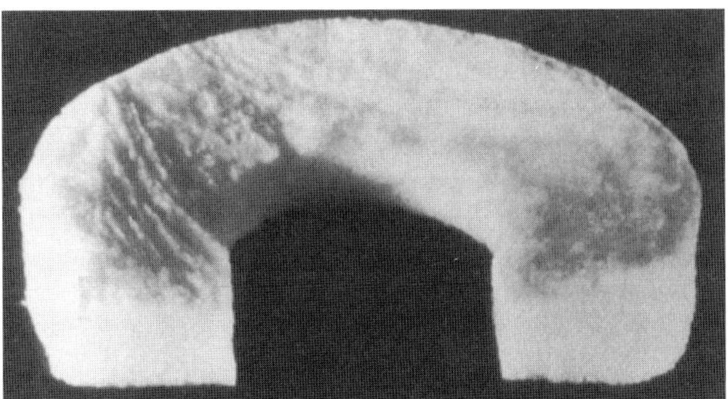

FIGURE 15.8. Photograph of the collagen meniscal implant. (From Stone KR, Steadman JR, et al. Regeneration of meniscal cartilage with use of a collagen scaffold. *J Bone Joint Surg Am* 1997;79:1770–1777, with permission.)

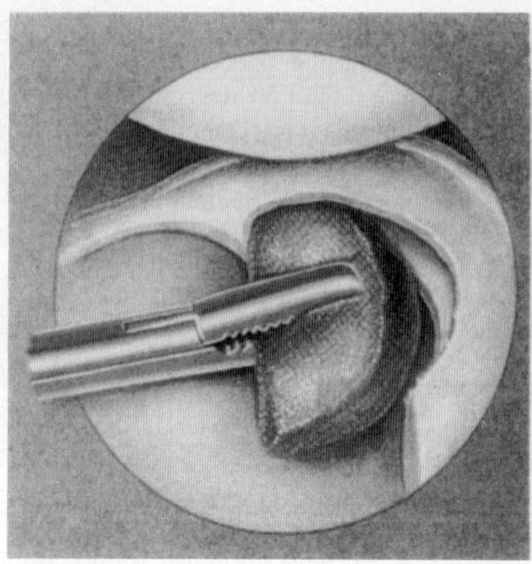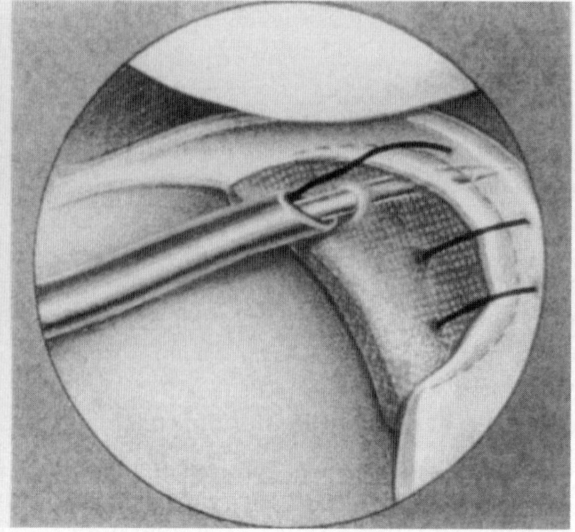

FIGURE 15.9. Drawings showing insertion and suturing of collagen meniscal implant. (From Stone KR, Steadman JR, et al. Regeneration of meniscal cartilage with use of a collagen scaffold. *J Bone Joint Surg Am* 1997;79:1770–1777, with permission.)

would migrate into the scaffolds, and whether the density of the material or the cross-linking would affect the depth of cellular penetration.

In vivo studies of meniscal regeneration followed (148), using a canine model consisting of an 80% subtotal meniscectomy followed by implantation of a collagen template that had been optimized from the *in vitro* studies. Substantial meniscal regeneration was found in 63% of the joints implanted with the collagen scaffold compared with 25% of the resection controls. More importantly, the gross appearance of the regenerated meniscus was not different from normal controls. Histologically, the regenerated fibrocartilage had viable chondrocytes and organized collagen bundles. Biochemically, regenerated menisci synthesized normal amounts of proteoglycan by 9 months.

A human clinical trial was initiated in 1993 (149). The implants were performed in 10 patients and evaluated over 3 years (Fig. 15.9). The scaffold was found to be safe over the 3-year period of the study with transient initial effusions that resolved spontaneously as the only problem. At second-look arthroscopy 6 months after implantation, gross and histologic examination revealed normal-appearing meniscal cartilage replacing the implant as it was resorbed. At 3 years, the patients in the study reported a decrease in symptoms, and magnetic resonance imaging (MRI) scans showed progressive maturation of the signal within the regenerated meniscus. The definitive success awaits the results of a prospective clinical trial with longer follow-up.

FUTURE DIRECTIONS

As we begin the 21st century, the future of meniscal repair may shift from the mechanical to the biochemical. The ability to use proteins such as fibronectin and chondronectin to manipulate meniscal repair may allow adhesion on a cellular level. Fibronectin can function as an adhesive between cells, and chondronectin has been described as an adhesive factor for articular chondrocytes (150,151). Growth factors are likely to play an important role in the future. Platelet-derived growth factor (152), endothelial cell growth factor (54), and angiogenin (153) are all being studied for healing potential of meniscal injuries. Growth factors described for articular chondrocytes include epidermal growth factor, basic fibroblast growth factor, and transforming growth factor beta (154). These may show some activity for the meniscal fibrochondrocyte as well. Autologous fibrochondrocytes grown in tissue culture may provide viable tissue for implantation (155) and eliminate the potential for disease transmission from the use of allografts. Probably the future of complex irreparable tears will be resection followed by replacement with cultured autologous fibrochondrocytes on biodegradable, resorbable scaffolds. These scaffolds will be contoured to the defect and bonded in place with fibronectin or chondronectin adhesives. Growth factors will be used as well to help stimulate healing. The treatment of meniscal pathology promises to be an exciting field for many years to come.

REFERENCES

1. Annandale T. An operation for displaced semilunar cartilage. *BMJ* 1885;1:779.
2. Sutton J. *Ligaments: their nature and morphology.* London: H. K. Lewis, 1897.
3. Jones R. *Notes on derangements of the knee.* London: AGT Fisher, 1909:969.
4. Gibson A. Regeneration of the internal semilunar cartilage after operation. *Br J Surg* 1931;19:302.
5. Smillie I. Observations on the regeneration of the semilunar cartilages in man. *Br J Surg* 1944;31:398.
6. King D. The function of semilunar cartilages. *J Bone Joint Surg Am* 1936;18:1069.

7. Fairbank T. Knee joint changes after meniscectomy. *J Bone Joint Surg Br* 1948;30:664.
8. Cox J, Nye C, et al. The degenerative effects of partial and total resection of the medial meniscus in dogs' knees. *Clin Orthop* 1975;109:178.
9. Jackson J. Degenerative changes in the knee after meniscectomy. *BMJ* 1968;2:525.
10. Allen P, Denham R, et al. Late degenerative changes after meniscectomy. *J Bone Joint Surg Br* 1984;66:666.
11. Baratz M, Fu F, et al. Meniscal tears: the effect of meniscectomy and of repair on intraarticular contact areas and stress in the human knee. *Am J Sports Med* 1986;14:270.
12. Baratz M, Rehak D, et al. Peripheral tears of the meniscus: the effect of open versus arthroscopic repair on intraarticular contact stresses in the human knee. *Am J Sports Med* 1988;16:1.
13. Burks R, Metcalf M, et al. Fifteen-year follow-up of arthroscopic partial meniscectomy. *Arthroscopy* 1997;13:673.
14. Burr D, Radin E. Meniscal function and the importance of meniscal regeneration in preventing late medial compartment osteoarthrosis. *Clin Orthop* 1982;171:121.
15. Cox J, Cordell L. The degenerative effects of medial meniscus tears in dogs' knees. *Clin Orthop* 1977;125:236.
16. Fauno P, Nielsen A. Arthroscopic partial meniscectomy: a long-term follow-up. *Arthroscopy* 1992;8:345.
17. Gear M. The late results of meniscectomy. *Br J Surg* 1987;54:270.
18. Hede A, Larsen E, et al. The long-term outcome of open total and partial meniscectomy related to the quantity and site of the meniscus removed. *Int Orthop* 1992;16:122.
19. Johnson R, Kettelkamp D, et al. Factors affecting late results after meniscectomy. *J Bone Joint Surg Am* 1974;56:719.
20. Jorgensen U, Sonne-Holm S, et al. Long-term follow-up of meniscectomy in athletes. *J Bone Joint Surg Br* 1987;69:80.
21. Krause W, Pope M, et al. Mechanical changes in the knee after meniscectomy. *J Bone Joint Surg Am* 1976;58:559.
22. Lanzer W, Komenda G. Changes in articular cartilage after meniscectomy. *Clin Orthop* 1990;252:41.
23. Radin E, de Lamotte F, et al. Role of the menisci in the distribution of stress in the knee. *Clin Orthop* 1984;185:290.
24. Roos H, Lauren M, et al. Knee osteoarthritis after meniscectomy. *Arth Rheum* 1998;41:687.
25. Shrive N, O'Connor J, et al. Load-bearing in the knee joint. *Clin Orthop* 1978;131:279.
26. Sommerlath K, Gillquist J. The long-term course of various meniscal treatments in anterior cruciate ligament deficient knees. *Clin Orthop* 1992;283:207.
27. Tapper E, Hoover N. Late results after meniscectomy. *J Bone Joint Surg Am* 1969;51:517.
28. King D. The healing of semilunar cartilages. *J Bone Joint Surg Am* 1936;18:333.
29. Heatley F. The meniscus: can it be repaired? *J Bone Joint Surg Br* 1980;62:397.
30. DeHaven K. Peripheral meniscus repair: an alternative to meniscectomy. *J Bone Joint Surg Am* 1981;63:463.
31. DeHaven K. Decision-making factors in the treatment of meniscus lesions. *Clin Orthop* 1990;252:49.
31. Clark C, Ogden J. Development of the menisci of the human knee joint: morphological changes and their potential role in childhood meniscal injury. *J Bone Joint Surg Am* 1983;65:539.
33. Fu F, Thompson W. Motion of the meniscus during knee flexion. knee meniscus: basic and clinical foundations. In: *Knee meniscus: basic and clinical foundations.* Mow V, Arnoczky S, Jackson D, eds. New York: Raven Press, 1992;75.
34. Thompson W, Thaete F, et al. Tibial meniscal dynamics using three-dimensional reconstruction of magnetic resonance images. *Am J Sports Med* 1991;19:210.
35. Aspden R, Yarker Y, et al. Collagen orientations in the meniscus of the knee joint. *J Anat* 1985;140:371.
36. Bullough P, Miunuera L, et al. The strength of the menisci of the knee as it relates to their fine structure. *J Bone Joint Surg Br* 1970;52:564.
37. Kummer B. Anatomie und Biomechanik des Kniegelenksmeniscus. *Langenbecks Arch Chir* 1987;372:241.
38. Wagner H. Die Kollagenfaserarchitektur der Menisken des menschlichen Kniegelenkes. *Z Mikrosk Anat Forsch* 1976;90:302.
39. Petersen W, Tillmann B. Collagenous fibril texture of the human knee joint menisci. *Anat Embryol* 1998;197:317.
40. Kurosawa H, Fukubayashi T, et al. Load-bearing mode of the knee joint: physical behavior of the knee joint with or without menisci. *Clin Orthop* 1980;149:283.
41. Arnoczky S, Warren R. Microvasculature of the human meniscus. *Am J Sports Med* 1982;10:90.
42. Arnoczky S, Warren R. The microvasculature of the meniscus and its response to injury. *Am J Sports Med* 1983;11:131.
43. Arnoczky S. Meniscus healing. *Contemp Orthop* 1985;10:31.
44. Arnoczky S, Warren R, et al. Meniscal repair using an exogenous fibrin clot. *J Bone Joint Surg Am* 1988;70:1209.
45. Webber R, York L, et al. Fibrin clot invasion by rabbit meniscal fibrochondrocytes in organ culture. *Trans Orthop Res Soc* 1987;12:470.
46. Webber R, Zitaglio T, et al. Serum-free culture of rabbit meniscal fibrochondrocytes: proliferative response. *J Orthop Res* 1988; 6:13.
47. Henning C, Lynch M, et al. Vascularity for healing of meniscus repairs. *Arthroscopy* 1987;3:13.
48. Fox J, Rintz K, et al. Trephination of incomplete meniscal tears. *Arthroscopy* 1993;9:451.
49. Zhang ZJ, Arnold, et al. Repairs by trephination and suturing of longitudinal injuries in the avascular area of the meniscus in goats. *Am J Sports Med* 1995;23:35.
50. Henning C. Current status of meniscus salvage. *Clinics Sports Med* 1990;9:567.
51. Jakob R, Staubli H, et al. The arthroscopic meniscal repair techniques and clinical experience. *Am J Sports Med* 1988;16:137.
52. Miller D. Arthroscopic meniscus repair. *Am J Sports Med* 1988;16: 315.
53. Nakhostine M, Gershuni D, et al. Effects of abrasion therapy on tears in the avascular region of sheep menisci. *Arthroscopy* 1990;6:280.
54. Hashimoto J, Kurosake M, et al. Meniscal repair using fibrin sealant and endothelial growth factor: an experimental study in dogs. *Am J Sports Med* 1992;20:537.
55. Henning C, Lynch M, et al. Arthroscopic meniscal repair using an exogenous fibrin clot. *Clin Orthop* 1990;252:64.
56. Henning C, Yearout K, et al. Use of the fascia sheath coverage and exogenous fibrin clot in the treatment of complex meniscal tears. *Am J Sports Med* 1991;19:626.
57. Nakhostine M, Gershuni D, et al. Effects of an in-substance conduit with injection of a blood clot on tears in the avascular region of the meniscus. *Acta Orthop Belgica* 1991;57:242.
58. Ishimura M, Tamai S, et al. Arthroscopic meniscal repair with fibrin glue. *Arthroscopy* 1991;7:177.
59. Ishimura M, Ohgushi H, et al. Arthroscopic meniscal repair using fibrin glue, I: experimental study. *Arthroscopy* 1997;13:551.
60. Ishimura M, Ohgushi H, et al. Arthroscopic meniscal repair using fibrin glue, II: clinical applications. *Arthroscopy* 1997;13:558.
61. Jitsuiki J, Ochi M, et al. Meniscal repair enhanced by an interpositional free synovial autograft: an experimental study in rabbits. *Arthroscopy* 1994;10:659.
62. Ochi M, Mochizuki Y, et al. Augmented meniscal healing with free synovial autografts: an organ culture model. *Arch Orthop Trauma Surg* 1996;115:123.
63. Shirakura K, Niijima M, et al. Free synovium promotes meniscal healing. *Acta Orthop Scand* 1997;68:51.
64. Dew D, Supik L, et al. Tissue repair using lasers: a review. *Orthopedics* 1993;16:581.
65. Forman S, Oz M, et al. Laser-assisted fibrin clot soldering of human menisci. *Clin Orthop* 1995;310:37.
66. Vangsness C, Akl Y, et al. The effects of the neodymium laser on meniscal repair in the avascular zone of the meniscus. *Arthroscopy* 1994;10:201.
67. Conteduca F, Ferretti A, et al. Chondromalacia and chronic anterior instabilities of the knee. *Am J Sports Med* 1991;19:119.
68. Irvine G, Glasgow M. The natural history of the meniscus in anterior cruciate insufficiency. *J Bone Joint Surg Br* 1992;74:403.
69. Kannus P, Jarvinen M. Conservatively treated tears of the anterior cruciate ligament. *J Bone Joint Surg Am* 1987;69:1007.
70. Keene G, Paterson R. Anterior cruciate instability: meniscal and chondral damage. *J Bone Joint Surg Br* 1987;69:162.
71. Keene G, Bickerstaff D, et al. The natural history of meniscal tears in anterior cruciate ligament insufficiency. *Am J Sports Med* 1993;21: 672.
72. Feagin J, Curl W. Isolated tears of the anterior cruciate ligament: five-year follow-up study. *Am J Sports Med* 1976;4:95.

73. Lynch M, Henning C, et al. Knee joint surface changes: long-term follow-up meniscus tear treatment in stable anterior cruciate ligament reconstructions. *Clin Orthop* 1983;172:148.

74. Cerabona F, Sherman M, et al. Patterns of meniscal injury with acute anterior cruciate ligament tears. *Am J Sports Med* 1988;16:603.

75. DeHaven K. Diagnosis of acute knee injuries with hemarthrosis. *Am J Sports Med* 1980;8:9.

76. Warren R. Meniscectomy and repair in the anterior cruciate ligament-deficient patient. *Clin Orthop* 1990;252:55.

77. Warren R, Marshall J. Injuries of the anterior cruciate and medial collateral ligaments of the knee: a retrospective analysis of clinical records—part 1. *Clin Orthop* 1978;136:191.

78. Wickiewicz T. Meniscal injuries in the cruciate-deficient knee. *Clin Sports Med* 1990;9:681.

79. Kornblatt I, Warren R, et al. Long-term follow-up of anterior cruciate ligament reconstruction using the quadriceps tendon substitution for chronic anterior cruciate ligament insufficiency. *Am J Sports Med* 1988;16:444.

80. Levy I, Torzilli P, et al. The effect of medial meniscectomy on anterior-posterior motion of the knee. *J Bone Joint Surg Am* 1982;64:883.

81. Levy I, Torzilli P, et al. The effect of lateral meniscectomy on motion of the knee. *J Bone Joint Surg Am* 1989;71:401.

82. DeHaven K, Lohrer W, et al. Long-term results of open meniscal repair. *Am J Sports Med* 1985;23:524.

83. Sommerlath K. Results of meniscal repair and partial meniscectomy in stable knees. *Int Orthop* 1991;15:347.

84. Asahina S, Muneta T, et al. Arthroscopic meniscal repair in conjunction with anterior cruciate ligament reconstruction: factors affecting the healing rate. *Arthroscopy* 1996;12:541.

85. Barber A, Click S. Meniscus repair rehabilitation with concurrent anterior cruciate reconstruction. *Arthroscopy* 1997;13:433.

86. Buseck M, Noyes F. Arthroscopic evaluation of meniscal repairs after anterior cruciate ligament reconstruction and immediate motion. *Am J Sports Med* 1991;19:489.

87. Hanks G, Gause T, et al. Repair of peripheral meniscal tears: open versus arthroscopic technique. *Arthroscopy* 1991;7:72.

88. Horibe S, Shino K, et al. Results of isolated meniscal repair evaluated by second-look arthroscopy. *Arthroscopy* 1996;12:150.

89. Jensen N, Riis J, et al. Arthroscopic repair of the ruptured meniscus: one to 6.3 years follow up. *Arthroscopy* 1994;10:211.

90. Morgan C, Wojtys E, et al. Arthroscopic meniscal repair evaluated by second-look arthroscopy. *Am J Sports Med* 1991;19:632.

91. Rubman M, Noyes F, et al. Arthroscopic repair of meniscal tears that extend into the avascular zone. *Am J Sports Med* 1998;26:87.

92. Hanks G, Gause T, et al. Meniscus repair in the anterior cruciate deficient knee. *Am J Sports Med* 1990;18:606.

93. Stone R, Van Winkle G. Arthroscopic review of meniscus repair: assessment of healing parameters. *Arthroscopy* 1986;2:77.

94. DeHaven K. Rationale for meniscus repair or excision. *Clin Sports Med* 1985;4:267.

95. Cannon W, Vittori J. The incidence of healing in arthroscopic meniscal repairs in anterior cruciate ligament-reconstructed knees versus stable knees. *Am J Sports Med* 1992;20:176.

96. Cannon W, Morgan C. Meniscal repair, II: arthroscopic repair techniques. *J Bone Joint Surg Am* 1994;76:294.

97. Tenuta J, Arciero R. Arthroscopic evaluation of meniscal repairs: factors that effect healing. *Am J Sports Med* 1994;22:797.

98. Torg J, Barton T, et al. Natural history of the posterior cruciate ligament-deficient knee. *Clin Orthop* 1989;246:208.

99. Ikeuchi H. Surgery under arthroscopic control. In: Proceedings of the Societe Internationale d'Arthrocopie: 1975;57.

100. Henning C. Arthroscopic repair of meniscal tears. *Orthopedics* 1983;6:1130.

101. Warren R. Arthroscopic meniscus repair. *Arthroscopy* 1985;1:170.

102. Schulte K, Fu F. Meniscal repair using the inside-to-outside technique. *Clin Sports Med* 1996;15:455.

103. Bach B, Jewell B, et al. Surgical approaches for medial and lateral meniscal repair. In: *Techniques in orthopedics*. Dorr LD, ed. Frederick, MD: Aspen Publications, 1993.

104. Scott G, Jolly B, et al. Combined posterior incision and arthroscopic intraarticular repair of the meniscus. *J Bone Joint Surg Am* 1986;68:847.

105. Rodeo S, Warren R. Meniscal repair using the outside-to-inside technique. *Clin Sports Med* 1996;15:469.

106. Morgan C. The "all-inside" meniscus repair. *Arthroscopy* 1991;7:120.

107. Mulhollan JS. Meniscus repair. In: *Techniques in therapeutic arthroscopy*. Parisien JS, ed. New York: Raven Press, 1993:1–11.

108. Newman A, Daniels A, et al. Principles and decision making in meniscal surgery. *Arthroscopy* 1993; 9:33.

109. Barber F, Gurwitz G. Inflammatory synovial fluid and absorbable suture strength. *Arthroscopy* 1988;4:272.

110. Barrett G, Richardson K, et al. The effect of suture type on meniscus repair. *Am J Knee Surg* 1997;10:2.

111. Rimmer M, Nawana N, et al. Failure strengths of different meniscal suturing techniques. *Arthroscopy* 1995;11:146.

112. Albrecht-Olsen P, Lind T, et al. Failure strength of a new meniscus arrow repair technique: biomechanical comparison with horizontal suture. *Arthroscopy* 1997;13:183.

113. Barrett G, Richardson K, et al. T-fix endoscopic meniscal repair: technique and approach to different types of tears. *Arthroscopy* 1995;11:245.

114. Dervin G, Downing K, et al. Failure strengths of suture versus biodegradable arrow for meniscal repair: an in vitro study. *Arthroscopy* 1997;13:296.

115. Escalas F, Quadras J, Caceres E, et al. T-fix anchor sutures for arthroscopic meniscal repair. *Knee Surg Sports Traumatol Arthrosc* 1997;5:72–76.

116. DeHaven K. Meniscus repair in the athlete. *Clin Orthop* 1985;198:31.

117. Fowler P, Pompan D. Rehabilitation after meniscal repair. *Tech Orthop* 1993;8:137.

118. Ryu R, Dunbar W. Arthroscopic meniscal repair with two-year follow-up: a clinical review. *Arthroscopy* 1988;4:168.

119. DowdyP, Miniaci A, et al. The effect of cast immobilization on meniscal healing. *Am J Sports Med* 1995;23:721.

120. Cooper D, Arnoczky S, et al. Meniscal repair. *Clin Sports Med* 1991;10:529.

121. Barber A. Accelerated rehabilitation for meniscus repair. *Arthroscopy* 1994;10:206.

122. Mariani P, Santori N, et al. Accelerated rehabilitation after arthroscopic meniscal repair: a clinical and magnetic resonance imaging evaluation. *Arthroscopy* 1996;12:680.

123. de Groot J, de Vrijer R, et al. Use of porous polyurethanes for mensical reconstruction and meniscal prostheses. *Biomaterials* 1996;17:163.

124. Messner K. Meniscal substitution with a Teflon-periosteal composite graft: a rabbit experiment. *Biomaterials* 1994;15:223.

125. Toyonaga T, Uezaki N, et al. Substitute meniscus of Teflon-net for the knee joint of dogs. *Clin Orthop* 1983;179:291.

126. Veth R, Den Heeten G, et al. An experimental study of reconstructive procedures in lesions of the meniscus. *Clin Orthop* 1983;181:250.

127. Veth R, Jansen H, et al. Experimental meniscal lesions reconstructed with a carbon fiber-polyurethane-poly(L-lactide) graft. *Clin Orthop* 1987;202:286.

128. Mankin H, Doppelt S, et al. Osteoarticular and intercalary allograft transplantation in the management of malignant tumors of bone. *Cancer* 1982;50:613.

129. Milachowski K, Weismeier K, et al. Homologous meniscus transplantation. *Int Orthop* 1989;13:1.

130. Shelton W, Dukes A. Meniscus replacement with bone anchors: a surgical technique. *Arthroscopy* 1994;10:324.

131. Stone K, Rosenberg T. Surgical technique of meniscal replacement. *Arthroscopy* 1993;9:234.

132. Arnoczky S, McDevitt C, et al. The effect of cryopreservation on canine menisci: a biochemical, morphologic, and biomechanical evaluation. *J Orthop Res* 1988;6:1.

133. Jackson D, McDevitt C, et al. Meniscal transplantation using fresh and cryopreserved allografts: an experimental study in goats. *Am J Sports Med* 1992;20:644.

134. Jackson D, Whelan J, et al. Cell survival after transplantation of fresh meniscal allografts. *Am J Sports Med* 1993;21:540.

135. Graham W, Smith D, et al. The use of frozen stored tendons for grafting: an experimental study. *J Bone Joint Surg Am* 1985;37:624.

136. Jackson D, Simon T. Biology of meniscal allograft. knee meniscus: basic and clinical foundations. In: *Knee meniscus: basic and clinical foundations*. Mow V, Arnoczky S, Jackson D, eds. New York: Raven Press, 1992;141.

137. Arnoczky S, Warren R, et al. Meniscal replacement using a cryopreserved allograft. *Clin Orthop* 1990;252:121.

138. Canham W, Stanish W. A study of the biological behaviors of the

meniscus as a transplant in the medial compartment of a dog's knee. *Am J Sports Med* 1986;14:376.

139. Fabbriciani C, Lucania L, et al. Meniscal allografts: cryopreservation vs deep-frozen technique. *Knee Surg Sports Traumatol Arthrosc* 1997;5:124.

140. Cummins J, Mansour J. Meniscal transplantation and degenerative articular change: an experimental study in the rabbit. *Arthroscopy* 1997;13:485.

141. Edwards D, Whittle S, et al. Radiographic changes in the knee after meniscal transplantation. *Am J Sports Med* 1996;24:222.

142. Paletta G, Manning T, et al. The effect of allograft meniscal replacement on intraarticular contact area and pressures in the human knee. *Am J Sports Med* 1997;25:692.

143. Veltri D, Warren R, et al. Current status of allograft meniscal transplantation. *Clin Orthop* 1994;303:44.

144. Cameron J, Saha S. Meniscal allograft transplantation for unicompartmental arthritis of the knee. *Clin Orthop* 1997;337:164.

145. Garrett J, Stevensen R. Meniscal transplantation in the human knee: a preliminary report. *Arthroscopy* 1991;7:57.

146. Kuhn J, Wojtys E. Allograft meniscus transplantation. *Clin Sports Med* 1996;15:537.

147. Stone K, Rodkey W, et al. Autogenous replacement of the meniscus cartilage: analysis of results and mechanisms of failure. *Arthroscopy* 1995;11:395.

148. Stone K, Rodkey W, et al. Meniscal regeneration with copolymeric collagen scaffolds. *Am J Sports Med* 1992;20:104.

149. Stone K, Steadman J, et al. Regeneration of meniscal cartilage with use of a collagen scaffold. *J Bone Joint Surg Am* 1997;79:1770.

150. Hewitt A, Kleinman H, et al. Identification of an adhesion factor for chondrocytes. *Proc Natl Acad Sci U S A* 1980;77:385.

151. Hewitt A, Varner H, et al. The isolation and partial characterization of chondronectin, an attachment factor for chondrocytes. *J Biol Chem* 1982;257:2330.

152. Webber R, Harris M, et al. Cell culture of rabbit meniscal fibrochondrocytes: proliferative and synthetic response to growth factors and ascorbate. *J Orthop Res* 1985;3:36.

153. King T, Vallee B. Neovascularisation of the meniscus with angiogenin. *J Bone Joint Surg Br* 1991;73:587.

154. Kollias S, Fox J. Meniscal repair: where do we go from here? *Clin Sports Med* 1996;15:621.

155. Ibarra C, Jannetta C, et al. Tissue engineered meniscus: a potential new alternative to allogeneic meniscus transplantation. *Transplant Proc* 1997;29:986.

CHAPTER 16

Experimental Design and Statistical Analysis

Richard L. Lieber

Improved understanding of the musculoskeletal system results from the search for general truths and the desire to understand the general laws that regulate the system. Building such an understanding requires that experiments be conducted to observe how the system operates under different conditions. The way such observations are made depends on the type of phenomenon observed. In certain circumstances, a phenomenon can be considered deterministic; that is, every time it is observed the outcome is the same. For example, a ball with a known size and weight dropped from a certain height will always hit the ground with the same force, no matter how many times it is observed. In this situation, only one observation is needed to know what the results will always be. However, certain phenomena may occur only sometimes; each time one of these phenomena occurs or is tested, different results can be obtained. Because these results occur with a certain probability, such phenomena are considered probabilistic. To determine whether there is some consistency in the effects produced, or whether relationships or associations occur, such phenomena must be observed many times, and the data obtained must be analyzed.

Analysis of such results must distinguish between causality and chance occurrence. These distinctions are made using statistical analysis. Inherent in this analysis is the fact that conclusions are reached by repeatedly observing a subset of members of an entire population. For example, members of the entire population of a given fish species must be examined many times to be sure that a color or design pattern is, indeed, inherent in that species. Observing one member of that species once would not necessarily provide such a conclusion. Because it is often either impractical, costly, or inefficient to examine the entire population, a representative group is selected, and the phenomenon is tested only the number of times with each representative member that suffices to ensure its validity. Statistics provides the objective methodology to assure adequate performance of this task.

The reliability of statistics and the conclusions drawn from it are based on the science of probability.

This chapter defines and describes many terms and techniques used in statistics. Its purpose is to provide the reader with the basis for understanding, appreciating, and evaluating conclusions that may be drawn from clinical or basic science studies. In addition, it will provide the reader with the means to recognize both the validity and limitations of the conclusions that are drawn. Not all statistical topics are covered in this chapter; it covers only those that are current or that more particularly demonstrate principles that apply to the extraction of valid conclusions for musculoskeletal system phenomena.

HYPOTHESIS TESTING

If we are to examine a phenomenon and try to extract information from observations of it, where the chance of its occurring each time it is observed is not 100%, we must first describe it in a quantitative form. We often have a preconceived notion of how a group of individuals will respond to a treatment. We thus formulate a hypothesis. A hypothesis, simply stated, is a supposition that appears to describe a phenomenon and acts as a basis of reasoning and experimentation. Hypotheses may be extremely basic—for example, growth factor binding to extracellular matrix proteins activates cellular protein synthesis—or very applied—for example, use of the patellar tendon for surgical reconstruction of the anterior cruciate ligament results in loss of quadriceps strength.

A hypothesis is an untested statement based on previous information, a hunch, or an intuition. It can be stated for any group of observations. However, to ensure that the observations noted are appropriate, the measurements made are accurate, the experiment is performed efficiently, and the conclusions drawn are accurate, the hypothesis must be stated in a quantitative form and in a specific manner. Clearly stating the hypothesis focuses attention on the central issues and assures that a given phenomenon can properly be evaluated and reexamined.

A hypothesis to be tested using statistical methodology is presented in terms of the null hypothesis. The null hypothesis states that experimental treatment has no effect; that is, is null. As an example, we could propose the following null hypothesis: There is no difference in ultimate tensile strength between a patellar tendon that is a surgically repaired substitute for the anterior cruciate ligament and a normal anterior cruciate ligament. To test this hypothesis, ultimate tensile strength from a control group that has no injury to the ligament is compared with ultimate strength from an experimental group that was surgically repaired using the patellar tendon.

In the earlier example, we would then test the null hypothesis that there is no difference in tensile strength between the patellar tendon autograft and normal ligament. If we find the hypothesis is not true, a difference exists; this is the most important thing we want to know. If we had chosen any other hypothesis; for example, there is a 25% loss in strength, and we found that this hypothesis was not true, we still would not know whether there may be a 50%, 25%, 10%, 5%, 4%, or no difference in strength. Without a great deal more testing and analysis, we would not have a significant conclusion.

In one of the most common embodiments, an experiment based on a null hypothesis is designed with a control group that receives no treatment, and one or more experimental groups that receive treatment (Fig. 16.1).

Four conclusions can be drawn from the use of the null hypothesis (Table 16.1). The null hypothesis can be either true or false. In addition, each of these can be accepted or rejected (that is, believed or not believed). Of the four potential decisions, two are correct and two are incorrect (Table 16.1). Suppose, in our ligament strength example, that the null hypothesis is true; that is, there really is no difference in ligament strength between experimental and control groups. But suppose also that, based on our analysis or limited sample, we choose to believe that there is a

TABLE 16.1. *Statistical errors related to the null hypothesis*

Null hypothesis	Null hypothesis	
	Accepted	Rejected
True	Correct decision	Type I error
False	Type II error	Correct decision

difference (that is, we reject a true null hypothesis). In statistics, rejection of a true null hypothesis is an incorrect conclusion known as type I error. In this experiment, committing type I error would imply that there is a significant effect of surgical repair when, in fact, there is not. In more clinical terms, this error can be viewed as a false positive (Table 16.2).

An alternate possibility is that the null hypothesis is false; that is, surgical repair has a significant effect on ligament strength. If, for similar reasons, we chose to believe that there was no effect on ligament strength, we would be falsely accepting the null hypothesis. Accepting a false null hypothesis is known as a type II error. In this experiment, committing a type II error would imply that surgery had no effect when, in fact, it actually had an effect. This can be viewed in clinical terms as a false negative (Table 16.2).

In the experiment described earlier, what would it mean clinically to commit a type I or type II error, and if one did commit such errors, how serious would they be? First, if we committed a type I error, we would state there is a difference in strength with surgical repair using the patellar tendon when, in fact, there is none. We would be stating something is different when it really is not. We then would probably try to find another tendon that showed no difference in strength, and we would modify our rehabilitation program when we used the patellar tendon in the procedure. We would continue to test different tendons until we found one that showed no difference in strength. However, if we kept committing the same type of error, we might never find the right tendon. Then we would be forced to accept a procedure as a compromise—a less than desirable condition. In spite of the time and expense involved in such experimentation, we still would be left with the incorrect conclusion.

If we made a type II error, we would be stating that there is no difference in strength when the patellar tendon is used, when in fact there is a difference. We would be missing something that is really there. This is a more serious error in this example, for it can lead not only to our

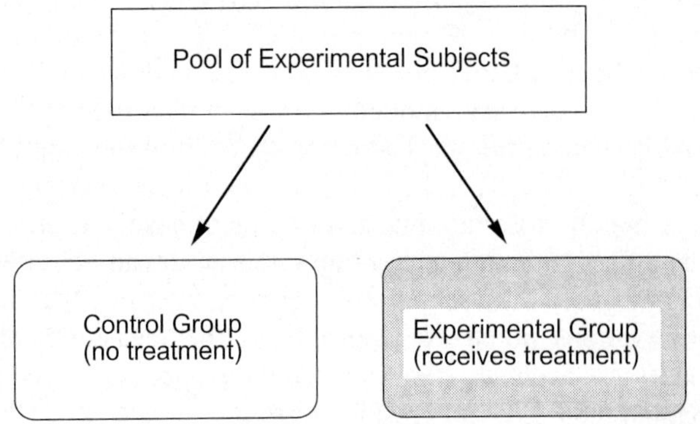

FIGURE 16.1. Schematic illustration of the simplest experimental design in which experimental subjects are divided into a control and an experimental group.

TABLE 16.2. *Interpretation and control of statistical error*

Condition	Greek symbol	Clinical meaning	Controlled using
Type I error	α	False-positive	Significance level
Type II error	β	False-negative	Statistical power

abandoning the attempt to find a better substitute, but also to our performing a procedure that could subsequently produce complications. Only after we knew of these complications and our patients have suffered the consequences, would we seek a substitute.

The seriousness of each type of error depends on the situation; in the best situation, we must try not to commit either type of error. If we cannot eliminate errors, we must at least try to reduce the chance of committing either type of error. The probability or chance of committing a type I error, that is, the probability of finding an effect when there really isn't one, is known as the significance level of a statistical test, termed alpha or α. The probability or chance of committing a type II error, that is, the probability of failing to find an effect when there really is one, is known as beta or β. In statistical testing, the term "significance level" is used to describe a type I error, and "statistical Power" (defined as 1 β) to describe a type II error. The calculation of α, β, or Power is based on the science of probability and need not be detailed here because it can readily be found in statistical tables and/or automatically calculated by a computer program. Its importance to readers of this text lies in the awareness that both types of errors can exist and in the understanding of how they are avoided. Now, let us consider many terms and definitions that are common in statistical analysis.

STATISTICAL DEFINITIONS AND DESCRIPTIONS OF OBSERVATIONS

Our ability to extract the truth from a set of observations rests on our ability to accurately describe the phenomenon and use the appropriate tools to analyze it. To do this, we must first describe the phenomenon in statistical terms, which are presented here.

Statistical Terms

Sample Versus Population

In statistics, a population is the entire collection of elements about which information is desired. A sample is a collection of observations representing the population or a collection of individual observations from the population selected by a specified procedure. Statistics are used to generalize from a sample to a population. In practice, a correct interpretation of these terms is related to a proper value for sample size; that is, the value for n.

It is important to define the "collection of elements" from which data are obtained. An example of a population could be the anterior compartment muscles of male humans in San Diego county. Additional qualifications such as age and health status might also be important. Having defined the population, it would only be appropriate to generalize from the analysis of our sample to other populations having similar traits. This fact has been recognized by the National Institutes of Health in their recent report on the paucity of scientific data that are applicable to women.

The sample concept refers both to the actual data obtained and to the procedure itself. An example of a sample is the maximum dorsiflexion torque from 40 male college-aged volunteers. Here the concept of sample includes the amount of data or number of observations or data points to be examined, termed n. This number must be explicitly determined to guard against erroneous generalizations or inflated significance levels.

Variable

A variable is the actual property measured by the individual observations. Using our example, a variable would be torque, measured in $N \cdot m$.

Variate

A variate is a single reading, score, or observation of a given variable. Thus, a sample is composed of a number of variates obtained for a selected number of variables. An example of a variate would be the value 142.2 $N \cdot m$ from subject A164.

Level

Level is the number of different values a grouping variable can have. For example, in an experiment where men's versus women's strength is compared, the grouping variable, sex, has two levels: male or female.

Precision

Precision is the closeness of repeated measurements of the same quantity.

Accuracy

Accuracy is the closeness of a measured variate to its true value. This definition implies that a standard is available against which a measure can be compared. A knowledge of accuracy determines the numbers of significant figures for the presentation of experimental results. Using an example, we might determine that a 2.000000-kg standard mass is shown on a balance scale as 2.011233 kg. This is probably an acceptable level of accuracy (within 1%), but it would be absurd to report mass to six decimal places. Although there is no problem in retaining all figures for intermediate calculations, the final data presentation must reflect the appropriate accuracy, in this case 2.01 or about 0.56%.

Accuracy and precision are often confused. Precision simply refers to the repeatability of a particular measurement. Thus, in our example above, the balance scale may read 2.011233 kg for one reading, 2.011210 for the next, and 2.011225 for the next. Our device is thus precise to 0.00002 kg in spite of the fact that it is only accurate to about 0.01 kg. In this age of computers and digital displays, it is important to vigilantly recall that high precision does not imply high accuracy.

It is important to ensure that accurate results are obtained to enable comparison of experimental data across laboratories. For example, a balance scale used to weigh samples in one laboratory might be precise but consistently read values that are greater than another balance scale down the hall. In such a case, the two laboratories will differ with respect to their interpretation of a particular phenomenon. In addition, if an experimenter uses both balances interchangeably, experimental variability will be needlessly increased.

Conversely, we should not be quick to discard measurements that are not very precise (for example, intraoperative measurements of nerve width) believing that they do not contain useful information. For example, intraoperative measurements with a standard ruler calibrated in millimeters can be read to a fraction of a millimeter. One of the beauties of multiple measurements of the same quantity is that random errors tend to cancel out. Thus, three measurements of nerve width might be 2.5 mm, 3.0 mm, and 3.0 mm. The average value of 2.83 mm is probably closer to the true value than any of the individual measurements. It is, therefore, possible to resolve smaller differences than are actually present on a measuring device by repeated measures with this "less precise" device!

Mean

The sample mean, designated $\overline{X}$, is the average of all variates for a sample and is an unbiased estimator of the population μ. The population mean is the most probable value within the population and the one that the investigator wishes to estimate based on the mean of its representative sample. The sample mean estimates the population mean if the population is normally distributed. The values within a normally distributed sample fit into the classic bell-shaped curve (Fig. 16.2). The shape of the normal distribution is very specific; the curve cannot be too tail heavy if it is to be considered normally distributed. Many natural measurements, such as length, height, and mass, are usually normally distributed, whereas many others, especially ratios and percentages, are almost never normally distributed. One of the first concerns in statistical analysis of experimental data is whether the sample variates are normally distributed.

The units of the mean are the same as the units of the variable. Sample mean is calculated as:

$$\overline{X} = \frac{\sum_{i=1}^{i=n} X_i}{n} \qquad [1]$$

where

$\sum_{i=1}^{i=n}$ = the arithmetic summation of all n values of X_i

X_i = the value of an individual variate (read as the "i^{th}" variate)

n = the sample size.

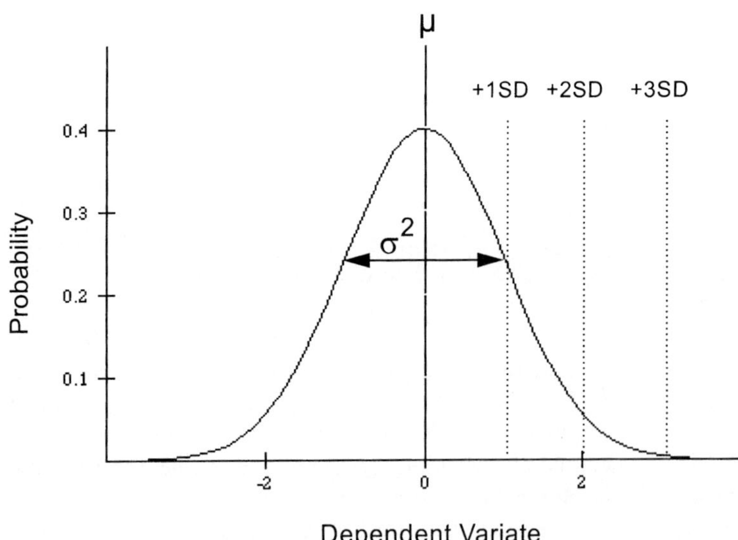

$$y = \frac{e^{\dfrac{-(x-\mu)^2}{2\sigma^2}}}{\sigma\sqrt{2\pi}}$$

Equation plotted for $\mu=0$ and $\sigma^2=1$

FIGURE 16.2. Graphic representation of the normal distribution. Note that the mean (μ) represents the most common value, whereas the variance (σ^2) represents the population variability.

An example of a sample mean would be 136.2 N · m of knee extension torque, calculated as the mean of 12 individual variates.

Median

The median is the value below which half of the values lie and above which the remaining half of the values lie. It is the middle or the fiftieth percentile of a normal distribution.

Variance

The sample variance s^2 is a measure of the spread of data about the sample mean and is an estimator of the population variance σ^2. As shown in Figure 16.1, each population not only has its most probable value, the mean μ, it also has a certain variability or variance σ^2 about that value. It is more difficult to extract the "truth" from a population with large variance because the likelihood of obtaining a variate near the mean is less when sample variability is high.

As an example, to determine whether a particular exercise caused an increase in quadriceps strength after surgery, two groups of individuals were used—one group receiving traditional therapy and one group receiving therapy using the new exercise. Average group strengths would be compared, and the results of the comparison would indicate whether the exercise was efficacious. Suppose that the results in one population were highly variable (Fig. 16.3). The high variability might make it difficult to determine whether the two samples are truly different because the exercised group has many values that overlap with the traditional therapy group. It is easy to detect a difference between the two means μ_1 and μ_2 in Figure 16.2 (top); however, with increased population variability (Fig. 16.2, bottom), this difference is less easy to demonstrate.

The proper units used to express variance are variable units squared. The calculation of variance uses a "sum of squared terms" as a type of expression.

$$\sigma^2 = \frac{\sum_{i=1}^{n}(\overline{X} - X_i)^2}{n-1} \qquad [2]$$

The variance term contains a squared difference between the sample mean and the individual variate. This squared difference, represents the "distance" from the mean to the value of a particular variate; it is squared to eliminate the sign of the difference (positive or negative) so that variability of either sign is summed over the entire sample. The entire summed, squared difference is divided by $(n - 1)$ to yield a sort of "average" difference. The term $n - 1$ is used instead of the more intuitively appealing n because, as sample size gets small, statisticians have determined that this mathematical expression tends to slightly overestimate population variance. An example of a population variance might be 44 N · m², which describes the variance of the mean of 12 individual knee extension torque variates.

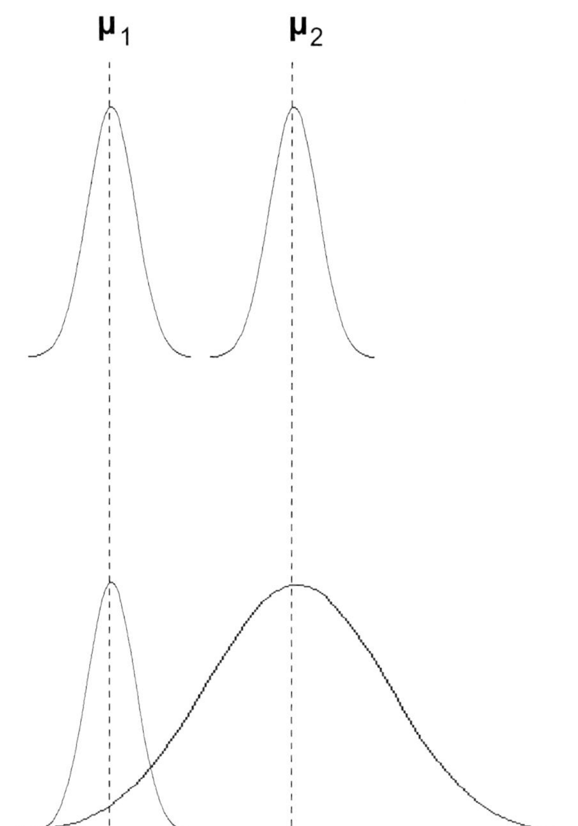

FIGURE 16.3. Graphic illustration of the difficulty in detecting a difference between the means of two populations when one population has a high variability (**bottom**) compared with when it has a lower variability (**top**).

Standard Deviation

Standard deviation (SD) is the square root of the sample variance. SD is more often used to describe population variability than sample variance because the units of SD are the same as the original variate units. An example of a SD is 6.6 N · m. This statement contains information as to the estimated population mean and has some information with respect to population variability.

The calculation of SD is simply:

$$SD = \sqrt{S^2} \qquad [3]$$

where
S^2 = the calculated sample variance

SD has a very useful property for normally distributed data in that 66% of the variates are within 1 SD of the mean, 95% of the variates are within 2 SDs of the mean, and 99% of the variates are within 3 SDs of the mean (Fig. 16.2). Because this value refers to the variability of the original sample, it can be used to make powerful predictions regarding the variability of the original population if the sample properly represents the entire population.

An example of this type of approach is a study by investigators who were interested in understanding the normal anatomic path of the superficial branch of the radial nerve (SBRN). It was important to know where the SBRN became subcutaneous from the interval between the brachioradialis and the extensor carpi radialis longus, because external fixator pins are frequently inserted in this area and thus surgical approaches must avoid the SBRN. The researchers measured, in cadaveric specimens, the distance between the subcutaneous SBRN and an external bony landmark such as the radial styloid process, which can be palpated. They found that this distance was mean ± SD = 9.0 ± 1.4 cm, which enabled them to conclude that, in 95% of the individuals from the general population, the subcutaneous SBRN region extended from 6.2 cm (mean − 2 SD) to 11.8 cm (mean + 2 SD) proximal to the radial styloid process. Knowledge of this 95% confidence interval has significant surgical implications.

Standard Error of the Mean

The standard error of the mean (SEM) is the variability associated with estimation of the population mean. This value is used to describe the level of confidence we have that the mean, which is determined from a sample of a given population, represents the mean of the entire population. It is calculated as

$$SEM = \frac{SD}{\sqrt{n}} \qquad [4]$$

where
SD = standard deviation
N = sample size

SD is a relatively constant estimate of population variability, whereas SEM changes with sample size and does not estimate the population variability at all. Because it actually represents the accuracy of a mean estimate, it is preferable to use SEM when comparisons are made between means. SD, which is related to population variability, is preferable when it is necessary to express the variability of the original population. For example, SD might be preferred when describing the baseline characteristics of a group of experimental subjects because it would provide the reader with an idea of the level of variability in the population from which the sample was obtained. However, when comparing a treatment group to a control group, SEM may be preferable because the accuracy of the individual mean values is of interest.

Coefficient of Variation

The coefficient of variation (CV) is a generic indicator of population variance. CV is calculated as

$$CV = \frac{SD}{\overline{X}} \cdot 100\% \qquad [5]$$

so that the CV is expressed without the original units of measurement. Because CV is independent of units and absolute variate magnitude, it provides a general feel for a population's variability. There is no acceptable level of variability for a particular population. Thus, in a clinical experiment involving complex treatment of individuals who have variable characteristics, a CV of 50% to 100% might be expected and accepted, whereas in a laboratory experiment involving a more homogeneous species and a clearly defined procedure, a CV of 10% to 25% would be more likely. It is much easier to determine whether significant effects of a particular treatment exist when the CV of the sample is low.

Choice of Significance and Power Values

Terms such as SD, SEM, and CV and the calculation of such parameters illustrate that an experiment does not always work the way we expect. It is the variation that these terms represent that causes us to question or believe the results we obtain, and these terms give us an indication of how much we can believe the conclusions drawn. However, there is no true or ideal answer to the question of how much variability or error we can accept before we will no longer believe or disbelieve the results. The investigator and reader must decide what to accept, and their decisions will vary depending on the nature of the study. Statistics provides a means of quantifying what we wish to accept. This is expressed in the p value and α and β levels.

The p value is simply the probability (denoted α) of committing type I error in a given experiment (Table 16.2). When a report states that the results were significant ($p < 0.05$), the investigator is saying that type I error has been committed less than 5% of the time. Often we conclude that if a type 1 error is committed only 5% of the time we can believe the results; that is, we expect the conclusions drawn to be found not just in the representative sample but in the entire population as well. The problem with this automatic use of p less than 0.05 as the level for statistical significance is that many times, especially in clinical situations, it may not be reasonable, nor even safe, to commit a type I error 5% of the time, whereas in other cases it might be acceptable to commit a type I error a greater percentage of the time. The significance level a should actually be determined based on its meaning in the context of the experiment performed.

The p level chosen by the investigator as determining significance for the results obtained from a particular experiment is called the critical p level; this level may be different from the one that actually is obtained when the study is run. While most investigators are familiar with setting limits for type I error by choosing a critical p value, they are not as familiar with limiting type II error. However, controlling type II error can be as important as, or more important than, controlling type I error, as described in the next example.

Many of us have observed presentations where a small sample size was used (for example, n = 3), statistical analysis was performed, and a *p* value greater than 0.05 was obtained. The speaker concluded that the treatment had no effect. Immediately, a protestor, believing the sample size to be too small, claimed that the speaker committed type II error.

In another presentation, we may observe a surgeon who performed an experiment using a small sample size in which he or she attempted to compare a new surgical technique to the standard technique. Based on a high *p* value, the surgeon concluded that there was no significant difference between the new and standard methods and that the new method should be used because it is easier and cheaper. Is this an appropriate conclusion?

Although this conclusion might be correct, we would also want to be sure that if a *p* value greater than 0.05 were obtained, we are not committing type II error by incorrectly accepting a false null hypothesis. In the example stated earlier, we may wish to design the experiment with a power of 95%. In that case, we would be 95% sure that if the surgical repair had an effect on ligament strength (the null hypothesis were false), we would not falsely conclude that it did not.

Several methods, which use graphs, tables, and equations, have been developed to allow the experimenter to set the significance level (α, the critical *p* value) and the statistical power for an experiment, and then to determine the sample size required to achieve that design. Using these methods, the experimenter chooses α and β, esti-

mates the σ sample variance, and anticipates the magnitude of the treatment effect (Fig. 16.4).

A survey of the scientific literature, especially that related to biology and medicine, reveals that an overwhelming majority of investigators set the critical α value to 0.05. It should be obvious that there is nothing magical about an α value of 0.05. This value simply indicates that the investigator is willing to accept committing type I error 5% of the time and still believe that the results obtained are true. However, there may be situations where the investigator is not willing to commit type I error 5% of the time or even 1% of the time. In such cases, the critical α value should be adjusted accordingly; that is, made lower. An example of this concept is an experiment in which the investigator attempts to demonstrate a significant decrease in knee laxity using a new surgical procedure compared with an established procedure. If the critical α value is 0.05, the investigator is willing to conclude 5% of the time that the new surgical procedure is more effective, even if it actually is not. If the new procedure represents an increased risk to the patient or a significant increase in expense or rehabilitation time, the surgeon may be willing to commit type I error only 1% of the time or a fraction of a percent of the time. In such a case, a critical α value of 0.05 may be too high.

At times, type II error may be more important to an investigator than type I error. For example, suppose that a safe experimental drug were administered to prevent

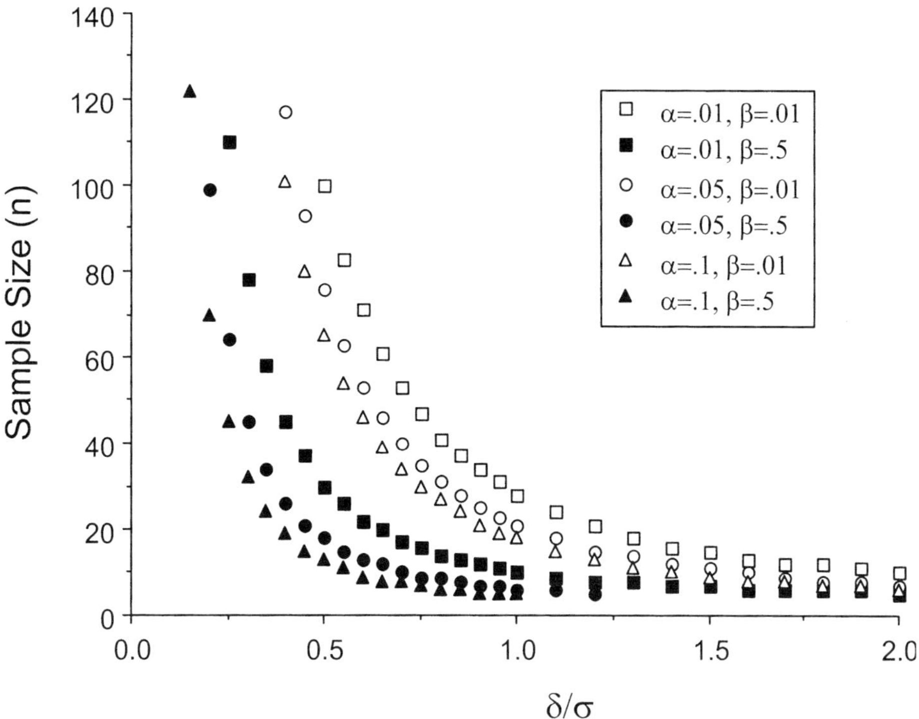

FIGURE 16.4. Relationship between sample size (n), type 1 error rate (α), type 2 error rate (β), and the ratio of δ/σ for a *t* test between two groups of data. Note that as α, β, and δ/σ decrease, sample size increases.

thrombophlebitis after knee surgery. In this case, type I error would indicate that the drug had an effect when in fact it did not. The detriment to the patient is that he or she would take a drug that had no effect and would be at risk for developing the problem that the drug was intended to avoid. However, suppose type II error were committed in the same study. Type II error would indicate that the drug had no effect when in fact it had an effect. In this case, an effective drug would be withheld from the patient, which could represent a large problem. It may be that in this example, the power of the test should be 99.9%, while the critical α value should only be 0.1. The interpretation of the meaning of the α value is therefore paramount in selecting its value and in guarding against cookbook application of statistical methods.

Calculation of Sample Size

To properly test a hypothesis and ensure that the conclusions drawn accurately represent the phenomenon, we infer that our sample adequately represents the behavior of the population. Clearly, the greater the n is for this sample, the greater is the likelihood that our conclusions will, in general, be correct. However, the greater the sample size, the greater the amount of testing and cost will be required to perform the investigation. Therefore, a balance must be struck between adequate representation and available resources.

A number of experimental methods have been developed to calculate sample size for various experimental designs. Each method is specific for the experimental model used. Several of these are presented in the "Suggested Readings." For purposes of illustration, we will consider the equation used for sample size calculation in the full factorial analysis of variance (ANOVA) model. This equation relates sample size to significance level and statistical power. In its most common form, the equation is represented as

$$n = 2 \cdot \left\{\frac{\sigma}{\delta}\right\}^2 \cdot \left\{t_{\alpha,\upsilon} + t_{2\beta,\upsilon}\right\}^2 \qquad [6]$$

where

  n = required sample size
  σ = population SD
  δ = difference desired to detect
  α = desired significance level (type I error rate)
  υ = *df*, which is related to sample size
  β = desired type II error rate
  $t_{\alpha,\upsilon}$ = *t* statistic corresponding to significance level α and *df*, υ
  $t_{2\beta,\upsilon}$ = *t* statistic corresponding to significance level 2β and *df*, υ

Both of these *t* values can be found in tables such as Table 16.3.

The meanings of σ, α, and β have already been discussed. The parameter δ represents the magnitude of the intended treatment effect. For example, in our previous discussion of quadriceps strength, the hypothesis might be that use of a particular tendon would be acceptable only if it increased strength over that of an unrepaired ligament by 30 N · m. Anything less than this would be considered as no difference. This experiment is a much different experiment than if the hypothesis were that a particular tendon would increase strength by 300 N · m. The point made here is that the value of δ is an implied part of the experimental design determined by clinical or scientific knowledge rather than statistical knowledge.

A number of observations follow from inspection of Equation 16.6 and Figure 16.4. First, as population variability σ increases, required sample size increases. Population variability can increase as a result of extrinsic variability; that is, poor technique, instrument measuring variability, and intrinsic variability (variability of the population itself). Thus, the investigator's techniques should be as clean as possible.

Second, to resolve very small differences δ relative to the population SD σ, it will be necessary to use a large sample size. Notice how the graph curves up to higher sample sizes as the ratio of δ/σ decreases (Fig. 16.4). Stated another way, big differences are easy to detect and do not require large population samples. Note in Equation 16.6 that one does not need to know the actual values for σ and δ, only their ratio δ/σ. This means that it is possible to predict the sample size needed for many combinations of α, β, and δ/σ (Table 16.4 and Fig. 16.4). Note that sample size must increase as the desired rates of type I and type II errors decrease (α and β, respectively) and/or with the attempt to resolve smaller and smaller differences (ratio of δ/σ increases).

Third, high statistical power (or low β) or low significance levels (low α), which provide greater assurance against committing type II or type I errors, require a concomitant increase in sample size (Fig. 16.4). The understanding of the relationship between the ratio δ/σ and sample size permits almost immediate evaluation of proposed experiments. For example, if an experiment is proposed for increasing tendon suture strength by 25 N in a system where the normal tendon strength variability is 20 N, this represents a design in which $\delta = 25$ N, $\sigma = 20$, and the ratio δ to σ is 1.25. Clearly, it would require a relatively small sample size to test this hypothesis (Table 16.4). Conversely, suppose it was hypothesized that using a new method would increase suture strength by 2 N. Now, the ratio δ/σ of 0.1 would require a sample size of several hundred, perhaps precluding the study entirely. Thus, before beginning an experiment, it is possible, and should be required, to know the amount of time, energy, and money that will be required to achieve the desired experimental design. This decision can be based only on very approximate pilot data in which estimates can be made for the parameters discussed.

TABLE 16.3. *Critical values of Student's t distribution*

df (υ)	Significance (α)								
	0.9	0.5	0.4	0.2	0.1	0.05	0.02	0.01	0.001
1	0.158	1.000	1.376	3.078	6.314	12.706	31.821	63.657	636.62
2	0.142	0.816	1.061	1.886	2.920	4.303	6.965	9.925	31.598
3	0.137	0.765	0.978	1.638	2.353	3.182	4.541	5.841	12.924
4	0.134	0.741	0.941	1.533	2.132	2.776	3.747	4.604	8.610
5	0.132	0.727	0.920	1.476	2.015	2.571	3.365	4.032	6.869
6	0.131	0.718	0.906	1.440	1.943	2.447	3.143	3.707	5.959
7	0.130	0.711	0.896	1.415	1.895	2.365	2.998	3.499	5.408
8	0.130	0.706	0.889	1.397	1.86	2.306	2.896	3.355	5.041
9	0.129	0.703	0.883	1.383	1.833	2.262	2.821	3.250	4.781
10	0.129	0.700	0.879	1.372	1.812	2.228	2.764	3.169	4.587
11	0.129	0.697	0.876	1.363	1.796	2.201	2.718	3.106	4.437
12	0.128	0.695	0.873	1.356	1.782	2.179	2.681	3.055	4.318
13	0.128	0.694	0.87	1.350	1.771	2.160	2.650	3.012	4.221
14	0.128	0.692	0.868	1.345	1.761	2.145	2.624	2.977	4.41
15	0.128	0.691	0.866	1.341	1.753	2.131	2.602	2.947	4.073
16	0.128	0.69	0.865	1.337	1.746	2.12	2.583	2.921	4.015
17	0.128	0.689	0.863	1.333	1.74	2.11	2.567	2.898	3.965
18	0.127	0.688	0.862	1.330	1.734	2.101	2.552	2.878	3.922
19	0.127	0.688	0.861	1.328	1.729	2.093	2.539	2.861	3.883
20	0.127	0.687	0.860	1.325	1.725	2.086	2.528	2.845	3.850
21	0.127	0.686	0.859	1.323	1.721	2.080	2.518	2.831	3.819
22	0.127	0.686	0.858	1.321	1.717	2.074	2.508	2.819	3.792
23	0.127	0.685	0.858	1.319	1.714	2.069	2.500	2.807	3.767
24	0.127	0.685	0.857	1.318	1.711	2.064	2.492	2.797	3.745
25	0.127	0.684	0.856	1.316	1.708	2.060	2.485	2.787	3.725
26	0.127	0.684	0.856	1.315	1.706	2.056	2.479	2.779	3.707
27	0.127	0.684	0.855	1.314	1.703	2.052	2.473	2.771	3.690
28	0.127	0.683	0.855	1.313	1.701	2.048	2.467	2.763	3.674
29	0.127	0.683	0.854	1.311	1.699	2.045	2.462	2.756	3.659
30	0.127	0.683	0.854	1.310	1.697	2.042	2.457	2.750	3.646
40	0.126	0.681	0.851	1.303	1.684	2.021	2.423	2.704	3.551
60	0.126	0.679	0.848	1.296	1.671	2.000	2.390	2.660	3.460
120	0.126	0.677	0.845	1.289	1.658	1.980	2.358	2.617	3.373
∞	0.126	0.674	0.842	1.282	1.645	1.960	2.326	2.576	3.291

Correct sample size determinations, which represent a balance between guarantees against committing errors and the costs in time, money, and ability to perform the experiment, are not statistical in nature; rather they are clinical or scientific decisions to be made based on the clinician's understanding of the comfort level with being wrong either as a false positive or false negative. However, reviewers of an investigator's work may have a different comfort level than the investigator. This means it is a good idea to be conservative in most cases.

The procedure used to calculate sample size using Equation 16.6 is an iterative one. It is initiated based on some information about the experiment. A first guess is made at sample size, and the expected sample size is calculated. A new, better guess at sample size is obtained, the process is repeated, and a new expected sample size is calculated. These steps continue until the repeated calculations of sample size converge on a particular value of *n*.

An example of such a process is taken from a study of the treatment of flexible flatfoot in children. Before performing the study, the investigators wished to determine the number of subjects required to determine whether three different treatment methods were effective. The experimental design included one control group and three experimental groups (Fig. 16.5). The investigators measured radiographic angles of the foot before and after treatment. Based on their previous experience with radiographic angle measurements on other children, they knew that the SD of radiographic angle within the general pediatric population was approximately 5 degrees. In their clinical judgment, they considered an improvement in the radiographic angle of 5° to be a significant effect of treatment. The null hypothesis in this experiment was that treatment had no effect on the radiographic angle. Type I error would conclude that the treatment had an effect when, in fact, it did not. Type II error would conclude that treatment had no effect when, in fact, it did. The investigators decided to accept a type I error frequency of 5% (a critical *p* value or significance level α of 0.05), and wished to make the power of the statistical test 90% ($p = 0.9$, $\beta = 0.1$).

TABLE 16.4. *Number of observations for* t *test of means between two groups*

β =	α = 0.01					α = 0.05					α = 0.1				
	0.01	0.05	0.1	0.2	0.5	0.01	0.05	0.1	0.2	0.5	0.01	0.05	0.1	0.2	0.5
0.05	—	—	—	—	—	—	—	—	—	—	—	—	—	—	—
0.1	—	—	—	—	—	—	—	—	—	—	—	—	—	—	—
0.15	—	—	—	—	—	—	—	—	—	—	—	—	—	—	122
0.2	—	—	—	—	—	—	—	—	—	99	—	—	—	—	70
0.25	—	—	—	—	110	—	—	—	128	64	—	—	139	101	45
0.3	—	—	—	134	78	—	—	119	90	45	—	122	97	71	32
0.35	—	—	125	99	58	—	109	88	67	34	—	90	72	52	24
0.4	—	115	97	77	45	117	84	68	51	26	101	70	55	10	19
0.5	100	75	63	51	30	76	54	44	34	18	65	45	36	27	13
0.55	83	63	53	42	26	63	45	37	28	15	54	38	30	22	11
0.6	71	53	45	36	22	53	38	32	24	13	46	32	26	19	9
0.65	61	46	39	31	20	46	33	27	21	12	39	28	22	17	8
0.7	53	40	34	28	17	40	29	24	19	10	34	24	19	15	8
0.75	47	36	30	25	16	35	26	21	16	9	30	21	17	13	7
0.8	41	32	27	22	14	31	22	19	15	9	27	19	15	12	6
0.85	37	29	24	20	13	28	21	17	13	8	24	17	14	11	6
0.9	34	26	22	18	12	25	19	16	12	7	21	15	13	10	5
$\frac{\delta}{\sigma}$ = 1	28	22	19	16	10	21	16	13	10	6	18	13	11	8	5
1.1	24	19	16	14	98	18	13	11	9	6	15	11	9	7	—
1.2	21	16	14	12	8	15	12	10	8	5	13	10	8	6	—
1.3	18	15	13	11	8	14	10	9	7	—	11	8	7	6	—
1.4	16	13	12	10	7	12	9	8	7	—	10	8	7	5	—
1.5	15	12	11	9	7	11	8	7	6	—	9	7	6	—	—
1.6	13	11	10	8	6	10	8	7	6	—	8	6	6	—	—
1.7	12	10	9	8	6	9	7	6	5	—	8	6	5	—	—
1.8	12	10	9	8	6	8	7	6	—	—	7	6	—	—	—
1.9	11	9	8	7	6	8	6	6	—	—	7	5	—	—	—
2	10	8	8	7	5	7	6	5	—	—	6	—	—	—	—
2.1	10	8	7	7	—	7	6	—	—	—	6	—	—	—	—
2.2	9	8	7	6	—	7	6	—	—	—	6	—	—	—	—
2.3	9	7	7	6	—	6	5	—	—	—	5	—	—	—	—
2.4	8	7	7	6	—	6	—	—	—	—	—	—	—	—	—
2.5	8	7	6	6	—	6	—	—	—	—	—	—	—	—	—
3	7	6	6	5	—	5	—	—	—	—	—	—	—	—	—
3.5	6	5	5	—	—	—	—	—	—	—	—	—	—	—	—
4	6	—	—	—	—	—	—	—	—	—	—	—	—	—	—

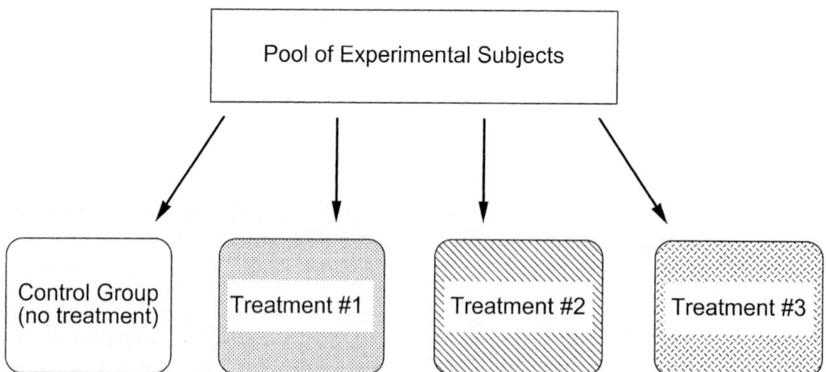

FIGURE 16.5. Schematic diagram of the experimental design used to test three different treatments against no treatment (control) to correct flexible flatfoot in children.

To calculate the required sample size given this problem, we first make a rough guess at sample size, for example, n =10. We then calculate the degrees of freedom, using the following equation:

$$\upsilon = a(n-1) \qquad [7]$$

where

υ = the degrees of freedom
a = the number of groups
n = the number of independent samples per group.

Because we have four groups, the degrees of freedom are $4(10 - 1) = 36$. We obtain from a statistical table (Table 16.3) the t value corresponding to a significance level of 0.05, 36 df, and a significance level of 0.2, 36 df. The corresponding t values are 2.031 and 1.308. We enter these values into Equation 16.6 and solve for n, obtaining n = 22.8 (Fig. 16.6). Based on this calculation, we now refine our guess of sample size to n = 25 and repeat the calculations. Now the degrees of freedom are $4(25 - 1) = 96$. The appropriate t values are 1.990 and 1.292. We recalculate the sample size and n = 27.3. We then repeat the calculations with n = 30 and find that the calculated n = 27.05. Thus, as we refined our guess, the number of samples converged on a particular number. We would probably decide to perform the experiment with at least 30 independent samples per group. This may require actually entering about 35 individuals per group to allow for attrition.

To summarize, in designing this experiment, we specified the type I error rate, or the acceptable probability that we will commit a false positive. We also established the type II error rate by specifying the power. We then computed sample size, given the experimental variability and our desired difference. Having specified both type I and type II errors, interpretation of the data is straightforward. If our p value exceeds 0.05, we conclude that the treatment has no effect. We can be sure that if it is greater than 0.05, it is so, not because we have too few samples, but because the null hypothesis is indeed false. In fact, this latter result was the study outcome. The authors concluded that the four different methods for treating flexible flatfoot (including *no treatment*) were equally effective.

Student's *t* Test

One of the simplest experimental designs involves the comparison of two groups—one that is treated experimentally and one that serves as an untreated control (Fig. 16.1). A characteristic of the experimental group is measured and is compared with the same characteristic of the control group to determine whether the particular treatment has had a significant effect. Consider a case in which the experimental sample represents the quadriceps extension strength from 15 individuals who have received conservative treatment for femoral fracture. At the end of 4 weeks of cast immobilization, quadriceps strengths of the treated individuals are measured and compared with quadriceps strengths of the normal legs of 15 untreated individuals. It is hoped that these individuals would be matched for physical and socioeconomic factors.

Suppose that the average strength of the immobilized leg was 210 ± 15 N $\pm$ m (mean $\pm$ SEM) and the average strength of the control leg were 240 ± 13 N·m. Are these leg strengths significantly different? When there are one or two experimental groups, the traditional statistical analysis involves the use of Student's t test. Note that ANOVA yields exactly the same results and is generally applicable to more than two groups and to designs that are more complex. It is, thus, preferable to learn ANOVA. However, for the sake of completeness, we present an example of the use of the t test.

The null hypothesis for the t test is that

$$H_o: \mu_1 = \mu_2$$

where μ_1 and μ_2 represent the means of the first and second groups, respectively. If the sample sizes are equal, the statistic used to compare the two means is the t-statistic, which is calculated as

$$t = \frac{\overline{X}_1 - \overline{X}_2}{\frac{s}{\sqrt{n}}} = \frac{\overline{X}_1 - \overline{X}_2}{\text{SEM}} \qquad [8]$$

where

$\overline{X}_1$ and $\overline{X}_2$ = the sample means for groups 1 and 2, respectively.

SEM = the average standard error of the mean for the two groups

If the sample sizes are not equal, the equation is only slightly modified and can be found in most statistical texts. Thus, the t-statistic calculates "how many" standard errors two means are apart from one another. Depending on the sample size, critical values of the t-distribution have been compiled (Table 16.3) and can be used to determine whether means are significantly different from one another. In the current example,

$$t = \frac{240 - 210}{14} = 2.14$$

The degrees of freedom for this experimental design is $a(n-1) = 2(14) = 28$, and the critical t value for a significance level of 0.05 is 2.048. Thus, the calculated t value of 2.14 is (barely) statistically significant at the 0.05 level. The two-sample t test is easily modified to treat the one sample case where a particular sample mean is compared with a hypothetical mean value. In this case, the t-statistic is calculated as

$$t = \frac{\overline{X} - \mu}{\text{SEM}} \qquad [9]$$

where

$\overline{X}$ = the sample mean
μ = the hypothetical mean to which the sample mean is compared

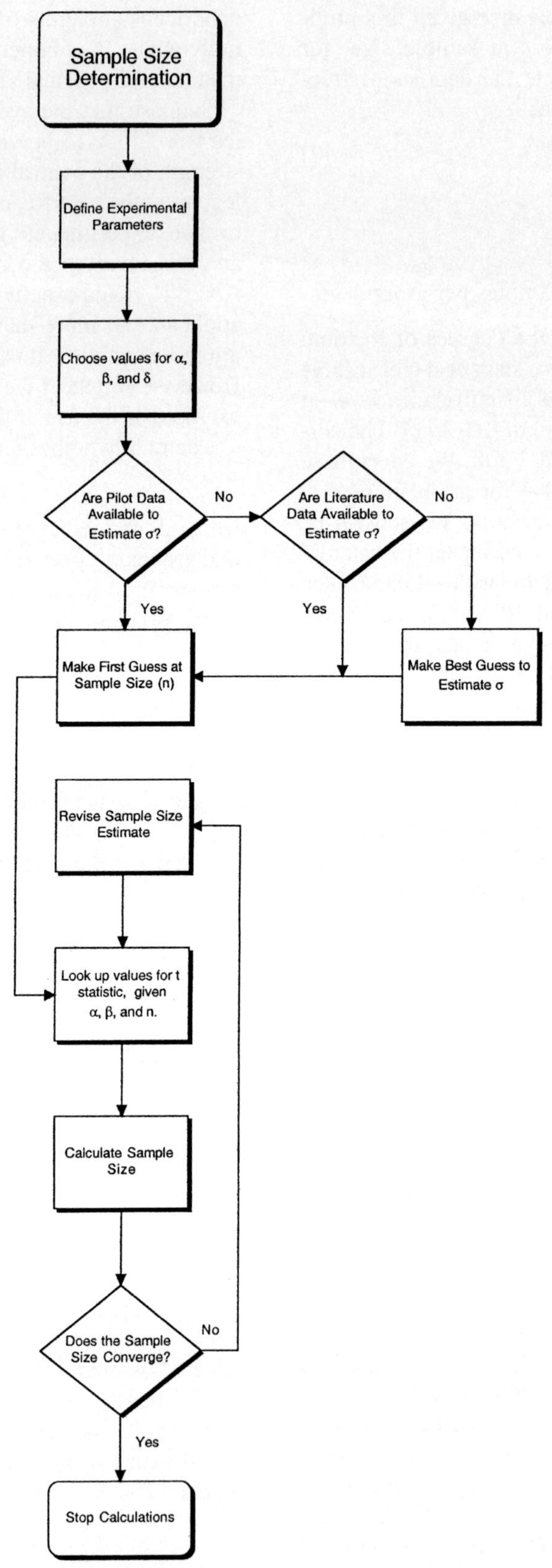

FIGURE 16.6. Logical progression for sample size calculation. Terms contained within symbols are defined in the text.

For the cases in which more than two groups are to be considered, ANOVA is required to properly extract the appropriate information.

Analysis of Variance

The purpose of ANOVA is to determine whether a significant difference exists between two or more sample means. This statistical test is often used in the experimental setting to determine whether an experimental treatment has a significant effect. In practice, this analysis tests the null hypothesis that the means of "a" groups are equal. In other words, the null hypothesis for ANOVA is that

$$H_o: \mu_1 = \mu_2 = \mu_3 = ... = \mu_a$$

where μ_a represents the mean of the ath group and H_o is the abbreviation for the null hypothesis.

When ANOVA involves only two groups, the analysis is mathematically equivalent to Student's t test and as such its description will follow the general ANOVA discussion.

Analysis of Variance Assumptions

ANOVA assumes that the various sample groups are normally distributed and that the variance between groups is equivalent. These assumptions are important because deviations from them can invalidate ANOVA results. As mentioned earlier, not all bell-shaped curves are normally distributed. A population that is normally distributed can be described in terms of its mean μ and its variance σ_2 (Fig. 16.2). The population mean of each group can be estimated by the arithmetic average and each sample variance describes each group's variability.

Analysis of Variance Table

An example is used to explain ANOVA and the ANOVA table. Suppose we are interested in determining whether there is a difference in average muscle fiber area between three quadriceps muscles. In this experiment, we would obtain three groups of data from, for example, the vastus medialis (VM), the vastus lateralis (VL), and the rectus femoris (RF) muscles. This experimental design is similar in concept to the one presented in Figure 16.5 for the flexible flatfoot problem in which the three different groups were the different treatments. These raw data are presented in Table 16.5 and plotted in Figure 16.7 as the mean ± SEM. In this example, we have three groups and six samples per group. The null hypothesis in this experiment is stated as

$$H_o: \mu_{VL} = \mu_{VM} = \mu_{RF}$$

where

μ_{VL} = the mean of the sample obtained from the vastus lateralis muscle

μ_{VM} = the mean of the sample obtained from the vastus medialis muscle

μ_{RF} = the mean of the sample obtained from the rectus femoris muscle

Calculation of the Analysis of Variance Statistics

To determine whether there is a difference in average muscle fiber area between the three muscles using ANOVA, we first calculate the variance *within* each group relative to its average by

$$\sigma_i^2 = \frac{\sum_{i=1}^{n} (Y_i - \overline{Y})^2}{} \qquad [10]$$

which is simply a modified form of the variance equation presented earlier. The variance of the *ith* group in Equation 16.10 is calculated as the difference between an individual observation Y_i and the mean of that $\overline{Y}$ sample. Those differences, which are calculated for each variate, are squared and summed, and the sum of squares (SS) is divided by the sample size in order to calculate variance within that group. (Actually, for mathematical reasons, the SS is divided by $n - 1$ to obtain the within-group variance.) This procedure in which an individual value is subtracted from another and squared is extremely common in statistical equations.

TABLE 16.5. *Fast muscle fiber area from three quadriceps muscles (μm^2)*

Animal ID	Muscle		
	Vastus lateralis	Vastus medialis	Rectus femoris
461	2265	2505	1961
463	2506	2305	2794
464	1918	1396	2077
467	2491	2065	2233
469	1717	1975	2682
472	1809	1905	2122
Mean fiber area	2118	2025	2311
SD	348	380	343
SE	142	155	140

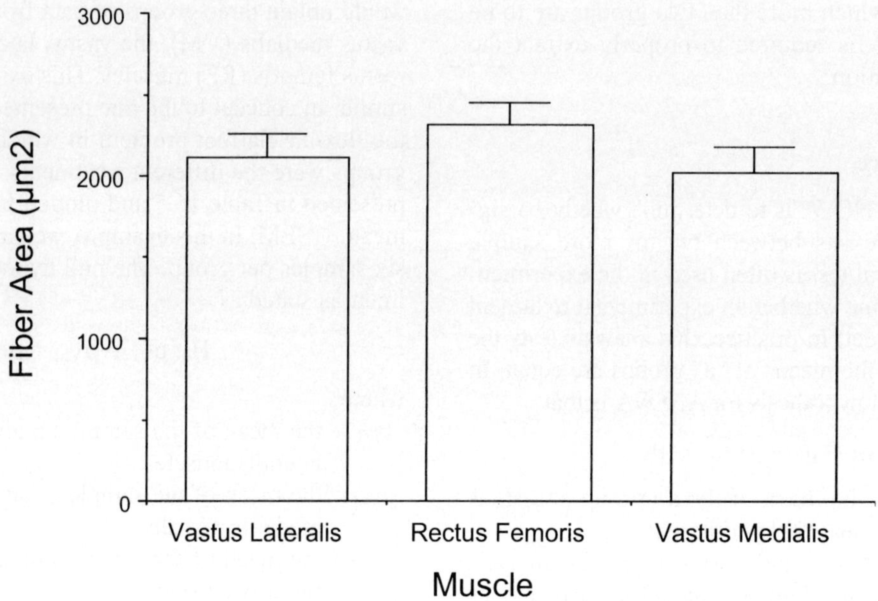

FIGURE 16.7. Bar graph of muscle fiber area from three different quadriceps muscles. Each bar represents the group mean ± SEM. One-way analysis of variance (ANOVA) reveals no significant difference between groups ($p > 0.3$; Table 16.6).

To estimate the overall variance of the entire data set including all three groups, the variances of all the individual groups are averaged. This variance is termed the *mean squared error* (MSE):

$$MSE = \frac{\sum\limits_{j=1}^{a} \left(\dfrac{\sum\limits_{i=1}^{n} (Y_{ij}-\overline{Y}_j)^2}{n-1} \right)}{a} \qquad [11]$$

where
 a = the number of groups
 n = the number of variates per group
 Y_{ij} = the *ith* variate in the *jth* group
 $\overline{Y}_j$ = the mean of the *jth* group

This value can be expressed more simply as:

$$MSE = \frac{1}{a(n-1)} \sum\limits_{j=1}^{a} \sum\limits_{i=1}^{n} (Y_{ij}-\overline{Y}_j)^2 \qquad [12]$$

In this equation, the value obtained from Equation 16.10 for each of the "a" groups has been added and divided by the total number of groups (three in this example).

In addition to the overall or average within group variance, the variance between the three groups can be calculated as shown:

$$MST = \frac{1}{(a-1)} \sum\limits_{j=1}^{a} (\overline{Y}_j - \overline{\overline{Y}})^2 \qquad [13]$$

where

$\overline{Y}_j$ = the mean of the *jth* group
$\overline{\overline{Y}}$ = the average of all of the means (grand mean)

Equation 16.13 again has a SS term, but this term is used to calculate the variability *between* groups because each group mean is compared with the grand mean. These squared differences are added, and the sum is divided by the number of groups minus one. This value is known as the *mean square for treatment* (MST) because this term is related to the magnitude of the treatment effect. Readers should note that the term treatment used here is a statistical term and does not specifically denote a medical treatment.

Equations 16.12 and 16.13 are used to estimate the variability within groups and between groups, respectively. Statisticians have determined that both of these terms are unbiased estimators of the population variance; that is, variability of the population from which these data were obtained.

Significance Level in Analysis of Variance

If data obtained from a sample population represent that population, any observation should be similar to any other. The MSE and MST would be similar, and their ratio would be unity. This is a key point. This ratio of the variability between groups to the variability within groups is defined as a statistic known as the *F* distribution. It is this *F* value that is tested for significance. From the *F* value, a *p* value is obtained using a computer program or statistical tables. (Elucidation of the theory behind the calculation of the *p* level from the *F* value is beyond the scope of this chapter.) In a typical ANOVA

TABLE 16.6. *One-way ANOVA table for control muscle example*

Source of variation	Sum of squares	df	Mean square	F	p
Between	256,228	2	128,114	1.001	0.391
Within	1,920,493	15	128,032	—	—

ANOVA, analysis of variance.

table (Table 16.6), all of the values that have been discussed are reported.

When the *F* value is not one, the ratio of the two mean squares (MSE and MST) reveals information relevant to our understanding of the existing variation in the study (Table 16.7). First, consider the within-group variance. It can be seen from Equation 16.12 that the within-group variance is calculated using the variability of an individual variate within a group relative to its group mean. In other words, this variance represents experimental variability, the variability in obtaining values from a given population. It is hoped that most of this variability results from the nature of the actual variability itself and not from other factors that could have been controlled, such as time of day, humidity, temperature, and so forth. That is why the SS term derived from Equation 16.12 is referred to as the *SSE*, which is the error associated with making repeated measurements from a particular population. This variability should be as small as possible. Each experimental group has its own SSE, and these are averaged to yield the MSE. ANOVA assumes that the variability of each of the groups is approximately equivalent. If it is not, other statistical tests that do not rely on equality of variance between groups are used. The MSE term does not depend on the absolute value of the mean for a particular group. For example, group 1 could have a mean value of approximately 1, group 2 could have a mean value of approximately 100, and group 3 could have a mean value of approximately 1,000. If the error variability of each group is the same, their individual SSE terms will be similar. The MSE term, thus, is not sensitive to the absolute mean value of the individual groups.

However, this is clearly not the case for the MST term. The MST represents the average between-group variability of the individual sample means around the grand mean. Thus, the MST term is very sensitive to differences between absolute mean values. In the previous hypothetical example, where the grand mean of the sample is the

average of 1, 100, and 1,000, which is 367, the MST term would be large.

At this point, the reader should realize that as the differences between group means becomes large, given the same experimental variability in each group, the MST becomes large; whereas, the MSE remains relatively unchanged. This is the manner in which ANOVA detects differences between group means by testing variances and, therefore, why it is termed *analysis of variance*. When the *F* value is close to unity, there is generally not a significant difference between group means. However, as the group means become significantly different, the *F* value increases dramatically because of the increased MST term. There is, thus, a high level of probability or statistical significance that the groups are different (low *p* value).

ANOVA, as described here, in which the variates are grouped by a single classification (from which type of muscle the sample was obtained, VL, VM, or RF) is known as *single classification* or one-way ANOVA. It is important to clarify that one-way ANOVA refers only to the way in which the data are classified, not to the number of parameters or groups to be analyzed. Thus, the current example is of a one-way ANOVA on fiber area between muscles, but it is also possible to perform a one-way ANOVA on such things as capillary density, fiber type percentage, area fraction of connective tissue, and so forth, simply using one-way ANOVA repeatedly for the analysis of each parameter.

With this strategy, any problem can be approached using essentially the same procedure modified for the experiment at hand.

Two-Way Analysis of Variance

As an extension of our previous example, consider the case in which each variate is classified based on two factors. This experiment, shown schematically in Figure 16.8, is undertaken to determine whether there is a sig-

TABLE 16.7. *Symbolic one-way ANOVA table*

Source of variation	Sum of squares	df	Mean square	F ratio
Between	SST	$\upsilon_1 = a-1$	MST = SST/υ_1	$F_{\upsilon1, \upsilon2}$ = MST/MSE
Within	SSE	$\upsilon_2 = a(n-1)$	MSE = SSE/υ_2	—

ANOVA, analysis of variance; SST, sum of squares for treatment; MST, mean square for treatment; SSE, sum of squares for error; MSE, mean squared error.

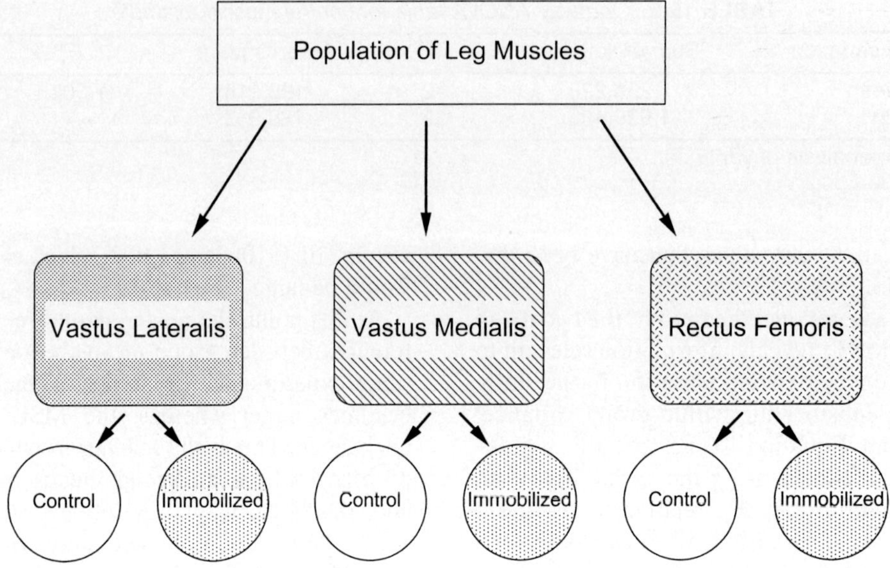

FIGURE 16.8. Schematic representation of the two-way analysis of variance (ANOVA) experimental design. Note that each variate is classified by two factors: The muscle from which it was obtained and the leg (immobilized or control) it came from.

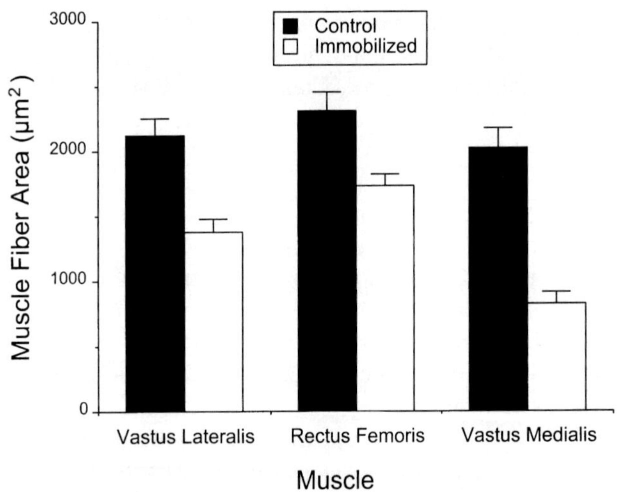

FIGURE 16.9. Graphic representation of mean ± SEM of fiber area (μm^2) from three different muscles (VL, VM, RF) and two types of leg (control and immobilized). This 2×3 two-way analysis of variance (ANOVA) design is shown schematically in Figure 16.8. Data are from Table 16.8.

nificant difference in fiber area among the three different muscles in immobilized and nonimmobilized legs (Figure 16.9). Whereas, in the previous example each variate was classified based only on the muscle from which it came (single classification), each variate is now classified by its muscle and whether or not the muscle was immobilized (two classifications). This is an example of a two-way ANOVA design (Table 16.8). Data are collected from each of three different types of muscle when each of these muscles is in a state of immobilization or mobilization; that is, six different combinations of the two factors need to be observed. In tabular form, data for six "cells" need to be obtained. Calculations involved in two-way ANOVA are analogous to those for one-way ANOVA. We have an MSE term, which is calculated for each group (now six) in the two-way ANOVA and, instead of a single MST term, we have two MST terms. One MST term refers to the variance between legs (immobilized versus nonimmobilized), and the other refers to the variance between muscles (VM vs VL vs RF).

TABLE 16.8. *Fast muscle fiber area from control and immobolized muscles (μm^2)*

	Muscle					
	Vastus lateralis		Vastus medialis		Rectus femoris	
Animal ID	Control	Immobilized	Control	Immobilized	Control	Immobilized
474	2,265	1,755	2,505	1,000	1,961	1,780
476	2,506	1,302	2,305	450	2,794	1,599
479	1,918	998	1,396	943	2,077	2,100
481	2,491	1,442	2,065	800	2,233	1,632
483	1,717	1,364	1,975	851	2,682	1,450
488	1,809	1,421	1,905	921	2,122	1,821

TABLE 16.9. *Two-way ANOVA table for immobilization example*

Source of variation	Sum of squares	df	Mean square	F ratio	p
Type	6331094.7	1	6331094.7	71.2	0.0001
Muscle	2126327.2	2	1063163.6	11.9	0.0002
Type*muscle	616367.1	2	308183.5	3.466	0.0442
Within	2667405.8	30	88913.5	—	—

ANOVA, analysis of variance.

The data that led to this analysis, expanded from our previous experiment, appear in Table 16.8. Note that instead of three cells or groups of data, we now have six. These six cells result from two factors (muscle and state of mobilization) and three levels for each factor (three different muscles). In experimental design, this commonly is described as a 3×2 level ANOVA design. (If six muscles and three states of mobilization for each muscle were to be examined, this would be considered a 6×3 level two-way ANOVA design).

For this analysis, we establish two null hypotheses (one for each classification):

$$H_1: \mu_{VL} = \mu_{VM} = \mu_{RF}, \text{ and}$$

$$H_2: \mu_{immobilized} = \mu_{controls}$$

In this example, it is possible that immobilization will have a different effect on fiber area, depending on which muscle is examined. To understand this effect, in addition to the two main null hypotheses above, there is a *very important* interaction term that also will be calculated. This will be described later.

In the two-way ANOVA, only one error term (MSE) is determined, but six groups will be used to calculate it. However, there are now two separate treatment effects: type and muscle. The equations describing these two treatment effects are completely analogous to the MST for a one-way ANOVA. The equations are:

$$MST_{Type} = \frac{1}{(b-1)} \sum_{k=1}^{b} (\overline{Y}_k - \overline{\overline{Y}})^2 \qquad [14]$$

where
$\overline{Y}_k$ = the mean of the *kth* type
b = the number of types
$\overline{\overline{Y}}$ = the grand mean

Similarly, the equation for the other MST is shown here:

$$MST_{Muscle} = \frac{1}{(c-1)} \sum_{j=1}^{c} (\overline{Y}_j - \overline{\overline{Y}})^2 \qquad [15]$$

where
$\overline{Y}_j$ = the mean of the jth muscle
c = the number of muscles
$\overline{\overline{Y}}$ = the grand mean

The two-way ANOVA table looks very much like the one-way table, except that it has a few more rows (Table 16.9).

Because two MST terms exist, two F values are needed to test for the significance of a Type effect and a Muscle effect. These values are calculated as follows:

$$F_{Type} = \frac{MST_{Type}}{MSE} \qquad [16]$$

$$F_{Muscle} = \frac{MST_{Muscle}}{MSE} \qquad [17]$$

so that, symbolically, the two-way ANOVA table (excluding the interaction row) looks like that shown in Table 16.10.

The Meaning of Statistical Interaction

In the current example, the data presented in Table 16.9 indicate there is a significant effect of immobilization, a significant effect of muscle, and a significant "interaction" term. This indicates that the effect of immobilization on fiber area depends on which muscle is examined, or, stated in statistical terms, the immobilization effect *interacts* with the muscle effect.

The interaction term demonstrates that each grouping factor or classification, whether it is the state of immobilization or which muscle is tested, is not independent of the other. From Figure 16.9 it can be seen that the VM shows a dramatic decrease in fiber area on immobilization, whereas the RF shows less decrease. Stated another

TABLE 16.10. *Symbolic two-way ANOVA table*

Source of variation	Sum of squares	df	Mean squares	F ratio
Between types	SST_Types	υ_T	$MST_T = SST/\upsilon_T$	$F_{\upsilon_T, \upsilon_E} = MST_T/MSE$
Between muscles	SST_Muscles	υ_M	$MST_M = SST/\upsilon_T$	$F_{\upsilon_T, \upsilon_E} = MST_M/MSE$
Within	SSE	υ_E	$MSE = SSE/\upsilon_E$	—

ANOVA, analysis of variance; SST, sum of squares for treatment; MST, mean square for treatment; MSE, mean squared error; SSE, sum of squares for error.

TABLE 16.11. *Symbolic two-way ANOVA table with interaction*

Source of variation	Sum of squares	df	Mean squares	F ratio
Between types	SST_{Types}	$\upsilon_T = b-1$	$MST_T = SST/\upsilon_T$	$F_{\upsilon T, \upsilon E} = MST_T/MSE$
Between muscles	$SST_{Muscles}$	$\upsilon_M = c-1$	$MST_M = SST/\upsilon_T$	MST_M/MSE
Type*muscles	SST_{MXT}	$\upsilon_{MXT} = (b-1)(c-1)$	$MST_{MXT} = \upsilon_{MXT}$	$F_{\upsilon MXT, \upsilon E} = MST_{MXT}/MSE$
Interaction within	SSE	υ_E	$MSE = SSE/\upsilon_E$	—

ANOVA, analysis of variance; SST, sum of squares for treatment; MST, mean square for treatment; MSE, mean squared error; SSE, sum of squares for error.

way, this study has demonstrated a muscle-dependent effect of immobilization.

The mean squared term for interaction represents the departure of the subgroup means from the values expected on the basis of additive combinations of data from the two grouping factors. This term is calculated from Equation 16.18 or 16.19.

The value $MST_{All\ Groups}$ represents the average MST for all six groups regardless of whether they are muscle groups or type groups. In this way, the interaction term increases as level-specific changes within a factor occur. The interaction mean squared term can be represented as

$$MST_{M \times T} = \{MST_{All\ Groups}\} - \{MST_{Muscle} + MST_{Type}\} \quad [18]$$

$$MST_{M \times T} = \left\{ \frac{1}{(a-1)(b-1)} \sum_{j=1}^{ab} (\overline{Y_j} - \overline{\overline{Y}})^2 \right\} - \quad [19]$$
$$\left\{ \frac{1}{(a-1)} \sum_{k=1}^{a} (\overline{Y_k} - \overline{\overline{Y}})^2 + \frac{1}{(b-1)} \sum_{m=1}^{b} (\overline{Y_m} - \overline{\overline{Y}})^2 \right\}$$

The complete symbolic two-way ANOVA table is shown in Table 16.11.

Multiple Comparisons of Subgroups

While it is important to determine the significance of main effects and interaction terms, sometimes comparisons between specific cells within the analysis are of interest. For example, in the previous two-way ANOVA example, it is possible to say that there is a significant effect of immobilization and a significant interaction term. However, the investigator may wish to determine whether there is a significant difference between the control and immobilized leg for each muscle, that is, to determine whether there is a significant immobilization effect on a muscle-by-muscle basis. It is important to understand that although such paired comparisons are made using the Student's *t* test, the number of comparisons and the specific comparisons to be made must be determined in the initial planning stages of the experiment. In the current example, the investigators wished to determine whether a significant immobilization effect was present for each muscle, and, therefore, were interested in paired comparisons between each muscle; that is, control versus immobilized leg. In addition, the inves-

tigators were interested in determining whether fiber areas between the immobilized legs were significantly different, but not in whether the control legs differed significantly. It is not possible to extract the same information from two one-way ANOVAs as from one two-way ANOVA, nor is it valid. In other words, it is not appropriate to analyze the experimental data that were presented earlier as two one-way ANOVAs. Results obtained from the one-way ANOVAs would lead to the erroneous conclusion that there was no significant difference between muscles and no significant effect of immobilization. The results would be misleading because the differences between muscles would have been averaged out across the immobilized and control legs. The interaction effect, which was a crucial aspect of this analysis, would have been impossible to extract from two parallel one-way ANOVAs.

The analysis thus involved six paired comparisons: control versus immobilized for each of the three muscles, and VM versus VL, VM versus RF, and VL versus RF for the three immobilized muscles. In such a situation, it is also not appropriate to simply perform six separate Student's *t* tests because as the number of *t* tests increases, so does the probability of obtaining a significant difference only because of chance. In other words, a correction must be made for performing this number of comparisons. One of the simplest methods for making this correction is to perform the Bonferroni approximation for multiple paired comparisons. To achieve an overall experimental significance level of 0.05, the critical *p* value for any individual test must be adjusted based on the number of comparisons as follows:

$$\text{New critical } p \text{ value} = \frac{\text{Experimental } p \text{ value}}{\text{Number of comparisons}} \quad [20]$$

In the current example, in which there are six paired comparisons, the experimental *p* value of 0.05 is divided by six to achieve a new critical *p* value of 0.0083. Then each individual *p* value obtained by Student's *t* test is compared with 0.0083 to determine whether there is a significant difference between groups at the desired 0.05 level.

To satisfy the mathematical assumption of random sampling, the specific comparisons to be made in multiple paired comparisons must be chosen based on the experimental design, not on viewing of the data. For example, it would have been inappropriate, after looking at the data (Fig. 16.9), to test whether there was a significant difference between the VM control leg and the VL immobilized leg using a Student's *t* test, although it appears from the figure that such a difference exists. However, if after performing the experiment and viewing the data, the investigators determined that this comparison was of interest, the paired comparison could be made using the Bonferroni approximation. However, it would be necessary to adjust the critical *p* value of 0.05 by the total number of possible paired comparisons in that entire data set. With six groups of data, the total number of possible paired comparisons is 15, which would make the critical *p* value 0.0033. In other words, it would be difficult to demonstrate a significant difference between these groups, but this is the price to be paid for making unplanned or a posteriori comparisons.

Potential Errors Using Analysis of Variance

As stated earlier, ANOVA assumes that the groups are independent, that they are normally distributed, and that their variances are similar. Any departure from these assumptions will affect the validity of the results. Specific statistical tests are available to test these assumptions in a given experiment. The concept of group independence is subtle and, in many situations, may be difficult to appreciate. The requirement of independence can be stated as "the knowledge of a value from one group should not allow us to predict a value from another group." One common example of when groupings are related occurs when values obtained are separated only by time. These should not be considered independent. Suppose that we measure a person's weight before and after a diet program. Generally, extremely heavy people will still be heavy following a diet program, even after losing weight. The groups before and after, separated only by time, are not independent but, instead, have a high degree of covariance. This analysis requires a separate type of ANOVA design, known as a repeated measures design, in which the different groups are expected to have some degree of covariance and the covariance is adjusted for in the analysis itself.

Another common mistake made using ANOVA is to use the significant ANOVA p values to make statements about individual groups. In the example earlier, there was a significant difference between control and immobilized legs, no significant difference between muscles, and a significant interaction term. Based on the null hypothesis, it is obvious that if any single leg were different from its control leg, there would be a significant difference between control and immobilized legs. To simply state, therefore, that immobilization causes muscle atrophy for all legs would be incorrect. The ANOVA must be followed with multiple paired comparisons in order to make specific statements about each leg or muscle.

Another more subtle problem associated with ANOVA arises when the within group variance (MSE) is artificially decreased. As can be appreciated from the *F* ratio, any factor that tends to decrease the MSE artificially will inflate the *F* value and produce significant results. This occurs most commonly when an n for a particular group is artificially high. Generally, this problem occurs when an investigator uses an n value that does not actually represent the number of independent samples obtained from a population, but rather represents the number of measurements that were made, which are not necessarily independent (for example, multiple weighing of a single sample). Repeated or replicate measurements from exactly the same sample only estimate the reproducibility of the measurement technique. Thus, repeated measurements of tumor mass obtained from the same subject simply serve to establish the mass of that tumor more accurately. No matter how many times that mass is measured, the mass of that particular tumor counts as n = 1 in the final tally because the population that we intend to generalize to is the mass of all tumors obtained from subjects. The total number of subjects in the sample must equal the sample size.

In summary, ANOVA is used to detect differences between group means. The mathematical procedure used relies on the fact that it is possible to obtain several estimates of the population variance. ANOVA tests only the null hypothesis that the group means are equal, and it generally is followed up by a multiple comparison that corrects for the number of paired comparisons made. The strength of ANOVA is in using it to design experiments in which the main and secondary effects will have great scientific meaning. These interaction terms can provide great insights into biologic and clinical phenomena but would be extremely difficult to obtain using a simple one-at-a-time experimental approach. Designs that incorporate multiple factors, as well as the investigation of interaction terms, should be encouraged.

The discussion of ANOVA has shown that ANOVA determines whether an effect is significant by creating an *F* ratio—a ratio of two variances. The steps generally used to test the significance of an effect are (a) define the variances of interest, (b) define the comparisons to be made, (c) calculate the appropriate *F* statistics, and (d) test the *F* values for significance levels.

The next sections will refine our understanding of ANOVA by describing several common variations on the theme presented earlier.

Fractional Factorial Designs

The discussion of ANOVA demonstrated the power of examining main effects and interactions to determine the relative contribution of each to the observed effect. However, when there is an interest in knowing the effect of many factors, our traditional, full-factorial ANOVA may become extremely cumbersome.

For example, suppose an investigator were interested in determining the optimal screw design for bone fixation, and 10 supposedly different factors of each screw needed to be considered, such as screw pitch, screw diameter, and so on. Performing this experiment using a full factor factorial model; that is, a 10-way ANOVA, would involve a lot of effort (Table 16.12). In fact, if only two different levels (values per factor) are used, multiple experiments would have to be performed, testing each value against every other value of every other factor. This would mean 1,024 experiments would have to be performed to obtain a single data point. Many investigations involve not two levels, but at least three or four levels per factor. For four levels, this could increase the number of experiments per data point to 4,096. Moreover, for a ten-factor design with two levels, to insure that an accurate mean value is obtained if five replications of each experiment are required 5 × 1,024 or 5,120 experiments would have to be performed. There must be a better way. Fractional factorial designs are that way.

Fractional factorial designs are based on the "sparsity of effects" principle, which states that any time there are more than about four factors, the system is probably driven by the main effects and a few of the low order interactions.

In ANOVA, replication generates the MSE term, which represents experimental error. In a full factorial experiment of k factors or groups and two levels per factor with n replicates per group, there are $_n2^k$ experiments required. How many are actually needed? In the 10-way ANOVA example, 5,120 experiments is overkill. In general, statisticians have shown that only about 30 to 35 experiments are really needed for a good estimate of MSE.

The downside of our decision to perform fewer experiments is our inability to calculate higher-order interaction terms. The sparsity of effects principle suggests that because such high-order interaction terms are likely to be unimportant, it is not necessary to go to all of the trouble to perform a full factorial 2^k experiment. Thus, when it is desirable to perform a smaller number of experiments, a different statistical methodology is needed to evaluate the results. This methodology is called fractional factorial analysis.

The key to the fractional factorial experiment is to perform enough experiments to generate a reliable MSE term and to eliminate unnecessary replication, which only serves to generate high-order interaction terms. While it is beyond the scope of this chapter to describe this methodology, awareness of it and an understanding of when it is useful are important to all readers of this text.

Nested Analysis of Variance Designs

Statistical methods of fractional factorial design can be used when a full factorial ANOVA would require such a large number of experiments that it would be impractical or too costly or time consuming to perform. In other cases, a full factorial ANOVA is not sufficient to describe the complexity of the phenomena or to fully extract all of the information from it regardless of how many experiments are performed. The nested ANOVA, sometimes referred to as a hierarchical ANOVA, is the statistical method to address this issue. In essence, it allows one or more factors to be subordinate to another factor.

In the full factorial model, the treatment effects (factors) may be either fixed (that is, defined by the investigator, as in the case of three specific surgical procedures) or random (that is, treatments chosen as interesting but not fully under the investigator's control, as in the case of three geographic locations in which blood pressure values are studied). An example of a full factorial ANOVA with two factors would be an experiment in which the investigators were interested in the effects of drug A and drug B on the blood pressure of males and females. The two factors are drug and sex. Each factor has two levels (drug A and B for the factor drug and male and female for the factor sex). This is thus commonly referred two as a 2 × 2 factorial design and is represented in Table 16.13.

Another example of a full factorial ANOVA would be the measurement of respiratory rate of both sexes of three species of rats at three temperatures. Each factor is a fixed effect with two levels of the factor sex and three levels each of species and temperature as shown in Table 16.14. This design is a 2 × 3 × 3 full factorial three-way ANOVA. The model is referred to as full factorial, because each level of each factor exists in combination with each level of every other factor. Statisticians would say that the model is "fully crossed." Also, low tempera-

TABLE 16.12. *Number of experiments required for n = 1 of a full factorial design*

No. of factors (k)	Levels per factor	No. of experiments (2^k)
2	2	4
3	2	8
4	2	16
5	2	32
6	2	64
7	2	128
8	2	256
9	2	512
10	2	1,024

TABLE 16.13. *Factorial design (2 × 2)*

	Factor 1 (sex)	
	Male	Female
Factor 2 (drug)	Drug A	Drug A
	Drug B	Drug B

TABLE 16.14. *Three-way ANOVA ($2 \times 3 \times 3$)*

Species no.	Male			Female		
1	Low temp	Medium temp	High temp	Low temp	Medium temp	High temp
2	Low temp	Medium temp	High temp	Low temp	Medium temp	High temp
3	Low temp	Medium temp	High temp	Low temp	Medium temp	High temp

ANOVA, analysis of variance; temp, temperature.

ture in one cell has exactly the same meaning as low temperature in any other cell. Finally, measurements in one cell of the ANOVA are independent of measurements in another cell. For example, if the investigator knows something about species 2 at low temperature, he or she does not necessarily know anything about species 3 at low temperature. These points may seem subtle now, but will be contrasted with the following example of nested ANOVA design.

Consider the experiment in which the investigator is interested in determining the effect of immobilization on muscle fiber area in three different muscles. The muscles themselves differ with respect to fiber orientation and fiber type distribution (that is, percentage of fast and slow muscle fibers). Muscle fiber area is measured twice from each of four different blocks of tissue from each muscle. In this experiment (Table 16.15), the dependent variable is fiber area, and the factors are muscle (three levels) and block (four levels).

In this case, measurement 2 from block 2 of the tibialis anterior will not have anywhere near the same meaning as measurement 2 from block 2 of the plantaris. Block 2 of the tibialis anterior does not have exactly the same meaning as block 2 of the plantaris because the anatomy of the two muscles is different. It, therefore, would not be appropriate to analyze these data as a full factorial two-way ANOVA (effect of immobilization or mobilization) because the meaning of a particular cell, in this instance, measurement 2 from block 2, needs to be expressed in terms of the hierarchical factors from which is it obtained. If the proper statistical technique is to be used to analyze these data, the physician must realize the relative importance or weight to be given to each factor and provide this information to the statistician. Statisticians cannot be expected to understand the subtleties of different medical factors. To illustrate the nested ANOVA and the importance of choosing the correct statistical methodology, data from this experiment will be statistically analyzed in three different ways.

In our first (incorrect) analysis of these fiber area data, each of the pairs of measurements is treated as a separate "treatment" and the data analyzed as a one-way full factorial ANOVA between 12 groups (Table 16.16). Each of the two measurements, from each of the four blocks from each of the three muscles, is considered from a separate group ($2 \times 2 \times 2$). When this analysis is performed, a highly significant difference between cells is found. The F ratio, which is MST/MSE, is calculated as 216.9/1.3. This suggests there is no statistical difference between immobilization and mobilization using these four sections in these three muscles as representative of the animals' muscles. However, the MSE of 1.3 is only a result of repeated measurement of areas from a given section, but the large MST is a result of several factors such as intermuscular differences and interblock differences. Underestimating the MSE term will lead to artificial inflation of the F values, resulting in a very low and untrue significance level. This is another way in which a type I error can be made—by choosing an incorrect analysis method for the experimental design. The current problem is that all of the effects (muscles, blocks, and repeat measurements) have been lumped together, which makes one very large effect that cannot be sorted out. For proper experimental analysis, the MST needs to be broken down into its components.

Now the analysis is rearranged (again incorrectly) by simply pooling all of the blocks and repeated measurements for a given muscle and comparing each of these pooled data from the three different muscles using a one-way ANOVA (Table 16.17). There is still a significant difference between muscles, but it is less than with the previous example. The within group variability measured is now increased. The MSE now is 82.6 whereas it was only 1.3 in the first example. The MSE term now includes all

TABLE 16.15. *Nested ANOVA example*

Block no.	Tibialis anterior		Gastrocnemius		Plantaris	
1	Measure 1	Measure 2	Measure 1	Measure 2	Measure 1	Measure 2
2	Measure 1	Measure 2	Measure 1	Measure 2	Measure 1	Measure 2
3	Measure 1	Measure 2	Measure 1	Measure 2	Measure 1	Measure 2
4	Measure 1	Measure 2	Measure 1	Measure 2	Measure 1	Measure 2

ANOVA, analysis of variance.

TABLE 16.16. *Sample ANOVA table obtained by incorrectly analyzing the nested problem as a one-way ANOVA with 12 independent groups*

Source	df	Sum of squares	Mean square	F	p
Cell No.	11	2386.353	216.941	166.664	0.0001[a]
Residual	12	15.620	1.302	—	—

ANOVA, analysis of variance.
[a]Highly significant difference between "cells."

TABLE 16.17. *Sample ANOVA table obtained by incorrectly analyzing the nested problem as a one-way ANOVA with three independent groups*

Source	df	Sum of squares	Mean square	F	p
Muscle	2	665.676	332.838	4.026	0.0331[a]
Residual	21	1736.298	82.681	—	—

ANOVA, analysis of variance.
[a]Significant effect of muscle, even when combining blocks.

TABLE 16.18. *Sample ANOVA table obtained by incorrectly analyzing the nested problem as a two-way ANOVA with two grouping factors*

Source	df	Sum of squares	Mean square	F	p
Muscle	2	665.676	332.838	2.56E2	0.0001[a]
Block	3	260.203	86.734	66.633	0.0001[a]
Muscle*block	6	1460.474	243.412	1.87E2	0.0001[a]
Residual	12	15.620	1.302	—	—

NOTE: Dependent, fiber area.
ANOVA, analysis of variance.
[a]Highly significant effects of muscle, block, and significant interaction.

TABLE 16.19. *ANOVA table obtained by correctly analyzing the repeated measures problem*

Source	df	Sum of squares	Mean square	F	p	Error term
Muscle	2	665.676	332.838	1.741	0.2295[a]	Block (muscle)
Block (muscle)	9	1720.677	191.186	146.878	0.0001	Residual
Residual	12	15.620	1.302	—	—	—

NOTE: Dependent, fiber area.
ANOVA, analysis of variance.
[a]Differences between muscles were not significant. Note that the description of the error term has been included for didactic reasons.

within group variability, which means that the MSE term has some between-block and between-section information within it. This leads to further breakdown of the model into its components.

The next (incorrect) approach to the phenomena could be to analyze the data as a two-way factorial ANOVA using blocks and muscles as the main factors (Table 16.18). The problem with this analysis is twofold. First, the F value for muscles can be calculated as the between-muscle variability divided by the MSE (332.8/1.3). This calculation is incorrect because the MSE term represents the error or variability associated with repeated measurements of different sections within a block. To know if there is a muscle effect, the between-muscle effect must be expressed relative to the next level of organization, which is the different blocks.

Finally, the data are analyzed correctly using a two-way nested ANOVA, and then the results are interpreted (Table 16.19). Note that the data, when analyzed correctly, actually show that there is no significant effect of muscle, but a highly significant block effect. In other words, it is not which muscle that is important, but the block from which the sample is taken. Between-block variability is actually the important factor in this experiment, not the particular muscle. This result may indicate, for example, that there is much more heterogeneity observed along a muscle in the proximal-distal direction than between different muscles. The experiment could thus be refined to ensure that the major source of variability in the data (between blocks) was accounted for in any experimental protocol. In this nested ANOVA, the F value for muscle is 1.74, which is the MST for muscle divided by the block (muscle) effect (read as blocks within muscles), or 332.8/191.2.

Use of the nested ANOVA has resulted in determination of the major sources of error in our experiment. The relative portion of each source of error can be quantified directly from the SS terms (MST and MSE) in Table 16.19. The total data variability is represented by the sum of all the SS terms, which, for our experiment, is:

Total variability	=	between muscle variability	+	between block variability	+	residual error

or

2,400	=	666	+	1,721	+	16

The relative contribution of each source to the total variability is thus: muscles, 27% (666/2,400); blocks, 72% (1,721/2,400); and repeated measurements, 1% (16/2,400). Thus, it makes no sense to spend the extra time and effort to make the repeated measurements when they are a minuscule part of the total variability. Conversely, the investigator may want to take several different blocks to try to understand the very large between-block variation.

This type of approach can be applied to any experimental system in which sample "aliquots" are nested. This is an excellent initial screening method for determining the major sources of experimental error in a system that is subdivided such as in this example. It is prudent not to waste time and energy "oversampling" at the levels with very low experimental variability. Thus, by understanding the need for use of a nested ANOVA here, not only is a proper understanding of where the variability lies acknowledged, but the number of experiments is reduced if all the factors are considered. Alternatively, it can allow a fractional factorial analysis to be considered, thereby eliminating repeated measures as one of the factors.

The incorrect analyses performed here illustrate an extremely important point in data analysis, which has been made even more important with the advent of microcomputer programs that make statistical analysis easy. Mathematically, the computer does not care about the numbers and will generate p values for just about any design that is input. In our examples, it was incorrect simply to provide block and muscle as individual factors that were assumed to be crossed. It is necessary to indicate to the computer program that blocks are nested within muscles and repeat measures nested within blocks.

The initial incorrect conclusion, that there were significant muscle effects, was obtained when the data were analyzed using the incorrect one-way ANOVA model in which each cell was considered a treatment. The incorrect conclusion was a result of testing the hypothesis that all group means were equal. This incorrect significant difference between muscles was determined because several of the cells were from different blocks, and difference between blocks really was the major source of variability.

Repeated Measures Analysis of Variance

The nested ANOVA model presented earlier is based on the premise that measurements are believed to be needed and are thought to be related because large heterogeneities or variabilities are thought to be present within a factor. Conversely, measurements are sometimes related just because they come from the same subject. For example, suppose we measured body mass of subjects before a diet program, and at 5 and 10 weeks after the diet program, which involved three different diet foods. There are two factors: type of diet food (three levels) and time (three levels). It would not be appropriate to treat the three levels of time as independent and perform a 3×3 factorial, two-way ANOVA because the weights of the same subjects were measured before and during the diet treatment. To make this a full factorial design, we would use three random samples of individuals obtained at different times. We would measure one group's mass before the diet, one group's mass at 5 weeks after the diet, and one group's mass at 10 weeks. This design satisfies the requirement

TABLE 16.20. *Repeated measures ANOVA example*

Food type	Timing of measurement (wk)		
Diet no. 1	0	5	10
Diet no. 2	0	5	10
Diet no. 3	0	5	10

ANOVA, analysis of variance.

for the full factorial design because the groups are independent-knowledge about the 5-week group on diet no. 1 would not carry over to the 10-week group on diet no. 1 because the subjects would be different. However, this design would be undesirable because it adds unnecessary variability to the data in that each person weighed at each interval has no relationship to the person weighed at a different time interval. The repeated measures ANOVA design is a way to minimize extraneous variability while providing an internal control for the experimental treatment. As with the nested ANOVA, the data to be obtained must be properly defined and the proper statistical methodology used to obtain meaningful results.

A typical repeated measures ANOVA data set might be set up as in Table 16.20 and the resulting ANOVA table might look like the one shown in Table 16.21. There is no significant effect of diet ($p > 0.1$), but there is a significant effect of the timing of the measurement ($p < 0.001$). Thus, all subjects probably improved, independent of the particular diet. Also note a significant timing × diet interaction term that represents a differential time-dependent effect of diet on weight loss. This term indicates that the time course of weight loss is different between the different diets.

Table 16.22 shows what the results might have looked like if this problem had been analyzed incorrectly as a two-way ANOVA. This situation leads to the conclusion that food type has a significant effect because the F value for food type is created using the MSE instead of the more appropriate MSE which includes variability between the subjects themselves. In this case, this type of incorrect analysis results in a type I error.

The lesson of these presentations of ANOVA models is that the ANOVA technique is a powerful one that can extract important information from a particular experiment. However, it is equally true that a computer does not care which type of model the investigator chooses and cannot distinguish between correct and incorrect deci-sions based on the experimental data alone. The investigator must choose the correct model based on his or her expertise, and the person reading the report of the research must evaluate the conclusions based on the analysis of the data. This exposure to various models should provide at least an appreciation for the nature of the problem, and should encourage the investigator to approach a biostatistician for technical advice. There are numerous ANOVA models available for use, and the reader is referred to several of the excellent experimental design texts listed in the "Selected Bibliography" for further information.

REGRESSION ANALYSIS

Another statistical test that is used in many experimental designs is regression analysis. The regression method is applied to a data set consisting of a group of independent variables that are measured exactly and a group of dependent variables. The analysis, known as the "least-squares" procedure, determines the equation that best fits the data and determines the relationship between the independent and dependent variables. This procedure can be performed selecting an exponential, logarithmic, polynomial, or any other equation to describe the relationship mathematically. In the interest of simplicity, we will illustrate regression analysis using linear regression; that is, best fit of the data to a straight line. The concepts learned using linear regression are applicable to other regression equations.

The most common reason for using linear regression is to test whether a relationship (not necessarily one of cause and effect) exists between two variables. This procedure may be as simple as determining the relationship between force and voltage output in the calibration of a force transducer or as complex as determining the relationship between drug dosage and a particular physiologic response in creating a dose-response curve. Once established, a functional relationship can be statistically analyzed.

In linear equation analysis, any data set can be fit to a line. Solving for the best-fit line is easily done on any type of data no matter how they appear, because the procedure simply consists of mathematical operations applied to a given data set. The pertinent questions to ask after performing linear regression are whether the data

TABLE 16.21. *ANOVA table (obtained from repeated measures problem illustrated in Table 16.20)*

Source	df	Sum of squares	Mean square	F	p
Diet	2	26.751	13.376	2.154	0.1370
Subject (group)	25	155.225	6.209	—	—
Time	2	19.121	9.560	8.874	0.0005
Time*diet	4	18.171	4.543	4.216	0.0051
Time*subject (group)	50	53.869	1.077	—	—

NOTE: Dependent variable measured is weight loss.

TABLE 16.22. *ANOVA table obtained by incorrectly analyzing the repeated measures problem as a two-way ANOVA with two grouping factors*

Source	df	Sum of squares	Mean square	F	p
Food type	2	26.751	13.376	4.798	0.0109
Measure time	2	19.121	9.560	3.429	0.0376
Food type*measure time	4	18.171	4.543	1.629	0.1757
Residual	75	209.095	2.788	—	—

NOTE: Dependent variable measured is weight loss.
ANOVA, analysis of variance.

provide a good fit to the line, and whether the relationship between the two variables is significant.

The first question, dealing with goodness of fit, is answered by inspection of the correlation coefficient r; the second question, dealing with significance, is answered using the p value. All of the concepts that will be used to discuss the r and p values follow directly from the previous discussion of ANOVA. Keep in mind that both the p and r values should be reported by a linear regression program. Beware of obtaining one value without the other using pocket calculators and the like.

Statistical Significance

The method for calculating the p value for a regression model is a simple modification of the methods learned in the one-way ANOVA: defining SS terms and calculating variance ratios. In the case of linear regression, the SS terms are the familiar variances within and between groups, here called the unexplained SS and the new explained SS. The schematic diagram in Figure 16.10 illustrates the source of these terms.

Following calculation of these terms, significance testing occurs in a manner similar to a one-way ANOVA in which the F value is the ratio of the two mean squares mentioned earlier. The data can be organized to look like an ANOVA table containing two mean squares, an F value, and a p value. The difference here relates only to what we call the terms. The MSE term used in ANOVA, here called the unexplained error, is simply the SS of the distances between the predicted data and actual observed points, or

$$\text{Unexplained variation} = \sum_{i=1}^{n}(y_i - \hat{y}_i)^2 \qquad [21]$$

where

Y_i = predicted value of y, given a particular value of X_i.

As the predicted line approaches the data points, this term becomes small. The reason that these points deviate from the line is not known and, thus, this is termed unexplained variability.

The second mean squared term, which in ANOVA analysis was called mean square treatment MST, is here called the explained source of variability. It is the difference between the predicted values y_i and the group mean:

$$\text{Explained variation} = \sum_{i=1}^{n}(\bar{y} - \hat{y}_i)^2 \qquad [22]$$

The F value is calculated as the ratio of the explained/unexplained mean squared terms. Thus, the total variation is partitioned into explained and unexplained terms rather than MSE and MST as in ANOVA. The statistical significance level is then obtained using a table or computer program, and these values are expressed as a p value.

Goodness of fit

In addition to tests of significance, linear regression calculates a goodness of fit statistic called the coefficient of determination r^2. The coefficient of determination is the fraction of the total variation that our model, which in this case is a linear model, explains. In other words,

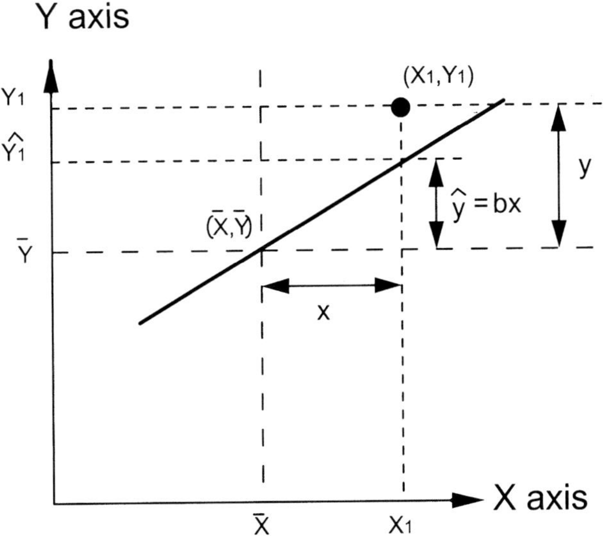

FIGURE 16.10. Graphic representation of the source of the sums of squares terms used in linear regression. *(X,Y)* represents the mean of all of the data, (X_1,Y_1) represents a typical data point, and *y* represents the predicted values for *y* given *x*.

$$r^2 = \frac{\sum_{i=1}^{n}(\bar{y} - \hat{y}_i)^2}{\sum_{i=1}^{n}(y_i - \bar{y})^2} = \frac{\text{Explained variation}}{\text{Total variation}} \qquad [23]$$

The total variation about the mean can be represented as:

$$\text{total variation} = \sum_{i=1}^{n} (y_i - \overline{y})^2 \qquad [24]$$

which can be partitioned as:

$$\sum_{i=1}^{n} (y_i - \overline{y})^2 = \sum_{i=1}^{n} (\overline{y} - \hat{y}_i)^2 + \sum_{i=1}^{n} (y_i - \hat{y}_i)^2 \qquad [25]$$

or

$$\text{Total variation} = \text{explained variation} + \text{unexplained variation}$$

Thus, the closer r^2 is to 1, the better is the fit of the data to the model; the relationship is represented as a line or a mathematical equation. If the fit is good, a quantitative relationship exists, which enables powerful statements to be made regarding the percentage of total experimental variability explained by a particular model. This percentage concept is equally valid for multiple regression (in which multiple independent parameters are used) as it is for simple regression.

Often the goodness of fit is expressed as a correlation coefficient rather than as the coefficient of determination. The correlation coefficient, r is simply defined as

$$r = \sqrt{r^2} \qquad [26]$$

where

$r > 0$ if the slope of the line is positive
$r < 0$ if the slope of the line is negative.

A correlation coefficient of -1 is a perfect fit to a negatively sloped line and a correlation coefficient of $+1$ is a perfect fit to a positively sloped line.

Linear Regression Example

As an example of the application of linear regression to experimental data, consider the data presented in Table 16.23, which were obtained from several different dogs.

TABLE 16.23. *Dog mass versus dorsiflexion torque (n = 15)*

Dog mass (kg)	Left leg torque (Nm)	Right leg torque (Nm)
9.2	2.38	2.51
14.1	3.50	3.61
13.9	2.25	2.41
14.0	2.71	2.81
21.1	2.50	2.70
23.1	3.11	3.45
23.1	2.75	2.95
23.0	2.50	2.84
24.0	3.51	3.71
28.0	4.55	5.15
28.1	3.22	3.55
30.0	4.53	4.74
31.1	3.66	3.84
32.1	3.78	3.98
33.1	4.00	4.11

In this particular experiment, the investigators wanted to know whether there was a significant relationship between dog mass and dorsiflexion torque so that they would be able to predict torque simply based on dog mass. For each dog, maximum dorsiflexion torque was measured (in N · m) from each leg along with dog mass (in kilograms). These data were entered into a computer, and the graph shown in Figure 16.11 was obtained. Note that there is a fair amount of scatter to the data. The best-fit equation and other relevant statistics from regression analysis were:

$$Y \ (\text{N•m}) = 0.072 \ (\text{N•m/kg}) \bullet \text{mass (kg)} + 1.605 \ (\text{N•m})$$
$$(p < 0.005, \ r^2 = 0.486) \qquad [27]$$

and the corresponding ANOVA table is shown in Table 16.24.

The table obtained from the regression analysis is completely analogous to the table we saw in the one-way ANOVA example. The coefficient of determination of these

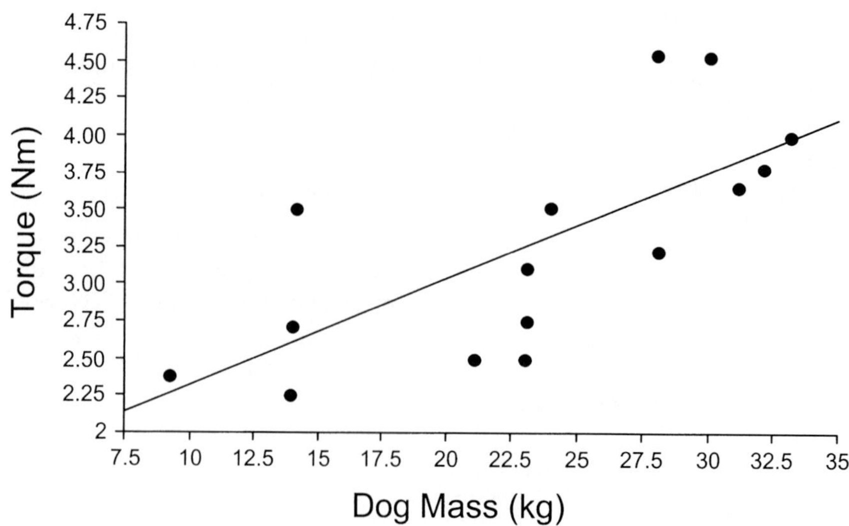

FIGURE 16.11. Scatter graph of the data in Table 16.17 along with linear regression best-fit line.

TABLE 16.24. *ANOVA table of torque (Nm) versus dog mass (kg)*

	df	Sum of squares	Mean square	F	p
Explained	1	4.030	4.030	13.496	0.0028
Unexplained	13	3.882	0.299[a]	—	—
Total	14	7.911	—	—	—

ANOVA, analysis of variance.
[a]Low unexplained error relative to explained error, yielding a high F value.

data, as calculated from Equation 16.25, is $3.882/7.991 = 0.49$. Thus, although the regression relationship is highly significant ($p < 0.005$), the linear relationship only explains 49% of the experimental variability. As a result, its use as a predictor of leg torque would be questionable.

Potential Problems with Regression Analyses

Although regression provides a powerful tool for data analysis, it is possible to be fooled by the statistics or to overstate the implications of the analysis. Such errors come from an incomplete understanding of the meaning of the p value and correlation coefficients. These potential problems are discussed briefly later, and a graph is shown that illustrates the problem.

Extrapolating Beyond the Independent Value for the Data Set

Clearly, the predictive value of curve-fitted data applies only to the range of independent values for which the original relationship was derived (Fig. 16.12, top left).

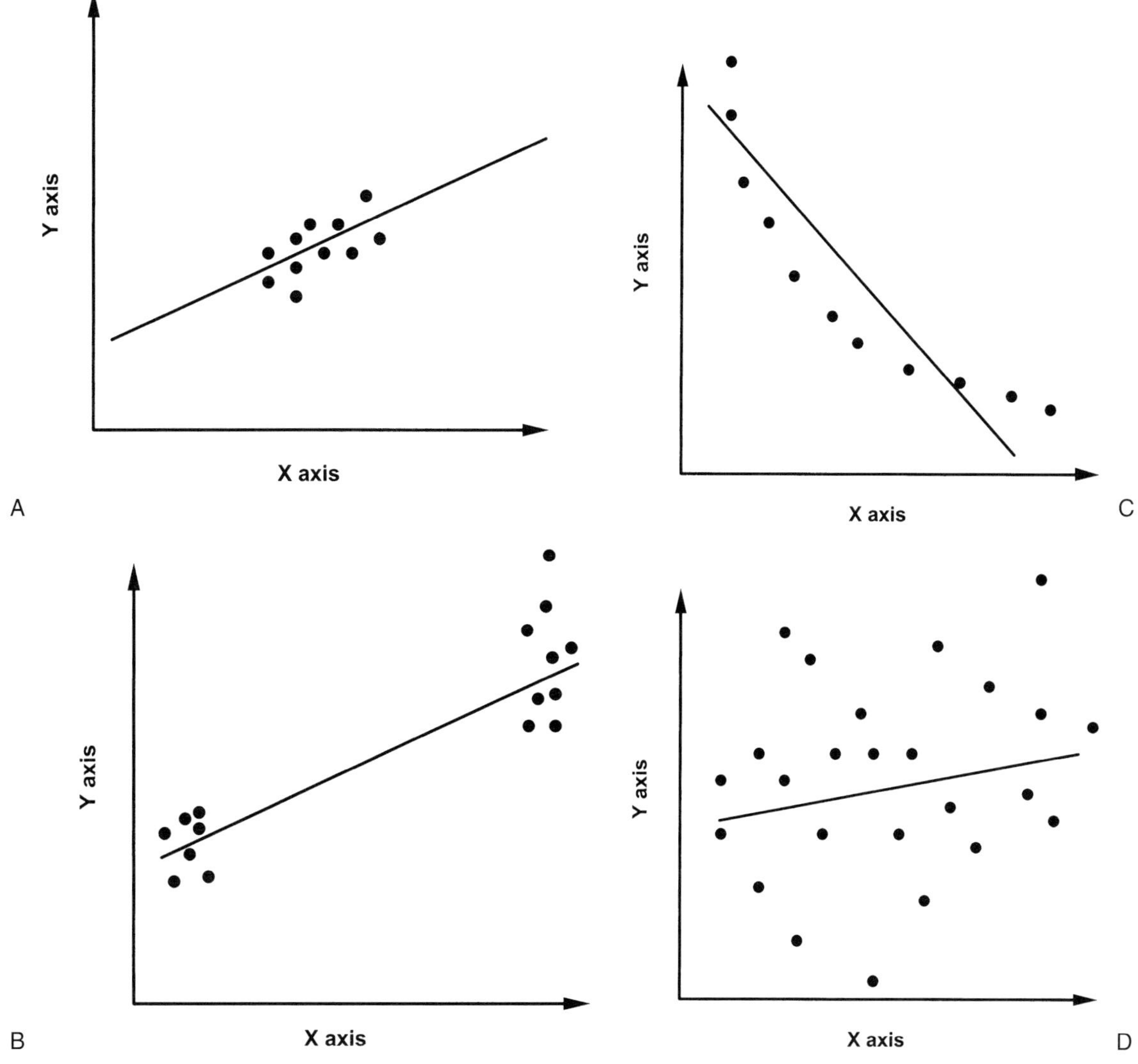

FIGURE 16.12. Schematic examples of errors that can be made using linear regression. **A:** Extrapolating beyond the range for which independent data values are available. **B:** Interpolating between two clusters of data to a region where no independent data are available. **C:** Missing a secondary trend superimposed on the linear trend. **D:** Using a regression equation when the p value is not significant.

Many complex functions, exponential and logarithmic, for example, are highly linear over restricted ranges. Extrapolation beyond the range for which data are available assumes incorrectly that the relationship between the two variables is invariant for all possible values of the independent variable.

Interpolating Into a Region That Contains No Data

Similar to the argument presented earlier, sometimes data are obtained that cluster into two regions (Fig. 16.12, top right). An excellent mathematical fit can be obtained to two clusters of data gathered at different values for the independent variable, in spite of the fact that no information is available for the intermediate values. Again, it is incorrect to assume a relationship for which no data are available; it is better to make two groups of data and use ANOVA.

Missing a Secondary Trend Superimposed Onto a Linear Trend in Linear Regression

Very good linear fits are possible for data that are not changing in a strictly linear fashion. In Figure 16.12 (bottom left), the linear fit is excellent although the overall behavior of the phenomenon has been missed. This mistake can be avoided by inspecting the residuals of the data that are obtained following analysis. Residuals are the individual errors for all of the data points. That is, the residual for a given data point is the unexplained error for that data point. If the linear fit is equally good across the entire data set, the residuals should appear as a sort of random cloud of data points. However, if an underlying trend has been missed, there will be a good deal of form to the residual plot.

Neglecting p Values and Implementing an Insignificant Equation

Any data set can be fit to a straight or curved line. Thus, if the p value is high, suggesting no significant relationship between the independent and dependent variables, there is no sense in using the regression equation for any purpose (Fig. 16.12, bottom right). The analysis should stop at this point. Often, a regression equation is used in the absence of knowledge of the p value, and inappropriate calculations are made using an irrelevant equation.

Neglecting r^2 and Overemphasizing a Significant p Value

The other extreme of misinterpretation is to rely only on the significant p value in deciding to implement a regression equation (Fig. 16.12, top right). As was seen in the dog leg example above, a highly significant linear relationship can still have an extremely small correlation coefficient and, thus, have no useful prognostic value.

ANOVA Versus Regression

The previous example has demonstrated a great deal of analytical and conceptual similarity between ANOVA and regression. In many cases, it is difficult to decide which type of analysis is more appropriate. When the data are gathered across a continual range, regression makes more sense than ANOVA because it would be difficult to define distinct independent variables, factors, or treatment groups for the ANOVA. However, if the data are gathered either at discrete intervals (for example, age) or in fairly well-defined subgroups (for example, old and young), the ANOVA model is more applicable. This type of question is more easily answered in the context of a specific experiment. It is this type of question that can be addressed by local statisticians, provided they are made aware of the inherent characteristics of the variables (factor, treatment groups).

ANALYSIS OF COVARIANCE

Introduction to Covariates

In contrast to ANOVA, analysis of covariance (ANCOVA) is used when the value of the dependent variable is affected by additional information related to the independent variable. In this case, the dependent variable is corrected for fluctuations in the independent variable, known as the covariate, before the analysis is performed. ANCOVA is thus similar to ANOVA in that it is used to test for equality among group means. In terms of calculations, ANCOVA actually represents the combination of ANOVA and linear regression.

ANCOVA often is used when it is not possible or practical to keep all things constant between groups. For example, in comparing muscle strength between two different groups of patients, patients of different weights might necessarily have been used. Because strength (dependent variable) is highly dependent on patient weight (independent variable), there will be scatter in the data solely as a result of variability in patient weight and unrelated to the actual diet treatments. This scatter will increase the MSE term, making it difficult to obtain statistically significant results. Therefore, ANCOVA is used to correct muscle strength for patient weight and then perform the statistical comparison. Although, at first, ANCOVA appears to be a panacea for decreasing sample variability, we must remember that ANCOVA is useful only when a detailed measure of the covariate property is available. This requires not only predicting the need for a covariate but also choosing the correct covariate, in this case patient weight. Such decisions typically should be made during pilot experiments.

As an example of the use of the ANCOVA model, suppose we were interested in comparing the pullout strength

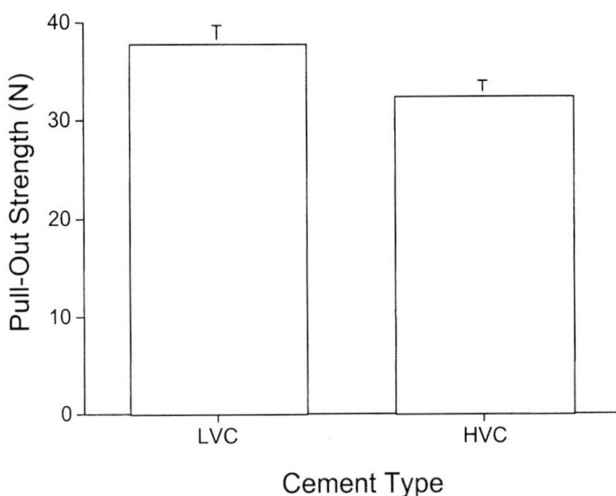

FIGURE 16.13. Bar graph of pull-out strength ± SEM of prostheses that were embedded in cadaveric femurs using high-viscosity cement (HVC) and low-viscosity cement (LVC).

of prostheses inserted into cadaveric specimens using two different bone cements—one with high-viscosity (HVC) and one with low-viscosity (LVC). Human cadaveric specimens are highly variable in their mechanical properties; therefore, we might predict that a covariate will be useful with regard to bone cement. Suppose the biomechanical experiments were performed and the data were obtained as shown in Figure 16.13.

Because there are two groups of data that are classified based on one factor (cement type), it is possible to compare pullout strength using a one-way ANOVA design (mathematically equivalent to an unpaired t test). When this analysis is performed (Table 16.25), no significant difference is found between groups ($p > 0.6$).

Note that almost all of the variability is unexplained (98% to be exact, calculated as residual error divided by total variability, 2,902/2,974). However, much of the residual error term variability is simply variability between specimens, which can be accounted for by using ANCOVA.

It is possible that the lack of significant difference between the LVC and HVC cements is being masked by variability resulting from some other factor, which must be measurable. This is particularly suited to ANCOVA. To perform the ANCOVA, an independent variable (the covariate) must be measured, which estimates something relevant about the specimen. In the present case, we might suspect that some of the variability between specimens may simply be a result of the quality of the tubercular bone. Thus, the bone density of the various specimens is measured independently, and the analysis is rerun using bone density as the covariate.

Analysis of Covariance Calculation Method

The first step in ANCOVA is to perform a linear regression on the pullout strength of each cement versus bone density to determine the precise relationship, if any, between the dependent and independent variables. All pullout strengths then are adjusted for bone quality based on the regression relationship. This is mathematically analogous to creating bones of similar bone density before the actual statistical test in order to decrease within-group variability. Finally, the two adjusted group means are tested for equality in a manner similar to ANOVA.

There is a very strong relationship between bone density and pullout strength for both types of cement (Fig. 16.14). Thus, bone density is a useful covariate in this experiment. In ANCOVA, it is important that the slopes of the two regression lines are not significantly different. In effect, then, the ANCOVA tests for differences between y-intercepts. The mean values for the HVC and LVC groups (arrows) are relatively close, but are smeared out because of variation in bone density (Fig. 16.14). Finally, and most importantly, the ANCOVA table (Table 16.26) shows a significant effect of cement type now that the variability due to bone density is accounted for as a covariate.

A comparison between Tables 16.25 and 16.26 reveals the basis for the initial inability to detect differences between cements. The MSE variability (residual) in Table 16.25 is 2,902; whereas, in Table 16.26, it is only 86. Where did it go? Note that the SS due to bone density is 2,815. Thus, of the initial 2,902 residual error, 2,815/2,902 or 97% simply was caused by variations in bone density. This can be seen in Figure 16.14 in which the change in pullout strength is large with respect to bone density, but relatively small due to cement type. Thus, while the effect of cement type is significant, it is of smaller magnitude than the bone density effect. If it were not for the existence of the ANCOVA method, the information would have been lost completely (Fig. 16.15).

TABLE 16.25. *ANOVA table from cement example analyzed without a covariate*

Source	df	Sum of squares	Mean square	F	p
Cement type	1	72.361	72.361	0.199	0.6670[a]
Residual	8	2902.384	362.798	—	—

NOTE: Dependent variable pull-out strength.
ANOVA, analysis of variance.
[a]No significant effect of cement type.

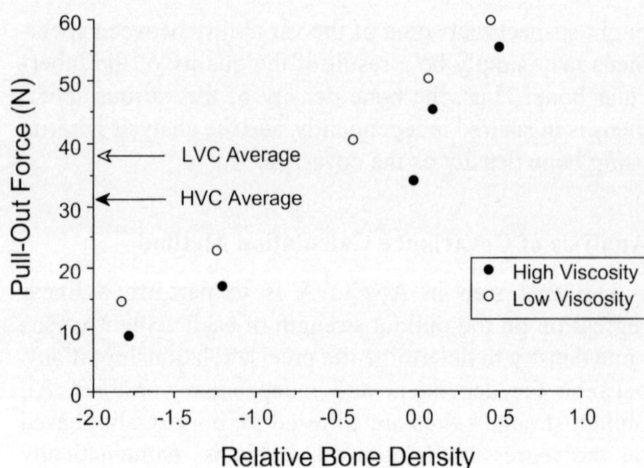

FIGURE 16.14. Scatter graph of pullout strength of prostheses that were embedded in cadaveric femurs using high-viscosity cement (HVC) and low-viscosity cement (LVC) as a function of bone quality (the covariate). Note the average value for HVC and LVC are rather close compared with the scatter in the data caused by altered bone quality.

Generalization of the Analysis of Covariance Model

The simple ANCOVA example described here can be extended to multiple covariates and multiple grouping factors. In fact, the basis for the general linear model (GLM) approach to ANOVA or regression, which now we see are essentially the same thing, simply requires that the experimenter choose, for a given dependent variable, any design that includes grouping variable(s), dependent variable, and independent variable(s), if any.

Judicious choice of experimental design can often demonstrate a significant effect that would otherwise be masked by unrelated variability, as seen in the above example, and can also demonstrate no significant effect of a grouping factor that is confounded by another, uncontrolled variable. Again, the importance of a clinical study of the data used in statistical analyses cannot be overemphasized.

Frequency Analysis

Sometimes there is interest in evaluating an effect that cannot be, or is not, measured using traditional, continu-ous variables. A continuous variable is one that can be measured to vary over a continuous range. For example, length, height, and weight are all continuous variables because they take on a continuous range of values. However, sometimes we are unable to measure continuous variables in an experiment and instead "measure" a discrete categorical variable that can only take on certain values (for example, surgical outcome of good, fair, or excellent; presence or absence of a disease state). In these examples, it would be inappropriate to apply ANOVA simply by assigning numbers to different portions of the scale. The assigned numbers would be completely arbitrary because the numbers in and of themselves have a distinct mathematical meaning or value different from what we arbitrarily assign to them, and this must be considered when it comes to using them for calculations. Use of such numbers in regression or ANOVA models is inappropriate. For example, an investigator might judge tissue healing on a rating scale and judge the tissues from 0 (the worst) to 5 (the best). It would be just as easy to make the scale from 0 to 100, but this would have different meaning using the various parametric statistics described earlier. Thus, for the case in which categorical or qualitative data are to be analyzed, traditional parametric statistics, such as ANOVA and regression analysis, are not appropriate.

Frequency tables are used to express qualitative and categorical data, and frequency analysis is used to test specific hypotheses regarding the data contained in these tables. Frequency tables can be one-way, two-way, or multiway, analogous to classification schemes in ANOVA.

Chi-Square (X^2) Test for Proportions

Sometimes we wish to compare a set of observed frequencies to an expected proportion. The classic examples come from genetics in which, for example, frequencies of two colors of flowers are compared with the expected proportions, 0.75 and 0.25, which represent dominant and recessive traits, respectively. A clinical example might be envisioned in which we wish to test patient choice regarding three different knee braces. The braces might differ with respect to size, shape, or color, but we

TABLE 16.26. *ANOVA table from cement example analyzed using bone density as a covariate*

Source	df	Sum of squares	Mean square	F	p
Cement type	1	109.595	109.595	7.671	0.0324[a]
Bone density	1	2815.795	2815.795	197.101	0.0001
Cement type	1	0.791	0.791	0.055	0.8218
Residual	6	85.716[b]	14.286	—	—

ANOVA, analysis of variance.
[a]Note the significant effect of cement now that bone density is included as covariate.
[b]Note the low residual (unexplained) error after including the bone density covariate.

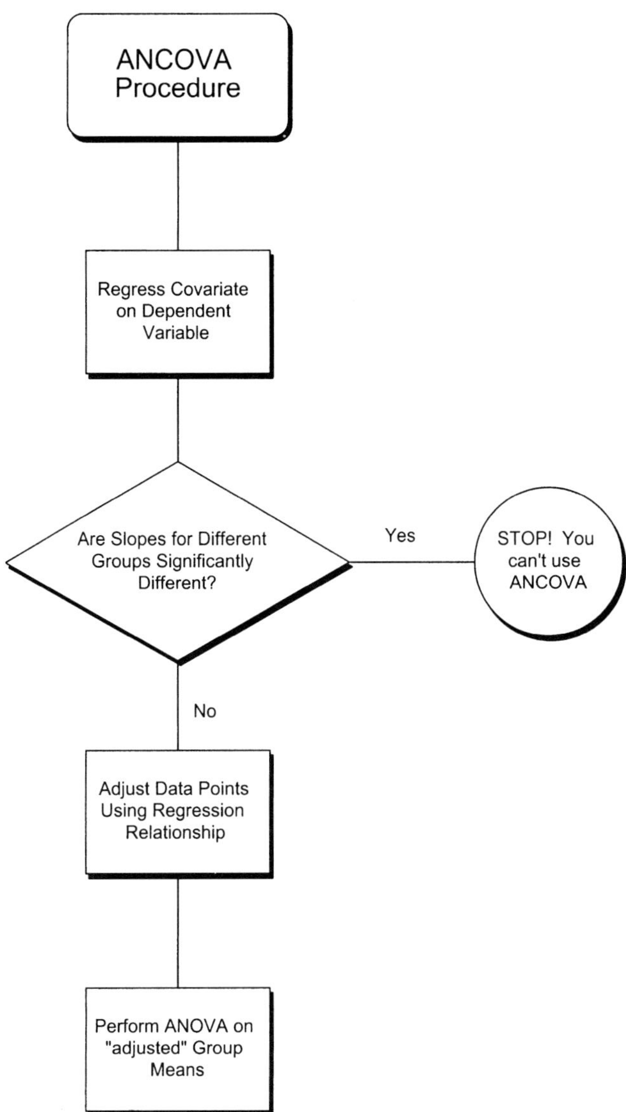

FIGURE 16.15. The flow of events included in the analysis of covariance (ANCOVA) procedure. Note that if group slopes are significantly different, the procedure cannot be applied.

are interested merely in knowing if one choice dominates over the other two. Suppose we asked 270 patients to state their choice regarding knee braces and obtained the data shown in Table 16.27. Note that 108 patients chose brace 2 over the other two. Does this indicate that patients choose brace 2 significantly more often? To answer this question, we use the method of X^2 analysis. As with other statistics we have seen, the X^2 statistic is used to measure

TABLE 16.27. *Observed and expected counts for knee brace preference*

Frequency	Brace no. 1	Brace no. 2	Brace no. 3
Observed	69	108	93
Expected	90	90	90

how far a particular distribution deviates from a theoretical distribution. It is calculated according to the equation

$$X^2 = \sum_{i=1}^{a} \frac{(f_i - \hat{f}_i)^2}{\hat{f}_i} \qquad [28]$$

where
f_i = the observed frequency of the *"ith"* group
$\hat{f}_i$ = the expected frequency of the *ith* group
a = the number of groups

Because we think each brace has an equal likelihood of being chosen, the expected frequency of observation for each of the braces, given 270 patients is 270/3 = 90. The X^2 statistic is calculated as

$$X^2 = \frac{(69 - 90)^2}{90} + \frac{(108 - 90)^2}{90} + \frac{(93 - 90)^2}{90}$$
$$= 4.9 + 3.6 + 0.1$$
$$= 8.6 \qquad [29]$$

Statisticians have compiled tables of calculated critical values for the X^2 distribution for various sample sizes and numbers of experimental groups. We look up in such a table that, for an experiment with a = 3 groups (that is, 2 *df*), the critical X^2 value corresponding to p less than 0.05 is 5.991. Because our value of 8.6 is much greater than 5.991, we reject the null hypothesis that our observed frequency equals our expected frequency (in fact, 8.6 exceeds the critical X^2 value corresponding to p less than 0.025). Note that in Equation 16.28, it makes sense that, the larger the value for X^2, the more probable it is that a significant difference exists between observed and expected frequencies. This is because the numerator of the statistic is calculated directly from the difference between observed and expected frequencies.

Single Classification Frequency Analysis

The general problem of numeric analysis of frequencies also can be illustrated using a basic science study in which a nerve was cut, repaired, and then allowed to grow back into a specific muscle and innervate individual muscle fibers. Before the transection, it was demonstrated that a normal muscle contained 50% fast and 50% slow fibers as judged using a histochemical reaction on tissue slices. Six months after nerve repair, 450 muscle fibers were examined on tissue sections; 290 turned out to be fast fibers and 160 were slow fibers.

The investigator wanted to know if the muscle fibers that were reinnervated were reinnervated randomly, or if there was some type of preferential innervation of either fast or slow muscle fibers. In effect, the investigator would state the null hypothesis that the proportion of fiber type after reinnervation would be the same as the proportion before surgical transection.

If muscle fibers, which initially were present in a 1:1 ratio, were randomly innervated, a 1:1 ratio of fiber types would also be expected after reinnervation. The actual

TABLE 16.28. *Expected and observed fiber type values*

Fiber type	Observed frequency	Observed proportion	Expected frequency	Expected proportion
Fast	290	0.64	225	0.5
Slow	160	0.36	225	0.5

ratio, however, was 290:160 = 1.81:1. Is this significantly different from what could happen if random reinnervation occurred? To answer this question, we apply simple ideas from probability theory to the specific numbers obtained from this experiment. First, we summarize both the data expected if reinnvervation were random and the observed data. The expected proportions for the fiber types were: fast = 0.50 and slow = 0.50. However, the observed proportions were fast = 290/450 = 0.64 and slow = 160/450 = 0.36. Using the terminology of frequency analysis, the expected frequency of fast fibers was E(fast) = 0.50 × 450 = 225 and the expected frequency of slow fibers was E(slow) = 0.50 × 450 = 225. The data are summarized in Table 16.28.

Calculation of the Likelihood Ratio

To use probability theory for determining the likelihood of the observed finding, we compare it to the expected finding. If the two results are very different, we may conclude that the observed frequency was not expected. If the two are similar, we may conclude that the observed result is expected and our hypothesis is true. Thus, probability theory is used here to test a null hypothesis. In this case, the investigator is testing the null hypothesis that E(fast) = E(slow) = 0.5, making use of the expected proportion. An investigator, who had previous knowledge regarding probabilities in another muscle where the normal muscle might contain 75% fast and 25% slow fibers, would choose another value.

To test this hypothesis, the investigator first calculates the probability of observing a 290:160 frequency given a probability of occurrence of 0.5. According to probability theory, the probability of observing x occurrences out of n trials given an expected success rate of p is given by the expression

$$E(x; n, p) = C(n, x)\, p^x\, (1 - p)^{n - x} \qquad [30]$$

where

$C(n,x)$ = the number of possible combinations from a sample of n taken x at a time

p^x = the probability of achieving x successes

$(1 - p)^{n - x}$ = the probability of achieving n − x failures.

This is a reasonable expression because, in order for the observed outcome to have occurred, we must first know the probability of 290 successes (that is, fast fibers innervated) and the probability of 160 failures (that is, slow fibers innervated) both occurring. This is represented by the expression $(1 - p)^{n - x}\, p^x$ because the probability of multiple events occurring is simply the product of their individual probabilities. Finally, this successful event can occur in $C(n,x)$ different ways. Therefore, the event probability is multiplied by the total number of different ways by which it can occur to arrive at Equation 16.30. In this example, the probability of obtaining the actual results when $p = 0.64$ is 0.1229, whereas the probability of obtaining the actual results when $p = 0.50$ is 0.01838.

Therefore, there is a greater probability that the observed frequencies would result if the odds of innervating a fast fiber were 0.64 than if the odds of innervating a fast fiber were 0.5. It follows that the greater the ratio between the observed and expected probabilities, the more likely it is that the observed data did not come from the hypothetical (expected) population. This is analogous to our ANOVA statistic F, in which the MST was compared with the MSE. The greater the ratio, the greater the probability of significant differences.

In frequency analysis, a statistical test based on such a ratio is called the likelihood ratio test. In this example, the likelihood ratio is L = 0.1229/0.01838 or 6.683, and it can be shown that this result is not quite significant ($p > 0.1$).

This example represents a single classification or one-way frequency analysis problem. Frequency analysis classifications can be based on one or multiple factors. In fact, a significant set of tools is available to analyze two-way frequency analysis problems.

Two-way Frequency Analysis

As a second example of a frequency analysis problem, suppose an investigator were interested in determining the best method for repair of a meniscus following a bucket-handle tear. Ideally, a continuous variable that characterizes the state of the meniscus (for example, meniscal compression or shear strength) should be measured. However, many times, the evaluation of the success of a procedure is more often based on intuitive or subjective interpretation of repair quality, such as a subjective rating of meniscal healing based on histologic evaluation of excised menisci from experimental animals. In the former case, ANOVA would suit the problem well, whereas in the latter case, frequency analysis must be used.

As an example, we can analyze the data from an experiment in which two types of surgical repairs were performed on a canine right medial meniscus. In one group of experimental animals, a core of tissue was removed to

TABLE 16.29. *Frequency analysis example (2 × 2)*

Method	Weightbearing	
	Yes	No
Flap	21	29
Core	11	39

promote vascular ingrowth from the meniscal periphery; in the other group, a section of synovial flap was sutured to the defect to promote vascular ingrowth. The measure of the success of the procedures was based on whether or not the animals were weightbearing after a certain time interval, whereupon it was assumed that the menisci of the weightbearing animals had been successfully repaired. If the repair method had no influence in whether or not the animal was bearing weight, the conclusion would be that the repair methods were not significantly different; that is, the repair method and weightbearing results were independent. However, if the surgical repair method influenced whether or not the animal was weightbearing, this result might indicate that one procedure was more effective than another. The data from this type of experiment could be scored and arranged as data shown in Table 16.29. Based on the numbers provided and analytical methods such as those mentioned earlier for one-way frequency analysis problems, the p value obtained was 0.24, which leads us to the conclusion that the surgical repair methods are equivalent in efficacy, at least as far as the experimental animals evaluated are concerned. The experimental conclusion is only as powerful as the variables measured. The methods may have significantly different abilities to cause tissue healing, but the weightbearing status of the experimental animals may not depend on whether the tissue is healed. The investigator must beware of choosing the correct variable to measure.

Ordered Two-Way Frequency Analysis

Another type of frequency analysis is useful when the observations are ordered. For example, an investigator might use two surgical treatments on a ligament and then assess tissue healing on a scale from 1 (least healed) to 3 (most healed), or poor, better, best. The scale itself is irrelevant as long as it is ordered. The data from such an experiment might be organized as shown in Table 16.30.

The usefulness of frequency analysis in this type of problem, in which one category is ordered and the other is dichotomous, is that it is possible not only to test for differences in the treatment methods (independence), but

TABLE 16.30. *Histologic appearance*

Method	Poor	Better	Best
Sutured	11	22	30
Not sutured	14	26	23

also to check to see if there are trends across proportions (analogous to determining whether a slope is significant in linear regression).

The level of complexity of frequency analysis problems is limited only by the investigator's creativity. The key, as a designer of experiments knows, is that this tool exists and should be used when appropriate. Frequency analysis should not be used when another parametric statistical method, such as ANOVA, would be more useful. Furthermore, the investigator should try to measure the variable that is most closely related to the experimental question.

NONPARAMETRIC STATISTICS

Why Use Nonparametric Statistics?

For many parametric statistical tests (for example, ANOVA), certain numeric assumptions about the sample distribution must be satisfied. However, in spite of the power of mathematic transformations and all of our sophisticated experimental designs, it is not always possible to meet these requirements. Before performing statistical analyses, the assumptions of the particular test must be tested. For example, in ANOVA, the assumptions are that the groups have equal variance and that the group data are normally distributed.

Nonparametric statistical tests must be used when the requirements of parametric statistical tests cannot be satisfied. Nonparametric methods are also called distribution-free methods, because they are not dependent on any distribution, such as the normal distribution. The word nonparametric is used because the null hypothesis is not concerned with specific parameters, such as the mean in ANOVA, but only with the distribution of the variates. This point is critical, because conclusions based on nonparametric statistics cannot address differences between means. Therefore, the investigator must be careful not to use a phrase such as "the old patients were significantly heavier than the young ones ($p < 0.05$) as demonstrated by the Mann-Whitney nonparametric statistical test," because heavier implies a greater average mass and refers to a mean (a parameter that cannot be used in this test).

Advantages and Limitations of Nonparametric Statistics

Nonparametric tests pose a trade-off in terms of utility. On the one hand, there are absolutely no limitations to the characteristics of the data set to be analyzed; in fact, the data need not even be numeric. Conversely, significant effects cannot be related back to any parametric property of the data set, such as the mean or variance.

Data that appear to be distributed as a bell-shaped curve may not be normally distributed. The two parameters usually checked in testing the normal distribution assumption are skew and kurtosis. Skew simply refers to the direction in which the data distribution leans. A normal distribution does not lean, but non-normal distributions may lean to the right or to the left. Both of these variations are shown in Figure 16.16, in which it should be emphasized that all distributions are bell-shaped but not all are normally distributed. Because normal distribution is an assumption for all parametric statistical tests, one of the first decisions to be made in analyzing data is whether the data set is normally distributed. If it is not, and cannot be made to be normally distributed, then nonparametric statistics are the only option (Fig. 16.17). Kurtosis refers to the distribution of variates in the sample. A normal distribution has a certain weight in the tail and hump regions. Thus, a sample with too much data near the tails is said to be platykurtotic, whereas one with too much data near the hump is said to be leptokurtotic.

Common Nonparametric Tests and Their Parametric Counterparts

The five most common nonparametric statistical tests and their corresponding parametric counterparts are shown in Table 16.31. Fortunately, there are really no

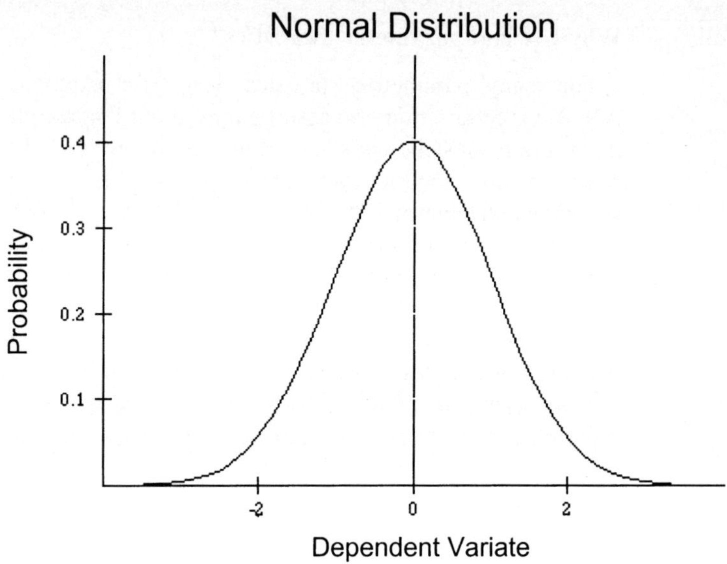

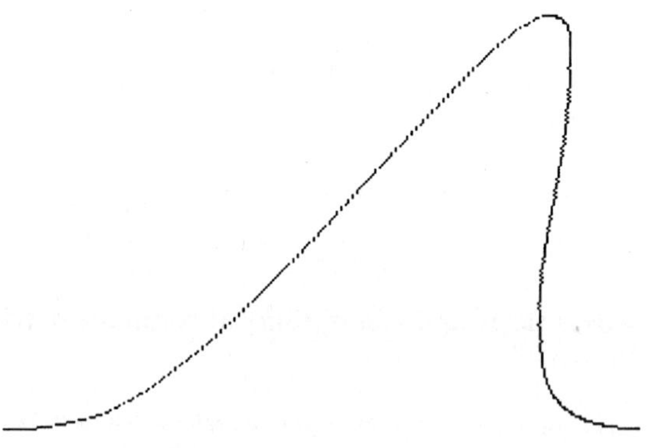

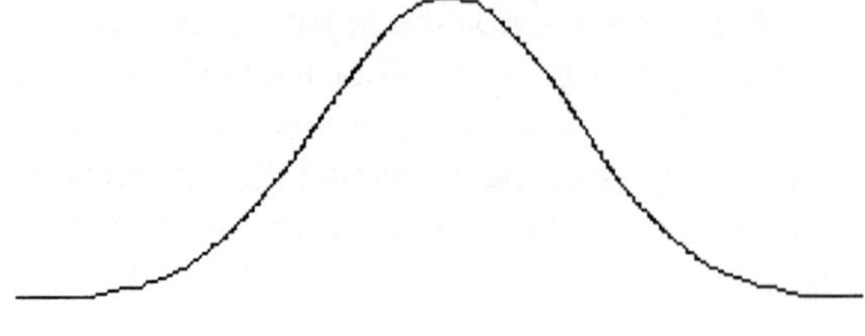

FIGURE 16.16. Alterations in the normal distribution which can be measured. **Top:** The normal distribution. **Middle:** A non-normal distribution skewed to the right. **Bottom:** A non-normal distribution that demonstrates leptokurtosis—too much weight in the tail region of the distribution.

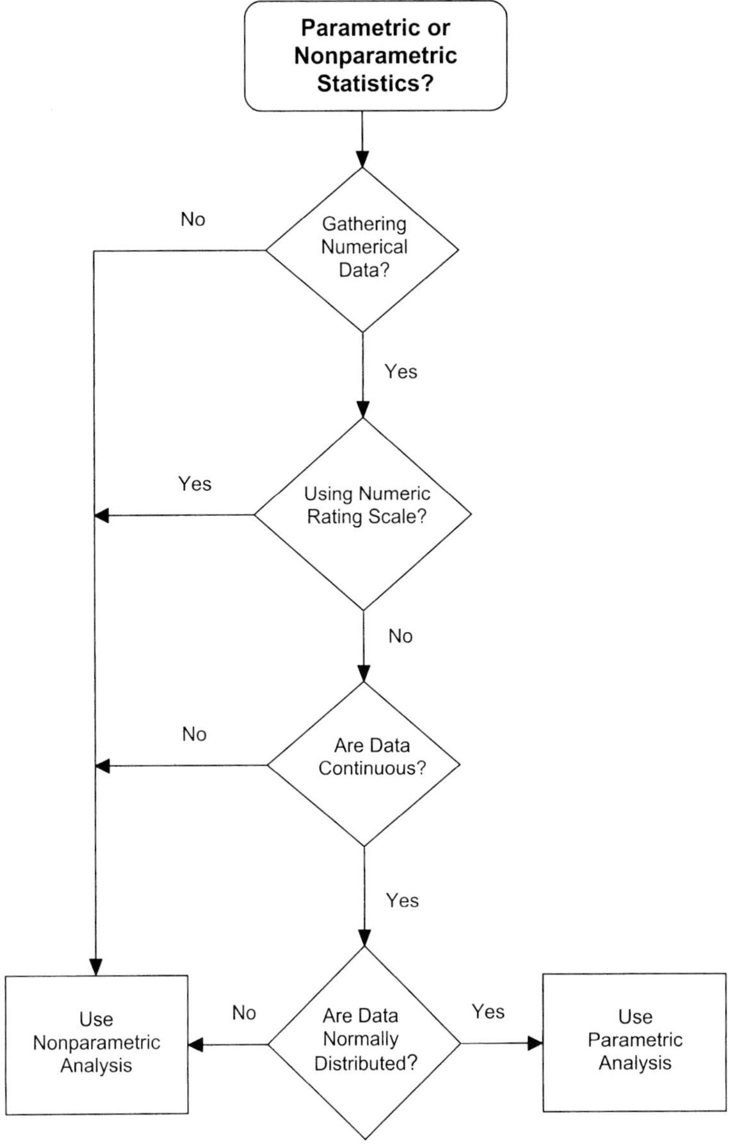

FIGURE 16.17. Logical algorithm used to decide between parametric and nonparametric statistical analysis methods.

new concepts to learn when choosing a nonparametric analytic tool. The classification schemes discussed in the ANOVA section above apply also to conditions in which nonparametric statistics are used. Thus, a perusal of Table 16.31 reveals that numerous nonparametric tests are available for one-way, two-way, and multiway

TABLE 16.31. *Corresponding parametric and nonparametric tests*

Nonparametric test	Parametric counterpart
Mann-Whitney *U*	Student *t*-test
Wilcoxon two-sample	Student *t*-test
Wilcoxon signed rank	Paired *t*-test
Kruskal-Wallis	One-way ANOVA
Friedman	Two-way ANOVA

ANOVA, analysis of variance.

classification experiments. The decision regarding the specific test is largely a matter of preference. The degree to which each type of test tends to be conservative is also a factor.

Wilcoxon Two-Sample Nonparametric Statistical Test

The Wilcoxon two-sample test is a good illustration of the basis for nonparametric testing. Many other nonparametric tests involve similar calculation methods, and the reader is referred to the "Selected Bibliography" for further examples.

Suppose an investigator wanted to compare femur lengths from individuals of the same age who live in either San Diego or Boston, and, in spite of heroic efforts, found that they were not normally distributed. The investigator chose to compare them anyway using the

TABLE 16.32. *Sample data for Wilcoxon two-sample test*

Boston sample		San Diego sample	
Femur length (mm)	Rank	Femur length (mm)	Rank
104	2	100	1
109	7	105	3
112	9	107	4.5
114	10	107	4.5
116	11.5	108	6
118	13.5	111	8
118	13.5	116	11.5
119	15	120	16
121	17.5	121	17.5
123	19.5	123	19.5
125	21	—	—
126	22.5	—	—
126	22.5	—	—
128	25	—	—
128	25	—	—
128	25	—	—

Wilcoxon two-sample test. The data are given in Table 16.32 and graphed as a histogram in Figure 16.18. Note that the raw data are given along with their "rank" relative to the total data set.

A good way to understand these tests is to examine the calculation procedure, which is relatively simple. First, we rank the variates from smallest to largest, independent of group. In the case of a tie, we split the difference. Then we calculate a statistic directly from the ranks, not the variates. In this case, it is the Wilcoxon C statistic. The equation for this statistic is

$$C = n_1 n_2 + \frac{n_2(n_2+1)}{2} - \sum_{i=1}^{n_2} R_i \qquad [31]$$

where
n_1 = the size of the larger sample
n_2 = the size of the smaller sample
R_i = the individual rank

This statistic is compared with $n_1 n_2 - C$, and the greater of the two quantities defined as the test statistic U.

In this example, we find a significant difference between femur lengths from San Diego versus Boston ($p = 0.0223$ using the Wilcoxon C statistic). However, looking at Figure 16.18 would not indicate exactly what is different about the distributions. These methods do not require each variate to be a precise measurement, as long as the observations can be ranked. The actual variate measured need not be related to a particular parameter because the calculations are made based on the observation's rank. Thus, typical observations might be: arrival time of patients for surgery, time of day casts are applied, or which flavor ice cream is ordered.

Multivariate Statistical Analysis

Univariate Versus Multivariate Tests

All analyses described up to this point have operated on a single dependent variable, and thus are referred to as univariate analysis methods. For example, the ANOVA example was used to measure the effects of immobilization on muscle fiber area, and the ANCOVA example to measure the effects of cement viscosity on prosthesis pullout strength. In both cases, the analysis was performed on a single variable, fiber area or pullout strength. What if the investigator had measured and was interested in the behavior of several dependent variables? How would the analysis proceed? Obviously, using univariate analysis would require performing numerous one-way ANOVAs on each variable and interpreting the results accordingly. Two problems could occur with the use of multiple univariate analyses. Because different dependent variables may contain different types of information, it is possible that multiple univariate analyses of experimental data would yield significant differences for different reasons. Many dependent variables behave in the same manner simply because they are indicators of the same underlying phenomenon. For example, in measurement of muscle compartment pressure, an investigator might also measure limb girth, mass, and temperature. Because all of these parameters would be expected to increase with a compartment syndrome, the investigator really would like to narrow the focus onto the one parameter that best characterized the phenomenon without the "dilution" of discussing the numerous other parameters. It would be nice to be able to evaluate all dependent variables simultaneously. To perform this type of simultaneous evaluation of multiple variables requires multivariate analysis.

Stepwise Linear Regression

There are several types of multivariate analyses, just as there are many types of univariate analyses. A stepwise linear regression problem will illustrate the general method.

In the stepwise linear regression method, simple linear regression analytic methods, such as those described earlier, are performed on a dependent variable, but multiple independent variables are included in the linear model in a stepwise fashion. At each step, only new information adds to the fit of the model and, thus, the investigator is assured that, by including multiple independent variables in the model, each has unique information. In addition, because the coefficient of determination is calculated after each step, it is possible to quantify the relative percentage to which each independent variable that is added affects the dependent variable.

As an example of stepwise regression applied to a musculoskeletal problem, consider the situation in which

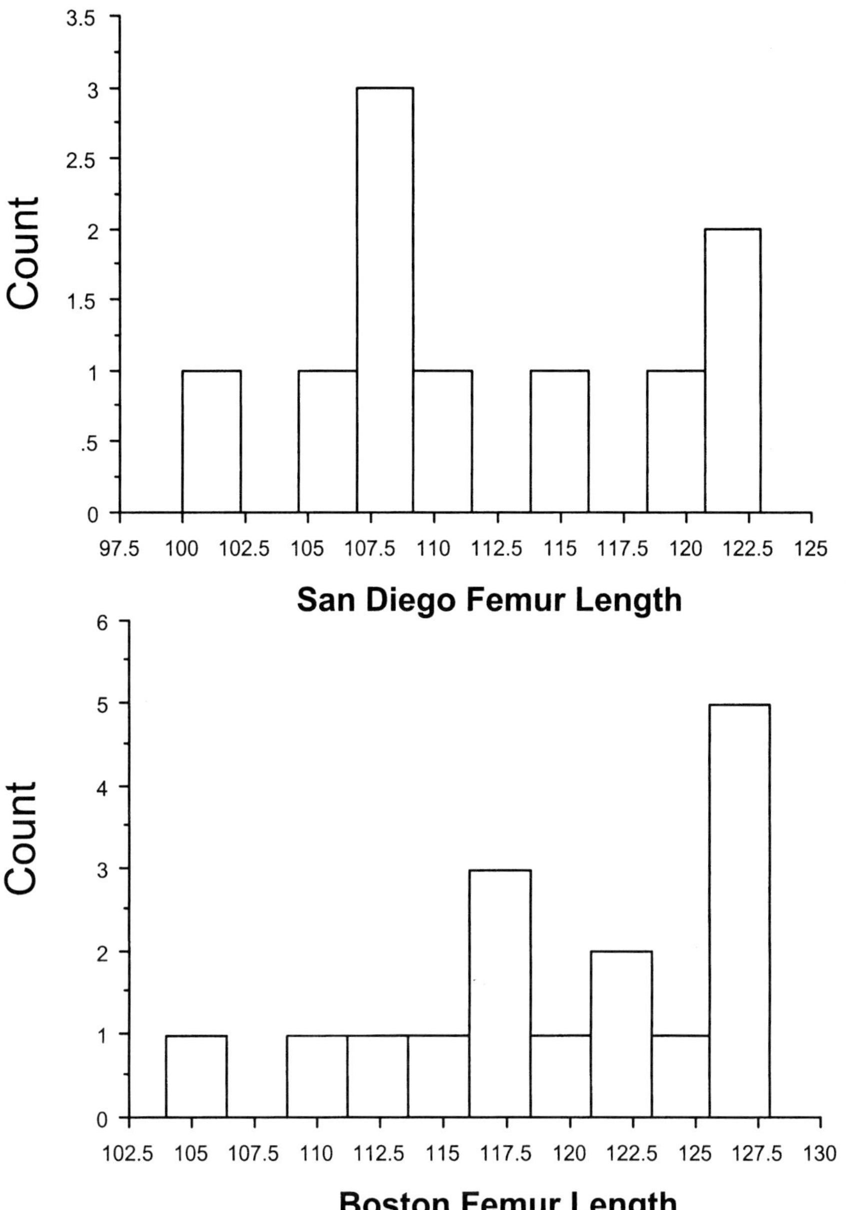

FIGURE 16.18. Histogram of data from Table 16.22 used in the Wilcoxon two-sample nonparametric statistical test. Nonparametric analysis reveals a significant difference between the distributions ($p < 0.03$).

the investigators want to know the factor or factors that contribute to muscle motor unit tension. It is known that some motor units develop high tensions (the dependent variable), and other units develop lower tensions. What are the anatomic factors that affect motor unit tension? It is possible to measure total motor unit muscle fiber area, number of muscle fibers per unit (innervation ratio), and muscle mass (all independent variables), as well as motor unit maximum tension (dependent variable). The raw data are presented in Table 16.33. The data are entered into a stepwise regression program.

By watching the stepwise process, it is possible to illustrate numerous concepts that were presented in the ANOVA and regression sections. New statistical methods are often simple extensions of familiar methods.

The first step in the analysis is to perform simple linear regression of each independent variable on the dependent variable. In statistical terminology, we regress each independent variable on the dependent variable to determine the one that accounts for the greatest explained variation. In our model, the dependent variable is maximum tension, and the independent variables are innervation

TABLE 16.33. *Sample data for multiple regression problem*

Unit no.	Maximum tension (mN)	Innervation ratio	Fiber area (μm^2)	Muscle mass (g)	Unit cross-sectional area (cm^2)	Specific tension (N/cm^2)
1	23.0	60	2149	6.40	0.001289	17.83
2	46.0	88	3007	5.80	0.002646	17.38
3	51.0	132	2296	7.40	0.003031	16.82
4	84.0	161	2234	5.40	0.003597	23.35
5	94.0	188	2451	8.00	0.004608	20.40
6	124.0	243	2607	6.70	0.006335	19.57
7	124.0	166	3239	6.00	0.005377	23.06
8	157.0	193	2953	4.30	0.005699	27.54
9	270.0	281	3694	6.10	0.010380	26.01
10	279.0	379	3287	6.50	0.012458	22.39
11	284.0	311	3483	6.90	0.010832	26.21

ratio (IR), fiber cross-sectional area (CSA), muscle mass, and specific tension (motor unit force/motor unit area). The initial regression table (Table 16.34) shows that the highest F ratio belongs to the variable IR ($F = 61.860$). Recall that in regression, F represents the explained variation (Eq. 16.22) divided by the unexplained variation (Eq. 16.21) and, thus, IR explains the most variability in tetanic tension of all variables. Also note that muscle mass is not a good predictor of tetanic tension with its very low F value.

Now, the typical simple linear regression analysis is performed and the appropriate ANOVA table generated (Table 16.35). Note that the relationship is highly significant ($p < 0.0001$) and the coefficient of determination $r^2 = 0.873$ (Table 16.35). Thus, IR accounts for 87.3% of the total experimental variability. This concludes step one of the procedure and, for many investigators, would conclude the entire experiment. However, additional interesting information can be extracted by proceeding to the next steps.

In step two, an analysis of covariance (ANCOVA) is performed using each remaining independent variable with IR as the covariate. The variable with the highest F value, CSA, is entered into the model (Table 16.36), an ANCOVA is performed, and the regression results are presented as before (Table 16.37).

TABLE 16.34. *Step 1: initial calculations*

	Partial correlation	F-to-Enter
IR	0.934	61.860
CSA	0.829	19.749
Muscle mass	−0.039	0.014
Calculated specific tension	0.737	10.685

NOTE: Initial calculation of F statistics for all dependent variables in the stepwise regression model. The higher the F value, the better the correlation between the independent variable shown and motor unit tetanic tension.

IR, innervation ratio; CSA, cross-sectional area.

Now the coefficient of determination has increased from 0.873 to 0.954 (Table 16.37), which means that the addition of CSA into the model has accounted for an additional 8.1% of the experimental variability. Because more than one independent variable contributes to the correlation coefficient, it is now termed a serial or multiple correlation coefficient. This added variability is, however, much less important than IR, which initially accounted for 87.3% of the variability.

The stepping process continues until one of two things happens: all variables are entered into the multiple regression equation or the remaining variables have F values that are lower than an arbitrary F value that is referred to as F-to-enter (representing the minimum F value required to enter the multiple regression model). In the current case, the next step included the specific tension variable and then the sole remaining variable (muscle mass) had an F value of 0.514, far lower than the F-to-enter value of 4.000, which we preselected. There is really no right or wrong F-to-enter value. This parameter can be varied and in many cases makes no difference as to the experimental outcome. Table 16.37 summarizes the stepping process for the stepwise regression model just described. In this case, it is clear that, unless the F-to-enter was decreased to 0.5, the same outcome would be obtained. It usually is possible, using most statistical programs, to force each variable into the equation to calculate just how much of the dependent variable can be accounted for by each independent variable.

The stepwise regression model, and simple variations of it are extremely useful in clinical settings in which we desire to know the relative influence of a number of risk factors. Each risk factor is entered as an independent variable and the relative influence determined by the percentage of data variability accounted for by it. The key in multivariate analysis is to go ahead and measure numerous factors. If they are unimportant, they will not enter the equation. If they are important, valuable insights can

TABLE 16.35. *Regression summary, step 1*

Count	11			
No. missing	0			
R	0.934			
R^2	0.873			
Adjusted R^2	0.859			
RMS residual	36.316			

	df	Sum of squares	Mean square	F	p
Regression	1	81584.867	81584.867	61.860	<0.0001
Residual	9	11869.679	1318.853	—	—
Total	10	93454.545	—	—	—

NOTE: Analysis of variance table generated following the first step of the multiple regression analysis. Even after entry of only a single variable into the equation, there is a highly significant effect of innervation ratio on maximum tetanic tension
RMS, root mean square.

Importance of Statistical Analysis

It is important to understand experimental design and statistical analysis in order to extract the "truth" from an experiment. The benefits of proper planning and analysis cannot be overstated. Many potentially superb ideas have not been realized because of poor experimental design. Similarly, the significance of numerous excellent experiments has not been extracted because of shoddy or qualitative analysis. Unfortunately, while many scientists and clinicians are trained in their specialty, very few are explicitly tutored in experimental design and statistical analysis. We are thus at risk of mixing well-conceived ideas with shoddy analysis and incorrect interpretation. Clearly, this compromises our pursuit of scientific truth and our ability to prescribe appropriate clinical treatment.

The purpose of this chapter has been to describe, by example, the basis for appropriate prospective experimental design and analysis. The two general classes of experimentation are prospective (experiments designed prior to their execution) and retrospective (experiments designed after the data have been gathered). Retrospective experiments are usually applied to clinical studies in which data from patients who have already been treated is analyzed. Retrospective experiments have two major advantages: they are relatively inexpensive and rapid to perform. These advantages exist because the time and money devoted to the experiment itself have already been spent. The investment consists of the time required to extract and analyze the data. The pitfall of retrospective clinical studies is that, because originally no experiment was envisioned, there is little control regarding the protocol used to record the data and important desired information may not be available. Because these are major drawbacks, numerous clinical journals will not publish retrospective studies and many clinicians view such studies with skepticism. For this reason, the majority of this chapter has been devoted to the description of methods used to design and analyze data from prospective studies, with the caveat that the methods discussed also allow comparisons to be made within data after they have been acquired as part of a prospective study.

Proper experimental execution consists of three steps: (a) planning and designing the experiment, (b) executing the experiment, and (c) analyzing and interpreting the data obtained from the experiment. The latter depends on the proper statistical techniques based on the proper size and clinical description of sample population and nature of dependent and independent variables. If these suggestions are followed, costs are decreased, direction is maintained, and the project retains continuity. Most importantly, the data ultimately have more impact because results are concisely and accurately presented.

The following steps will help the investigator choose among the various models presented and help the reader to evaluate the research and the results presented.

1. Describe the dependent variable
2. Define the factors
3. Define the levels of each factor
4. State whether the factors are fixed or random
5. Describe the appropriate statistical method along with a rationale for your choice

Applying these steps to the various models will be helpful to both the prospective investigator and evaluator.

TABLE 16.36. *Step 2: second set of* F *calculations*

Variable	Partial correlation	*F*-to-enter
CSA	0.799	14.145
Muscle mass	−0.414	1.652
Calculated specific tension	0.667	6.403

NOTE: *F* statistics calculated following step 2 of the multiple regression analysis. The next independent variable to enter the regression model is cross-sectional area (CSA).

TABLE 16.37. *Regression summary, step 2*

Count	11				
No. missing	0				
R	0.977				
R^2	0.954				
Adjusted R^2	0.943				
RMS residual	23.152				

	df	Sum of squares	Mean square	F	p
Regression	2	89166.580	44583.290	83.178	<0.0001
Residual	8	4287.966	535.996	—	—
Total	10	93454.545	—	—	—

Analysis of variance table of stepwise regression analysis after step 2. Note that the residual error (4287.966) has decreased from that shown in Figure 16.18 (11869.679) due to addition of cross-sectional area into the regression model. Note also that serial correlation coefficient has increased from 0.87 in step 1 to 0.94 in step 2. RMS, root mean square.

SUGGESTED READINGS

General Statistical Texts

Altman DG. *Practical statistics for medical research.* Chapman & Hall, 1991.

Bliss CI. *Statistics in biology.* Vol. I. New York: McGraw-Hill, 1967.

Bliss CI. *Statistics in biology.* Vol. II. New York: McGraw-Hill, 1970.

Bowerman BL, O'Connell RT. *Linear statistical models: an applied approach.* 2nd ed. Boston: PWS-Kent, 1990.

Cochran WG, Cox GM. *Experimental designs.* 2nd ed. New York: Wiley, 1957.

Dawson–Saunders B, Trapp RG. *Basic and clinical biostatistics.* Norwalk, CT: Appleton & Lange, 1990.

Dixon WJ, Massey FJ Jr. *Introduction to statistical analysis.* 3rd ed. New York: McGraw-Hill, 1969.

Draper NR, Smith H. *Applied regression analysis.* 2nd ed. New York: John Wiley & Sons, 1981.

Dunn OJ, Clark VA. *Applied statistics: analysis of variance and regression.* New York: John Wiley, 1974.

Fleiss JL. *The design and analysis of clinical experiments.* New York: John Wiley & Sons, 1986.

Fleiss JL. *Statistical analysis for rates and proportions.* New York: John Wiley & Sons, 1981.

Montgomery DC. *Design and analysis of experiments.* New York: Wiley, 1966.

Mostellar F, Tukey JW. *Data analysis and regression: a second course in statistics.* Reading, MA: Addison-Wesley, 1977.

Shuster JJ. *Handbook of sample size guidelines for clinical trials.* Boca Raton, FL: CRC Press, 1990.

Snedecor GW, Cochran WG. *Statistical methods.* 6th ed. Ames, IO: Iowa State University Press, 1967.

Sokal RR, Rohlf FJ. *Biometry.* 2nd ed. San Francisco: W.H. Freeman, 1981.

Tatsuoka MM. *Multivariate analysis.* New York: John Wiley, 1971.

Zar JH. *Biostatistical analysis.* 2nd ed. Englewood Cliffs, NJ: Prentice-Hall, 1974.

Some Details of Statistical Methodology

Bishop YMM, Fienberg SE, Holland PW. *Discrete multivariate analysis: theory and practice.* Cambridge, MA: MIT Press, 1975:557.

Cramer EM. Significance tests and tests of models in multiple regression. *Am Stat* 1975;26:26–30.

Fisher RA. *Statistical methods for research workers.* 12th ed. Edinburgh: Oliver & Boyd, 1954.

Fleiss JL. Confidence intervals vs significance tests: quantitative interpretation. *Amer J Pub Health* 1986;76:587–591.

Freiman JA, Chalmers TC, Smith HS Jr, et al. The importance of beta, the type II error and sample size in the design and interpretation of the randomized controlled trial: survey of 71 "negative" trials. *N Engl J Med* 1978;299:690–694.

French S. How significant is statistical significance? *Physiotherapy* 1988; 74:266–268.

Godfrey K. Simple linear regression in medical research. *N Engl J Med* 1985;313:1629–1636.

Grubbs FE. Procedures for detecting outlying observations in samples. *Technometrics* 1969;11:1–21.

Gurland J, Tripathi RC. A simple approximation for unbiased estimation of the standard deviation. *Am Stat* 1971;25:30–32.

Ku HH, Kullback S. Log-linear models in contingency table analysis. *Amer Stat* 1974;28:115–122.

Nelissen RG, Brand R, Rozing PM. Survivorship analysis in total condylar knee arthroplasty. *J Bone Joint Surg Am* 1992;74:383–389.

Poole C. Beyond the confidence interval. *Am J Public Health* 1987;77: 195–199.

Ratain J, Hochberg MC. Clinical trials: a guide. *Arthritis Rheum* 1990;33: 131–139.

Ricker WE. Linear regression in fishery research. *J Fish Res Board Can* 1993;30:409–434.

Rudicel S, Esdaile J. The randomized clinical trial. *J Bone Joint Surg Am* 1985;67:1284–1293.

Seal H. *Multivariate statistical analysis for biologists.* New York: John Wiley, 1964.

Sokal RR, Braumann CA. Significance tests for coefficients of variation and variability profiles. *Syst Zool* 1980;29:50–66.

Spector P. Post-hocs vs. contrasts: a look at the strengths and weaknesses of both types of means comparisons. *Abacus News.* Fall, 1990.

Student (Gossett, WS). On the error of counting with a haemacytometer. *Biometrika* 1907;5:351–360.

Thompson WD. On the comparison of effects. *Am J Public Health* 1987;77:491–493.

Thompson WD. Statistical criteria in the interpretation of epidemiologic data. *Am J Public Health* 1987;77:191–194.

Tsutakawa RK, Hewett JE. Comparison of two regression lines over a finite interval. *Biometrics* 1978;34:391–398.

Welsch RE. Stepwise multiple comparison procedures. *J Am Stat Assoc* 1977;72:566–575.

Examples of Statistics Applied to Biology and Medicine

Bodine SC, Roy RR, Eldred E, et al. Maximal force as a function of anatomical features of motor units in the cat tibialis anterior. *J Neurophys* 1987;6:1730–1745.

Frank C, McDonald D, Lieber R, et al. Biochemical heterogeneity within the maturing rabbit medial collateral ligament. *Clin Ortho Rel Res* 1988;236:279–286.

Golbranson FL, Wirta RW, Kuncir EJ, et al. Volume changes occurring in postoperative below-knee stumps. *J Rehab Res Dev* 1988;25:11–18.

Lieber RL. Invited opinion: Statistical significance and statistical power in hypothesis testing. *J Orthop Res* 1990;8:304–309.

Lieber RL, Brown CG. Quantitative method for comparison of skeletal muscle architectural properties. *J Biomech* 1992;25:557–560.

Lieber RL, Blevins FT. Skeletal muscle architecture of the rabbit hindlimb: functional implications of muscle design. *J Morphol* 1989;199:93–101.

Lieber RL, Fridén JO, Hargens AR, et al. Differential response of the dog quadriceps muscle to external skeletal fixation of the knee. *Mus Nerve* 1988;11:193–201.

Lieber RL, Jacobson MD, Fazeli BM, et al. Architecture of selected muscles of the arm and forearm: anatomy and implications for tendon transfer. *J Hand Surg* 1992;17:787–798.

Wenger DRD, Maulden D, Speck G, et al. Effect of corrective shoes and inserts on flexible flat foot in children—a prospective randomized trial. *J Bone Joint Surg* 1989;71:800–810.

GLOSSARY TERMS

α (significance level): The probability of type 1 error in an experiment involving hypothesis testing.

Analysis of covariance (ANCOVA): The analytical technique that compares mean values between groups after adjusting for an independent covariate.

Analysis of variance (ANOVA): The analytical method for determining whether means obtained from various samples are equivalent.

Average ($\overline{X}$): A value calculated from a sample that estimates the population mean.

β: The probability of type 2 error in a hypothesis testing experiment.

c^2 statistic: The statistic used in frequency analysis to compare expected proportions.

Coefficient of determination (r^2): The "goodness of fit" statistic which represents the total fraction of the data explained by the linear relationship.

Correlation coefficient (r): The "goodness of fit" statistic which represents the degree to which the experimental data fits a line. Square root of coefficient of determination. Positive for positive slopes and negative for negative slopes.

Descriptive statistics: Numerical expressions which serve to describe a sample. Example, mean (X).

F statistic: The statistic created by the ratio of two variances which can be used in ANOVA to compare whether a number of means are equivalent.

Frequency analysis: The analytical technique which determines the probability that certain numbers of frequencies of observations are independent.

Kurtosis: The degree to which the variability of a distribution matches the variability of a normal distribution.

Leptokurtotic: A distribution property in which a greater number of observations are obtained near the tails of the distribution rather than near the mean.

Linear regression: The analytical technique whereby a line is fit through a data set yielding a correlation coefficient and a p value.

Mean (μ): The most common observation within a population.

Multivariate analysis: An analytical technique that operates on a number of variables simultaneously. Example, stepwise linear regression.

Normal distribution: The probability distribution described by the function which has the following form:

$$y = e^{-\frac{(x-\mu)^2}{2\sigma^2}} \Big/ \sigma\sqrt{2\pi}$$

that represents the probability of obtaining an observation a certain distance away from the mean within a standard sample.

Outcomes research: A type of clinical research in which specific outcomes (such as range of motion, patient satisfaction, or subjective pain) are used as measures of the success of a particular clinical treatment.

p value: The probability obtained from a statistical analysis that type 1 error will occur.

Platykurtotic: Kurtosis of a distribution in which a greater number of samples are obtained near the mean than near the tails of the distribution.

Prospective study: An experimental study in which the data are acquired after the experimental design is proposed.

Repeated measures: Measurements that are taken from a population from the same sampling element. Example, measuring blood pressure in the same individuals over time.

Retrospective study: An experiment in which the data are already acquired by the time the specific experiment is designed.

Sample size (n): The number of independent observations that make up a sample. Sample size is related to statistical power in hypothesis testing.

Significance level (α): The probability of type 1 error in an experiment involving hypothesis testing.

Skew: The property of a distribution that "leans" either to the right or to the left. Skewed distributions are, by definition, not normally distributed.

Standard deviation (s): The square root of the sample variance. A measure of population variability that is expressed in terms of the original measurement units.

Standard error of the mean (SEM): The error associated with estimating the mean value of a sample.

Statistical power (1-β): The probability that if a negative result is obtained that it truly represents a negative result and not simply inadequate sample size.

t statistic: The statistic used to compare two means obtained from two different samples.

Univariate analysis: Any statistical analytical technique which operates on a single variable at a time. Example, one-way analysis of variance.

Variance (s^2): The variance measure of the spread of data about the sample mean and is an estimator of the population variance s2. As shown in Figure 16.1, each population not only has its most probable value, the mean μ, it also has a certain variability or variance s^2 about that value.

CHAPTER 17

In Vivo Measurement of Anterior Cruciate Ligament and Anterior Cruciate Ligament Graft Strain

Braden C. Fleming, Bruce D. Beynnon, Per A. Renström, and Robert J. Johnson

THE ANTERIOR CRUCIATE LIGAMENT PROBLEM

Anterior cruciate ligament (ACL) disruptions have reached epidemic proportions. The annual incidence has been reported as high as 0.6 injuries occurring for every 1,000 people in the United States (1). This is particularly disturbing because an ACL tear is a disabling injury that has been shown to predispose individuals to the early onset of osteoarthritis even when treated conservatively (2–12). ACL disruption results in abnormal kinematics such as pivot shift or giving-way episodes. Thus, the contact stress on the articular surfaces and menisci are increased in response to different joint loadings. The change in load distribution and repetitive joint trauma are thought to initiate and accelerate the degenerative process in the ACL deficiency (13).

For the young and active patient, ACL reconstruction is currently the procedure of choice (14). Although ACL reconstruction has been touted as a successful procedure from a functional standpoint, universally acceptable results have yet to be obtained. Thirty percent to 70% of patients who underwent ACL reconstruction continue to report pain and swelling (15,16). Changes in knee laxity over time have also been observed in many patients (15,17–21) as well as the continued progression of osteoarthritis (17,18,22,23).

The ACL plays a primary role in controlling the kinematics of the knee. It functions as a primary restraint to anterior tibial motion with respect to the femur, and as a secondary restraint to axial rotation and varus-valgus angulation (24). It also works in conjunction with the other ligaments and articular surfaces to guide flexion–extension motion of the knee. An example of this contribution is the simple four bar cruciate linkage used to describe the kinematics of the tibiofemoral joint during flexion motion (25). To eliminate the processes of functional instability and articular surface degeneration, it is essential that the kinematics of the knee be restored to its preinjury state. There are several variables that contribute to the outcome of reconstructive surgery including graft type, intraarticular graft position, initial graft tension, graft remodeling, and rehabilitation. At this time, there is no grafting material that duplicates the geometry or structural properties of the normal ACL. Likewise, the intraoperative variables such as placement and initial graft tension required to restore the normal function of the ACL, and hence the tibiofemoral joint, remain controversial. Thus, it is not possible to directly reproduce or replicate the behavior of the normal ACL. However, since an autogenous graft is a viable structure, it may have potential to approximate the ACL once healing is complete. It is through rehabilitation that the mechanical strain environment of the ACL may be controlled to optimize its healing potential while minimizing failure.

When loads are applied to the leg, they are transmitted to the joint, which in turn initiate motion. These motions are controlled by the interaction of ligamentous structures, contact surfaces, and muscles. Because ligaments are passive stabilizers, tensile forces are generated in the ligament when they become strained. A ligament that is supporting a tensile load is acting as a restraint to bony motion. Thus, measurement of ligament strain provides insight into its function. A method for measuring both ACL and ACL graft force *in vivo* does not currently exist. Although measurements of ACL graft forces have been performed *in vivo* (26,27), these methods are not applicable to the normal ACL. Thus, it is difficult to compare the biomechanical response of the ACL graft to that of the normal ACL. It is possible, however, to measure ACL and ACL graft displacements *in vivo*, which can then be used to determine their strain responses (28–38).

CHAPTER OBJECTIVE

Using an arthroscopically implantable displacement sensor, it is possible to measure strain and elongation in ACL and ACL grafts, *in vivo*. The activities that can be evaluated using this technology are less restricted when measuring strain in the normal ACL since the experiment may be performed while the patient is under local anesthesia and normal muscle function is maintained. Displacement measurements in the ACL graft have been limited to passive loading conditions because the surgery and experimental measurements must be performed while the patient is under spinal, epidural, or general anesthesia. It is the intent of this chapter to review the displacement response of an ACL graft *in vivo* and compare this response to that of the intact ACL. Data on the normal ACL are necessary to provide an objective database for the comparison, and to provide insight into the possible displacement response of a properly positioned ACL graft under different muscle loading conditions. Currently, these conditions have not been directly tested in the ACL graft.

There are several aims to this chapter. First, the instruments and techniques to measure ACL and ACL graft displacements are described (28,38). Second, the ACL strain data for passive flexion–extension motion are presented to provide a baseline for later comparisons to that of the ACL graft (28). Third, the initial elongation response of a bone-patellar tendon-bone reconstruction will be discussed (30,36). This includes a description of graft seating that occurs immediately after fixation, the elongation response of the graft during passive flexion–extension motion, and a comparison to that of the normal ACL. Graft elongation at time of fixation can also be used to validate isometers for predicting graft placement (36). Fourth, the elongation response of the graft measured 1 year following the initial reconstruction procedure is compared with that measured at the time of surgical reconstruction of the ligament (39). The importance of graft elongation is illustrated by examining the relationship between initial graft elongation at the time of surgical reconstruction and the change of anterior–posterior laxity of the knee (40). Finally, the ACL strain response during commonly prescribed rehabilitation activities following ACL reconstruction is presented (28,34,41). These results will then be compared with other *in vivo* investigations of ACL or ACL graft biomechanics.

LIGAMENT STRAIN MEASUREMENT TECHNIQUES

Displacement measurements for the calculation of strain have been commonly performed to determine the biomechanical function of ligaments and their replacements. Ligament strains (ε) have been typically calculated using the engineering strain formulation;

$$\varepsilon = [(L - L_o)/L_o]*100$$

where L is the length of the ligament measured by the transducer under a particular loading condition, and L_o is a reference length used to standardize the displacement across patients. Previous investigations of ligament displacement *in situ* have selected reference lengths based on the slack-taut transition of the ligament (28,37,38,42), anatomically based references such as the transducer length that corresponding to a particular knee flexion angle (43,44), or based on a particular external loading condition (45,46). A reference that identifies the slack-taut transition length provides an absolute strain reference, whereas one that is based on an arbitrary joint position, or loading condition, or both, provides a relative strain reference (or elongation reference). The concepts of these strain references and their interpretation will be elaborated on later in the chapter.

Bone to bone displacement measurements have been performed using many methods including liquid metal strain gages (42,46–49), plethysmographic transducers (50), digitization of the origin and insertions to calculate ligament elongation (51–54), bone-to-bone displacement measured by a materials testing system (55), displacement of a wire in a tube (45), and clip gauges (56,57). These transducers span the entire ligament and measure the change in distance between the proximal and distal ligament insertion sites. They do not differentiate between the strain levels in the midsubstance or at the insertion sites. The invasive nature of these techniques limits their use for *in vivo* human research.

Other transducers and techniques have been used to map out the strain of the ligament midsubstance. These techniques include placing pins along the ligament and digitizing their location under specific loading conditions (53,58), using optical techniques to map surface strains (55,59-61), clip gauges (44), Hall effect transducers, or differential variable reluctance transducers (DVRT; MicroStrain, Inc. Burlington, VT) (28,38,43,62,63). Digitization methods are currently not possible *in vivo* because structures must be cut to gain access to ACL or ACL graft to digitize anatomic landmarks (i.e., ligament insertion sites). Video systems are advantageous for evaluating surface strain measurements particularly during high rate tests. Video techniques also facilitate biaxial strain analyses if desired (59). However, optical methods are currently limited for ACL or ACL graft strain analyses in cadavers since these structures are located within the intra-articular space and are blocked from view during *in vivo* testing. Miniature implantable displacement transducers such as the Hall effect transducer and the DVRT have been successfully used for *in vivo* use and are the focus of this chapter (28,30,32–34,39).

IN VIVO STRAIN MEASUREMENT

In vivo ACL and ACL graft strain measurements have been performed using either the Hall effect transducer or the DVRT. The Hall effect transducer and DVRT are similar in form and function. However, the DVRT has a greater measurement range and improved sensitivity compared with the Hall effect transducer. Both of these transducers have been used in the different studies reviewed in this chapter; those prior to 1995 used the Hall effect transducer, while those after 1995 used the DVRT.

The body of the DVRT consists of two stainless steel tubes, one that slides within the other (Fig. 17.1). The outer tube is approximately 1.5 mm in diameter and the overall length of the transducer is less than 6 mm. A force less than 0.5 g is sufficient to initiate displacement between the two tubes. Consequently, the size and compliance of the gage has the advantage of not interfering with normal joint mechanics, ACL, or ACL graft function throughout most of the range of knee flexion–extension motion.

Fixation barbs, approximately 3 mm long, are mounted to the outer end of each tube. The surface of each barb contains several hooks which inter-digitate with the tissue. Sutures are attached to the DVRT body near the barbs to facilitate transducer removal. The DVRT is attached to soft tissue structures by pressing the two barbs into its surface. As the length of the structure changes due to externally applied or muscle induced

loads, the tubes that comprise the body of the DVRT move relative to one another.

The DVRT uses a differential change in the reluctance of two coils to measure displacement. Two coils are located within the outer tube of the body and are wired into two arms of a Wheatstone bridge. A magnetically permeable core is fixed within the free sliding inner tube. When the bridge is excited by a high-frequency alternating-current signal, movement of the core causes the reluctance of one coil to increase while the other decreases. This response alters the amplitude of the input signal that may be measured across the bridge output using a synchronous demodulator. The change in amplitude is related to the change in position of the core. Since each tube of the DVRT is securely attached to tissue through its fixation barb, the output may be calibrated to the relative change in length between the two barbs. The DVRT output signals are delivered through a lightweight and flexible polyamide and copper cable that is coupled to the DVRT within epoxy to eliminate problems due to moisture. The root mean square error for the DVRT is 7 μm (as compared with 12 μm for the Hall effect transducer) (64).

DIFFERENTIAL VARIABLE RELUCTANCE TRANSDUCER IMPLANTATION

The implantation procedures for the DVRT onto the normal ACL and ACL graft have been described in detail by Howe et al. (38) and Beynnon et al. (30), respectively. For both procedures, the patient is positioned supine on the operating table with the knee at 45° flexion. The ACL (or ACL graft) is viewed through the arthroscope that is placed in the medial parapatellar portal. The DVRT is then introduced into the knee joint capsule through a tube placed within the lateral parapatellar portal using a cus-

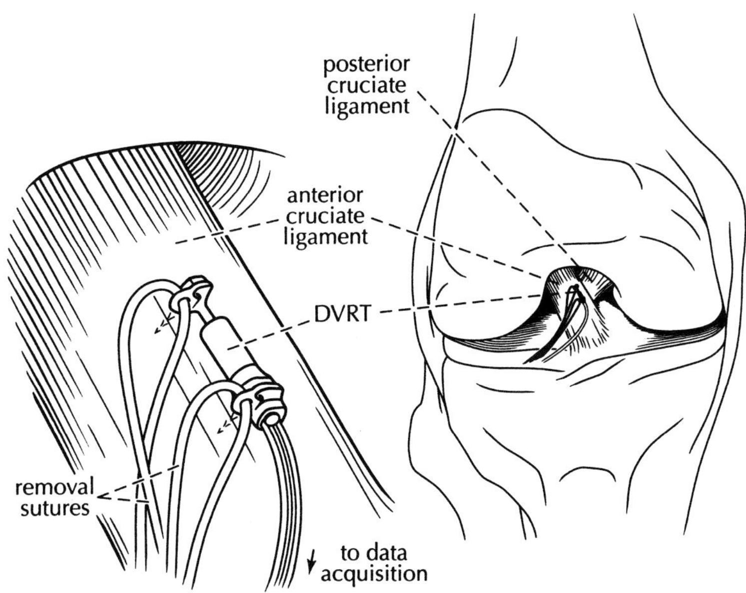

FIGURE 17.1. The differential variable reluctance transducer (DVRT) is a small, highly compliant transducer that may be arthroscopically applied to the anterior cruciate ligament (ACL) or ACL graft as shown. The gauge is oriented collinear with the ligament or graft fibers. Fixation is achieved by the two small barbs that penetrate the tissue. (From Fleming BC, Beynnon BD, Renstrom PA, et al. The strain behavior of the anterior cruciate ligament during bicycling: an in vivo study. *Am J Sports Med* 1998;26:109–118, with permission.)

tom designed insertion tool. The long axis of the DVRT is oriented collinear with the anterior fibers of the ligament or graft and the fixation barbs are pressed into the tissue (Fig. 17.1). The electrical cables and removal sutures of the DVRT course through the lateral portal and are strapped to the side of the thigh for stress relief. The joint irrigation fluid is evacuated, the arthroscopic portals are closed, and the patient is ready for testing. After the test protocol is completed, the portals are opened, and the DVRT removed by pulling on the removal sutures.

STRAIN VERSUS ELONGATION CALCULATIONS

The DVRT is a displacement sensor that can be used to determine length changes in an ACL or ACL graft. Ligament strains are commonly defined using the engineering strain formulation in an effort to standardize the length change with that of the initial length of the ligament. Previous studies of ligament or graft displacement have utilized different reference lengths for the calculation of strain. If the slack-taut transition length of the ligament or graft can be identified then an absolute strain value may be calculated. Thus, a positive strain value is indicative of a loaded ligament or graft. Conversely, a strain value that is equal to or less than zero corresponds to a ligament or graft that is unloaded. When an arbitrary reference is utilized, such as a ligament length corresponding to a particular knee position or externally applied loading condition, a relative strain or "elongation" value is determined. It is important to remember that a positive or negative elongation value does not specify the graft loading state.

In vivo studies of the normal ACL strain response have utilized a reference that was based on the slack-taut transition length. The reference length was selected using the "inflection point method" that was previously described (28,38) and since validated (37). The overall objective of these experiments was to obtain displacement measurements for the calculation of strain under a variety of different loading conditions, such as passive flexion–extension (muscle relaxed and motion provided by examiner) or quadriceps dominated (active) flexion–extension motion of the lower leg. Before and after each loading condition, an instrumented Lachman test was performed where anteroposterior directed shear loads were applied to the proximal tibia using a load cell while the knee was supported at 30° of knee flexion. An anterior–posterior (A/P) load was then plotted as a function of DVRT displacement (Fig. 17.2). A tangent line was drawn through the lax (or horizontal) region of the curve to determine the inflection point. The length of the DVRT that corresponded to the inflection point was used as the strain reference (L_o) (Fig. 17.2). This method of selecting a reference has been shown to correspond to the slack-taut transition of the ligament through ligament palpation (38) and objectively validated using an implantable force transducer (37).

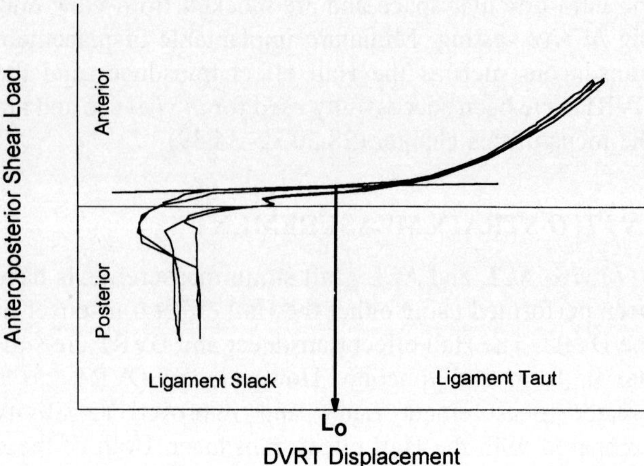

FIGURE 17.2. The slack-taut transition length of the anterior cruciate ligament (ACL) was used as a strain reference and was determined from the relationship between the anterior–posterior directed shear loads and the differential variable reluctance transducer (DVRT) output during an instrumented Lachman test. A line was drawn tangent to the lax region of the curve to mark the inflection point. The length of the transducer (L_o) corresponding to the inflection point served as the reference length. (From Fleming BC, Beynnon BD, Nichols CE, et al. An in vivo comparison between intraoperative isometric measurement and local elongation of the graft after reconstruction of the anterior cruciate ligament. *J Bone Joint Surg Am* 1994;76A:520–531, with permission.)

Unfortunately, we were unable to identify the slack taut transition of the graft (bone-patellar tendon-bone graft) during the instrumented Lachman test (30). Unlike the normal ACL, the force-strain relationship for an ACL graft is dependent on several different variables including the intra-articular graft placement and the initial tension applied to the graft at the time of fixation (65–67). These factors obscured our ability to define the slack-taut transition. Thus, without an absolute strain reference, we were unable to express the length change of the graft as absolute strain. Instead, the engineering strain formulation was employed using an anatomical reference; the length of the transducer when the knee was passively extended to 10° of flexion. It is important to note that this provided a relative strain value, which we termed "elongation" to avoid confusion with the absolute strain value. A positive elongation value refers to an increase in graft length relative to the reference position (10° passive flexion) while a negative value indicates that the graft is shorter than that of the reference position. In this chapter, graft displacement measurements are presented as elongation values instead of strain values to prevent confusion.

TEST SUBJECTS

The patient volunteers for the normal ACL strain studies were typically candidates for arthroscopic partial meniscectomy performed under local anesthesia, allowing the patients to retain full control of their musculature. Hence, a variety of different loading conditions involving the musculature were tested. Subjects had no history of knee ligament trauma, normal knee ligaments as documented by clinical examination and arthroscopic visualization, and exhibited normal range of knee motion. All patients granted their informed consent before participation. Following the knee surgery, the DVRT was implanted and the patient underwent the experimental protocols. After testing was complete the strain gage was removed.

The patients who participated in the studies of ACL graft measurement at the time of fixation were volunteers who required arthroscopically assisted surgical reconstruction of the ACL. All reconstructions were performed using a bone-patellar tendon-bone graft under epidural or spinal anesthesia. Thus, only passive loading conditions could be evaluated in the ACL graft studies. Preoperatively, the patients had no clinically detectable laxity of the posterior cruciate, medial collateral and lateral collateral ligaments. Patients with concomitant meniscal lesions were included.

ANTERIOR CRUCIATE LIGAMENT STRAIN DURING PASSIVE FLEXION–EXTENSION MOTION

After the transducer was inserted into the ACL, the patient was seated at the end of the operating table on a custom designed seat. The femur was horizontal and the tibia hung over the end of the table. Prior to recording ACL displacements during passive flexion–extension, an instrumented Lachman test was performed. This test was then repeated after the flexion–extension data was recorded. Data obtained from the Lachman tests served two functions: (a) to provide the slack-taut reference length for the strain calculation using the inflection point technique as previously described, and (b) as a repeated normal to ensure the integrity of the transducer-ligament interface. For the instrumented Lachman test, the lower leg was strapped to an adjustable t-bar that supported the knee at 30° of knee flexion. The anteroposterior shear loads were applied via a load cell to determine the relationship between shear force and ACL strain. The lower leg was then removed from the t-bar support. The examiner then supported the patient's calcaneus and flexed and extended the knee from 10° to 110°.

The mean strain response of the ACL as a function of knee flexion angle during knee extension is plotted in Figure 17.3. The minimum strain value of -4.1% occurred when the knee was at 50° of knee flexion. The negative value indicates that the ACL was slack. As the knee was passively extended, the mean strain increased to a maximum value of 0.1% ± 0.9% at 10° of flexion. Full extension was avoided to prevent transducer impingement against the roof of the intercondylar notch. As the knee

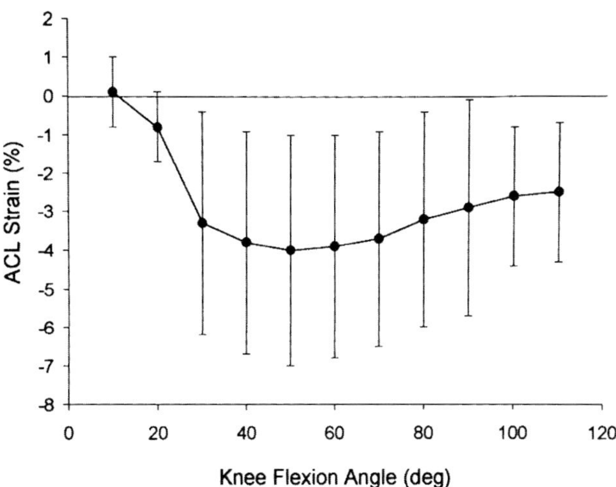

FIGURE 17.3. Average anterior cruciate ligament (ACL) strain response during passive extension of the knee (n = 10). As the knee nears extension, the strain increases. The ligament becomes load-bearing at 11° of knee flexion. (From Beynnon BD, Howe JG, Pope MH, et al. Anterior cruciate ligament strain, in vivo. *Int Orthop* 1992;16:1–12, with permission.)

approached 10°, the ACL became load bearing (a positive strain value). As the patient's limbs were flexed from the minimum strain position of 50°, the mean strain increased slightly but did not become load bearing (28).

ANTERIOR CRUCIATE LIGAMENT GRAFT ELONGATION DURING PASSIVE FLEXION–EXTENSION MOTION AT IMPLANTATION

For this study, the ACL reconstructions were performed by one of two surgeons. Patients who were operated on by surgeon one were considered group one, while those receiving treatment by surgeon two were group two. Standard arthroscopic examination of the joint was performed followed by appropriate removal of irreparable fragments of torn menisci when necessary. A standard two-incision technique was used. Eight- to 10-mm-wide ACL grafts were harvested from the central third of the patellar tendon. The graft size was dependent on the size of the patient and the tendon available. Bone blocks were removed from the tibial tubercle and patella. After the appropriate tunnels were drilled, the graft was passed through the tibial and femoral tunnels. The proximal bone block was fixed with either an interference fit screw or with three number five Mersiline sutures secured by a 6.5-mm AO cancellous bone screw and washer driven across the femur proximal to the external portion of the femoral tunnel. The surgeon tensioned the graft manually. The tension applied to the graft was not measured and was left to the clinician's judgment. At the time the study was performed, the clinicians create an A/P laxity of the knee less than that of the normal contralateral control knee to compensate for the initial stress relaxation that occurs in the graft after fixation. The distal bone block was then fixed with an interference screw in all patients. The wounds were then closed except for the arthroscopic portals, and the strain transducer was prepared for implantation.

For all study patients the initial passive flexion–extension motion cycles applied to the knee, immediately after graft fixation, produced a seating response of the graft. The seating response was defined as the change in graft length at specified knee flexion angles over the 20 flexion–extension cycles with respect to the transducer length at 10° of flexion during the first cycle. Thus, the seating behavior quantified the cyclic response by plotting the change in transducer length as a function of cycle number at specified knee flexion angles (20° and 80°). Two different cyclic responses were observed. In some patients, the cyclic response of the graft was characterized by a positive value, indicating that the length of the graft increased through the multiple cycles of passive knee motion (Fig. 17.4). Conversely, other patients produced a negatively directed cyclic response, indicating that the length of the graft decreased through the multiple cycles of passive knee motion (Fig. 17.4). In all cases, the cyclic response became asymptotic in approximately 15 cycles. Although there was a trend indicating that one of the surgeons obtained a positive cyclic response and the other a negative response, a statistical comparison indicated that there was no difference between patient groups.

A comparison of the elongation behavior of the graft during passive flexion–extension motion was also made between surgeons after the graft seating (30). For this portion of the analysis, the elongation response of the 20th cycle was referenced to the 10° of flexion position of the 20th cycle. The mean elongation patterns of the graft for the 20th cycle of passive knee motion were found to be similar between the two patient groups (Fig. 17.5). Group 2 demonstrated a greater magnitude of elongation, on average, in comparison to group 1 (Fig. 17.5). There were, however, no statistically significant differences in elongation values between groups 1 and 2.

A comparison between elongation values of the normal ACL and the ACL graft after fixation during passive flexion–extension was also performed (30). To directly compare the elongation values of the graft with those of the normal ACL, the strain values calculated for the ACL (as described previously) were recalculated using the elongation reference; which was based on the transducer length with the knee passively flexed to 10°. The mean graft elongation data, for the reconstructed patients (groups 1 and 2) were similar in pattern to that of the normal ACL. However, the overall elongations were less for the graft data (Fig. 17.5). An effective way to compare elongation values between the ACL graft and that of the normal ACL was to plot the difference in elongation values and their corresponding 95% confidence limits at common knee angles. The mean difference between the normal ACL and ACL graft elongation values was always positive, indicating that the graft demonstrated less elongation than the ACL. In addition, the 95% confidence levels were found to span zero, demonstrating that there were no significant differences between the bone-patella ten-

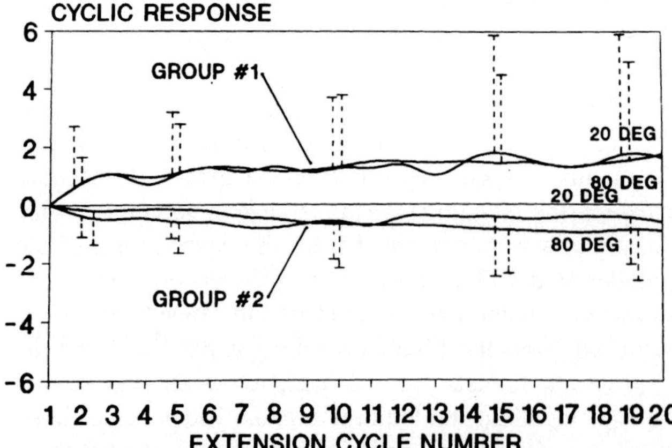

FIGURE 17.4. The mean cyclic response of the knee when the knee passed through the 20° and 80° of flexion position over the 20 initial flexion–extension cycles following graft fixation. The results are plotted for each of the two surgeons who participated in the study. (From Beynnon BD, Johnson RJ, Fleming BC, et al. The measurement of elongation of anterior cruciate ligament grafts in vivo. *J Bone Joint Surg Am* 1994;76:511–519, with permission.)

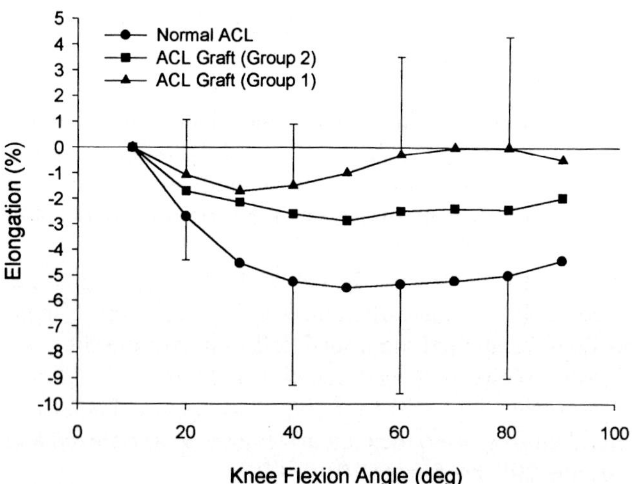

FIGURE 17.5. The elongation response of the anterior cruciate ligament (ACL) and bone-patellar tendon-bone ACL grafts (two different surgeons) during the twentieth cycle of passive knee joint extension. Error bars represent the 95% confidence intervals. There were no statistical differences between the elongation response of the normal ACL or the ACL grafts. (From Beynnon BD, Johnson RJ, Fleming BC, et al. The measurement of elongation of anterior cruciate ligament grafts in vivo. *J Bone Joint Surg Am* 1994;76:511–519, with permission.)

don-bone ACL graft and the normal ACL over the range of knee flexion angles tested.

A method that measures graft elongation can be used to determine the effectiveness of isometers at predicting graft placement (36). An isometer is a device designed to measure the change in displacement between a pair of potential tibial and femoral insertion sites during passive flexion–extension motion of the knee before drilling the actual insertion tunnels for the graft. In nine of the patients who participated in the *in vivo* investigation of the graft elongation response at the time of surgery, a commercially available isometer system was used. Comparisons were made between the graft elongation prediction of the isometer and the actual graft elongation response produced after graft implantation. From 10 to 30° of knee flexion, the isometer elongation and the local graft elongation demonstrated a similar decrease in length. However, the elongation responses deviated at flexion angles greater than 40°. On average, the isometer predicted that the length change of the graft would increase in flexion relative to extension. In contrast, the graft did not. Furthermore, there was no significant correlation between the isometer prediction and the actual graft healing response ($r^2 = 0.05$). The study demonstrated that isometers may not provide an accurate representation of the graft elongation response.

ANTERIOR CRUCIATE LIGAMENT GRAFT ELONGATION DURING PASSIVE FLEXION–EXTENSION MOTION AT FOLLOW-UP

All of the patients who participated in the ACL graft strain study at the time of fixation were invited back for voluntary arthroscopic surgery. It was our intent to reapply the displacement transducer on the graft 1 year following the original reconstructive procedure. Seven subjects agreed to participate in this study. All subjects underwent a moderately aggressive rehabilitation program and returned to full activity within 1 year.

Second look arthroscopy was performed and the transducer was reattached to the healed graft in the approximate location of the first measurement. A comparison of the 1-year postoperative elongation data during passive flexion–extension motion was made to that obtained immediately following graft fixation during the reconstruction surgery. The mean difference between elongation values at both time intervals and the corresponding 95% confidence limits at each knee flexion angle were calculated and plotted.

Across all knee flexion angles, the local elongation behavior of the graft at the time of implantation was not significantly different in comparison to the local elongation response measured at the 1-year follow-up ($p < 0.1$) (Fig. 17.6). Although not statistically significant, there was a trend suggesting that the remodeling process of the

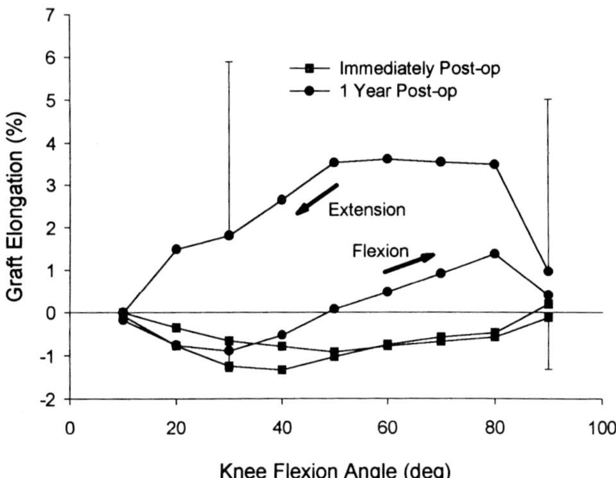

FIGURE 17.6. Elongation response of the bone-patellar tendon-bone graft during passive flexion–extension motion of the knee at the time of anterior cruciate ligament (ACL) reconstruction and 1 year after surgery (n = 7). There was a trend indicating that the elongation response changed over time.

graft could potentially change its elongation pattern. Furthermore, there was an increase in the hysteresis between the elongation values produced during flexion–extension motion.

Although it is not possible to make definitive conclusions from this study due to the low sample size, it appears that the graft remodeling process and rehabilitation may initiate changes in the healing ACL graft. On average, there was greater graft elongation evident in the 1-year follow-up data compared with that of the time of surgery. This result may explain in part the common clinical finding of an increase in anterior translation of the tibia with respect to the femur that results during the ACL graft healing period. The 1-year follow-up data also have a greater variability associated with the elongation patterns than those recorded immediately after graft fixation. This may be attributed to differences in intra-articular graft placement, initial graft tension, and the variability associated with rehabilitation noncompliance during rehabilitation. This study suggests that remodeling may play an important role in graft biomechanics and hence the outcome of ACL reconstructive surgery.

RELATIONSHIP BETWEEN GRAFT ELONGATION AND ANTERIOR–POSTERIOR KNEE LAXITY

The elongation response of the graft is an important parameter of ACL reconstruction. We performed a clinical follow-up of the patients who participated in the study involving the elongation measurements of the bone-patellar tendon-bone ACL graft immediately following surgical reconstruction (30,40). In 19 of the subjects, the antero-

TABLE 17.1. *Outcome measures of the patients whose initial elongation values fell within the 95% confidence intervals of the normal ACL (group 1) compared with those who fell outside the 95% confidence intervals (group 2)*

Outcome	Group 1	Group 2	p
Postoperative KT-1000	−2.6 (0.7) mm	−1.7 (1.0) mm	0.49
Follow-up KT-1000	1.2 (0.7) mm	4.7 (0.6) mm	0.004
Lysholm score	99.7 (0.3)	98.6 (1.3)	0.43
Tegner score	5.3 (0.9)	5.3 (0.7)	0.97
One-legged hop test	5.6 (5.8) cm	−1.8 (2.2) cm	0.60

The KT-1000 and one-legged hop test values are presented as injured minus the contralateral control knee. Numbers in parentheses are standard deviations.

posterior knee laxity of both knees were measured immediately following the surgical procedure using the KT-1000 Knee Arthrometer (MedMetrics, San Diego, CA) to document the initial laxity conditions achieved by the reconstructive procedure. Fifteen of the 19 subjects returned at a mean of 62 months (range, 58–69 months) for a follow-up examination. Two of the 15 subjects were excluded from further analysis because they had injured the ACL of their normal control knee since their surgical procedure was performed. At the 5-year follow-up visit, the KT-1000 was used to measure the A/P laxity of both knees. In addition the Lysholm, Tegner, and one-legged hop test were performed to determine the functional ability and activity level of the subject at the 5-year follow-up.

Subjects were divided into two groups by comparing the elongation values of the graft with that of the normal ACL as previously described. The first group (n=6) comprised those subjects in which the graft elongation pattern fell within the 95% confidence intervals of the normal ACL elongation pattern. The second group consisted of patients whose graft elongation patterns fell outside those confidence intervals. Immediately following surgical reconstruction, the A/P laxity values of both groups were similar (Table 17.1). The bone-patellar tendon-bone grafts whose elongation values at the time of surgery closely matched those of the normal ACL had A/P laxity values that were similar to the contralateral normal knee (side to side difference of 1.2 mm). In contrast, A/P laxity values of the knees whose ACL graft elongation patterns fell outside the confidence limits of the ACL demonstrated significantly greater A/P laxity values in comparison to that of the contralateral side at the 5-year follow-up (side to side difference of 4.7 mm). There were no differences in Lysholm, Tegner, and one-legged hop test scores between the two patient groups (Table 17.1). These observations support our previous findings using the canine model (68).

ANTERIOR CRUCIATE LIGAMENT STRAIN DURING REHABILITATION EXERCISES

Ideally, it would be interesting to measure graft strain during different rehabilitation activities that are commonly prescribed following ACL reconstruction. Although the strain values that are detrimental to graft healing remain unknown, strain data obtained during different rehabilitation exercises would determine which activities produce high strain values on the graft and those that do not. These data would be essential in developing aggressive and conservative rehabilitation programs that could then be used to design prospective, randomized studies of ACL graft rehabilitation programs to determine the optimal treatment. Because the graft displacement measurements must be taken immediately following the reconstructive procedure, the patient would be at risk of graft failure. At the time of graft implantation, the forces applied to the graft would be supported at the fixation site, which has been shown to be significantly weaker than the graft itself (69,70). Also, it would be difficult to perform the reconstructive surgery under local anesthesia. However, insight into graft strain values may be obtained by evaluating the strain response of the normal ACL during different rehabilitation activities. These data could then be transferred to the ACL graft with the following two assumptions: the displacement response of the ACL graft is similar to that of the normal ACL, and the graft is correctly positioned within the knee and tensioned appropriately.

Following a similar ACL strain measurement protocol that was previously described for passive flexion–extension motion, various rehabilitation activities were evaluated and compared (28). These data were then rank-ordered by peak ACL strain values (Table 17.2). These include the quadriceps-dominated activities, hamstring-dominated activities, and exercises that involve quadriceps and hamstring muscles co-contraction with and without weight bearing.

We have found that exercises that produce low ACL values are dominated by the hamstring muscle group (isometric hamstring muscle contraction) (Fig. 17.7), incorporate contraction of the quadriceps muscle group with the knee flexed at 60° or greater (isometric contraction of the quadriceps, simultaneous quadriceps and hamstrings contraction) (Fig. 17.7), or involve active flexion–extension of the knee between 35° and 90° (Fig. 17.8). Quadriceps dominated activities with the knee between 50° and full extension strain the ACL (Fig. 17.9). Active extension of the knee produced by contraction of the dominant quadriceps muscles produce substantial increases in ACL strain values.

TABLE 17.2. *Rank comparison of peak ACL strain values during commonly prescribed rehabilitation activities (mean ± 1 standard deviation)*

Rehabilitation activity	Peak strain	Number of subjects
Isometric quads contraction at 15° (30 Nm extension torque)	4.4 (0.6)%	8
Squatting with sport cord	4.0 (1.7)%	8
Active flexion-extension of the knee with 45 N weight boot	3.8 (0.5)%	9
Lachman test (150 N of anterior shear load; 30° flexion)	3.7 (0.8)%	10
Squatting	3.6 (1.3)%	8
Active flexion-extension (no weight boot) of the knee	2.8 (0.8)%	18
Simultaneous quads and hams contraction at 15°	2.8 (0.9)%	8
Isometric quads contraction at 30° (30 Nm of extension torque)	2.7 (0.5)%	18
Anterior drawer (150 Nm of anterior shear load; 90° flexion)	1.8 (0.9)%	10
Stationary bicycling	1.7 (1.9)%	8
Isometric hams contraction at 15° (to 10 Nm of flexion torque)	0.6 (0.9)%	8
Simultaneous quads and hams contraction at 30°	0.4 (0.5)%	8
Passive flexion-extension of the knee	0.1 (0.9)%	10
Isometric quads contraction at 60° (30 Nm of extension torque)	0.0%	8
Isometric quads contraction at 90° (30 Nm of extension torque)	0.0%	18
Simultaneous quads and hams contraction at 60°	0.0%	8
Simultaneous quads and hams contraction at 90°	0.0%	8
Isometric hams contraction at 30°, 60°, and 90° (to -10 Nm of flexion torque)	0.0%	8

From Fleming BC, Beynnon BD, Renstrom PA, et al. The strain behavior of the anterior cruciate ligament during bicycling: an in vivo study. *Am J Sports Med* 1998;26:109–118, with permission.

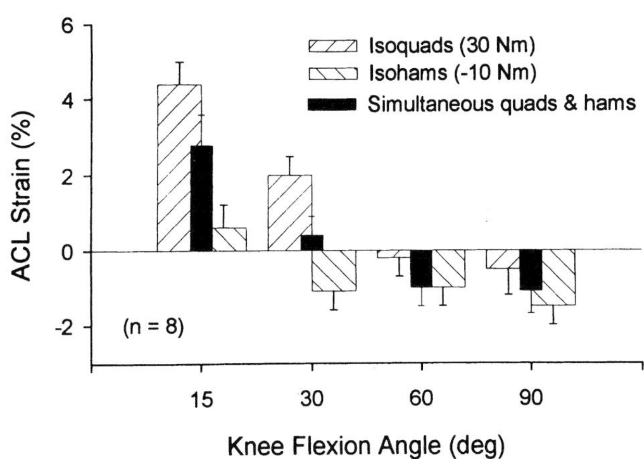

FIGURE 17.7. The mean anterior cruciate ligament (ACL) strain response created by isometric contraction of the quadriceps (isoquads), isometric contraction of the hamstrings (isohams), and simultaneous contraction of the quadriceps and hamstrings (simultaneous quads and hams). An isometric quadriceps contraction which produced a 30 N torque produced significant ACL strain values (relative to the relaxed state) when the knee was flexed to 15° and 30° but did not strain the ACL at 60° and 90° of flexion. Isometric contraction of the hamstrings that produced a flexion moment of –10 N did not significantly strain the ACL at any flexion angle tested. Simultaneous contraction of the quadriceps and hamstrings strained the ACL at 15° but not at 30°, 60°, or 90° of knee flexion. The mean strain produced at 15° was less than that produced during the pure isometric quadriceps contraction. (From Beynnon BD, Fleming BC, Peura GD, et al. An *in vivo* investigation of anterior cruciate ligament strain: The effect of functional knee bracing and attachment strap tension. *Trans Orthop Res Soc* 1995;20:1994, with permission.)

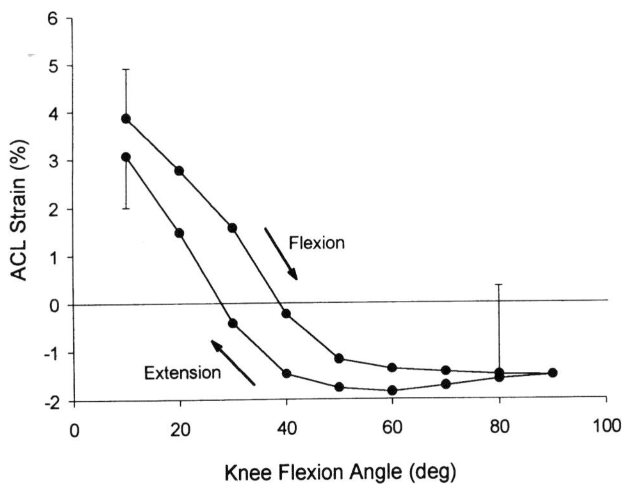

FIGURE 17.8. Knee extension motion produced by contraction of the dominant quadriceps muscle group (active extension) strained the anterior cruciate ligament (ACL) from approximately 35° to near full extension. The ACL was not strained from 35° to 90° of flexion. (From Beynnon BD, Johnson RJ, Fleming BC, et al. The strain behavior of the anterior cruciate ligament during squatting and active flexion-extension: a comparison of an open- and a closed-kinetic-chain exercise. *Am J Sports Med* 1997;25:823–829, with permission.)

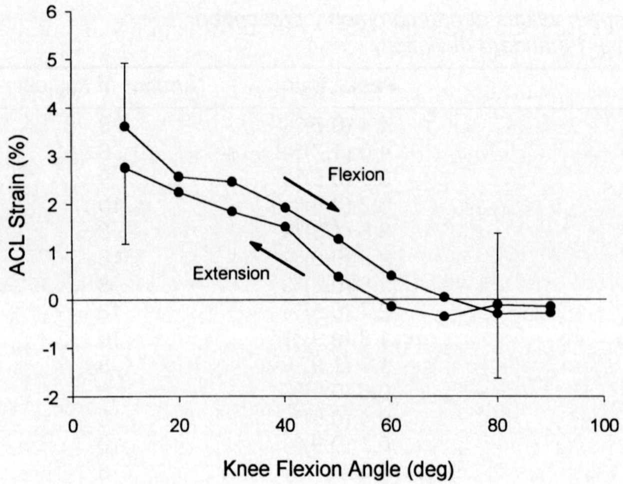

FIGURE 17.9. The mean anterior cruciate ligament (ACL) strain values produced during a simple squat. As the knee was extended the ACL became strained from 55° to near full extension.

More recently, we determined that the maximum ACL strain values produced during squatting; a closed-kinetic-chain exercise, are similar to those produced during active flexion–extension of the knee (Fig. 17.9); an open-kinetic-chain exercise. The similarity of ACL strain response during these two common rehabilitation exercises calls into question whether or not we should consider exercises to be either safe or unsafe based on the commonly used closed- and open-kinetic-chain terminology during rehabilitation of an ACL graft (33). In addition, we determined that ACL strain values produced by squatting were unaltered with the application of an elastic resistance (the Sport Cord) that increased the muscle activity about the knee (33). This finding demonstrates that increasing resistance with the Sport Cord (producing a moderate increase in muscle activity) to strengthen the leg muscles during the squat exercise does not necessarily produce a significant increase in ACL strain values. This is in contrast to our earlier investigations that revealed increasing resistance during open-kinetic-chain active flexion–extension of the leg created a significant increase in ACL strain values (41).

The safe limits of ACL graft strain during healing are currently unknown; therefore it is not possible to identify which exercises are safe or harmful to a healing graft. However, the peak strain values produced during the quadriceps-dominated exercises (Table 17.2) could conceivably produce damaging effects if used too early during rehabilitation, if they are performed at improper knee flexion angles, or if they are advanced to more challenging levels of muscle contraction.

DISCUSSION

The DVRT has been shown to be an accurate means to measure the strain and elongation biomechanics of both the normal ACL and bone-patellar tendon-bone ACL grafts, respectively. The DVRT is an ideal tool for strain measurement since it attaches directly to the soft tissue, it can be easily calibrated on the bench top, and is applicable to testing both the ACL or ACL graft.

The first *in vivo* elongation measurements of grade II ACL sprains were performed by Henning et al. (45) in two patients. A hooked wire probe was secured to the ACL approximately 1 cm from the tibial insertion. The wire was inserted through a tube that was rigidly fixed to the tibia. The displacement of the wire relative to the tube was measured using a displacement gage. As the two patients performed different activities of daily living and commonly prescribed rehabilitation exercises the displacement of the wire within the tube was recorded. The authors did not attempt to report absolute strain values. They normalized their ACL displacement data by assigning 100 units to the change in wire position in response to a 350 N anterior directed load applied to the proximal tibia. The elongation values of all other rehabilitation activities that they tested were reported relative to this scale. Although a direct comparison between the elongation values reported in their study to those measured using the DVRT is limited due to differences in ACL status, measurement techniques, and activities tested, the same general rank ordering of values was obtained as those listed in Table 17.2. In an attempt to measure ACL force, Henning et al (45) also recorded the deflection of the bone immediately beneath the tibial insertion of the ACL by drilling out a tunnel beneath the ACL attachment site in one of the patients. Unfortunately, these procedures were only applied to two patients who had severely damaged ACLs and were candidates for arthroscopic reconstruction. This was the first successful attempt at measuring the biomechanical response of the ACL *in vivo*.

Several attempts have been made to measure either the ACL or ACL graft force, *in vivo*. In 1994, Roberts et al. (71) used the arthroscopically implantable force transducer (AIFP) to measure ACL force in a patient with a normal ACL. The AIFP is a sensor that is implanted between the fibers of the ACL. The device works on the following principle. As a tensile force is applied to the ligament, the fibers that are deflected about the sensor place a compressive load on the device. Unfortunately, it was not possible to directly calibrate the ACL force to the transducer output. The investigators indirectly calibrated the AIFP using data derived from cadaveric specimens. The relationships between AIFP output and ligament force were described using regression analysis on a set of cadaveric specimens where ligaments could be cut to isolate the ligament *in situ*. However, there are several problems inherent to implantable force transducers and their calibration (71–78). These include the sensitivities of implantable force transducers to transducer placement and orientation, transducer size, flexion angle dependencies, temperature sensitivity, and reproducibility problems with repeated transducer application within the same tissue. During passive extension motion, Roberts and associates determined that the ACL was unloaded from 90° to approximately 15° of flexion. From 15° to full extension, the force increased linearly from 0 N to approximately 100 N in one patient. These data are similar to our strain data obtained during passive flexion–extension where the ACL became load bearing at a mean flexion angle of 10° (28).

Shino et al. (26) measured the forces produced in a hamstring tendon graft using an extra-articular approach. Before fixing the graft to the tibia, the distal end of the graft was attached to a load cell via sutures. The load cell was then mounted to the proximal calf via an ankle brace. Limitations of this technique were the skewed alignment of the measurement axis of the transducer with the axis of the graft, no accountability for the friction losses at the bone-tunnel interface, and the compliance of the sutures and soft tissue connections of the graft to the load cell and the load cell to the ankle. During passive flexion–extension motion of the knee, they reported a mean maximum increase of 18 N as the knee was brought into extension. Only the peak force value was presented. The greatest strains measured during passive flexion–extension in our study also occurred at full extension. During these experiments, the patients were awakened from the general anesthesia and asked to walk. Peak forces of 84 ± 28 N were recorded during gait (26).

At the University of California, Wallace et al. (27) used four extraarticular load cells to measure the forces, *in vivo*, in each band of a quadrupled stranded hamstrings tendon graft during passive flexion–extension of the knee. They used an improved force measurement technique that aligned the measurement axis of the load cell with the long axes of each strand. They also reduced the length of the sutures that were required to connected the graft strands to the load cells which would improve accuracy by reducing suture line compliance. They reported a mean peak graft tension value of 142 ± 59 N as the knee was passively brought into full extension. They also reported a slight increase in graft force relative to the minimum at 30° of flexion as the knee was flexed to 90°. The strain patterns recorded for the patellar tendon graft in our study were similar to the force patterns observed in the semitendinosus graft. The investigators are currently developing a load cell that is incorporated into the femoral fixation device that will measure graft force after fixation, which will eliminate the effects of a compliant graft-transducer interface and errors due to tunnel friction (79). As yet, no *in vivo* data have been reported using this technology.

The DVRT provides an efficient way to measure ACL strain and ACL graft elongation. It is limited, however, to measuring soft tissue displacements in the anteromedial band of the ACL or anterior aspect of the ACL graft. Unfortunately, it is not possible to attach the DVRT to other regions of the ACL without disrupting or cutting other structures. Although it would be interesting to measure ACL strain value in multiple regions of the ACL or ACL graft, we believe that the measurements of the anterior bundle are sufficient. Surgeons generally strive to recreate the function of the anteromedial band of the ACL when performing a reconstructive procedure (14).

It should be noted that the strain data of the "normal" ACL were acquired from patients who were undergoing arthroscopic meniscectomy under local anesthesia. Using clinical examination techniques, the function of the knee was determined normal except for meniscal pathology. It was assumed that the meniscectomy should have little effect on the ligament strains since previous cadaver studies have shown that a meniscectomy in an ACL intact knee has little effect on knee joint kinematics (80–82). It has also been shown that local anesthesia has little effect on knee joint proprioception (83). These investigations suggest that the normal knee assumption for our normal subjects is appropriate.

It is currently not possible to convert the strain or elongation values established in these *in vivo* studies to force magnitudes. Although strain values can distinguish between the loaded and unloaded state, it is inappropriate to predict ligament forces from the strain values. The material properties of the graft have been shown to vary along ACL fibers and between the fibers. The moduli near the insertion sites were less than the midsubstance (84). The moduli in the anterior bundle have also been shown to be greater than the posterior bundle (55,85). Thus, a constitutive equation relating strain to stress would be extremely complicated and would have to be based on several geometrical parameters. Furthermore, the load distribution across the cross section of the ACL is not constant. The load-bearing portion of the ACL changes with knee joint motion. Thus, the effective load bearing area of the ligament would remain unknown. Even if the stress were known, it would not be possible to calculate the force. The elongation values reported here have the same limitations. The problem of relating force to graft elongation is exacerbated since elongation values do not differentiate between the loaded and unloaded graft.

An increase in variability was noted for the ACL grafts as compared with the normal ACL. This increase was expected due to the potential increase in variables that would effect graft tension due to the operative procedure. A recent evaluation of the accuracy and repeatability of the DVRT indicated that errors up to 30% were introduced to the displacement measurements by removing and reinserting the DVRT into a tissue (86). We controlled these sources of variability by making measurements without removing the DVRT from the tissue within each subject. However, this error may influence the comparison between the ACL graft elongation measurements taken at the time of surgical reconstruction and those at the 1-year postoperative follow-up visits. Despite the increase in variability, a trend was observed between the elongation values between time points that suggests that changes in the biomechanical elongation response of the graft is possible due to rehabilitation and remodeling. Unfortunately, additional patients were not willing to participate in the second look arthroscopy. Further research is necessary to determine the impact of rehabilitation on graft healing. This can only be done through carefully controlled, prospective, randomized clinical studies.

CONCLUSIONS

The DVRT provides an accurate means to measure elongation in the bone-patellar tendon-bone ACL graft during passive flexion–extension motion of the knee.

Immediately after fixation, the graft exhibited a seating response over the first 15 passive flexion–extension cycles of the knee. By the 20th cycle, the elongation response of the knee was reproducible.

Commercially available isometers do not provide an accurate prediction of the graft elongation response.

At the time of reconstruction, there was no significant difference in elongation values between the bone-patellar tendon-bone ACL grafts and that of the normal ACL.

There was a trend indicating that the initial graft elongation response (immediately following graft implantation) changed over time during the healing process. A change in elongation pattern and hysteresis were observed 1 year following the surgical procedure. These data may support the increase in laxity that is observed over time in many subjects following ACL reconstruction.

Patients who demonstrate an elongation response that fell outside the 95% confidence intervals of the normal ACL at the time of implantation demonstrated a much greater increase in knee laxity five years following the surgical procedure than those patients whose elongation patterns were within the 95% confidence intervals.

Quadriceps-dominated rehabilitation activities produced high strains on the ACL (and therefore the ACL graft) when the knee was flexed between 50° and full extension.

Hamstrings dominated rehabilitation activities produced low or no strains on the ACL (and hence the ACL graft) over the entire range of flexion–extension motion.

Activities involving co-contraction of the hamstrings and quadriceps muscle groups reduced but did not necessarily eliminate ACL strain. No distinction was found between the strain values produced when comparing open kinetic chain exercises with closed kinetic chain exercises.

ACKNOWLEDGMENTS

This work was supported by the National Institutes of Health, grant nos. AR39213 and AR40174; the Department of Orthopaedics and Rehabilitation at the University of Vermont, Burlington VT; and the Department of Orthopaedics, Sports Medicine and Arthroscopy at the Karolinska Institute, Stockholm Sweden.

REFERENCES

1. Hirshman HP, Daniel DM, Miyasaka KC. The fate of unoperated knee ligament injuries. In: Daniel D, AkesonW, O'Connor J, eds. *Knee ligaments: structure, function, injury, and repair.* New York: Raven Press, 1990:481–503.
2. Noyes FR, Mathews CS, Mooar PA, et al. The symptomatic anterior cruciate deficient knee. Part 2: the results of rehabilitation, activity modification, and counseling on functional disability. *J Bone Joint Surg Am* 1983;65:163–174.
3. Fetto JF, Marshall JL. The natural history and diagnosis of anterior cruciate ligament insufficiency. *Clin Orthop* 1980;147:29–38.
4. Hawkins RJ, Misamore GW, Merritt TR. Follow-up of the acute nonoperated isolated anterior cruciate ligament tear. *Am J Sports Med* 1986;14:205–210.
5. Hefti FL, Kress I, Fasel J, et al. Healing of the transected anterior cruciate ligament in the rabbit. *J Bone Joint Surg Am* 1991;73:373–383.
6. Kannus P, Jarvinen M. Conservatively treated tears of the anterior cruciate ligament. Long term results. *J Bone Joint Surg Am* 1987;69A:1007–1012.
7. Kannus P, Jarvinen M. Post traumatic anterior cruciate ligament insufficiency as a cause for osteoarthritic in a knee joint. *Clin Rheumatol* 1989;8:251–260.
8. Liljedahl S, Nordstrand A. Injuries to the ligaments of the knee. *Injury* 1969;2:17–24.
9. McDaniel WJ, Dameron TB. The untreated anterior cruciate ligament rupture. *Clin Orthop* 1983;172:90–92.
10. Roos H, Adalberth T, Dahlberg L, et al. Osteoarthritis of the knee after injury to the anterior cruciate ligament or meniscus: the influence of time and age. *Osteoarthritis Cartilage* 1995;3:261–267.
11. Roos H, Lauren M, Adalberth T, et al. Knee osteoarthritis after meniscectomy: prevalence of radiographic changes after twenty-one years, compared with matched controls. *Arthritis Rheum* 1998;41:687–693.
12. Sommerlath K, Lysholm M, Gillquist J. The long term course after treatment of cute anterior cruciate ligament rupture: a 9-16 year follow-up. *Am J Sports Med* 1991;19:156–162.
13. Brandt KD, Braunstein EM, Visco DM, et al. Anterior (cranial) cruciate ligament transection in the dog: a bona fide model of osteoarthritis, not merely of cartilage injury and repair. *J Rheumatol* 1991;18:436–446.
14. Johnson RJ, Beynnon BD, Nichols CE, et al. The treatment of injuries of the anterior cruciate ligament. *J Bone Joint Surg Am* 1992;74A:140–151.
15. Seto JL, Orofino AS, Morrissey MC, et al. Assessment of quadriceps/hamstring strength, knee ligament stability, functional and sports activity levels five years after anterior cruciate ligament reconstruction. *Am J Sports Med* 1988;16:170–180.
16. Wilk KE, Romaniello WT, Soscia SM, et al. The relationship between subjective knee scores, isokinetic testing, and functional testing in the ACL-reconstructed knee. *J Orthop Sports Phys Ther* 1994;20:60–73.
17. Johnson RJ, Eriksson E, Haggmark T, et al. Five- to ten-year follow-up evaluation after reconstruction of the anterior cruciate ligament. *Clin Orthop* 1984:122–140.
18. Howe JG, Johnson RJ, Kaplan MJ, et al. Anterior cruciate ligament reconstruction using quadriceps patellar tendon graft. Part I. Long-term followup. *Am J Sports Med* 1991;19:447–462.
19. Paschal SO, Stone KR, Steadman JR. Changes in knee stability after bone-patellar tendon-bone graft anterior cruciate ligament reconstruction and iliotibial band tenodesis. *Am J Knee Surg* 1991;4:173–178.
20. Shelbourne KD, Nitz P. Accelerated rehabilitation after anterior cruciate ligament reconstruction. *Am J Sports Med* 1990;18:292–299.
21. Wachtl SW, Imhoff A. Retrospective comparison of four intra-articular anterior cruciate ligament reconstructions using three evaluation systems. *Arch Orthop Trauma Surg* 1994;114:25–31.
22. Daniel DM, Stone ML, Dobson BE, et al. Fate of the ACL-injured patient: a prospective outcome study. *Am J Sports Med* 1994;22:632–644.
23. Fink C, Hoser C, Benedetto KP. Development of arthrosis after rupture of the anterior cruciate ligament. A comparison of surgical and conservative therapy. *Unfallchirurg* 1994;97:357–361.

24. Markolf KL, Gorek JF, Kabo JM, et al. Direct measurement of resultant forces in the anterior cruciate ligament. *J Bone Joint Surg Am* 1990;72:557–567.

25. Zavatsky AB, O'Connor JJ. A model of human knee ligaments in the sagittal plane. Part I.: Response to passive flexion. *J Engineering Med* 1992;206:125–134.

26. Shino K, Hamada M, Tanaka M, et al. In vivo direct measurement of load applied to ACL grafts. *Trans Orthop Res Soc* 1993;18:2.

27. Wallace MP, Howell SM, Hull ML. In vivo tensile behavior of a four-bundle hamstring graft as a replacement for the anterior cruciate ligament. *J Orthop Res* 1997;15:539–545.

28. Beynnon BD, Howe JG, Pope MH, et al. Anterior cruciate ligament strain, in vivo. *Int Orthop* 1992;16:1–12.

29. Beynnon BD, Pope MH, Wertheimer CM, et al. The effect of functional knee braces on anterior cruciate ligament strain, in vivo. *J Bone Jt Surg Am* 1992;74:1298–1312.

30. Beynnon BD, Johnson RJ, Fleming BC, et al. The measurement of elongation of anterior cruciate ligament grafts in vivo. *J Bone Joint Surg Am* 1994;76:511–519.

31. Beynnon BD, Fleming BC, Peura GD, et al. An *in vivo* investigation of anterior cruciate ligament strain: The effect of functional knee bracing and attachment strap tension. *Trans Orthop Res Soc* 1995;20:1994.

32. Beynnon BD, Johnson RJ, Fleming BC, et al. The effect of functional knee bracing on the anterior cruciate ligament in the weight bearing and non-weight bearing knee. *Am J Sports Med* 1997;25:353–359.

33. Beynnon BD, Johnson RJ, Fleming BC, et al. The strain behavior of the anterior cruciate ligament during squatting and active flexion-extension: a comparison of an open- and a closed-kinetic-chain exercise. *Am J Sports Med* 1997;25:823–829.

34. Fleming BC, Beynnon BD, Renstrom PA, et al. The strain behavior of the anterior cruciate ligament during bicycling: an in vivo study. *Am J Sports Med* 1998;26:109–118.

35. Fleming BC, Beynnon BD, Nichols CE, et al. An in vivo comparison of anterior tibial translation and strain in the anteromedial band of the anterior cruciate ligament (ACL). *J Biomech* 1993;26:51–58.

36. Fleming BC, Beynnon BD, Nichols CE, et al. An in vivo comparison between intra-operative isometric measurement and local elongation of the graft after reconstruction of the anterior cruciate ligament. *J Bone Joint Surg Am* 1994;76A:520–531.

37. Fleming BC, Beynnon BD, Tohyama H, et al. The determination of a zero strain reference for the anteromedial band of the anterior cruciate ligament. *J Orthop Res* 1994;12:789–795.

38. Howe JG, Wertheimer CM, Johnson RJ, et al. Arthroscopic strain gauge measurement of the normal anterior cruciate ligament. *Arthrosc J Arthrosc Relat Surg* 1990;6:198–204.

39. Beynnon BD, Fleming BC, Johnson RJ, et al. Anterior cruciate ligament graft elongation at the time of implantation and one year post-operatively. *Trans Orthop Res Soc* 1994;19:612.

40. Uh BS, Beynnon BD, Johnson RJ, et al. The elongation behavior of the anterior cruciate ligament graft in vivo: a long term follow-up study. *Trans Orthop Res Soc* 1998;23:68.

41. Beynnon BD, Fleming BC, Johnson RJ, et al. Anterior cruciate ligament strain behavior during rehabilitation exercises *in vivo*. *Am J Sports Med* 1995;23:24–34.

42. Berns GS, Hull ML, Patterson HA. Strain in the anteromedial bundle of the anterior cruciate ligament under combined loading conditions. *J Orthop Res* 1992;10:167–176.

43. Arms SW, Pope MH, Johnson RJ, et al. The biomechanics of anterior cruciate ligament rehabilitation. *Am J Sports Med* 1984;12:8–18.

44. Durselen L, Claes L, Kiefer H. The influence of muscle forces and external loads on cruciate ligament strain. *Am J Sports Med* 1995;23:129–136.

45. Henning CE, Lynch MA, Glick KR. An in vivo strain gage study of elongation of the anterior cruciate ligament. *Am J Sports Med* 1985;13:22–26.

46. Draganich LF, Vahey JW. An in vitro study of anterior cruciate ligament strain induced by quadriceps and hamstrings forces. *J Orthop Res* 1990;8:57–63.

47. Brown TD, Sigal L, Njus GO, et al. Dynamic performance characteristics of the liquid metal strain guage. *J Biomech* 1986;19:165–173.

48. Edwards RG, Lafferty JF, Lange KO. Ligament strain in the human knee joint. *J Basic Engineering* 1970:131–136.

49. Kennedy JC, Haskins RJ, Willis RB. Strain gauge analysis of knee ligaments. *Clin Orthop* 1977;129:225–229.

50. Kurosawa H, Yamakoshi K-I, Yasuda K, et al. Simultaneous measurement of changes in length of the cruciate ligaments during knee motion. *Clin Orthop* 1991;265:233–240.

51. Hefzy MS, Grood ES. Sensitivity of insertion locations on length patterns of anterior cruciate ligament fibers. *J Biomech Eng* 1986;108:73–82.

52. Sidles JA, Larson RV, Garbini JL, et al. Ligament length relationships in the moving knee. *J Orthop Res* 1988;6:593–610.

53. Wang CJ, Walker PS, Wolf B. The effects of flexion and rotation on the length patterns of the ligaments of the knee. *J Biomech* 1973;6:587–596.

54. Warren LF, Marshall JL, Girgis F. The prime static stabilizer of the medial side of the knee. *J Bone Joint Surg Am* 1974;56:665–674.

55. Butler DL, Kay MD, Stouffer DC. Comparison of material properties in fascicle-bone units from human patellar tendon and knee ligaments. *J Biomech* 1986;19:425–432.

56. Mutchler W, Burri C, Claes L. Dept. of Traumatology, University of Ulm, West Germany, 1979.

57. White AA, Raphael IG. The effect of quadriceps loads and knee position on strain measurements of the tibial collateral ligament. *Acta Orthop Scand* 1972;43:176.

58. Butler DL, Martin ET, Kaiser AD, et al. The effects of flexion and tibial rotation on the 3-D orientations and lengths of human anterior cruciate ligament bundles. *Trans Orthop Res Soc* 1988;13:59.

59. Weiss JA, France EP, Bagley AM, et al. Measurement of 2-D strains in ligament under uniaxial tension. *Trans Orthop Res Soc* 1992;17:662.

60. Woo SL-Y, Gomez MA, Seguchi Y, et al. Measurement of mechanical properties of ligament substance from a bone-ligament-bone preparation. *J Orthop Res* 1983;1:22–29.

61. Woo SL-Y, Hollis JM, Adams DJ, et al. Tensile properties of the human femur-anterior cruciate ligament-tibia complex: the effect of specimen age and orientation. *Am J Sports Med* 1991;19:217–225.

62. Fischer RA, Arms SW, Johnson RJ, et al. The functional relationship between the posterior oblique ligament to the medial collateral ligament of the knee. *Am J Sports Med* 1985;13:390.

63. Renstrom P, Arms SW, Stanwyck TS, et al. Strain within the anterior cruciate ligament during hamstring and quadriceps activity. *Am J Sports Med* 1986;14:83–87.

64. Beynnon BD, Fleming BC. Anterior cruciate ligament strain in-vivo: A review of previous work. *J Biomech* 1998;31:519–525.

65. Bylski-Austrow DI, Grood ES, Hefzy MS, et al. Anterior cruciate ligament replacements: A mechanical study of femoral attachment location, flexion angle at tensioning, and initial tension. *J Orthop Res* 1990;8:522–531.

66. Penner DA, Daniel DM, Wood P, et al. An in vitro study of anterior cruciate ligament graft placement and isometry. *Am J Sports Med* 1988;16:238–243.

67. Fleming BC, Beynnon BD, McLeod WD, et al. Effect of tension and placement of a prosthetic anterior cruciate ligament on the anteroposterior laxity of the knee. *J Orthop Res* 1992;10:177–186.

68. Beynnon BD, Johnson RJ, Tohyama H, et al. The relationship between anterior-posterior knee laxity and the structural properties of the patellar tendon graft. A study in canines. *Am J Sports Med* 1994;22:812–820.

69. Kurosaka M, Yoshiya S, Andrish JT. A biomechanical comparison of different surgical techniques of graft fixation in anterior cruciate ligament reconstruction. *Am J Sports Med* 1987;15:225–229.

70. Daniel DM, Robertson DB, Flood DL, et al. Soft tissue fixation to bone. *Am J Sports Med* 1986;14:398–403.

71. Roberts CS, Cummings JF, Grood ES, et al. In vivo measurement of human anterior cruciate ligament forces during knee extension exercises. *Trans Orthop Res Soc* 1994;19:84.

72. Fleming BC, Good L, Peura GD, et al. Calibration and application of an intra-articular force transducer for the measurement of patellar tendon graft forces: An in situ evaluation. *J Biomech Eng* 1999;121:393–398.

73. Rupert M, Grood E, Byczkowski T, et al. Influence of sensor size on the accuracy of in vivo ligament and tendon force measurements. *J Biomech Eng* 1998;120:764–769.

74. Herzog W, Archambault JM, Leonard TR, et al. Evaluation of the implantable force transducer for chronic tendon-force recordings. *J Biomech* 1996;29:103–109.

75. Herzog W, Hasler EM, Leonard TR. In-situ calibration of the implantable force transducer. *J Biomech* 1996;29:1649–1652.

76. Holden JP, Grood ES, Cummings JF. Factors affecting sensitivity of a transducer for measuring anterior cruciate ligament force. *J Biomech* 1995;28:99–102.

77. Markolf KL, Willems MJ, Jackson SR, et al. In situ calibration of miniature sensors implanted into the anterior cruciate ligament part II: force probe measurements. *J Orthop Res* 1998;16:464—471.

78. Peura GD, Fleming BC, Beynnon BD. Measurement of load in soft tissue with the Arthroscopically Implantable Force Probe. Presented at the 2nd Combined Meeting of the Orthopaedic Research Societies, November 6–8, 1995, San Diego.

79. Ventura CP, Wolchak J, Hull ML, et al. An implantable transducer for measuring tension in an anterior cruciate ligament graft. *J Biomech Eng* 1998;120:327–333.

80. Bargar WL, Moreland JR, Markolf KL, et al. In vivo stability testing of post meniscectomy knees. *Clin Orthop* 1980;150:247–252.

81. Levy IM, Torzilli PA, Gould JD. The effect of lateral meniscectomy on motion of the knee. *J Bone Joint Surg Am* 1989;71:401–406.

82. Levy IM, Torzilli PA, Warren RF. The effect of medial meniscectomy on anterior-posterior motion of the knee. *J Bone Joint Surg Am* 1982;64:883–888.

83. Barrack RL, Skinner HB, Brunet ME. Functional performance of the knee after intra-articular anesthesia. *Am J Sports Med* 1983;11:258–261.

84. Butler DL, Sheh MY, Stouffer DC, et al. Surface strain variation in human patellar tendon and knee cruciate ligaments. *J Biomech Eng* 1990;112:38–45.

85. Butler DL, Guan Y, Kay MD, et al. Location-dependent variations in the material properties of the anterior cruciate ligament. *J Biomech* 1992;25:511–518.

86. Markolf KL, Willems MJ, Jackson SR, et al. In situ calibration of miniature sensors implanted into the anterior cruciate ligament part I: strain measurements. *J Orthop Res* 1998;16:455–463.

Injury and Repair: Clinical

CHAPTER 18

Epidemiology of Knee Ligament Injuries

William M. Ohara, Elizabeth W. Paxton, and Donald C. Fithian

The epidemiology of knee ligament injuries has attracted greater interest with the shift toward population-based health and prevention that has occurred in the medical community at large over the past decade. Particularly with increasing participation of older individuals in high-level sporting activities, more participation by women and younger patients that previously were not considered at particular risk for knee injuries, the growth of "extreme" or high-velocity sports, and increasing attention to the socioeconomic "burden" of these injuries to society, prevention has taken on new and increasing urgency.

Ligamentous injuries of the knee are extremely common, with an estimated 50,000 to 80,000 ACL disruptions occurring each year in the United States alone. Griffin (1) estimated the cost of ACL injuries in the United States at approximately $1 billion per year, making prevention and treatment a significant public health concern. The incidence of anterior cruciate ligament injury is highest among a relatively narrow segment of the population: individuals aged 15 to 25 years of age who participate in sports that involve jumping and hard pivoting (the so-called level 1 and 2 sports [2]) (1,3). Yet despite a better understanding of the causes and mechanisms of injury, the number of reported knee ligament injuries is still increasing (4–7). These are often devastating injuries that may require long periods of recovery and necessitate significant time off work. For the athlete, ligament disruptions will result in extended time away from sports for recuperation (8), and may even signify the end of a career (8–10). We have developed a much better understanding of ligament injuries, but the majority of our attention has focused on diagnosis and treatment of ligament injuries, and less attention has been paid toward their frequency and associated risk factors.

In reviewing the vast literature on knee injuries, relatively few studies can be found that have examined the incidence of ligament disruptions; fewer still address risk factors and preventive measures. The majority of published articles on knee ligament injury are retrospective in nature and have presented data on various knee injuries based on review of insurance claims, self-reporting questionnaires, mail-in surveys, and medical records–surgical logs, clinic records, and hospital records. These studies often fail to identify the population at risk, and as such, are unable to determine the actual incidence of injury. Those studies that have calculated injury rates have, for the most part, focused specifically on individual sports such as soccer, basketball and football, or high-risk recreational activities, such as skiing. There have been very few prospective studies that have reported the incidence of knee ligament injuries in an unselected segment of the general population (11,12).

This chapter begins with a description of the methodology that qualifies studies as suitable for evaluating epidemiology of knee ligament injuries. As background for discussion, we report epidemiological data on knee ligament injuries collected at San Diego Kaiser Permanente during a 13-year period. We also review the published literature that has been most influential in establishing our current understanding of knee ligament injury frequency, risk, and prevention. Where appropriate, results of population-based studies will be compared with our own data to illuminate the discussion.

EPIDEMIOLOGIC METHODS IN KNEE LIGAMENT INJURY RESEARCH

Determining the risk for knee ligament injuries requires an understanding of several basic epidemiologic principles (13). Epidemiology is defined as the study of the distribution of diseases and other health related conditions in defined populations. It is concerned with the frequencies and types of illnesses and injuries that occur in groups of people, and with the factors that influence their distribution. The measurements of disease commonly used in epidemiologic research include incidence and prevalence rates. Incidence measures the probability that healthy people will develop a disease during a specified time; hence it is the number of new cases of a disease in a population over time. The formula for incidence is:

$$incidence = \frac{number\ of\ new\ cases}{population\ at\ risk\ over\ time}$$

The prevalence rate measures the number of people in a population who have the disease at a given time.

$$prevalence = \frac{number\ of\ existing\ cases}{total\ population}$$

Of the two, incidence rates provide a more direct measure of the rate at which individuals in a given population develop disease, and thus provide a basis for statements about the probability or risk for disease.

To determine incidence, it is necessary to follow prospectively a defined group of people and to determine the rate at which new cases of disease appear. Certain basic requirements must be met if incidence rates are to be calculated.

1. **Knowledge of the Health Status of the Study Population**. There must be adequate grounds on which to assess the health of individuals in a population and to classify people as diseased or not diseased. This requires a clear definition of the condition being studied, and the ability to diagnose the condition in question (see number 3).
2. **Time of Onset**. Determination of the date of onset is necessary for studies of incidence.
3. **Specification of Numerator**. The outcome being measured must be well defined (14,15), and effective means of data collection must be utilized (15,16).
4. **Specification of Denominator**. The denominator must consist of a defined population, accurately enumerated.
5. **Period of Observation**. Incidence rates must always be stated in terms of a definite period of time. Injuries within a general population may be reported as the number of injuries per thousand population per year. When reporting on the incidence of injury in a specific sport, the period of observation should be sufficiently long to provide a representative sample of *all types of exposure* that the sport may involve. For example, preseason training, early competitive and late competitive phases of the season all may involve different rates of injury. Junge and Dvorak (15) have recommended that the reporting period should include an entire year if one's intention is to draw general inferences about injury risk among those participating in competitive soccer.
6. **Exposure**. In calculating incidence rates for injuries in a general population, the preceding five elements

are all the investigator needs. However, with respect to sports injuries, there is the additional consideration that athletes may be up to 1,000 times more susceptible to injury than the general population (3). Furthermore, athletes do not spend 100% of their time "at risk," even at the height of the season, and not all players get the same amount of playing time in game situations, where the risk for traumatic injury is highest (15,16). Authors control for this in various ways, by recording the amount of time spent in training and in games, the amount of time skiers spend "at the slopes" (usually in units of days), or the (vertical) distance covered by skiers. There is at present no single standard for reporting "time at risk" for injury during sport. However, some conventions are emerging for individual sports such as soccer and skiing, which will be discussed below (see sport-specific studies). While it clearly is desirable to develop consistent standards, it is unlikely that a single approach will be appropriate for all sports activities, both because of specific questions that are of interest for particular sports, and due to the logistical challenges one may encounter in recording data such as injuries, time of exposure, and the population at risk.

The application of epidemiologic concepts to the study of knee ligament injuries can provide important insights into their frequency and distribution. These studies can tell us much about who sustains knee ligament injuries and how often these injuries occur. This information would be invaluable in planning the allocation of medical resources for a specific population. More importantly, they can also shed light on potential risk factors for knee injury, and subsequently lead to the development and testing of preventative measures for injury. Interventional measures that will likely reduce the risks of injury can then be introduced, and their effects can be monitored as new incidence rates are determined.

THE SAN DIEGO KAISER EXPERIENCE

The Kaiser-Permanente Medical Center in San Diego serves the Kaiser Health Plan members in the greater San Diego area. This population represents a segment of the local population, which is selected by choice of health plan only. Because of the nature of the health plan, members receive virtually all of their care at San Diego Kaiser facilities. During the period from 1985 to 1997, the San Diego Health Plan grew from 292,000 to 457,800 members, averaging 353,754 members.

Patients who present to the Kaiser Emergency Department with a soft tissue knee injury are referred to the Knee Injury Clinic of the Department of Orthopaedic Surgery if they have at least one of the following: an effusion, pathologic joint motion, or disability that prevents the patient from working. Patients with fractures (except minor avulsions) or tibial-femoral dislocations are evaluated by an orthopedic surgeon in the emergency room and are not referred to the clinic.

For various reasons, some patients receive emergency care at non-Kaiser facilities. Because the Knee Clinic is a referral clinic, these patients still should receive their orthopedic follow-up care at the clinic after they present to our primary care offices. Patients who receive initial care at out-of-plan facilities would be expected to submit a claim for reimbursement of the expenses of outside care. We surveyed all claims submitted for out-of-plan emergency care during the year 1996. We identified all diagnosis-related groups (DRGs) relevant to injuries of the thigh, knee, or leg and reviewed by hand the charts of all patients seen at outside facilities for indications that might represent knee injuries. A total of 45 claims were identified which represented encounters satisfying the criteria for referral to the Knee Injury Clinic. Of those, 34 patients had been referred to the Knee Injury Clinic, as expected, on presentation to our facilities subsequent to the original outside encounter. Only 11 patients did not receive a referral to Knee Injury Clinic for whom such a referral would have been appropriate. Two of the 11 patients were not referred to the clinic because of knee dislocation (one patient) or fractures with multiple ligamentous knee injuries (one patient), both of which were admitted to our hospital for immediate operative care. The total of 11 cases not seen in the Knee Clinic represents only 1.1% of all 981 San Diego Kaiser Health Plan members sustaining knee injuries during the course of that year. We concluded that the Knee Injury Clinic database represents approximately 99% of all knee injuries sustained by Kaiser Health Plan members on a yearly basis.

Statistics in this review are based on the initial San Diego Kaiser Knee Injury Clinic diagnosis. This diagnosis was based on a standard clinical examination and radiographs. Patients suspected of having knee ligament injuries underwent instrumented measurements with the KT-1000 knee ligament arthrometer. Collateral ligament injuries were graded on a scale of 1 to 3 as follows:

1 = Pain or tenderness without opening to varus or valgus stress, that is, no pathologic motion
2 = Abnormal joint space opening, but a firm end point
3 = Abnormal joint space opening and a soft end point.

Cruciate ligament injuries were diagnosed by ligament arthrometry (KT-1000, MedMetric, San Diego, California). Pathologic anterior motion was defined as a 3 mm anterior displacement difference between the injured and the uninjured (I-N) knee with a 20-lb, 30-lb, or manual maximum displacement force with the knee in 30° of flexion. Pathologic posterior motion was defined as anterior tibial motion greater than 2 mm at the quadriceps neutral angle (QNA) with the quadriceps active test (QAT) (17), or a corrected posterior displacement difference (I-N) greater than 2 mm with a posteriorly directed load of 20 lb (17). (For details on diagnostic criteria or techniques, see Chapter 19, Part C, "Diagnosis of Knee Ligament Injury: Arthrometry.")

Overall Incidence

During the 13-year period of this review, 11,710 patients were evaluated in the San Diego Kaiser Knee Injury Clinic. Of these, 2,235 (19%) had knee ligament injuries with pathologic motion (i.e., grade II or grade III). This represents an injury rate of 0.49 per 1,000 health plan members per year. Injury rates fluctuated from year to year (range 0.38–0.64). The yearly injury rates are presented in Table 18.1.

Anterior Cruciate Ligament

Disruption of the ACL was the most common ligament injury. There were a total of 1,379 ACL injuries, resulting in an injury rate of 0.30 per 1,000 per year. The yearly fluctuations in ACL injury rate are noted in Table 18.1. The majority of ACL disruptions were isolated injuries (73%), while combined ACL/MCL disruptions represented 24% of the total ACL disruptions (Table 18.2). These two groups made up 97% of all ACL injuries.

Isolated ACL disruptions represented 45% of all ligament injuries, and were clearly the most common type of ligament injury. Seventy-one percent of isolated ACL injuries occurred during sports activities, and were evenly distributed between four sports: skiing, football, basketball, and soccer. Similarly, 70% of the ACL/MCL injuries were sustained during sports activities. However, in contrast to the isolated ACL injury, there was one sport that

TABLE 18.1. *Incidence of ligament injuries with pathologic motion (injuries per 1,000 members per year)*

Year	ACL	MCL	PCL	LCL	Overall
		Incidence of injury			
1985	0.23	0.15	0.041	0.017	0.38
1986	0.34	0.24	0.024	0.003	0.52
1987	0.32	0.29	0.021	0.021	0.54
1988	0.25	0.18	0.036	0.039	0.43
1989	0.26	0.18	0.031	0.006	0.38
1990	0.28	0.27	0.029	0.021	0.49
1991	0.39	0.34	0.031	0.028	0.64
1992	0.30	0.29	0.016	0.008	0.53
1993	0.28	0.26	0.019	0.011	0.50
1994	0.35	0.26	0.028	0.017	0.53
1995	0.41	0.28	0.038	0.014	0.62
1996	0.28	0.20	0.044	0.007	0.45
1997	0.22	0.14	0.015	0.000	0.33
Total	0.30	0.24	0.029	0.015	0.49

ACL, anterior cruciate ligament; LCL, lateral collateral ligament; MCL, medial collateral ligament; PCL, posterior cruciate ligament.

TABLE 18.2. *Acute knee ligament injuries with pathologic motion (n = 2,235)*

	Ligament injury			
ACL	MCL	PCL	LCL	Number
X				1006
	X			710
		X		80
			X	37
X	X			328
X		X		7
X			X	19
	X	X		24
	X		X	4
		X	X	1
X	X	X		16
X		X	X	3
Total 1379	1082	131	64	2235

ACL, anterior cruciate ligament; LCL, lateral collateral ligament; MCL, medial collateral ligament; PCL, posterior cruciate ligament.

clearly stood out as the most common activity at the time of injury—skiing (Table 18.3).

Medial Collateral Ligament

There were 1,082 MCL disruptions, resulting in an injury rate of 0.24 per 1,000 members per year. The majority of MCL disruptions were isolated injuries (710, 66%). These isolated injuries made up 32% of the total ligament injuries. Combined ACL/MCL injuries accounted for 30% of the total MCL disruptions. Thus, isolated MCL and combined ACL/MCL injuries together accounted for the vast majority of MCL disruptions (96%). Sixty-three percent of the isolated MCL and ACL/MCL combined injuries occurred during sports activities. Of these sports-related injuries, the most common activity at the time of injury was skiing (20%), followed by football (11%) and soccer (8%). The incidence of MCL injury among males was twice the incidence among females (0.36 vs. 0.18).

Posterior Cruciate Ligament

Posterior cruciate ligament disruption was a fairly uncommon injury, accounting for only 6% of all ligament injuries (Table 18.2). The rate of injury was 0.029 per 1,000 per year. The year-to-year variations in PCL injury rate are noted in Table 18.1. The majority of PCL disruptions were isolated injuries (61%), while the most common combined PCL injury was disruption of the PCL, ACL, and MCL (16, 12% of PCL injuries). Obvious dislocations of the knee were either evaluated in the emergency room by an orthopaedic surgeon and thus not referred to the clinic, or sent to outside trauma centers due to the mechanism of injury. Consequently, the number of three- and four-ligament disruptions presented here does not represent its true incidence among the Kaiser Health Plan membership in San Diego.

The most common mechanism of PCL injury was sports (53%) while vehicular accidents accounted for 21% of the ligament disruptions. Fifteen of the 27 PCL disruptions (56%) resulting from vehicular accidents were combined ligament injuries, reflecting the high amount of energy responsible for these injuries.

Lateral Collateral Ligament

The lateral collateral ligament (LCL) group included all lateral ligament injuries, as well as injuries of the posterolateral corner. These injuries were the least common of the ligament disruptions, with an injury rate of 0.015 per 1,000 per year. The yearly fluctuations in lateral ligament injury rate are shown in Table 18.1. These injuries made up only 2.8% of the total ligament disruptions. Of the 64 documented lateral ligament injuries, over half (58%) were isolated disruptions (Table 18.2). The most common combined injuries were the ACL/LCL and ACL/PCL/LCL tears, accounting for 30% and 25%, respectively, of the total lateral ligament injuries. Fifty-eight percent of the lateral ligament injuries occurred during sports activities (Table 18.3). Although the general

TABLE 18.3. *Acute knee ligament injuries with pathologic motion activity at the time of injury*

Ligament injury	Ligament injury								
	Ski	Football	Basketball	Soccer	Baseball	Other sports	Vehicle	Misc	Number
ACL single ligament	123 (12%)	118 (12%)	140 (14%)	120 (12%)	83 (8%)	127 (13%)	39 (4%)	256 (25%)	1006
MCL single ligament	109 (15%)	77 (11%)	33 (5%)	59 (8%)	57 (8%)	90 (13%)	42 (6%)	243 (34%)	710
MCL/ACL combined	100 (30%)	31 (9%)	22 (7%)	24 (7%)	14 (4%)	37 (11%)	23 (7%)	77 (23%)	328
PCL injury	8 (6%)	7 (6%)	6 (5%)	8 (6%)	16 (13%)	22 (17%)	27 (21%)	33 (26%)	127
LCL injury	6 (9%)	4 (6%)	8 (13%)	5 (8%)	5 (8%)	9 (14%)	6 (9%)	21 (33%)	64
Total	346 (15%)	237 (11%)	209 (9%)	216 (10%)	175 (8%)	285 (13%)	137 (6%)	630 (28%)	2235

ACL, anterior cruciate ligament; LCL, lateral collateral ligament; MCL, medial collateral ligament; PCL, posterior cruciate ligament.

TABLE 18.4. *Incidence of ligament injuries with pathologic motion (1990–1997): Gender distribution (injuries per 1,000 members per year)*

Sex	ACL	MCL	ACL/MCL	PCL	LCL	Total
			Incidence of injury			
Females	0.16	0.11	0.06	0.017	0.0047	0.36
Males	0.32	0.24	0.10	0.039	0.022	0.72
Total	0.24	0.17	0.08	0.028	0.013	0.53

ACL, anterior cruciate ligament; LCL, lateral collateral ligament; MCL, medial collateral ligament; PCL, posterior collateral ligament.

incidence of ligament disruptions among males was twice that of females, the incidence of lateral ligament disruptions was almost five times higher in males than in females (Table 18.4).

Combined Ligament Injury

By far the most common multiple ligament injury was a combined disruption of the ACL and MCL, representing 24% of all ACL injuries, and 15% of all ligament injuries with pathologic motion (Table 18.2). The remaining combined ligament disruptions represented only 3% of all ligament injuries. In order, the next most common combined injuries were PCL/MCL, ACL/LCL, and ACL/PCL/MCL (Table 18.2). Again, as noted previously, there was a subset of patients that sustained multi-ligament injuries treated outside of our institution, and were thus not included in this review.

Activity at the Time of Injury

Although the nature and circumstances of each injury are recorded in our clinic data sheets, the computerized database does not differentiate between specific injury mechanisms such as contact with other persons, whether the injury occurred during jumping, landing or cutting, whether the foot was in contact with the playing surface, the type of playing surface, or other information that could be of interest with respect to the incidence of knee injuries in our population. For purposes of this discussion, only the activity at the time of injury is presented.

Sixty-seven percent of the acute ligament injuries with pathologic motion were sustained in sports activities (Table 18.3). The majority of the isolated ACL (71%), isolated MCL (60%), and combined ACL/MCL (68%) injuries were sustained in sports activities. Skiing accounted for the highest number of acute ligament injuries [346] in the San Diego population, followed by football [237], soccer [216], basketball [209], and baseball [175]. These five sports were responsible for 81% of the sports injuries, and 53% of the total injuries. Football, soccer, and baseball seemed to produce similar profiles of knee ligament injury (Table 18.4). However, there were several notable differences when the various sports were compared. Basketball produced more isolated ACL injuries and fewer MCL injuries, while skiing resulted in fewer isolated ACL injuries and more combined ACL/MCL injuries when compared with the other sports.

Although the proportion of ligament injuries attributable to these various sports could be calculated, the incidence rate of knee ligament injury for each specific sport could not be determined due to a lack in information regarding the number of health plan members participating in each sport. Other studies in the literature have focused specifically on individual sports in reporting knee ligament injury rates, and they will be reviewed later in this chapter.

Vehicular accidents produced a very different profile of injuries (Table 18.5). Isolated ACL and MCL injuries each represented approximately one-third of the total, while isolated and combined PCL injuries accounted for one fifth. In fact, although vehicular accidents were

TABLE 18.5. *Acute knee ligament injuries with pathologic motion injury profile for activity at time of injury*

Activity	ACL	MCL	ACL/MCL	PCL isolated and combined	LCL isolated and combined	Total
			Ligament injury			
Ski	123 (36%)	109 (32%)	100 (29%)	8 (2%)	6 (2%)	346
Football	118 (50%)	77 (32%)	31 (13%)	7 (3%)	4 (2%)	237
Basketball	140 (67%)	33 (16%)	22 (11%)	6 (3%)	8 (4%)	209
Soccer	120 (56%)	59 (27%)	24 (11%)	8 (4%)	5 (2%)	216
Baseball	83 (47%)	57 (33%)	14 (8%)	16 (9%)	5 (3%)	175
Vehicle	39 (28%)	42 (31%)	23 (17%)	27 (20%)	6 (4%)	137

ACL, anterior cruciate ligament; LCL, lateral collateral ligament; MCL, medial collateral ligament; PCL, posterior cruciate ligament.

TABLE 18.6. *Acute knee ligament injuries with pathologic motion: Age distribution*

Age	ACL	MCL	ACL/MCL	PCL isolated and combined	LCL isolated and combined	Total
0–14	36 (47%)	28 (36%)	3 (4%)	6 (8%)	4 (5%)	77
15–29	524 (49%)	313 (29%)	143 (13%)	64 (6%)	34 (3%)	1078
30–44	345 (44%)	256 (33%)	117 (15%)	43 (6%)	19 (2%)	780
>44	101 (34%)	113 (38%)	65 (22%)	14 (5%)	7 (2%)	300
Total	1006 (45%)	710 (32%)	328 (15%)	127 (6%)	64 (3%)	2235

ACL, anterior cruciate ligament; LCL, lateral collateral ligament; MCL, medial collateral ligament; PCL, posterior cruciate ligament.

responsible for only 6% of the knee ligament injuries, they resulted in 21% of the PCL injuries. Thus, in the vehicular group, ACL injuries are less frequent and PCL injuries more frequent than when we consider all knee injury mechanisms together. It is worth remembering that there is a small subset of members that sustained knee dislocations by this mechanism that were not included in this review.

Age Distribution

The age distribution of ligament disruptions with pathologic motion is shown in Table 18.6. Although only 19% of the membership was between 15 and 29 years of age, almost one-half of the knee ligament injuries (48%) were found in this group. Data regarding the age distributions of the general population was only available between the years 1990 and 1997. Incidence rates for the various age groups were thus only calculated within this period of time (Table 18.6). The overall incidence of knee ligament injury within the 15- to 29-year-old group was almost twice that of the 30 to 44 year old group (1.3 vs. 0.72 per 1,000). The incidence of knee ligament injury was lowest in the 0 to 14 year old group (0.093 per 1,000 members). It is important to

note, however, that this group included infants and young children who were not at risk for significant ligament injury. The patterns of ligament injury were similar for the three age groups younger than 45 years of age (Table 18.7). Isolated ACL disruptions were the most common injury in these three groups, followed by isolated MCL injuries. In the group of individuals older than 44 years of age, isolated MCL injuries were the most common injury, followed by isolated injuries of the ACL. Thus, while age seems to be a factor influencing the incidence of acute knee ligament injuries with pathologic motion, age does not seem to influence dramatically the specific pattern of ligament injury within the injured group, particularly in those groups younger than 45 years.

Gender Differences

Of those individuals sustaining knee ligament injuries with pathologic motion 1,506 (67%) were male and 729 (33%) were female. Data regarding gender in our general population was only available for the years 1990 to 1997. Thus, as with the age group calculations, the incidence of injuries among the two gender groups was calculated only for this period of time. The incidence of

TABLE 18.7. *Incidence of ligament injuries with pathologic motion (1990–1997): Age distribution (injuries per 1,000 members per year)*

Age	ACL	MCL	ACL/MCL	PCL isolated and combined	LCL isolated and combined	Total
0–14	0.043	0.035	0.0048	0.0064	0.0032	0.093
15–29	0.63	0.39	0.18	0.072	0.042	1.3
30–44	0.32	0.24	0.11	0.036	0.013	0.72
>44	0.084	0.090	0.054	0.011	0.0030	0.24
Total	0.24	0.17	0.08	0.028	0.013	0.53

ACL, anterior cruciate ligament; LCL, lateral collateral ligament; MCL, medial collateral ligament; PCL, posterior cruciate ligament.

ligament injuries with pathologic motion was 0.36 per 1,000 females per year and 0.72 per 1,000 males per year (Table 18.4). The gender differences for the various knee ligament injuries are also listed in Table 18.4. In general, for most ligament injuries, the incidence among males was twice that of females. However, the incidence of lateral ligament injuries was almost five times higher in males than in females.

REVIEW OF THE LITERATURE

The literature on knee injuries is so extensive as to seem overwhelming. However, relatively few studies have examined the frequency of knee ligament disruptions. The majority of the published data are comprised of tallies of ligament injuries without any reference to the population at risk. These case counts are often derived from the office records of individual practitioners, hospital records, surgical logs, or insurance claims. The absolute number of cases can provide useful information regarding the relative frequency of specific ligament injuries when compared with other ligament injuries. Such studies also provide valuable information regarding characteristics of various ligament injuries, particularly when such injuries are rare and individual experience with a particular injury may be limited. However, without reference to the population at risk, these case counts cannot provide useful information regarding the risk or probability of sustaining an injury. In contrast, those studies that have calculated the incidence have provided a direct measure of the rate at which individuals in a given population sustain injuries, and thus have provided a basis for statements about probability or risk for injury.

Many of the studies that have calculated the frequency of knee ligament injuries are retrospective in nature, and have used one of several methodological approaches in collection of their data. Most commonly, archival methods (past records, participation rosters, hospital charts, etc.) or post hoc questionnaires have been used to acquire injury data. Direct interviews have also been used to obtain information. Unfortunately, methods relying either on retrospective recall or on information that may have been recorded for another purpose are subject to inaccuracies and bias. This emphasizes the importance of prospective data collection for accurate determination of rates of injury. In a study of methodology in documenting soccer injuries, Junge and Dvorak (15) found that athletes recalled fewer than one third of moderate injuries and only 10% of mild injuries when answering follow-up questionnaires. Although shorter duration of symptoms and longer time to follow-up were associated with poorer recall, even severe injuries such as fractures were forgotten by athletes when completing the questionnaires. The importance of prospective data collection in detection of injuries cannot be overstated.

Knee Ligament Injuries in the General Population

There are only a handful of studies that have attempted to determine the frequency of knee ligament injuries in a general population. These studies, for the most part, have relied on knee injury data prospectively collected at emergency departments (12,18) and outpatient clinics (11,19,20). In some cases, the authors have not determined the population at risk, and their results have thus not included rates of knee ligament injury.

O'Beirne et al. (18) prospectively evaluated a group of patients presenting acutely to a casualty department following a knee injury. Overall, 233 patients with acute knee injuries were identified during a 4-month period. The authors identified 34 knees with ligament injuries, including seven complete ligament injuries. Among these seven complete ligament tears were four isolated MCL injuries, one isolated ACL injury, one isolated PCL injury, and one combined ACL/PCL/MCL injury. The total population served by this hospital was not reported, and incidence rates were not calculated.

Similarly, Jensen et al. (19) prospectively evaluated a group of patients presenting to a sports medicine center with acute knee injury. A total of 225 acute knee injuries were identified during a 32-month period. They recorded 44 ACL injuries, 30 MCL injuries, 1 PCL injury, and 2 LCL injuries. Seventy-four percent of the ligament injuries were sports related. As with the prior study, no incidence rates were reported.

Natri et al. (21) analyzed 450 ACL ruptures treated at a university hospital in Finland from 1980 to 1989. These included only surgically treated ACL lesions, and the number of nonsurgically treated patients was unknown. Although the authors noted that this hospital served approximately 400,000 people, the exact population at risk was not defined, and hence, incidence rates were not calculated. In their analysis, they noted that 63% of the ACL ruptures occurred in males, and that 54% of the injuries were sustained in sports activities. Fifty-one percent of the injuries were isolated ACL injuries, while 38% were ACL/MCL injuries, and 6% were combined ACL/PCL injuries. The authors also noted that there was a 247% increase in the number of surgically treated ACL injuries over the 10 years of the study, although it was not clear if this was the result of an increase in population, a change in surgical indications, or improvements in diagnostic abilities. The proportion of injuries sustained by females in this study (37%) was similar to the Kaiser study (33%). A higher proportion of isolated ACL injuries was noted in the Kaiser study (73% vs. 51% in this study), while a higher proportion of injuries were sustained in sports activities in the Kaiser study (67% vs. 54% in this study).

Without a description of the population at risk, the calculation of incidence rates becomes impossible. Failure to define the population at risk may reflect the inherent difficulties in accurately defining the population served by any one emergency department or outpatient clinic. Several authors have determined the population at risk in collecting data on knee injuries, and have thus calculated rates of knee ligament injury for a general population (11,12,20) (Table 18.8). Miyasaka et al. (11) reviewed the rate of knee ligament injuries in the San Diego Kaiser population between 1985 and 1988. The annual incidence of knee ligament injuries with pathologic motion was 0.6 per 1,000 members per year. With the exception of combined ACL/MCL injuries, which constituted 12% of the ligament injuries with pathologic motion, combined ligament injuries were uncommon. Seventy-two percent of the patients with acute ligament injuries were male and 28% were female. Sixty-five percent of the injuries were sustained in sports activities. The population at risk was the same Kaiser population presented earlier in this chapter. The incidence of knee ligament injury was slightly higher in the earlier review (0.60 vs. 0.49). Overall, the patterns of injury and their distribution among the various age groups and genders were similar.

Nielsen and Yde (12) reviewed all acute knee injuries presenting to two emergency departments in Aarhus, Denmark over a period of 1 year. These emergency departments served a community consisting of 253,753 inhabitants. The number of acute knee injuries that were either treated outside of these two hospitals or were never even seen was unknown. The authors did state, however, that in Denmark most patients with acute knee injuries are treated at emergency departments. There were 265 knee ligament ruptures, and the overall rate of knee ligament injury was 1.04 injuries/1,000 inhabitants/year. This was twice the rate of ligament injury noted in our study. The rate of ACL injury was 0.30 injuries per 1,000 inhabitants per year, with isolated ruptures comprising the majority of these injuries (63%). The incidence of ACL injury was thus identical to the Kaiser experience. There were only 5 PCL tears, with an injury rate of 0.02 per 1,000 inhabitants per year, which again was similar to our experience. Of the 198 collateral ligament injuries, only 5 were stated to be lateral collateral ligament ruptures. Presumably, the remaining collateral ligament injuries (193) were MCL tears, and the rate of MCL injury was thus

0.76 per 1,000 inhabitants per year. This was three times the incidence of the Kaiser population and would account for the higher overall incidence of ligament injuries in their study. In addition, 65% of the ligament injuries were sustained in sports activities. The rate of ACL injury was 0.4 per 1,000 males and 0.2 per 1,000 females.

Kannus and Jarvinen (20) prospectively recorded all visits to physicians due to knee injuries over 1 year starting in July 1985 in a well-defined population in Finland. Due to an unavailability of private practitioners or medical specialists, the 13,700 inhabitants in this region almost without exception sought medical treatment in a community health center, allowing the authors to capture all knee injuries that occurred within this population. One hundred forty-eight knee injuries were recorded during this 1-year period, resulting in an incidence rate of 1.1%, or 1.1 injuries per 100 inhabitants. The authors noted that knee ligament injuries comprised 43% of the total, but an incidence rate was not reported. Extrapolating from these data, the incidence of ligament injury in this population was approximately 0.47 per 100 inhabitants.

The majority of the literature on knee ligament injuries has focused primarily on disruptions of the anterior cruciate ligament. Because of its relative infrequency, posterior cruciate ligament injuries have received much less attention, and consequently, rates of injury are not well reported. In reviewing the literature, there is considerable variability in the reported incidence of PCL disruptions, ranging from 1% to 44% of all knee ligament injuries. The range of reported injury rates seems to result from the differences in the population of individuals examined. Our reported PCL injury rate of 0.029 per 1,000 members per year is very similar to the 0.02 per 1,000 per year rate reported by Nielsen (12) in his study of a general population in Denmark. Their PCL disruptions constituted 2% of all ligament injuries. In addition, only one of their 5 PCL injuries was a combined ligament injury (20%). In contrast, in Fanelli's report (22) of 61 acute knee injuries with hemarthrosis that presented to a tertiary care center over an 11-month period, 44% of the ligament injuries were PCL disruptions. In addition, 25 of the PCL injuries (93%) were combined ligament disruptions. Twenty-two of the injuries were the result of trauma, whereas only 5 (18.5%) were related to sports. In a follow-up study,

TABLE 18.8. *Review of the literature: Incidence of ligament injury in the general population (injuries per 1,000)*

Reference	Overall	ACL	MCL	PCL	LCL
Kaiser (1985–1997)	0.49	0.30	0.24	0.029	0.015
Miyasaki (11)	0.60	0.38	0.26	0.044	0.023
Nielsen (12)	1.04	0.30		0.02	
Kannus (20)	0.47				
Griffin (1)		0.57			

ACL, anterior cruciate ligament; LCL, lateral collateral ligament; MCL, medial collateral ligament; PCL, posterior cruciate ligament.

Fanelli and Edson (23) presented 222 acute knee injuries with hemarthrosis that presented to the same regional trauma center over a period of 48 months. There were 85 PCL injuries, making up 38% of the knee injuries. The vast majority of these PCL disruptions were combined ligament injuries (96%). Forty-three of these injuries (51%) were the result of motor vehicle accidents, and 28 (33%) were sports related. No incidence rates were reported in this study. The higher proportion of PCL injuries in this study when compared with others is clearly a reflection of the population of patients seen at the authors' regional trauma center, and of the author's tertiary trauma care practice. It likely did not reflect the incidence in a general population.

Similarly, Lu et al. (24) reported the results of a prospective study of victims of road traffic accidents who presented with acute hemarthroses. These 46 patients with 47 hemarthroses subsequently underwent knee arthroscopy. There were 24 ACL injuries (51%), although 15 were described as partial tears. The remaining nine ACL injuries (15%) also included five tibial avulsions. There were 18 (38%) PCL injuries, 3 of which were partial tears. The remaining 15 injuries (32%) included 9 tibial avulsions. Overall, they found a higher proportion of PCL injuries compared with injuries of the ACL. A higher proportion of PCL injuries were also seen amongst our patients involved in vehicular accidents. As mentioned earlier, the true incidence of PCL injuries in our population would expected to be higher because those individuals involved in high-energy accidents are brought to the nearest trauma center and would not present to our Acute Knee Injury Clinic.

Effect of Gender on Knee Ligament Injuries

Our data confirm other studies that suggest ACL injuries in the general public occur more commonly among men than among women. However, none of these studies have closely inspected the portion of the population at highest risk. Knee ligament injury risk is activity-specific, so data on gender-specific injury rates must take into account hours of sports activity (13). Therefore, the influence of gender is examined in greater detail in the section that follows.

Summary of Evidence on Knee Ligament Injuries in the General Population

In a consensus paper sponsored by the AOSSM, OREF, NATAREF, and NCAA, Griffin et al. (1) estimated that in the 3 decades of life from age 15 to 45, there is 1 ACL injury per 1,750 persons per year (0.57 per 1,000 persons per year). Review of the Kaiser population has confirmed that knee ligament injuries resulting in pathologic motion are common in a general population. The incidence is highest in a relatively narrow segment of the population—those individuals between the ages of 14 and 30—and in our general population, the rate of injury is higher in males than in females. ACL disruptions are the most common injury, although the incidence of MCL injuries is not far behind. At present, very few other studies have examined the incidence of knee ligament injuries in a general population (12,20). This more than likely reflect the difficulties inherent in conducting such an investigation. It requires a well-defined population that can accurately be enumerated. More importantly, there must be some mechanism to allow for the identification of all ligament injuries that occur within the population. These difficulties not withstanding, the Kaiser Health Plan has provided an ideal situation for conducting this type of population based epidemiologic study. The membership represents a segment of the local population that is well defined, and the Knee Injury Clinic has provided a mechanism by which the majority of these injuries can be captured and identified. This has resulted in incidence rates based on large sample sizes and many years of data collection.

A large sample size allows one to make more precise statements regarding the population at large, as reflected in the calculation of confidence intervals. A confidence interval is a range of values for a study variable specifying the probability that the true value of the variable is included within the range (25). By convention, the confidence interval is usually chosen at 95% or 99%. A 95% confidence interval means that 95% of all sample means based on a given sample size will fall within 1.96 standard errors of the population mean. As sample size increases, the size of the confidence interval decreases, and as the confidence interval becomes more narrow, the data becomes more precise. In Table 18.9, confidence

TABLE 18.9. *Review of the literature: Incidence of ligament injury in the general population (per 1,000)*

Reference	Overall		ACL		MCL		PCL	
	Incidence	95% CI	Incidence	95% CI	Incidence	95% CI	Incidence	95% CI
Kaiser Permanente	0.49	0.47–0.50	0.30	0.29–0.31	0.24	0.22–0.25	0.029	0.024–0.033
Nielsen (11)	1.04	0.92–1.16	0.30	0.24–0.36	0.76	0.71–0.81	0.02	0.00–0.04
Kannus (12)	4.7	3.9–5.5						
Griffin (1)			0.57					

ACL, anterior cruciate ligament; LCL, lateral collateral ligament; MCL, medial collateral ligament; PCL, posterior cruciate ligament; CI, confidence interval.

intervals for the Kaiser population have been calculated. Also included in this table are two other studies that determined incidence of knee injury in a general population.

Sport-Specific Studies

In the Kaiser population, 67% of the acute knee ligament injuries with pathologic motion were sustained in sports activities. In this population, the number of health plan members participating in each sport was unknown. The number of injuries observed therefore probably reflects the popularity of different sports within the population (15,26), not the risk for injury. Thus, although the proportion of ligament injuries attributable to various sports could be calculated (Tables 18.3, 18.4), the risk for knee ligament injury for each specific sport could not be determined. But even if one documents the total number of *participants* (i.e., the portion of the population with reasonable chance of injury), as Sandelin (27) did for Finnish soccer players, he still cannot assume that all participants have the same level of exposure to risk. For example, Sandelin could not know how much time Finnish women spent in soccer unless he measured it specifically. This is because cultural and societal influences affect not only how many women play soccer, but also the amount of time they spend playing games and training, and what levels of competition are available. The study by Roaas (28) based on insurance records of all Norwegian football players is similarly flawed.

Exposure

After a comprehensive review of the literature and a review of insurance data sources covering one decade of sports injuries in Switzerland, de Loes (29) recommended enhancements of both the quantity and the quality of Swiss research in the field. Given that knee ligament injuries commonly are associated with specific sporting activities (2), epidemiologic studies must pay careful attention to variables such as time of exposure (15,26) to yield useful information. In the last dozen years numerous studies in the literature have focused specifically on the epidemiology of sports injuries. Many of these articles have reported rates of knee injury. These studies provide insight into the pattern and frequency of knee injuries associated with specific sports, which may then lead to the development of preventative measures to minimize the risks of injury.

One of the difficulties in comparing the frequency of knee injuries reported in the sports literature has been a lack of agreement in the method of calculating the incidence of injury. To identify the amount of time actually spent at risk for injury, investigators must define some measure of activity-specific exposure (13)—time spent in games and/or practice sessions (15,16,26,30–32), exposure events (a practice session or game) (33,34), or in the case of skiing, (vertical) distance skied (35) or days of participation (36). Meaningful comparisons can be difficult to make when different units of exposure are used, and there is as yet no single standard for reporting exposure. For competitive sports where the proportion of training and competitive situations vary considerably, it seems advisable to record injuries and exposure separately for games and training (8,37–39) so that risk for injury can be compared across skill levels, and between regular season and tournaments (15,39).

Soccer

Soccer is the world's most popular sport, and the fastest-growing team sport in the United States. Current estimates put participation at 200 million, 40 million of whom are women (40). On average, organized soccer participation results in 1 to 2 injuries per player per year (26,38). A conservative estimate of the economic burden for medical treatment of soccer-related injuries based on this estimate is about $30 to $60 billion per year (16), not considering the cost of follow-up or late sequelae (38,41,42). Hawkins (3) showed that the risk for injury among professional football players is around 1,000 times higher than for industrial occupations generally regarded as high risk. After an exhaustive study and review of the epidemiologic literature on soccer, Inklaar justifiably concluded that in countries where soccer is very popular, the health care and social security systems are taxed considerably (26).

Sixty-five percent to 90% of soccer injuries involve the lower extremities (26,27,43–51). The most frequently injured joints are the knee and ankle (52–54), with knee injuries accounting for about one-third to one-half of all traumatic injuries (8,38,54). Knee injuries account for more than half of all soccer injuries requiring surgery (43). Of all soccer injuries, Nielsen (55) found knee injuries caused the most serious long-term effects. Only one in three elite soccer players returns to an elite level of play within 18 months after sustaining a major knee injury (8). One in three players quit soccer altogether after an ACL rupture, because of poor knee function or concern about further injury (9). Most of those wishing to return to play will require reconstruction (9), despite which their careers likely will be foreshortened (10). Clearly, there is much to be gained by a careful examination of knee injury mechanisms and potential strategies for injury prevention.

Sandelin (27) reviewed the insurance records of all acute soccer injuries during 1 year in Finland. All soccer players in Finland participating in games arranged by their national soccer association have obligatory insurance coverage. There were 35,500 registered soccer players during this time. Overall, there were 460 acute knee injuries, 185 of which were ligamentous injuries. The calculated incidence of ligamentous knee injury for that 1 year was 5.2 per 1,000 players. Sandelin estimated that there were approximately 70,000 in over 4,000 in Finland. Thus, this report accounted for approximately half of the soccer participants in the country.

Bjordal et al. (9) retrospectively reviewed all ACL injuries sustained while playing soccer during a 10-year period in Hordaland, Norway. As standard procedure, all patients with suspected ACL injuries were admitted to one of three hospitals in Hordaland, and all ACL injuries were verified by arthroscopic or surgical evaluation. The rate of ACL injury was calculated in terms of exposure time. The average annual exposure time was 32.8 game hours per player, with an annual average of 8,030 players per year. There were 176 ACL injuries during this time period, and the overall incidence rate of ACL injury was 0.063 per 1,000 game hours. Interestingly, the incidence rate was 0.10 per 1,000 game hours for women and 0.057 for men.

Nielsen (55) prospectively evaluated the injuries sustained among a group of soccer players participating at various levels of competition for a single Danish soccer club during a single season in 1986. The injury rate was calculated based on the number of hours of participation. There were three MCL and one ACL injury sustained during the season. Based on the overall injury rates of 3.6 per 1,000 practice hours and 14.3 per 1,000 game hours, the calculated MCL and ACL injury rates were 0.18 and 0.06 per 1,000 combined game and practice hours.

Luthje (43) prospectively recorded injuries sustained by elite level Finnish soccer players over the course one season (1993). There were 7 ACL injuries sustained among the 263 soccer players over the course of the season, resulting in a calculated ACL injury rate of 2.7 per 100 soccer players for the season.

It is widely believed that the risk for injury in soccer, calculated per hour of exposure, may be influenced by age, gender, and skill level (16,26). Other factors that may be important in determining the mix of injuries include the proportion of time spent in training and in games, and the time of season. Blaser noted the highest injury rate at the beginning of training (56), as did Ekstrand (57). Engstrom (8) reported that overuse injuries were more commonly the result of practice and occurred during preseason or at the end of the season, whereas traumatic injuries were more common in games and occurred throughout the regular season. Although some studies have reported differences in the risk for injury based on position (10,53,58,59), they do not agree on which positions carry increased risk. Most studies have found no difference in injury rates among the field positions (60,61). To eliminate bias in studies on the etiology of soccer injuries, Inklaar (62), Poulsen (63), Junge (15) and others (30) have recommended that epidemiologic studies should control for age, skill level, gender, and the number of hours and injuries should be calculated separately for training and games.

Youth players (under 18 years of age) are reported by some authors to experience fewer injuries than adult players (30,48,49,55,60,64–66). Injury rates among youth players clearly increase with advancing age, rising abruptly among 14 to 16 year olds compared with younger players (26,48,49). In a review of the literature and a comparison study of youth players from two regions of Europe, Junge (67) concluded that the injury rate among 14 to 18 year olds ranges from 0.9 to 4.9 per 1,000 hours of exposure, with the older (16–18 year old) players showing injury rates similar to adults. The distribution of injuries between game and training situations, proportion of overuse and traumatic injuries, the severity of injuries, and the distribution of injuries by body part appeared similar to published figures for adult players (16,26,38,61). In Junge's study, 22% of injuries involved the knee (67).

In a comparison study of 264 youth and adult soccer players representing low and high skill levels, Peterson et al. found that 14 to 16 year olds had more injuries per 1,000 hours of exposure than 16 to 18 year olds (38). Skill level exerted a much greater influence than age: less skilled players in the 14 to 16 year range were twice as likely to sustain injuries, and knee injuries in particular, compared with highly skilled players in the same age group, and less skilled players among the 14 to 16 year olds had the highest rate of injury (including knee injury) of all groups studied (38). The authors stressed the apparent need to enforce proper training and technique among youth players. These findings support the observation by Backous (64) that boys who were skeletally mature but muscularly weak had the highest injury rates among youth male players.

Injury rates have been compared between male and female soccer players (9,30,33,45,48,49,68–70). It is not clear whether the overall risk for injury in soccer differs for males and females. Sandelin analyzed all acute soccer injuries in Finland in 1980 and found no differences in the population based on gender (27). Of course, without calculating the hours of exposure, the study could not determine whether the risk for injury was the same, or whether their data merely reflected less participation by women in soccer. Lindenfeld noted similar rates of overall injury among male and female indoor soccer players during a 7-week period of an indoor soccer season (70), as did Putukian during an indoor soccer tournament (68). On the other hand, in studies of youth soccer players Kibler (69), Schmidt-Olsen (48), and Sullivan (65) all noted higher injury rates among girls than among boys. Could this be another manifestation of the role of conditioning in adolescent athletes, or does it reflect the rather liberal definition of "injury" in studies limited to youth soccer? Consider that among elite female outdoor soccer players, Engstrom (45) recorded injury rates of 7 per 1,000 hours of practice and 24 per 1,000 hours of competitive play, similar to injury rates among similarly trained men (37,38). Methodologic differences among these studies, including sampling, playing conditions, records of exposure, definitions of injury, and periods of study, make it difficult to compare their findings.

But whether or not overall injury rates differ, the evidence seems clear that the rate of knee injury, and specifically ACL injury, is higher among women than among men when exposure is taken into account. Arendt reported ACL injury rates (33) were twice as high among collegiate women soccer and basketball players than among their male counterparts (0.31 per 1,000 exposures vs. 0.13 per 1,000 exposures). Bjordal (9) analyzed 176 soccer players with arthroscopically verified ACL injuries. The incidence of ACL rupture was 0.10 per 1,000 game hours for women and 0.063 per 1,000 game hours for men. In Lindenfeld's study of indoor soccer players, despite a similar rate of injuries overall, females suffered knee ligament injuries at a rate more than three times that seen in males (0.87/100 hours vs. 0.29/100 hours). In a study of insurance records of soccer players in Sweden, Roos (10) found female soccer players had a higher relative risk for ACL tear, and tended to be injured at a younger age than male players.

Studies differ on whether the level of competition influences the risk for injury among adult players (26,30,38,55,56,63). In studies on the epidemiology of knee injuries in soccer the risk for ACL injury seems to be higher among elite players (9,10). Roos (10) reported an odds ratio of 3.3 for ACL injury among elite players. This was higher than the odds for ACL injury among women (10). In Bjordal's study the incidence of ACL tear for men in the top 3 divisions of Norwegian soccer, 0.41 per 1,000 game hours, was the highest among all groups studied (including women).

Engstrom's 1-year study of 3 elite male soccer teams reported that the incidence of major knee ligament injury during games was 13 per 1,000 hours, while the incidence during training was 3 per 1,000 hours (8). The rates in Engstrom's study approach one third of all injuries reported in studies of soccer injuries in general. On its face, this evidence suggests a very high risk for knee ligament injury among very highly skilled players. However, Engstrom noted that three of seven ACLs examined arthroscopically were chronic. This raises the question of whether Engstrom was truly identifying new ACL injuries, or reinjuries of previously ACL-deficient knees. If the chronic ACL tears represented ACL deficient knees presenting at the time of reinjury, then the actual incidence (number of *new* cases per study period) would have been only 7.4 per 1,000 game hours and 1.7 per 1,000 practice hours. While this is still a high rate of injury, it is in closer agreement with the studies by Bjordal (9) and Roos (10).

As stated earlier in this chapter, it is a requirement of all studies of incidence that the date of onset of the disease in question be known. When this principle is violated, risk is overestimated. The problem is further compounded when the pre-existing condition has a bearing risk for reinjury. Pre-existing ACL rupture clearly places the knee at risk for further injury when participating in high-level sports such as soccer (16,37,62,71,72) (see Chapter 20). Together, these factors would combine to bias the data toward poorer outcomes among participants with a longer playing history.

To assess the extent of this problem in the literature, several studies have examined the prevalence of pre-existing knee problems among soccer players (37,61,73). Arnason classified 58% of all joint sprains as reinjuries, but they did not separate out ACL tears. Chomiak et al. reported on severe knee injuries (those resulting in an absence of more than 4 weeks) that occurred in a population of European soccer players during a 1-year period (61). The presence of knee instability was documented by physical examination at the outset of the study. Of a total of 29 severe knee injuries, 7 were total or partial ACL ruptures. Seven of 18 knees injured by noncontact mechanisms had pre-existing instability documented on the baseline examination. Of 11 knee injuries resulting from contact with another player, none had pre-existing instability and only one had suffered a previous injury. In Junge's study of male soccer players, all patients underwent a Lachman test by a skilled examiner. The rate of anterior instability was 2.5% to 8.0%, and the highest prevalence of anterior instability was among adult amateur players. Almost one fourth of the players (134, 23%) had a pathologic finding in either the right or left knee. They recommended that further research should address the prevalence of pathologic findings and complaints in soccer players as well as the secondary structural changes that may occur as the result of playing soccer (73). These studies confirm that previous knee injuries are an important factor predisposing to risk for injury during a season of play. Pre-existing instability of the knee that is not documented at baseline examination will falsely elevate the incidence of knee injury and predispose to further injuries during play.

Indoor Soccer

Epidemiologic studies of indoor soccer are not as numerous as those on outdoor soccer. Because of the playing surface (37,74), shoes, and perhaps greater frequency of direction changes and player contact due to the smaller playing area, indoor soccer is associated with more injuries than outdoor soccer (26,60). Chomiak et al. (61) did not record higher rates of injury on artificial turf or during indoor competition, but they acknowledged that their documentation of these variables was not good enough to warrant firm conclusions. Hoff found that the incidence of injuries among youth (under age 16) indoor soccer players was 4.5 to 6.1 times greater than that of outdoor soccer players in the same age group. Injuries were uncommon among players under age 10 in either setting. Medical assistance was required for 6.5% of the injuries among outdoor players and for 24.3% among indoor players. Overall, 66.6% of the injuries were the result of physical contact between players. No relationship was observed between the risk for injury and playing position, conduct of warm-up exercises, or the team having a licensed coach (60).

Lindenfeld (70) registered all injuries occurring during a 7-week period at a local indoor soccer arena, calculating injury rates as the number of injuries per 100 player-hours. The overall injury rates for male and female players were similar, 5.04 and 5.03, respectively. The most common injury types were sprains and muscle contusions, both occurring at a rate of 1.1 injuries per 100 player-hours, and the most common injury mechanism overall (31% of the total) involved collisions with other players. Female players had a significantly higher rate of knee ligament injuries compared with men (0.87 vs. 0.29 per 100 player hours).

Putukian (68) prospectively recorded injuries in 824 players competing in open men's, open women's, over-30 men's, and mixed divisions during an indoor soccer tournament. The overall rate of injury per 100 player hours was 4.44, with a rate of 5.79 in the open men's, 4.74 in the open women's, 2.73 in the over-30 men's, and 1.54 for the mixed divisions. The differences in injury rates for men versus women and men versus older men were not statistically significant. Combined ligamentous injuries to the knee were the most common severe injuries. As the injuries increased in severity, they were more likely to be noncontact injuries.

Handball

Yde (66) compared the risk of participation by adolescents in soccer, handball, and basketball. The rates of injury were 5.6, 4.1, and 3.0 per 1,000 playing hours respectively. There was only 1 ACL injury recorded among 302 players and a total of 119 injuries. Soccer resulted in the most severe injuries and the longest periods of rehabilitation after injury. Unlike soccer, where the majority of injuries occurred during tackling and contact with other players, injuries in handball and basketball were caused by contact with the ball and running. In a larger study based on Swiss insurance records of acute injuries treated by physicians, de Loes (75) compared injury rates among several organized youth sports (ice hockey, handball, soccer, wrestling, hiking and basketball, skiing, volleyball, and rock climbing). Among both girls and boys, handball was among the highest risk activities (75).

Nielsen and Yde (76) reported the overall injury incidence to be 4.6 per 1,000 playing hours and 11.4 per 1,000 game hours, with the upper extremity most commonly involved. They did not find knee injuries to be particularly common, and the authors did not discuss in much detail the severity of the injuries reported during the study. On the other hand, Andren-Sanberg thought that ACL injury was probably the most serious risk of participation in handball (77). In 1998 Seil (78) reported on players from two male team handball senior divisions who were observed prospectively for 1 season to study the injury incidence in relation to exposure in games and practices (78). Ninety-one injuries were recorded. Injury incidence was evaluated at 2.5 injuries per 1,000 player-hours, with a significantly higher incidence in game injuries (14.3 injuries per 1,000 game-hours) compared with practice injuries (0.6 injuries per 1,000 practice-hours). Practice injury incidence was higher in the lower performance level group, and game injury incidence was higher in the high-level group. The upper extremity was involved in 37% of the injuries, and the lower extremity in 54%. The knee was the most commonly injured joint, followed by the finger, ankle, and shoulder. Knee injuries were also the most severe injuries, and they were more frequent in high-level players. There was an increase in the severity of injury with respect to performance level. The injury mechanism revealed a high number of offensive injuries, one-third of them occurring during a counterattack. In other words, the knee appears to be not only the most common joint injured among senior amateur male handball players, but also the most serious injury for which they are at risk.

Strand (79) reported a retrospective study of 144 anterior cruciate ligament injuries sustained during team handball. The incidence of ACL injury was 1.8% per year or 0.82 injuries per 1,000 playing hours in female athletes playing at a high division level. The risk was higher for women than among men, and higher on synthetic surfaces than on parquet. Analysis of injury mechanisms indicated that a high degree friction between shoes and playing surface was a major risk factor for injury. Two thirds of the injuries were by noncontact mechanisms (mostly cutting and jumping), and only 10% were caused by foul play.

Myklebust (80) recorded all cruciate ligament injuries occurring in the three top divisions of men's and women's team handball during the 1989 to1990 and 1990 to 1991 seasons in Norway. A total of 3,392 players participated at these levels during the period of study. They reported 93 cruciate ligament injuries: 87 ACL and 6 PCL. The injury rate among women was 1.8% compared with 1.0% among men. First division players had a higher risk for cruciate ligament injury (4.5%). Taking all three levels together, there were 0.97 cruciate ligament injuries per 100 playing hours. Seventy-five percent of the injuries occurred during games. Ninety-five percent were noncontact injuries. More than one half of the injuries were attributed to significant friction between shoe and floor. Contact with another player accounted for only 5% of injuries. No significant association was observed between the type of flooring (parquet, Pulastic, and other synthetic surfaces) and the risk for injury to the cruciate ligaments.

Myklebust (81) examined gender differences, injury mechanisms, and risk factors for ACL injuries in a population of high-level team handball players. The prospectively designed study covered the 1993 to1994, 1994 to 1995, and 1995 to 1996 seasons. They found 28 ACL injuries, 23 among women (incidence: 0.31/1,000 player-hours) and 5 among men (0.06 per 1000). The risk ratio for women compared with men was 5.0. Of the 28 injuries, 24 occurred during competition (0.91/1,000 hours; women: 1.60/1,000 hours; men: 0.23/1,000 hours; risk ratio: 7.0). Injuries during practice were less common (0.032/1,000 hours). The risk ratio of games to practice was 29.9. Twenty-five injuries occurred in noncontact situations when the players performed high-speed plant-and-cut movements, which is a common maneuver in handball (82).

Volleyball

Because of the jumping and pivoting involved, volleyball is considered a high-risk activity with respect to knee injuries (2,83). In 1990, Ferretti (84) reported the results of a retrospective study based on cases (ten men and 42 women) of ACL rupture treated from 1979 to 1989. There were 37 amateurs (continuous and regular participation without economic benefit) and 15 professionals (top level with economic benefit). The injured patients included ten setters and 42 spikers—14 of them specialized centers, that is, mainly engaged in blocking. Injury occurred during smashing (an offensive maneuver) in 38 cases, while blocking (a defensive maneuver involving jumping) in 10, and during other defensive situations in 4 patients. In 48 of 52 cases, injury occurred during a phase of jumping: during the landing phase in 38 cases and during take-off in 7. Only two injuries were the result of contact with another player. Injuries occurred during games in 32 cases, and during training in 20. The frequency was higher for women than men, although actual injury rates could not be determined given the way in which the injuries were recorded. The ACL injury was associated with serious MCL injuries in seven, and with partial MCL tears in three. Surgical exploration revealed injury to the anterolateral and/or posterolateral capsule in six cases. One patient sustained a femoral detachment of the PCL associated with damage to the ACL, injury to the surface and deep fasciae of the medial collateral ligament, and serious disorders in the entire lateral compartment. Centers, setters, and spikers had higher than average relative risk for knee injury in this study. It is clear

from this study that concern about knee injuries in volleyball is justified, but the study itself does not allow us to assess the incidence of knee injury.

Watkins (85) reported an overall injury rate of 0.52 per player during the 1989 to 1990 Scottish National Volleyball League Season, but the retrospective study design did not allow detailed analysis of injury rates or exposure. The distribution of injuries in volleyball reflects the specific tasks involved. Overuse injuries are fairly common in the shoulder due to repetitive overhead use of the arm (86–88). Overuse injuries in the knee are related primarily to training and occur most commonly in the knee extensor mechanism (83,86,88). Aagaard reported 3.8 injuries per 1,000 player hours among Danish elite divisions. The overall injury rate was the same for men and women (86). The highest risk for injury was associated with defense (blocking) and spiking, and it involved the upper extremity (fingers and shoulder) as well as the lower extremity (ankle and knee) (87).

Schafle (89) registered injuries occurring during the 1987 United States Volleyball Association's national tournament. Before the tournament, the participants' history was taken, and during the week of participation, records were kept of every player who presented with an injury. Players ranged in age from 17 to 60 and competed in five age/gender groups. There were 154 injuries in 1,520 participants during 7,812 hours of play. The injury rate was 19.7 per 1,000 hours of play. Females had an injury rate of 2.3 and males had an injury rate of 1.7. The highest injury rate was seen in the men's open division, ages 17 to 35 (2.7), and the lowest rate was seen in the men's Golden Masters, ages 46 and up (1.5). Seventy-nine percent of the injuries occurred during the tournament and 21% were considered to be chronic injuries with an acute exacerbation. The knee accounted for only 11% of injuries. Only eight (5.2%) injuries resulted in more than 5 days of time loss. Two of these injuries involved the knee. The authors concluded that because so many of the injuries were minor, studies that rely on retrospective methods for data collection would result in an overestimation of the proportion of knee and ankle injuries and the proportion of severe injuries. They concluded that coverage for a high-level volleyball tournament should provide for a preponderance of minor injuries occurring in a variety of anatomical locations.

Bahr (90) undertook a study to examine the incidence and mechanisms of acute volleyball injuries in the top two divisions of the Norwegian Volleyball Federation. Records were kept of exposure time and all acute volleyball injuries resulting in at least 1 day off. Eighty-nine injuries were recorded among 272 players during 51,588 player hours (45,837 hours of training and 5,751 hours of match play). The injury incidence was 1.7 per 1,000 hours of total exposure, 1.5 per 1,000 hours of training and 3.5 per 1,000 hours of match play. The ankle (54%) was the most commonly injured region, followed by the lower back (11%), knee (8%), shoulder (8%) and fingers (7%). These injury rates are about one tenth those reported for soccer (38,67).

Basketball

Basketball traditionally has not been associated with high rates of injury, even at the professional level (91). In Yde's study of adolescents, basketball had a lower rate of injury than soccer and handball (66), with a rate of 3.0 injuries per 1,000 hours of play. De Loes (75) reported rates of about 0.4 for boys and girls playing basketball, and it ranked below soccer and handball for both sexes with respect to the risk for injury per 1,000 hours of exposure. In a comparison study of basketball and netball among female athletes in Australia, McKay (34) reported 18.22 injuries per 1,000 exposures in basketball. The ankle, hand and knee were the body parts injured most frequently and most severely. Major or severe injuries occurred at an average of 1 injury every 625 games in female basketball. Colliander (92) reviewed all injuries among Swedish male and female basketball players during the 1981 to 1982 season by means of interviews with the players. Fifty-eight percent of the male and 62% of the female players reported injuries. The injury frequency was 2.5 injuries/1,000 activity-hours in male and 2.85 injuries/1,000 hours of activity in female players. This corresponds to 8.6 injuries/male team/season and 7.5 injuries/female team/season. Ankle sprains were the most common injuries (52%), and knee injuries occurred in 18%.

Despite lower overall injury rates in basketball, Engel (93) felt that ligamentous injuries of the knee were more common in basketball than in soccer players. They concluded that age and height affected the injury pattern, but they did not account for the effect of player position or proportion of time spent in training and in games. In a review by Hickey of all injuries reported to the sports medicine clinic at an elite Australian girls' basketball training institute during a 6-year period, the knee was the most common site of injury (94). Evidence suggests that the sport-specific pattern of injury in basketball includes a high proportion of knee injuries (32,34,91,95).

A higher susceptibility for knee ligament injury among female basketball players has been recognized for over 15 years (95). In a survey of 76 female basketball-related injuries seen at a sports medicine clinic, Gray (95) observed that the knee was the most common site of injury (72%), and ACL injury accounted for 25% of all injuries seen. Compared with males presenting with a total of 151 basketball-related injuries during the same period, of which only 4 were ACL ruptures, the authors noted a much higher relative risk for ACL injury among women than among men. Gray evaluated the injured patients for the effects of age, height, weight, alignment, mechanism of injury, playing position, experience, train-ing and history of previous injuries. Gray postulated that player position, joint laxity, weak quadriceps or hormonal influences may have been responsible of the higher rate of injury among women.

Subsequent studies have confirmed Gray's data. Several recent studies have reported injury rates among high school students categorized by sport and the gender of participants. Messina (32) undertook a prospective study to determine the incidence of injury among high school basketball players and to examine the differences in injury type, incidence, rate, and risk between male and female athletes. During successive basketball seasons, injury surveys of girls' and boys' varsity teams at 100 class 4A and 5A high schools in Texas were conducted. Athletic trainers collected data on each reportable injury and reported the data weekly to the University Inter-scholastic League. A reportable injury was defined as one that occurred during a practice or a game, resulted in missed practice or game time, required physician consul-tation, or involved the head or the face. The boys' and girls' data were compared and statistically analyzed. The rate of injury was 0.56 among the boys and 0.49 among the girls. The risk for injury per hour of exposure was not significantly different between the two groups. In both groups, the most common injuries were sprains, and the most commonly injured area was the ankle, followed by the knee. Female athletes had a significantly higher rate of knee injuries including a 3.79 times greater risk for anterior cruciate ligament injuries. For both sexes, the risk for injury during a game was significantly higher than during practice. Powell (96) used varsity team ros-ters for boys' and girls' basketball, soccer, (boys') base-ball, and (girls') softball to compare injury rates for these sports in high school athletes. They found that the knee injury rates per 100 players for girls' basketball (4.5) and girls' soccer (5.2) were higher than for their male coun-terparts. Major injuries occurred more often in girls' bas-ketball (12.4%) and soccer (12.1%) than in boys' basket-ball (9.9%) and soccer (10.4%). They also noted more surgeries, particularly knee and anterior cruciate ligament surgeries, for female basketball and soccer players than for boys or girls in other sports.

Arendt (33) performed a 5-year evaluation of anterior cruciate ligament injuries in collegiate men's and women's basketball programs using the National College Athletic Association Injury Surveillance System. Their results showed significantly higher anterior cruciate liga-ment injury rates in women's basketball than in the men's sport (0.29 vs. 0.07/1,000 exposures). Noncontact mech-anisms were the primary cause of anterior cruciate liga-ment injury in both female sports. No other knee struc-ture examined (collateral or posterior cruciate ligament and patella or patellar tendon) exhibited such a distinctive difference in injury rates. The authors pointed out that even in the female group ACL injuries were relatively infrequent in the college environment. They estimated the

ACL injury rate among NCAA collegiate basketball programs to be 1 ACL injury every 952 activity sessions for men and 1 ACL injury every 247 activity sessions for women. Both men and women were three times more likely to have an ACL injury in a game as compared with a practice.

Football

With respect to perceptions on the risk for injury, American football enjoys a certain notoriety among sports. A striking feature of studies on the epidemiology of American football played in Europe is that authors seemingly go out of their way to remark on the absence of fatal or catastrophic injuries (97–99). This caution is to some extent justified by the violent nature of the contact between players. As many as 1.2 million football-related injuries are reported annually among an estimated 1.5 million participants in the United States (100). American football is perhaps more accurately described as a collision sport than as a contact sport, and this distinction undoubtedly affects both the pattern and frequency of injuries that have been reported. Canale (101) registered all injuries in an American collegiate football team over a 5-year period, from 1975 to 1979. They calculated the injury rate for a single football player over to be 1.07 over a 5-year period, 0.99 over 4 years, and 0.47 for a single year of collegiate play. The exposure was not calculated specifically for each athlete, so these statistics probably represent about half the actual risk of participation in games. Defensive linemen, particularly defensive ends, were at greatest risk (101).

But there is evidence that the risk for injury in football has declined over the past 25 to 35 years (100,102). In a comprehensive review of the documentation on football injuries in the United States, Saal (100) attributed the reduction in injuries (catastrophic cranial and cervical injuries in particular) since 1975 to a combination of rule changes, equipment improvements, and better coaching and training techniques. Fifty-one percent of injuries occurred at training; contact sessions were 4.7 times more likely to produce injuries than controlled sessions. Injury rates were reduced by wearing shorter cleats and with better preseason conditioning. Overall, lower extremity injuries accounted for 50% of all injuries (with knee injuries accounting for up to 36%). Upper extremity injuries accounted for 30%. In general, sprains and strains account for 40% of injuries, contusions 25%, fractures 10%, concussions 5% and dislocations 15% (100).

Nicholas documented injuries during regular season games for a single American professional football team over a 26-year period (102). Significant injuries were defined as those resulting in at least two consecutive games' absence from play, and major injuries caused at least 8 weeks out of play. The rate of significant injuries averaged 0.89 per game and major injuries 0.35 per game for the entire 26 years. There was a reduction in the risk for significant injury after 1965, and subsequent injury rates were episodic. The rate of major injuries declined during the study period. Since 1969 there has been a decline in major knee injuries and a decline in major injuries incurred during special-teams play. The team began playing games on synthetic surfaces in 1968, with no significant difference in the rates of significant injuries per game (0.57 vs. 0.67) or major injuries per game (0.22 vs. 0.33) between games played on grass or artificial turf, respectively. The authors concluded that over the period of study the risk of missed games due to injury decreased, but they did not attribute the reduced risk to specific interventions, such as rule changes (100,103), equipment modification (100,104–109), or training (100,110).

Current epidemiologic studies suggest that risk for injury in football is comparable with that in other contact sports. In a prospective study of two professional German teams spanning two seasons, Baltzer reported an overall injury rate of 15.7 per 1,000 hours of total exposure (practice plus games) (97). They noted that this injury rate was comparable to handball and soccer. Bauer (111) registered all injuries in major league American football in southern Germany in 1991. They reported injury rates comparable to German soccer and hockey. Karpakka (99) reported that injury rates in Finland were similar to those reported in the United States.

DeLee (112) noted an injury rate of 0.51 per player during a single season among 100 varsity high school football programs. Calculated by time of exposure, the injury rate was 3 per 1,000 total hours of play. The rate of severe injuries was 0.031 per player per year. Again, these rates are similar to rates for soccer and handball. On the other hand, in a survey of injuries among scholastic athletic programs in the United States, Landry (113) found that at the high school and collegiate levels football had the highest injury rate, followed by wrestling and gymnastics. Despite improvements, football still is considered a high-risk sport.

Age influences the pattern and frequency of injuries in American football. In a study of youth players (ages 8 to 15) Goldberg (114) reported an overall rate of significant injury of 0.05 per year, with 61% classified as moderate and 38.9% as major injuries. No catastrophic injuries occurred, and it was rare for a permanent disability to result from any injury. Unlike most studies of adult players, in Goldberg's study the upper extremity was most likely to be injured, and fractures were more common than soft tissue injuries of any kind. They remarked that the rate, site, and type of injuries experienced by the pre-adolescent and early adolescent players differed from the pattern for older players at higher levels of competition, even within their sample. Variables related to an increased risk for injury included participation in the older and heavier divisions, heavier weight, and involvement in contact activities.

Cahill investigated the effects of training on injury rates in football. In an 8-year study comparing two groups of high school varsity football players, the number of knee injuries, and the severity of knee injuries that do occur may be significantly reduced by a preseason regimen focused on total body conditioning (110). In a second study, five football teams from major colleges were surveyed during practices and games in the 1976 season. Injury exposure rate was calculated as a ratio of injuries to minutes of exposure in 14 categories (12 specific drills, practice games, and other activities). Practice games carried the highest risk for injury among training activities. After reviewing the epidemiological literature, Halpern (115) made the following recommendations to reduce the incidence of injury: (a) optimum maintenance of playing fields; (b) use of the soccer-style shoe; (c) noncontact and controlled activities in practice sessions; and (d) increased vigilance over technique during injury-prone preseason practices.

The knee accounts for the majority of injuries in most studies (97,99–101,112), representing as much as 30% of all significant injuries (98,99). As has been noted in epidemiological studies on knee injuries in soccer, as many as 27% of reported knee injuries in football probably represent reinjuries (116). Of the 2,228 total injuries registered in DeLee's study (112), there were 445 knee injuries. Thirty-eight knee ligament injuries were treated surgically. The authors stated that these 38 injuries accounted for all of the ligament disruptions. Given this fact, the calculated rate of knee ligament injury was 0.86 per 100 athletes per year. In breaking down the individual ligament injuries, the authors noted that there were 37 ACL repairs/reconstructions, and 1 posterior cruciate ligament repair. Although it would seem unlikely that there were no MCL injuries during the course of the football season, no note is made of any collateral ligament injuries.

Powell (117) calculated knee injury rates based on data collected by athletic trainers at each National Football League club from 1980 to 1989, hoping to determine if there was a difference in injury rates between games played on natural grass and on artificial surfaces. The exposure unit used in this study was the team-game. All game-related knee sprains were recorded, in addition to MCL and ACL sprains. The authors did not define the criteria required to meet inclusion into the knee sprain groups, and thus it is not clear if these injuries included only those knees with pathologic motion. The general injury rate for knee sprains was 0.21 per team-game. The MCL sprain injury rate was 0.14 per team-game, while the ACL sprain injury rate was 0.02 per team-game.

Hewson (103) reviewed a group of collegiate football players at one university to compare the effects of prophylactic bracing with nonbracing on the incidence of knee injury. They compared the incidence of knee injury during a 4-year period when preventative braces were worn by all players at risk with a 4-year period when no braces were worn. During the 4-year period when no braces were worn, the incidence of ACL injury was 2.65 per season per 100 players at risk, while the incidence of MCL and combined ACL/MCL injury was 1.77 and 10.62, respectively. Numerous studies of brace use have failed to provide compelling evidence that prophylactic braces prevent or mitigate knee ligament injuries among football players (108,109,118–126).

Skiing

The knee is a common site of injury among alpine skiers. In 1981 Schaffer (127) reported that knee ligament injuries represented 24% of all injuries requiring medical attention at Jackson Hole, MCL sprains being the most common knee injury. Johnson (128) evaluated injured skiers that presented to a ski injury clinic at the base lodge of a large northern Vermont ski area over a 4-year period between 1972 to 1976. Overall, there were 1,052 injured skiers with 1,141 injuries. There were 246 knee ligament injuries, the majority of which (213, 86.2%) were medial collateral ligament sprains with or without anterior cruciate sprain. Other knee ligament injuries included 21 lateral collateral ligament sprains, six posterior cruciate sprains, and six anterior cruciate sprains. Although there were six isolated ACL sprains, some of the other ACL injuries were grouped together with the MCL injuries and the total number of ACL injuries is thus unknown. In a study of 420 ski-related knee injuries in northern Sweden, Edlund reported more injuries among cross-country and distance skiers than among downhill skiers, but the cohorts were dissimilar in the distribution of age and sex among subjects, and non-alpine skiers used nonrelease bindings (129). Edlund made no attempt to control for the popularity of Nordic skiing in northern Sweden. None of these early studies attempted to record the amount of exposure, so injury risk could not be calculated.

Epidemiologic studies of skiing have used a variety of approaches to control for the amount of exposure associated with injuries, including (vertical) distance skied (35) or days of participation (36). Another technique, used by Johnson and Pope (130), expressed the incidence of injury in terms of mean days between injury (MDBI = skier visits/number of injuries). This is essentially an inverse of the conventional equation, and was used to avoid changing the base to 10,000 or 100,000 for relatively rare injury groups. There is as yet no single standard for reporting exposure, and it is not a trivial matter to impose such a standard. Furthermore, exposure to injury in alpine skiing is related not only to the amount of time spent skiing, but to the course rating, type of terrain and quality of snow, none of which is easily controlled in studies of recreational skiers. It is simpler to measure exposure among training athletes because total time spent skiing, and the type of skiing done (racing, slalom, moguls, jumping), can be recorded. But for recreational skiers, a skier day for one person may involve two or three times as much time on the slopes or vertical distance skied as it would for someone else. Presumably, better skiers cover more vertical distance and use more challenging runs than inexperienced skiers, so the effects of training and experience cannot be studied using skier day as the measure of exposure. From the point of view of precision and accuracy then, the Swiss method (35) seems best. But for various reasons the majority of studies still use skier days as the measure of exposure.

Feagin et al. (131) observed 1.2 knee injuries per 1,000 skier days at a single ski area. Sixty percent included an ACL injury, 65% of which were isolated injuries by clinical examination. Tapper (36) reviewed all ski injuries occurring at a single facility during a 4-year period from 1972 to 1976. Overall, 4,227 injuries were noted, resulting in 3.2 injuries per 1,000 skier days. Eight hundred twenty-eight knee injuries, categorized as medial and lateral knee sprain, lateral knee sprain, and internal derangement, were observed during this period, for an incidence of 0.63 injuries per 1,000 skier days. The use of the term internal derangement reflects the state of clinical examinations at that time and the author's ability in accurately making the diagnosis of cruciate ligament ruptures. More recently, however, improved examination techniques using ligament arthrometry (see Chapter 19) as well as ancillary tests such as magnetic resonance imaging have made it easier to obtain a more accurate and complete diagnosis at the time of injury.

Currently, the knee is reported to be the most common site injured among adult skiers (132). Warme (133) retrospectively reviewed all skiing injuries that occurred over a 12-season period at Jackson Hole ski resort. The overall rate of injury, based on 2.55 million skier-days, was 3.7 injuries per 1,000 skier-days. There were 2,935 ligamentous knee injuries. Ligamentous knee injuries comprised 30% of this total. Although injury rates were not calculated for the individual ligament disruptions, the authors did note that there were 1,761 MCL sprains, 1,615 ACL injuries, and 675 combined ACL/MCL lesions.

On the basis of epidemiologic data from several different countries, the specific risk of knee injury among alpine skiers appears to be increasing (21,35,130, 134–137) even as overall injury rates among skiers are declining (135,138). During the period 1980 to 1989, Natri noted a 247% increase in the frequency of ACL injuries treated annually at the University Hospital of Tampere, Finland (21). Most authorities on this subject have attributed the rise to newer boot designs that protect against lower leg fracture. In a series of papers summa-

rizing their experience treating nearly 30,000 winter sport injuries at the hospital in Davos, Holzach and Bruesch noted that 85% of all injuries were caused by alpine skiing (35,134,139). Currently 1 in 4 ski injuries (35,139), or half of all injuries to the lower extremities (134), treated at Davos Hospital involve the knee ligaments. They reported that the increase in knee injuries over two decades of study corresponded to the reduction in fractures of the leg, which the authors attributed directly to changes in boot design. They also noted that ski areas favored by beginning skiers referred three times as many injuries as other resorts.

In studies performed at the University of Vermont the incidence of ACL injuries as a percentage of all injuries associated with skiing in northern Vermont rose from 4.5% in 1972 to 19.3% in 1999 (137). In an earlier paper on a portion of this cohort, Johnson and Pope (130) reported on ski-related injuries seen over the 15-year period between 1972 and 1987. There were 5,701 injuries and 1,690,000 skier visits over the period of the study. Knee sprains were subdivided into two groups. The incidence of grade I and II knee sprains decreased from year 1 of the study (1,121 mean days between injury) to year 15 (3,945). In contrast, grade III knee sprains, usually involving the anterior cruciate ligament, increased from 6,669 to 2,452 mean days between injuries. This increase in higher grade knee ligament injuries occurred at a time when overall injury rates were decreasing, and equipment design and adjustment were improving (138). Nevertheless as many as 80% of knee ligament injuries were thought to be equipment-related (138). The Vermont group has applied its experience toward exploring preventative measures such as improvements in equipment (140) and training (141) to reduce rates of knee ligament injury. Johnson (140) has argued that smarter bindings and better standards for their adjustment are needed if a reduction in injury rates are to be achieved among elite skiers.

Overall injury rates in some studies appear to be higher in school-age children (142,143) than in adults, but this seems to be due primarily to higher rates of head (143) and upper extremity (144) trauma. Deibert (132) prospectively gathered data on skiing injuries sustained at two ski areas during a 22-year period. Injured skiers were evaluated at a base-lodge clinic, and data were collected to determine the frequency and pattern of injury in three age groups—children (1–10 years old), adolescents (11–16 years old), and adults (older than 16 years). Ligamentous knee injuries recorded during the period of data collection included grade III sprains of the anterior cruciate ligament and grade I or II sprains of the medial collateral ligament. Based on the data presented in this study, the overall calculated ACL injury rate was 0.398 per 1,000 skier days, while the ACL injury rate among the children, adolescents, and adults was 0.024, 0.125, and 0.458, respectively. Similarly, the overall MCL injury rate was

0.334 per 1000 skier-days, whereas the injury rate in the three age groups was 0.565, 0.271, and 0.336, respectively.

No clear consensus has emerged regarding the effect of gender on ski-related injuries. Methodological differences in study design probably account for inconsistent findings reported in the literature. De Loes (145) collected standardized Swiss national insurance and participation data on youth subjects (ages of 14 and 20 years) playing 12 different sports including alpine skiing. Enrollment averaged 370,000 subjects annually. They identified 3,864 knee injuries from all sports during the 7 years of study. Females were significantly more at risk in downhill skiing than males, particularly for injuries to the knee ligaments.

Stevenson and colleagues (146) sent a questionnaire to all members of the Vermont Alpine Racing Association and several New England NCAA Division I ski racing programs in 1995. Of 404 responses, 27% reported a history of a knee injury. Female racers were 2.3 times more likely to have sustained a knee injury than male racers. One in 5 female alpine racers (22%) reported an ACL disruption, and females were 3.1 times more likely to sustain an ACL injury in comparison to their male counterparts. The authors also noted that the risk for repeat surgery for failed ACL reconstruction among women respondents was higher than among men (27% vs. 13%), although the difference was not statistically significant.

Viola (147) reported a retrospective study of anterior cruciate ligament injuries among professional alpine skiers. Preparticipation records were available for 7,155 ski patrollers or instructors (4,537 men and 2,618 women) to identify pre-existing knee conditions before each ski season from 1991 to 1997. Screening involved a ski history questionnaire, a knee injury history questionnaire, and a knee physical examination. Any patient with an equivocal Lachman or pivot shift test was evaluated by KT-1000 arthrometry. A manual maximum side-to-side difference was 3 mm or more excluded subjects from the study so that presumably the study sample was limited to subjects with intact anterior cruciate ligaments at the beginning of each season. Skiers injured during the study were identified through mandatory workers' compensation claims. Each injured skier was reevaluated using an injury questionnaire and physical examination. The men skied an average of 110 days per year (499,070 skier-days) and the women skied an average of 87 days per year (227,766 skier-days). Thirty-one skiing-related anterior cruciate ligament injuries were diagnosed, 21 in men and 10 in women. The incidence of ACL disruption was 4.2 injuries per 100,000 skier-days in men and 4.4 injuries per 100,000 skier-days in women. These data suggest that the incidences of anterior cruciate ligament injuries among male and female professional alpine skiers are similar.

Children, Sports, and Knee Injuries

Over the past two decades, the number of children and adolescents participating in both organized and recreational sports has increased significantly (113,148,149). It is estimated that 45 million children engage in scholastic and organized sports annually (150). In soccer alone, an estimated 6 million children in the United States under the age of 12 played on some form of soccer team in 1990 (151). As one might expect, this increase in sports participation has resulted in an increase in sports-related injuries (152).

Numerous studies have examined the incidence of sports injuries in young athletes (38,66,114,148,151, 153). For the most part, these are cross-sectional, retrospective surveys that are often limited to a specific type of sport and do not give a true representation of the young population. The incidence of knee ligament injuries in the pediatric population has been reported by only a handful of authors. This may be due, in part, to the fact that disruptions of knee ligaments are relatively rare injuries in children and adolescents. Ligaments are stronger than the adjacent growth plates (154), and for this reason, epiphyseal plate injuries or long bone fractures tend to occur before ligamentous failure (155–158). When ligamentous injuries do occur in children, they usually will consist of an avulsion fracture at the insertion site (155–157).

In the Kaiser population, the rate of knee ligament injuries in children less than 15 years of age was 0.093 per 1,000 members. This was much lower than the overall incidence of 0.49 injuries per 1,000 members. However, this pediatric group also included infants and young children who were probably not at risk for significant ligament injury. The youngest individual with a ligament injury was 10 years of age. If only those children and adolescents 10 years and older were to be considered, the incidence of injury would be expected to be higher. Unfortunately, the number of children in the Kaiser population that were 10 to 14 years of age was not available, and consequently, incidence rates for this subgroup could not be calculated.

Anterior cruciate ligament tears, with the exception of avulsion fractures of the intercondylar eminence, appear to be rare injuries in children. In the Kaiser population, the incidence of ACL injury in the pediatric population was 0.043 per 1,000. Although ACL injuries in children have been reported in the literature, incidence rates have been not calculated. Clanton et al. (156), in reviewing 1,749 cases of ligament injury, found only 9 cases of ACL injuries in children under 14 years of age. McCarroll et al. (159) reported on 57 patients 14 years of age or younger with ACL injuries out of a total of 1,722 ACL injuries treated over 5½ years. Between 1977 and 1983, Lipscomb and Anderson (160) operated on 710 patients with tears of the ACL. This included 24 athletes between the ages of 12 and 15 years that underwent ACL reconstruction. DeLee and Curtis (157) reported 3 cases of ACL injury in children ages 9, 11, and 12 during a 3-year period in which they treat 338 knee ligament injuries. Kannus and Jarvinen (161) reviewed a group of 33 adolescents aged 10 to 18 with grade II or III knee ligament injuries. Included in this group were 12 injuries of the ACL, 7 isolated and 5 combined ACL/MCL injuries. Injury rates were calculated in none of the above reports.

Skak (158) recorded knee injuries in children ages 0 to 14 years that presented to three hospitals in Denmark. The number of children that lived in the areas served by these hospitals was known to the authors and used to calculate the annual incidence of various knee injuries. There were twenty cruciate ligament avulsions overall (18 ACL and 2 PCL), with an annual incidence of 3.0 per 100,000. There were 5 collateral ligament injuries (four medial and one lateral) and the overall annual incidence was 0.7 per 100,000.

Zaricznyj et al. (162) documented all sports-related injuries to school-aged children in Springfield, Illinois during a 1-year period beginning in November 1974. The authors obtained the cooperation of the principals and coaches of all the schools, supervisors of community sports programs, hospital emergency rooms, schools' accident insurance company, and local physicians in compiling sports-related accident reports for all children from kindergarten to high school. There were 25,512 school-aged children over-all. Eight torn knee ligaments were reported, although no specific breakdown of the individual ligaments injured was noted. Although knee injury incidence rates were not calculated by the authors, based on the data that they provided, the rate of knee ligament injury was 0.31 per 1,000 children.

More recently, Deibert et al. (132) prospectively gathered data on skiing injuries sustained at two Vermont ski areas over a 22-year period to document rates of injury in children, adolescents, and adults participating in alpine skiing. Children were younger than 11 years old, while adolescents were 11 to 16 years of age. Grade III ACL injuries were the most common injury in adults, while they were only the eighth most common injury in adolescents. Interestingly, ACL injuries did not even make the top ten among injuries in children. Based on the data presented in this study, the overall calculated ACL injury rate was 0.398 per 1,000 skier days, while the ACL injury rate among the children, adolescents, and adults was 0.024, 0.125, and 0.458, respectively. Similarly, the overall MCL injury rate was 0.334 per 1,000 skier-days, while the injury rate in the three age groups was 0.565, 0.271, and 0.336, respectively.

Despite the abundance of literature on sports-related injuries in children, specific data regarding the incidence of knee ligament injuries are sorely lacking. Until the epidemiology of knee ligament disruptions in the pediatric population is better defined, measures to prevent these injuries cannot be developed.

Gender-Specific Studies

Women's participation in intercollegiate athletics has increased dramatically in recent years. Greater participation has increased awareness of health and medical issues specific to the female athlete. The adoption in 1972 of Title IX, a U.S. Federal entitlement that legislates equal opportunities and benefits to both sexes in all student services, academic programs, and employment, was a significant factor in the explosion of women's athletic programs. In 1994, Nattiv and Arendt (163) reported that girls' participation in high school sports had increased 600% in the period after Title IX was adopted, compared with a 20% increase in boys' participation during the same time.

Levy (164) sent a questionnaire to 50 female collegiate rugby clubs, and calculated injury rates based on the 810 female collegiate rugby players from the 42 clubs that responded. Injury rates were determined based on the number of exposures, which included games and practices. All diagnoses were confirmed by either arthroscopic evaluation or magnetic resonance imaging. The incidence of ACL tear was 0.36 per 1,000 exposures, while the rate of MCL and PCL injury was 0.39 and 0.03 per 1,000 exposures, respectively. This paper provided no data for comparison of injury rates between male and female rugby players.

Hickey et al. (94) retrospectively reviewed the medical records of female basketball players on scholarship at the Australian Institute of Sport from 1990 to 1995. Overall, there were 2.9 injuries per basketball player per year. Although the incidence of knee ligament injuries was not reported, the authors did record four ACL injuries. Based on this information, the calculated rate of ACL injury was 5.1 per 100 basketball players per year. Like the study by Levy, no data were provided for comparison to injury rates in male athletes.

The explosion in women's participation in competitive sports has prompted closer examination of relative injury rates between the sexes (Table 18.10). These studies, for the most part, have noted a higher incidence of knee injuries, particularly ACL disruption, among female athletes when compared with their male counterparts (9,32,33,81,146,165–167). Arendt and Dick (33) reviewed data from the National Collegiate Athletic Association (NCAA) Injury Surveillance System (ISS) to determine the relative differences in knee injury pattern among men and women in collegiate basketball and soccer. They recorded gender-specific knee injuries during a 5-year period from 1989 to 1993 sustained while playing soccer and basketball. These two sports were chosen specifically because they were the only two monitored by the ISS that offered similar rules and playing conditions for both male and female competitors. The rates of injury were expressed in units of athlete-exposure. An athlete-exposure was defined as one athlete participating in one

TABLE 18.10. *Review of the literature: Incidence of anterior cruciate ligament injury gender comparisons*

Reference	Sport	Overall	Female	Male	Unit (per)
Kaiser, 1985–1997	General population	0.49	0.36	0.72	1,000 members per year
Arendt and Dick (33)	Soccer		0.31	0.13	1,000 athlete-exposures
	Basketball		0.29	0.07	1,000 athlete-exposures
Harmon and Dick (165)	Soccer		0.321	0.123	1,000 exposures
	Basketball		0.297	0.080	1,000 exposures
Messina et al. (32)	Basketball	0.008	0.012	0.004	Athlete per season
	Basketball	0.052	0.09	0.024	1,000 player-hours
Myklebust et al. (81)	Handball		0.31	0.06	1,000 player-hours
Gwinn et al. (166)	Naval Academy		0.0135	0.0055	Athlete per year
	Basketball, soccer, and rugby		0.511	0.129	1,000 athlete-exposures
Bjordal et al. (9)	Soccer	0.063	0.10	0.057	1,000 game hours
Viola et al. (147)	Skiing		4.4	4.2	100,000 skier-days
Levy et al. (164)	Rugby		0.36		1,000 exposures
Hickey et al. (94)	Basketball		5.1		100 players per year

practice or game where he or she is exposed to the possibility of an athletic injury. In soccer, the incidence of ACL injury in women was 0.31 per 1,000 athlete-exposures, which was more than double the incidence in men (0.13). In contrast, the incidence of collateral ligament injury (women 0.62, men 0.51) and PCL injury (women 0.04, men 0.04) between sexes was similar. Similar results were noted in basketball. The incidence of ACL injury in women's basketball (0.29) was more than four times that of men's basketball (0.07). Again, as in the sport of soccer, the incidence of collateral ligament and PCL injury was similar between the sexes.

Harmon (165) also reviewed data from the NCAA Injury Surveillance System to examine gender differences among athletes participating in basketball and soccer. The period of review was from 1989 to 1996. Overall, they found that the ACL injury rate for women basketball players was 0.297 per 1,000 exposures, while the injury rate for men was 0.080. Thus, women basketball players had a 3.7 times greater incidence of ACL injury than their male counterparts. Similar results were found among the collegiate soccer players. The overall ACL injury rate in women's soccer was 0.321, while the rate in men's soccer was 0.123. As expected, these results are similar to those of Arendt and Dick (33) because the same database was used.

Messina (32) undertook a prospective study to determine the incidence of injury among high school basketball players and to examine the differences in injury type, incidence rate and risk between male and female athletes. Injury data were collected from a group of public high schools in Texas during a single basketball season. All information was recorded by certified athletic trainers from the participating schools. The ACL injury rate was 0.008 per athlete per season. However, when the athletes were divided by gender, the injury rate for the boys was 0.004 per athlete per season, and for girls was 0.012. Injury risk was also calculated in terms of player-hours of exposure. The overall ACL injury risk was 0.052 per

1,000 player-hours. Again, when gender differences were examined, the risk for ACL injury among boys was 0.024, and for girls was 0.09.

Similar gender-related differences in the rate of ACL injury have been reported for other sports as well. Myklebust (81) prospectively examined gender differences in the incidence of ACL injury in a population of elite Norwegian team handball players. The rate of ACL injury among women players was 0.31 per 1,000 player hours, while the incidence among men was 0.06 per 1,000 player hours.

In 1995 Stevenson (146) surveyed all members of a statewide alpine racing association and several regional NCAA Division I ski racing programs to determine the prevalence of knee ligament insufficiency. Four hundred four (40%) of subjects responded. Twenty-seven percent of respondents reported having sustained a knee injury. Women were 2.3 times as likely as men to have had a knee injury. Twenty-two percent of female racers reported having sustained an ACL disruption, a rate more than three times that of male racers. In contrast, Viola (147) retrospectively reviewed the incidence of ACL injuries among professional alpine skiers, noting that the incidence of ACL disruption was 4.2 injuries per 100,000 skier days in men and 4.4 injuries per 100,000 skier days in women.

Gwinn et al. (166) compared ACL injury rates between male and female midshipmen at the US Naval Academy from 1991 to 1997. ACL injuries were defined as "tears requiring surgical intervention as identified by physical examination and confirmed at arthroscopy." Data were collected at the time of injury, and all ACL injuries were identified by orthopaedic surgeons during "sick call." In addition to calculating the overall injury rate, the authors also reported incidence rates for similar men's and women's intercollegiate sports, intramural/recreational sports, and military training. The overall incidence rate was calculated as injury cases per athlete per year, while incidence rates for the subgroups were calculated as the number of injury cases divided by the total number of athlete-exposures. An exposure was defined as any practice or game in which the athlete was exposed to the possibility of an athletic injury.

The overall incidence rate of ACL injury for the female and male midshipmen was 0.0135 and 0.0055 per athlete per year, respectively. Thus, the female midshipmen sustained ACL injuries at over twice the rate of their male counterparts. The results were similar when the various subgroups were also examined. When the incidence of injury was compared in intercollegiate basketball, soccer, and rugby, in every instance, the rate of ACL injury was higher among the female midshipmen. When comparing these sports collectively, the rate of ACL injury among the women and men was 0.511 and 0.129 per 1,000 athlete-exposures, respectively, suggesting that the female varsity athlete was almost four times more likely to sustain an ACL injury than her male counterpart.

Higher ACL injury rates among female athletes have been attributed largely to one of three factors: hormonal influences (81,168–170), anatomic differences (smaller notch width or notch width index (171–173), valgus limb alignment (174), increased ligamentous laxity (175–177), or inferior levels of strength/conditioning compared with male athletes (176). However, there is no conclusive explanation for the higher frequency among women, and more than likely, the cause is multifactorial. Further study will be required to determine the gender-specific factors associated with ACL injury and eventually develop preventative measures based on these findings.

PREVENTION OF KNEE LIGAMENT INJURIES

Recognizing that any attempt at reducing the incidence of sports injuries requires a well-structured plan of preventative measures, Backx et al. (148) described a four-step plan to meet these goals. The first step consists of acquiring data regarding the nature, extent, and severity of sports injuries. The second step involves the identification of etiologic factors involved in sports injuries. The third step is applying one or more measures, based on identified etiologic factors, to prevent sports injuries or reduce their severity. The last step involves evaluating the applied preventative measure to determine whether there was any effect on the incidence and severity of injury. Most studies to date have not proceeded beyond the second step, although there are now a few studies that have evaluated the effect of preventative measures (141,178).

The first step in developing any preventative program requires data acquisition regarding the incidence of injury. In the United States, the NCAA has taken an active role in supporting research on the epidemiology of injuries in college athletes (33). The NCAA ISS was developed in 1982 to provide current and reliable data on injury trends in intercollegiate athletics. Injury data are collected yearly from a representative sample of NCAA member institutions, and the resulting summaries are reviewed by the NCAA Committee on Competitive Safeguards and Medical Aspects of Sports. The Committee's goals include reduction of injury rates through suggested changes in rules, protective equipment, or coaching techniques based in part on data provided by the ISS. The ISS can be used not only to identify injury rates, but to monitor the effects of preventative measures.

In recognition of the enormous economic and public health impact of any activity practiced on such a scale, several national and international sporting associations (33,40) have begun to take an active role in assessing and managing risk of participation in soccer, or football as it is called outside North America. The Fédération Internationale de Football Association, the international governing body of soccer, has sponsored a comprehensive study of risk factors and injury prevention that was published as a supplement to the 2000 American Journal of Sports Medicine (40). The authors of these studies reported several remarkable findings, some of which were summarized in the section on soccer injuries. Taken as a whole, the supplement is a benchmark in epidemiological research on soccer injuries and should serve as a blueprint for the assessment of risks and identification of preventive measures in any other competitive sport.

Prior to considering potential strategies for preventing knee ligament injuries, the risk factors for injury must first be established. Griffin et al. (1) divided risk factors for noncontact ACL injuries into four categories: environmental, anatomic, hormonal, and biomechanical. Other authors have drawn a distinction between factors extrinsic to the athlete (e.g., injury activity, contact, playing surface or shoe wear) and those that are intrinsic to the individual or the knee (knee anatomy, muscular activation, level of conditioning, gender) (33,179,180). Once the risk factors and mechanisms of injury are well understood, strategies for injury prevention can be developed. Dvorak (40) and others (1) have suggested specific interventions for reducing the rate of athletic injuries. Emerging data indicate that some prevention strategies may be effective in reducing the risk for ACL injury (141,178), while others may not (82). In the final section of this chapter, we shall summarize approaches that have shown promise for the prevention of knee ligament injury.

Mechanisms of Knee Injury

A firm understanding of the mechanisms of knee injury is essential to the development of preventative strategies. In the case of ACL injury, there are two basic mechanisms—direct contact and noncontact. The literature is not in complete agreement on the proportion of knee injuries that result from these two mechanisms. Most authors have suggested that the majority of ACL disruptions are the result of noncontact injuries. Boden et al. (181), in a report on 100 knees that sustained rupture of the ACL as a result of athletic activity other than skiing, found that 72% were injured through a noncontact mechanism. Other authors have reported a similar proportion of noncontact injuries (Noyes 78% [183], McNair and Marshall 70% [182], Griffin 70% [1]) (1,182,183). In studies of skiing and volleyball, the majority of ACL injuries are reported to occur without contact with another person. However, in well-designed, prospective studies of soccer injury rates, direct contact with another player was responsible for over half of all injuries. Arendt et al. (33) reported that 50% of ACL injuries sustained by men playing intercollegiate soccer were the result of direct contact. It may be concluded that injury mechanisms, like injury rates, are activity-specific.

Injuries of the ACL that involve direct contact usually are the result of an excessive valgus force to the knee (184). In Boden's (181) series of 100 ACL ruptures, the most common mechanism of direct contact injury was a contact blow to the lateral aspect of the leg or knee, resulting in valgus collapse. This mechanism accounted for 13% of all ACL injuries, and 46% of the contact ACL injuries. Contact from a medial blow resulting in varus collapse occurred in 6% of all ACL injuries.

Because contact injuries occur with the foot in a planted position, more force is required to displace the tibia relative to the femur (184). This has been proposed as an explanation for the increased rate of associated injuries seen with contact injuries. O'Donoghue's unhappy triad has been classically described as a combined ACL, MCL, and medial meniscus injury resulting from a clipping-injury to the lower extremity in football. Shelbourne (185) has reported that combined ACL and MCL injuries are more commonly associated with lateral meniscus tears rather than medial tears. In soccer, contact injuries of the ACL are as common as noncontact injuries among male collegiate soccer players (33). These injuries are often the result of a slide-tackle, when an opponent strikes the lateral aspect of the player's knee. Rule changes that enforce proper slide-tackling technique may have a dramatic effect in reducing the incidence of these injuries.

Noncontact mechanisms are clearly responsible for a substantial number of knee injuries. These knee injuries are of particular interest because they are believed to hold a key to understanding how factors intrinsic to an individual or a knee can lead to ACL injury (1). A better understanding of these noncontact mechanisms may allow preventative strategies to be developed (179).

Sudden decelerations and abrupt changes in direction on a fixed foot are felt to be crucial elements in producing noncontact ACL injuries (1,186). Video analysis of noncontact ACL injuries (1,181) has revealed that these injuries often occur during a sharp deceleration or landing maneuver with the knee at a flexion angle between 30° and full extension. These decelerations at low knee flexion angles will result in strong eccentric contractions of the quadriceps, placing measurable strains on the ACL (1,187–190). Ground contact in the flat foot position has also been noted in many of these injuries. A flat-footed position will place the center of gravity behind the knee and subsequently stimulate a quadriceps contraction in order to bring the trunk forward, again resulting in an anteriorly directed tibial force (1). Valgus knee moments, which may further stress the ACL (178,187,191), have also been noted on these videotapes (181).

It is important to note that the hamstrings, in contrast to the quadriceps, are ACL agonists, and provide a posterior shear force that may protect the ligament (188,190,192,193). Athletes with excessive hamstring flexibility may lose some of the protective ability of this muscle, predisposing them to ACL injury. Based on this information, it has been hypothesized (1) that a neuromuscular training program may prevent noncontact ACL injuries sustained in pivoting sports. Such a program should seek to keep the center of gravity forward and the athlete on his or her toes, and should encourage better lower-extremity rotational and angular control.

Observed differences in ACL injury rates between males and female have focused attention on neuromuscular responses as a possible mechanism for higher injury rates among women. Gender differences have been observed in the patterns of quadriceps and hamstring contractions in response to anterior tibial translations, possibly explaining the higher incidence of ACL injuries among female athletes (176,191). Huston and Wojtys (176) performed physiologic testing on a group of elite athlete and nonathlete males and females to determine if there were any differences between genders that could account for the disproportionate number of ACL injuries seen in women. They found that female athletes relied more on the quadriceps to resist anterior tibial translation, while males recruited the hamstrings for initial knee stabilization more frequently. The female athletes also took significantly longer to generate peak hamstring torques when compared with males during isokinetic testing. These physiologic differences may contribute to the higher incidence of ACL injury among women athletes, and suggest that a specific training regimen tailored toward addressing these differences may reduce the risk for injury.

Arnason (37) investigated the frequency, cause and location of injuries in Icelandic elite soccer in 1991. Strains occurred mainly during sprinting, sprains by tackling, and contusion during other contact. Significantly more injuries occurred on artificial turf than on grass or per number of hours spent in games and practices. Teams who had the longest preseason preparation period obtained significantly fewer injuries during the season.

The mechanisms of ACL injury in alpine skiing seem to be distinct from other injury mechanisms. Through analysis of both the Vermont database and videotapes of skiers sustaining ACL injuries, the most common mechanisms of ACL injury in alpine skiing have been identified and divided into three categories (137,141). The valgus-external rotation mechanism occurs when the medial edge of the ski tip engages the snow and propels the skier downhill. This results in an external rotation torque with the leg in an abducted position. It is hypothesized that the MCL in the primary ligament injured by this mechanism, with the ACL injury occurring secondarily. The anterior drawer mechanism results when the top of the ski boot drives the tibia forward, placing an anteriorly directed force on the ACL. This mechanism occurs during hard landings following a jump by off-balance skiers. The flexion-internal rotation, or phantom foot mechanism is thought to be the most common cause of ACL injury in alpine skiing at this time (Fig. 18.1). The skier typically loses balance and falls backward, resulting in a sudden internal rotation of the hyperflexed knee.

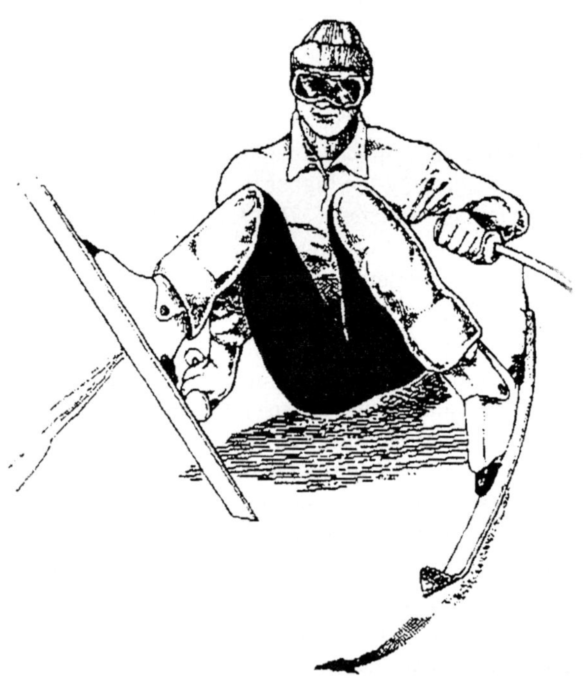

FIGURE 18.1. "Because this injury involves the tail of the ski, a lever that points in a direction opposite that of the human foot, we have termed this mechanism of injury the phantom-foot ACL injury mechanism and believe it to be the most common and insidious ACL injury scenario in alpine skiing today. In all the cases we have observed in our video analysis, the skier is off balance to the rear, with all his or her weight on the inside edge of the tail of the downhill ski and the uphill ski unweighted. The hips are below the knees with the upper body generally facing the downhill ski. The uphill arm is back and the injury is sustained in each case by the downhill leg." (From ACL Awareness Training-Phase II, Copyright Vermont Safety Research 1994. Illustration is copyrighted by William Hamilton, 1988, with permission.)

Return to Activity After Injury

Return to activity after a prior injury has been viewed as a potential risk factor for subsequent reinjury, particularly noncontact injury (37,39,44,52,55,71). The prevalence of prior knee injuries among competitive athletes may be fairly significant. Brynhildsen (52) noted a high prevalence of symptoms related to prior knee injuries among female players at the start of a new season. Twenty of these 150 athletes (13%) had a history of knee sprain, and 11 of these 20 had persistent symptoms at the start of the season. These previous injuries predispose the athletes to subsequent injuries. In a 1-year prospective study of 180 male adult soccer players, Ekstrand (44,71) observed that 35% of all moderate or major injuries were preceded by a minor injury. The authors considered inadequate rehabilitation to be an important contributor to risk for significant injury. There were 18 moderate or major traumatic knee injuries. Seven were noncontact injuries, while 11 occurred during a collision. Five of the 7 (71%) noncontact injuries occurred in players with histories of knee injury, compared with 1 of the 11 (9%) knee collision injuries.

Nielsen and Yde (55), in a prospective investigation of soccer injuries in a Danish soccer club, found that in 41% of injured players, there was an injury of the same type and location during the preceding year. Arnason (37) reviewed the frequency and cause of injuries in Icelandic male elite soccer players during one season, and found that the overall frequency of reinjury was markedly high. Forty-four percent of the strains and 58% of the sprains were registered as reinjuries. There were five knee strains, two of which were considered reinjuries.

Clearly, a history of knee injury will predispose an athlete to subsequent reinjury. Successful return to sport after an injuries requires thorough evaluation and management of the original injury, especially if the injury predisposes the athlete to reinjury, as ACL tears do. Furthermore, current evidence suggests that athletes who are inadequately rehabilitated after injuries are also at increased risk, probably because of fatigue and poor technique. Future investigations examining the length of time and degree of effort devoted to rehabilitation before returning to play after a knee injury may shed some light on this subject and offer better guidelines for return to play.

Skill, Training, and Risk for Knee Ligament Injury

Regardless of the sport, skill level has been considered extensively in relation to injury rates (9,27,28,33,38,78,165). Previous findings concerning the influence of skill level on the incidence of sports injuries, particularly severe knee injuries, are conflicting (8,10,44). Some authors have found no difference in injury rates among athletes at different skill levels (63,165).Harmon (165) reviewed ACL injury rates from National Collegiate Athletic Association (NCAA) Division I, II, and III level men's and women's basketball and soccer players. They observed no association between the NCAA Division level and rates of ACL injury for either men or women athletes. Poulsen et al. (63), in a prospective study of soccer injuries in Denmark, found that lower-skilled players had a higher injury rate than highly skilled players. However, they found that the lower level players participated in more games that the high level players. When this was taken into account and the injury rates were stratified into game and practice injuries, the injury rates were very similar.

In contrast, Nielsen and Yde (55), in a prospective study on Danish soccer players, noted that upper level players had a higher incidence of injury during games, while lower level players sustained more practice injuries. Similarly, Seil et al. (78), in a prospective study that examined sports injuries in team handball, found that the overall incidence of game-injury was higher in the high-level group, while practice injury incidence was higher in the lower performance group. In addition, knee injuries tended to be more frequent in the higher level group. The authors thought that a higher exposure to pivoting stresses with growing performance level could have been responsible for the higher incidence of injury. Similarly, Roos et al. (10) reported that more ACL injuries were registered in elite soccer players than in lower-skill players.

Other authors have proposed that higher level athletes are more skilled and better conditioned, and should thus have lower rates of injury (8,26,71) Peterson et al. (38), in a prospective study on the incidence of soccer-related injuries among players of different ages and skill levels, found that low-level players had a higher incidence of injuries per player, especially in relation to severe injury. Low-level players had twice as many severe injuries as high-level players. They suggested that better conditioning, techniques, and tactics among the high-level players resulted in their lower injury rates. Similarly, Chomiak et al. (61) prospectively analyzed the factors related to the occurrence of severe soccer injuries in the Czech Republic and found that the overall incidence of severe injuries was twice as high in the low-skill group as in the high-skill group. The incidence of severe knee injuries, however, was similar in the lower- and higher-skilled players with the exception of ACL injuries, the majority of which occurred among the lower-skill players. The higher incidence of injury among female athletes may also be due to lower levels of playing technique and skills (33,45,47,48,187).

The term skill can have many different meanings, and this may account for the discrepancy among the various studies. Unfortunately, the quality of documentation among those studies considering skill as a risk factor has been inconsistent, and these divisions may be based on age, years of experience, technical ability, or a combination. Until the term "skill" is better defined, the effect of skill level in the incidence of knee injury cannot be determined.

PREVENTATIVE STRATEGIES

Based on previous studies of injury mechanisms, Ekstrand et al. (194) developed an injury prevention program that attempted to reduce the incidence of soccer related injuries. This was a multi-pronged approach toward injury prevention that consisted of seven parts. Overall, the program was designed to encourage appropriate training and rehabilitation techniques, to provide protective equipment and taping, to instruct athletes on the potential mechanisms of injury, and to exclude those athletes with knee instability that were at high risk for injury. In a randomized study, those teams that used the prophylactic program had 75% fewer injuries than the control group that did not follow the program. In particular, there were fewer "knee sprains" in the test group when compared with the control group. Unfortunately, because of the diverse approach that was in this program, it is impossible to determine which part of the program was effective at preventing injury. This early study did demonstrate, however, that a preventative strategy based on known injury mechanisms and risk factors could alter the incidence of sports injury.

An understanding of those risk factors that predispose to knee ligament injury have resulted in several suggested interventions for reducing the incidence of knee ligament injury. These preventative strategies can be divided into two general categories—those related to changes in training or technique, and those related to introducing or changing athletic equipment.

Training/Technique and Risk for Knee Ligament Injury

The current understanding of the mechanisms of knee injury has led to the development of several preventative programs designed to alter these biomechanical risk factors. These programs have attempted either to alter preexisting techniques, or to introduce novel neuromuscular training methods to reduce the risk for injury.

From a review of ACL injury tapes and data at a Vermont ski resort, Ettlinger et al. (141) determined that the majority of ACL injuries in recreational skiing resulted from the "phantom foot" mechanism. This involves internal rotation of the tibia with the knee flexed well beyond 90°. Based on these observations, the authors initiated a prevention program and subsequently performed a controlled study to determine the effect of training in reducing knee injuries among their on-slope staff. Training sessions included review of videotaped scenes of actual injuries as they occurred, and subsequent discussions on the potential mechanisms of injury. The participants were also provided with guidelines to avoid high-risk behavior. The treatment group consisted of ski patrollers and instructors from 20 ski areas who participated in the training program during the 1993 to 1994 season. Knee injury data were recorded and compared with injury data for the same season among the staff of 22 ski areas who did not participate in the training program. Further data on injury rates at all 42 sites during the 2 previous winters (1991–1993) were compared with the injury data for the treatment group during the 1993–1994 season. A total of 179 serious knee sprains were identified. The trained skiers experienced a 62% reduction in the incidence of serious knee sprains compared with the two previous seasons. No decline in injuries was observed in the untrained subjects. As an extension of the Ettlinger (141) study, the Vermont Ski Research Safety Group has produced a teaching videotape designed for viewing by the general public, with the goal of increasing general awareness of injury mechanisms and strategies for avoiding knee injuries (1). The effectiveness of this approach in reducing injury rates in the skiing public has not been verified to date, however.

Neuromuscular training for the purpose of preventing injury has been reported by several authors. The results to date have been mixed, although several promising training programs have been described. Based on the assumption that the side-step cutting maneuver caused the greatest risk for ACL injury in the sport of team handball, Bencke et al. (82) attempted a prophylactic co-contraction training program for team handball players to reduce the risk for injury. There is evidence that cutting maneuvers may result in significant anterior displacement of the tibia, placing the ACL at risk for injury (195). Experience had shown the program to be successful in generating hamstring co-contraction among ACL-deficient patients. However, the authors were not successful with their training program in increasing co-contraction about the knee joint in healthy athletes during side-step cutting.

Griffin et al. (1) credited Henning with establishing the first training program designed to teach proper technique for reducing risk for ACL injury. The program involved videotapes of actual noncontact ACL injuries as they occurred in play situations, and drills designed to enhance protective reflexes. Preliminary data using this training strategy demonstrated an 89% decrease in ACL injury rate among NCAA Division I basketball players.

Based on evidence that proprioceptive training is effective in preventing ankle injuries, Caraffa et al. (196) developed a proprioceptive training program to reduce the incidence of ACL injury in soccer players. In a prospective controlled study of 600 soccer players in 40 semiprofessional or amateur teams, they studied the preventative effect of a progressive proprioceptive training program using four different types of wobble-boards during three soccer seasons. Both the trained and control groups were observed for three whole soccer seasons, and possible ACL lesions were diagnosed by clinical examination, diagnostic imaging, and arthroscopy. There was an incidence of 1.15 ACL injuries per team per season in the control group, compared with an incidence of 0.15 in the proprioceptively trained group. The authors concluded that proprioceptive training could significantly reduce the incidence of ACL injuries in soccer players.

Hewett et al. (191) developed a jump-training program designed to decrease landing forces by teaching neuromuscular control of the lower limb during landing, and to increase joint stability by increasing the strength of the knee joint musculature. They hypothesized that such a training program would potentially reduce the incidence of knee injury. The program consisted of three phases, each approximately 2 weeks in duration. Phase I was the technique phase, when proper jump technique was demonstrated and drilled. The fundamentals phase (phase II) concentrated on the use of proper technique to develop strength, power, and ability. Phase III was the performance phase, which focused on maximizing vertical jump height. In a group of female high school volleyball players, this training program was shown to reduce the peak landing forces by 22%, as well as to reduce knee adduction and abduction moments. The program also enhanced hamstring strength and hamstring-to-quadriceps peak torque ratios, and reduced side-to-side hamstring strength differences. The authors speculated that these changes, in particular, would reduce anterior shear forces on the ACL and reduce its risk for injury.

Having established the ability of the jump-training program to address potential neuromuscular deficits that were risk factors for ACL injury, Hewett et al. (178) next performed an intervention study on high school female athletes in order to test the effectiveness of this program in reducing the incidence of knee injury. A group of female high school athletes participating in soccer, volleyball, and basketball completed the 6-week preseason neuromuscular training program. They were compared with a similar group of female athletes that did not participate in the program, and also to a group of untrained male athletes that served as a control population. When all serious knee injuries were considered, the untrained group demonstrated a significantly higher incidence of injury than the male control group. There was no difference, however, between the trained group and male controls. The incidence of all knee injuries was 0.43 injuries per 1,000 exposures in the untrained group, 0.12 in the trained group, and 0.09 in the male control group. The incidence of noncontact knee injury demonstrated a similar pattern. The authors concluded that neuromuscular training was effective in reducing the risk for knee injury in female athletes. Female athletes demonstrate a marked imbalance between hamstring and quadriceps muscle strength before training (176,191). The authors suggested that neuromuscular training should be undertaken by female athletes as a preventative measure to reduce the incidence of serious knee injury.

Equipment

Ski Boots and Bindings

The overall incidence of ski injuries has deceased during the past 25 years (133). Much of this can be attributed to advances in ski equipment, particularly in the design of boots and bindings (130). These changes have been especially effective in protecting the skier from ankle and tibia fractures (137). Unfortunately, modern ski bindings have not been effective in protecting the knee from ligament injury, and the incidence of knee ligament injury remains alarmingly high. The primary purpose of the release properties of modern binding systems is to prevent mid-shaft tibia fractures, which can result when the ski acts as a lever to twist the tibia, and even an optimally adjusted ski binding may be incapable of preventing a knee injury (137). Currently, there are no binding designs or settings that can protect the knee from ligament sprains, and no innovative changes in binding design appear to be on the horizon (137). In fact, some have suggested that the development of a boot-binding system that is capable of protecting against serious knee injury may not be feasible (137). Given these difficulties, preventative measures may have to rely more on behavioral modifications and training programs to decrease the risk for knee injury.

Shoe Wear and Playing Surface

Given the volume of evidence on mechanisms of knee injury, it should not be surprising that the risk for knee injury is influenced by playing surface, shoe design, and the interactions between the two. Clearly, a significant percentage of noncontact knee injuries are torque-related, and are due primarily to foot fixation resulting from either cleats catching on the turf or from excessive friction between the shoe and the playing surface. Myklebust et al. (80), in a prospective study on the incidence ACL injuries in the sport of team handball, suggested that the friction between shoes and playing surface was a major factor in noncontact ACL injury. Ekstrand and Nigg (74) speculated that two thirds of all noncontact soccer injuries were due to excessive shoe-surface friction. Studies have implicated specific shoe designs (106,197,198), playing surfaces (117,197), and playing conditions (197,199) as being responsible for a higher risk for knee injury.

Based on the assumption that noncontact knee injuries are often torque-related, several investigators have examined the torques generated by different shoe types on various playing surfaces (106,198,200-203). Earlier studies (198,203) consistently demonstrated that the conventional seven-post shoe with ¾-inch-long cleats developed greater torque on natural grass than other shoe-surface combinations. In contrast, the molded sole soccer -type shoe with fifteen cleats ½ inch long was deemed "safe" because less force was necessary to release an engaged shoe-surface interface (198). Bostingl et al. (203), testing 11 different shoe types on artificial turf and natural grass, noted that other factors also played a role in the development of torque at the shoe-surface interface. They found that a heavier person was exposed to a larger torque than a lighter person, and that torque was higher in a foot-stance position when compared with a toe-stance position. As expected, noncleated shoes resulted in less torque than cleated shoes on both artificial and natural turf.

Andreasson et al. (201) measured torques for 25 different shoes while simulating sliding conditions on artificial turf. In contrast to Bostingl et al. (203), they concluded that the torque resulting from a foot-stance position was lower than the corresponding torque for the toe-stance position. They suggested that a balanced shoe sole could be designed with more material on the heel surface compared with the toe surface that would result in zero torque while sliding.

The presence of multiple variables that could potentially affect the shoe-surface interface has made the development of a universally safe shoe especially difficult. Preventative measures must also take into account the changes in performance that may take place as shoe designs are altered. Unfortunately, the safest shoe may not necessarily allow optimal athletic performance. Recent laboratory studies have examined more contemporary shoe designs that have claimed to enhance athletic performance. Lambson et al. (106) tested four basic types of cleat designs to determine their torsional resistance on artificial and natural turf. Of the four designs tested, the Edge cleat design produced significantly greater torsional resistance than the other three designs (Flat, Screw-in, and Pivot disk) on both artificial and natural turf. The Edge cleat consisted of longer irregular cleats placed at the peripheral margin of the sole with a number of smaller pointed cleats positioned interiorly. The Flat shoe consisted of cleats of the same height and shape, such as those found on the soccer-style shoe, while the Screw-in shoe consisted of seven ½-inch screw-in cleats with a diameter of ½ inch. The Pivot disk shoe consisted of a 10-cm circular edge on the sole of the forefoot with a single central cleat. No significant difference in torsional resistance was noted among the other three cleat designs.

Heidt et al. (202) evaluated 15 different football shoes on various playing surfaces and conditions, and recognized that there was significant variability in frictional and torsional resistance at the shoe-turf surface interfaces. Shoes tested in conditions for which they were not designed exhibited excessive or extreme minimal friction characteristics that could place the knee at risk for injury. They suggested the shoe manufacturers display suggested indications and playing surface conditions for which their shoes are recommended.

Because the incidence and severity of knee injuries has been significant among American football players (112), clinical studies on the relationship between shoe design, playing surface, and knee ligament disruption have frequently focused on injuries that occur on the football field. In these studies, shoe design has been linked to the risk for ACL injury (104,106). Torg and Quendenfeld (104) compared two types of shoes to determine the effect of shoe type on the incidence and severity of knee injuries among high school football players in Philadelphia. They compared conventional shoes with seven ¾-inch length cleats and soccer type shoes with molded soles containing 14 ⅜-inch length cleats, and found that there was a marked decrease in both the incidence and severity of knee injuries when the players wore the multi-cleated soccer type shoes. They felt that foot fixation was responsible for many of the knee injuries sustained by football players, and the soccer-type shoe with multiple shorter cleats allowed forces to be distributed over a larger cleat tip surface area with less depth of penetration of the turf. Halpern et al. (115), in their epidemiologic survey of the literature on risk factors associated with high school football injuries, also concluded that use of the soccer-style shoe reduced the incidence of knee injury.

Recognizing that rigid cleats exposed the athlete to a higher risk for knee and ankle injury, Cameron et al. (204) developed the swivel football shoe to minimize the rate of torque-related injuries. These shoes were designed with four forefoot cleats mounted on a rotating turntable that was intended to reduce fixation on the ground. This allowed the athlete to be "cleated yet relatively protected from injury." The heel consisted of a cleatless platform with a beveled notch. A group of high school football players wearing the swivel shoe was then compared with a control group wearing conventional shoes. Fewer overall knee injuries were noted in the group wearing the swivel shoes (2.14%) when compared with the control group (7.54%). The authors, however, did not distinguish between the various types of knee injuries.

More recently, Lambson et al. (106) conducted a 3-year prospective study evaluating 3,119 high school football players. They documented both the type of football cleats worn by each player and the number of arthroscopically documented ACL tears they sustained. Because their previous laboratory study had demonstrated no difference in torsional resistance between the Flat, Screw-in, and Pivot disk designs, they were combined to form a non-Edge group. The overall injury rate was 13.5 per 1,000 players over the 3-year period. There was a significantly greater ratio of ACL injuries in the group of players who wore the Edge-type cleats when compared with the non-Edge group. The authors concluded that cleat design can have a significant influence on the risk for significant knee injury, and recommended the use of non-Edge cleat designs to minimize the risk for knee injury.

Sports such as American football and soccer were originally played on natural grass. However, the development of covered indoor stadiums, the desire to make these sports less dependent on external influences such as weather, and the need to reduce operating and maintenance costs all prompted the subsequent development of artificial turf surfaces. The first installation of artificial turf was in the field house of Moses Brown School, Providence, Rhode Island in 1964 (205,206). The first artificial turf surface for a major American football team was installed in the AstroDome in 1966 (205,206). Since then,

arguments both for and against the use of artificial surfaces have been voiced by various authors concerned with the prevention of sports injuries. Despite these arguments, both natural and artificial surfaces continue to be used at all levels of athletic competition. Nigg and Segesser (205), in their review of the influence of playing surfaces on American football injuries, analyzed 32 publications on this topic. There clearly was no consensus regarding the relative risk for knee injury when artificial turf was compared with natural grass, particularly when severe lower extremity injuries were considered. Fourteen percent of the reports claimed more injuries on natural grass, 41% suggested that the frequency of injury was higher on artificial turf, and 45% suggested that the rate of injury was about the same on natural grass and on artificial turf.

Skovron et al. (206), in their critical assessment of the literature on the epidemiology of injuries related to artificial grass, reviewed the available information provided by injury surveillance data bases collected from all levels of competitive football. This included the National Athletic Injury/Illness Reporting System (NAIRS), which collects data on injuries in high school and collegiate sports, as well as the NCAA and the NFL. They concluded that play and practice on an artificial surface was probably responsible for an increase in relative risk for injury to the lower extremity, which they estimated at 1.3 to 1.5.

Similarly, Powell et al. (117) examined the game-related knee injuries that occurred in the National Football League during the 1980 to 1989 seasons. They found that there was a significant increase in the number of knee sprains, particularly ACL sprains, when athletes played on AstroTurf as opposed to natural grass. No distinction was made, however, between contact and non-contact injuries, and the type shoes worn by the players was not addressed. Nicholas et al (102), on the other hand, followed a single professional football team for 26 years from 1960 to 1985, and found no difference in the rate of game-related football injuries when games played on grass and artificial turf were compared.

Various surface conditions have also been examined as they relate to the risk for knee ligament injury. Wet surface conditions, in particular, have been associated with a lower risk for ACL injury (197,199,207). Scranton et al. (197) reviewed all noncontact ACL injuries sustained during five seasons of the National Football League, and found that the preponderance of injuries (93.4%) occurred under dry conditions. Presumably, wet conditions decrease both friction and torsional resistance at the shoe-surface interface. Orchard et al (199) recorded all noncontact ACL injuries that occurred between 1992 and 1998 in the Australian Football League to determine if weather conditions affected the risk for ACL tear. High water evaporation in the month before and low rainfall in the year before an AFL match conferred an increased risk for ACL injury. The authors speculated that a higher soil moisture content and softer surface resulted in lower shoe-surface "traction", decreasing the risk for knee injury. Based on these results, they suggested watering grounds during times of lower rainfall and covering them during times of increased sunshine. Torg et al (200), in a laboratory study, examined the effect of ambient temperature on the torsional resistance of various shoe types on dry AstroTurf. For all shoes that were tested, the release coefficient was greater at the higher temperatures, suggesting a higher torsional resistance.

Based on biomechanical and clinical investigations, recommendations have been made regarding the optimal shoe designs and playing surfaces that will minimize the risks of knee injuries. However, these recommendations have not always taken into consideration the fact that a certain amount of friction is necessary to run quickly, start, stop, and make changes in motion, and that higher levels of friction between the shoe and the surface are generally associated with better performance (1). Thus, any recommendations must strike a balance between optimal performance and maximal safety. Levy identified this dilemma when he stated "An athlete's skills are limited by the quality of the fixation of that player to his present playing surface...But there is a trade off. An increase in fixation increases the risk of injury" (208).

Bracing

Bracing has traditionally been used to provide protection for a previously injured or surgically treated knee. However, braces have also been used for the purpose of preventing knee injuries. Prophylactic braces are defined as those designed to prevent or reduce the severity of knee injuries. The most commonly used prophylactic brace is the lateral knee guard worn by athletes participating in contact sports. It is designed to protect the knee from lateral impacts that can result in MCL and cruciate ligament injuries (209). In 1979, Anderson (210) described the use of a single-sided, double-hinged lateral knee brace (the Anderson Knee Stabler) in nine players who had sustained MCL injuries. These players were able to play a combined 29 games without reinjury. This prompted the authors to state, "Its use as a preventative device by athletes in vulnerable positions seems highly applicable." Following this report, the use of prophylactic bracing became widespread. Initially, there was very little clinical evidence to support the use of these braces. Then, during the mid-1980's, several reports appeared in the literature examining the use of prophylactic bracing to prevent knee injuries (103,120,211,212). Since bracing was seen as a means to prevent contact-related injuries, these early studies focused primarily on the use of prophylactic braces to prevent football injuries. The majority of these reports used collegiate football teams as their study populations.

The Anderson Knee Stabler was one of the earliest prophylactic knee braces. Its use among football players at University of Southern California was examined by

Hansen et al. (213) in a retrospective study that reviewed the medical records of all players that underwent knee surgery from 1980 to 1984. They made note of which players were wearing braces at the time of injury and which were not. Overall, fewer knee ligament injuries were noted among players who used the brace (1.4% of players) when compared with those that did not (5.2%). The number of players the sustained ligament injuries but did not undergo surgery was not given.

Hewson et al. (103) reviewed the records of the University of Arizona football team to determine the effectiveness of prophylactic bracing in preventing significant knee injuries. They compared a 4-year period (1981–1985) in which prophylactic bracing was used by all high risk players with a 4-year period (1977–1981) when no braces were used. During the 4-year bracing period, all high-risk players (linemen, linebackers, and tight ends) were required to use a brace (the Anderson Knee Stabler) for all practices and games. The overall incidence of MCL injury in the nonbrace group was 18.14 per 100 players at risk per season, compared with 14.73 in the brace group. This difference was not found to be significant. The incidence of ACL and combined ACL/MCL injuries was also found to be similar in both the nonbrace and brace groups.

In a similar study by Rovere et al. (108), the Anderson Knee Stabler was used during two quarters by all players on the Wake Forest University football team. The braces were worn during every practice session and every game. The incidence of knee injury among these braced players was then compared with a similar 2-year period in which prophylactic bracing was not used. Overall, the incidence of knee injuries was higher when the braces were worn (7.5 injuries per 100 players) when compared with a similar period when braces were not worn (6.1). There was also a higher incidence of grade I MCL injuries during the period that braces were used. The incidence of other ligament injuries was not calculated. Both this and the previous study by Hewson et al. (103) are similar in design in that they compare distinct period of bracing with periods of nonbracing. However, factors such as changes in coaching, technique, or league rules can affect different time periods and make the result of this type of longitudinal study difficult to interpret. Ideally, these investigations should be prospective and should randomize the assignment of brace wear within a similar group of players during the same time.

In a more extensive review, Teitz et al. (120) reported the results of a survey of athletic trainers undertaken following the 1984 and 1985 football seasons covering more than 60 NCAA Division I football teams. This study included over 11,000 collegiate football players. Brace use varied from institution to institution, with most schools reporting that only a portion of the players had used a prophylactic brace. Overall, there were significantly more injuries to the MCL among the players who wore braces. However, there was no difference in the severity of MCL injury when the two groups were compared. When injuries of the ACL were analyzed, there was no difference noted between the braced and unbraced groups. They concluded that "so-called preventative braces are not preventative and may in fact be harmful."

The effectiveness of prophylactic bracing in high school football players was examined by Grace et al. (212) in a study that matched each athlete who wore a prophylactic brace with a comparable participant who did not wear a brace. Two types of prophylactic braces were used—a single upright, single hinged brace, and a single upright, double-hinged brace. Incidence rates were not calculated by the authors. They noted that the group that wore the single hinged braces had significantly more knee injuries than the control group. Although the group that wore the double hinged braces also had a higher rate of knee injury than their matched controls, the difference was not significant. Thus, this study also suggested that prophylactic bracing increased the rate of knee injury and recommended that they not be used as a preventative device.

Most of these early studies demonstrated little or no benefit to the use of prophylactic bracing, and some even suggested an increased risk for knee injury with brace use (120,211,214). This led to a position statement issued by the American Academy of Orthopaedic Surgeons (AAOS) in 1987 against the use of prophylactic knee braces. This statement read in part:

> The American Academy of Orthopaedic Surgeons believes that the routine use of prophylactic braces currently available has not been proven effective in reducing the number or severity of knee injuries. In some circumstances, such braces may even have the potential to be a contributing factor to injury.

Perhaps referring to deficiencies in the studies that had been performed up to that point, the statement also added that "there remains a need for further epidemiological, biomechanical, and performance research studies with unbiased evaluation" (118).

Since the AAOS position statement was first published, several studies have shown that prophylactic knee braces may indeed help prevent knee injuries. Sitler et al. (119), in a prospective randomized study performed at West Point, evaluated the efficacy of a prophylactic knee brace in reducing knee injuries among cadets participating in an intramural tackle football program. At the beginning of each of two seasons, the cadets were randomly assigned to either a braced or nonbraced group. The brace was a double-hinged single-upright off-the-shelf model (DonJoy Protector Knee Guard), and was used by the brace group for all practices and games. This well-designed study attempted to control such variables as playing surface, type of athletic shoe, exposure, and compliance. The incidence of injury was calculated per 1,000 athlete-exposures. The knee injury rate was 1.50 per 1,000 athlete exposures in the brace group, and 3.40 in the nonbrace control group. Incidence rates were not calculated for individual ligament injuries. The authors did find, however, that a significantly greater number of MCL injuries occurred in the control group than in the brace group. A greater number of ACL injuries also occurred in the control group, although no statistical analysis could be performed due to a small sample size. There was also a trend toward a higher proportion of less severe MCL and ACL injuries in the brace group.

Albright et al. (121,215) conducted a 3-year prospective multi-institutional study of collegiate football players in the Big Ten Conference to assess the effectiveness of prophylactic bracing on injuries of the MCL. Players chose whether or not to use a brace, and the type of brace was based on personal preference. For each study participant, the use or nonuse of a prophylactic knee brace was recorded on a daily basis. The authors also recorded the player's position, the session (practice vs. game), and whether the player was a starter, a regular substitute, or a bench-player (nonplayer). The term "knee exposure" was used to express the number of opportunities the knees were exposed to a sports-related risk for injury.

Over the 3-year period, there were 55,722 knee exposures, 50.7% of which were with prophylactic knee braces. In the nonbraced group, the rate of MCL injury was highest among the interior linemen, particularly during the games (0.532 per 1,000 exposures). This was almost twice as high as the rate among linebackers and tight ends (0.290), and over twice as high as the skill position players (0.227). In general, the rate of injury was much higher during games when compared with practices. The effectiveness of prophylactic bracing was examined by comparing players within the same position groups during the same sessions. In general, injury rates were lower in the braced players when compared with the nonbraced group. This held true for the most part when the various position groups were compared. During games, the rate of MCL injury was lower among the braced linemen when compared with their nonbraced counterparts (0.437 vs. 0.532). Similar results were noted when the braced linebacker-tight end group was compared with the nonbraced group (0.186 vs. 0.290). However, among the skill position players, the rate of MCL injury during games was higher in the braced group (0.606 vs. 0.227).

Currently, there is still no consensus regarding the need or effectiveness of prophylactic bracing. Most biomechanical and clinical studies indicate that braces can be beneficial in reducing the number of MCL injuries due to lateral blows to the knee, especially at or near full extension (209). However, the evidence is still not conclusive. The AAOS reissued the position statement on the use of knee braces in 1997, but did not change its recommendation against the routine use of prophylactic knee bracing.

Again citing the lack of adequate research, they stated that "There is no credible, long-term, scientifically conducted study that supports using knee braces on otherwise healthy people."

REFERENCES

1. Griffin LY, et al. Noncontact anterior cruciate ligament injuries: risk factors and prevention strategies. *J Am Acad Orthop Surg* 2000;8: 141–150.
2. Hefti F, Muller W. (Current state of evaluation of knee ligament lesions. The new IKDC knee evaluation form). *Orthopade* 1993;22: 351–362.
3. Hawkins RD, Fuller CW. A prospective epidemiological study of injuries in four English professional football clubs. *Br J Sports Med* 1999;33:196–203.
4. Balkfors B. The course of knee-ligament injuries. Acta *Orthop Scand Suppl* 1982;198:1–99.
5. Clancy WG Jr. Knee ligamentous injury in sports: the past, present, and future. *Med Sci Sports Exerc* 1983;15:9–14.
6. Kannus P, Jarvinen M. Long-term prognosis of conservatively treated acute knee ligament injuries in competitive and spare time sportsmen. *Int J Sports Med* 1987;8:348–351.
7. Pickett JC, Altizer TJ. Injuries of the ligaments of the knee. A study of types of injury and treatment in 129 patients. *Clin Orthop* 1971;76: 27–32.
8. Engstrom B, et al. Does a major knee injury definitely sideline an elite soccer player? *Am J Sports Med* 1990;18:101–105.
9. Bjordal JM, et al. Epidemiology of anterior cruciate ligament injuries in soccer. *Am J Sports Med* 1997;25:341–345.
10. Roos H, et al. Soccer after anterior cruciate ligament injury—an incompatible combination? A national survey of incidence and risk factors and a 7- year follow-up of 310 players (see comments). *Acta Orthop Scand* 1995;66:107–112.
11. Miyasaka KC, et al. The incidence of knee ligament injuries in the general population. *Am J Knee Surg* 1991;4:3–8.
12. Nielsen AB, Yde J. Epidemiology of acute knee injuries: a prospective hospital investigation. *J Trauma* 1991;31:1644–1648.
13. Kuhn JE, Greenfield ML, Wojtys EM. A statistics primer. Prevalence, incidence, relative risks, and odds ratios: some epidemiologic concepts in the sports medicine literature. *Am J Sports Med* 1997;25:414–416.
14. Noyes FR, Lindenfeld TN, Marshall MT. What determines an athletic injury (definition)? Who determines an injury (occurrence)? *Am J Sports Med* 1988;16(suppl 1):S65-S68.
15. Junge A, Dvorak J. Influence of definition and data collection on the incidence of injuries in football (in process citation). *Am J Sports Med* 2000;28(5 suppl):S40-S46.
16. Dvorak J, Junge A. Football injuries and physical symptoms. A review of the literature (in process citation). *Am J Sports Med* 2000;28(5 suppl):S3-S9.
17. Daniel DM, et al. Use of the quadriceps active test to diagnose posterior cruciate- ligament disruption and measure posterior laxity of the knee. *J Bone Joint Surg Am* 1988;70:386–391.
18. O'Beirne J, et al. The diagnosis of knee injuries in casualty—a prospective study. *Injury* 1984;15:232–235.
19. Jensen JE, et al. Systematic evaluation of acute knee injuries. *Clin Sports Med* 1985;4:295–312.
20. Kannus P, Jarvinen M. Incidence of knee injuries and the need for further care. A one-year prospective follow-up study. *J Sports Med Phys Fitness* 1989;29:321–325.
21. Natri A, et al. Changing injury pattern of acute anterior cruciate ligament tears treated at Tampere University Hospital in the 1980s. *Scand J Med Sci Sports* 1995;5:100–104.
22. Fanelli GC. Posterior cruciate ligament injuries in trauma patients. *Arthroscopy* 1993;9:291–294.
23. Fanelli GC, Edson CJ. Posterior cruciate ligament injuries in trauma patients: part II. *Arthroscopy* 1995;11:526–529.
24. Lu KH, Hsiao YM, Lin ZI. Arthroscopy for acute knee haemarthrosis in road traffic accident victims. *Injury* 1996;27:341–343.
25. Szabo RM. Principles of epidemiology for the orthopaedic surgeon. *J Bone Joint Surg Am* 1998;80:111–120.
26. Inklaar H. Soccer injuries. I: incidence and severity. *Sports Med* 1994; 18:55–73.
27. Sandelin J, Santavirta S, Kiviluoto O. Acute soccer injuries in Finland in 1980. *Br J Sports Med* 1985;19:30–33.
28. Roaas A, Nilsson S. Major injuries in Norwegian football. *Br J Sports Med* 1979;13:3–5.
29. de Loes M, Marti B. On the epidemiology of sports injuries in Switzerland. *Schweiz Z Sportmed* 1992;40:123–129.
30. Keller CS, Noyes FR, Buncher CR. The medical aspects of soccer injury epidemiology. *Am J Sports Med* 1987;15:230–237.
31. Lindenfeld TN, Noyes FR, Marshall MT. Sports injury research. Components of injury reporting systems. *Am J Sports Med* 1988;16(suppl 1):S69–S80.
32. Messina DF, Farney WC, DeLee JC. The incidence of injury in Texas high school basketball. A prospective study among male and female athletes. *Am J Sports Med* 1999;27:294–299.
33. Arendt E, Dick R. Knee injury patterns among men and women in collegiate basketball and soccer. NCAA data and review of literature. *Am J Sports Med* 1995;23:694–701.
34. McKay GD, et al. A comparison of the injuries sustained by female basketball and netball players. *Aust J Sci Med Sport* 1996;28:12–17.
35. Holzach P, Bruesch M, Matter P. (Epidemiology of internal knee injuries in Alpine skiing). *Helv Chir Acta* 1994;60:531–537.
36. Tapper EM. Ski injuries from 1939 to 1976: the Sun Valley experience. *Am J Sports Med* 1978;6:114–121.
37. Arnason A, et al. Soccer injuries in Iceland. *Scand J Med Sci Sports* 1996;6:40–45.
38. Peterson L, et al. Incidence of football injuries and complaints in different age groups and skill-level groups (in process citation). *Am J Sports Med* 2000;28(5 suppl):S51–S57.
39. Dvorak J, et al. Risk factor analysis for injuries in football players. Possibilities for a prevention program (in process citation). *Am J Sports Med* 2000;28(5 suppl):S69–S74.
40. Dvorak J, et al. Editorial (in process citation). *Am J Sports Med* 2000; 28(5 suppl):S1–S2.
41. Roos H, et al. The prevalence of gonarthrosis and its relation to meniscectomy in former soccer players. *Am J Sports Med* 1994;22:219–222.
42. Larsen E, Jensen PK, Jensen PR. Long-term outcome of knee and ankle injuries in elite football. *Scand J Med Sci Sports* 1999;9: 285–289.
43. Luthje P, et al. Epidemiology and traumatology of injuries in elite soccer: a prospective study in Finland. *Scand J Med Sci Sports* 1996;6: 180–185.
44. Ekstrand J, Gillquist J. Soccer injuries and their mechanisms: a prospective study. *Med Sci Sports Exerc* 1983;15:267–270.
45. Engstrom B, Johansson C, Tornkvist H. Soccer injuries among elite female players. *Am J Sports Med* 1991;19:372–375.
46. Fried T, Lloyd GJ. An overview of common soccer injuries. Management and prevention. *Sports Med* 1992;14:269–275.
47. Nilsson S, Roaas A. Soccer injuries in adolescents. *Am J Sports Med* 1978;6:358–361.
48. Schmidt-Olsen S, et al. Soccer injuries of youth. *Br J Sports Med* 1985;19:161–164.
49. Schmidt-Olsen S, et al. Injuries among young soccer players. *Am J Sports Med* 1991;19:273–275.
50. Gaulrapp H, Siebert C, Rosemeyer B. (Injury and exertion patterns in football on artificial turf). *Sportverletz Sportschaden* 1999;13: 102–106.
51. Cromwell F, Walsh J, Gormley J. A pilot study examining injuries in elite gaelic footballers. *Br J Sports Med* 2000;34:104–108.
52. Brynhildsen J, et al. Previous injuries and persisting symptoms in female soccer players. *Int J Sports Med* 1990;1:489–492.
53. McGregor JC, Rae A. A review of injuries to professional footballers in a premier football team (1990-93). *Scot Med J* 1995;40:16–18.
54. Muckle DS. Injuries in professional footballers. *Br J Sports Med* 1981;15:77–79.
55. Nielsen AB, Yde J. Epidemiology and traumatology of injuries in soccer. *Am J Sports Med* 1989;17:803–807.
56. Blaser KU, Aeschlimann A. (Accidental injuries in soccer). *Schweiz Z Sportmed* 1992;40:7–11.
57. Ekstrand J, et al. Incidence of soccer injuries and their relation to training and team success. *Am J Sports Med* 1983;11:63–67.
58. McMaster WC, Walter M. Injuries in soccer. *Am J Sports Med* 1978; 6:354–357.

59. Hawkins RD, Fuller CW. Risk assessment in professional football: an examination of accidents and incidents in the 1994 World Cup finals. *Br J Sports Med* 1996;30:165–170.
60. Hoff GL, Martin TA. Outdoor and indoor soccer: injuries among youth players. *Am J Sports Med* 1986;14:231–233.
61. Chomiak J, et al. Severe injuries in football players. Influencing factors (in process citation). *Am J Sports Med* 2000;28(5 suppl):S58–S68.
62. Inklaar H. Soccer injuries. II: aetiology and prevention. *Sports Med* 1994;18:81–93.
63. Poulsen TD, et al. Injuries in high-skilled and low-skilled soccer: a prospective study. *Br J Sports Med* 1991;25:151–153.
64. Backous DD, et al. Soccer injuries and their relation to physical maturity. *Am J Dis Child* 1988;142:839–842.
65. Sullivan JA, et al. Evaluation of injuries in youth soccer. *Am J Sports Med* 1980;8:325–327.
66. Yde J, Nielsen AB. Sports injuries in adolescents' ball games: soccer, handball and basketball. *Br J Sports Med* 1990;24:51–54.
67. Junge A, Chomiak J, Dvorak J. Incidence of football injuries in youth players. Comparison of players from two European regions (in process citation). *Am J Sports Med* 2000;28(5 suppl):S47–S50.
68. Putukian M, et al. Injuries in indoor soccer. The Lake Placid Dawn to Dark Soccer Tournament. *Am J Sports Med* 1996;24:317–322.
69. Kibler WB. Injuries in adolescent and preadolescent soccer players. *Med Sci Sports Exerc* 1993;25(12):1330–1332.
70. Lindenfeld TN, et al. Incidence of injury in indoor soccer. *Am J Sports Med* 1994;22:364–371.
71. Ekstrand J, Gillquist J. The avoidability of soccer injuries. *Int J Sports Med* 1983;4:124–128.
72. Daniel DM, et al. Fate of the ACL-injured patient. A prospective outcome study (see comments). *Am J Sports Med* 1994;22:632–644.
73. Junge A, et al. Medical history and physical findings in football players of different ages and skill levels (in process citation). *Am J Sports Med* 2000;28(5 suppl):S16–S21.
74. Ekstrand J, Nigg BM. Surface-related injuries in soccer. *Sports Med* 1989;8:56–62.
75. de Loes M. Epidemiology of sports injuries in the Swiss organization youth and sports 1987-1989. Injuries, exposure and risks of main diagnoses. *Int J Sports Med* 1995;16:134–138.
76. Nielsen AB, Yde J. An epidemiologic and traumatologic study of injuries in handball. *Int J Sports Med* 1988;9:341–344.
77. Andren-Sanberg A, et al. (Low incidence of injuries in handball. Knee injuries demand the longest therapeutic intervention). *Lakartidningen* 1981;78(49):4444–44445.
78. Seil R, et al. Sports injuries in team handball. A one-year prospective study of sixteen men's senior teams of a superior nonprofessional level. *Am J Sports Med* 1998;26:681–687.
79. Strand T, et al. (Anterior cruciate ligament injuries in handball playing. Mechanisms and incidence of injuries). *Tidsskr Nor Laegeforen* 1990;110(17):2222–2225.
80. Myklebust G, et al. Registration of cruciate ligament injuries in Norwegian top level team handball. A prospective study covering two seasons. *Scand J Med Sci Sports* 1997;7:289–292.
81. Myklebust G, et al. A prospective cohort study of anterior cruciate ligament injuries in elite Norwegian team handball. *Scand J Med Sci Sports* 1998;8:149–153.
82. Bencke J, et al. Motor pattern of the knee joint muscles during side-step cutting in European team handball. Influence on muscular coordination after an intervention study (see comments). *Scand J Med Sci Sports* 2000;10:68–77.
83. Ferretti A, Papandrea P, Conteduca F. Knee injuries in volleyball. *Sports Med* 1990;10:132–138.
84. Ferretti A, et al. Knee ligament injuries in volleyball players. *Am J Sports Med* 1992;20:203–207.
85. Watkins J, Green BN. Volleyball injuries: a survey of injuries of Scottish National League male players. *Br J Sports Med* 1992;26:135–137.
86. Aagaard H, Jorgensen U. Injuries in elite volleyball. *Scand J Med Sci Sports* 1996;6:228–232.
87. Aagaard H, Scavenius M, Jorgensen U. An epidemiological analysis of the injury pattern in indoor and in beach volleyball. *Int J Sports Med* 1997;18:217–221.
88. Briner WW Jr, Kacmar L. Common injuries in volleyball. Mechanisms of injury, prevention and rehabilitation. *Sports Med* 1997;24:65–71.
89. Schafle MD, et al. Injuries in the 1987 national amateur volleyball tournament. *Am J Sports Med* 1990;18:624–631.
90. Bahr R, Bahr IA. Incidence of acute volleyball injuries: a prospective cohort study of injury mechanisms and risk factors. *Scand J Med Sci Sports* 1997;7:166–171.
91. Henry JH, Lareau B, Neigut D. The injury rate in professional basketball. *Am J Sports Med* 1982;10:16–18.
92. Colliander E, et al. Injuries in Swedish elite basketball. *Orthopedics* 1986;9: 225–227.
93. Engel J, Baharav U, Modan W. (Epidemiology of basketball injuries). *Harefuah* 1990;119(5-6):121–124.
94. Hickey GJ, Fricker PA, McDonald WA. Injuries of young elite female basketball players over a six-year period. *Clin J Sport Med* 1997;7:252–256.
95. Gray J, et al. A survey of injuries to the anterior cruciate ligament of the knee in female basketball players. *Int J Sports Med* 1985;6:314–316.
96. Powell JW, Barber-Foss KD. Sex-related injury patterns among selected high school sports. *Am J Sports Med* 2000;28:385–391.
97. Baltzer AW, et al. American football injuries in Germany. First results from Bundesliga football. *Knee Surg Sports Traumatol Arthrosc* 1997;5:46–49.
98. Bauer A, et al. (American football in Germany—aspects of trauma surgery). *Unfallchirurgie* 1993;19:27–32.
99. Karpakka J. American football injuries in Finland. *Br J Sports Med* 1993;27:135–137.
100. Saal JA. Common American football injuries. *Sports Med* 1991;12:132–147.
101. Canale ST, et al. A chronicle of injuries of an American intercollegiate football team. *Am J Sports Med* 1981;9:384–389.
102. Nicholas JA, Rosenthal PP, Gleim GW. A historical perspective of injuries in professional football. Twenty-six years of game-related events. *JAMA* 1988;260:939–944.
103. Hewson GF Jr, Mendini RB, Wang JB. Prophylactic knee bracing in college football. *Am J Sports Med* 1986;14:262–266.
104. Torg JS, Quedenfeld T. Effect of shoe type and cleat length on incidence and severity of knee injuries among high school football players. *Res Q* 1971;42:203–211.
105. Garrick JG, Requa RK. Football cleat design and its effect on anterior cruciate ligament injuries (letter; comment). *Am J Sports Med* 1996;24:705–706.
106. Lambson RB, Barnhill BS, Higgins RW. Football cleat design and its effect on anterior cruciate ligament injuries. A three-year prospective study (see comments). *Am J Sports Med* 1996;24:155–159.
107. Hardin GT, Farr J, Stiene HA. Prophylactic knee braces for football: do they work? *Indiana Med* 1993;86:308–311.
108. Rovere GD, Haupt HA, Yates CS. Prophylactic knee bracing in college football. *Am J Sports Med* 1987;15:111–116.
109. Deppen RJ, Landfried MJ. Efficacy of prophylactic knee bracing in high school football players. *J Orthop Sports Phys Ther* 1994;20:243–246.
110. Cahill BR, Griffith EH. Effect of preseason conditioning on the incidence and severity of high school football knee injuries. *Am J Sports Med* 1978;6:180–184.
111. Bauer FC, Wredmark T, Isberg B. Krogius tenoplasty for recurrent dislocation of the patella. Failure associated with joint laxity. *Acta Orthop Scand* 1984;55:267–269.
112. DeLee JC, Farney WC. Incidence of injury in Texas high school football. *Am J Sports Med* 1992;20:575–580.
113. Landry GL. Sports injuries in childhood. *Pediatr Ann* 1992;21:165–168.
114. Goldberg B, et al. Injuries in youth football. *Pediatrics* 1988;81:255–261.
115. Halpern B, et al. High school football injuries: identifying the risk factors. *Am J Sports Med* 1987;15:316–320.
116. Stocker BD, et al. Results of the Kentucky high school football knee injury survey. *J Ky Med Assoc* 1997;95:458–464.
117. Powell JW, Schootman M. A multivariate risk analysis of selected playing surfaces in the National Football League: 1980 to 1989. An epidemiologic study of knee injuries. *Am J Sports Med* 1992;20:686–694.
118. Albright JP, Saterbak A, Stokes J. Use of knee braces in sport. Current recommendations (editorial). *Sports Med* 1995;20:281–301.
119. Sitler M, et al. The efficacy of a prophylactic knee brace to reduce

knee injuries in football. A prospective, randomized study at West Point. *Am J Sports Med* 1990;18:310–315.

120. Teitz CC, et al. Evaluation of the use of braces to prevent injury to the knee in collegiate football players. *J Bone Joint Surg Am* 1987;69:2–9.

121. Albright JP, et al. Medial collateral ligament knee sprains in college football. Effectiveness of preventive braces (see comments). *Am J Sports Med* 1994;22:12–18.

122. Garrick JG, Requa RK. Prophylactic knee bracing. *Am J Sports Med* 1987;15:471–476.

123. Johnston JM, Paulos LE. Prophylactic lateral knee braces. *Med Sci Sports Exerc* 1991;23:783–787.

124. Paluska SA, McKeag DB. Knee braces: current evidence and clinical recommendations for their use. *Am Fam Physician* 2000;61:411–418, 423–424.

125. Requa RK, Garrick JG. A review of the use of prophylactic knee braces in football. *Pediatr Clin North Am* 1990;37:1165–1173.

126. Baker BE. The effect of bracing on the collateral ligaments of the knee. *Clin Sports Med* 1990;9:843–851.

127. Schaffer DJ. Knee ligament injuries induced by skiing. *Ann Emerg Med* 1981;10(9):472–475.

128. Johnson RJ, et al. Knee injury in skiing. A multifaceted approach. *Am J Sports Med* 1979;7:321–327.

129. Edlund G, Gedda S, Hemborg A Knee injuries in skiing. A prospective study from northern Sweden. *Am J Sports Med* 1980;8:411–414.

130. Johnson RJ, Pope MH. Epidemiology and prevention of skiing injuries. *Ann Chir Gynaecol* 1991;80:110–115.

131. Feagin JA Jr, et al. Consideration of the anterior cruciate ligament injury in skiing. *Clin Orthop* 1987;(216):13–18.

132. Deibert MC, et al. Skiing injuries in children, adolescents, and adults. *J Bone Joint Surg Am* 1998;80:25–32.

133. Warme WJ, et al. Ski injury statistics, 1982 to 1993, Jackson Hole Ski Resort. *Am J Sports Med* 1995;23:597–600.

134. Holzach P, et al. (Incidence and treatment of fresh connective tissue injuries of the knee in winter sports). *Helv Chir Acta* 1989;56:581–585.

135. Rohrl S, et al. (Pattern of injuries in skiing worldwide. Can current guidelines for adjusting ski bindings reduce injuries in the future?). *Sportverletz Sportschaden* 1994;8:73–82.

136. Sherry E, Fenelon L. Trends in skiing injury type and rates in Australia. A review of 22,261 injuries over 27 years in the Snowy Mountains. *Med J Aust* 1991;155:513–515.

137. Natri A, et al. Alpine ski bindings and injuries. Current findings. *Sports Med* 1999;28:35–48.

138. Johnson RJ, et al. Trends in skiing injuries. Analysis of a 6-year study (1972 to 1978). *Am J Sports Med* 1980;8:106–113.

139. Bruesch M, Holzach P. (Epidemiology, treatment and follow-up of acute ligamentous knee injuries in Alpine skiing). *Z Unfallchir Versicherungsmed* 1993;(suppl 1):144–155.

140. Johnson SC. Anterior cruciate ligament injury in elite Alpine competitors. *Med Sci Sports Exerc* 1995;27:323–327.

141. Ettlinger CF, Johnson RJ, Shealy JE. A method to help reduce the risk of serious knee sprains incurred in alpine skiing. *Am J Sports Med* 1995;23:531–537.

142. Moreland MS. Skiing injuries in children. *Clin Sports Med* 1982;1:241–251.

143. Macnab AJ, Cadman R. Demographics of alpine skiing and snowboarding injury: lessons for prevention programs. *Inj Prev* 1996;2:286–289.

144. Ungerholm S, et al. Skiing injuries in children and adults: a comparative study from an 8-year period. *Int J Sports Med* 1983;4:236–240.

145. de Loes M, Dahlstedt LJ, Thomee R. A 7-year study on risks and costs of knee injuries in male and female youth participants in 12 sports. *Scand J Med Sci Sports* 2000;10:90–97.

146. Stevenson H, et al. Gender differences in knee injury epidemiology among competitive alpine ski racers. *Iowa Orthop J* 1998;18:64–66.

147. Viola RW, et al. Anterior cruciate ligament injury incidence among male and female professional alpine skiers. *Am J Sports Med* 1999;27:792–795.

148. Backx FJ, et al. Injuries in high-risk persons and high-risk sports. A longitudinal study of 1818 school children. *Am J Sports Med* 1991;19:124–130.

149. Kvist, M, et al. Sports-related injuries in children. *Int J Sports Med* 1989;10:81–86.

150. Stanitski CL. Pediatric and adolescent sports injuries. *Clin Sports Med* 1997;16:613–633.

151. Metzl JD, Micheli LJ. Youth soccer: an epidemiologic perspective. *Clin Sports Med* 1998;17:663–673.

152. Sandelin J, et al. Sports injuries in a large urban population: occurrence and epidemiological aspects. Int J Sports Med 1988;9:61–66.

153. Watkins J, Peabody P. Sports injuries in children and adolescents treated at a sports injury clinic. *J Sports Med Phys Fitness* 1996;36:43–48.

154. Salter RB, Hu WR. Injuries involving the epiphyseal plate. *J Bone Joint Surg Am* 1963;45:587–622.

155. Bradley GW, Shives TC, Samuelson KM. Ligament injuries in the knees of children. *J Bone Joint Surg Am* 1979;61:588–591.

156. Clanton TO, et al. Knee ligament injuries in children. *J Bone Joint Surg Am* 1979;61:1195–1201.

157. DeLee JC, Curtis R. Anterior cruciate ligament insufficiency in children. *Clin Orthop* 1983;172:112–118.

158. Skak SV, et al. Epidemiology of knee injuries in children. *Acta Orthop Scand* 1987;58:78–81.

159. McCarroll JR, Rettig AC, Shelbourne KD. Anterior cruciate ligament injuries in the young athlete with open physes. *Am J Sports Med* 1988;16:44–47.

160. Lipscomb AB, Anderson AF. Tears of the anterior cruciate ligament in adolescents. *J Bone Joint Surg Am* 1986;68:19–28.

161. Kannus P, Jarvinen M. Knee ligament injuries in adolescents. *J Bone Joint Surg Br* 1988;70:772–776.

162. Zaricznyj B, et al. Sports-related injuries in school-aged children. *Am J Sports Med* 1980;8:318–324.

163. Nattiv A, Arendt E. Female athletes. In: Griffin LY, ed. *Orthopaedic knowledge update: sports medicine*. Chicago: American Academy of Orthopaedic Surgeons, 1994:361–366.

164. Levy AS, et al. Knee injuries in women collegiate rugby players. *Am J Sports Med* 1997;25:360–362.

165. Harmon KG, Dick R. The relationship of skill level to anterior cruciate ligament injury. *Clin J Sport Med* 1998;8:260–265.

166. Gwinn DE, et al. The relative incidence of anterior cruciate ligament injury in men and women at the United States Naval Academy. *Am J Sports Med* 2000;28:98–102.

167. Wirtz PD. High school basketball knee ligament injuries. *J Iowa Med Soc* 1982;72:105–106.

168. Liu SH, et al. Primary immunolocalization of estrogen and progesterone target cells in the human anterior cruciate ligament. *J Orthop Res* 1996;14:526–533.

169. Slauterbeck J, et al. Estrogen level alters the failure load of the rabbit anterior cruciate ligament. *J Orthop Res* 1999;17:405–408.

170. Wojtys EM, et al. Association between the menstrual cycle and anterior cruciate ligament injuries in female athletes (see comments). *Am J Sports Med* 1998;26:614–619.

171. Muneta T, Takakuda K, Yamamoto H. Intercondylar notch width and its relation to the configuration and cross-sectional area of the anterior cruciate ligament. A cadaveric knee study. *Am J Sports Med* 1997;25:69–72.

172. Shelbourne KD, Davis TJ, Klootwyk TE. The relationship between intercondylar notch width of the femur and the incidence of anterior cruciate ligament tears. A prospective study. *Am J Sports Med* 1998;26:402–408.

173. Souryal TO, Freeman TR. Intercondylar notch size and anterior cruciate ligament injuries in athletes. A prospective study (published erratum appears in *Am J Sports Med* 1993;21:723). *Am J Sports Med* 1993;21:535–539.

174. Shambaugh JP, Klein A, Herbert JH. Structural measures as predictors of injury basketball players. *Med Sci Sports Exerc* 1991;23:522–527.

175. Anderson AF, et al. Instrumented evaluation of knee laxity: a comparison of five arthrometers. *Am J Sports Med* 1992;20:135–140.

176. Huston L, Wojtys EM. Neuromuscular performance characteristics in elite female athletes. *Am J Sports Med* 1996;24:427–436.

177. Rozzi SL, et al. Knee joint laxity and neuromuscular characteristics of male and female soccer and basketball players. *Am J Sports Med* 1999;27:312–319.

178. Hewett TE, et al. The effect of neuromuscular training on the incidence of knee injury in female athletes. A prospective study. *Am J Sports Med* 1999;27:699–706.

179. Kirkendall DT, Garrett WE Jr. The anterior cruciate ligament enigma. Injury mechanisms and prevention. *Clin Orthop* 2000;372:64–68.

180. Huston LJ, Greenfield ML, Wojtys EM. Anterior cruciate ligament injuries in the female athlete. Potential risk factors. *Clin Orthop* 2000; 372:50–63.

181. Boden BP, et al. Mechanisms of anterior cruciate ligament injury (in process citation). *Orthopedics* 2000;23:573–578.

182. McNair PJ, Marshall RN, Matheson JA. Important features associated with acute anterior cruciate ligament injury. *NZ Med J* 1990;103(901): 537–539.

183. Noyes FR, et al. The symptomatic anterior cruciate-deficient knee. Part I: the long-term functional disability in athletically active individuals. *J Bone Joint Surg Am* 1983;65:154–162.

184. Delfico AJ, Garrett WE Jr. Mechanisms of injury of the anterior cruciate ligament in soccer players. *Clin Sports Med* 1998;17: 779–785.

185. Shelbourne KD, Nitz PA. The O'Donoghue triad revisited. Combined knee injuries involving anterior cruciate and medial collateral ligament tears (see comments). *Am J Sports Med* 1991;19:474–477.

186. Feagin JA Jr, Lambert KL. Mechanism of injury and pathology of anterior cruciate ligament injuries. *Orthop Clin North Am* 1985;16: 41–45.

187. Hewett TE. Neuromuscular and hormonal factors associated with knee injuries in female athletes. Strategies for intervention. *Sports Med* 2000;29:313–327.

188. More RC, et al. Hamstrings—an anterior cruciate ligament protagonist. An in vitro study. *Am J Sports Med* 1993;21:231–237.

189. Arms SW, et al. The biomechanics of anterior cruciate ligament rehabilitation and reconstruction. *Am J Sports Med* 1984;12:8–18.

190. Renstrom P, et al. Strain within the anterior cruciate ligament during hamstring and quadriceps activity. *Am J Sports Med* 1986;14:83–87.

191. Hewett TE, et al. Plyometric training in female athletes. Decreased impact forces and increased hamstring torques. *Am J Sports Med* 1996;24:765–773.

192. Draganich LF, Vahey JW. An in vitro study of anterior cruciate ligament strain induced by quadriceps and hamstrings forces. *J Orthop Res* 1990;8:57–63.

193. Markolf KL, et al. Combined knee loading states that generate high anterior cruciate ligament forces. *J Orthop Res* 1995;13:930–935.

194. Ekstrand J, Gillquist J, Liljedahl SO. Prevention of soccer injuries. Supervision by doctor and physiotherapist. *Am J Sports Med* 1983;11: 116–120.

195. Colby S, et al. Electromyographic and kinematic analysis of cutting maneuvers. Implications for anterior cruciate ligament injury. *Am J Sports Med* 2000;28:234–240.

196. Caraffa A, et al. Prevention of anterior cruciate ligament injuries in soccer. A prospective controlled study of proprioceptive training. *Knee Surg Sports Traumatol Arthrosc* 1996;4:19–21.

197. Scranton PE Jr, et al. A review of selected noncontact anterior cruciate ligament injuries in the National Football League. *Foot Ankle Int* 1997;18(12):772–776.

198. Torg JS, Quedenfeld TC, Landau S. The shoe-surface interface and its relationship to football knee injuries. *J Sports Med* 1974;2:261–269.

199. Orchard J, et al. Rainfall, evaporation and the risk of non-contact anterior cruciate ligament injury in the Australian Football League. *Med J Aust* 1999;170:304–306.

200. Torg JS, Stilwell G, Rogers K. The effect of ambient temperature on the shoe-surface interface release coefficient. *Am J Sports Med* 1996; 24:79–82.

201. Andreasson G, et al. Torque developed at simulated sliding between sport shoes and an artificial turf. *Am J Sports Med* 1986;14:225–230.

202. Heidt RS Jr, et al. Differences in friction and torsional resistance in athletic shoe-turf surface interfaces. *Am J Sports Med* 1996;24: 834–842.

203. Bonstingl RW, Morehouse CA, Niebel BW. Torques developed by different types of shoes on various playing surfaces. *Med Sci Sports* 1975;7:127–131.

204. Cameron BM, Davis O. The swivel football shoe: a controlled study. *J Sports Med* 1973;1:16–27.

205. Nigg BM, Segesser B. The influence of playing surfaces on the load on the locomotor system and on football and tennis injuries. *Sports Med* 1988;5:375–385.

206. Skovron ML, Levy IM, Agel J. Living with artificial grass: a knowledge update. Part 2: Epidemiology. *Am J Sports Med* 1990;18: 510–513.

207. Adkison JW, Requa RK, Garrick JG. Injury rates in high school football. A comparison of synthetic surfaces and grass fields. *Clin Orthop* 1974;99:131–136.

208. Levy IM, Skovron ML, Agel J. Living with artificial grass: a knowledge update. Part 1: Basic science. *Am J Sports Med* 1990;18: 406–412.

209. France EP, Paulos LE. Knee Bracing. *J Am Acad Orthop Surg* 1994;2: 281–287.

210. Anderson G, Zeman SC, Rosenfeld RT. The Anderson Knee Stabler. *Physician Sportsmed* 1979;7:125–127.

211. Rovere GD, Bowen GS. The effectiveness of knee bracing for the prevention of sport injuries. *Sports Med* 1986;3:309–311.

212. Grace TG, et al. Prophylactic knee braces and injury to the lower extremity. *J Bone Joint Surg Am* 1988;70:422–427.

213. Hansen BL, Ward JC, Diehl RC. The preventive use of the Anderson Knee Stabler in football. *Physician Sportsmed* 1985;13(9):75–81.

214. Grace JN, Rand JA. Patellar instability after total knee arthroplasty. *Clin Orthop* 1988;237:184–189.

215. Albright JP, et al. Medial collateral ligament knee sprains in college football. Brace wear preferences and injury risk (see comments). *Am J Sports Med* 1994;22:2–11.

CHAPTER 19

Diagnosis of Ligament Injury

Part A: History and Physical Examination

William F. Luetzow

The history and physical examination remains the core of the clinician's diagnostic expertise. The clinician must focus not only on the extent of injury, but particularly on the various ways in which the individual patient's injury affects his or her life circumstances. While imaging modalities evolve, a thorough history and physical examination will allow diagnosis of ligament injury in the vast majority of cases without the need for routine magnetic resonance imaging. On-site or emergency department examinations are obviously necessary to rule out fracture, gross instability or neurovascular injury. However, the environment offered by the office setting often allows for a more thorough evaluation. An important aspect of the historical data includes an assessment of the patient's athletic and/or vocational exposure to the risks of reinjury. The International Knee Documentation Committee has divided sports into levels 1-3 based on presumed risk for major knee injury. Sports participation can be quantified, for example, in terms of hours per week and weeks per year participated. In our clinic we have found the total sports hours per year, particularly of level 1 and 2 sports, to be a useful and statistically significant predictive measure for comparison amongst patients in determining risk for reinjury. A detailed understanding of past knee injury and/or surgery is certainly important and a review of prior records, especially surgical, is in order. The patient's general health status must be understood. A precise history is taken in regards to the mechanism of the acute or most recent injury.

HISTORICAL FEATURES OF SPECIFIC KNEE LIGAMENT INJURY

Anterior Cruciate Ligament Rupture

The patient with no prior injuries who presents with a history of a significantly traumatic pivoting or decelera-tion injury, associated with a sense of a painful "pop," giving way, and swelling within a few hours has a greater than 70% chance of having sustained an anterior cruciate ligament (ACL) injury (1). The above presentation is also the typical history associated with an ACL tear. It must be kept in mind, however, that some patients will present with no "pop" or little swelling. Occasionally a patient is able to, for example, ski down the rest of the run after an acute ACL injury. Sports injuries account for approximately 70% of ACL injuries in our knee injury clinic. The differential diagnosis of an acute traumatic hemarthrosis must also include fracture, peripheral meniscal tear, posterior cruciate injury and extensor mechanism derangement such as patellar dislocation. Meniscal tears occur in over 50 percent of acute primary ACL injuries, though not all will require treatment (2). In many patients the pain and swelling resolves quickly and the patient may not present for the first time until after their ACL deficient knee develops further episodes of instability or a symptomatic meniscal tear. Such patients may have functioned reasonably well (coped) with their prior ACL injury. Treating the newly symptomatic meniscal tear may or may not be all that is required to allow the patient to return to coping status. Therefore the past history must be thorough enough to detect the likelihood of coping with a previous ACL injury, and this information plays an integral role in treatment recommendations.

Posterior Cruciate Ligament Rupture

If a PCL rupture is missed on the history and physical examination, the abnormal anterior-posterior motion in the knee can be wrongly attributed to the more commonly injured ACL. The classic presentation, a direct blow or fall on the proximal tibia with the knee flexed, occurs in over half of our patients with PCL disruption. Sports injuries account for only about half of PCL ruptures, the bulk of the remainder being from falls or dashboard type injury. Although the PCL is extrasynovial, injury can result in hemarthrosis (3). The chronic PCL deficient knee is unlikely to present with giving way; nor are meniscal tears typical sequelae of PCL insufficiency, in contrast to ACL insufficiency. Although no pure natural history study is available, several studies indicate that anterior and medial compartment loading is increased in the chronic state of PCL deficiency and therefore pain in those areas are historical elements of importance (4–8).

Medial Collateral Ligament Injury

The isolated medial collateral ligament (MCL) injury has a wide range of severity. A valgus stress causing localized pain and a highly variable but typically limited amount of swelling is the usual history. It must be kept in mind that pain at the MCL origin on the medial epicondyle can also be from an injury to the medial patellofemoral ligament. MCL injuries with minimal valgus laxity can mimic the presentation of a locked meniscal tear with the patient reporting difficulty achieving full extension. Another finding from our clinic is not intuitive: A high grade (presumably complete) tear of the MCL often presents with much less pain than lower grade MCL injuries. However, there is typically more medial swelling in the complete tear than with a partial tear. It is important to understand that the MCL has considerable capacity for healing. Isolated significant MCL laxity is rare and isolated MCL injuries rarely cause chronic symptoms. MCL injuries often occur in association with ACL injuries. Chronic symptoms of valgus instability should alert the clinician to a combined cruciate injury, most likely involving the ACL (9).

Lateral Structures

Isolated lateral collateral ligament (LCL) injuries are likely quite rare and rarely reported. However, according to cutting studies by Gollehon and others an isolated transection of the LCL may not be detectable to clinical stress testing (10,11). Combined LCL and posterolateral ligament complex (PLC) injuries do rarely occur in the absence of ACL or PCL injuries, but more commonly are combined with cruciate injury. The classic mechanism would involve a varus stress with extension and external rotation, such as a direct blow to the anteromedial knee (12). However, LCL/PLC injury can also occur with flexion and external rotation such as with the classic slide tackle in soccer. The combined ACL/LCL/PLC injury is most likely to occur with hyperextension (13).

PHYSICAL EXAMINATION OF THE KNEE LIGAMENTS

General

A careful manual examination of joint motion will reveal most ligament disruptions. Patient relaxation is paramount. For ligament testing the patient should lie supine on a firm but comfortable examining table with the limb supported. The motion resulting from a clinical test depends on the position of the limb at the initiation of the test, the force applied, the point of application of the force, and manner of detection of the displacement.

It is important to understand that knee joint motion or laxity varies considerably within the normal population, but there is little side-to-side variation in a normal subject. There is a difference to the terms laxity and instability. Laxity can be defined as the state of looseness of a particular joint motion. The degree of laxity can be normal or abnormal for a given patient or population. Instability is the pathological or symptomatically abnormal increased motion of a joint. Ligaments limit knee motion and define the joint's laxity. Abnormal ligament laxity can result in instability.

When 120 *normal* subjects' knees were examined with the KT 1000 arthrometer, single knee manual maximum anterior displacement varied from 4.5 to 15 mm (14) (see Part C later in this chapter). *In vitro* ligament sectioning studies have documented that disruption of a specific ligament results in a characteristic change in motion. For example, in a cadaver study anterior displacement increased with ACL sectioning by an average of 6.7 mm, as measured by the KT 1000 (15). However, one standard deviation included a range of 4.3 to 9.1 mm, and the entire range for the specimens was 2.8 to 13.0 mm (Fig. 19.1).

In a patient with a unilateral knee injury, the laxity of the injured knee should be compared to that of the normal knee. To effectively compare the two limbs the examination conditions must be constant. These conditions include starting position, applied force, and site of motion measurement. Placing a bolster or platform under both thighs with the patient supine will keep the measurement angle constant and allow for relaxation of the muscles surrounding the joint. In our clinic, we have standard sized platforms that support most thighs in 20° to 30° of flexion available for every knee examination. Holding the femur still and measuring the motion of the tibia relative to the femur is another important technique. The examiner places one hand on the distal femur to stabilize it. The thumb and index finger of the same hand are placed on the joint line to assess motion while the other hand applies the testing force. The relaxation and tactile sensation afforded by a bolster can help the examiner determine a sense of motion across the joint as well as the presence or absence of an endpoint. The starting position is the neutral resting position with the joint surfaces in

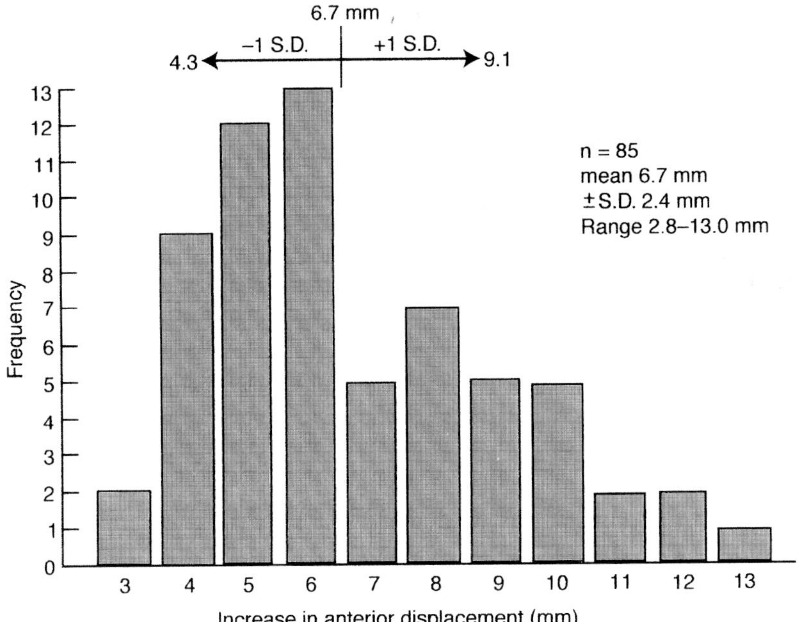

FIGURE 19.1. Effect of anterior cruciate ligament (ACL) sectioning on anterior displacement. Anterior displacement measurements with the MEDmetric KT-2000 were performed on 65 fresh cadaveric specimens with the ligaments intact and after sectioning the ACL. The difference between the ligament-intact state and the ACL-sectioned state for each specimen is presented.

contact. Maintaining constants in the knee examination is essential to comparing serial examinations and examinations by different observers.

While many tests are involved in examining a patient with a possible ligament injury, certain tests are most useful because the pathologic laxity resulting from them are associated with a specific ligament injury. Injury of other ligaments may increase the pathologic motion being tested, provided that the primary ligament is disrupted. These are termed secondary restraints (16). For a given direction of testing, disruption of a secondary restraint will not result in pathologic motion if the primary restraint is intact.

Gait, limb alignment, and range of motion (ROM) are important general initial elements of any knee ligament examination.

Approach to the Examination of the Acutely Injured Knee

The examination begins with inspection noting the general appearance of the patient, the gait or ambulatory status, the lower extremity alignment, skin condition, and neurovascular status. The knee is examined for effusion, which can be graded as 1) slight, with fluid wave, 2) moderate with ballotable patella, 3) tense. ROM is assessed and documented. The prone heel height difference is an excellent way to reproducibly measure flexion contracture (Fig. 19.2). The joint line and surrounding structures are carefully palpated for tenderness. A significant effusion or flexion contracture can limit the ability to assess ligament stability. An aspiration and injection of local anesthetic may be necessary to help

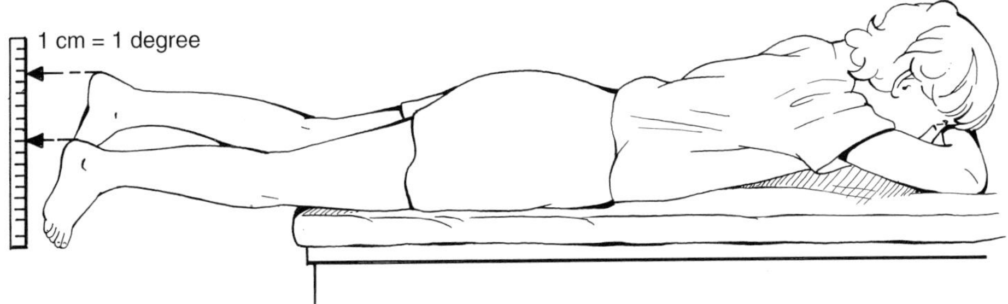

FIGURE 19.2. The prone heel height measurement is an easy and reliable way to quantitate and document flexion contracture relative to the normal knee. The patient lays prone with the end of the examination table a few inches proximal to the patella and relaxes both lower extremities. One centimeter of heel height difference equals roughly 1° of flexion contracture.

the patient relax for ligament testing. The presence of a hemarthrosis indicates ACL disruption, peripheral meniscus tear, extensor mechanism injury, osteochondral fracture, or PCL disruption. Palpating the extensor mechanism and assessing for extensor sag are important so quadriceps or patellar tendon ruptures are not missed. Fat droplets indicate fracture. Radiographs should be assessed to rule out fracture with any substantial knee injury. While more common in children, ACL avulsion fractures of the tibial eminence do occur in all ages. If possible, it is best in the office setting to review radiographs before stressing the ligaments, so as not to displace a nondisplaced avulsion. Stress radiographs are useful in documenting and quantifying displacement, especially in varus and valgus injuries. Physeal injuries must always be considered in the skeletally immature, and varus/valgus stress radiographs can document physeal opening when clinically suspected.

Posterior Cruciate Ligament

Because increased total anterior-posterior laxity is much more likely to be from an ACL disruption, the less common PCL injury can be missed. Therefore the examination of the cruciate ligaments begins with the evaluation of the PCL. The disrupted PCL causes posterior tibial sag, most pronounced at 90° flexion. To determine whether the ACL or the PCL is disrupted, one must be able to determine the neutral position in the anterior-posterior plane. In a supine patient, the neutral position is the resting position of the tibia supported by the intact PCL. The neutral position can be determined when the patient is lying supine with the knee at 90° of flexion. In comparison with the normal knee the tibia will sag posteriorly if the PCL is disrupted. To assess for posterior sag the examiner views the knee in profile from the side, and palpates the medial prominence or "step-off" between the tibia and the femur. The medial tibia step-off is usually approximately 1 cm anterior relative to the medial femoral condyle. Swelling or osteophytes can complicate this assessment. The 90° quadriceps active test, or "PCL screen" is used (17). With the knee 90° flexed, contraction of the quadriceps muscle pulls the tibia anteriorly when there is tibial sag. While it is often difficult to flex an acutely injured knee to 90°, this examination must be done in at least 70° flexion to allow the patellar tendon to impose an anteriorly directed vector force on a posteriorly sagged tibia (Fig. 19.3A). The examiner supports the thigh and assesses hamstring relaxation with one hand while the other resists the foot as the patient is instructed to attempt to slide the foot down the examination table. The KT 1000 can be used to quantitate the side-to-side difference. The technique for doing so is described in the chapter on instrumented measurements.

The posterior drawer test (Fig. 19.3B) is performed with the knee flexed 90° and the foot resting on the examination table. The examiner places both hands around the knee with thumbs on the joint line. While palpating the joint line the knee is translated posteriorly briskly. The examiner palpates for translation and endpoint. The examination may not demonstrate posteriorly directed increased translation if the tibia is already sagged back, and a step-off can be difficult to determine in a swollen knee; hence, the importance of the 90° quadriceps active test, or PCL screen. The sense of total anterior-posterior translation and presence or absence of an endpoint should be noted. Relaxation of the hamstrings is of utmost importance in performing these maneuvers. If necessary the examiner may sit on the patient's foot while performing the posterior drawer test. Another assistant may support the thigh if necessary for relaxation.

Anterior Cruciate Ligament

Lachman Test

After sectioning of the anterior cruciate ligament *in vitro*, the increased anterior translation of the knee is greatest when tested at 20° to 30° flexion. To perform the Lachman test, the knee is placed in 20° to 30° flexion with the patient supine. Placing a support under the thigh just proximal to the gastrocnemius insertion assists in muscular relaxation and reproducible patient positioning. The use of a thigh support frees both of the examiners hands. One hand palpates the joint line while stabilizing the distal femur against the thigh support. The other hand applies an anteriorly directed force to the proximal calf just below the joint line, without enhancing or restraining axial rotation. The examiner senses the tibial displacement and the firmness of the endpoint. If either the tibial anterior displacement or the endpoint is abnormal the test is positive. The displacement should be graded in millimeters and compared side to side (Fig. 19.4). The end point is graded as firm (normal), marginal, or soft. Loss of secondary restraints such as the MCL or posterior horn of the medial meniscus will increase anterior laxity.

Knee Ligament Arthrometry

As indicated by instrumented measurement studies an estimated right-left difference of 3 mm or greater is classified as pathologic, and in the absence of a PCL disruption indicates an ACL disruption. (The mean side to side KT 1000 instrumented manual maximum difference for 125 patients studied in our clinic with arthroscopically confirmed ACL disruption was 6.2 mm [18].) Examiners are generally better able to detect end-point differences

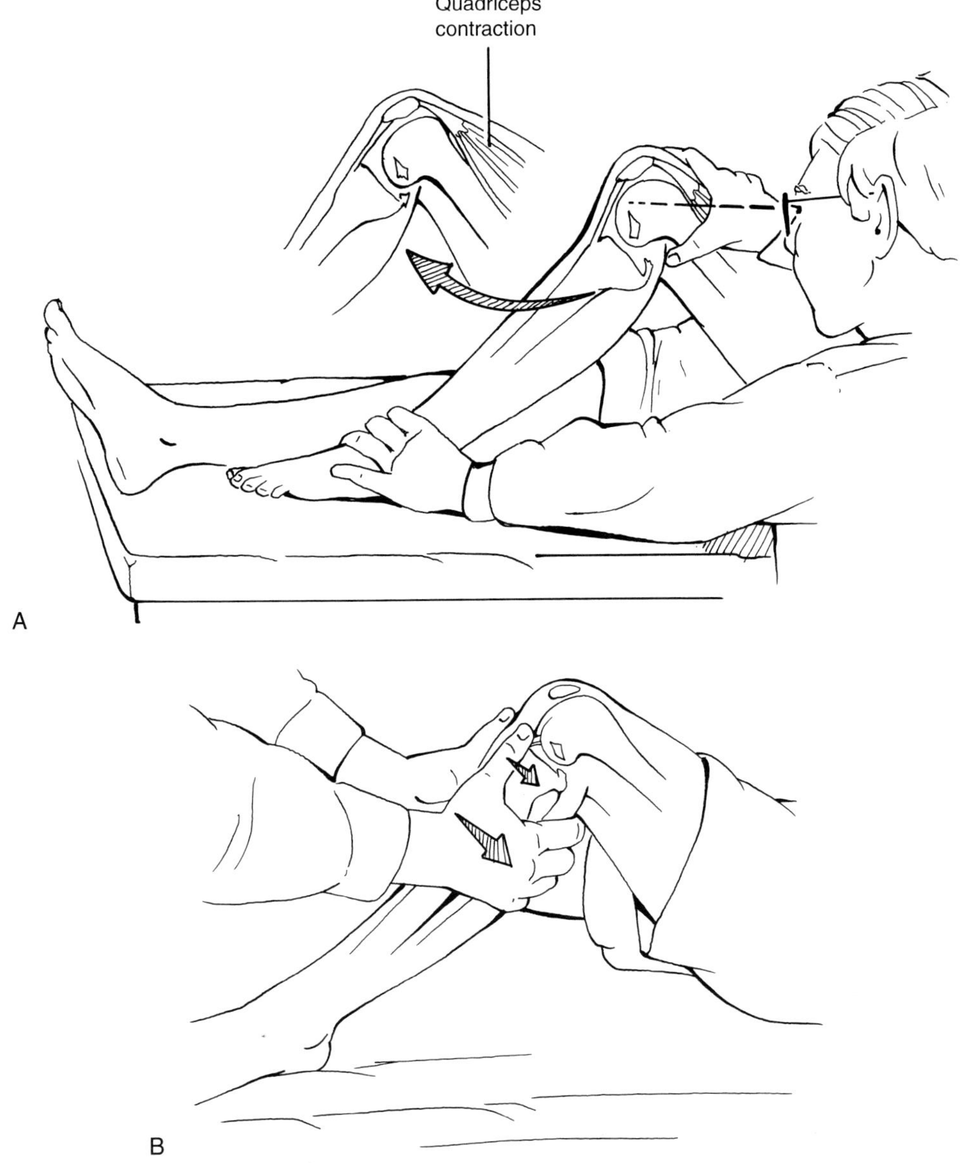

FIGURE 19.3. Tests for posterior cruciate ligament (PCL) laxity. **A:** The PCL sag test. With the knee at 90° flexion, the examiner stabilizes the foot and ankle with one hand and the distal thigh with the other. The patient is encouraged to relax and the examiner confirms this with the hand on the thigh. The examiner views the knee from the side and looks for a sagging back of the tibial tubercle relative to the normal knee. The patient is instructed to attempt to slide the foot down the table against the examiner's resistance and the examiner confirms contraction of the quadriceps, and not the hamstrings, by palpation. In the PCL-deficient state, the pull of the quadriceps will translate the tibial tubercle anteriorly toward its preinjury position. **B:** The posterior drawer test. The examiner can sit on the patient's foot if necessary to stabilize the extremity at 90° flexion. The examiner places both hands on the tibia with the thumbs on the joint line. The presence or lack of a normal medial tibial plateau step off is noted. With the patient relaxed a posterior force is applied to the proximal tibia. The presence or absence of an end point feel is noted as well as the translation. In the PCL-deficient knee, the tibia is typically already sagged posteriorly relative to the femur when the knee is in 90° flexion. Therefore, the posterior drawer test is not likely to accurately measure posterior laxity.

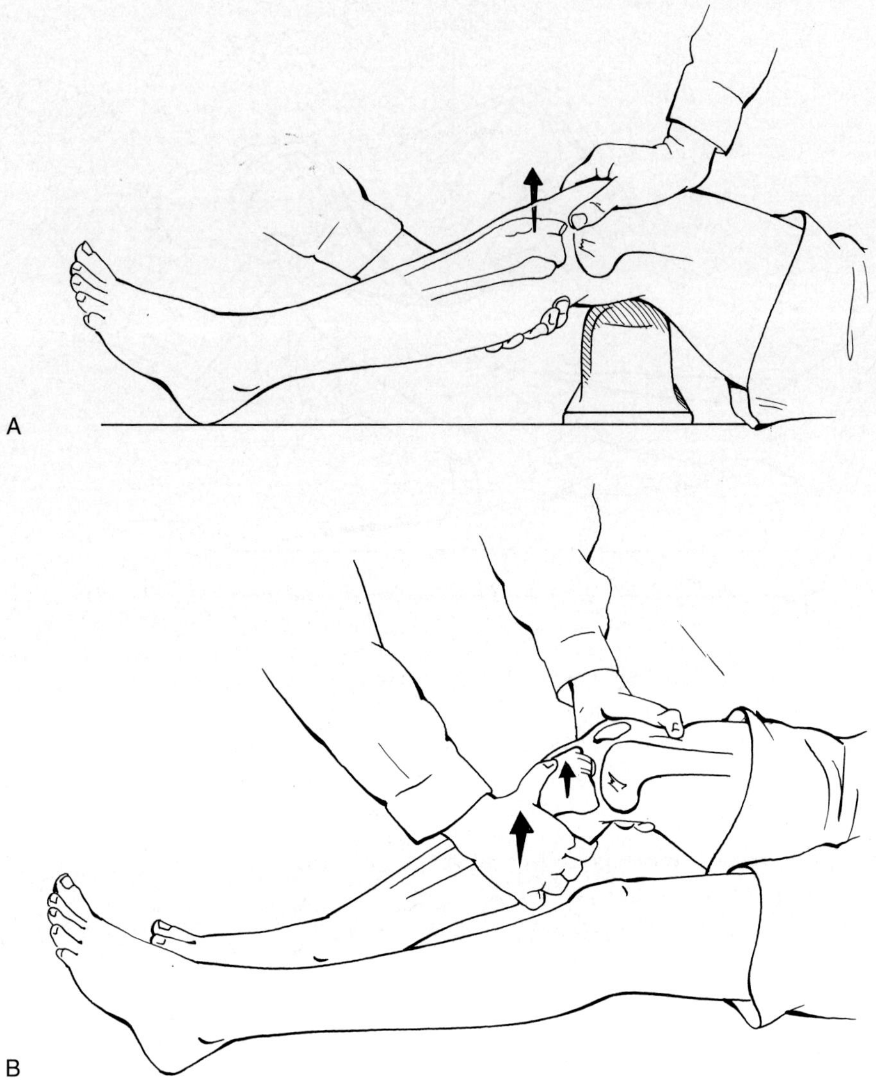

FIGURE 19.4. Tests for anterior cruciate ligament (ACL) laxity. **A:** The Lachman test using a bolster. The Lachman test is most accurately and reproducibly performed with the patient's distal thighs relaxed on a bolster at 20° to 30° flexion. The examiner palpates the joint line with the proximal hand while stabilizing the distal femur. The distal hand is placed behind the proximal calf and an anterior translation is applied. Translation and end point feel are noted. **B:** The traditional Lachman test. The traditional Lachman test lacks the elements of patient relaxation, reproducibility of positioning, and palpation of the joint line.

than subtle (3–4 mm) displacement differences. For example, an experienced clinician will usually correctly diagnose an ACL disruption even when there is only a 4-mm right-to-left displacement difference. However, when an end point is present such as after ACL reconstruction even experienced examiners will often sense a normal Lachman test when there is a 3- to 4-mm side-to-side displacement difference documented by instrumented measurement. Patient guarding or flexion contracture will often result in decreased measured anterior laxity. Because it accurate and well tolerated, as well as predictive of outcome (2) we have found knee ligament

arthrometry indispensable in the diagnosis and treatment of acute ACL injuries.

Pivot Shift

Many versions of pivot shift tests have been described. The tests share the common finding that an ACL disruption allows the tibia to subluxate anteriorly in early flexion with a manual force directed anteriorly and with the tibia in neutral to internal rotation. The posterior pull of the iliotibial tract reduces the tibia at 20° to 40° of flexion (Fig. 19.5). The test can be performed in the relaxed

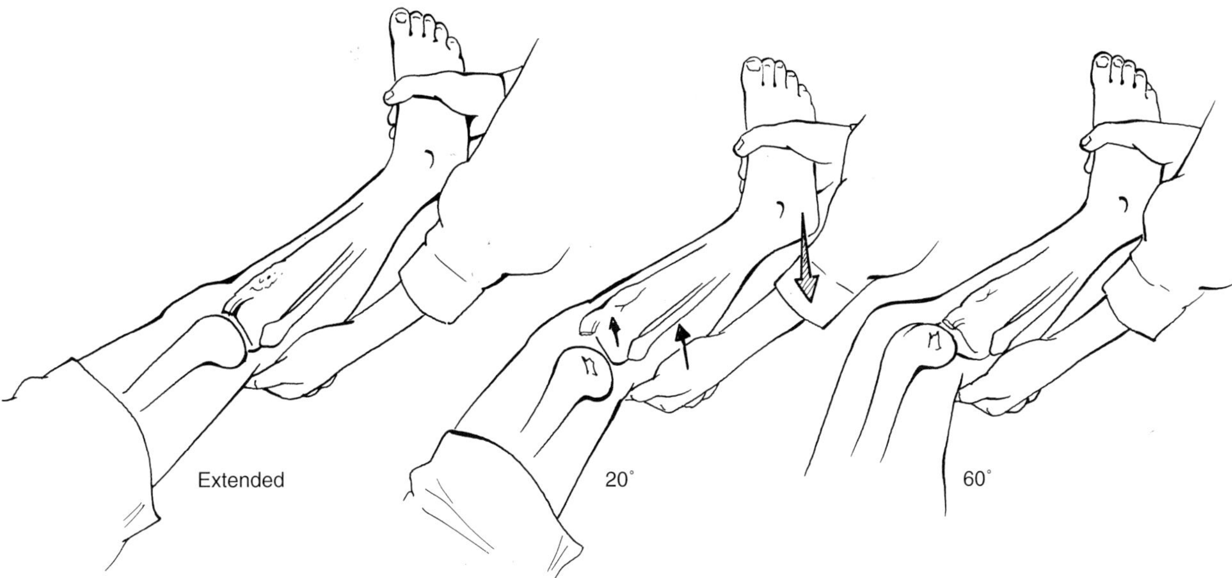

FIGURE 19.5. The pivot shift test. Starting with the knee extended, the examiner simply applies an anterior force to the proximal lateral tibia. In the anterior cruciate ligament–deficient knee this translates the proximal tibia forward. As the knee is flexed the tibia then reduces posteriorly with a "shift" around 20° to 40° of knee flexion. This occurs due to the iliotibial band causing a posterior force in the flexed knee.

patient by lifting the tibia with the knee extended, allowing the femur to fall posteriorly. One hand is placed behind the proximal fibula and the other supports the foot. A valgus force is applied. As the knee is flexed, the examiner relaxes the anterior force. The iliotibial tract tightening in flexion moves the tibia from a position anterior to the axis of knee flexion to a position posterior to the to the axis of knee flexion. It is the relocation event that the clinician grades. The pivot shift can be graded as 0 (absent), 1+ (slight slip), 2+ (moderate slip or jump), or 3+ (momentary locking). Normal knees are typically grade 0, rarely 1+ in lax individuals. If the tibia is internally rotated or the hip adducted, the IT band will tighten causing the tibia to reduce in less flexion and the apparent pivot shift grade is typical reduced. Disruption of the MCL allows the limb to go into valgus alignment and relax the iliotibial tract. The reduction in the iliotibial tract tone will result in a decrease in the pivot shift reduction event. The clinical usefulness of the pivot shift test is limited in the acutely injured, painful, or otherwise unrelaxed knee. The pivot shift is consistently positive in the relaxed patient with a chronic ACL disruption and in the acutely injured anesthetized patient with an ACL disruption.

Medial Collateral Ligament

The valgus stress test evaluates the MCL. The patient lies supine with the knees supported in 20° to 30° flexion and neutral axial rotation (Fig. 19.6). With one hand the

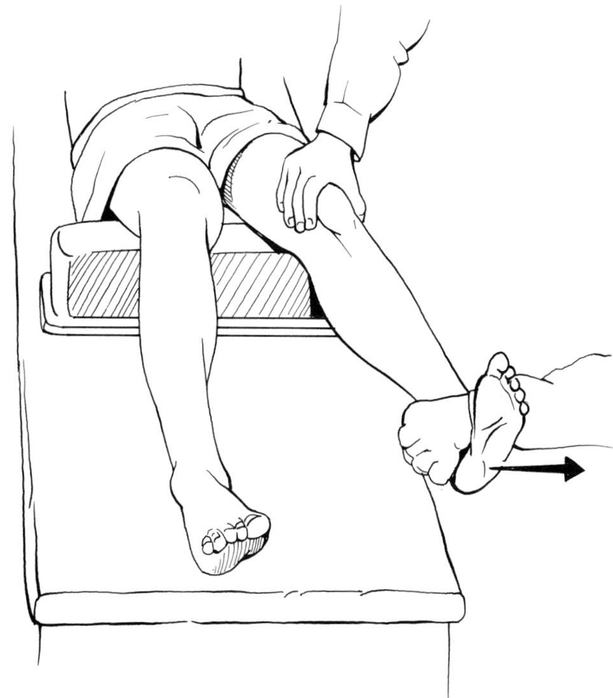

FIGURE 19.6. Valgus stress test. With both distal thighs relaxed on a bolster in 20° to 30° flexion, the examiner places the proximal hand to stabilize the distal femur and palpate the joint line. The neutral position is noted when joint contact feels distributed between medial and lateral compartments. Medial opening is detected as a valgus force is applied distally, without torque, to the tibia. Varus stress is applied (not shown) and lateral opening is palpated. Right to left knee comparison is critical as always.

examiner stabilizes the distal femur on the thigh support and palpates the medial joint line. The other hand on the distal tibia, the examiner exerts an axial load to place the joint surfaces in contact. The leg is abducted while constraining axial rotation. The medial joint space opening is estimated in millimeters and the stiffness of the motion limit evaluated. The findings are compared to the patient's contralateral normal knee. The test is graded 0 to 3. In the grade 1 injury, there is pain and tenderness at the site of the ligament injury, the end point is firm and the medial opening is the same as that in the normal knee. In grade 2 injury, there is increased opening up to 5 mm greater than the contralateral knee. In grade 3 injury, the end point is soft and the joint space opens more than 5 mm greater than the normal knee. Because of the subjective nature of such grading, valgus stress radiographs are often used in our clinic to quantitate MCL laxity.

Medial joint opening to valgus stress at full extension indicates additional injury to the posteromedial capsule and at least one of the cruciate ligaments. Some clinicians refer to valgus opening in full extension as a "grade 4" MCL injury.

Lateral Collateral Ligament

The lateral collateral ligament can often be palpated with the knee in the "figure of four" position. The varus stress test evaluates the lateral collateral ligament and posterolateral structures. The patient lies supine with the knees supported in 20° to 30° of flexion and the examiner stabilizes the distal thigh and palpates the lateral joint line. With the other hand on the distal leg, the examiner first exerts an axial load to place the joint surfaces in contact to determine the starting position for the test. The leg is then adducted while constraining axial rotation. The lateral joint space opening, as well as the stiffness of the end point, is estimated in millimeters. The grading system of injury is the same as for injuries to the MCL. One must keep in mind that sectioning studies indicate that it may take more than a complete isolated rupture of the LCL to generate clinically determinable increases in varus laxity.

Posterolateral Ligament Complex

Axial Rotation

As documented by cutting studies in cadavers, most knee ligament injuries will affect axial rotation in addition to other motions. The accurate determination of internal and external rotation is quite difficult clinically due to problems discerning the true neutral starting position (19). The rotational position of the tibia can be determined by reference to the tibial tubercle, the malleolar axis, and the foot. However, the precise position of the femur relative to the tibia cannot be determined.

The PLC—which includes the popliteus tendon and its attachment to the fibula and lateral meniscus, the arcuate ligament, and variably occurring other structures—limits external rotation of the tibia. To evaluate the PLC, the examiner must evaluate axial rotation and/or the posterior displacement of the lateral compartment. The dial test (Fig. 19.7) can be done with the patient supine with the knee again supported by a platform in 20° to 30° of flexion, or prone. Both femora must be stabilized while the examiner rotates the feet and evaluates tibial rotation by noting the external rotation of the tibial tubercle and the foot. Normal subjects can vary up to 10° side to side with this test (13). Therefore a positive test result is defined as greater than a 10° side-to-side difference. This test should also be performed in 90° of flexion, and if also positive, a combined injury of the PLC and the PCL is likely. Palpating the tibial compartments while externally and internally rotating the leg can determine rotational compartment subluxation (Fig. 19.8). The examiner can then try to assess whether the rotational abnormality is from posterior subluxation of the lateral tibial plateau as in a PLC

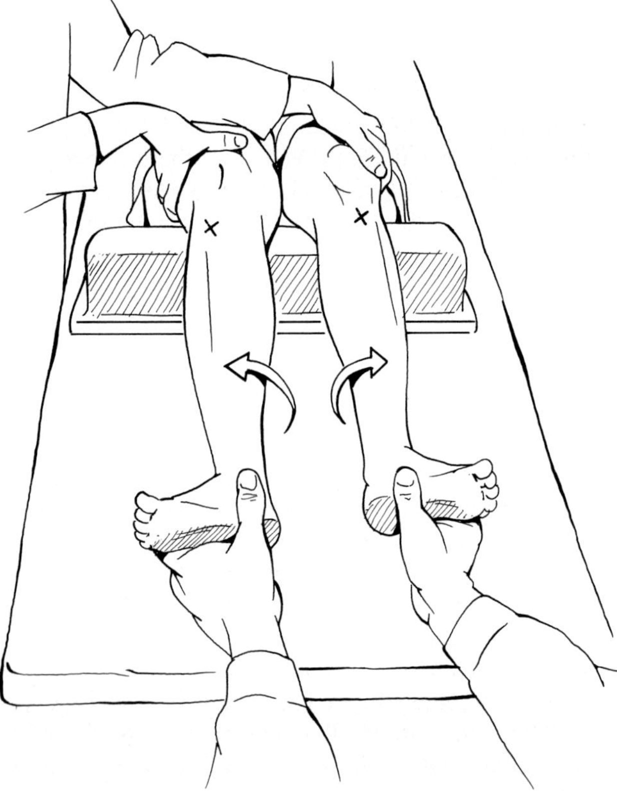

FIGURE 19.7. The dial test. With both distal thighs supported on a bolster in 20° to 30° flexion, the distal femur is stabilized and an external rotation force and then an internal rotation force are applied to the tibia through the feet. An increase in external rotation greater than 10° relative to the normal knee associated with a posterolateral subluxation of the knee joint indicates tearing of the PLC structures. This test may also be performed with the patient prone.

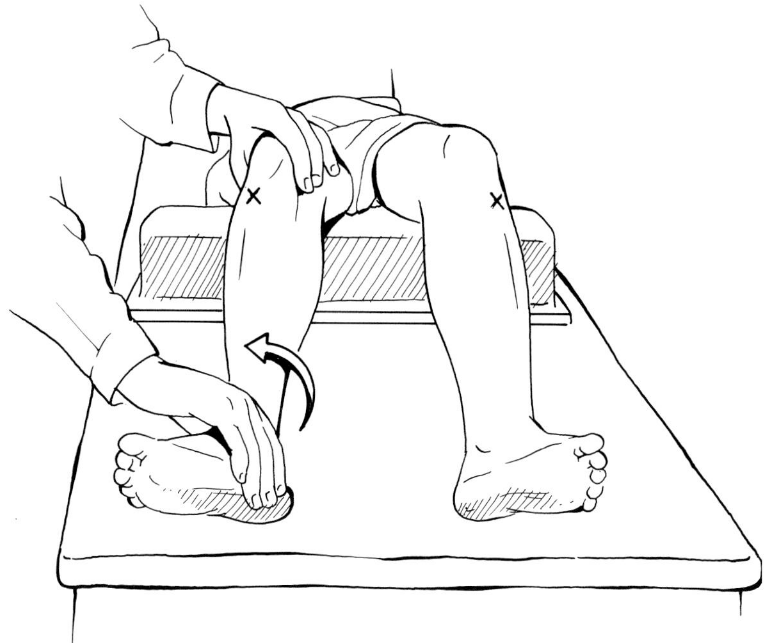

FIGURE 19.8. Evaluation of compartment subluxation. If the axial rotation test illustrated in Figure 19.7 is positive, the examiner holds the thigh and palpates the tibial compartments while an external rotation torque is applied. This allows the examiner to discern if the rotation movement is caused by posterior subluxation of the lateral tibial plateau or by anterior movement of the medial tibial plateau.

injury or from anterior subluxation of the medial tibial plateau as in an ACL/MCL injury.

Because the popliteus muscle-tendon unit is an active internal rotator of the knee, one can test for its function by asking the patient to actively internally rotate the leg while sitting with the knee flexed 90°.

Reverse Pivot Shift

The reverse pivot shift is probably the most reliable of the clinical tests of the posterior lateral ligament complex (Fig. 19.9). The test is started in the same position as described for a pivot shift. With a mild valgus stress, the knee is flexed. In a positive test result, at approximately

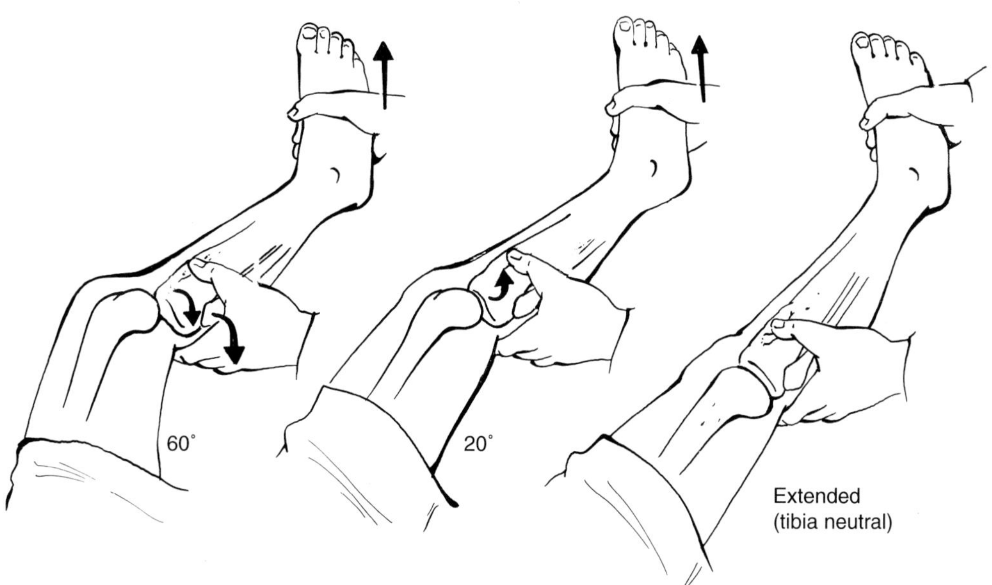

FIGURE 19.9. The reverse pivot shift test. The knee is flexed and the examiner applies a posterior force to the proximal lateral tibia. The knee is then slowly extended through the neutral to externally rotated foot while the proximal force is released. The test is positive if the change in directional force of the iliotibial band causes a sudden reduction anteriorly of the proximal lateral tibia. Although this test is an excellent measurement of abnormal posterolateral laxity, it is rarely positive in the unanesthetized acutely injured patient.

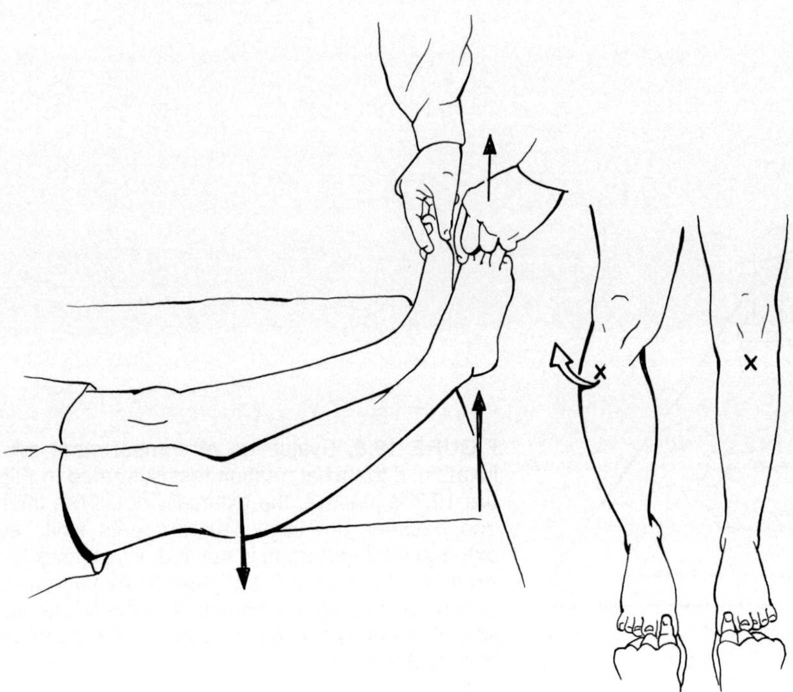

FIGURE 19.10. External rotation recurvatum test. With the patient supine, the examiner holds the patient's lower extremities up by the great toe or heel. The examiner observes for hyperextension and external rotation of the proximal tibia at the knee in comparison with the normal side. A markedly positive test indicates combined injury to the posterior capsule, posterior cruciate ligament, posterolateral ligament complex, and lateral collateral ligament.

20° to 30° of flexion, the tibia will externally rotate, and the lateral tibial plateau will displace posteriorly and will remain in this position during further flexion. When the knee is then extended, the tibia will reduce. In the standard pivot shift the tibia is anteriorly displaced in early flexion and then reduces between 20° and 40° of flexion. In the reverse pivot shift, the tibia is initially reduced and then the lateral tibial plateau displaces posteriorly at 20° to 30° of flexion. In the combined ACL and PLC, one may observe the tibia go from an anterior position to a reduced position and then on to a posterior position. The reverse pivot shift unfortunately requires considerable relaxation and is difficult to achieve in the painful or acutely injured knee.

Hyperextension/Recurvatum External Rotation Test and Observation of Gait

With the patient supine and the examiner supporting the weight of the limb by the heel or great toe, the knee is observed in comparison to the other side to be in hyperextension and external rotation (Fig. 19.10). In chronic cases of PLC insufficiency, particularly when accompanied by ACL deficiency, the patient may walk with a varus thrust gait.

Combined Ligament Injuries

Anterior Cruciate Ligament/Posterior Cruciate Ligament

The combined ACL/PCL-injured knee will demonstrate both a posterior sag (positive PCL screen) and increased anterior-posterior laxity with a soft end point to anterior translation. It is important to perform the quadriceps active test on each injured knee to not miss the posterior contribution to what is likely to be considerable laxity in the anterior-posterior plane. The KT 1000 can be used to quantitate the relative contributions of anterior and posterior laxity. The technique for doing so is illustrated in Part C of this chapter.

Anterior Cruciate Ligament/Medial Collateral Ligament

The MCL is a secondary restraint to anterior translation. This means that while isolated disruption of the MCL does not cause measurable increased anterior laxity, the combined ACL/MCL disruption will result in a greater increase in anterior laxity than a disruption of the ACL alone. As the MCL heals, the measured laxity often decreases (20). Opening to valgus stress in full extension indicates a combined complete MCL tear including the posterior oblique capsular portion and one of the cruciate ligaments (21).

Anterior Cruciate Ligament/Posterior Cruciate Ligament or Posterior Cruciate Ligament/Posterolateral Ligament Complex

Most LCL and PLC injuries occur in combination with a cruciate ligament injury. It is important to carefully assess the varus stress test and dial test in acutely injured patients so this uncommon combined injury is not missed. Acute repair is indicated for most LCL/PLC injuries with pathologic motion, thus the necessity to make the diagnosis early. In chronic ACL/PLC pathologic laxity a varus thrust may be seen with gait. This portends a poor prognosis for any reconstructive procedure (22).

Meniscus and Hyaline Cartilage Injuries Associated with ACL Injury

In a study involving early arthroscopic evaluation of 190 previously normal, acutely injured knees with KT 1000 documented increased anterior laxity, 25% of the knees had medial and 35% had lateral meniscus tears (2). Physical examination findings of joint line tenderness and pain with the McMurray test are not predictive of meniscal tears after acute ACL injury (2,23). In Daniel's study 6% of the 190 knees had tears that were deemed repairable. Hyaline cartilage injury was also frequently noted.

Other Diagnostic Tests

Plain films are essential to the workup of any patient presenting with knee injury or instability complaints. Alignment, avulsion fractures, degenerative changes, loose bodies, bone quality, and of course tumors or tumor like conditions must be noted. Stress radiographs can help quantitate laxity, confirm diagnostic impressions and guide patient management decisions.

Magnetic resonance imaging (MRI) is extremely useful for delineating knee injuries, especially when the diagnosis is in doubt (24). It is expensive and often not necessary for diagnosis. Expense and certain shortcomings, for example, in terms of distinguishing repairable from non-repairable meniscal tears and insensitivity to hyaline cartilage injury limit the routine use of MRI. A chronic ACL tear in continuity may not appear abnormal on MRI. Instrumented knee arthrometer measurements have proved more useful in quantitatively assessing anterior and posterior knee laxity. Based on KT 1000 (MEDmetric Corp, San Diego) measurements and knowledge of a patient's pre-injury activity level, treatment recommendations can be made for acutely injured ACL deficient knees exclusive of MRI findings (2) (see also Part C of this chapter). MRI is very useful in planning acute posterolateral corner repairs, although special imaging sequences are recommended with increased imaging in the coronal and oblique plane of the popliteus (25). Bone bruises are frequently seen on MRI after major ligament injury but the long-term clinical significance remains in doubt (26).

Diagnostic arthroscopy is a valuable tool, although rarely required. It is the best method for diagnosing hyaline cartilage damage and determining whether a meniscal tear is unstable or repairable. With a thorough history and physical examination, ligament disruptions may be diagnosed on manual examination by an experienced clinician with 90% accuracy. Instrumented measurements of ACL and PCL laxity are vital aspects of a complete knee ligament examination.

REFERENCES

1. Noyes FR, et al. Knee sprains and acute knee hemarthrosis: misdiagnosis of anterior cruciate ligament tears. *Phys Ther* 1980;60: 1596–1601.
2. Daniel DM, et al. Fate of the ACL-injured patient. A prospective outcome study (see comments). *Am J Sports Med* 1994;22:632–644.
3. Fanelli GC. Posterior cruciate ligament injuries in trauma patients. *Arthroscopy* 1993;9:291–294.
4. Andrews JR, Edwards JC, Satterwhite YE. Isolated posterior cruciate ligament injuries. History, mechanism of injury, physical findings, and ancillary tests. *Clin Sports Med* 1994;13:519–530.
5. Bickerstaff DR. Posterior cruciate ligament injuries. *Br J Hosp Med* 1997;58:129–133.
6. Dejour H, et al. The natural history of rupture of the posterior cruciate ligament. *Rev Chir Orthop* 1988;74:35–43.
7. Miller MD, et al. Posterior cruciate ligament injuries. *Orthop Rev* 1993; 22:1201–1210.
8. Shelbourne KD, Rubinstein RA Jr. Methodist Sports Medicine Center's experience with acute and chronic isolated posterior cruciate ligament injuries. *Clin Sports Med* 1994;13:531–543.
9. Kannus P. Long-term results of conservatively treated medial collateral ligament injuries of the knee joint. *Clin Orthop* 1988;226: 103–112.
10. Gollehon DL, Torzilli PA, Warren RF. The role of the posterolateral and cruciate ligaments in the stability of the human knee. A biomechanical study. *J Bone Joint Surg Am* 1987;69:233–242.
11. Nielsen S, et al. Rotatory instability of cadaver knees after transection of collateral ligaments and capsule. *Arch Orthop Trauma Surg* 1984; 103:165–169.
12. Veltri DM, Warren RF. Posterolateral instability of the knee. *Instr Course Lect* 1995;44:441–453.
13. Veltri DM, Warren RF. Anatomy, biomechanics, and physical findings in posterolateral knee instability. *Clin Sports Med* 1994;13:599–614.
14. Daniel DM, et al. Instrumented measurement of anterior laxity of the knee. *J Bone Joint Surg Am* 1985;67:720–726.
15. Shoemaker SC, Daniel DM. The limits of knee motion. In vitro studies. In: Daniel DM, Akeson WH, O'Connor JJ, eds. *Knee ligaments: structure, function, injury, and repair.* New York: Raven Press, 1990: 153–161.
16. Noyes FR, et al. Knee ligament tests: what do they really mean? *Phys Ther* 1980;60:1578–1581.
17. Daniel DM, et al. Use of the quadriceps active test to diagnose posterior cruciate-ligament disruption and measure posterior laxity of the knee. *J Bone Joint Surg Am* 1988;70:386–391.
18. Daniel DM, Stone ML. Instrumented measurement of knee motion. In: Daniel DM, Akeson WH, O'Connor JJ, eds. *Knee ligaments: structure, function, injury, and repair.* New York: Raven Press, 1990: 421–426.
19. Daniel DM. Assessing the limits of knee motion. *Am J Sports Med* 1991;19:139–147.
20. Hillard-Sembell D, et al. Combined injuries of the anterior cruciate and medial collateral ligaments of the knee. Effect of treatment on stability and function of the joint. *J Bone Joint Surg Am* 1996;78:169–176.
21. Reider B. Medial collateral ligament injuries in athletes. *Sports Med* 1996;21:147–156.
22. Noyes FR, et al. The anterior cruciate ligament-deficient knee with varus alignment. An analysis of gait adaptations and dynamic joint loadings. *Am J Sports Med* 1992;20:707–716.
23. Shelbourne KD, et al. Correlation of joint line tenderness and meniscal lesions in patients with acute anterior cruciate ligament tears. *Am J Sports Med* 1995;23:166–169.
24. Sanchis-Alfonso V, Martinez-Sanjuan V, Gastaldi-Orquin E. The value of MRI in the evaluation of the ACL deficient knee and in the postoperative evaluation after ACL reconstruction. (Published erratum appears in *Eur J Radiol* 1993;16(3):255.) *Eur J Radiol* 1993;16: 126–130.
25. LaPrade RF, et al. The magnetic resonance imaging appearance of individual structures of the posterolateral knee. A prospective study of normal knees and knees with surgically verified grade III injuries. *Am J Sports Med* 2000;28:191–199.
26. Johnson DL, et al. The effect of a geographic lateral bone bruise on knee inflammation after acute anterior cruciate ligament rupture. *Am J Sports Med* 2000;28:152–155.

Part B: Imaging

Paul N. Grooff, Jean P. Schils, and Donald L. Resnick

After the initial patient history and physical examination, diagnostic imaging is an increasingly important aspect in the accurate assessment of internal derangements of the knee. Routine and advanced imaging techniques can define the extent of ligamentous injuries of the knee, and provide important information regarding additional knee injuries in the setting of ligamentous injury. This section will review the normal and abnormal imaging findings in patients with acute and chronic ligamentous knee injuries, with increased emphasis given to MRI. The imaging evaluation of the postoperative knee in a patient with ACL repair will also be addressed.

IMAGING TECHNIQUES

Typically, conventional radiography is the initial step in diagnostic evaluation of the injured knee. The routine radiographic examination of the knee consists of multiple projections (1). In evaluating acute knee injuries, the anteroposterior and lateral views are routinely obtained. Complete assessment with conventional radiography may require supplemental projections, including tunnel, Merchant, oblique, and cross-table lateral views. Routine radiographs, by themselves, do not allow direct visualization of injured ligaments or tendons, unless they are surrounded by fat. It is the associated alterations in the bone or soft tissue (or both) that can provide clues to accurately diagnose ligamentous injuries. Soft tissue abnormalities that may accompany tendinous or ligamentous injury of the knee include swelling, joint effusion, and change in contour or configuration of an injured tendon or ligament. A bloody effusion, often associated with intraarticular ligament damage, is detected as a soft tissue density in the suprapatellar pouch on the lateral projection. The presence of fat in the effusion, a lipohemarthrosis, suggests an osseous injury and is identified as a fat-fluid level on a cross-table lateral projection. Although fat globules are occasionally seen in other types of effusion, the accumulation of fat is much greater in cases of trauma (2). Stress views for acute ligamentous injuries of the knee are often cited as helpful, but may be difficult to obtain following acute trauma secondary to patient pain and muscle spasm and, therefore, may require anesthesia to perform successfully (3).

Extensive fractures around the knee are readily demonstrated by standard radiography, but more careful radiographic analysis may be required to detect avulsion injuries at the attachment sites of ligaments or tendons. This is particularly true among children, in whom cruci-ate injuries are commonly of the avulsion type. The osseous fragment at either the femoral or tibial insertion may consist of a thin flake of bone, although occasionally larger bony fragments are present.

Advanced imaging techniques, and in particular MRI, has become a common, accurate, and cost-effective method for diagnosis of ligamentous knee injuries (4). In the United States, MRI has all but replaced arthrography, conventional tomography, and computed tomography (CT) in the assessment of internal knee derangements. Conventional or CT play a role in the further assessment of suspected or diagnosed fractures of the knee on routine radiographs, although are less helpful in the diagnosis of ligamentous or tendinous injuries without associated fractures. Ultrasound is noninvasive, requires no ionizing radiation, and is relatively inexpensive when compared to CT and MRI. Ultrasound is a useful technique for the detection and characterization of abnormalities of the popliteal fossa, as well as those of the quadriceps and patellar tendons. Ultrasound has also been applied with some success to the evaluation of ligaments, menisci, and hyaline cartilage, although ultrasound use in the setting of ligamentous injury has not gained widespread use.

The excellent tissue characterization, high resolution, lack of ionizing radiation, and multiplanar capabilities of MRI have led to its rapid acceptance in the workup of patients with suspected ligamentous injury. Indeed, MRI is playing an increasingly large role in the diagnosis of many musculoskeletal abnormalities.

When a sample of tissue is placed in an external magnetic field, some hydrogen nuclei line up parallel to the lines of force. In this situation, the tissue sample exhibits magnetization. Nuclei aligned against the magnetic field are in a slightly higher energy state than those aligned parallel to the field. Nuclei can be shifted from parallel to antiparallel alignment by exposing the tissue to a pulse of radiofrequency energy, with the frequency corresponding to the energy difference between the two alignment states. When the radiofrequency pulse is terminated, the nuclei return to their original alignment, giving up energy in the form of a radiowave. The radiowave is detected by an antenna and converted by computer to a representative image in a fashion similar to that of a CT scanner. The final signal obtained by the computer is related to the selected time of repetition (TR) and time to echo (TE), the number of hydrogen protons contained in the tissue volume of interest, and both the tissue T1 and T2 relaxation times. T1 and T2 are inherent properties of the tissue that reflect the chemical and molecular composition of the tissue, as well as the motion of hydrogen protons within the tissue. Therefore, T1 and T2 are parameters that are fixed, whereas the operator can select TR and TE.

To achieve an image with optimal T1-weighting, the operator sets a short TR and a short TE. T2-weighting is achieved with a long TR and a long TE, and intermediate-weighting is achieved with a long TR and a short TE. On T1-weighted images, subcutaneous fat and bone marrow have the highest signal. Hyaline cartilage is intermediate in signal intensity, and muscle has even less intensity. Fluid has little signal on T1-weighted images. On T2-weighted images, effusions have the brightest signal, followed in decreasing order by subcutaneous fat, bone marrow, and muscle. Because fluid has high signal intensity on T2-weighted images, these images are useful to detect areas of abnormality by identifying high signal edema. Normal ligaments, tendons, menisci, and cortical bone remain low in signal intensity on both T1- and T2-weighted images.

Multiple protocols using variable pulse sequences and imaging planes are used in the MRI evaluation of the knee. The precise protocol that is chosen is dependent on the specific clinical situation, and can be tailored by the radiologist or technologist monitoring the examination. In general, in the evaluation of ligamentous injury, T1-, intermediate-, and T2-weighted images are useful, and imaging in both the coronal and sagittal planes is obtained. Further evaluation of the bone marrow and hyaline cartilage with more complex MR techniques is often helpful and may include fat signal suppression, gradient echo imaging, or use of inversion recovery techniques.

CENTRAL SUPPORTING STRUCTURES

Both the ACL and PCL are largely composed of dense fibrous tissue, and are of low signal intensity (dark) on both T1- and T2-weighted MRI images. The sagittal plane allows best visualization of these central supporting structures, although both coronal and transverse imaging aid in their assessment. The patient is placed within the MRI scanner in a supine position with the leg in a neutral position or in slight external rotation. The sagittal plane of section is obtained parallel to the long axis of the ACL so that the ligament is usually identified completely on one image. On the intermediate- or T2-weighted images, the ACL appears as a straight, well-defined structure of low signal intensity coursing through the intercondylar notch parallel to or with an angle slightly greater than the intercondylar roof (Fig. 19.11A) (5–7). The PCL, which generally is wider than the ACL, is also usually seen on one sagittal image and demonstrates a slight curvature convex posteriorly (Fig. 19.12A) (6,8). The cruciate ligaments attach to the femur and tibia as a collection of individual fascicles, rather than at a single attachment site (9). The meniscofemoral ligaments of Humphry and Wrisberg are highly variable in appearance and extend from the posterior horn of the lateral meniscus and cross anterior and posterior to the PCL, respectively, to insert on the medial femoral condyle (Fig. 19.13).

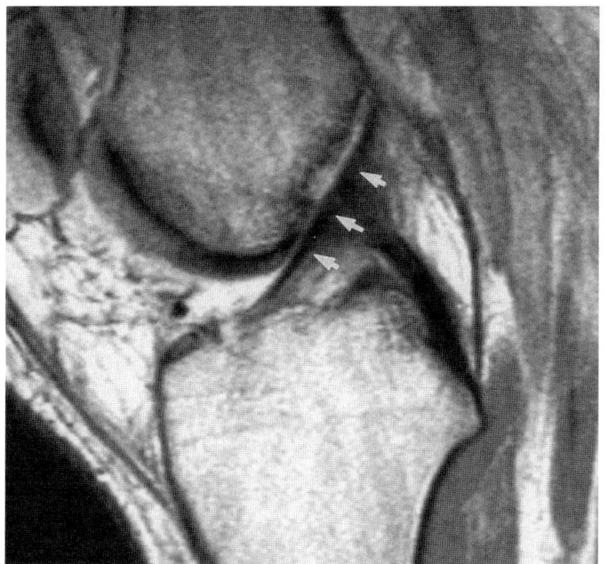
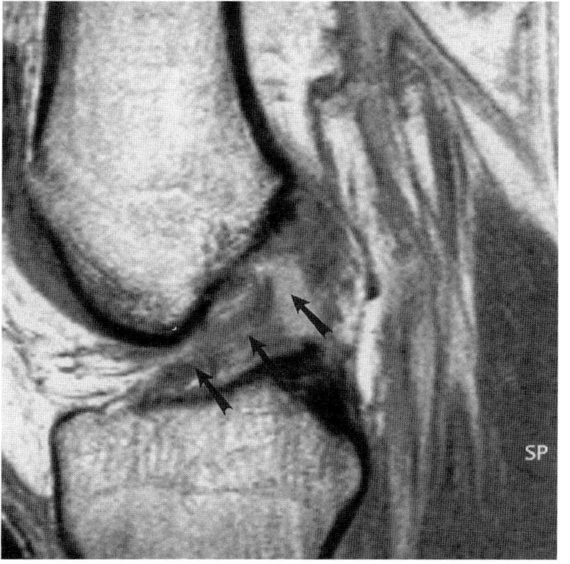

A B

FIGURE 19.11. A: Normal anterior cruciate ligament (ACL). Sagittal intermediate-weighted magnetic resonance image (MRI) demonstrates the ACL as a smooth, thin, low-signal intensity structure within the intercondylar notch (*arrows*). **B:** Acute ACL tear. Sagittal intermediate-weighted MRI demonstrates disruption of the ACL, with surrounding intermediate signal intensity giving the appearance of an amorphous mass (*arrows*).

(Continued on next page)

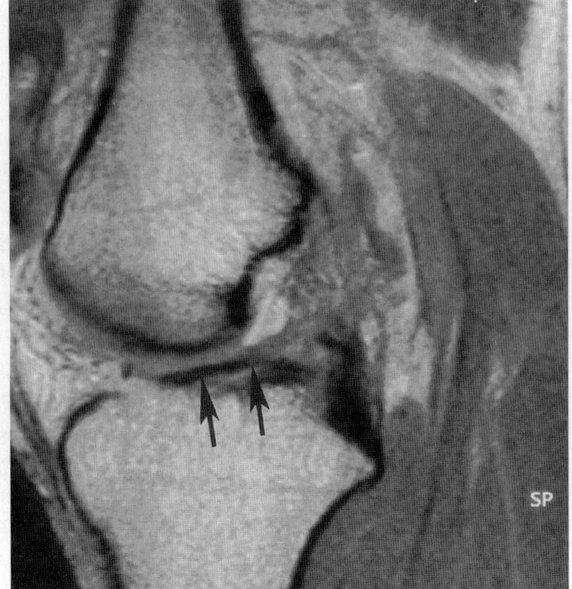

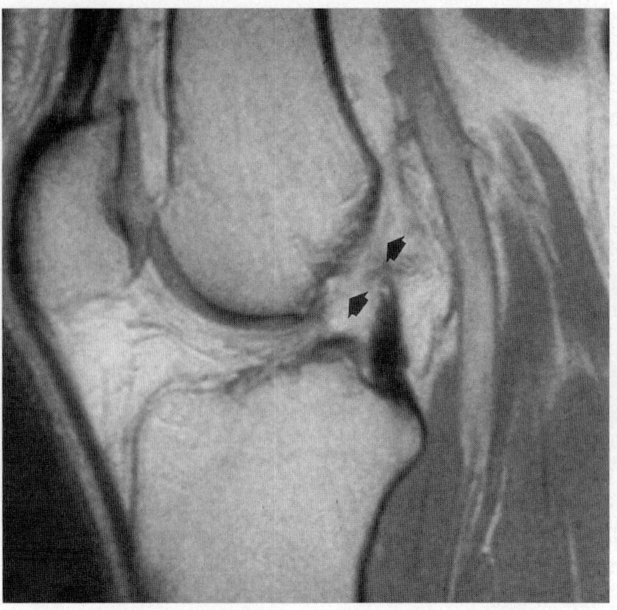

FIGURE 19.11. *Continued.* **C:** Chronic ACL tear. Sagittal intermediate-weighted MRI demonstrated a retracted ACL, with a decreased slope, laying on the tibial spines (*arrows*) in this patient with a chronic ACL tear. **D:** Chronic ACL tear. Sagittal intermediate-weighted MRI demonstrates nonvisualization of the ACL in its expected location (*arrows*) in this chronically ACL-deficient knee.

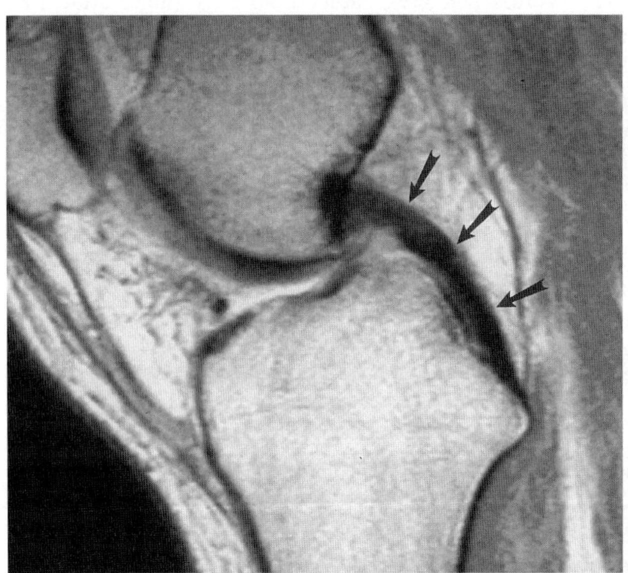

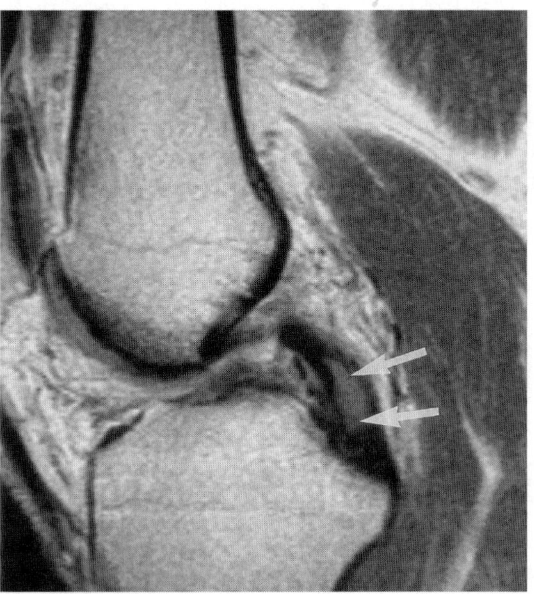

FIGURE 19.12. A: Normal posterior cruciate ligament (PCL). Sagittal intermediate-weighted magnetic resonance image (MRI) demonstrates a normal, low-signal intensity PCL within the intercondylar notch with a slightly convex posterior course (*arrows*). **B:** Acute PCL tear. Sagittal intermediate-weighted MRI demonstrates thickening and increased signal intensity within the mid and distal PCL (*arrows*) in this patient with acute interstitial tearing of the PCL.

(Continued on next page)

C
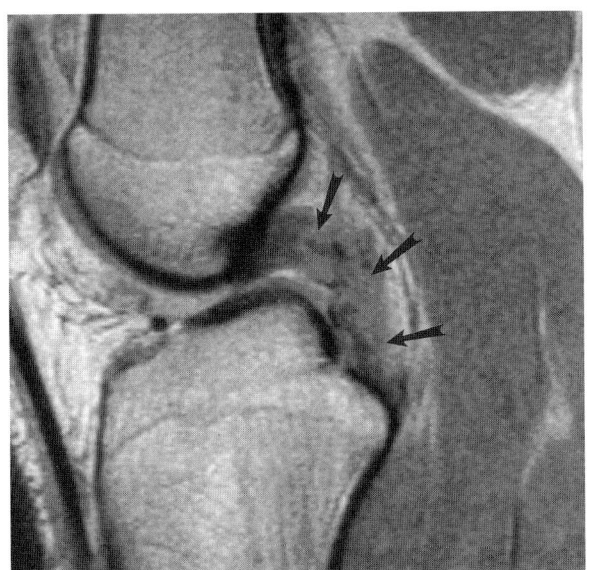
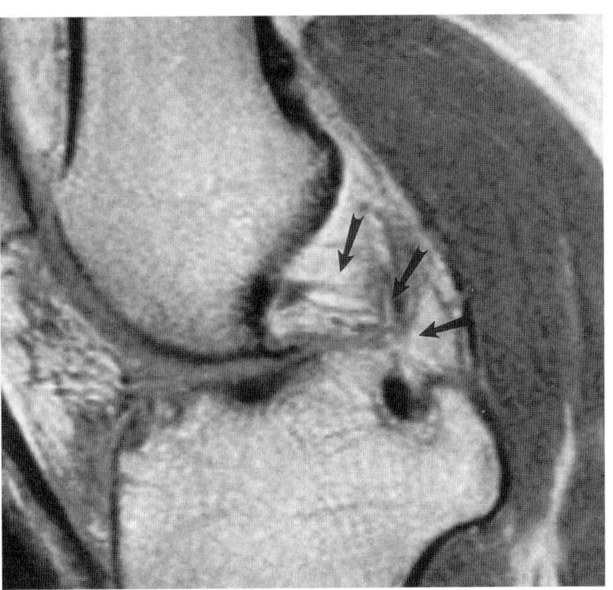
D

FIGURE 19.12. *Continued.* **C:** Acute PCL tear. Sagittal intermediate-weighted MRI demonstrates tearing of the PCL with increased signal intensity of the PCL fibers and thickening of the PCL (*arrows*), giving the appearance of an amorphous mass. **D:** Chronic PCL tear. Sagittal intermediate-weighted MR image demonstrates absence of the PCL (*arrows*) in this patient with chronic PCL deficiency.

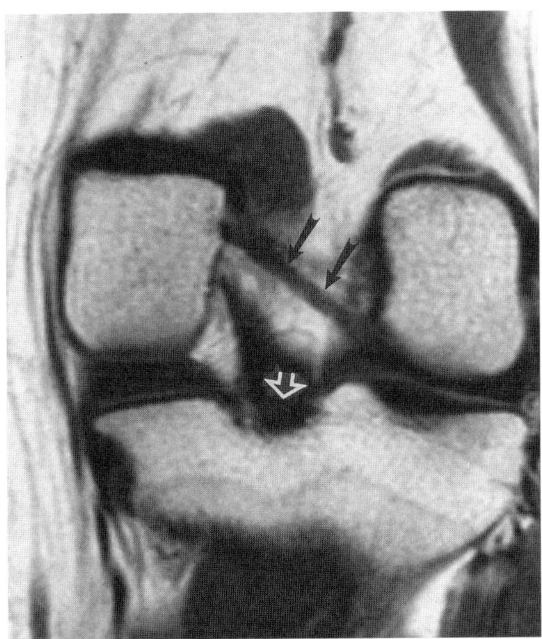

FIGURE 19.13. Meniscofemoral ligament of Wrisberg. Coronal T1-weighted magnetic resonance image demonstrate a normal meniscofemoral ligament extending from the lateral meniscus to the medial femoral condyle (*arrows*). Note the proximity of the meniscofemoral ligament to the posterior cruciate ligament (*open arrow*) as it inserts on the tibia.

ABNORMALITIES OF THE ANTERIOR CRUCIATE LIGAMENT

Acute Ligamentous Injuries

Initial radiography of a patient with an acute ACL injury may be normal or may demonstrate such nonspecific signs as a joint effusion or soft tissue swelling. More specific indicators of an ACL injury include an avulsion fracture of the anterior tibial eminence, a lateral tibial rim fracture (Segond fracture), an osteochondral impaction fracture of the lateral femoral condyle (Fig. 19.14) or a posterior fracture of the lateral tibial plateau (10). An avulsion of the insertion of the ACL is diagnosed on the lateral view by identification of the displaced fragment superior and anterior to the tibial spines. The fragment can also be observed on the tunnel view (11). The Segond fracture, although variable in size, is usually several millimeters in diameter and is located posterior to Gerdy's tubercle (12–14). This vertically oriented fracture results from excessive tension on the lateral capsular ligament of the knee. The fragment is identified lateral to the lateral tibial plateau on the anterior–posterior (A/P) radiograph (Fig. 19.15A). The Segond fracture, or lateral capsular sign, is invariably associated with an ACL injury.

The accuracy of MRI in detecting ACL tears is high, ranging from 92% to 100% in the literature (15–17), which explains the increasing use of this noninvasive technique in the assessment of ligamentous injuries. The appearance of the injured ACL on MRI depends of the time elapsed since the injury and the extent of associated injuries. The most important finding in the diagnosis of an ACL tear with MRI is discontinuity of the ligament in the sagittal plane. The tear is usually seen in the proximal aspect of the ligament, near its femoral insertion. In the case of an acute ACL injury, increased signal on either intermediate- or T2-weighted sequences is present within the ligamentous substance (presumably representing both edema and local hemorrhage), giving the ligament the appearance of an amorphous mass (Fig. 19.11B). These findings can be accompanied by a change (decrease) in the slope of the ACL. Effects of anterior translocation of the tibia with respect to the femur may also be present and include "buckling" of the PCL (Fig. 19.16) and "uncovering" of the undersurface of the posterior horn of the lateral meniscus (Fig. 19.17) (18,19). A specific pattern of bone marrow edema, or bone bruising, can result from the bone impaction forces during the course of the ACL injury. Bone marrow edema within the anterior

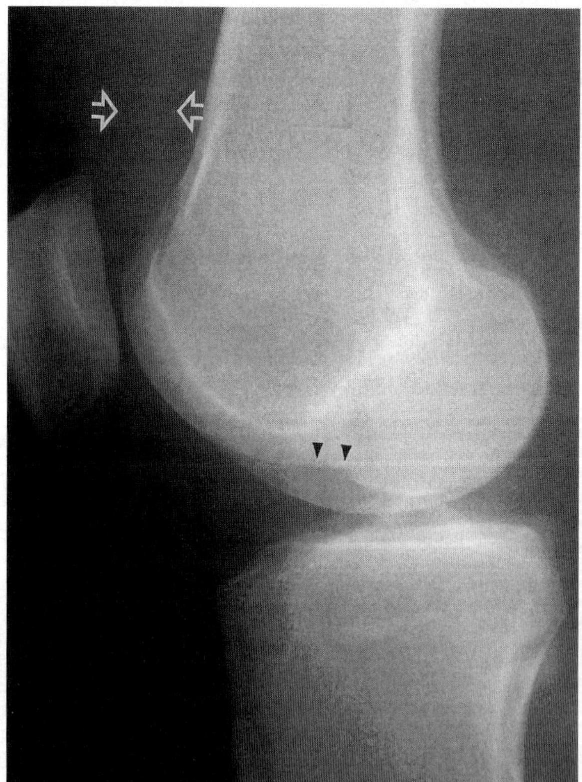
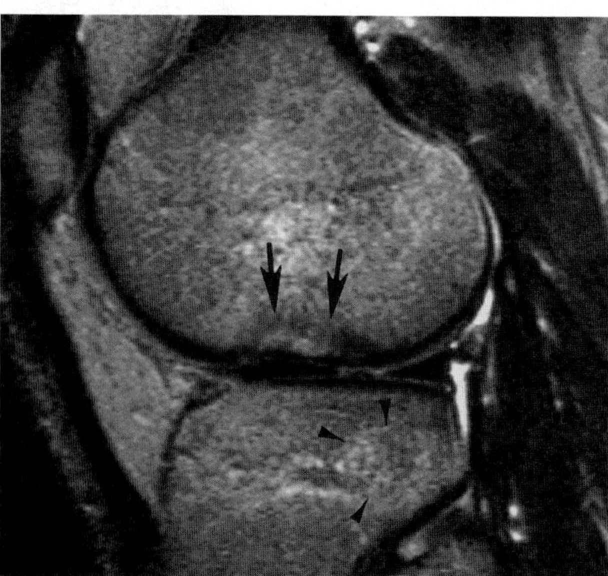

FIGURE 19.14. A: Lateral femoral condyle impaction fracture. Lateral radiograph of the knee demonstrates an osteochondral impaction fracture of the lateral femoral condyle (*arrowheads*) in this patient who is status postacute anterior cruciate ligament tear. A joint effusion is seen as added density in the suprapatellar pouch (*open arrows*). **B:** Lateral femoral condyle impaction injury. T2-weighted sagittal magnetic resonance image demonstrates curvilinear low signal within the lateral femoral condyle (*arrows*) representing an impaction fracture. There is surrounding high-signal intensity edema within the femoral condyle and within the posterior tibia (*arrowheads*) representing bone bruising.

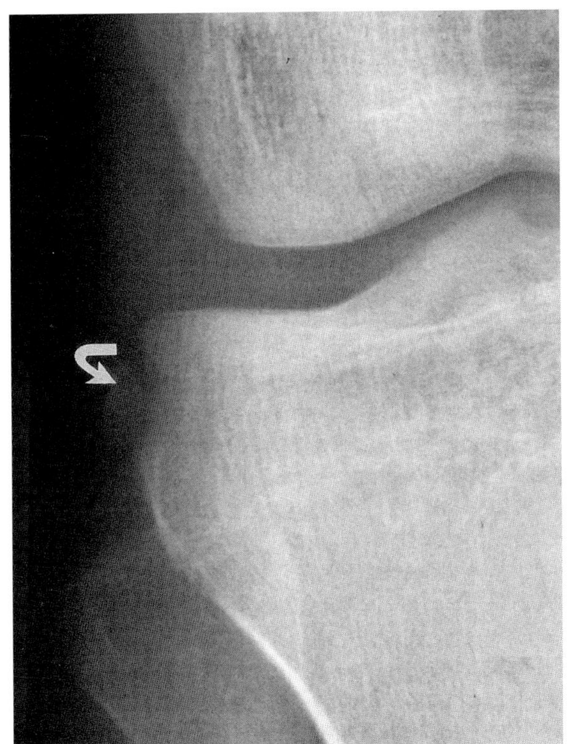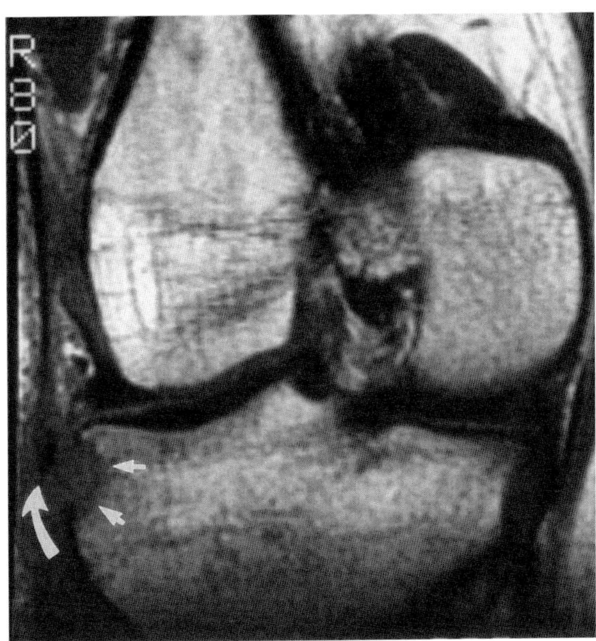

FIGURE 19.15. **A:** Segond fracture. The anterior–posterior radiograph demonstrates the capsular avulsion fragment (*curved arrow*) immediately lateral to the lateral tibial plateau. **B:** Segond fracture. Coronal T1-weighted magnetic resonance image demonstrates the defect within the lateral tibia (*arrows*) and the small adjacent avulsion fracture fragment (*curved arrow*).

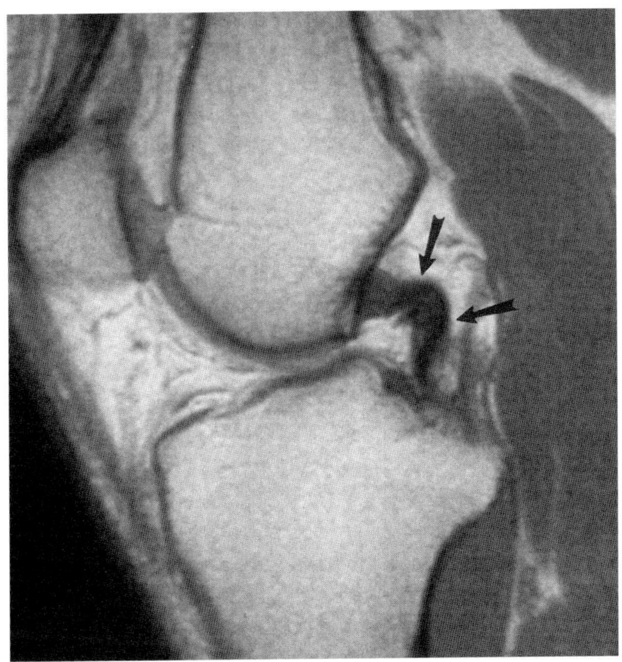

FIGURE 19.16. Buckling of the posterior cruciate ligament (PCL). Sagittal intermediate-weighted magnetic resonance image demonstrates a more acute posteriorly convex curve of the posterior cruciate ligament as the tibia translocates anteriorly (*arrows*). This is an indirect sign of acute or chronic ACL injury.

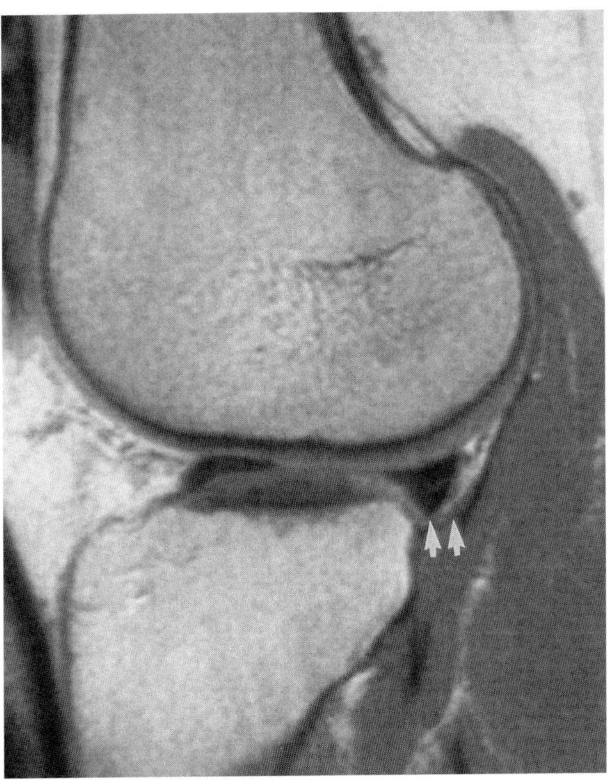

FIGURE 19.17. Uncovering of the undersurface of the lateral meniscus. Sagittal intermediate-weighted magnetic resonance image demonstrates the posterior horn of the lateral meniscus positioned posterior to the anteriorly translocated tibia (*arrows*). This is an indirect sign of acute or chronic anterior cruciate ligament injury.

aspect of the lateral femoral condyle and in the postero-lateral proximal tibia is suggestive of an ACL tear (Fig. 19.14B) and is secondary to anterior subluxation of the tibia. Detection of bone bruising is improved using inversion recovery techniques or T2-weighted imaging with fat signal suppression, seeking areas of high signal corresponding to the bone marrow edema.

Partial tears of the ACL may demonstrate relatively intact fibers with focal areas of increased signal intensity or subtle angulation deformities of the ACL in a clinically stable knee. The diagnosis of partial ACL tears remains difficult on MRI and clinical correlation is often needed to diagnose partial ACL tears correctly (20).

An additional benefit of MRI in the assessment of ligamentous injury is the discovery of associated injuries, which might confound the physical examination. Tears of the medial supporting structures, tears of the menisci, avulsion fractures, and Segond fractures (Fig. 19.15B) can be demonstrated by MRI. Medial meniscal tears accompany 40% to 80% of cases of ACL tears and should be sought out in the setting of ACL injury (21). Lateral meniscal tears are also associated with injuries of the ACL, although occur less commonly than medial meniscal tears. In 5% of ACL injuries, there may be an avulsion fracture at the tibial insertion (Fig. 19.18) with an intact ACL (22). As mentioned, these types of injuries occur

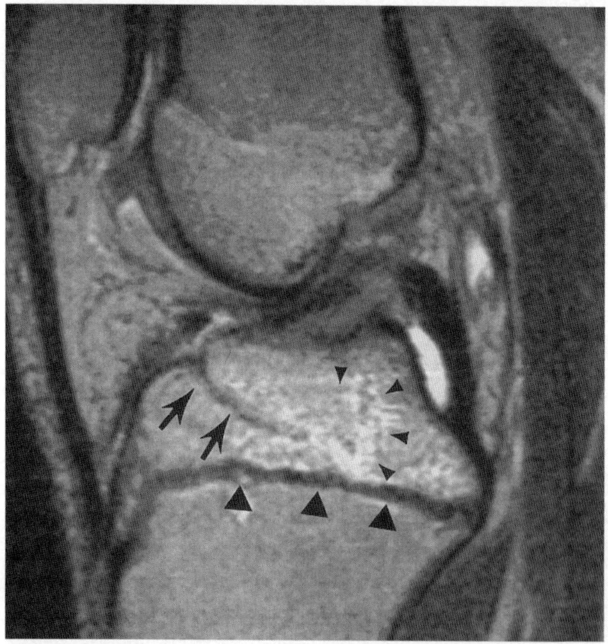

FIGURE 19.18. Anterior cruciate ligament (ACL) avulsion fracture. Sagittal T2-weighted magnetic resonance image demonstrates a low-signal intensity avulsion fracture of the proximal tibia at the insertion of the ACL (*arrows*). There is adjacent high-signal intensity bone marrow edema (*small arrowheads*). This type of injury occurs more commonly in pediatric patients. Note the open physeal plate (*large arrowheads*).

with greater frequency in children. MRI identification of the avulsion fracture fragment is often difficult, because there may be surprisingly little bone marrow edema associated with the site of avulsion.

CHRONIC LIGAMENTOUS INJURIES

A careful history and physical examination are the most crucial elements in the diagnosis of chronic instability of the knee. The purpose of radiography in this clinical situation is to allow identification of the sequelae of an unstable knee and to assist the surgeon in determining the most appropriate treatment.

Most authors agree that if untreated, osteoarthritic change will develop in the unstable knee secondary to a ligamentous injury. No prospective study of the evolution of the traumatized knee has firmly established this relationship, however (23–27). According to McDaniel (25), there appears to be a definite relationship between varus deformity, medial meniscectomy, and the development of medial joint narrowing and osteoarthritis in cases of untreated ACL rupture. In an extensive clinical and radiographic study of 127 ACL injuries of the knee, the effect of meniscal injury, meniscectomy, or both, in the presence of ligamentous insufficiency, was correlated with radiographic signs. The degree of degeneration appears to be influenced by the absence of the meniscus and associated collateral ligament damage and that progressive functional deterioration correlates with radiographic evidence of degenerative change (27). In another study related to the natural evolution of ACL-deficient knees, osteoarthritis involved the medial femorotibial compartment with genu varum and, in advanced cases, lateral subluxation of the tibia. Bicompartmental osteoarthritis was also recognized with no deviation in the frontal plane. Osteoarthritis of the lateral femorotibial compartment was very uncommon (28).

An area of controversy involves the optimal choice of projections to assess all of these radiographic signs. Generally, although multiple views are obtained, the protocols are inconsistent from one institution to another (29,30). A comparative study of both knees must be obtained, and the two following projections are required for the examination of the femorotibial joint: (i) a frontal unipodal weight-bearing view in slight flexion; and (ii) a lateral view, with the patient supine and with 30° of knee flexion. The first of these, the weight-bearing view, is obtained for detecting early degenerative change of the femorotibial joints, particularly to assess the degree of joint space narrowing (8,31,32). Biomechanical studies have demonstrated that the highest pressure about the femorotibial joint occurs with slight flexion (walking) and that the posterior part of the articular surface is principally involved. These data explain why the weight-bearing view must be obtained in slight flexion, so that the x-ray beam is tangent to this critical posterior joint surface where osteoarthritis begins. This view can also detect osteophytes along the condylar portion of the femur.

Many radiographic findings associated with the ACL-deficient knee have been described (5,23,28,33): intercondylar tubercle beaking, intercondylar eminence spurring and hypertrophy; inferior patellar facet osteophyte; joint space narrowing with buttressing osteophytosis; intercondylar notch narrowing; posterior osteophyte of the medial tibial plateau; and lateral notching of the lateral femoral condyle. Intercondylar notch narrowing, well seen on the frontal examination, is characterized by proliferative changes of the tibial spine and the intercondylar area of the femoral condyle with secondary stenosis of the notch. It represents a reliable sign of chronic instability when it is observed in a knee without significant joint space narrowing, and should be recognized by an orthopedic surgeon who is considering a notchplasty before an intraarticular ligamentous reconstruction (23). A posteromedial osteophyte of the medial plateau, identified on the lateral view, also is an early sign of chronic instability when the knee radiograph is otherwise normal. This osteophyte represents a response to repetitive stress at the insertion of the posterior component of the MCL, and it is indicative of a deficient ACL (28,33).

On a lateral radiograph of the knee, a groove in the middle third of the lateral femoral condyle is a constant normal finding. In some cases, it is very large (30,34,35). This groove and a less constant groove in the anterior part of the medial femoral condyle reflect the position of the anterior part of the corresponding tibial plateau when the knee is fully extended (35). The lateral notch sign is an exaggeration of this normal indentation and represents an abnormal finding when it is greater than 2 mm in depth on the lateral radiograph (5). This alteration may be seen in chronic and acute ACL-deficient knees, and results from anterior subluxation of the lateral tibial plateau secondary to impingement upon the lateral or posterolateral tibial margin. These findings can be compared to the Hill-Sachs lesion affecting the posterolateral aspect of the humeral head in patients with anterior glenohumeral dislocations.

With the exception of the weight-bearing A/P view of the knee (which can be considered a stress view), stress radiography has not been widely used. Views obtained with application of varus or valgus stress or with anterior or posterior "drawer" maneuvers to indirectly assess ligamentous integrity can be obtained with fluoroscopic guidance.

Magnetic resonance imaging allows direct visualization of the injured ACL, as well as the osteoarthritic changes that occur is the chronically ACL-deficient knee. With chronic tears of the ACL, edema and hemorrhage about the ACL have resolved. Typical MRI appearances of a chronically torn ACL include a retracted, atrophic ligament lying on the tibial spines (Fig. 19.11C) or complete nonvisualization of the ACL (Fig. 19.11D) (20). The bone marrow edema seen with the initial injury will have resolved, however an osteochondral impaction defect of the lateral femoral condyle, corresponding to the lateral notch sign on a radiograph, supports previous ACL injury. Recent advances in MRI imaging of articular cartilage now allow direct assessment of focal chondral and osteochondral defects seen with posttraumatic osteoarthritis.

ABNORMALITIES OF THE POSTERIOR CRUCIATE LIGAMENT

Routine radiography rarely contributes to the diagnosis of a posterior cruciate ligament injury and may demonstrate nonspecific signs such as a joint effusion or soft tissue swelling. An avulsion at the tibial insertion of the PCL is uncommon; however, it may be identified on routine radiographs (Fig. 19.19). The detection of this often subtle finding is important because surgery may be indicated in the setting of an acute PCL avulsion. MRI can be used to accurately diagnose PCL injuries, and can well demonstrate both PCL avulsions and the more common midsubstance PCL tears, which are often treated nonoperatively.

Acute tears of the PCL occur most commonly in the midsubstance of the ligament. The appearance is similar to ACL tearing, with increased signal intensity on the intermediate- and T2-weighted scans and thickening of the affected area (Figs. 19.12B, C). PCL tears differ from ACL tears in that an acute PCL injury typically exhibits

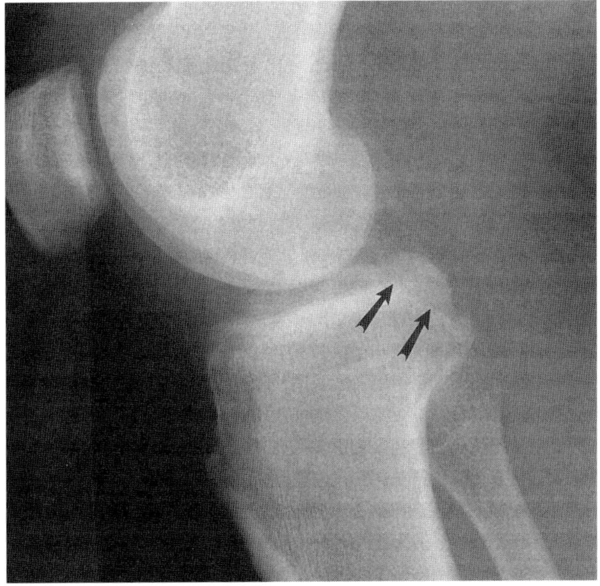

FIGURE 19.19. Posterior cruciate ligament (PCL) avulsion fracture. A lateral radiograph demonstrates linear radiolucency along the posterior proximal tibia (*arrows*) representing an avulsion fracture of the tibia at the insertion of the PCL.

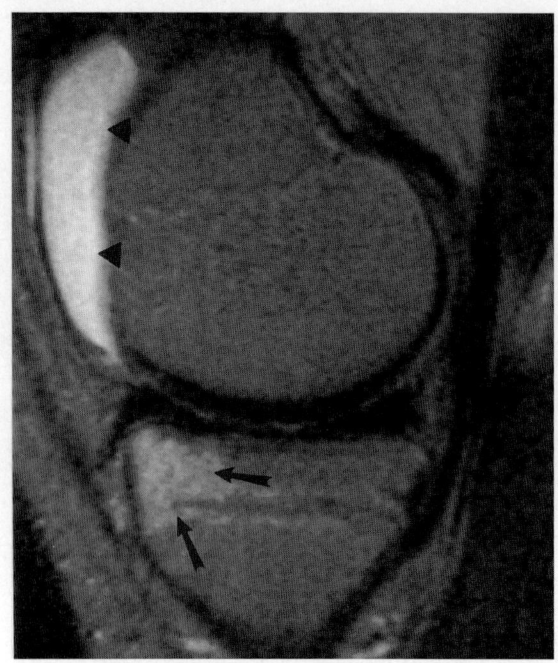

FIGURE 19.20. Bone bruising in a patient with an acute posterior cruciate ligament (PCL) tear. Sagittal T2-weighted magnetic resonance image demonstrates high-signal intensity bone marrow edema within the anterior and medial aspect of the proximal tibia (*arrows*) in this patient who is status postacute PCL injury. Also note the high signal intensity joint effusion (*arrowheads*) accompanying the acute injury.

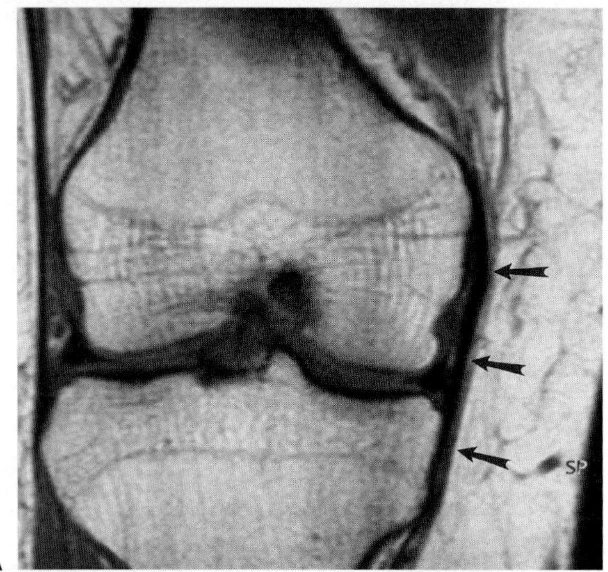

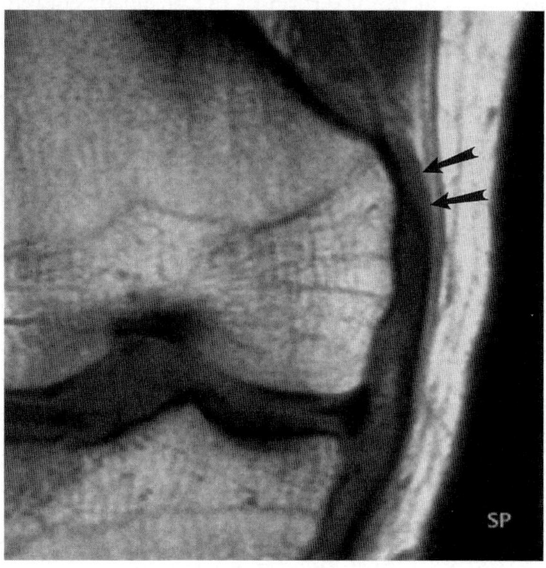

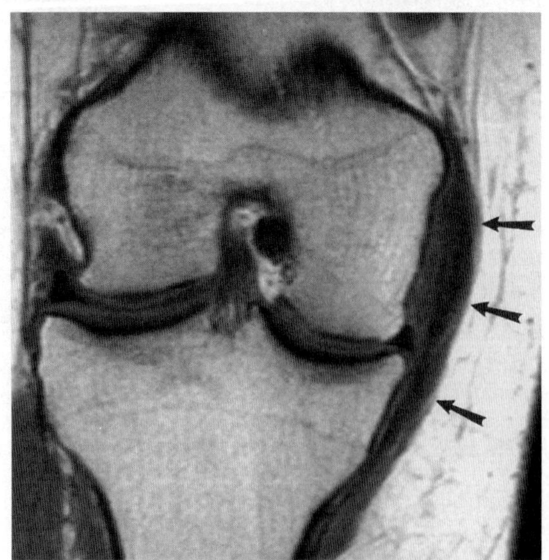

FIGURE 19.21. A: Normal medial collateral ligament (MCL). T1-weighted coronal magnetic resonance image (MRI) demonstrates the low-signal intensity normal MCL extending from the medial femoral condyle to the proximal tibia (*arrows*). **B:** Acute MCL sprain. T1-weighted coronal MRI demonstrates discontinuity of the proximal MCL fibers (*arrows*) and low-signal intensity edema about the MCL (*arrowheads*). These MR findings could be seen in both grade II and grade III MCL sprains. **C:** Chronic MCL tear. T1-weighted coronal MRI demonstrates diffuse thickening of the MCL (*arrows*), a finding seen in patients with previous or chronic MCL injuries.

interstitial ligament tearing, rather than disruption or avulsion of the ligament (8,36). Because the force producing a PCL tear is great, ACL and collateral ligament injuries, bone bruising, and meniscal injuries often occur in association with a PCL tear. Bone bruising of the anterior proximal tibia is typical (Fig. 19.20).

Because the initial PCL injury is typically interstitial, the MRI appearance of chronic PCL tears usually demonstrates an intact ligament with subtle signal alterations. Occasionally the chronically injured PCL may be attenuated or atrophied (Fig. 19.12D), but more typically the PCL will demonstrate areas of thickening or an irregular contour.

MEDIAL SUPPORTING STRUCTURES

The architectural arrangement of the medial collateral ligaments has been described previously in this book. Although MRI cannot delineate all of the individual components of the medial supporting structures, the MCL is identified on T1-, intermediate-, and T2-weighted images. The normal ligament is best seen in the coronal plane as a thin dark band extending from the femoral epicondyle to the medial portion of the tibia (Fig. 19.21A) (8,9). A portion of this signal presumably originates from the capsular ligament, as this structure becomes indistinguishable anatomically from the overlying oblique extension of the MCL in the posterior third of the capsule (posterior oblique ligament). The two fiber bundles of the MCL (vertical and oblique) cannot be differentiated with routine MRI. The ligament is often separated from the meniscus by an area of high signal intensity that represents an intraligamentous bursa. This bursa should not be mistaken for evidence of a meniscocapsular separation.

ABNORMALITIES OF THE MEDIAL COLLATERAL LIGAMENT

Soft tissue swelling in the medial part of the knee is often the only radiologic finding in cases of acute injury of the MCL. Rarely, an avulsion at the sites of ligamentous insertion may be evident. The MRI findings of acute MCL injury depend on the degree of injury (37,38). Grade 1 injuries show periligamentous edema as high signal intensity on T2-weighted images with an intact MCL. More severe injuries (grades 2 and 3) are difficult to distinguish as partial or complete disruption of the MCL on MRI. Grade 2 and 3 MCL tears demonstrate loss of continuity of the ligament fibers accompanied by focal or diffuse increased signal intensity on T2-weighted images (edema) and deformity of the ligament (Fig. 19.21B). Severe injuries of the MCL are often associated with injury of the cruciate ligaments and menisci. Bone bruising can be present in the lateral femoral condyle and the adjacent tibial plateau (Fig. 19.22).

Sequelae of an old injury affecting the MCLs may be evident on routine radiographs. A common finding is

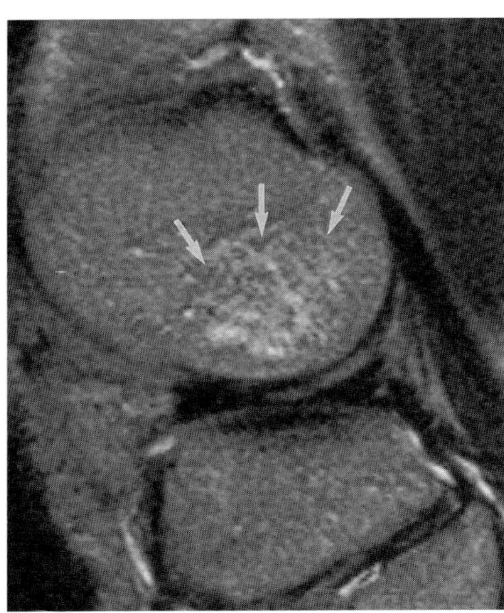

FIGURE 19.22. Bone bruising in a patient with an acute medial collateral ligament (MCL) tear. T2-weighted sagittal magnetic resonance image demonstrates high-signal intensity bone marrow edema within the lateral femoral condyle (*arrows*) after acute MCL injury.

ossification in the soft tissue adjacent to the upper pole of the medial condyle (the Pelligrini-Steida syndrome) (Fig. 19.23), which results from injury to the MCL at its femoral insertion. An associated varus deformity can also be seen. On MRI, the chronic MCL tear often regains

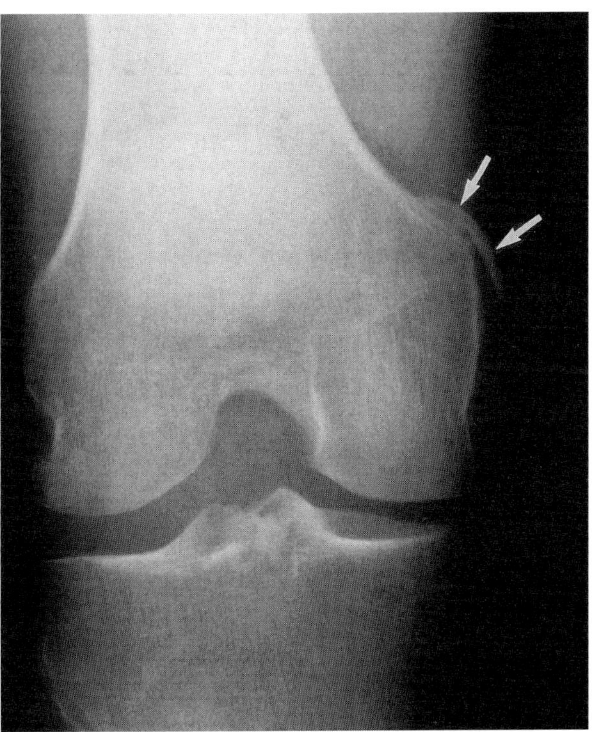

FIGURE 19.23. Pelligrini–Steida. Anterior–posterior radiograph demonstrates ossification of the proximal medial collateral ligament (MCL) at its insertion on the medial femoral condyle (*arrows*). This finding is frequently seen in patients with remote MCL injuries.

apparent continuity, appearing as a thick band of low-signal scar tissue on coronal images (Fig. 19.21C). A thickened MCL may also be present in a patient with medial compartment osteoarthritis and an intact MCL (8).

LATERAL SUPPORTING STRUCTURES

MRI allows delineation of the iliotibial band, the biceps femoris tendon in layer I, and the patellar retinaculum in layer II. The lateral (fibular) collateral ligament lies in the third layer and can also be identified with MRI (Fig. 19.24A). It inserts on the fibular head along with the biceps femoris tendon as the conjoined tendon. This insertion is evident on coronal and sagittal MR images, whereas the joint capsule itself is not reliably observed (8). Routine imaging of the knee often does not accurately demonstrate the posterolateral ligamentous structures. When there is concern for injury to the posterolateral ligamentous structures, additional imaging with an obliquely oriented coronal plane greatly increased the conspicuity of the arcuate ligament, the fabellofibular ligament, and the fibular origin of the popliteal muscle (39).

ABNORMALITIES OF THE LATERAL COLLATERAL LIGAMENT

Routine radiographs in the setting of lateral collateral ligament (LCL) injury rarely show focal soft tissue swelling laterally or avulsion of the fibula at the insertion of the conjoined tendon. The diagnostic criteria for disruption of the LCL by MRI are similar to those for the medial side of the knee. Acute disruption of the LCL demonstrates

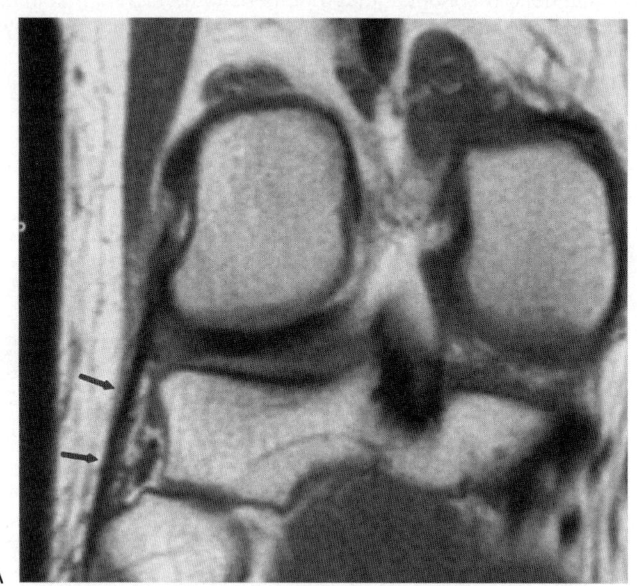

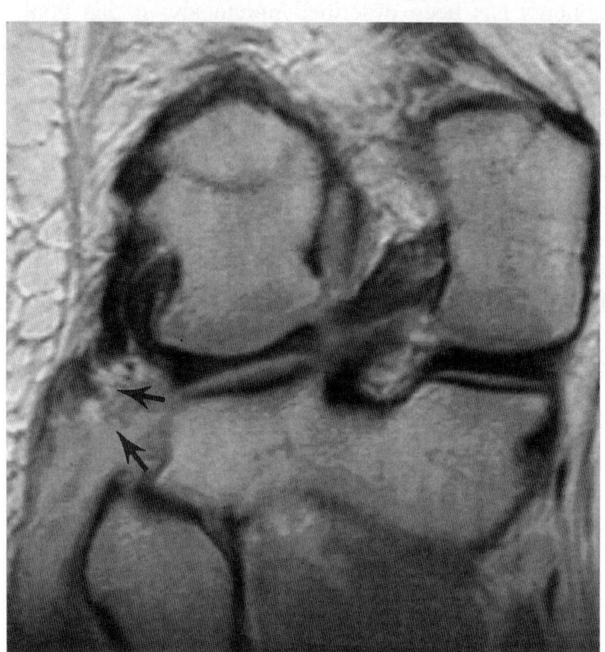

FIGURE 19.24. A: Normal lateral collateral ligament (LCL). T1-weighted coronal magnetic resonance image (MRI) demonstrates the low-signal intensity lateral (fibular) collateral ligament coursing from the lateral femoral condyle to the fibular head (*arrows*). **B:** Acute LCL tear. T1-weighted coronal MRI demonstrates disruption and disorganization of the soft tissues at the expected location of the LCL insertion on the fibula (*arrows*). An intact LCL is not identified. **C:** Acute LCL tear. T2-weighted coronal MRI demonstrates high signal intensity fluid extending through the lateral support structures (*arrows*) in this patient with an acute LCL tear. Also note the high-signal intensity bone marrow edema (*open arrows*) within the medial femoral condyle.

interruption of the normal ligament with increased signal within and around the ligament on T2-weighted coronal images (Figs.19.24B, 19.24C). Alternatively, the LCL may remain intact with an avulsion fracture of the fibular head. Because isolated injury to the LCL is extremely rare, MRI has the additional advantage of evaluating associated lesions involving the ACL and PCL. Indeed, the most common MRI appearance of injury to the lateral supporting structures is complex signal abnormalities and disorganization of the soft tissues in the region of the supporting structures associated with other findings or internal derangement (4). Bone bruising is commonly seen involving the medial joint compartment.

Isolated injuries involving the biceps femoris and iliotibial band demonstrate similar MRI alterations as those described for the lateral collateral ligament. An avulsion fracture of Gerdy's tubercle may be seen at the insertion of the iliotibial band. An acute injury of the popliteus tendon or muscle typically occurs near the musculotendinous junction and demonstrates intratendinous areas of increased signal intensity on T2-weighted images.

Chronic injuries to the lateral supporting structures are occasionally encountered on MRI. Again, the injured ligaments may appear thickened secondary to scar formation or may appear attenuated or absent. The iliotibial band friction syndrome may demonstrate thickening of the iliotibial band with a small amount of fluid about the band (40).

ADDITIONAL STRUCTURES AND FINDINGS

The normal anatomy of both menisci is demonstrated well on MRI. The normal internal substance of the menisci produces no significant signal on either T1- or T2-weighted images (Fig. 19.25A). Meniscal tears appear

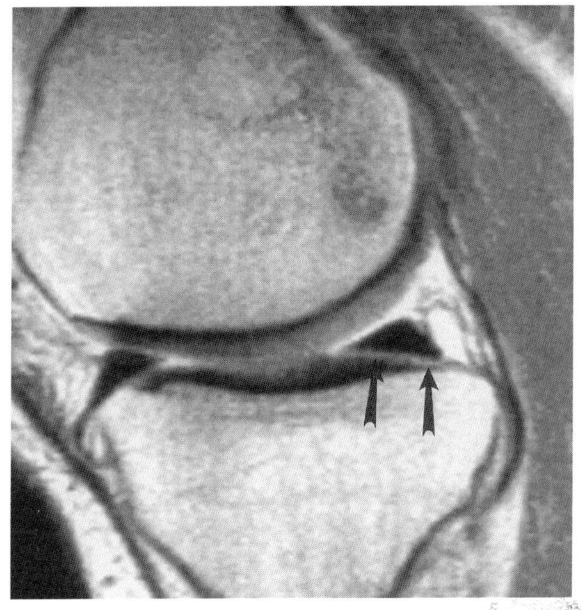

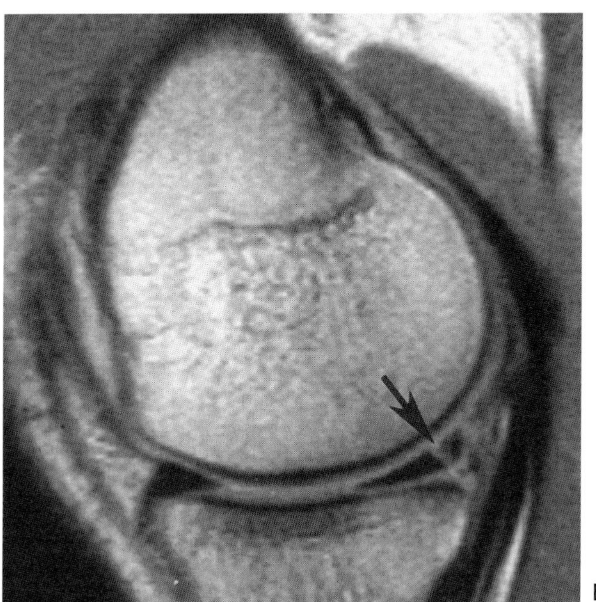

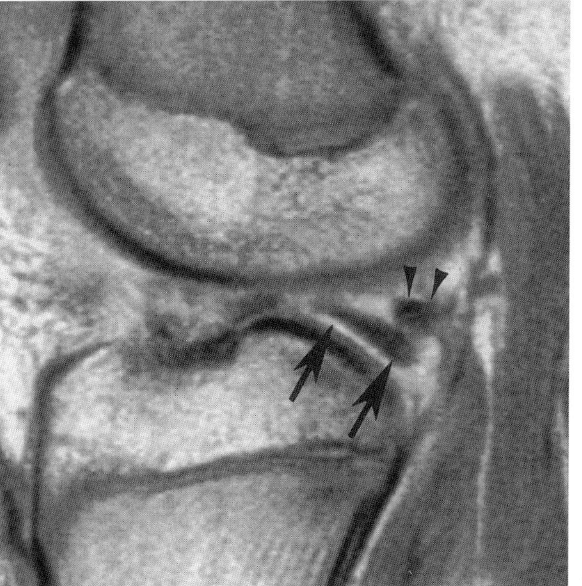

FIGURE 19.25. A: Normal medial meniscus. Sagittal intermediate-weighted magnetic resonance image (MRI) demonstrates the normal dark triangular appearance of the posterior horn of the medial meniscus (*arrows*). **B:** Medial meniscal tear. Sagittal intermediate-weighted MRI in a patient with an acute anterior cruciate ligament tear demonstrates a linear, vertically oriented high-signal intensity tear of the posterior horn of the medial meniscus (*arrow*). **C:** Bucket-handle lateral meniscal tear. Sagittal intermediate-weighted MRI in a pediatric patient demonstrates a bucket-handle meniscal tear with a low-signal intensity displaced meniscal fragment (*arrowheads*) positioned superior to the posterior horn of the lateral meniscus (*arrows*).

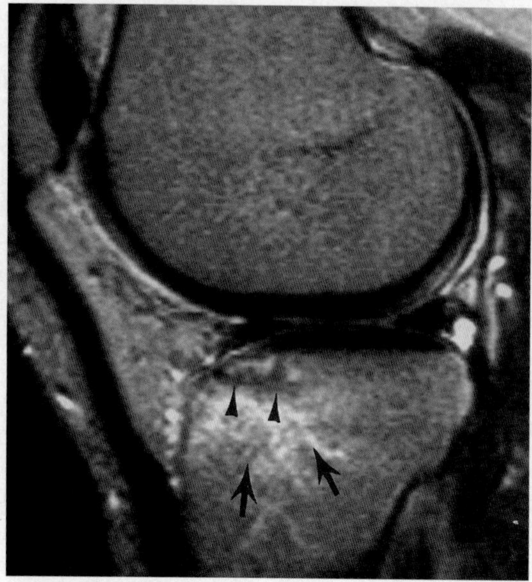

FIGURE 19.26. Subchondral fracture. Sagittal T2-weighted magnetic resonance image well demonstrates a radiographically occult proximal lateral tibia fracture in a patient with suspected ligamentous injury. The linear low-signal intensity fracture line (*arrowheads*) is identified within the anterior tibia with surrounding high signal intensity bone marrow edema (*arrows*).

as focal areas of increased signal intensity on MRI that extend to an articular surface (Fig. 19.25B) (41–43). Similar areas of increased signal intensity that do not communicate with an articular margin do not represent macroscopically evident tears and explain the negative arthroscopic

findings that may be encountered in patients with abnormal MR meniscal signal (44). Histologically, intrameniscal signal is associated with myxoid change. Coronal and sagittal scans allow identification of the exact morphology of meniscal tears (Fig. 19.25C).

Plain radiographs remain the preferred study for the evaluation of those osseous lesions that are associated with acute ligamentous injuries; however, MRI allows detection of bone abnormalities prior to, or in the absence of, their appearance on conventional radiographs (Fig. 19.26) (45). These "occult" osseous findings presumably represent a form of subchondral or epiphyseal fracture, and may explain the patient's symptoms in the absence of ligamentous injury.

POSTOPERATIVE KNEE

MRI of patients with ACL reconstruction is recommended for evaluation of complications following ACL reconstruction or other causes of joint pain. Routine radiographs are useful in the assessment of hardware failure and postoperative degenerative joint changes. However, MRI has the advantage of allowing direct visualization of the ACL graft (Figs. 19.27A, B) as well as direct visualization of the menisci, as discussed previously.

An intact ACL graft should be of low signal intensity on all pulse sequences and should not contact the intercondylar roof (4). Although controversy exits regarding the role of MR imaging is the evaluation of graft impingement, the alignment of both the femoral and tibial tunnels can be

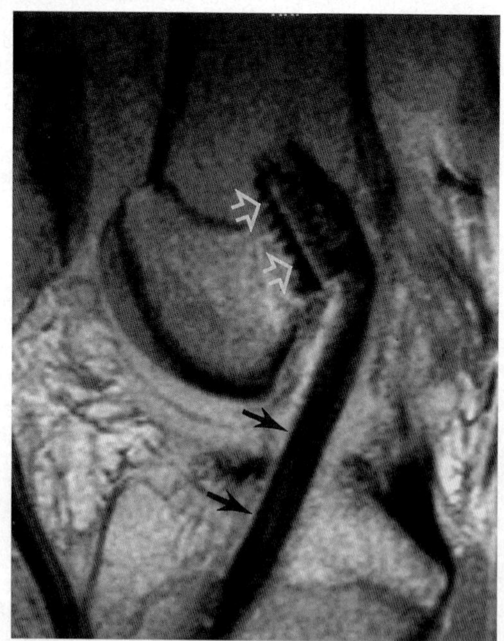

A

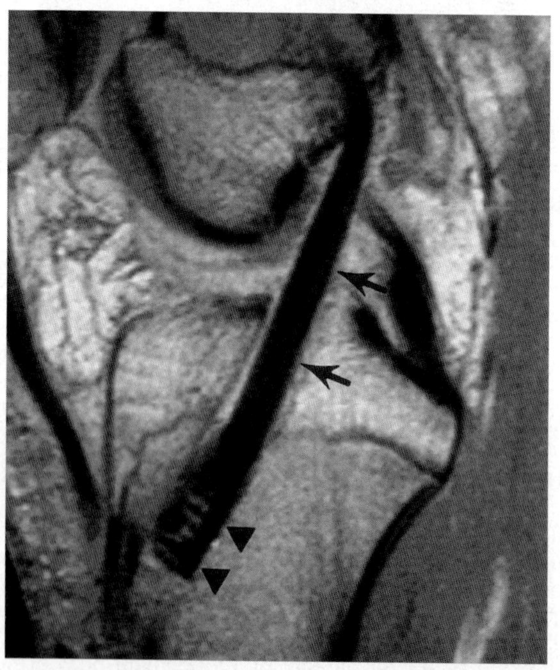

B

FIGURE 19.27. A: Intact anterior cruciate ligament (ACL) graft. Sagittal intermediate-weighted magnetic resonance image (MRI) demonstrates the femoral interference screw (*open arrows*) and the normal low-signal intensity ACL graft (*arrows*). **B:** Intact ACL graft. Adjacent sagittal intermediate-weighted MRI demonstrates the ACL graft coursing into the tibial tunnel (*arrows*). Note the tibial interference screw (*arrowheads*) securing the ACL graft.

(Continued on next page)

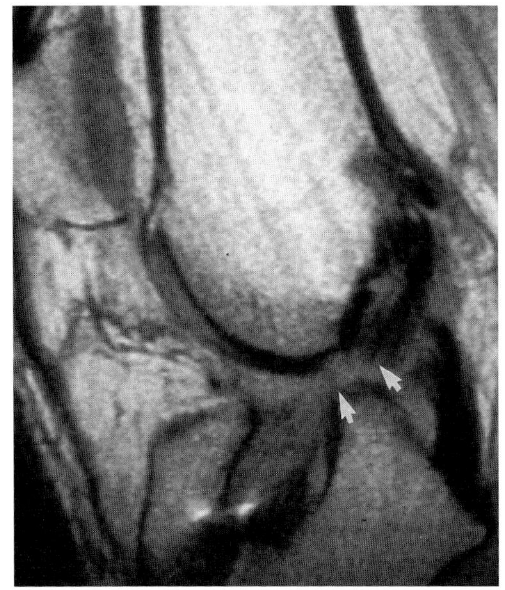
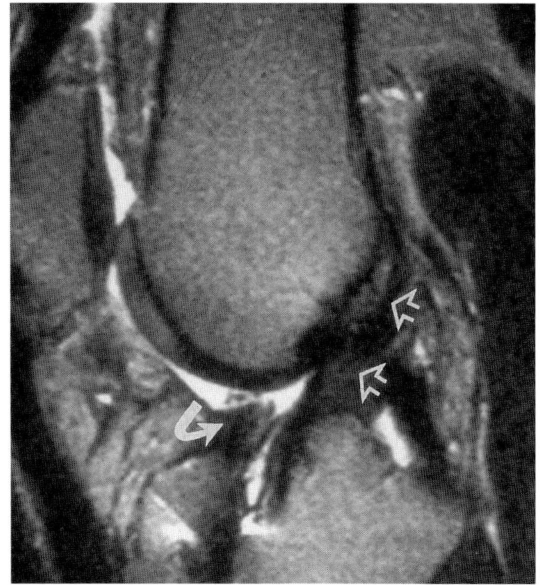

C

D

FIGURE 19.27. *Continued.* **C:** ACL graft impingement. Sagittal intermediate-weighted MRI demonstrates increased signal intensity within the midportion of the ACL graft in a clinically stable knee (*arrows*). The tibial tunnel is positioned anterior to the slope of the intercondylar roof. The patient experienced pain and decreased extension clinically. **D:** Cyclops lesion: Sagittal T2-weighted MRI demonstrates localized low-signal intensity fibrous tissue (*curved arrow*) anterior to the ACL graft (*open arrows*). Clinically the patient experienced decreased mobility and decreased knee extension.

assessed with MRI. On a sagittal image, the tibial tunnel should be parallel to the slope of the intercondylar roof in full knee extension and should be posterior to the intercondylar roof to allow graft isometry (46). In cases of graft impingement, the tibial tunnel frequently is anterior to the intercondylar roof and there is increased signal intensity or disruption of the graft fibers (Fig. 19.27C). Graft impingement may progress to graft failure.

Localized or diffuse arthrofibrosis can also cause morbidity in patients with ACL reconstruction, and may present as decreased range of motion, typically decreased knee extension (47). Localized anterior arthrofibrosis, or cyclops lesion, can be heterogeneous in signal intensity, although generally of low signal on both T1- and T2-weighted images. The cyclops lesion can be demonstrated within the intercondylar notch, anterior the ACL graft on sagittal images (Fig. 19.27D).

The postoperative appearance of a surgically resected or repaired meniscus on MR often has areas of increased signal intensity (48). As a result, routine MR is not reliable for the detection of recurrent meniscal tears. Improved detection of recurrent meniscal tears can be achieved with the use of MR imaging with intraarticular contrast material (MR arthrography).

REFERENCES

1. Cockshott WP, Racoveanu NT, Burrows DA, et al. Use of radiographic projections of the knee. *Skeletal Radiol* 1985;13:131–133.
2. Resnick D, Goergen TG, Niwayama G. Physical injury. In: Resnick D, Niwayama G, eds. *Diagnosis of bone and joint disorders*, 2nd ed. Philadelphia: WB Saunders, 1988:2756–3008.
3. Warren RF. Acute ligament injuries. In: Insall JN, Ed. *Surgery of the knee*. New York: Churchhill Livingstone, 1984:261–294.
4. Irizarry JM, Recht MP. MR imaging of the knee ligaments and the postoperative knee. *Radiol Clin North Am* 1997;35:45–76.
5. Back BR, Warren RF. Radiographic indicators of the anterior cruciate ligament injury. In: Feagin JA Jr, ed. *The crucial ligaments*. New York: Churchill Livingstone, 1988:317–327.
6. Reicher MA, Rauschning W, Gold RH, et al. High resolution magnetic imaging of the knee: normal anatomy. *AJR* 1985;145:895–902.
7. Turner DA, Prodromas CC, Petasnick JP, et al. Acute injury of the knee: magnetic resonance evaluation. *Radiology* 1985;154:711–722.
8. Mink JH. The cruciate and collateral ligaments. In: Mink JH, Reicher MA, Crues JV, eds. *Magnetic resonance imaging of the knee*. New York: Raven Press, 1993.
9. Arnoczky SP, Warren RF. Anatomy of the cruciate ligaments. In: Feagin JA, ed. *The crucial ligaments: diagnosis and treatment of ligamentous injuries about the knee*, second ed. New York: Churchill Livingstone, 1994:269.
10. Resnick D, Heung SK. Knee. In: Resnick D, Heung SK. *Internal derangements of joints: emphasis on MR imaging*. Philadelphia: WB Saunders, 1997:555–785.
11. Pavlov H. The radiographic diagnosis of the anterior cruciate ligament deficient knee. *Clin Orthop* 1983;172:57–63.
12. Segond P. Recherches cliniques et expérimentales sur les épanchements sanguins du genou par entorse: *Progres Med (Paris)* 1879;7:379–381.
13. Dietz GW, Wilcox DM, Montgomery JB. Segond tibial condyle fracture: lateral capsular ligament avulsion: *Radiology* 1986;159:467–469.
14. Woods GW, Stanley RF, Tullos HS. Lateral capsular sign: X-ray clue of a significant knee instability. *Am J Sports Med* 1979;7:27–33.
15. Barry KP, Mesagarzadeh M, Moyer R, et al. Patterns and accuracy of diagnosis of anterior cruciate ligament tears with MR imaging. *Radiology* 1991;181:303.
16. Lee JK, Yao L, Phelps CT, et al. Anterior cruciate ligament tears: MR imaging compared with arthroscopy and clinical tests. *Radiology* 1988;166:861.
17. Mink JH, Levy BA, Crues JV. Tears of the anterior cruciate ligament and menisci of the knee: MR imaging evaluation. *Radiology* 1988;167:769.
18. Vahey TN, Broome DR, Kayes KJ, et al. Acute and chronic tears of the anterior cruciate ligament: Differential features at MR imaging. *Radiology* 1991;181:251
19. Vahey TN, Hunt JE, Shelbourne KD. Anterior translocation of the tibia

at MR imaging: a secondary sign of anterior cruciate ligament tear. *Radiology* 1993;187:817.

20. Vahey TN, Hunt JE, Shelbourne KD, et al. MR imaging of anterior cruciate ligament injuries. *Magn Res Imaging Clin North Am* 1994;2:365.

21. DeSmet AA, Graf BK. Meniscal tears missed on MR imaging. Relationship to meniscal tear patterns and cruciate ligament tears. *AJR* 1994;162:905.

22. Zobel MS, Borrello JA, Siegel MJ, et al. Pediatric knee MR imaging: patterns of injuries in the immature skeleton. *Radiology* 1994;190:397.

23. Feagin JF Jr, Cabaud HE, Curl WW. The anterior cruciate ligament: radiographic and clinical signs of successful and unsuccessful repairs. *Clin Orthop* 1982;164:54–58.

24. Lynch MA, Henning CE, Glick KG. Knee joint surface changes. Long-term follow-up meniscal tear treatment in stable anterior cruciate ligament reconstruction. *Clin Orthop* 1983;172:148–153.

25. McDaniel WJ Jr, Dameron TB Jr. The untreated anterior cruciate ligament rupture. *Clin Orthop* 1983;172:158–163.

26. Segal P, Lallement JJ, Raguet M, et al. Les lésions ostéo-cartilagineuses de la laxité antéro-interne du genou. *Rev Chir Orthop* 1980;66:357–365.

27. Sherman MF, Warren RF, Marshall JL, et al. A clinical and radiographic analysis of 127 cruciate insufficient knees. *Clin Orthop* 1986;227:229–237.

28. Dejour H, Walch G, Deschamps G, et al. Arthrose du genou sur laxité chronique antérieuure. *Rev Chir Orthop* 1987;73:157–170.

29. Cockshott WP, Racoveanu NT, Burrows DA, et al. Use of radiographic projections of the knee. *Skeletal Radiol* 1985;13:131–133.

30. Malghem J, Maldague B. Le profil du genou. Anatomie radiologique différentielle des surfaces articulaires. *J Radiol* 1986;67:725–735.

31. Ahlback S. Osteoarthritis of the knee. *Acta Radio (Stockh)* 1968;277:1–72.

32. Marklund T, Myrnerts R. Radiographic determinations of cartilage height in the knee joint. *Acta Orthop Scand* 1974;45:752–755.

33. Lemaire M. Les instabilités chroniques antérieures et internes du genou. Etude théorique. Diagnostic clinique et radiologique. *Rev Chir Orthop* 1983;69:3–16.

34. Danzig LA, Newell JD, Guerra J, et al. Osseous landmarks of the normal knee. *Clin Orthop* 1981;156:201–206.

35. Harison RB, Wood MB, Keats TE. The grooves of the distal articular surface of the femur. A normal variant. *AJR* 1976;126:751–754.

36. Sonin AH, Fitzgerald SW, Friedman H, et al. Posterior cruciate ligament injury: MR imaging diagnosis and patterns of injury. *Radiology* 1994;190:455.

37. Garvin Gj, Munk PL, Vellet AD. Tears of the medial collateral ligament: magnetic resonance imaging findings and associated injuries. *J Can Assoc Radiol* 1993;44:199.

38. Schweitzer ME, Tran D, Deely DM, et al. Medial collateral ligaments injuries: evaluation of multiple signs, prevalence and location of associated bone bruises, and assessment with MR imaging. *Radiology* 1995;194:825.

39. Yu JS, Salonen DC, Hodler J, et al. Posterolateral aspect of the knee: improved MR imaging with a coronal oblique technique. *Radiology* 1996;198:199–204.

40. Murphy BJ, Hechtman KS, Uribe JW, et al. Iliotibial band friction syndrome: MR imaging findings. *Radiology* 1992;185:569.

41. Mandelbaum BR, Finerman GA, Reicher MA, et al. Magnetic resonance imaging as a tool for evaluation of traumatic knee injuries. *Am J Sports Med* 1986;14:361–370.

42. Reicher MA, Hartzman S, Bassett LW, et al. MR imaging of the knee: Part I, traumatic disorders. *Radiology* 1987;162:547–551.

43. Reicher MA, Hartzman S, Duckwiler G, et al. Meniscal injuries: detection using MR imaging. *Radiology* 1986;159:547–551.

44. Stoller DW, Martin C, Crues JV, et al. Meniscal tears: pathologic correlation with MR imaging. *Radiology* 1987;163:731–735.

45. Mink JH. Pitfalls in interpretation. In: Mink JH, ed. *Magnetic resonance imaging of the knee.* New York: Raven Press, 1987:141–155.

46. Howell SM, Clark JA. Tibial tunnel placement in anterior cruciate ligament reconstruction and graft impingement. *Clin Orthop* 1992;283:187.

47. Recht MP, Piraino DW, Cohen MAH, et al. Localized anterior arthrofibrosis (cyclops lesion) after reconstruction of the anterior cruciate ligament: MR imaging. *AJR* 1995;165:383–385.

48. Applegate GR, Flannigan BD, Tolin BS. MR diagnosis of recurrent tears in the knee: value of intraarticular contrast material. *AJR* 1993;161:821–825.

Part C: Instrumented Laxity Studies

Donald C. Fithian, Mary Lou Stone, and Mark D. Shaieb

Ligaments limit joint motion. *In vitro* ligament sectioning studies have documented that disruption of a specific ligament results in a characteristic change in motion. ACL disruption results in an increase in anterior displacement of the tibia with respect to the femur in response to an anteriorly directed force (Fig. 19.28) (1–4). Traditionally, ACL instability was evaluated clinically using the anterior drawer test (5) and the Lachman test (6). Although the anterior drawer sign has become less common due to concerns about both its sensitivity and specificity (5,7–11), the Lachman test appears quite sensitive and specific for ACL deficiency in most studies (7,9–13). In assessing the integrity of the ACL by the Lachman test, examiners appear to be better able to detect end-point differences than displacement differences (12). An experienced examiner usually can correctly diagnose an ACL disruption even when there is only a small right-left displacement difference, because of the alteration in end-point stiffness. However, the accuracy of the clinical examination has been shown to be dependent upon examiner experience (14,15). The Lachman test has only moderate reproducibility, even among the most experienced examiners (2,12–14).

An isolated ACL injury can produce a range of anterior laxity (7,13,16,17). *In vitro* studies have confirmed that isolated ACL sectioning does not result in a specific amount of increased laxity, but produces a fairly wide distribution of changes (Fig. 19.28) (2,4,18–20). It has been suggested that variations of individual anatomy may make some knees more dependent upon the ACL for controlling anterior displacement. It certainly is clear that some patients are disabled after isolated ACL injury, while others are relatively unaffected (21–25). Daniel (23,24) and others (26,27) have shown a link between measured laxity and outcomes following ACL injury. Outcomes of "partial ACL tears" discov-

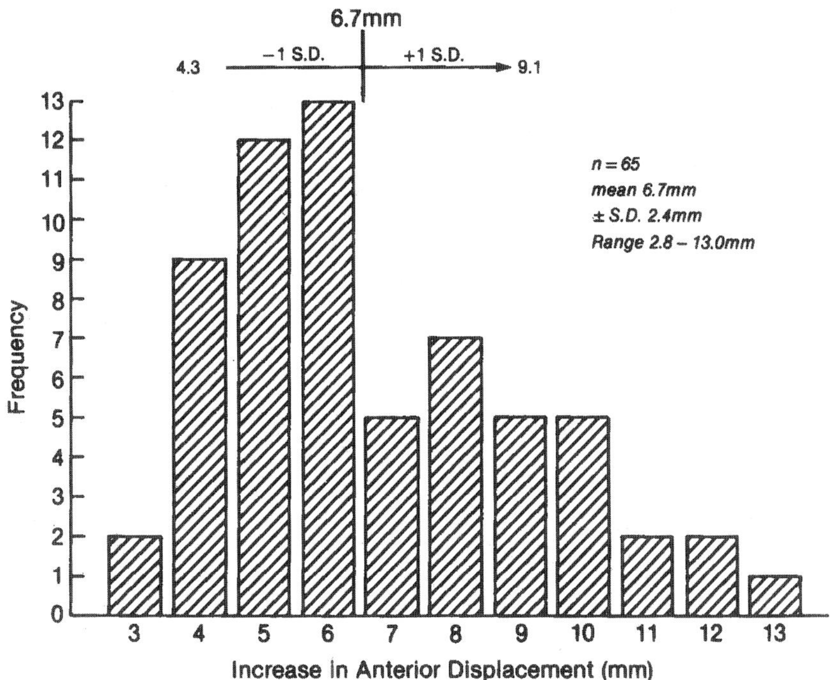

FIGURE 19.28. Effect of anterior cruciate ligament (ACL) sectioning on anterior displacement. Anterior displacement measurements with the MEDmetric KT-2000 were performed on 65 fresh cadaveric specimens with the ligaments intact and after sectioning the ACL. The difference between the ligament intact state and ACL-sectioned state for each specimen is presented.

ered on arthroscopy or with MRI also have been linked to the amount of laxity resulting from the initial injury (22,24). Furthermore, following ACL surgery, clinicians frequently state that a knee has a negative Lachman test when a normal end-point and a 4-mm right-to-left displacement difference is documented by instrumented measurement (28). It is desirable therefore to use objective means of quantifying anterior knee stability, both to assess the amount of anterior laxity in the ACL-deficient knee and to evaluate the effects of surgical reconstruction.

Instrumented measurement of joint motion can be used to assist the clinician in diagnosing ligament disruptions by detecting pathologic motion, to document the amount of pathologic motion and to measure the success of ligament surgery in re-establishing the normal motion limits. Instrumented joint motion measurement consists of 1) positioning the limb in a specified manner, 2) applying a displacing force, and 3) measuring the resultant joint motion. Early reports of instrumented testing consisted of positioning the limb, applying a standard displacement force, and documenting any change in joint position by comparing photographs (29) or radiographs (30–33) taken of the knee before and during the application of stress. Indeed, stress radiography is simply a specific technique of instrumented measurement. Although stress radiography techniques are widely known to clinicians, they have not been widely used for the diagnosis of knee

injuries. This may be due to concerns about radiation exposure, the expense of multiple radiographs, or the need for careful patient positioning and measurement.

Instrumented measurement systems that document anterior-posterior tibial displacement by tracking the tibial tubercle in relation to the patella or femur have become popular in the orthopedic community over the past twenty years. Markolf (34), Shino (35), Edixhoven (36), and Johnson (37) developed stationary testing systems. Portable testing systems that are commercially available have been developed by Cannon and Lamoreux (Knee Laxity Tester, Stryker Ligament Tester), Malcolm and Daniel (KT-1000, MEDmetric, San Diego, California) (1,17,38) and Jakob (Rolimeter, Aircast, Summit, New Jersey) (39). The Dyonics dynamic cruciate tester (DCT, Dyonics, Andover, Massachusetts) is a portable computerized device that, like the KT-1000 and Stryker, measures only A/P motion (40,41). Commercial devices have also been introduced that simultaneously measure motion in several directions (Genucom, Faro Medical Technologies, Champlain, New York; and KSS, Acufex, Norwood, Massachusetts; or CA-4000, OSI, Hayward, California) (42).

Many investigators have reported instrumented testing to be a useful clinical tool (1,7,17,39,43,44). As a result, instrumented testing has become a standard requirement for published outcome studies of knee ligament injury. But in studies comparing the accuracy and reliability of individual test instruments and diagnostic criteria, results are not uniformly good. Fleming nicely summarized the variability of results among published studies of instrumented knee laxity testing (45). A careful review of the available evidence clearly shows that designs and recommended techniques do not produce equivalent results for the different devices that are available (Table 19.1). Reliability of instrumented testing in normal and ACL-injured knees is dependent upon both examiner experience (46–48) and the device used (2,7,12,13,49).

While it obviously is important to use tools properly, if a clinical test or device is only effective in the hands of the most experienced examiners or most gifted technicians, then it is of little general use. Simplicity and ease of use, reliable measurements and a quick learning curve are important characteristics of any clinical tool. Even among devices that have these characteristics, examiner training and experience with the device have been shown to affect the reliability of knee ligament testing (46–48). A clinician that does not use a device regularly, or who has not devoted sufficient time and attention to attaining proficiency, should not expect reliable measurements with it. We have found that the development of proficient "testers" depends on proper instruction and practice. Several weeks of concentrated, supervised practice in the knee clinic is usually required for residents and fellows to produce reliable measurements of anterior instability. Two to 3 months of practice are needed to develop proficiency in the evaluation of posterior instability, largely due to the fact that PCL injury is less common.

In this chapter, we discuss the principles of instrumented measurement, noting important technical aspects and assumptions of testing, as well as common pitfalls. We include suggestions on how to get examiners "up to speed" and how to test the quality (i.e., reliability) of their measurements. We summarize the design as well as the testing protocol recommended for the KT-1000, the most commonly used and thoroughly tested instrument for measuring anteroposterior laxity in the knee. Other devices that are commercially available are discussed, along with the results of reliability and comparison tests, and considerations of design variation.

PRINCIPLES OF INSTRUMENTED TESTING

Accurate motion measurements depend on:

1. Joint position at the initiation of the test.
2. Motion constraints imposed by the testing system.
3. Displacing force.
4. Measurement system.
5. Muscle activity.
6. The passive motion constraints.

The role of the testing device is to minimize the variability between factors 1 through 5 so that the difference in measurements between two knees or one knee tested at intervals indicates a true change in the passive motion constraints. Examples of how variables 1 through 5 may affect the displacement measurements are presented below.

JOINT STARTING POSITION

Flexion

The joint flexion angle affects the orientation of the ligament with respect to the applied force and may affect the distance between the ligaments attachment sites. The changing orientation of the cruciate ligaments with joint flexion is illustrated in Figure 19.29. From a review of these figures, the ACL is better oriented to resist an anterior displacement force when the knee is flexed to 90° than when the knee is extended. The PCL is better oriented to resist a posterior displacement force with the knee in full extension than it is in 90° of flexion. This observation is consistent with the clinical experience that anterior tibial displacement in the uninjured knee is less at 90° of flexion than at 30° (34,50,51). However, when the ACL is disrupted, there is a greater increase in anterior displacement with the knee in 30° of flexion than in 90° of flexion (50–52). When the PCL is disrupted, there is a greater increase in displacement at 90° of flexion than at 30° of flexion (53). With the cruciate ligaments sectioned, other structures become the primary anterior-posterior displacement constraints. The effects of joint position on these structures vary. For example, the anterior

TABLE 19.1. *Comparison of anterior/posterior instrumented testing device in normal and ACL-injured knees*

Device	Flexion	Force	Anterior displacement	Total A/P displacement	Authors
Genucom	20	89–93	1.6–7.8	5.5–9.0	Highgenboten, McQuade, Steiner
	30	90–93	4.3–5.5	7.6–12.2	Emery, Fleming, McQuade, Torzelli, Wroble
KSS	20–30	89	4.7–5.2	7.5–7.9	Fleming, Riederman, Steiner
	20–30	178	7.5	10.7	Riederman
KT-1000	20–30	89	3.9–7.0	6.6–7.1	Anderson, Daniel, Feibert, Forster, Highgenboten, McLaughlin, McQuade, Myer, Sherman, Steiner, Torzelli, Wroble
	20–30	134	6.1–8.6		Highgenboten, McQuade, Wroble
Stryker	20	89	2.4–3.0	5.6–7.0	Anderson, Boniface, Emery, Highgenboten
	20	190	5.0	10.0	Anderson

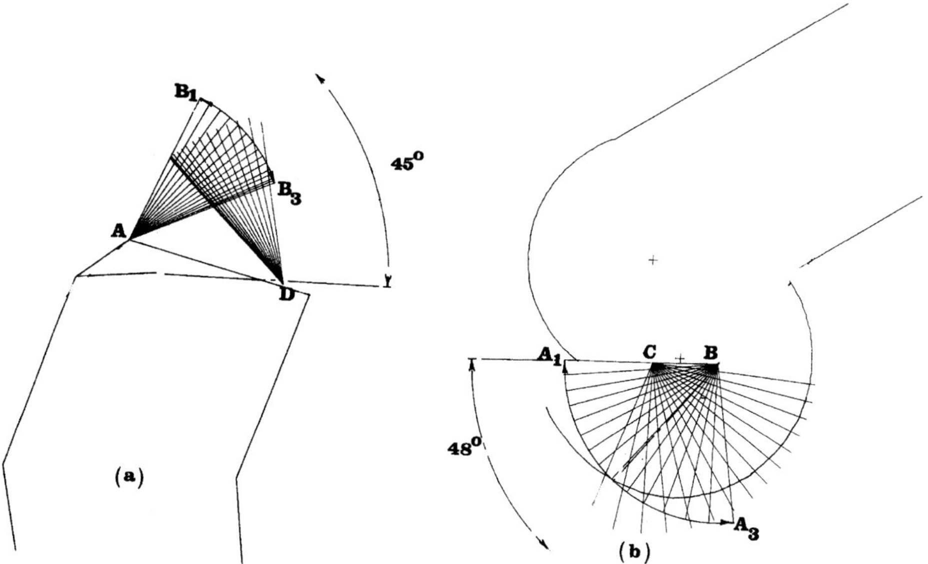

FIGURE 19.29. Diagrams of the tibia *(a)* and the femur *(b)* with the range of positions occupied by the anterior cruciate ligament from full extension to 140° of flexion when the ligament moves *(a)* from AB_1 to AB_3 relative to the tibia and *(b)* from A_1B to A_3B relative to the femur.

fibers of the MCL tighten with knee flexion. If the menisci are intact, and the tibia is displaced anteriorly, the femoral condyles ride up on the wedge-shaped meniscus and tension the capsule and collateral ligaments (52), thereby constraining anterior tibial displacement.

Joint flexion also affects the practical measurement of tibiofemoral motion. For devices that measure displacement of the tibia relative to the patella, such as the KT-1000, Stryker, DCT and Rolimeter, the patella must remain in secure contact with the femur. This requires a minimum flexion angle of 25° to 30° during testing. More flexion may be required in patients with severe patella alta or patellar instability (54). Other factors that affect patellofemoral contact, such as knee effusion (20) and variations in patellar pressure during measurement (54,55), must also be addressed. McQuade (56) reported that the Genucom system was highly sensitive to flexion changes of as little as 10°. Similarly, Andersson (57) found raw measurements obtained with the Stryker laxity tester were sensitive to knee flexion changes of 10° (15° vs. 25° flexion). Andersson did not state whether flexion affected side-to-side comparisons, however. It is clear that for best results when comparing side-to-side differences, both knees should be positioned in the same amount of flexion.

Resting Position of the Knee

The resting position refers to the relative position of the tibia with respect to the femur before any load is applied. Markolf (34,52) and others (2,57) have reported sagittal plane translation as total anterior-posterior translation. Others have divided the motion into anterior and posterior excursions. Shino (35) reported anterior translation as anterior motion from the knee resting position. Daniel (1,17,44) and Edixhoven (36) have referenced measurements to the position of the limb after a posterior displacing force is applied and then released.

If the PCL is intact, the resting position is determined by the weight of the leg resting against tension in the PCL. In that case, it may be assumed that any significant increase in anterior displacement will be due to ACL deficiency. If the PCL is not intact, Daniel recommended using the quadriceps active test to determine a reference point from which corrected anterior and posterior displacements could be calculated (58). Whether or not the PCL is intact, we have found that checking the KT-1000 dial at the resting position after each cycle of loading allows us to confirm that the knee is actually returning to a consistent position, and that the patient remains relaxed.

We define the "zero position" as the resting position of the leg after application of several gentle 20lb posteriorly directed loads. The loads are repeated until the tibia consistently returns to the same position. The dial is then set to zero at that position. Each subsequent loading cycle is completed with a 20-lb posterior force. If a patient is not relaxed or if the orientation of the arthrometer on the limb is changing (most commonly because of rotation), the dial will not return to zero. This provides feedback on the consistency of measurements.

Rotation

Rotation of the tibia affects the distance between the ligaments' attachment sites and anterior displacement measurements (52,59,60). Markolf (34,52) reported that 15° of

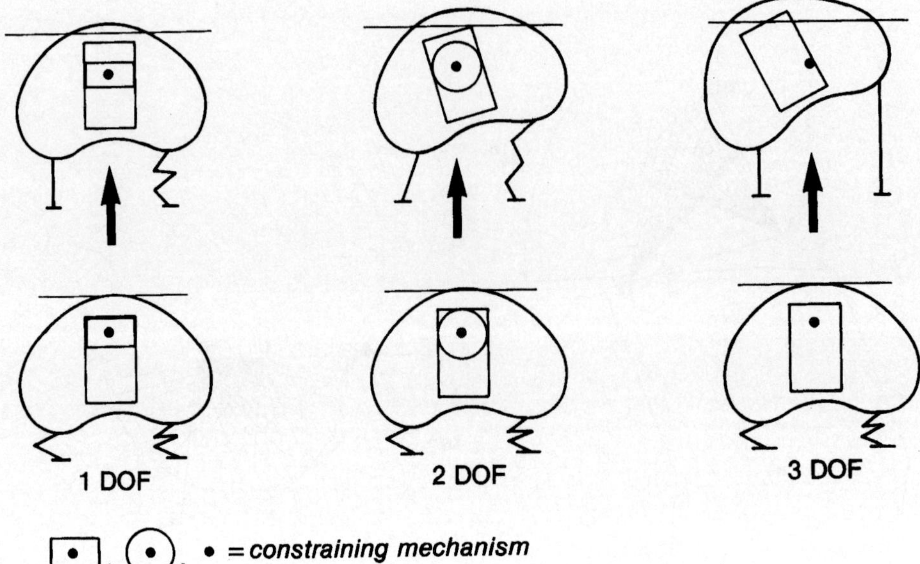

FIGURE 19.30. Influence of motion constrains on anterior translation in structures with two restraining tethers of different lengths. A structure shaped like the surface of the tibia is drawn with a central rectangular window. When the structure is placed over a rectangular peg the same width of the window, the structure can only translate anteriorly and posteriorly, there is 1 degree of freedom (DOF). When the structure is placed over a large circular peg, it has 2 DOF, anterior–posterior translation, and rotation about the peg. When the structure is placed over a small peg, there is anterior–posterior translation, medial–lateral translation, and rotation around the peg (3 DOF). The anterior translation of the structure is restrained by two tethers of different lengths. When there is only 1 DOF the structure can move only as far as the shorter tether will allow; when the structure has 2 DOF, the anterior translation increases; and when there is 3 DOF the structure can move forward until the two tethers are taut.

external rotation results in the greatest anterior knee laxity *in vivo*. However, as is discussed below, constraint of the tibia in 15° external rotation throughout the test will actually reduce overall motion because of the effects of coupled motion in the unconstrained knee (61) (Fig. 19.30).

Limb rotation also affects the orientation of the laxity tester as it is mounted on the leg, the effects of gravity, and numerous other variables. When testing anterior knee laxity, the patellae of both knees should be facing forward and the feet should be slightly externally rotated in a relaxed position. For the most reliable results of laxity measurement, care should be taken to position the both limbs as consistently as possible.

Sagittal Plane Translation

Flexion of the knee relaxes the posterior capsule. In a supine patient the posterior cruciate then supports the weight of the leg. If the PCL is disrupted, the tibia will sag posteriorly (Fig. 19.31). When the patient is prone, the tibia translates anteriorly and the anterior cruciate ligament supports the leg. The joint resting position depends on patient position and intact structures.

Markolf (34,52), Wroble (62-64) and Andersson (57) reported sagittal plane translation as total anterior-posterior translation. Others have divided the motion into anterior and posterior excursions. Shino (35) reported ante-

rior translation as anterior motion from the knee resting position. Daniel (1,17) and Edixhoven (36) have referenced measurements to the position of the limb after a posterior displacing force is applied and then released. Before assuming that the joint resting position in a supine patient is a physiologic position, the posterior cruciate screen (Fig. 19.32) should be used to confirm that the PCL is intact (58).

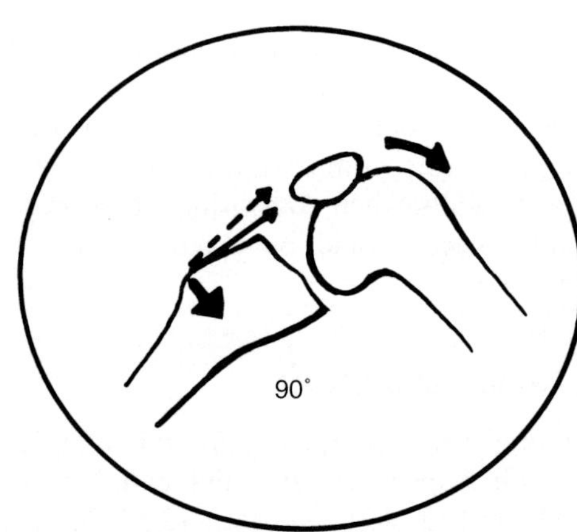

FIGURE 19.31. At the quadriceps neutral angle the quadriceps active position (tibial femoral position when the quadriceps is contracted) is independent of the cruciate ligaments.

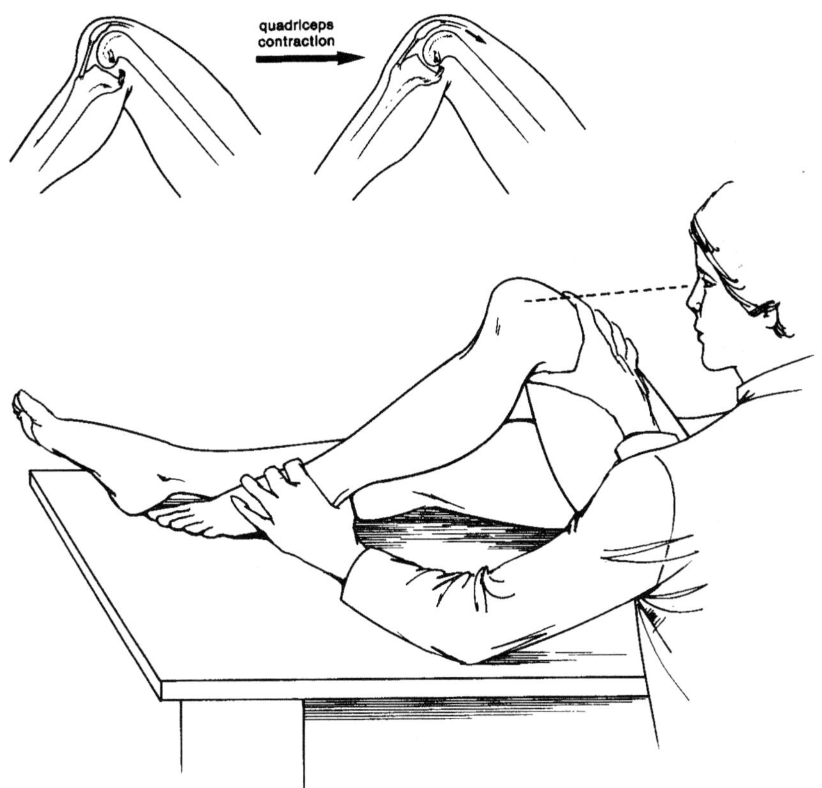

FIGURE 19.32. The 90° quadriceps active test keeping the eyes at the level of the patient's flexed knee, the examiner rests the elbow on the table and uses the ipsilateral hand to support the patient's thigh and to confirm that the thigh muscles are relaxed. The foot is stabilized by the examiner's other hand, and the subject is asked to slide the foot gently down the table. Tibial displacement resulting from the quadriceps contraction is noted.

MOTION CONSTRAINTS IMPOSED BY THE TESTER OR THE TESTING SYSTEM

An unconstrained testing system allows 6 degrees of freedom (*df*); that is, rotation around and translation along each of the three axes (Fig. 19.33). Many motions are linked or coupled to one another. For example, anterior translation and internal rotation are normally paired, as are posterior translation and external rotation (Fig. 19.34). When motions are coupled, constraint of one of the motions will limit the other. This concept is illustrated in Figure 19.30. The comparison of two *in vitro* ACL section-

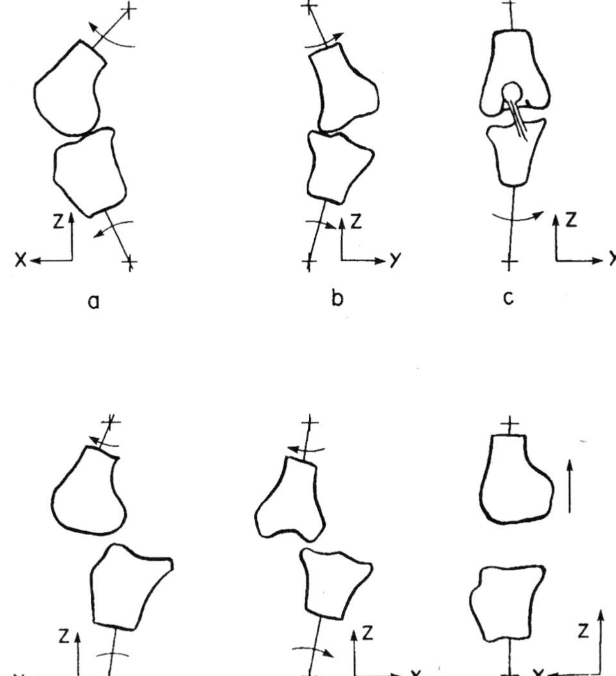

FIGURE 19.33. Motions of the Oxford rig to allow 6 basic degrees of freedom (*df*). The 6 basic *df* are three rotations and three translations. The Oxford rig allows five rotations and one translation, and thus no simple one-to-one correspondence exists. **A:** Rotation about *y* flexion is accomplished by the hip flexion axis rotation and the ankle flexion axis rotation. **B:** Rotation about *x* abduction–adduction causes the hip fore-aft axis to rotate one way while causing the ankle to rotate the other way. **C:** Rotation about *z*-rotation appears as motion of the tibial rotation of the *z* ankle axis. **D:** Translation along *x* occurs when the femur flexes forward and the tibial segment flexes backward, or vice versa. **E:** Translation along *y* mediolateral motion involves rotation above the fore-aft axis or above the hip or ankle. **F:** Translation along *z*-distraction of interpenetration is accomplished by movement of the slider. Knee flexion and tibial rotation can be obtained more or less directly. Other motions in this rig usually require mathematic analysis for interpretation.

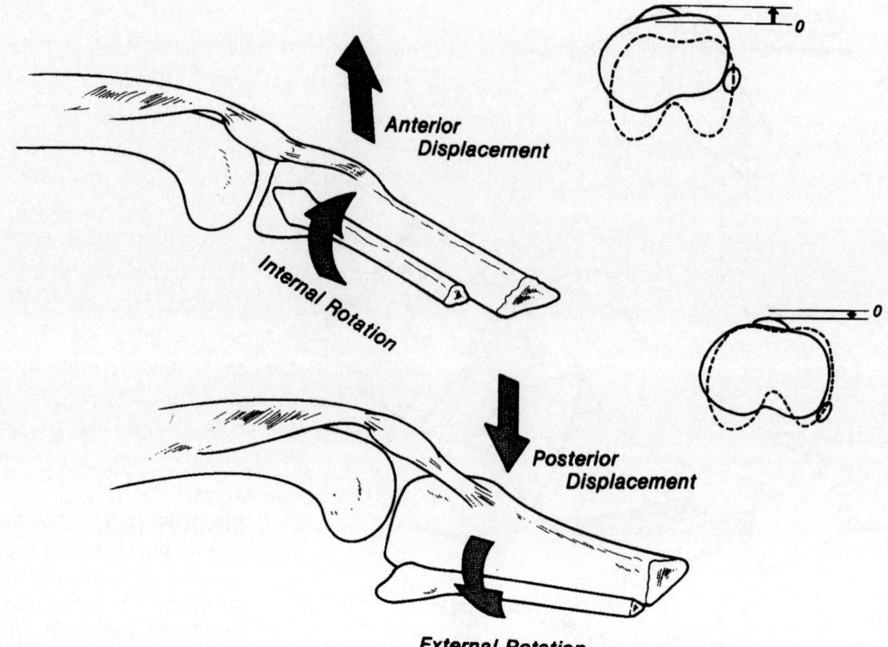

FIGURE 19.34. Coupled motion. Anterior drawer testing shows combined anterior translation and external rotation. Posterior drawer shows combined posterior translation and external rotation.

ing studies demonstrates the effect of the testing apparatus on anterior displacement measurements. In a 1-*df* system, anterior displacement after sectioning the ligament was 5 mm (65) while in a 5-*df* system, the tibial displacement was 15 mm (51). In a cadaver study of nine intact knees, Fukubayashi observed that anterior-posterior displacement increased by 30% when the tibia was allowed to rotate freely about its neutral rotation position (61).

In vivo, a 1-*df* measurement system is probably neither desirable nor attainable. In the modestly constrained anterior-posterior testing system reported by Edixhoven (36,66), pulling the tibia anteriorly resulted in 6° to 11° of knee flexion and 11° to 13° of internal tibia rotation. The KT-1000 testing system was designed to constrain knee motion as little as possible while measuring anterior-posterior translation. Perhaps one of the reasons that Sherman (67) measured greater displacements with the KT-1000 than with the UCLA testing device is because the UCLA device provides greater limb constraint.

DISPLACEMENT FORCE

Magnitude

The soft tissue constraints of the knee lengthen when loaded. In a compliant system such as the knee joint, the greater the displacement force, the greater the displacement (Fig. 19.35) (68). Ligament deficiency creates an

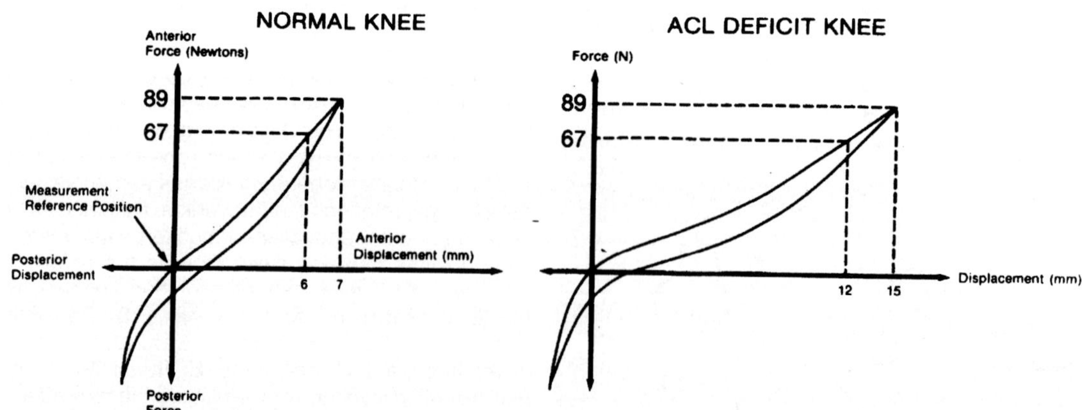

FIGURE 19.35. Force-displacement curves for normal knee (*left*) and for anterior cruciate deficit knees (*right*). The compliance index is the displacement between the 67 and 89 N anterior-force levels. On this curve, the compliance index for the normal knee is 1 mm; it is 3 mm for the knee with an anterior cruciate deficit.

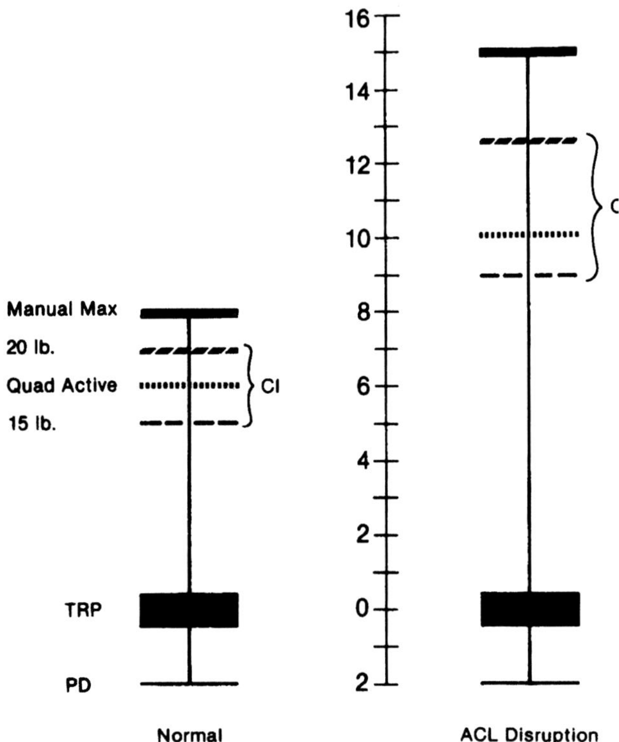

FIGURE 19.36. The relationship between displacement measurements in a typical patient with a unilateral anterior cruciate ligament (ACL) disruption. CI, compliance index: 30° anterior–posterior displacement. PD, posterior displacement; TRP, testing reference position.

even more compliant system, so that the load-response curve is even "flatter" than that in normal knees (Fig. 19.35) (17,52). Accordingly, differences between injured and uninjured knees are greater when compared at higher applied loads (Fig. 19.36). Instrumented systems allow us

to control the force applied in order to standardize displacement measurements. However, because leg size and shape varies among individuals, application of a uniform force does not necessarily produce a uniform net displacing force. Figure 19.37 illustrates factors to consider when calculating the displacing force.

The net load displacing the tibia forward when the patient is supine represents the magnitude of the displacing force minus the mass of the limb (36). When loads are applied to the proximal leg, the limb rotates around the ankle as shown in Figure 19.37. However, all loads applied to the leg produce a moment about the knee as well as a moment about the ankle. If large loads are applied at a distance below the knee joint line, the foot will rise off the examining table, invalidating the displacement measurements. Therefore, in a testing system that does not constrain the leg, there is a maximum force that can be applied to the leg without changing the knee flexion angle. This maximum depends on the mass of the leg and the distance (moment arm) below the knee at which the point is applied. Below this maximum, the magnitude of which varies from knee to knee, a range of forces have been used to standardize measurements as much as possible.

For large limbs, smaller forces in the range of 67 N to 89 N may not generate enough net load to produce abnormally high displacements even if the ACL is torn. The ability to distinguish normal from pathologic motion depends on reducing the overlap between the distributions of measurements obtained in normal and ACL deficient knees (Fig. 19.38). Higher applied forces generate greater displacement, particularly among unstable knees (Fig. 19.36) (17,52,68). Markolf observed greater diagnostic accuracy with a higher applied force when

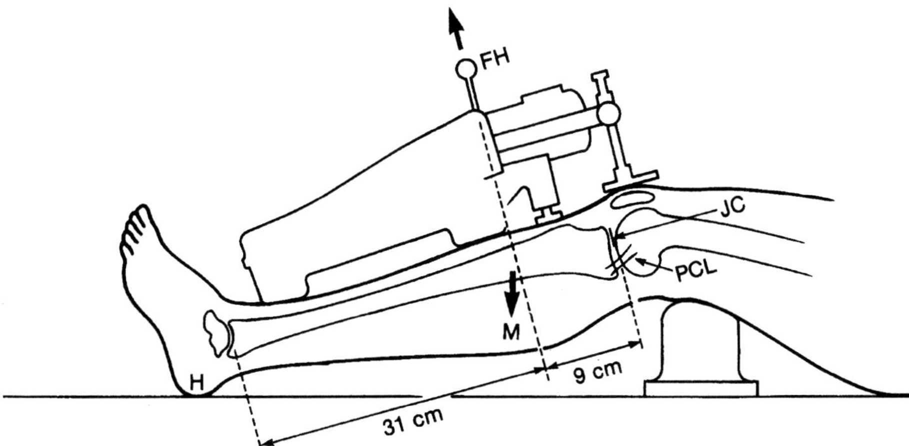

FIGURE 19.37. The patient is supine. The testing instrument is mounted on the front of the leg. The mass of the leg and the testing device *(M)* are supported by tension in the soft tissues, represented by the posterior cruciate ligament *(PCL)*, compression force at the joint surface *(JC)*, and compression at the heel *(H)*. When an anterior force is applied through the force handle *(FH)*, the weight of the leg and testing device are first lifted to unload the joint structures and then as further force is applied the anterior constraining soft tissues are placed under tension.

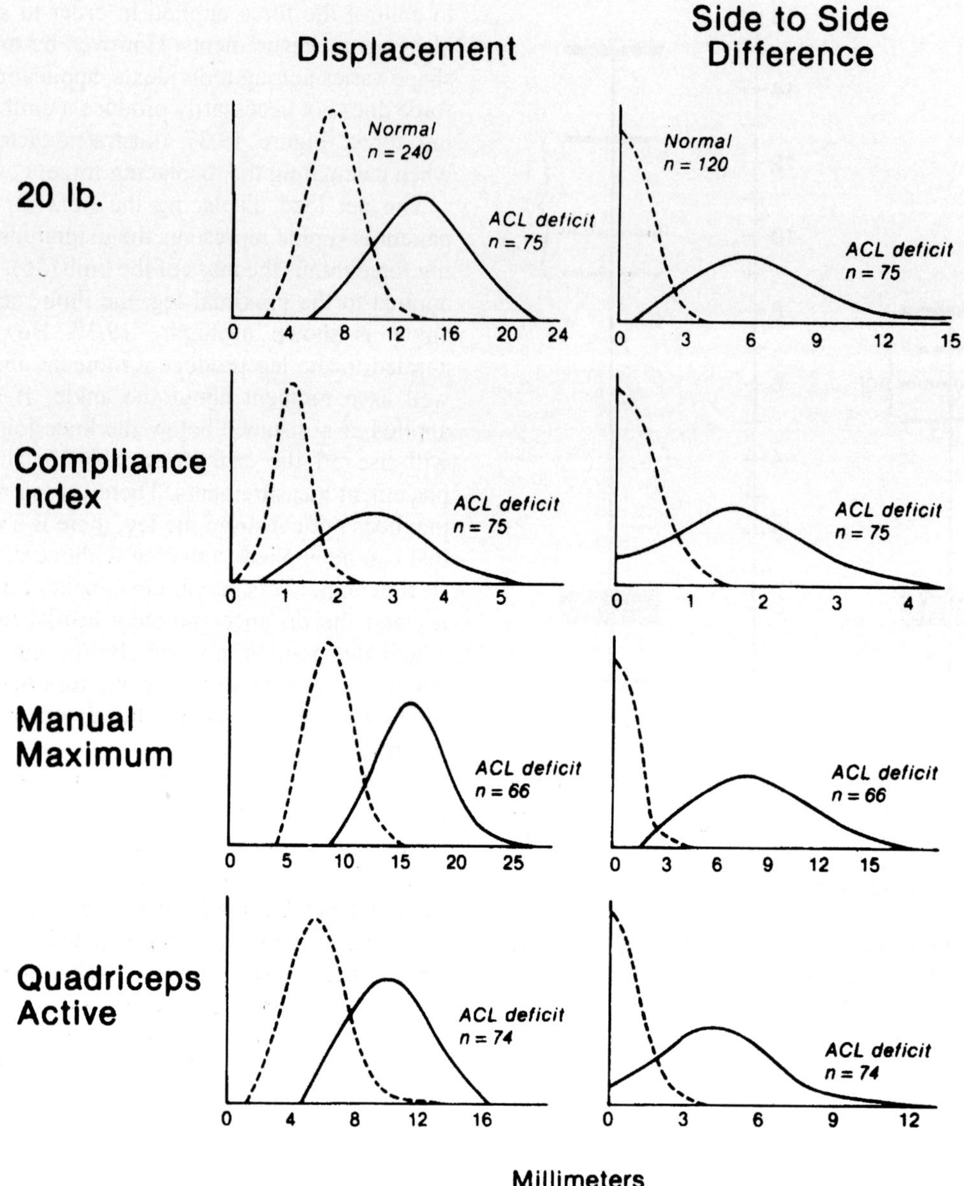

FIGURE 19.38. Anterior displacement measurements of 120 normal subjects (240 knees) and a group of patients with a chronic anterior cruciate ligament (ACL) disruption. Frequency distribution: 30° of knee flexion.

comparing normal to chronically ACL-deficient knees (52).Daniel and co-workers improved their diagnostic accuracy with the KT-1000 from 62% to 92% by increasing the load from 89 N to manual maximum force (17). The Genucom and Stryker systems allow application of 40 lb to the upper leg through the devices. Anderson estimated that the load applied during manual maximum testing with the KT-1000 or KT-2000 is in the range of 30 to 40 lb (40). In pilot testing at our facility using the KT-2000, loads between 30 and 40 lb sometimes caused the foot to lift off the table. Since the late 1980s, all KT-1000 arthrometers have been designed to include a beep at 30 lb (134 N). The straps on the KT-1000 are several

centimeters below the knee flexion crease (Fig. 19.39), making it difficult to apply more than 30 lb through the device handle without lifting the leg unless the leg is fairly massive. Myer et al. (68) were able to apply 40 lb consistently using the KT-2000. They did not comment on the occurrence of knee extension during loading. They did however report greater measurement error at 40 lb than at either 30 lb or manual maximum loads. Interestingly, the mean anterior displacement was slightly greater at 40 lb than at manual maximum load (68), which is consistent with our experience and estimates in the literature that manual maximum loads are between 30 and 40 lbs (7).

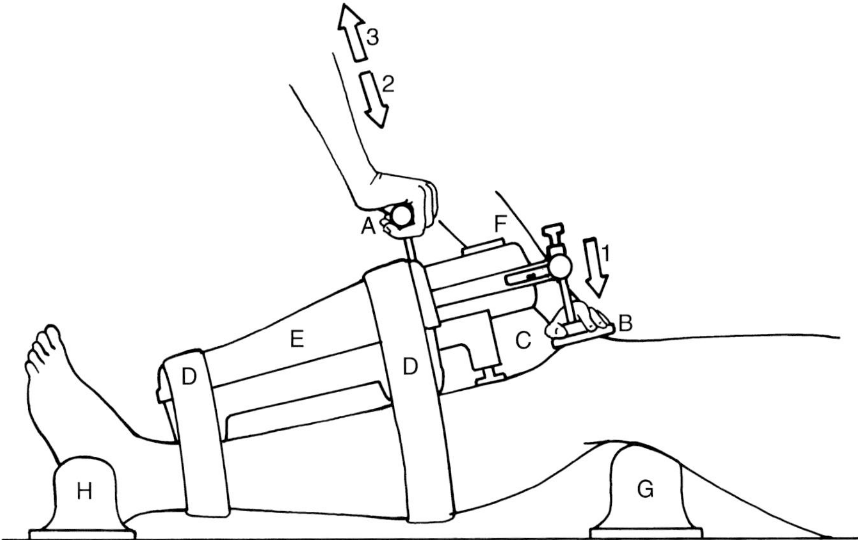

FIGURE 19.39. KT-1000 Arthrometer. **A:** Force handle (posterior force or anterior force is applied). **B:** Patellar sensor pad (a constant force is applied to stabilize the patellar sensor pad). **C:** Tibial sensor pad. **D:** Velcro straps. **E:** Arthrometer body. **F:** Displacement dial. **G:** Thigh support. **H:** Foot support.

The ligaments are viscoelastic tissues, so the rate of load application will affect ligament deformation. However, Markolf (34) and Edixhoven (36,66) have reported that the rate of load application in clinical testing did not affect the force/displacement curve. In practice, one needs to avoid "jerking" the leg or applying loads too quickly, which can cause the patient to become apprehensive and to contract the muscles involuntarily. Smooth, steady force application is the most effective way to test the compliance of the passive knee motion limits. Edixhoven recommends that one testing cycle be performed to condition the joint prior to measuring displacement. In general, it seems to be a good idea to repeat the load application cycle until the displacement is reproduced on several repetitions.

Point of Application

Up to the manual maximum load which, when applied to the proximal leg will raise the foot off the table, an anteriorly directed force applied to the upper leg results in a moment which rotates the leg around the foot and ankle. The rotational moment about the ankle is dependent on the distance of the point of force application from the ankle. Andersson reported that the point of tibial load application affected measurements obtained with the Stryker knee laxity tester. More distal load application produced less displacement at a constant force of 180 N. At 10 cm below the tibial tubercle, anterior translation was reduced 46%. In Figure 19.37, the rotational moment about the ankle is applied through a 31-cm moment arm. Applying the load as close as possible to the knee joint flexion crease maximizes the moment at the ankle *and*

minimizes the moment at the knee, thereby maximizing the anterior displacement at the knee joint.

Direction

If the displacement load is directed so that in addition to imparting an anterior force, a joint distraction or compression force or a rotational movement is applied, the resulting anterior displacement will be affected. An internal rotation moment on the tibia will increase anterior joint displacement and an external rotational moment will increase posterior joint displacement. A joint compression force will increase joint stiffness (67,69–71). The examiner should concentrate on pulling in line with the handle of the KT-1000 (Fig. 19.39).

MEASUREMENT SYSTEM

Measurement Location

The purpose of laxity testing is to evaluate the integrity of the ligaments. By measuring the relative motion between two bony landmarks, we can draw inferences about the condition of the ligaments responsible for constraining that motion. The tibial tubercle and patella are accessible subcutaneous landmarks, but the soft tissue envelope surrounding the femur makes it difficult to stabilize and locate by direct methods. The different laxity systems employ a variety of techniques for controlling and monitoring tibial and femoral motion. Anterior-posterior knee displacement has been evaluated by stabilizing the femur with a clamp and measuring A/P displacement of the tibial tubercle (34,67), measuring the

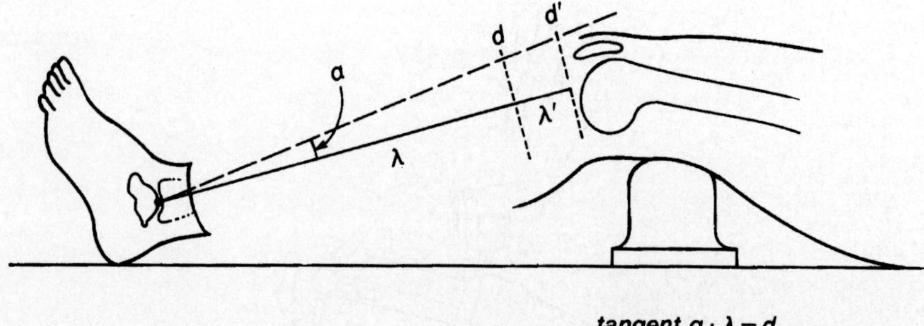

$$tangent\ a \cdot \lambda = d$$
$$tangent\ a\ (\lambda + \lambda') = d'$$

FIGURE 19.40. An anterior force applied to the proximal tibia rotates the tibia around the ankle. The anterior tibial displacement is dependent on the change in flexion angle and the distance from the ankle that the displacement is measured. The greater the distance, the greater the measured displacement.

differential displacement between the patella and the tibial tubercle (1,17,35,36,38,39,66) or by an "instrumented Lachman" using a cable system attached to the thigh and leg (37). During a standard A/P displacement test, the patella and femur are maintained in a constant position and the foot rests on the examining table. When a displacement force is applied to the proximal segment of the leg, the leg rotates around the foot and ankle. Using the KT-1000, the displacement measurement is dependent on the distance at which the measurement is taken with respect to the ankle (Fig. 19.40). Most devices display the displacement at the tibial tubercle (31,34,35,39,66,67). The KT-1000 displays the displacement occurring at the site of the arrow on the device, which should be placed on

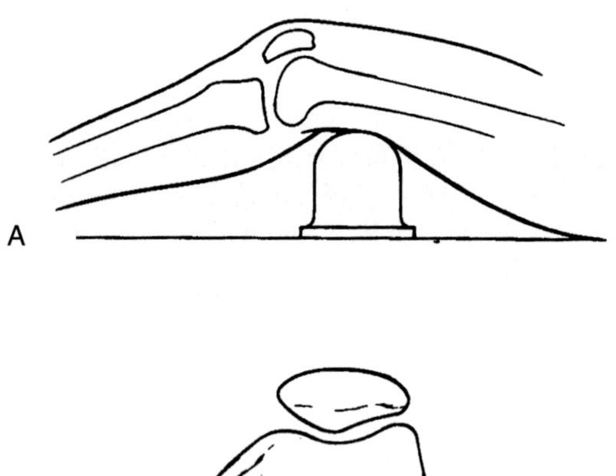

A

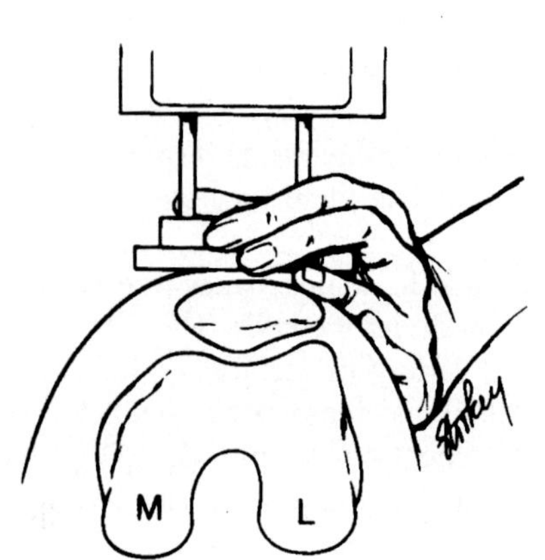

B

C

FIGURE 19.41. The knee is supported in a flexed position to engage the patella in the femoral trochlea. In some patients, the thigh support must be raised an additional 3 to 6 cm to provide sufficient knee flexion to engage the patella in the femoral trochlea. This may be done by placing a board under the thigh support. The thigh should be supported so the patella is facing up. Occasionally a thigh strap is used to accomplish this task (Fig. 19.37). The examiner stabilizes the patellar sensor with manual pressure. The stabilizing hand should rest against the lateral thigh and apply 2 to 5 lb pressure on the patellar sensor pad. The hand position, patellar sensor position, and patellar sensor pressure must remain constant throughout the test. Varying the pressure on the patellar sensor pad and/or rotation of the pad are common causes of measurement error.

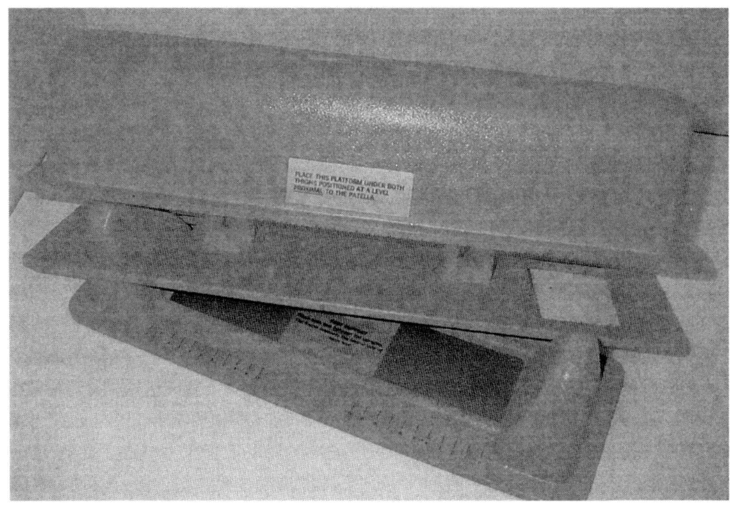

FIGURE 19.42. MEDmetric adjustable thigh support.

the joint line. In a subject with a tibia 40 cm in length, the A/P displacement measured at the tibial tubercle (34-36,66,67) 5 cm distal to the joint line will be 15% less than the displacement measured at the joint line (KT-1000). Whatever system is used, it is incumbent that the practitioner know the literature and understand the design characteristics of the device he or she uses.

For devices that measure motion of the tibia relative to the patella, the precision of A/P displacement measurements are dependent on a standardized method of placing the measuring device on the leg and securely stabilizing the patella in the femoral trochlea as shown in Figure 19.41. The knee must be flexed to 25° to 30° to engage the patella in the femoral trochlea. In patients with patella alta it may be necessary to flex the knee as much as 40° or more by placing a board under the thigh support or using the MEDmetric adjustable thigh support (Fig. 19.42). The hand stabilizing the patellar sensor pad must stabilize the patella in the trochlea and control femoral rotation (Fig. 19.41). The device is applied to the leg so that pressure applied through the patellar pad seats the patella directly against the femur. This usually positions the device handle parallel with the foot axis. While

watching the dial, patellar pressure should be applied until the dial motion stops. If the patella cannot be securely stabilized, the knee should be flexed in order to bring the patella farther down into the femoral groove. Daniel et al. (55) evaluated seven examiners using a modified KT-1000 with a pressure sensor located in the patellar pad. All examiners increased the patellar pad pressure as they increased the force applied to the force handle (Fig. 19.43). The authors' recommendation was that because it is difficult to maintain consistent pressure on the patella throughout the load cycle (55), one must apply and maintain at least enough pressure to keep the patella firmly in contact with the femur at all times during the evaluation. As long as the patella is kept firmly stabilized against the femoral trochlea, changes in pressure will not affect the accuracy of measurements.

In the setting of acute knee injury, pain, swelling, and guarding can all affect the accuracy and reproducibility of instrumented measurement. Effusion, in particular, can make it more difficult to stabilize the patella. Wright (20) studied five cadaver knees to determine the threshold volume at which KT-1000 measurements would be affected. Knee circumference increased linearly with the volume

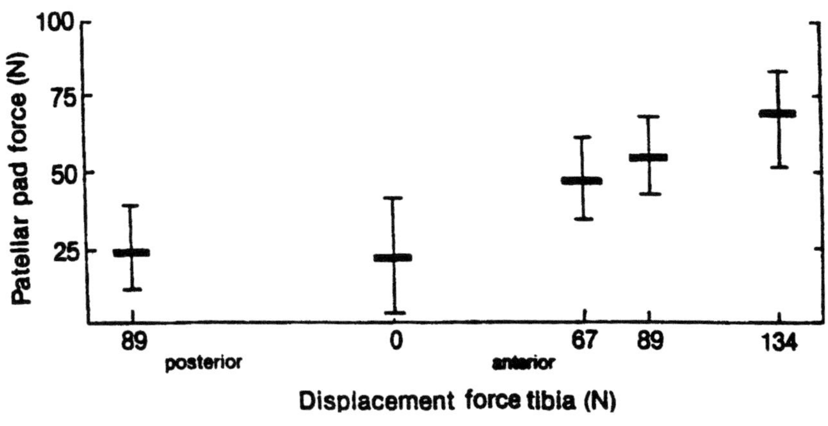

FIGURE 19.43. Patellar pad force versus force applied through the force handle. The mean and range at four force handle levels recorded by seven examiners testing the same patient.

of saline injected into the knee, ranging from 1.0 to 2.4 cm increased circumference at 70 mL. Measurable increases in displacements were noted in intact knees at injected volumes below 50 mL. An injected volume of 70 mL produced an average 3-mm increase in measured displacements. They recommended that a ballotable patella or a difference in knee circumference of at least 1 cm should be aspirated to avoid a false diagnosis of ACL tear based on falsely elevated instrumented laxity measurements.

Two devices are commercially available that were designed to measure several motions simultaneously. The CA-1000 (Orthopedic Systems, Inc., Hayward, California), formerly marketed as the Knee Signature System (KSS) through Acufex (Norwood, Massachusetts), uses an electrogoniometer attached via straps to the thigh and leg to monitor relative motion as displacements are applied to the leg by means of a load cell. The device measures four motions: anteroposterior translation and rotation in the sagittal, axial, and coronal planes. The Genucom (Faro Medical Technologies, Inc., Montreal, Canada) device uses an electrogoniometer and a computerized digitization system to monitor the external loads applied to the knee as well as motion in 6 *df*. The subject's thigh is clamped into the device and the computer attempts to predict the amount of motion artifact that will result from soft tissue motion about the femur and tibia. The theory behind these devices is that they allow control of externally applied loads and displacements that can affect A/P laxity measurement, which presumably would improve reproducibility of measurements. However, their superiority over simpler devices has not been shown. In

fact, many studies have reported that the Genucom produced less reliable measurements compared to other devices (12,13,40,49,72). Whatever theoretical concerns are addressed in the design of a measurement system, measurements must be both accurate and reproducible if the device is to be useful.

Soft Tissue Motion

Using the KT-1000, anterior-posterior displacement measurements are performed by tracking the tibial tubercle motion in relation to the patella. There is a relatively thin layer of soft tissue between these structures and the skin. *In vitro* studies by Daniel (Fig. 19.44) (1,17) and Edixhoven (36,66) documented little discrepancy between displacements measured by skeletal pin motion (1,17) or radiographic techniques (36). Both the KT-1000 and Edixhoven's system (Fig. 19.45) measure tibial tubercle motion independently of leg motion in attempt to limit the influence of the soft tissues. In contrast, Shino (35) reported relatively large measurement errors secondary to soft tissue deformation using a custom device that measured leg motion as a whole. The measurement of varus-valgus and internal-external rotations with surface-based testing devices pose even greater potential error from soft tissue motion. The technique for dealing with the soft tissue deformation utilized by the Genucom system (73) is to measure the stiffness of the soft tissue sleeve of the thigh and then, with computer assistance, subtract the predicted soft tissue motion from the measured motion. Accuracy and reproducibility of these devices is discussed below.

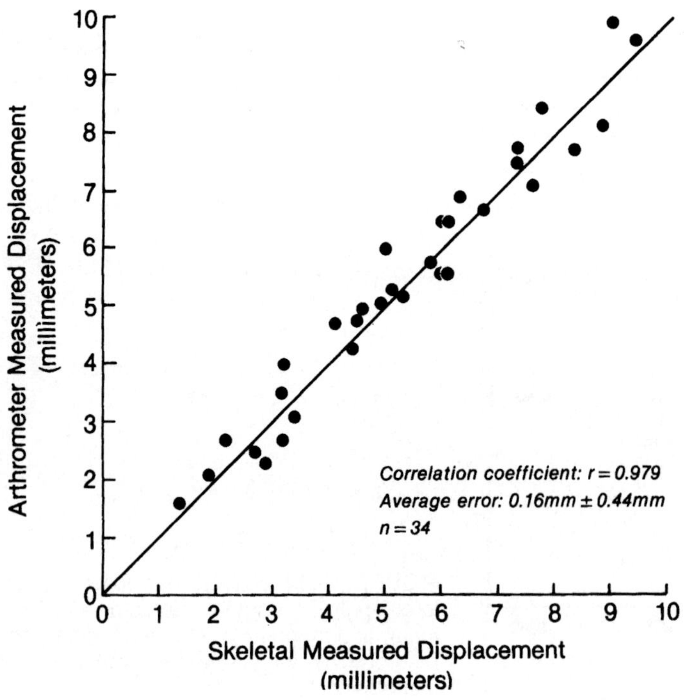

FIGURE 19.44. Arthrometer measurement (KT-2000) versus skeletally mounted measurement system in two cadaver specimens.

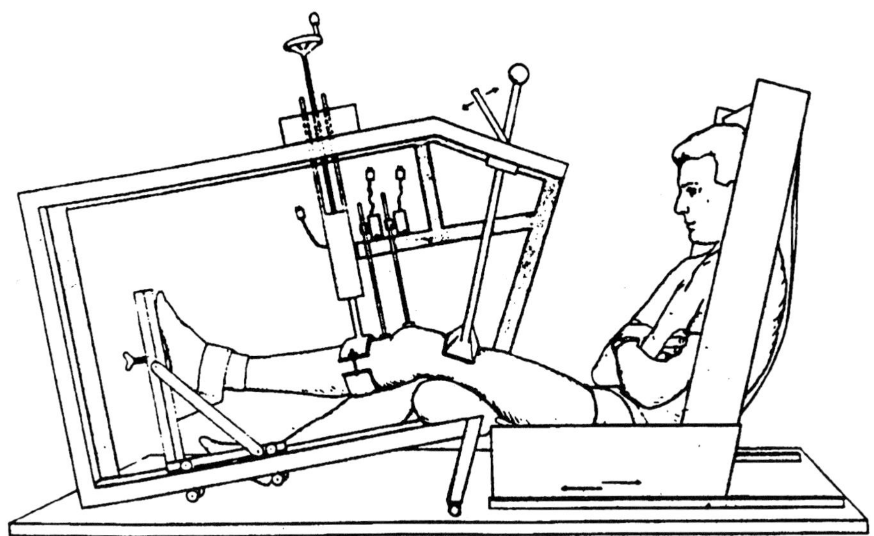

FIGURE 19.45. Edixhoven's measurement system. Schematic drawing of the anterior–posterior drawer test.

MUSCLE ACTIVITY

Muscle activity is probably the most significant variable in the measurement of motion limits (34-36,53,66). Activation of muscles crossing joints not only increases the joint stiffness, but also affects the joint resting position (36,53,66). Testing should be comfortable and conducive to muscle relaxation. Anderson hypothesized that the lower overall displacement values and relative imprecision of measurements produced with the Genucom device were due to discomfort and anxiety caused by clamping the femur (40). Several authors have suggested that the lower measured laxity reported in acute ACL injuries reflects pain and difficulty relaxing the muscles of the involved limb. No matter what device is used, and whatever the acuity of injury, the tester should continually monitor muscle tone and encourage patient relaxation to achieve the most reliable measurements.

KT-1000 KNEE LIGAMENT ARTHROMETRY

In a 1992 survey of trends in knee ligament surgery, Campbell (74) reported that only 21% of respondents relied entirely on the manual examination for the clinical diagnosis of ligament injury. Of the instrumented systems used, the KT-1000 was by far the most common (61% of all respondents). We have used the KT-1000 arthrometer in our clinic to measure anterior-posterior displacement since 1982. Measurements are routinely performed on patients with acute injuries and chronic instabilities. Patients who have knee ligament surgery are measured in the clinic at the preoperative examination, under anesthesia before surgery, and under anesthesia after wound closure. Postoperative displacement measurements are performed at 6 weeks, 3 months, 6 months, 9 months, and then yearly. We have used instrumented measurements to diagnose a cruciate ligament disruption, to document the amount of pathologic laxity, and to evaluate the success of cruciate ligament reconstruction surgery. In this section we discuss our testing technique, which takes into account the principles outlined above as well as our extensive experience with the device, noting potential pitfalls of KT-1000 data interpretation.

The KT-1000 and KT-2000 are essentially the same device, which is available either as a completely portable arthrometer that registers beeps corresponding to standard forces applied through the handle, or as an arthrometer attached to an X-Y plotter that registers continuous force-displacement output during examination. A version is also available to record force-displacement data directly onto a laptop computer.

TESTING TECHNIQUE

The arthrometer is placed on the anterior aspect of the leg and held with two circumferential Velcro straps (Fig. 19.39). There are two sensor pads: one in contact with the patella and the other in contact with the tibial tubercle. These move freely in the anterior-posterior plane in relation to the arthrometer case. The instrument detects the relative motion in millimeters between the two sensor pads and, therefore, motion of the arthrometer case (as the calf compresses under the Velcro straps) does not affect the instrument output. The design should also eliminate any effect of soft tissue compression as the leg is lifted and released. An exception to this may occur in a massively obese leg, in which pannus motion can cause false readings due to soft tissue motion directly under the patellar or tibial sensor pad. Displacement loads are applied through a force-sensing handle, which is located 10 cm distal to the joint line.

The precision of A/P displacement measurements depends on a standardized method of placing the measuring device on the leg and securely stabilizing the patella in the femoral trochlea. With adequate patellar stabilization, tibial tubercle motion relative to the patella accurately reflects the motion of the tibia relative to the femur. It is necessary to flex the knee 20° to 30° to engage the patella in the femoral trochlea. In patients with patella alta or lateral tracking patella, the knee may need to be flexed to 40°. The patella is stabilized in the femoral trochlea by direct pressure, which should be oriented to seat the patella (Fig. 19.41). The hand stabilizing the patella in the femoral trochlea should rest on the lateral thigh and prevent the instrument from rotating during the test (Fig. 19.41). To facilitate patella stabilization, the femur should be positioned so the patella is facing up or in slight external rotation. If there is excessive rotation, the thigh should be supported with a thigh strap (Fig. 19.46). The foot support of the KT-1000 is designed to assist in the consistent positioning of the legs and feet. Marks on the foot support allow the examiner to confirm that leg rotation is the same bilaterally. In our experience, consistent limb orientation using the thigh support, thigh strap, and foot support helps improve the reliability of laxity measurements particularly among inexperienced users.

The anesthetized patient represents a special case. When testing the anesthetized patient, additional care must be taken to adequately stabilize the patella in the femoral trochlea. The lower limbs usually lie in an externally rotated position in the anesthetized patient. A thigh strap (provided) or tape is required to internally rotate the limbs and position the patella anteriorly (Fig. 19.46). In many patients the knee must be flexed 35° to 40° to stabilize the patella (75). If tape is used to internally rotate the thigh, it should be applied no lower than 10 cm above

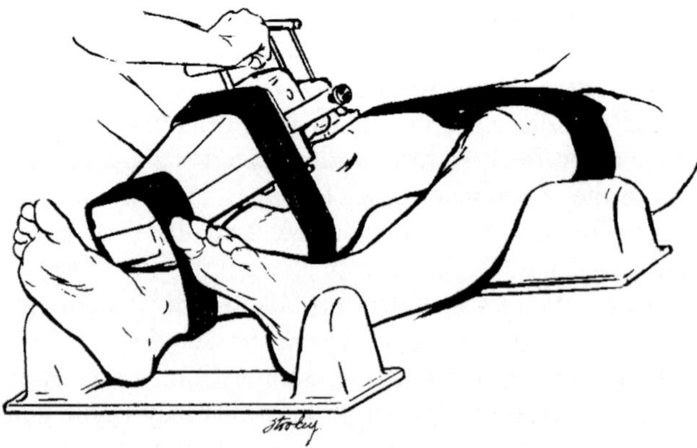

FIGURE 19.46. A 7-cm strap is used to support the thigh from excessive external rotation. The optimum limb position places the patella facing upward or in slight external rotation as shown in this figure. The foot support should not be used to internally rotate the limb, it is simply to support the feet.

the patella because of its potential effects on patellofemoral contact.

Posterior Cruciate Ligament Screen

Before performing 30° displacement measurements, the 90° active quadriceps test is performed to determine if there is posterior tibial subluxation. The examination is performed with the patient supine. The examiner sits lightly on the patient's foot to stabilize the limb with the knee flexed 90° as when performing a 90° Drawer test. The arthrometer is placed on the leg. The hand that stabilizes the arthrometer patella sensor pad also supports the patient's knee to prevent external rotation at the hip, so that the patient may completely relax the leg musculature (Fig. 19.47A). When examining larger patients we frequently have an assistant sit by the side of the table and support the limb, as shown in Figure 19.47B. In Figure 19.47B, the assistant's left hand prevents the patient's foot from moving, while the right hand supports the limb and monitors hamstring and quadriceps activity. Alternatively, an adjustable PCL limb holder (Fig. 19.48) (MEDmetric, San Diego, California) can assist in supporting large limbs for PCL testing if an assistant is not readily available. Hand position for a single examiner performing a PCL screen is as shown in Figure 19.47B with the following modifications: 1) the examiner's right hand replaces the assistant's right hand, which is positioned to detect both quadriceps and hamstring activity; and 2) the examiner's left hand then must be used to stabilize the patellar sensor pad and control the rotational orientation of the arthrometer on the limb. It is not necessary during the PCL screen to keep one hand on the force applicator handle of the KT-1000, because the PCL screen is an active test. It is, however, critical that the muscles crossing the knee are completely relaxed between cycles. The testing reference position is established: it is the resting position after a 20-lb posterior force is applied and then released several times with the right hand until the tibia consistently returns to the same position. The dial is rotated to mark this as the "zero" position. The right hand is then repositioned to support and monitor the thigh. The patient then performs an isolated quadriceps contraction. We have found the most helpful command to tell the patient is "Gently try to slide your foot down the examining table." The examiner palpates the hamstring and quadriceps tendons to confirm that there is no hamstring contraction. After the patient relaxes, a 20-lb posterior load is applied and the tibia is allowed to return to the "zero" position. If the dial does not return to zero after the 20-lb posterior load, the test is repeated. The test is repeated until the patient performs an isolated quadriceps contraction without concomitant knee extension, and without hamstring contraction. The arthrometer documents the presence and amount of anterior or posterior tibial displacement. Anterior tibial motion greater than 1

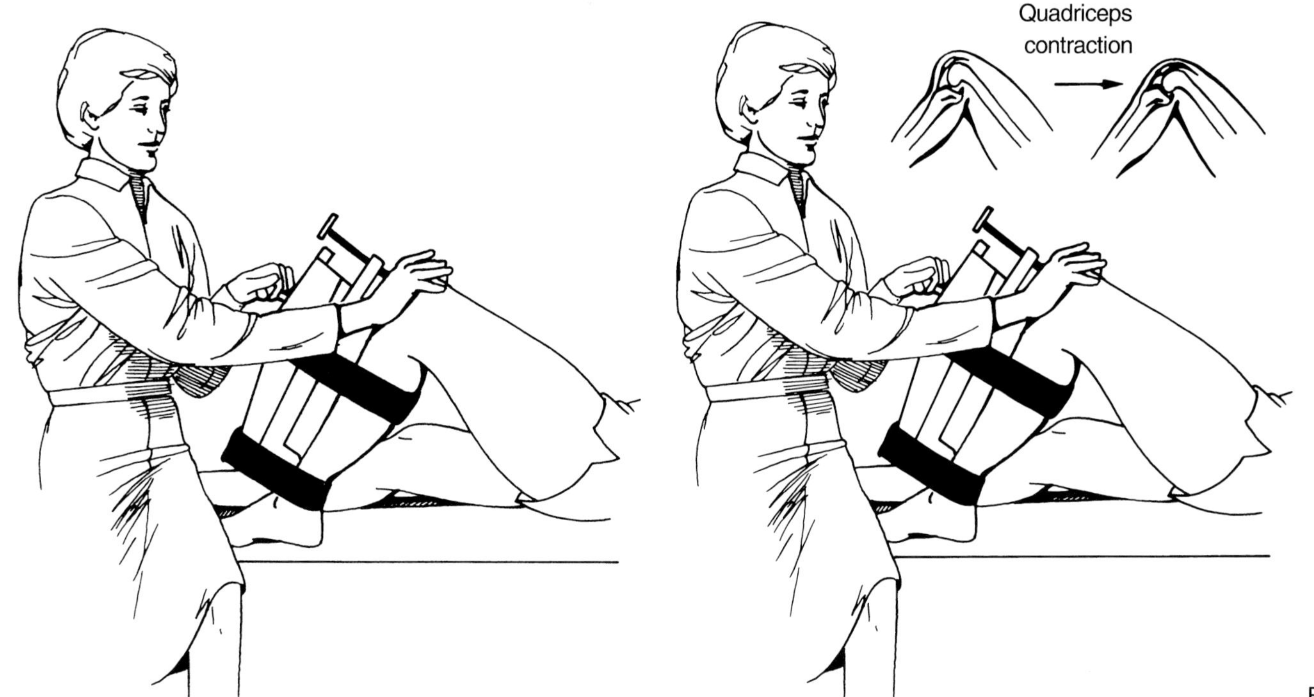

A

B

FIGURE 19.47. A: Measurement of anterior and posterior displacement using a knee ligament arthrometer and an 89 N displacing force. The examiner supports the subject's limb by sitting lightly on the foot and stabilizing the knee laterally. **B:** Alternatively, an assistant may support the limb (as seen in Figure 19.32). The support must be comfortable to ensure complete relaxation. The quadriceps neutral angle in the normal knee is located and measured. Anterior and posterior displacement are measured at this angle using the displacing force. The injured knee is then supported at the angle that has been identified as the quadriceps neutral angle in the normal knee. A posterior displacing force is applied and released to establish a reproducible reference position. Anterior and posterior displacement from the reproducible reference position are measured using the displacement force. The quadriceps active test is used to measure posterior subluxation of the tibia at the reproducible reference position.

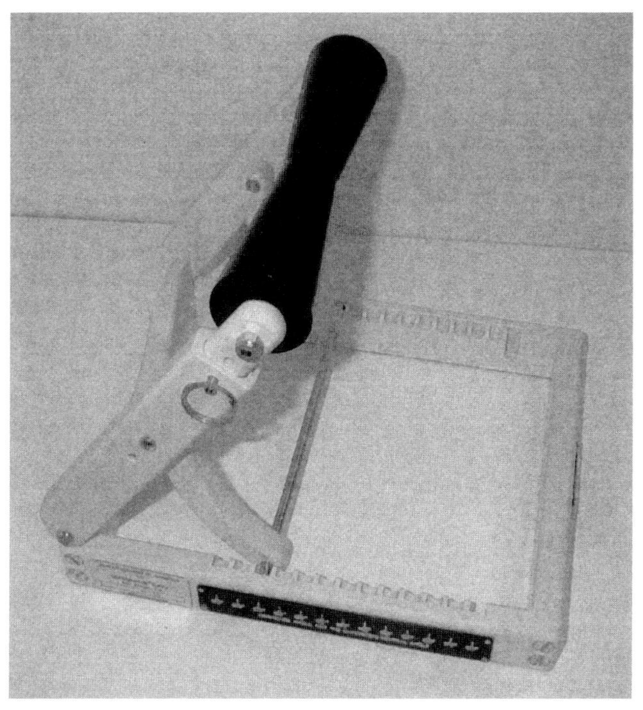

FIGURE 19.48. MEDmetric PCL thigh holder.

mm is abnormal and probably indicates a PCL injury. If the anterior tibial motion is greater than 1 mm, then the quadriceps neutral angle should be determined in the (opposite) uninjured knee. This is described later in this chapter. If there is no anterior tibial motion, the tibial position is normal and the examination should proceed to the 30° tests.

Passive 30° Tests

An ACL disruption is best revealed by testing the patient with the knee in slight flexion (34,50,51). To minimize measurement errors secondary to patellar motion, it is necessary to engage the patella in the femoral trochlea. This requires 20° to 40° of knee flexion (Fig. 19.41).

An 11-cm thigh support and a footrest positions both limbs in an equal position of flexion (30 + 5°) and limb rotation (10–30° of external rotation). With older models of the KT-1000, if insufficient flexion is obtained by the thigh support to stabilize the patella in the femoral trochlea, further knee flexion can be obtained by placing a board under the thigh support. In newer models, the height of the thigh support is adjustable (Fig. 19.42). If the limb lies in an externally rotated position with the patella facing laterally, the thigh should be internally rotated and supported with a restraining strap, to face the patella anteriorly (Fig. 19.46). Positioning the limb to place the patella anteriorly and engaged in the femoral trochlea optimizes stabilization of the patella in the femoral trochlea. The foot support helps the clinician orient the feet and legs without constraining motion.

The patient should be comfortable and relaxed. Gentle manual A/P oscillation of the thigh and/or leg typically will assist in obtaining muscle relaxation (Fig. 19.49). The arthrometer is applied to the leg and oriented so that pressure on the patellar sensor pad will stabilize the patella within the femoral trochlea (Fig. 19.41). This usually places the force handle parallel to the foot axis. Firm pressure is then applied to the patellar sensor pad until the patella is seated in the femoral trochlea. If the patella does not seat firmly, more knee flexion is needed. Rangger showed that it is impossible to maintain constant pressure on the patellar pad during instrumented measurement (Fig. 19.43) (54,55). Therefore enough pressure must be applied throughout the examination to keep the patella in contact with the femur to avoid spurious measurements. Several complete anterior-posterior cycles are performed to condition the joint, repeating until the displacements are reproducible. After the first cycle, the instrument dial is set at 0. After each successive cycle, the measurement reference position is once again obtained by applying and releasing a 20-lb posterior load. The reading on the dial should not differ by more than 0.5 mm from one cycle to the next if the reference position remains stable. If the dial indicates that the reference position is not stable within 0 + 0.5 mm, the instrument orientation on the leg may be changing or the quadriceps may not be fully relaxed. After two or three complete cycles, if the dial indicates that consistent displacements are being produced at 15-, 20-, and 30-lb force, the measurements are read directly from the dial. The mean of three tests rounded to the nearest 0.5 mm is recorded as the measurement at each force level. Confirmation of a stable reference position should be performed after the manual maximum test, the quadriceps active test, and those tests where the anterior load is applied through the force handle.

Five passive displacement measurements are recorded for each limb at 30°. In addition, anterior joint compliance may be measured by calculating the anterior displacement between any two load levels recorded in the same cycle. For theoretical considerations, Fleming thought it best to measure compliance at low force levels (45). We have recorded the displacement difference between the 15- and 20-lb anterior load as illustrated in Figure 19.35. However, as we shall see, this calculation does not seem to have much utility in practice. With the KT-2000, measurements are read from the x-y plot at the corresponding force. In the KT-1000 a specific tone (beep) corresponds to each of four loads (one posterior and three anterior) when applied through the device handle:

1. **20 lb (89 N) posterior displacement:** posterior excursion from the measurement reference position with a 20-lb posterior push.
2. **15 lb (67 N) anterior displacement:** anterior excursion from the measurement reference position with a 15-lb anterior pull.
3. **20 lb (89 N) anterior displacement:** anterior excursion from the measurement reference position with a 20-lb anterior pull.
4. **30 lb (134 N) anterior displacement:** anterior excursion from the measurement reference position with a 30-lb anterior pull.
5. **Manual maximum anterior displacement:** anterior displacement with a high anterior force applied directly to the proximal calf just distal to the posterior knee joint flexion crease (Fig. 19.50).

The configuration of the hands is very similar to the hand position for the Lachman test. The manual maximum test produces greater anterior displacement than loads applied through the device handle due to greater magnitude of the applied load and a more proximal

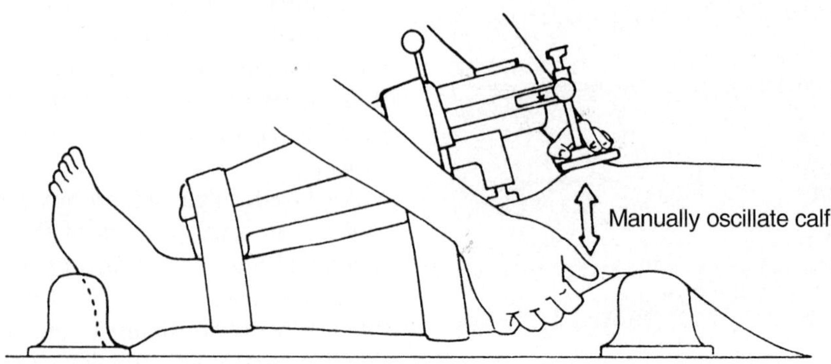

FIGURE 19.49. Gentle manual oscillation of the leg may assist in obtaining muscle relaxation.

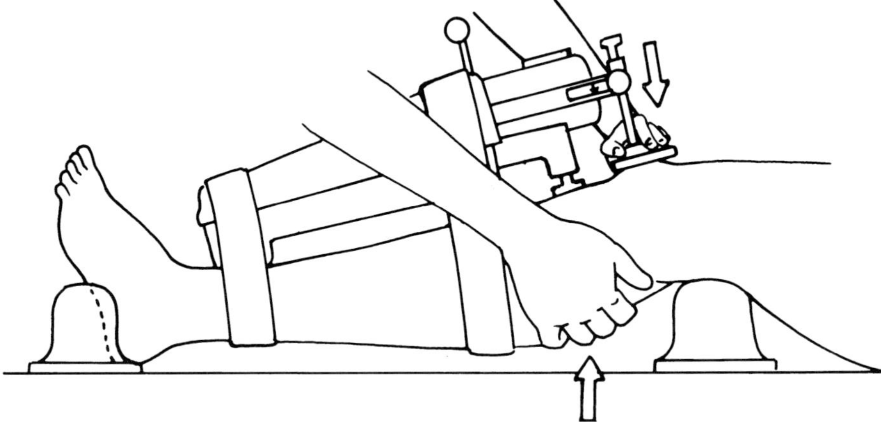

FIGURE 19.50. The limbs are positioned with the support system, the arthrometer applied and the testing reference position obtained in the standard way. While the patellar sensor pad is stabilized with one hand, the other hand then applies a strong anterior displacement force directly to the proximal calf to produce the maximum anterior displacement. Care is taken that the knee is not extended. The tibial displacement is read off the dial.

point of load application. Anteriorly directed load is applied until the heel begins to rise off the foot rest. In other words, the manual maximum load actually represents the load which, when applied to the upper leg, exactly neutralizes the flexion moment exerted at the knee by the force of gravity on the leg segment (Fig. 19.37). Application of the load close to the joint line reduces the moment applied to the knee, permitting a greater anterior force without lifting the foot off the examining table. In our clinic, manual maximum loads are estimated to be 30 to 40 lbs. The greater force, combined with a more proximally located point of application, results in a greater moment, which produces greater anterior displacement than is observed at 20 or 30 lb force (Fig. 19.37).

Summary of KT-1000 Arthrometry Technique

It is important to establish the precision of a testing system before using it in decision making. The manufacturer recommends monthly monitoring of the KT-1000 instrument to confirm accuracy of the load sensing handle and the displacement sensors. The important indicator of pathology is side-to-side difference. The same machine must be used on both sides to minimize the significance of small calibration errors in the machine itself. The crucial element in the testing process is to duplicate the testing technique on the second knee that was used on the first knee. Important points are:

1. Muscle relaxation.
2. Similar limb orientation (rotation and flexion angle).
3. Similar arthrometer placement on the leg in respect to the instrument marker at the joint line and instrument rotation in relation to the patella.
4. Consistent patella pad pressure technique.
5. Establishing the testing reference position.
6. Similar speed of force application.

The two greatest sources of measurement errors with the arthrometer are lack of muscle relaxation and inability to stabilize the patellar sensor pad (pressure *and* rotation).

Quadriceps Active Tests

Orthopedic surgeons have routinely evaluated the integrity of knee ligaments by estimating or measuring the amount and direction of motion between the tibia and femur due to manually applied external forces such as drawer tests, varus and valgus stress tests, and pivot shift tests (76). These are *passive* tests, as the displacing force is applied by the examiner. Another method of assessing ligamentous and capsular integrity is to measure the change in joint position which result from active contraction of the patient's muscles. These are *active* tests, as the patient's muscle contraction provides the joint displacement force.

At full extension, as the patellar tendon runs from the tibial tubercle to the patella, it lies anterior to a reference line drawn perpendicular to the surface of the tibial plateau and passing through the tibial tubercle (76–82). As the knee flexes, the femur rolls posteriorly on the tibia guided by the cruciate ligaments (83). The orientation of the patellar tendon changes continuously from anterior to posterior relative to the reference line (Fig. 19.51) (81,82, 84,85). Thus, the resultant shear force produced by the pull of the patellar tendon on the tibial tubercle also changes from anterior to posterior with increasing flexion angle. The crossover from anterior to posterior shear

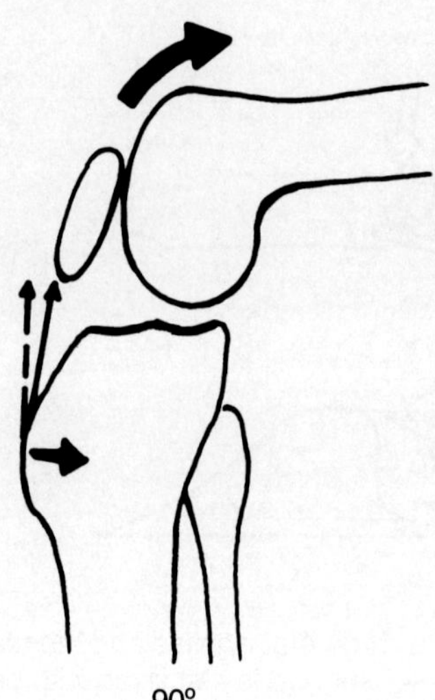

FIGURE 19.51. The patellar tendon force can be resolved into two components, a normal component that is perpendicular to the tibial plateau and a shear component that is parallel to the tibial plateau. When the patellar tendon is anterior, the shear component tends to slide the tibia forward on the femur; when directed posteriorly it tends to slide the tibia backward on the femur.

occurs between 60° and 90° in the normal knee (77,81,82,85,86). The angle of flexion at which the crossover occurs in the normal knee is termed the "quadriceps neutral angle," or QNA, and is defined as the angle of flexion at which the tibia does not shift anteriorly or posteriorly when the quadriceps is contracted in the normal knee. At this angle, the force in the patellar tendon is parallel to the reference line, therefore no net shear occurs at the tibio-femoral interface. Daniel determined the QNA to be at 71° flexion on average.

At angles less than the QNA, quadriceps contraction produces anterior movement of the tibia due to an anteriorly angled patellar tendon. This anterior motion should be constrained by a normal anterior cruciate ligament. Similarly, at angles greater than the quad neutral angle,

quadriceps contraction produces backward motion of the tibia resulting from a posteriorly angled patellar tendon. Posterior motion should be constrained by the posterior cruciate ligament (Fig. 19.31).

Anterior subluxation of the tibia with contraction of the quadriceps in the anterior cruciate ligament deficient knee can be documented with the 30° quadriceps active test. The limbs are supported with the thigh support and foot rest as performed for the 30° passive tests. The testing reference position is established and the instrument dial set at 0. The patient is then asked to gently lift the heel off of the table. The greatest anterior displacement observed as the patient extends the knee is recorded as the quadriceps active displacement (Fig. 19.52). Thirty-degree quadriceps active data are presented in Figure 19.38 and Tables 19.2 through 19.5.

A PCL rupture is diagnosed by using the quadriceps active test to demonstrate the posterior tibial subluxation. This maneuver is referred to as the "PCL screen." At 90° of flexion, the patellar tendon in the *normal* knee is oriented slightly posterior to the reference line and contraction of the quadriceps results in no movement or a slight posterior shift. If the PCL is ruptured, the tibia sags into posterior subluxation and the patellar tendon is then directed anteriorly (Fig. 19.31).

Every knee ligament instrumented examination begins with the PCL screen (see p. 384). The screening quadriceps active test is qualitative: it is intended to identify only the direction of displacement, if any. No shift or a slight posterior shift of the tibia on contraction of the quadriceps indicates an intact posterior cruciate ligament, allowing the examiner to proceed with testing at 30° of knee flexion. However, an anterior shift of the tibia of at least 1 mm from its sagging position of posterior subluxation indicates an injured posterior cruciate ligament. If the PCL screen indicates posterior knee laxity in the injured knee, the examiner proceeds directly to the uninjured (opposite) knee to determine the quadriceps neutral angle (QNA) and measure anterior and posterior displacement.

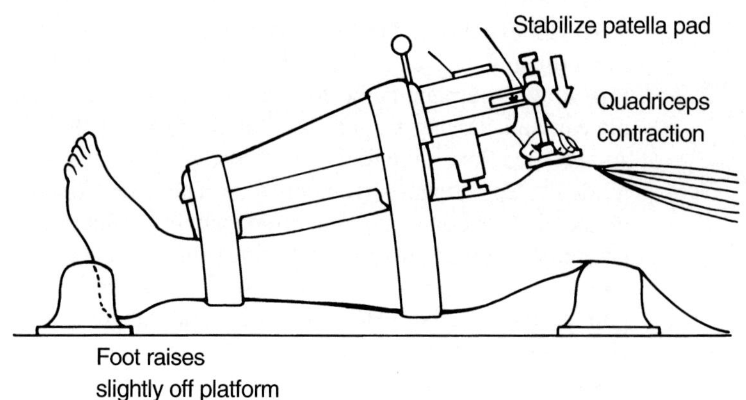

FIGURE 19.52. The thigh is supported in about 30° of flexion. The patellar sensor pad is stabilized and the testing reference position is established by pushing with a 20-lb load posteriorly and then releasing the force. The patient is then asked to gently lift the heel off the table. The anterior displacement as the heel lifts off the table is recorded.

TABLE 19.2. *Normal A/P displacement measurements*

Test	Range		Mean	SD	95% cutoff
	Low	High			
Displacement (n = 240)					
20 lb posterior	1	6	2.8	0.9	4.5
20 lb anterior	3	14	7.2	2.0	10
20 lb A/P	5	18	10.0	2.4	12
Manual maximum anterior	4.5	15	8.6	2.1	12
Quadriceps active displacement	2	12.5	5.7	1.8	9
Right minus left (n = 120)					
20 lb posterior	0	2	0	0.7	1.0[b]
20 lb anterior	−0.2	−3.5	2	1.0	2.0[b]
20 lb A/P	−4	4	0.2	0.9	2.5[b]
Manual maximum anterior	−4	3	−0.3	1.1	2.0[b]
Quadriceps active displacement	−3	2	−0.4	1.0	2.0[b]

[b]Right—left difference.
SD, standard deviation; A/P, anterior–posterior.

Using the KT-1000 to Measure Posterior Laxity

Total A/P laxity can be measured accurately in the PCL-deficient knee at 30°, as can end point compliance in response to anterior and posterior loads. But the specific contributions of ACL and PCL injuries to the overall displacement cannot be ascertained unless the "zero" position of the knee can be established. As stated previously, measurement of anterior laxity at 30° flexion assumes that the PCL is intact. If the PCL is not intact, and the clinician wishes to evaluate the individual contributions of the ACL and PCL to knee instability, he or she must measure displacement after positioning the knee at the quadriceps neutral angle, or QNA. The quadriceps active test (QAT) is used to determine the QNA in the normal knee, as well as to determine the amount of sag and the degree of correction needed for anterior and posterior measurements in the injured knee. Figure 19.53 presents a normal, ACL-disrupted knee and a PCL-disrupted knee tested at the quadriceps neutral angle. Note that only the quadriceps active position is common to all three conditions.

TABLE 19.3. *Evaluation of 34 high school football players: comparison of two examiners' displacement measurements*

Test	Millimeters of displacement (mean ± SD)	
	Examiner MLS	Examiner DMD
Right 20 lb posterior	3.5 ± 1.0	3.6 ± 0.8
Right 20 lb anterior	8.1 ± 1.2	5.7 ± 1.4
Right manual maximum anterior	8.8 ± 1.4	6.9 ± 1.7
Right quadriceps active	6.1 ± 1.6	5.2 ± 1.4
Mean right minus left difference		
20 lb posterior	−0.4 ± 1.2	0.2 ± 0.7
20 lb anterior	−1.1 ± 1.6	−0.7 ± 0.7
Manual maximum anterior	−1.0 ± 1.2	−0.5 ± 1.0
Quadriceps active	−1.0 ± 1.2	−1.4 ± 1.0
Number of subjects with R-L difference >2.5 mm (no subject had R-L difference >3.5 mm)		
20 lb anterior	3	0
Manual maximum anterior	2	1
Quadriceps active	1	2
Right minus left difference between examiners		
20 lb anterior	0.9 ± 0.8	
Manual maximum anterior	1.1 ± 0.9	
Quadriceps active	1.0 ± 0.6	

Measurements were obtained with the KT-1000. The knee flexion angle was 20° to 35°.

TABLE 19.4. *KT-1000 measurements of unilateral chronic ACL disruption at 20° to 35°; injured minus normal (I − N) displacement difference*

Clinical examination and author	n	Mean	Percent ≥3.0
20-lb test			
Anderson A	50	5.05	82
Anderson A (1989)	20	4.3	76[a]
Bach	153	—	79
Daniel (1985)	89	5.6	96
3M LAD	297	6.1	89
Neuschwander	16	6.3	—
Rangger	159	5.4	85
Sherman	19	5.1	95
Steiner	15	3.6	—
Manual maximum test			
Anderson	50	8.6	100
Bach	153	—	72
KSD	177	8.5	99
3M LAD	297	7.8	96
Neuschwander	16	7.8	—
Rangger	159	8.6	99
Quadriceps active test			
KSD	177	4.3	70
3M LAD	258	4.4	76
Examination under anesthesia before reconstruction 20-lb test			
KSD	223	5.6	87
3M LAD	297	6.9	96
Rangger	159	5.9	87
Examination under anesthesia before reconstruction manual maximum test			
KSD	223	8.9	97
3M LAD	297	8.9	99
Rangger	159	9.4	98
Examination under anesthesia after reconstruction 20-lb (I - N)			
KSD	223	−1.4	5

[a]Both acute and chronic.

TABLE 19.5. *Evaluation of 29 patients with a unilateral ACL injury: Comparison of two examiners' displacement measurements*

	Millimeters of anterior displacement (mean ± SD)	
Test	Examiner MLS	Examiner DMD
Normal 20 lb	6.9 ± 2.5	6.6 ± 2.1
Injured minus normal		
20 lb	4.2 ± 2.2	4.4 ± 2.5
Manual maximum	6.8 ± 3.5	6.7 ± 3.3
Quadriceps active	3.7 ± 2.2	3.9 ± 2.7
Subjects with R-L difference >2.5 mm		
20 lb	25 (86%)	22 (76%)
Manual maximum	29 (100%)	29 (100%)
Quadriceps active	21 (72%)	21 (72%)
Injured minus normal difference between examiners		
20 lb	1.2 ± 0.9	
Manual maximum	1.5 ± 1.7	
Quadriceps active	1.1 ± 1.1	

The knee flexion angle was 20° to 35°.

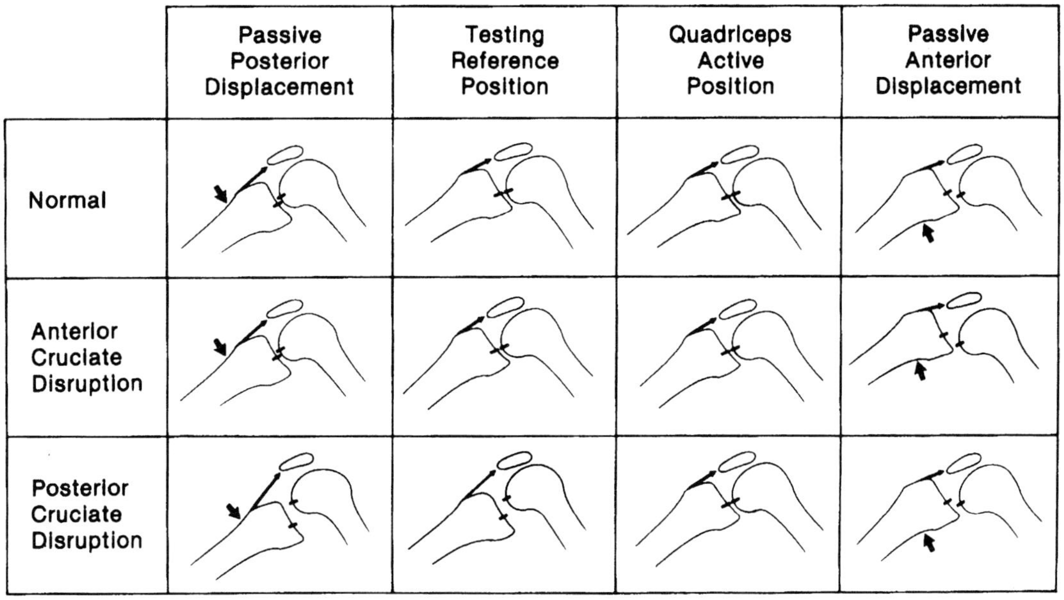

	Passive Posterior Displacement	Testing Reference Position	Quadriceps Active Position	Passive Anterior Displacement
Normal				
Anterior Cruciate Disruption				
Posterior Cruciate Disruption				

FIGURE 19.53. Measurements at the quadriceps neutral angle ($x = 70°$). Note that the quadriceps active test position (at the quadriceps neutral) is the only condition in which the joint is in the same position for all three states: the normal knee, the anterior cruciate ligament–injured knee, and the posterior cruciate ligament–injured knee.

The QNA of the knee is the flexion angle at which anterior and posterior tibial displacement can be measured when posterior instability is present. The instrumented QAT is used to establish the QNA. The QNA is determined in the *normal* knee. Daniel determined that the quadriceps neutral angle ranges from 60° to 90° with a mean of 71° (53). To determine the quadriceps neutral angle, the patient is placed on the examining table in the supine position with the uninjured knee flexed to approximately 90°. The quadriceps is actively contracted and the tibial motion is observed. Recall that we are testing the normal knee, so that any motion observed will be in the posterior direction. The angle of knee flexion is reduced toward 70° until there is no observable posterior tibial shift. This flexion angle represents the quadriceps neutral angle for that patient. Hand position is important to: (a) stabilize and support the limb, (b) support and maintain the orientation of the arthrometer, and (c) monitor muscle activity. A single examiner supports the limb as shown in Figure 19.47A. If help is necessary to perform any of these tasks, especially for a large patient, an assistant may be required to support the leg and monitor quadriceps and hamstring activity, Figure 19.47B. Figure 19.48 shows a device that can be used to hold the limb during testing if no assistant is available. Having determined the quadriceps neutral angle in the normal knee, the injured knee is then positioned at that angle in preparation for displacement measurements.

At the quadriceps neutral angle, passive anterior and posterior tibial displacements are recorded for the normal knee first (Fig. 19.54). Note that by definition, the QAT at the QNA in the *normal* knee is zero. The injured knee is then flexed to the QNA. The device is secured to the leg. After several passive oscillations to relax the knee, the zero position is determined by applying a posteriorly directed force of 20 lb, then releasing the load and setting the dial to zero. The quadriceps is then contracted and the amount of (active) anterior displacement of the tibia is determined. The quadriceps active test is repeated for two to three cycles. After each cycle, a posteriorly directed force of 20 lb is applied. The dial should return to the zero position to confirm that the patient is relaxing fully and the knee is returning to its original resting position. Passive displacements at 89 N anterior and posterior force are then recorded. The anterior and posterior displacements must then be corrected to account for the posterior sag. Note that when the tibia sags, a percentage of the posterior displacement occurs naturally, due to gravity. Thus, measurements taken from the resting position will tend to underestimate posterior laxity and overestimate anterior displacement. To correct the measurements, the millimeters of anterior shift during the QAT is added to the measured posterior tibial displacement in the injured knee and subtracted from the measured anterior tibial displacement (Fig. 19.54B). The side-to-side differences are then determined in the usual way by subtracting the values in the uninjured knee from the *corrected* mea-

INJURED KNEE

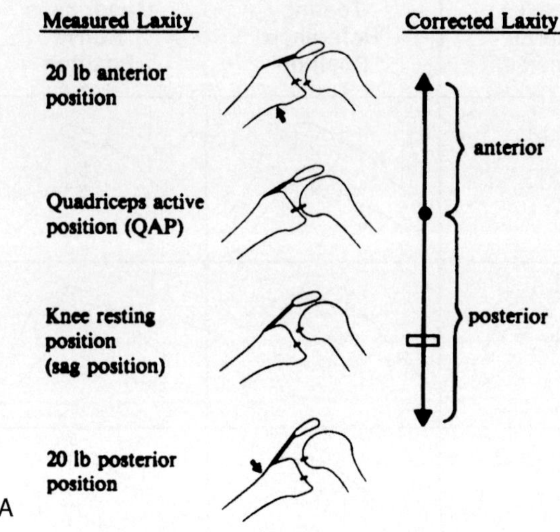

	Normal knee measured	Injured knee measured	Injured knee corrected	Injured corrected minus normal
20 lb anterior	4	10	10-5=5	5-4=1
20 lb posterior	2	3	3+5=8	8-2=6
Quadriceps active displacement	0	+5		

B

FIGURE 19.54. A: In the injured knee, the measured anterior tibial displacement is the distance from the resting position (*rectangle*) to the *superior arrowhead* (10 mm). The measured posterior displacement is from the resting position to the *inferior arrowhead* (3 mm). With contraction of the quadriceps, the tibia moves forward from the resting position to the quadriceps active position (*dark circle*). **B:** Determinations of the laxity are calculated from the quadriceps active position (corrected laxity).

surements in the injured knee (Fig. 19.54B). By convention, a corrected anterior side-to-side difference 2.5 mm or greater at the quadriceps neutral angle is indicative of ACL deficiency; a corrected posterior side-to-side difference 2.5 mm or greater at the quadriceps neutral angle is indicative of PCL deficiency (58).

Daniel reported that contraction of the quadriceps at the quadriceps neutral angle in the posterior cruciate ligament-deficient knee results in an average anterior shift of the tibia of 6 mm in the chronic PCL-injured knee and 4.2 mm in acute PCL-injured knees (53). Figure 19.55 present the right-left displacement difference for all subjects in that study. Note that uncorrected posterior displacements (the portion of the vertical bars below the resting position) are small even when significant posterior instability exists.

INSTRUMENTED MEASUREMENT AND THE DIAGNOSIS OF LIGAMENT INJURY

The definition of knee laxity, and the parameters used in its measurement, have evolved somewhat over the past 20 years. Laxity has been defined by Noyes (87) as "some amount of motion that results from the application of forces and moments." Figure 19.35 shows the typical sigmoidal passive force-displacement curves for normal and ACL-deficient knees. Instrumented devices have been used to measure laxity in response to both passive (externally applied) and active (internally applied, usually by quadriceps activation) loads. Daniel introduced the instrumented quadriceps active test at 30° flexion (Fig. 19.38) (88) as a functional test, hypothesizing that it might correlate with symptoms of functional instability

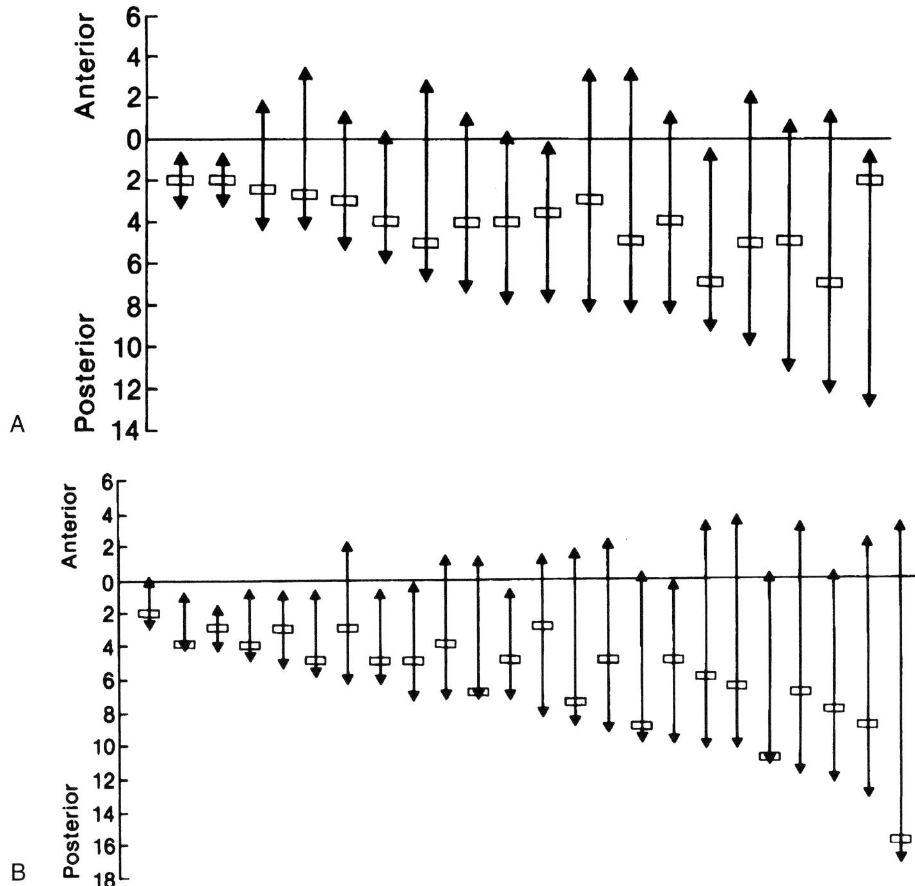

FIGURE 19.55. R-L displacement difference for patients with a posterior cruciate ligament (PCL) disruption. **A:** Unilateral acute PCLs (n = 18). **B:** Unilateral chronic PCL (n = 24). Each *vertical line* represents one patient. The zero mark is the knee neutral position (quadriceps active test position at the quadriceps neutral angle). The *rectangle* indicates the injured limb resting position, or posterior sag position. Note that in many of the patients there was a small posterior displacement from the resting position.

during functional quadriceps contraction. In fact, he initially called it the "voluntary quadriceps shift." Some authors have also measured stiffness (34,35,45,52), or compliance index (1,36,88), which represent the slope of the load-displacement curve within a given range (Fig. 19.35). Although useful for heuristic or academic purposes, neither of these parameters has been shown to have much practical value in diagnosing or managing knee ligament injuries. To facilitate comparisons between studies, the majority of investigators have measured laxity as tibial displacement in response to set loads, which have become more or less standardized to include some combination of 89 N (20 lb, both anterior and posterior) (1,7, 17,40,57,63,68,89-93), 134 N (30 lb) anterior (13,63,68, 88,94), 178 N (40 lb) anterior (57,68), and manual maximum anterior loads (17,68,92,93).

Ligament arthrometers are not tests. They are devices that measure the relationship between force and displace-

ment. Arthrometers have varying degrees of accuracy and precision that affect our ability to distinguish normal from ACL-injured knees (13,45). But it is not appropriate to discuss diagnostic accuracy, correctness, sensitivity or specificity of a device without specifying all the elements that affect the distribution of measurements, as well as the ranges of displacement that are to be considered "normal" or "abnormal." In addition to millimeters of displacement, interpretation of arthrometer measurements depends on knowing what force is being applied, whether side-to-side comparisons are being made, and what displacement value is being applied as the diagnostic threshold. In Figure 19.38, the distributions of the measured laxity of the two populations, uninjured and ACL-deficient, resemble relatively symmetric normal distributions. But the distributions of measured displacements of injured and uninjured knees vary under the different conditions presented. The distributions and their overlapping areas are determined by 1) the magnitude of the applied force, and 2) calculation of side-to-side differences. Inclusion of all this information represents an instrumented test; it is a hypothesis applied to the sample distributions and is exactly analogous to setting alpha and beta values in a statistical analysis. For example, injured-minus-normal displacement difference at 20 lb force with a diagnostic threshold of 3 mm or more constitutes an instrumented test: the two populations will have predictable distributions with a certain amount of overlap, and a cut-off value of 3 mm results in a predictable and measurable degree of diagnostic error. For such a test, determination of diagnostic accuracy, correctness, sensitivity and specificity has meaning.

Reliability of Instrumented Measurement

The reliability of measurements obtained with instrumented laxity systems has been tested extensively. Reliability can be assessed either as accuracy or as reproducibility. Accuracy is defined as the ability of a device to conform to a known standard. Studies of measurement accuracy have compared instrumented devices against direct measurement of bone displacements in cadaver knees, and against radiographic measurements in cadavers and in living subjects. Daniel (1) reported a correlation coefficient of .97 and a standard error of 0.4 mm comparing the KT-2000 against concurrent skeletal pin displacements in cadaver knees (Fig. 19.44). Edixhoven and co-workers (36) compared their custom laxity system to highly accurate roentgen stereo photogrammetric measurements concurrently in two postmortem leg specimens. Like Daniel (1), they observed that the effects of relative motion between patella and femur were negligible. In addition to A/P shifts, significant knee flexion and tibial rotations occurred, although the foot and the thigh were fixed as well as possible. The ability of the laxity measurement system to isolate and measure only the relative A/P motion of the patella and tibia was effective in circumventing this problem. Measurement error of their custom laxity system was reported as 0.4 to 1.0 mm at 180 N force (36). The studies reported by Daniel and Edixhoven represent ideal conditions for evaluating measurement error, because simultaneous measurement by both techniques eliminated potential error caused by repositioning or differences in the application of load. Shino compared measurements of a custom testing system in cadaver knees before and after all soft tissues were removed (35). In contrast to Daniel and Edixhoven, Shino observed that soft tissue deformation accounted for significant measurement error with his device. Fleming (2) evaluated the accuracy of the Genucom and KSS systems in cadaver knees. The standard used for comparison was displacement measured on a Materials Testing System, or MTS (MTS Systems, Eden Prairies, Minnesota). After

displacement measurements with the two laxity systems, the knees were positioned on the MTS and direct measurements of motion during Lachman and anterior drawer tests were taken. The Genucom registered displacements not significantly different from the MTS, while the KSS consistently registered lower displacements. These studies show that some devices can produce highly accurate measurements of tibiofemoral displacement. They also demonstrate that measurement accuracy is variable and depends to a large extent on the design characteristics of individual laxity measurement systems.

Accuracy has been tested *in vivo* using stress radiography as the standard of comparison. For such comparisons to represent true tests of accuracy, the measurement technique used as the standard must have greater documented accuracy than the instrumented system being evaluated. Due to a variety of design flaws, no *in vivo* study comparing stress radiography to instrumented measurement has satisfied this requirement. Staubli (32) found no correlation between stress radiographs and KT-1000 arthrometry at 89 N force. Fleming (45) has pointed out that because the radiographic method did not include a stereo measurement technique using precise bony landmarks, the study does not represent an assessment of error, but merely a comparison of two methods for documenting joint laxity. Staubli concluded that the two methods had, in fact, similar diagnostic accuracy in detecting ACL deficiency.

For an ideal test of accuracy, measurements should be recorded with both methods concurrently under identical loads (1,36). Jonsson (95) used a highly accurate stereo radiographic technique with tantalum beads embedded in the femur and tibia. Average KT-1000 arthrometer displacements (89 N anterior force) were similar to stereophotogrammetric displacements (150 N anterior, 80 N posterior force) in the normal knee, but underestimated true displacements by 2.5 mm in the injured knee. Because the larger loads were applied during the radiographic measurements, it is to be expected that the radiographs would have recorded larger displacements, particularly among unstable knees, which are more compliant. It is not clear from this study whether the arthrometer recorded less displacement because it was inaccurate or because lower loads were applied during KT-1000 testing.

Reproducibility is a measure of agreement between successive examinations, either by a single examiner at two times (test-retest, or intra-tester variation) or by two different examiners (inter-tester variation). An important difference between a device that is clinically useful and one that is only a research tool is that a clinically useful device must be reliable enough to make decisions about an individual patient. This implies that the device is not only accurate, but that the results of an individual examination can be reproduced by the same or another examiner under similar conditions. As a general rule, the mea-

TABLE 19.6. *95% confidence intervals (in millimeters) for right leg anterior laxity and side-to-side differences*

	Force (N)				
Variables	67	89	134	178	MM[a]
Right leg: any tester/any day	±1.32	±1.56	±1.93	±2.17	±1.81
Right leg: same tester/any day	±1.12	±1.30	±1.65	±1.94	±1.71
Side-to-side difference: any tester/any day	±1.11	±1.16	±1.42	±1.68	±1.49
Side-to-side difference: same taster/any day	±1.11	±1.16	±1.42	±1.68	±1.46

[a]Manual maximum.

surements should be reproducible within some range deemed to be clinically relevant, such as the threshold used to distinguish normal from abnormal knees (13,45). Of the devices tested by Steiner (13), only the Genucom registered variations that did not allow a high degree of diagnostic correctness. Myrer has documented the 95% confidence intervals for passive measurements with the KT-2000 (Table 19.6). To document the test/retest variation by a single skilled examiner, author MLS examined ten normal subjects on 5 different days without reference to her previous examinations. The test/retest variations were seldom greater than a millimeter (Fig. 19.56). MLS has tested patients with a unilateral ACL disruption at 6- to 12-month intervals for 3 years. The first examination was performed within 2 weeks of injury. Table 19.7 presents the test/retest variation of the displacement in the normal knee between the patient's first examination and last examination. The test/retest variation is less than 2.5 mm in 87% of patients with the 89 N test and 83% of subjects with the manual maximum test.

Forster and colleagues (96) tested reliability of the KT-1000 in 10 inpatients, four of whom had no history of knee problems and six of whom had a diagnosis of ACL instability. Four examiners (two experienced surgeons and two novices) examined all ten patients twice on the same day, and five of the six patients with unilateral anterior laxity were re-examined under anesthesia a few days later. The trial produced 320 measurements of ACL laxity in 10 conscious subjects, each having two knees examined at two forces by four surgeons on two occasions. They reported substantial inter- and intraexaminer variation in the measurements both of absolute displacement in single knees and of side-to-side differences between pairs of knees. However, careful analysis of their data show that only nine of 80 re-tests by experienced examiners varied by more than 2 mm, while 22 of 80 re-tests by novice examiners varied by more than 2 mm. Four of 40 re-tests of side-to-side difference were greater than 2 mm for the experienced examiners, while 12 of 40 re-tests exceeded 2 mm for the novices. This article

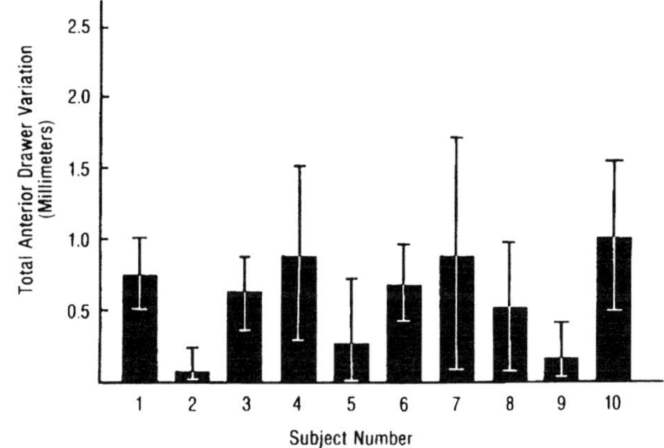

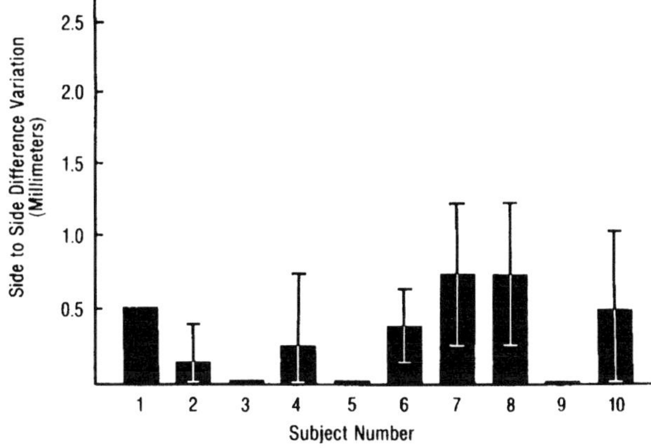

FIGURE 19.56. A single examiner (MLS) tested 10 normal subjects once a day on 5 different days. **A:** The 30°/20-lb anterior displacement test–retest variation for each subject. **B:** The 30°/20-lb anterior displacement right–left difference test–retest variation for each subject.

TABLE 19.7. *Test–retest variation of the displacement in the normal knee in ACL-injured patients*

	Percent of patients	
Millimeters of difference	20-lb test	Manual maximum test
≤1.0	60	59
≤2.0	87	83
≤3.0	97	94
≤4.0	100	100

The test interval was 6 to 36 months; n = 134.

underscores the importance of documenting reliability of any device, and any examiner, whose measurements are to be used for clinical care or research.

Queale et al. (49) investigated the reliability of knee laxity measurements using three different instrumented devices: the KT-2000, the Knee Signature System (KSS), and the Genucom Knee Analysis System to aid in the interpretation of instrumented laxity measurements during rehabilitation. Ten subjects with unilateral ACL deficiency were examined by two testers on two separate days. Measurement error was calculated as the minimum difference required to assume a true change in laxity between two measurements ($p < 0.05$). Between-day reliability was relatively high for both the KSS and the KT-2000 (0.95 and 0.83, respectively) but substantially lower for the Genucom (0.22). Intertester reliability was 0.92 for the KT-2000, 0.78 for the KSS, and 0.27 for the Genucom. The authors recommended that for monitoring changes in anterior laxity of ACL deficient knees, the following error values were determined necessary to assume a true difference between successive measurements: KT-2000, 2.0 mm; KSS, 4.2 mm; and Genucom, 5.9 mm.

Diagnosing Ligament Injury

Studies have shown considerable variation in anterior knee laxity among the normal population and among the uninjured knees of unilateral ACL-deficient patients (1,34,35,52,57,97). In a published report of A/P displacement testing with the KT-2000 (1), a single examiner measured 338 normal subjects (150 females and 188 males) between the ages of 15 and 45, and 87 patients with a unilateral ACL-disrupted knee. No significant differences were observed based on age or gender as illustrated in Figure 19.57. In another study, 6 different examiners each examined both knees of 20 normal subjects between the ages of 15 and 45 (10 males and 10 females) to produce the values for 240 individual examinations with the KT-1000 (Table 19.2, Fig. 19.58) (17).

ACL injuries do not always cause the same degree of anterior laxity. It was presumed that knees with greater laxity represented a greater degree of injury, either to the ACL alone or to a combination of other ligaments in addition to the ACL. But clinical studies have documented that isolated ACL injury can produce a wide range of laxity. Studies in cadaver knees have confirmed that surgical sectioning of the ACL produces a range of laxity that closely resembles the range of increases seen in clinical studies of isolated ACL injury (2,4,18–20). Figure 19.28 shows the distribution of increased laxity among cadaver knees after ACL sectioning (4). The variation in measured laxity in ACL-deficient knees exceeds the variability of ACL-intact knees. The clinical utility of knee laxity measurement systems for diagnosing and managing ACL injury depends on the distributions of

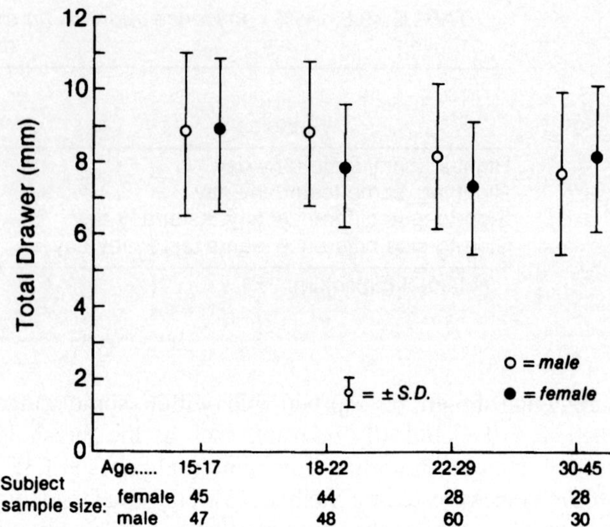

FIGURE 19.57. Total anterior–posterior displacement with an 89 N (20 lb) displacement force (in the normal population). Measurements were obtained with the KT-2000. The device is similar to the KT-1000. The displacement is printed on an X-Y plotter as a load-displacement curve.

both the injured and the non-injured population, and the overlap between the two.

Let us assume that a system produces measurements that are both accurate and reproducible. To maximize its value clinically, it may be desirable to refine the technique further or to perform computations on the raw measurements in order either to narrow the distributions of normal and abnormal values or to minimize the overlap between the two populations. Investigators have evaluated a number of approaches for this purpose. Figure 19.38 presents the normal and pathologic distributions of several parameters that have been used in evaluating ACL deficiency. The distributions represent actual data from 120 normal subjects and a group of unilateral ACL-deficient patients. The figure shows that the variability of the injured knees is greater than that observed in normal knees for all parameters. For the purpose of distinguishing the two populations from one another with as little overlap as possible, not all parameters have the same value. For example, the compliance index, or stiffness, and the quadriceps active test at 30° flexion are two parameters with little clinical utility because, as can be seen in Figure 19.38, they offer no advantage over the simpler and more easily reproduced displacement at 89 N passive force. Recording total A/P laxity has also been advocated by some authors because of concerns about locating the zero position during testing (36,57,62,98), but the practice is not widespread. Two approaches have been uniformly successful, and have become widely accepted. They are a) increasing the applied force (17,52,57,94), which generates greater displacements, particularly in ACL-deficient knees; and b) recording side-to-side differences (1,17,34,43,52,57).

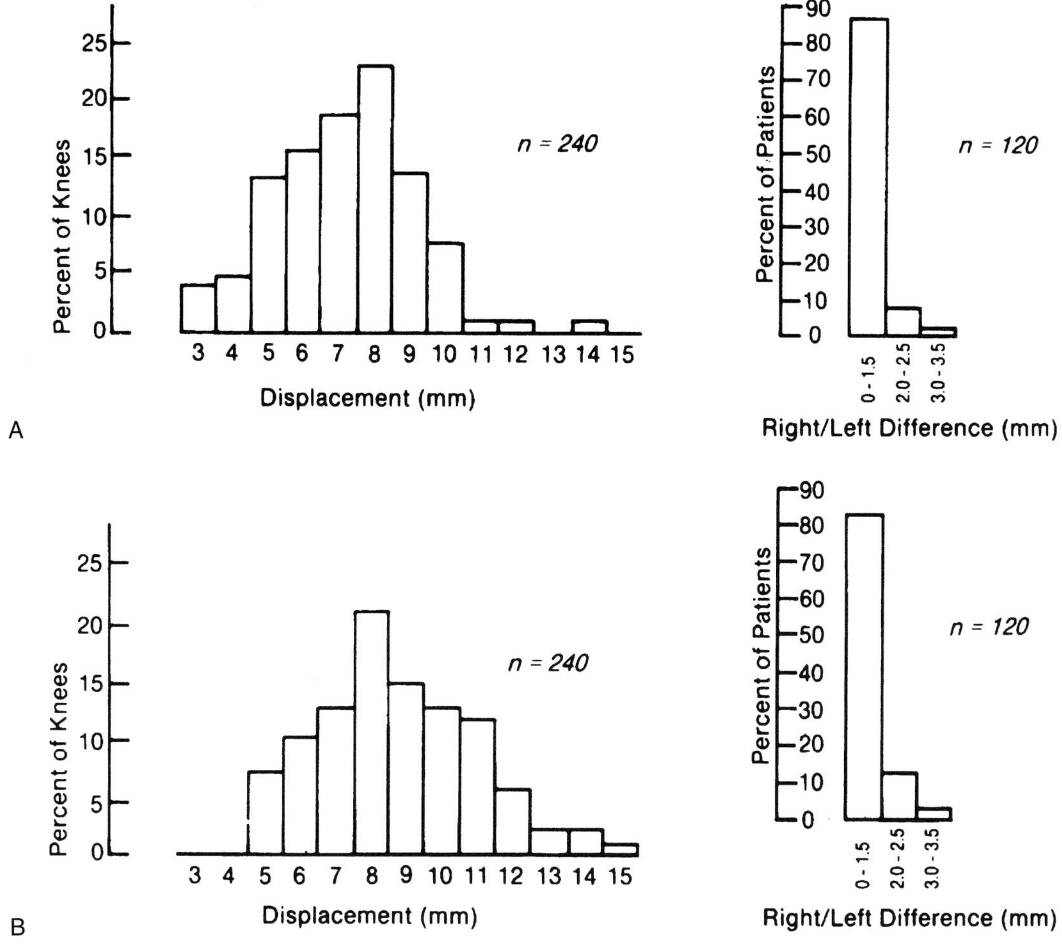

FIGURE 19.58. Displacement measurements in normal subjects. Six examiners each examined different patients—10 healthy males and 10 healthy females, between 15 and 45 years old. There were a total of 120 normal subjects. **A:** 30°/20-lb. anterior displacement. **B:** 30°/manual maximum test.

Increasing the force applied to the knee takes advantage of differences in compliance between normal and ACL-deficient knees. The ACL-deficient knee is more compliant, i.e., less stiff, in response to anterior tibial force than an intact knee (Fig. 19.35). Normal knees show only slight incremental displacement in response to loads greater than 89 N. In their study of KT-2000 arthrometry in 30 healthy adults, Myer and co-workers noted approximately 1 mm additional displacement for each incremental increase in applied force between 67 N and manual maximum force in normal knees (68). Markolf et al. reported an increase from 5.5 to 10 mm total anteroposterior laxity with an increase in applied force from 100 N to 200 N (52). Furthermore, they noted that differences in laxity between normal and chronic ACL-deficient knees were more reliably demonstrated at 200 N force than at 100 N force. Daniel also observed that manual maximum force resulted in greater measured displacements, greater side-to-side displacement differences, and was more effective than 89 N force in correctly identifying patients with ACL rupture (17). Figure

19.36 shows typical responses to increasing displacement loads of normal and ACL-deficient knees. Note that, whether side-to-side comparisons or raw displacement measurements are used, greater force results in greater pathologic motion, and less overlap between normal and ACL-deficient patients (Fig. 19.38).

The second approach is to compare the injured knee to the contralateral uninjured knee. Obviously, this approach is only applicable to patients with at least one uninjured knee. But in such cases, side-to-side comparisons are now firmly established as the most effective way to control for individual variation, reduce measurement error and optimize diagnostic correctness. Among a group of high school players examined by MLS and the late Dale Daniel (Table 19.3) (88), no subject had a right-left difference of greater than 2.5 mm in more than one examination by either examiner. Results of KT-1000 arthrometry in normal subjects have been reported by Sherman (67), Daniel (1,17), Bach (99), Steiner (13). For all tests reported by these investigators, greater than 95% of normal subjects had a right-left difference of less than 3 mm.

Six different examiners each examined 20 normal subjects between the age of 15 and 45 (ten males and ten females) to produce the values for 120 normal subjects tested with the KT-1000 reported by Daniel (Table 19.2, Fig. 19.58) (1,17). One hundred sixteen of the 120 patients (97%) had a right-left difference of less than 3 mm on all anterior displacement tests (20 lb, manual maximum, and quadriceps active). Several studies have reported the likelihood of observing more than 2.5 mm displacement difference comparing knees in normal individuals using the KT-1000 is less than 5% (Fig. 19.58) (17,67,99). Rangger et al. studied right-left differences among 120 normal individuals, reporting it to be less than 3 mm in 98% for the 89 N test and 97% for the manual maximum test (44). The authors recommended that an evaluation should always include testing of both limbs, so that side-to-side differences may be calculated. Figure 19.38 also presents measurements in a sample of patients with chronic unilateral ACL disruption.

Liu (92) and Strand (93) evaluated clinical examination and ligament arthrometry using the KT-1000 in diagnosing acute ACL injuries. Both papers reported a higher percentage of subjects with greater than 3-mm side-to-side displacement difference at manual maximum than at 89 N force. In Liu's study, diagnostic sensitivity was increased from 87% to 97%; Strand reported an increase from 24% to 88%. It is recommended for greatest diagnostic accuracy to apply manual maximum force and use 3-mm side-to-side displacement difference as the minimum diagnostic threshold for identifying complete ACL rupture.

Normal Subjects

It has been extremely useful to measure the limits of normal knee laxity *in vivo*. For example, it has been established that the laxity in the uninjured knee of unilateral ACL-deficient patients does not differ significantly from the measured laxity in the normal population (1,13, 17,35,40,57,62,64,99). This fact allows the uninjured knee to serve as the patient's own control when evaluating an individual with a unilateral knee injury. Because there is considerable variability among uninjured knees in the normal population, the ability to compare the injured knee to the uninjured knee allows us to establish a range of "normal" laxity (95% confidence interval) that is unique for an individual patient. As we shall see below, this improves the reliability and diagnostic accuracy of most instrumented devices.

Examination of normal control subjects and patients' uninjured knees also provides our best opportunity for evaluating the reliability of instrumented devices. Because it is difficult and costly to check accuracy, most studies rely heavily on measures of precision in evaluating these instruments (13,39,40,41,63,64,68,99). Normal control and uninjured knee laxity have been shown to be stable over time using a variety of different arthrometry systems (41,64,68,91) (Fig. 19.59). Therefore, the repro-

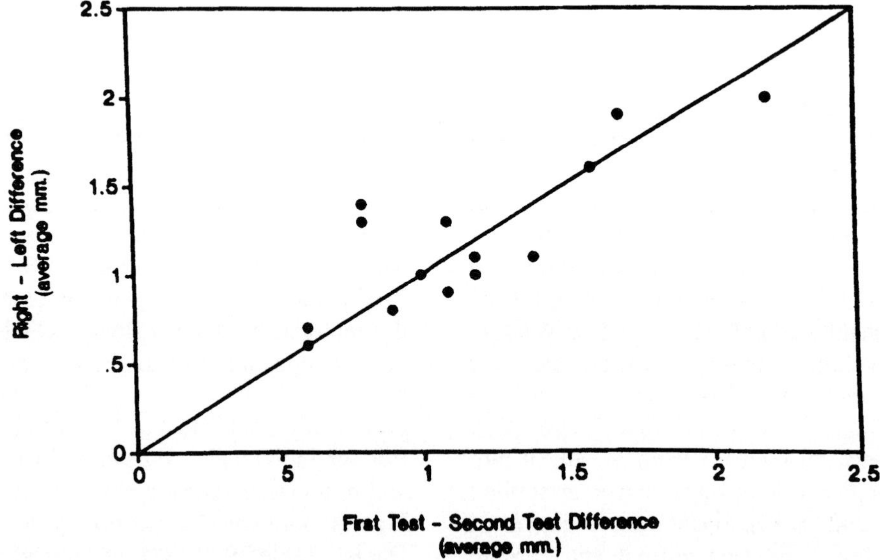

FIGURE 19.59. For normal subjects only, the difference in displacement between the right and left knee is plotted relative to the difference in displacement between the first and second tests on the same knee. Each point is the average measurement for a particular device, direction of displacement (anterior or posterior), and force (89 N or 133 N). The difference in displacement between the right and left knees tended to increase when a test or device had poorer reproducibility of measurement. In the normal subjects, the difference in displacement between the right and left knees increased as the test variability increased (correlation coefficient $= 0.743$, $p < 0.01$).

ducibility of measurements in normal knees provides perhaps the best measure of reliability routinely available to investigators and clinicians. Using measurements obtained in normal knees, Steiner and co-workers made an important discovery that unfortunately has gone largely unnoticed in subsequent literature. The authors examined the relationship between side-to-side differences of normal subjects, and the test-to-test variation of measurements in the same knee of those same subjects. Their findings, summarized in Figure 19.59, showed a strong correlation between side-to-side difference and test-retest variability. That is, side-to side difference in the normal population is a measure of instrument precision. By comparing these parameters among the devices used, they were able to show that some devices registered higher side-to-side differences among normal knees. These same devices were inferior in their ability to distinguish normal from ACL-injured patients, and demonstrated higher test-retest variability than other devices. In other words, examining normal knees with instrumented devices provides practical feedback on the utility and reliability of the devices being used. It may be more convenient to study knee laxity among patients with no ligament injury, and the side-to-side comparisons provide information very similar to that provided by serial examination of uninjured knees over time. Table 19.1 summarizes the variability of measured side-to-side differences in normal populations in several published studies of commercial devices. The results support the finding by Steiner that the KT-1000 and Stryker systems are superior to other systems with respect to the precision of anteroposterior laxity measurement.

This approach can also be used to evaluate the proficiency of an individual examiner such as a clinician. Again, Steiner (13) observed that for each device the variability of side-to-side comparisons in normal knees correlated strongly with the variability over time in normal knees. This implies that measuring side-to-side differences in a sample of subjects with normal knees can provide a quality measure, a test of proficiency, for an examiner with a given device.

It seems reasonable to suggest that an examiner's measurements in *uninjured* knees should be stable within 2.5 mm over time if their measurements are to be presented as outcome data. To document the test-retest variation by a single skilled examiner with the KT-1000, author MLS examined 10 normal subjects on five different days without reference to her previous examinations. The test/retest variations were seldom greater than a millimeter (Fig. 19.56). MLS has tested patients with a unilateral anterior cruciate ligament disruption at 6- to 12-month intervals for 3 years. The first examination was performed within 2 weeks of injury. Table 19.7 presents the test/retest variation of the displacement in the normal knee between the patient's first examination and last examination. The test/retest variation is less than 2.5 mm

in 87% of patients with the 89 N test and 83% of subjects with the manual maximum test. Author MLS and the late Dale M. Daniel each independently examined a 34-player high school football team (Table 19.3). MLS consistently recorded higher displacements than did DMD. All three examinations (89 N anterior displacement, manual maximum anterior displacement, QAT) were performed by both examiners on all patients. Myrer determined absolute and relative reliability of the KT-2000 ligament arthrometer (68). The results of that study are summarized in Table 19.6, and which gives 95% confidence intervals for various load levels. These data allow us to extrapolate from published studies or from our practice the range of possible laxity values for a given knee on any given day by any given examiner.

Unilateral Chronic Anterior Cruciate Ligament Disruption

A number of authors have reported the results of instrumented testing of patients with ACL injury with commercially available devices. Some of the reports are presented in Table 19.4. Table 19.5 presents the results of two examiners independently testing patients with a unilateral ACL disruption. Both examiners recorded a right-left difference of greater than 2.5 mm on all patients by at least one examination. The recorded mean right-left displacement differences were similar. The same two examiners also examined independently 23 patients with a unilateral ACL disruption that had been reconstructed (Table 19.8). The mean right-left differences and number of patients with a right-left difference of greater than 2.5 mm for the two examiners were similar. We have routinely tested patients having ACL surgery in the clinic at the time of their preoperative evaluation (Fig. 19.60) and again under anesthesia before surgery. Data from our clinic as well as data from ten centers participating in the LAD ACL reconstruction study are presented in Table 19.4. At the conclusion of the surgical procedure, after

TABLE 19.8. *Evaluation of 23 ACL-reconstructed patients: comparison of two examiners' displacement measurement*

Test	Millimeters of anterior displacement (mean ± SD)	
	Examiner MLS	Examiner DMD
20 lb		
Reconstructed knee	11.0 ± 2.5	8.7 ± 2.7
Contralateral knee	8.3 ± 1.9	6.3 ± 2.5
R-L difference	2.7 ± 1.8	2.4 ± 2.7
Number >2.5 mm	13 (56%)	10 (43%)
Manual maximum		
R-L difference	3.7 ± 2.1	3.2 ± 2.3
Number >2.5 mm	15 (65%)	16 (70%)

Measurements were obtained with the KT-1000. The knee flexion angle was 20° to 35°.

Acute R-L difference (mm)
mean = 2.7mm

	< 2	2.0-2.5	3-5	5.5-7.5	> 7.5
< 2	26	5	2		
2.0-2.5	10	4	9		
3-5	6	10	33	9	
5.5-7.5	3	3	11	8	
> 7.5				2	2

(Row labels: Follow up R-L difference (mm), mean - 3.4mm)

Acute R-L difference (mm)
mean = 4.9mm

	< 3	3-5	5.5-7.5	8-10	> 10
< 3	29	5			
3-5	3	17	13	6	2
5.5-7.5	1	12	17	6	3
8-10	1	5	4	7	2
> 10	1	2	3	3	1

(Row labels: Follow up R-L difference (mm), mean - 5.0mm)

FIGURE 19.60. One hundred forty-three patients with a unilateral acute knee injury. Measurements were made in the clinic within 14 days of injury. Follow-up measurements were made 6 to 60 months after injury (mean = 19 months). The right–left difference measured acutely is compared with the R-L difference measured at follow-up examination. **Top:** 20-lb test. **Bottom:** Manual maximum test.

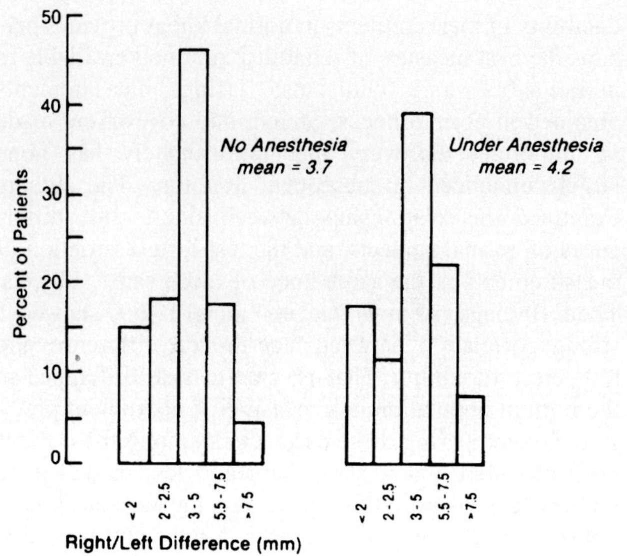

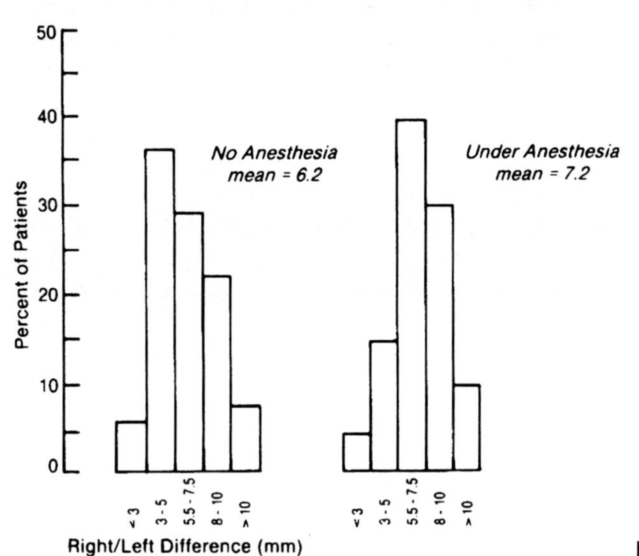

FIGURE 19.61. Examination of 125 patients with a unilateral acute anterior cruciate ligament disruption confirmed at arthroscopy. **A:** 30°/20-lb displacement force. **B:** 30°/manual maximum displacement force.

wound closure, we apply a sterile adhesive plastic drape to isolate the knee, and repeat the displacement measurements using the KT-1000 (Table 19.4). If the side-to-side difference is 3 mm or greater, the graft is re-tensioned and re-fixed.

Unilateral Acute Anterior Cruciate Ligament Disruption

We routinely perform KT-1000 measurements in the clinic on patients with suspected ACL disruptions. To allow better stabilization of the patella, we aspirate the knee before testing if we estimate that the patient has an effusion of greater than 50 mL. Frequently the examiner must spend a little time coaching the patient to relax and demonstrating that the examination is not going to be painful. Patients who have received an injury to the patella may not tolerate the pressure needed to stabilize the patella sensor. The normal knee is tested prior to testing the injured knee. Data on 125 confirmed acute ACL disruptions is presented in Figure 19.61. In a report from

The Hospital for Special Surgery, Bach (99) reported the clinic measurements of 107 acute ACL disruptions revealed a side-to-side difference of 3 mm or greater in 69% of patients on the 20-lb test and 87% on the manual maximum. In 1985 we added a 30 lb anterior force to our testing routine. This test reveals greater displacement than the 20 lb, but less than the manual maximum (Fig. 19.62). If the injured minus normal knee displacement difference on any of the four tests routinely performed (20 lb, 30 lb, manual maximum and QAT) is 3 mm or greater, the likelihood of a cruciate ligament disruption is greater than 95%. Both an ACL-injured knee and a PCL-injured knee may result in an increased anterior displacement measured from the supine 30° resting position (53). An ACL-injured knee will have an increased anterior

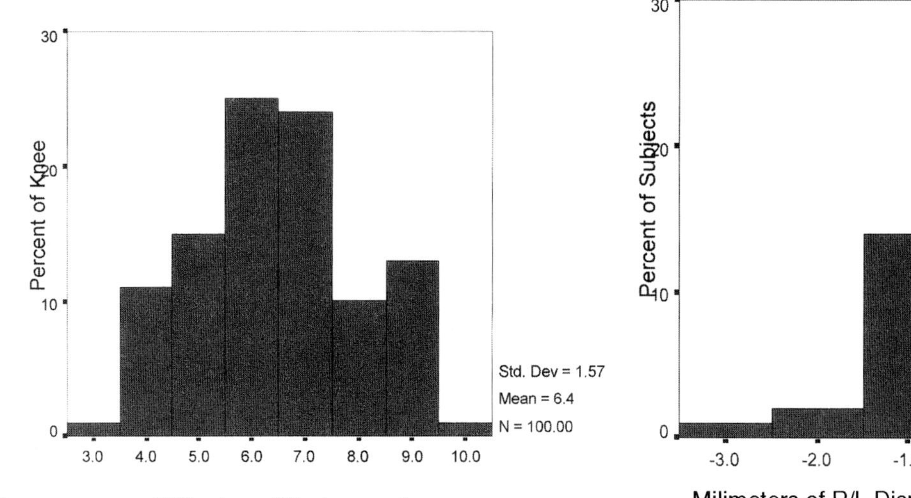

FIGURE 19.62. KT-1000 30-lb anterior force test on normal knees/degree flexion on normal knees.

compliance and a PCL-injured knee will have increased posterior compliance. The most diagnostic sign of a PCL disruption is demonstration of posterior sag in 90° of flexion and demonstration of an increased posterior displacement from the anatomic position at or near the quadriceps neutral angle. Figure 19.61 presents follow-up examinations on 143 patients with acute traumatic hemarthrosis. Not all of the patients had an ACL tear and none have undergone knee reconstruction. Eighty-five percent (65/76) with an acute 20-lb right-to-left (R-L) difference of 3 mm or greater acutely had a R-L difference of 3 mm or greater at follow-up. Ninety-five percent (103/108) with a manual maximum R-L difference of 3 mm or greater acutely had a follow-up R-L difference of 3 mm or greater.

Foreman (86) reviewed 30 patients with arthroscopically confirmed partial ACL tears from our clinic. On acute examination, 14 patients had normal displacement measurements (the R-L difference on the 20 lb, manual maximum, and QAT was less than 3 mm on all tests), and 16 had pathologic displacement measurements (on at least one test the R-L difference was 3 mm or greater). Follow-up measurements 1 year after injury revealed 13 of 14 patients with normal acute displacement measurements had normal measurements at follow-up and all patients with pathologic measurements acutely had pathologic measurements at follow-up. The function in the patients with normal measurements was better than those with pathologic measurements. Figure 19.63 compares the displacement measurements in patients who are coping with an ACL disruption to those who are not coping. The 20-lb (89 N) load was selected as a standard test by Malcom and Daniel in 1980 (1,17) because it was a low load that, in cadaveric studies, consistently revealed an increase in anterior tibial displace-

ment after the ACL was disrupted (Fig. 19.28), yet was well tolerated by acutely injured patients.

Instrumented Measurement in Children

ACL disruption has been reported with increasing frequency among patients with open growth plates. Whereas patients under 12 years old usually experience avulsion of the tibial eminence, in the adolescent patient, ACL rupture usually represents a mid-substance ACL tear. Ligament arthrometry is thought to be useful not only in establishing the diagnosis of ACL injury, but for documenting the amount of knee instability resulting from the disruption (100). Lo recommended the routine use of ligament arthrometry in evaluating knee injuries among children and adolescents (100). Unfortunately, there are only limited data available on the range of laxity normally present in this population. It may not be valid to extrapolate from studies of adult knee laxity when diagnosing ligament injuries in immature patients.

The design of the KT-1000 assumes a tibial length of at least 31cm. A modified version, called the KT-1000 Jr. is designed for use in smaller patients, where the tibial length is at least 27 cm. The tibia is at least 27 cm in 98% of all subjects (boys and girls) aged 10 years or older. For a significant proportion of patients younger than 10 years of age, even the KT-1000 Jr. will be too large. Theoretically at least, other devices such as the Stryker Laxity Tester can be used for any sized knee. However, all existing commercially available devices would require specific modifications for use in this age group also because of the supports and frames used to stabilize the limb, the location of measurement, and so on. Age-specific testing is also needed to define the limits of normal anteroposterior knee motion.

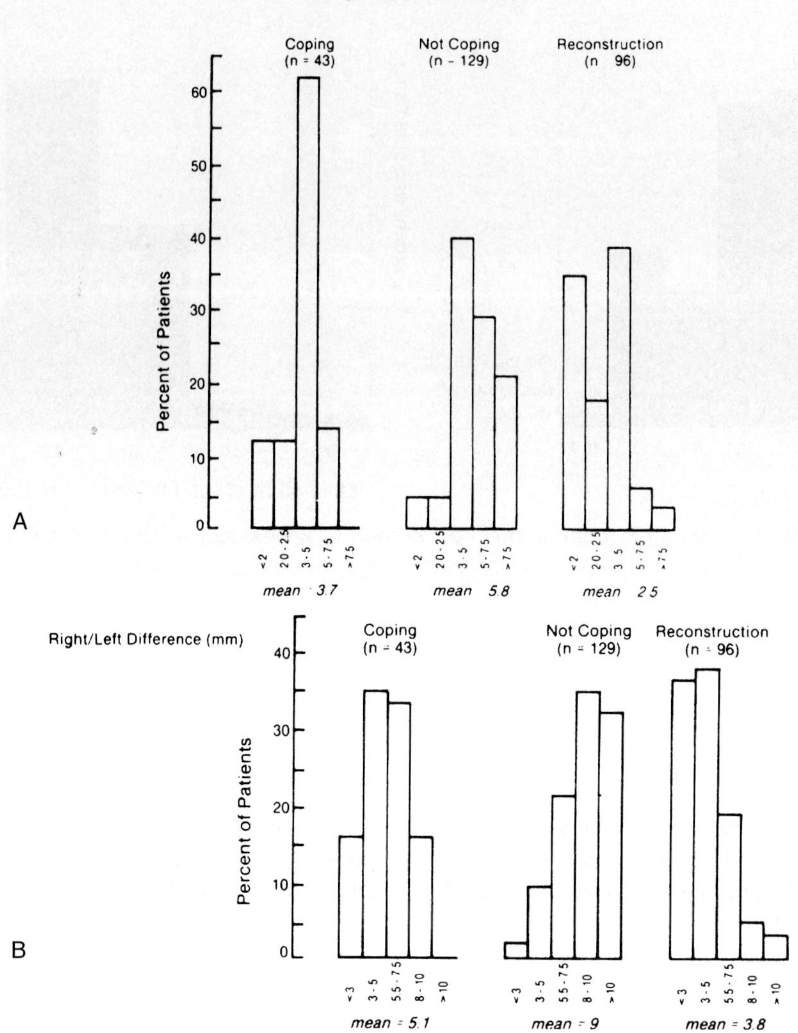

FIGURE 19.63. Measurements in three populations with a chronic anterior cruciate ligament (ACL) disruption. **A:** 20-lb test. **B:** Manual maximum test. The coping patients are patients with a unilateral chronic ACL disruption who are participating in a running sport, having none or infrequent giving way episodes and are not asking for an ACL reconstruction. The not coping patients have a chronic unilateral ACL disruption and are asking for a reconstruction. The reconstruction patients are 2 years post-ACL reconstruction. Note that most coping patients have 20-lb R-L difference of 0 to 5 mm and a manual maximum R-L difference of 0 to 7.5 mm. In contrast, half of the not coping have a 20-lb R-L difference of greater than 5 mm and most have a manual maximum R-L difference greater than 7.5 mm.

Flynn reported examining 300 knees in 150 normal children aged 6 to 18 years old to assess variations in anteroposterior knee laxity by age and gender. Paired measurements with the full-sized KT-1000 and the KT Jr. showed no difference in laxity measurements between the two devices. No difference was observed between males and females. There was a slight negative correlation between laxity and age. The effect was gradual throughout the age range studied. The authors concluded that younger children had slightly greater laxity than older children. Flynn reported the side-to-side (Right-minus-Left) difference only at 30 lb force. The standard error of

the mean was only 1.27 mm, indicating that the mean R-L difference should be less than 3 mm in greater than 98% of subjects. It may be concluded from their data that a side-to-side difference of 3 mm may be used as the diagnostic threshold for children.

Flynn emphasized the importance of patient relaxation in achieving reliable measurements in children. This cannot be overemphasized regardless of the age of subjects, but it can be particularly problematic in children. Flynn's study excluded an unspecified number of subjects whose "inability to relax and cooperate precluded an accurate, reproducible KT1000 evaluation" (101).

Posterior Testing

In 1988, Daniel introduced instrumented measurement for the detection of posterior knee instability (58). Early reports by Daniel (58) and Anderson (40) demonstrated the KT-1000 to be both sensitive and specific in diagnosing PCL rupture. Later studies have supported the diagnostic value of KT-1000 testing in PCL deficiency (102,103), and a number of studies of surgically treated PCL deficient knees have reported results of instrumented testing (104–112). Yet instrumented measurement still is not commonly used for evaluating PCL deficiency. Today, use of instrumented systems for evaluation of PCL injury remains controversial and limited to only a few centers. There are several reasons why ligament arthrometry has not caught on for the clinical evaluation of PCL deficiency. First, the technique requires practice as well as an above-average understanding of knee kinematics. Second, there are lingering questions about measurement precision and accuracy, and diagnostic accuracy, compared to stress radiography. Finally, there is some question as to whether objective laxity, measured with the KT-1000, in PCL-deficient patients is related to subjective patient outcomes (113).

The literature presents conflicting data as to whether the KT-1000 is as accurate as stress radiography in *diagnosing* PCL ruptures. Mathiak et al. (103) evaluated 18 patients with KT-1000 and stress x-ray 2 to 13 years after surgical treatment for ruptures of the PCL. Knee arthrometer testing was done at 90° knee flexion, with loads of 67 N and 89 N. Stress radiographs used a lateral projection at 90° knee flexion, with an applied force of 134 N. Results were classified only as "normal" and "PCL deficient." Both methods yielded good diagnostic accuracy for detecting residual posterior laxity, and the diagnostic results corresponded in 89% of patients. The authors found no difference in the diagnostic accuracy of the techniques, and recommended ligament arthrometry because it does avoids ionizing radiation.

Hewett et al. (114) compared stress radiography to KT-1000 arthrometry in 21 patients with unilateral partial (11 patients) and complete (ten patients) posterior cruciate ligament tears diagnosed by arthroscopy or MRI. For stress radiographic measurements, an 89 N posterior load was applied to the proximal tibia at 70° of flexion. The relative amount of sagittal translation (involved minus noninvolved) was determined at both the medial and lateral tibial plateaus from the radiographs. Arthrometric measurements with the KT-1000 were done according to the method of Wroble (64), which places the knee at 25° of knee flexion. The mean relative posterior translation measured radiographically averaged 12.2 ± 3.7 mm for knees with complete tears. Arthrometer testing of the same knees showed 7.6 ± 2.5 mm of increased translation. Stress radiographic side-to-side differences were statistically similar to the differences in electrogoniomet-

ric measurements before and after PCL section in an unspecified number of cadaveric knees. KT-1000 testing with their testing protocol consistently underestimated the amount of posterior translation compared to stress radiographs. It is not clear whether this was due to measurement error inherent to the testing device, or to differences in the positioning of the knees between the radiographic and arthrometric protocols. The authors did not state whether radiographic magnification was corrected as part of the protocol, and correlation of measurement results between the two methods was not analyzed in order to derive a conversion factor. Arthrometric measurements were not compared to electrogoniometric measurements in the cadaver knees, which is unfortunate. In studies comparing measurement accuracy with two different techniques, it is essential for all parameters except the measurement itself be kept constant. From this study it cannot be said which is the more accurate technique to evaluate posterior knee laxity, only that greater displacements were recorded with the stress x-ray technique.

Measurement accuracy of the KT-1000 at the QNA has not been studied. Huber (102) assessed the reliability of the device at the QNA in the knees of 22 subjects with posterior cruciate ligament tears or reconstructions. Two testers, one experienced and the other a novice, made two measurements for each study subject. The intraclass correlation coefficient values for the novice, experienced, and inter-tester reliability were 0.67, 0.79, and 0.62, respectively, for corrected posterior translation. Ninety-five percent confidence intervals for the novice, experienced, and inter-tester reliability were ±2.95, ±2.53, and ±3.27 mm, respectively, for corrected posterior translation. The KT-1000 arthrometer was found to be a moderately reliable tool for the measurement of tibial translation in patients with PCL tears and reconstructions. Huber's data indicate that an experienced tester's measurements are precise enough to diagnose PCL rupture and estimate the degree of instability resulting from the injury. This is the only study that reports measurement precision (intra-tester and inter-tester reliability) with the knee position and measurement protocol as was originally described by Daniel (58).

Finally, a clear link between the degree of posterior instability and subjective symptoms has not been established for injuries involving the PCL. While it is not essential, it obviously would be desirable to document a correlation between the degree of posterior instability and the severity of patients' symptoms. Shelbourne et al. (113) observed 68 patients for an average of 5.4 years (range, 2.3–11.4) after acute isolated PCL rupture. There was no change in objective laxity from initial injury to follow-up. Objective laxity measurements with the KT-1000 and stress radiography were correlated with an ordinal scale (115) used to grade posterior laxity. No correlation was found between radiographic joint space narrowing and grade of laxity. Patients with higher laxity grades did not have worse subjective scores. Regardless of the grade of laxity, one half of the patients returned to the same sport at the same or higher level, one third returned to the same sport at a lower level, and one sixth did not return to the same sport. The researchers concluded that patients with acute isolated PCL tears treated nonoperatively achieved a level of objective and subjective knee function that is independent of the grade of laxity. It is uncertain whether the results of the analysis were affected by the authors' reliance on the rough, three level ordinal scale described by Rubinstein. The sequelae that may follow ligament injury, such as subjective instability, sports disability, and degenerative changes are complex and multifactorial in etiology. One would expect any relationship with the degree of laxity, if indeed it exists, to be relatively weak. It may nevertheless be significant. Further research is needed before a relationship is entirely ruled out. More quantitative measures of instability, such as ligament arthrometry or stress radiography, may prove more powerful in delineating such a relationship.

In the absence of clear and immediate benefits to the clinician, instrumented testing is often not used for the evaluation and management of PCL-injured patients. Given these lingering questions, most examiners use an ordinal grading scale of 0 to 3+ to record laxity in PCL deficiency (116). Rubinstein reported that orthopedists should be able to diagnosis PCL insufficiency with a high degree of diagnostic accuracy (115). Nevertheless it would be a mistake not to continue to refine methods for instrumented measurement. There can be little doubt that instrumented measurement has had a profound influence on the way we think about anterior knee instability. Progress in treatment of PCL insufficiency will be facilitated if we investigate techniques that allow us to measure, as accurately as possible, the relationship between PCL injury and knee function. It seems self-evident that some form of objective measurement, either by arthrometry or stress radiography, should be included in all clinical research on PCL injury and treatment if subjective outcomes are to be compared in any way to knee stability. More studies are needed to determine exactly what the level of accuracy is for stress radiographic and arthrometric laxity measurement.

SUMMARY

It would be fair to say that instrumented measurement of knee joint laxity has changed the way surgeons think about, document, and manage ligament injuries. Early in the development of instrumented measurement systems, the load needed to demonstrate joint instability was not known. A low load was selected to make the examination easy to perform, comfortable for the patient, and to minimize the risk for injury to repaired or reconstructed structures. However, it soon became apparent that a greater displacement force reveals a greater level of pathology. Especially in the acutely injured patient with a large limb, an anterior displacement force greater than 20 lb is often needed to reveal pathology. At follow-up after knee ligament surgery, low displacement force of 20 lb will not reveal the extent of pathologic motion that will be revealed by larger loads (Table 19.8).

Further testing has revealed that a 178 N load (40 lb) anterior displacement force applied through the KT-1000 handle frequently lifts the foot off the table, producing measurement error. A 134 N load (30 lb), we have found, improves anterior displacement diagnostic accuracy and is well-tolerated by the testing system, tester and patient. We continue to use the manual maximum test. Manual application of force to the proximal calf is more proximal than the force applied by pulling through the arthrometer handle. A more proximally applied load provides a greater rotation moment at the ankle, and therefore a greater anterior displacement. The examiner applies the force until the displacement stops, the knee begins to extend (foot rises off the table), or the patient begins to tighten the limb musculature. Performed by an experienced clinical examiner, the test produces the greatest anterior displacement of the standard arthrometer tests. However, the precise test load is not known and there is greater risk for inadvertently applying axial rotation moments to the limb than when loads are applied through the force handle.

KT-1000 measurements may be used to document the anterior-posterior knee motion and to diagnose cruciate ligament disruptions. The test begins with the assessment of posterior tibial sag at 90° of flexion which indicates a PCL disruption. If the PCL is disrupted, measurements are then performed at the quadriceps neutral angle. If the PCL is intact, measurements are performed at 30° of flexion to evaluate the ACL. Measurements at 30° of flexion are performed under five loading conditions: 15 lb, 20 lb, 30 lb, manual maximum and quadriceps contraction to lift the weight of the leg and testing device. In a unilaterally injured patient, a R-L difference less than 3 mm is classified as normal motion and a R-L difference on any test of 3 mm or greater is classified as pathologic motion. To obtain the greatest diagnostic accuracy and testing reproducibility, the patient must be relaxed, the instrument properly positioned, the patellar sensor stabilized against the patella, and the patella in the femoral trochlea. After each test a posterior load is applied and then released, after which the knee should return to the zero resting position. It is recommended that physicians, nurses, therapists, and technicians who plan to do KT-1000 testing receive formal instruction in KT-1000 testing and document their own test/retest reproducibility by testing a number of patients on different days.

For obtaining reliable measurements with any laxity measuring system, the importance of training and quality assessment cannot be overstated. For gaining experience and checking reliability, the value of testing normal knees, and repeat testing of both knees of injured patients. To document proficiency, users should measure side-to-side differences in a sample of subjects with normal knees and monitor the measurements of uninjured and injured knees in unilateral ligament-injured patients over time.

Instrumented measurement of knee laxity has undergone extensive scientific testing. It clearly has value both to the clinician and to the scientist studying ligament injuries. Yet all systems are not equivalent in their accuracy or precision, and there is room for improvement in even the most useful devices. New devices have been introduced that have not been tested thoroughly at this time. They should be examined in the laboratory and in the clinic. History has shown us certain design principles that work, but the accuracy of new devices cannot be considered a foregone conclusion. The clinical validation of these systems is not a trivial affair.

REFERENCES

1. Daniel DM, et al. Instrumented measurement of anterior laxity of the knee. *J Bone Joint Surg Am* 1985;67:720–726.
2. Fleming BC, et al. Clinical versus instrumented knee testing on autopsy specimens. *Clin Orthop* 1992;282:196–207.
3. Markolf KL, Mensch JS, Amstutz HC. Stiffness and laxity of the knee—the contributions of the supporting structures. A quantitative in vitro study. *J Bone Joint Surg Am* 1976;58:583–594.
4. Shoemaker SC, Daniel DM. The limits of knee motion. In vitro studies. In: Daniel DM, Akeson WH, O'Connor JJ, eds. *Knee ligaments: structure, function, injury, and repair.* New York: Raven Press, 1990: 153–161.
5. Fetto JF, Marshall JL. The natural history and diagnosis of anterior cruciate ligament insufficiency. *Clin Orthop* 1980;147:29–38.
6. Torg JS, Conrad W, Kalen V. Clinical diagnosis of anterior cruciate ligament instability in the athlete. *Am J Sports Med* 1976;4:84–93.
7. Anderson AF, Lipscomb AB. Preoperative instrumented testing of anterior and posterior knee laxity. *Am J Sports Med* 1989;17: 387–392.
8. DeHaven KE. Arthroscopy in the diagnosis and management of the anterior cruciate ligament deficient knee. *Clin Orthop* 1983;172:52–56.
9. Donaldson WF, Warren RF, Wickiewicz T. A comparison of acute anterior cruciate ligament examinations. Initial versus examination under anesthesia. *Am J Sports Med* 1985;13:5–10.
10. Jonsson T, et al. Clinical diagnosis of ruptures of the anterior cruciate ligament: a comparative study of the Lachman test and the anterior drawer sign. *Am J Sports Med* 1982;10:100–102.
11. Katz JW, Fingeroth RJ. The diagnostic accuracy of ruptures of the anterior cruciate ligament comparing the Lachman test, the anterior drawer sign, and the pivot shift test in acute and chronic knee injuries. *Am J Sports Med* 1986;14:88–91.
12. Daniel DM. Assessing the limits of knee motion. *Am J Sports Med* 1991;19:139–147.
13. Steiner ME, et al. Measurement of anterior-posterior displacement of the knee. A comparison of the results with instrumented devices and with clinical examination. *J Bone Joint Surg Am* 1990;72:1307–1315.
14. Marks JS, et al. Observer variation in examination of knee joints. *Ann Rheum Dis* 1978;37:376–377.
15. Pope M, et al. Variations in the examination of the medial collateral ligament of the knee. *Clin Biomech* 1987;2:71–73.
16. Bach B, et al. KT-100 evaluation of normal, acute and chronic anterior cruciate ligament deficient knees. *J Bone Joint Surg* 1990;72A:9.
17. Daniel DM, et al. Instrumented measurement of anterior knee laxity in patients with acute anterior cruciate ligament disruption. *Am J Sports Med* 1985;13:401–407.
18. Hole RL, et al. Increased tibial translation after partial sectioning of the anterior cruciate ligament. The posterolateral bundle. *Am J Sports Med* 1996;24:556–560.
19. Lintner DM, et al. Partial tears of the anterior cruciate ligament. Are they clinically detectable? (see comments). *Am J Sports Med* 1995;23: 111–118.
20. Wright RW, Luhmann SJ. The effect of knee effusions on KT-1000 arthrometry. A cadaver study (see comments). *Am J Sports Med* 1998; 26:571–574.
21. Clancy WG Jr, Ray JM, Zoltan DJ. Acute tears of the anterior cruciate ligament. Surgical versus conservative treatment. *J Bone Joint Surg Am* 1988;70:1483–1488.
22. Daniel DM, Fithian DC. Indications for ACL surgery. *Arthroscopy* 1994;10:434–441.
23. Daniel DM, et al. A ten-year prospective outcome study of the ACL-injured patient. OREF Clinical Research Award, 1995.
24. Daniel DM, et al. Fate of the ACL-injured patient. A prospective outcome study (see comments). *Am J Sports Med* 1994;22:632–644.
25. Meunier A, et al. Osteoarthritis after surgical or conservative treatment of the acutely torn anterior cruciate ligament—a randomized study with 15 years follow-up. *Acta Orthop Scand* 1999;suppl 287.
26. Chick RR, Jackson DW. Tears of the anterior cruciate ligament in young athletes. *J Bone Joint Surg Am* 1978;60:970–973.
27. Kannus P, Jarvinen M. Knee ligament injuries in adolescents. Eight year follow-up of conservative management. *J Bone Joint Surg Br* 1988;70:772–776.
28. Markolf KL, et al. Instrumented measurements of laxity in patients who have a Gore-Tex anterior cruciate-ligament substitute. *J Bone Joint Surg Am* 1989;71:887–893.
29. Sprague RB, Asprey GM. Photographic method for measuring knee stability: a preliminary report. *Phys Ther* 1965;45:1055–1058.
30. Jacobsen K. Stress radiographical measurement of the anteroposterior, medial and lateral stability of the knee joint. *Acta Orthop Scand* 1976; 47:335–343.
31. Kennedy JC, Fowler PJ. Medial and anterior instability of the knee: an anatomical and clinical study using stress machines. *J Bone Joint Surg Am* 1971;53:1257–1270.
32. Staubli HU, Jakob RP. Anterior knee motion analysis. Measurement and simultaneous radiography. *Am J Sports Med* 1991;19:172–177.
33. Torzilli PA, Greenberg RL, Insall J. An in vivo biomechanical evaluation of anterior-posterior motion of the knee. Roentgenographic measurement technique, stress machine, and stable population. *J Bone Joint Surg Am* 1981;63:960–968.
34. Markolf KL, Graff-Radford A, Amstutz HC. In vivo knee stability. A quantitative assessment using an instrumented clinical testing apparatus. *J Bone Joint Surg Am* 1978;60:664–674.
35. Shino K, et al. Measurement of anterior instability of the knee. A new apparatus for clinical testing. *J Bone Joint Surg Br* 1987;69: 608–613.
36. Edixhoven P, et al. Accuracy and reproducibility of instrumented knee-drawer tests. *J Orthop Res* 1987;5:378–387.
37. Johnson RJ, Eriksson E, Haggmark T, et al. Five- to ten-year follow-up evaluation after reconstruction of the anterior cruciate ligament. *Clin Orthop* 1984;183:122–140.
38. Malcom LL, et al. The measurement of anterior knee laxity after ACL reconstructive surgery. *Clin Orthop* 1985;196:35–41.
39. Balasch H, et al. Evaluation of anterior knee joint instability with the Rolimeter: a test in comparison with manual assessment and measuring with the KT-1000 arthrometer (see comments). *Knee Surg Sports Traumatol Arthrosc* 1999;7:204–208.
40. Anderson AF, et al. Instrumented evaluation of knee laxity: a comparison of five arthrometers. *Am J Sports Med* 1992;20:135–140.
41. Steele JR, Roger GJ, Milburn PD. Reproducibility of knee laxity assessment results using the dynamic cruciate tester. *J Sci Med Sport* 1998;1:245–259.
42. Oliver JH, Coughlin LP. Objective knee evaluation using the Genucom knee analysis system: clinical implications. *Am J Sports Med* 1987;15:571–578.
43. Markolf KL, Amstutz HC. The clinical relevance of instrumented testing for ACL insufficiency: experience with the UCLA clinical knee testing apparatus. *Clin Orthop* 1987;223:198–207.
44. Rangger C, et al. Diagnosis of an ACL disruption with KT-1000 arthrometer measurements. *Knee Surg Sports Traumatol Arthrosc* 1993;1:60–66.
45. Fleming BC, Beynnon BD, Johnson RJ. The use of knee laxity testers for the determination of anterior-posterior stability of the knee. Pitfalls in practice. In: Jackson DW, et al., eds. *The anterior cruciate ligament: current and future concepts.* New York: Raven Press, 1993: 239–250.

46. Berry J, et al. Error estimates in novice and expert raters for the KT-1000 arthrometer. *J Orthop Sports Phys Ther* 1999;29:49–55.

47. King JB, Kumar SJ. The Stryker knee arthrometer in clinical practice (see comments). *Am J Sports Med* 1989;17:649–650.

48. Werlich T, et al. (The knee arthrometer KT-1000: value of instrumental measurement in diagnosis of complex anterior knee instability). *Aktuelle Traumatol* 1993;23:43–49.

49. Queale WS, et al. Instrumented examination of knee laxity in patients with anterior cruciate deficiency: a comparison of the KT-2000, knee signature system, and Genucom. *J Orthop Sports Phys Ther* 1994;19: 345–351.

50. Nielsen S, et al. Instability of cadaver knees after transection of capsule and ligaments. *Acta Orthop Scand* 1984;55:30–34.

51. Sullivan D, et al. Medial restrains to anterior-posterior motion of the knee. *J Bone Joint Surg Am* 1984;66:930–936.

52. Markolf KL, Kochan A, Amstutz HC. Measurement of knee stiffness and laxity in patients with documented absence of the anterior cruciate ligament. *J Bone Joint Surg Am* 1984;66:242–252.

53. Daniel DM, et al. A measurement of lower limb function. The one-leg-hop-for-distance. *Am J Knee Surg* 1988;1:212–214.

54. Rangger C, Daniel DM, Stone ML. (Instrumented measurement of ruptures of the anterior cruciate ligament). *Unfallchirurg* 1994;97: 462–466.

55. Daniel DM, Stone ML, Rangger C. Instrumented measurement of anterior-posterior knee motion. In: Aichroth PM, Cannon WD, Patel DV, eds. *Knee surgery: current practice.* 1992:188–205.

56. McQuade KJ, Sidles JA, Larson RV. Reliability of the Genucom knee analysis system. A pilot study. *Clin Orthop* 1989;245:216–219.

57. Andersson C, Gillquist J. Instrumented testing for evaluation of sagittal knee laxity. *Clin Orthop* 1990;256:178–184.

58. Daniel DM, et al. Use of the quadriceps active test to diagnose posterior cruciate-ligament disruption and measure posterior laxity of the knee. *J Bone Joint Surg Am* 1988;70:386–391.

59. Bargar WL, et al. The effect of tibia-foot rotatory position on the anterior drawer test. *Clin Orthop* 1983;173:200–203.

60. Noyes FR, et al. Advances in the understanding of knee ligament injury, repair, and rehabilitation. *Med Sci Sports Exerc* 1984;16:427–443.

61. Fukubayashi T, et al. An in vitro biomechanical evaluation of anterior-posterior motion of the knee. Tibial displacement, rotation, and torque. *J Bone Joint Surg Am* 1982;64:258–264.

62. Riederman R, et al. Reproducibility of the knee signature system. *Am J Sports Med* 1991;19:660–664.

63. Wroble RR, et al. Reproducibility of Genucom knee analysis system testing. *Am J Sports Med* 1990;18:387–395.

64. Wroble RR, et al. Repeatability of the KT-1000 arthrometer in a normal population. *Am J Sports Med* 1990;18:396–399.

65. Butler DL, Noyes FR, Grood ES. Ligamentous restraints to anterior-posterior drawer in the human knee. A biomechanical study. *J Bone Joint Surg Am* 1980;62:259–270.

66. Edixhoven P, Huiskes R, de Graaf R. Anteroposterior drawer measurements in the knee using an instrumented test device. *Clin Orthop* 1989;247:232–242.

67. Sherman OH, Markolf KL, Ferkel RD. Measurements of anterior laxity in normal and anterior cruciate absent knees with two instrumented test devices. *Clin Orthop* 1987;215:156–161.

68. Myrer JW, Schulthies SS, Fellingham GW. Relative and absolute reliability of the KT-2000 arthrometer for uninjured knees. Testing at 67, 89, 134, and 178 N and manual maximum forces. *Am J Sports Med* 1996;24:104–108.

69. Hsieh HH, Walker PS. Stabilizing mechanisms of the loaded and unloaded knee joint. *J Bone Joint Surg Am* 1976;58:87–93.

70. Markolf KL, et al. The role of joint load in knee stability. *J Bone Joint Surg Am* 1981;63:570–585.

71. Shoemaker SC, Markolf KL. Effects of joint load on the stiffness and laxity of ligament-deficient knees. An in vitro study of the anterior cruciate and medial collateral ligaments. *J Bone Joint Surg Am* 1985; 67:136–146.

72. Torzilli PA, et al. Measurement reproducibility of two commercial knee test devices. *J Orthop Res* 1991;9:730–737.

73. Baxter MP. Assessment of normal pediatric knee ligament laxity using the genucom. *J Pediatr Orthop* 1988;8:546–550.

74. Campbell JD. The evolution and current treatment trends with anterior cruciate, posterior cruciate, and medial collateral ligament injuries. *Am J Knee Surg* 1998;11:128–135.

75. Moore HA, Larson RL. Posterior cruciate ligament injuries. Results of early surgical repair. *Am J Sports Med* 1980;8:68–78.

76. Henning CE, Lynch MA, Glick KR Jr. An in vivo strain gage study of elongation of the anterior cruciate ligament. *Am J Sports Med* 1985; 13:22–26.

77. Daniel DM, et al. The quadriceps anterior cruciate interaction. *Orthop Trans* 1982;6:199–200.

78. Grood ES, et al. Biomechanics of the knee-extension exercise. Effect of cutting the anterior cruciate ligament. *J Bone Joint Surg Am* 1984; 66:725–734.

79. Lindahl O, Movin A. The mechanics of extension of the knee-joint. *Acta Orthop Scand* 1967;38:226–234.

80. Morrison JB. Bioengineering analysis of force actions transmitted by the knee joint. *Biomed Eng* 1968;3:164–170.

81. Nisell R. Mechanics of the knee. A study of joint and muscle load with clinical applications. *Acta Orthop Scand Suppl* 1985;216:1–42.

82. Smidt GL. Biomechanical analysis of knee flexion and extension. *J Biomech* 1973;6:79–92.

83. Goodfellow J, O'Connor J. The mechanics of the knee and prosthesis design. *J Bone Joint Surg Br* 1978;60-B(3):358–369.

84. Kapandji IA. *The physiology of the joints: annotated diagrams of the mechanics of the human joints.* 2nd ed. London: E & S Livingstone, 1974.

85. O'Connor JJ, et al. Mechanical interactions between the muscles and the cruciate ligaments in the knee. *Trans Orthop Res Soc* 1985;9:271.

86. Barnett P, et al. Posterior cruciate ligament/quadriceps interaction. *Orthop Trans* 1984;8:258.

87. Noyes FR, Grood ES, Torzilli PA. Current concepts review. The definitions of terms for motion and position of the knee and injuries of the ligaments (see comments). *J Bone Joint Surg Am* 1989;71:465–472.

88. Daniel DM, Stone ML. Instrumented measurement of knee motion. In: Daniel DM, Akeson WH, O'Connor JJ, eds. *Knee ligaments: structure, function, injury, and repair.* New York: Raven Press: 1990: 421–426.

89. Fiebert I., et al. Comparative measurements of anterior tibial translation using the KT-1000 knee arthrometer with the leg in neutral, internal rotation, and external rotation. *J Orthop Sports Phys Ther* 1994; 19:331–334.

90. Hanten WP, Pace MB. Reliability of measuring anterior laxity of the knee joint using a knee ligament arthrometer. *Phys Ther* 1987;67: 357–359.

91. Highgenboten CL, Jackson A, Meske NB. Genucom, KT-1000, and Stryker knee laxity measuring device comparisons. Device reproducibility and interdevice comparison in asymptomatic subjects. *Am J Sports Med* 1989;17:743–746.

92. Liu SH, et al. The diagnosis of acute complete tears of the anterior cruciate ligament. Comparison of MRI, arthrometry and clinical examination. *J Bone Joint Surg Br* 1995;77:586–588.

93. Strand T, Solheim E. Clinical tests versus KT-1000 instrumented laxity test in acute anterior cruciate ligament tears. *Int J Sports Med* 1995;16:51–53.

94. Highgenboten CL, et al. KT-1000 arthrometer: conscious and unconscious test results using 15, 20, and 30 pounds of force. *Am J Sports Med* 1992;20:450–454.

95. Jonsson H, Karrholm J, Elmqvist LG. Laxity after cruciate ligament injury in 94 knees. The KT-1000 arthrometer versus roentgen stereophotogrammetry. *Acta Orthop Scand* 1993;64:567–570.

96. Forster IW, Warren-Smith CD, Tew M. Is the KT1000 knee ligament arthrometer reliable? *J Bone Joint Surg Br* 1989;71:843–847.

97. Boniface RJ, Fu FH, Ilkhanipour K. Objective anterior cruciate ligament testing. *Orthopedics* 1986;9:391–393.

98. Mononen T, et al. Instrumented measurement of anterior-posterior translation in knees with chronic anterior cruciate ligament tear. *Arch Orthop Trauma Surg* 1997;116:283–286.

99. Bach BR Jr, et al. Arthrometric evaluation of knees that have a torn anterior cruciate ligament. *J Bone Joint Surg Am* 1990;72:1299–1306.

100. Lo IK, et al. The outcome of operatively treated anterior cruciate ligament disruptions in the skeletally immature child. *Arthroscopy* 1997; 13:627–634.

101. Flynn JM, et al. Objective evaluation of knee laxity in children. *J Pediatr Orthop* 2000;20:259–263.

102. Huber FE, et al. Intratester and intertester reliability of the KT-1000 arthrometer in the assessment of posterior laxity of the knee. *Am J Sports Med* 1997;25:479–485.

103. Mathiak G, Wening JV, Jungbluth KH. (Examinations with the KT-1000 knee arthrometer in injuries of the posterior cruciate ligament in comparison with stress roentgen images in the Scheuba positioning device). *Unfallchirurgie* 1995;21:118–123.

104. Aroen A, Strand T, Molster A. (Primary suture of the posterior cruciate ligament). *Tidsskr Nor Laegeforen* 1992;112:1582–1584.

105. Becker R, Ropke M, Nebelung W. (Clinical outcome of arthroscopic posterior cruciate ligament-plasty). *Unfallchirurg* 1999;102:354–358.

106. Fanelli GC, Giannotti BF, Edson CJ. Arthroscopically assisted combined anterior and posterior cruciate ligament reconstruction. *Arthroscopy* 1996;12:5–14.

107. Fanelli GC, Giannotti BF, Edson CJ. Arthroscopically assisted combined posterior cruciate ligament/posterior lateral complex reconstruction. *Arthroscopy* 1996;12:521–530.

108. Fowler PJ, Messieh SS. Isolated posterior cruciate ligament injuries in athletes. *Am J Sports Med* 1987;15:553–557.

109. Kim SJ, Kim HK, Kim HJ. Arthroscopic posterior cruciate ligament reconstruction using a one-incision technique. *Clin Orthop* 1999;359:156–166.

110. Lipscomb AB Jr, et al. Isolated posterior cruciate ligament reconstruction. Long-term results. *Am J Sports Med* 1993;21: 490–496.

111. Mariani PP, et al. Comparison of surgical treatments for knee dislocation. *Am J Knee Surg* 1999;12:214–221.

112. Wu JK, et al. Instrumented laxity test for the evaluation of posterior cruciate ligament reconstructed knee. *Kao Hsiung I Hsueh Ko Hsueh Tsa Chih* 1992;8:306–311.

113. Shelbourne KD, Davis TJ, Patel DV. The natural history of acute, isolated, nonoperatively treated posterior cruciate ligament injuries. A prospective study. *Am J Sports Med* 1999;27:276–283.

114. Hewett TE, Noyes FR, Lee MD. Diagnosis of complete and partial posterior cruciate ligament ruptures. Stress radiography compared with KT-1000 arthrometer and posterior drawer testing. *Am J Sports Med* 1997;25(5):648–655.

115. Rubinstein RA Jr, et al. The accuracy of the clinical examination in the setting of posterior cruciate ligament injuries. *Am J Sports Med* 1994;22:550–557.

116. Hughston JC, et al. Classification of knee ligament instabilities. Part I. The medial compartment and cruciate ligaments. *J Bone Joint Surg Am* 1976;58:159–172.

The Anterior Cruciate Ligament–Deficient Knee

Natural History and the Effects of Nonsurgical Treatment

Donald C. Fithian, David H. Goltz, and T. Tadashi Funahashi

NATURAL HISTORY OF THE ANTERIOR CRUCIATE LIGAMENT–DEFICIENT KNEE

To understand the effects of treatment of any condition, we must first understand the natural history of the condition itself. Once we have a firm grasp of the consequences of neglect or nontreatment, we can draw up reasonable guidelines and expectations for what is to be gained by intervention. Furthermore, we can weigh the effects of various levels of intervention, such as surgical or nonsurgical treatment, against the chances of failure or complications. The ideal natural history study of any specific acute knee ligament injury would identify all the patients who sustained this injury within a population. It would document definitively the presence of this injury and exclude or subcategorize patients with additional injuries (including other ligament injuries, fractures, chondral injuries, and meniscal injuries). It would follow up these patients over a long time without intervention and finally, it would assess the status of all these patients objectively, subjectively, and functionally at the conclusion. Of course, no such study has been done. Indeed, it may be surprising to see how far we are from the ideal. Nevertheless, there is much to be learned from the literature if we can understand the limitations imposed by study design and interpret results within the context of those limitations.

Like most problems encountered in clinical practice, anterior knee instability frequently presents as part of a complex of findings. Patients may present acutely or after failing to recover from the initial injury. They may seek help because of a sudden change in symptoms after a reinjury or because of nagging but infrequent "giving-way" with specific activities. Patients who are predisposed to avoid contact with surgeons may delay consultation until they are disabled beyond the point of coping. In some cases, given time to consider their disability, patients may "shop" for an "expert" in knee surgery or sports medicine. In this way, the most demanding patients may seek out more prominent anterior cruciate ligament (ACL) surgeons. In so far as each of these scenarios represents a unique clinical problem, each has its own value for purposes of assessing outcomes. Nevertheless, each patient sample is representative only of its own type, and therefore the results in a given subgroup are not easily generalized to ACL-deficient patients in general. Furthermore, if the study sample includes a mixture of patients from different categories, the results may be confusing or misleading.

Unlike the laboratory, where it is often possible to distill a problem to its essential elements by controlled experimentation, in clinical research it is difficult or impossible to control every variable. The outcome of the ACL-deficient knee involves the complex interplay of so many variables that only an enormous study could possibly answer all questions at the same time with reasonable statistical power. Therefore, it is appropriate for an individual study to focus on one or two important issues, using sampling methods (enrollment criteria) designed to flesh out the specific hypotheses. Because the patient cohort in each published report represents a unique sample, the conclusions of any study based on an individual clinical practice can at best be described as one author's experience. Retrospectively identified samples are partic-

TABLE 20.1. *Problems noted in natural history studies of the ACL-deficient knee*

Many undocumented and undiagnosed ACL injuries
Patients specifically selected for nonsurgical treatment from a larger group
Acute and chronic injuries mixed together
High percentage of patients lost to follow-up
Patient age and activity level not accounted for
Frequency of associated injuries varies from group to group
Nonsurgical treatment is variable (rehabilitation, brace, etc.)
No consistent method for reporting results

ACL, anterior cruciate ligament.
From Wojtys EM. *The ACL deficient knee.* American Academy of Orthopaedic Surgeons Monograph Series, Rosemont, IL: American Academy of Orthopaedic Surgeons, 1994:3.

ularly prone to overinterpretation and false conclusions because the influence of associated conditions or bias is often impossible to evaluate. Prospectively designed studies can at least properly characterize the sample and identify the presence of confounding variables, even if not all the variables are controlled. However, prospective studies are also subject to bias in sampling, treatment decisions, and other important areas. The main advantage of such studies is that such bias is easier to identify than in retrospective series, so that their limitations are more immediately apparent. The most common flaws in studies of the ACL-deficient knee are listed in Table 20.1 (1). The following discussion is an attempt to interpret the literature while taking into account the limitations imposed by the design of each individual study.

Historical Background

Interest in the outcome of anterior cruciate injuries dates back at least to Stark's article (2) on cruciate ligament injuries treated by bracing in 1850. After World War II, O'Donoghue (3) emphasized study of knee ligament injuries. He pointed out poor results in patients with unrepaired ACLs and contrasted these patients with his operative results. He did not provide systematic follow-up of an unselected group of nonoperatively treated patients. In 1965, Liljedahl et al. (4) again gave anecdotal reports of poor results including osteoarthritis in patients in whom ACL lesions were untreated. Jacobsen (5) reported observing articular cartilage damage in more than half of the knees of patients who had sustained anterior cruciate injuries at least 6 months before the time of arthrotomy. Of course, only symptomatic patients underwent arthrotomy. Liljedahl et al. did point out, however, that almost half of the patients with chondral changes had intact menisci, suggesting that ligamentous laxity alone could lead to joint dysfunction. However, they did not exclude collateral ligament injuries in their study group.

In a classic article published in 1976, Feagin and Curl (6) reported the 5-year follow-up of 32 West Point cadets who had sustained "isolated" anterior cruciate injuries. All of the patients underwent surgical repair of the ligament. The results of surgery were so poor that Feagin and Curl regarded the data as "similar to the natural history of the unrepaired ACL," although they did not furnish any natural history data. Of the 32 patients, 17 had sustained significant reinjury within 5 years, 12 requiring reoperation. In these 12, 10 had medial meniscus tears, and 1 had a lateral meniscus tear. Twenty-four of the 32 were impaired in athletic endeavors and 12 had impairment in "ordinary" activities. If this did approximate natural history data, the prognosis appeared poor, but the assertion that the prognosis of a knee with a failed operation is identical to the prognosis of an unoperated knee is open to question.

Youmans (7) made the well-known assertion about ACL injury that "in the case of a skilled athlete, it may well be the beginning of the end of his career," although he provided little direct evidence to substantiate his assertion. In the same year, Chick and Jackson (8) presented a much more optimistic assessment of the prognosis of ACL injury. They studied 30 patients with "minimum to mild anterior instability." These patients were competitive athletes younger than 30 years old whose ACL tear was confirmed at the time of meniscectomy. Eighty-three percent returned to full activity with mean follow-up of 2.6 years, although 20% had intermittent effusion, 33% experienced occasional "slipping of the knee" during sports, and 56% had some radiographic changes on follow-up x-ray films. The sample in the study by Chick and Jackson represented only patients without severe laxity, which may have contributed to the relatively good results reported in their series. This was the first evidence to suggest that the degree of "instability" or pathologic motion resulting from an ACL injury may affect the outcome.

Acute Knee Hemarthrosis

Following up on the study by Gillquist et al. (9), published in 1977, regarding arthroscopy in acute injuries of the knee joint, DeHaven (10) published an article in 1980 that furnished important data for the analysis of literature on the natural history of ACL injuries. DeHaven reported the results of arthroscopies on 113 consecutive athletes who had sustained "significant acute trauma to the knee with immediate disability and the early onset of hemarthrosis but who did not have demonstrable clinical laxity." In many cases, standard clinical tests could not be performed because of pain and splinting. All patients underwent arthroscopy within 21 days of injury. ACL injures were found in 81 (71%). In 68 cases, these ACL lesions were judged to be acute. Of these 68 cases, 44 (65%) had significant meniscal tears (Table 20.2).

In 1980, Noyes et al. (11) also published an article on the results of arthroscopy of the knee in patients with acute hemarthrosis and "absent or negligible instability

TABLE 20.2. *Meniscal injuries accompanying ACL tears*

Study	n	Meniscal tear (%)	Medial meniscal tear only (%)	Lateral meniscal tear only (%)	Medial and lateral meniscal tear (%)
Acute ACL injury					
DeHaven (10)	68	65	13	34	18
Noyes (11)	61	62	21	38	3
Woods (16)	99	45	18	20	7
Indelicato (51)	44	68	36	9	10
Daniel (13)	190	59	25	35	11
Total	462	47	23	30	10
Chronic ACL injury					
Woods (16)	122	88	48	17	23
Indelicato (51)	56	91	55	11	25
Fowler (50)	51	72	35	35	2
Total	229	84	48	21	17

ACL, anterior cruciate ligament.

on clinical examination" in the office. As in DeHaven's study, all patients underwent arthroscopy within 3 weeks of injury. In contrast to DeHaven, however, Noyes et al. excluded patients who were found to have chronic ACL injuries. Of 85 patients, 61 (72%) had complete or partial ACL tears. Of these 61 patients, 38 (62%) had meniscal tears; 13 (21%), medial only; 23 (38%), lateral only; and 2 (3%), medial and lateral. These findings are in substantial agreement with those of DeHaven (Table 20.2). In the group with ACL injuries, Noyes et al. noted six (10%) with femoral chondral fractures and six (10%) with significant fibrillation of the chondral surface, usually on the lateral side.

Hardaker et al. (12) reviewed the findings of 132 arthroscopies done within 21 days of injury in patients presenting with acute traumatic knee hemarthrosis. No patient reported a previous injury to the knee. Patients with history or clinical findings of patellar dislocation were excluded. Patients with obvious fractures or gross instability of the knee were also excluded. At arthroscopy, 101 patients (77%) had partial or complete tears of the ACL (Table 20.2). In knees with ACL injury, 62% of the tears were complete and 38% were partial. Sixty-one percent of the 101 knees with ACL injury had meniscal tears, 40% had collateral ligament injuries, and 16% had chondral or osteochondral fractures.

Daniel et al. (13) reported initial findings in 292 patients with acute traumatic hemarthrosis presenting a mean of 4 days after injury. Fifty-six patients were stable by KT-1000 testing (side-to-side difference less than 3 mm with 89 N and manual maximum force) and 236 were KT-unstable. Instability on KT-1000 testing was believed to indicate ACL rupture. Arthroscopy was performed within 12 weeks of injury in 190 patients with unstable knees, 188 (99%) of whom had either partial or complete ACL tear documented at arthroscopy. There were 47 (25%) medial meniscus tears and 66 (35%) lateral meniscus tears in 92 (48%) patients. Ten meniscus repairs and

50 partial meniscectomies were performed in 54 patients. As had been reported previously, approximately half of patients with acute ACL disruptions had associated meniscal tears (11,12,14–16). However, many of these tears may not have required surgery. The incidence of meniscal tears in the patient with an acute ACL injury is high, but the incidence of reparable meniscal injuries is low. Daniel et al. noted a higher incidence of reparable meniscal tears among patients undergoing late ACL reconstruction than among patients presenting with an acute ACL injury. Forty-four patients (23%) had hyaline cartilage lesions confirmed by arthroscopy, compared with previous reports of 10% to 16% (Table 20.2) (11,12).

Bomberg and McGinty (17) reported their findings in 45 patients presenting with an acute knee injury followed by a posttraumatic hemarthrosis. All patients were evaluated before surgery followed by examination under anesthesia and arthroscopy of the knee. Most patients, 32 (71%), had an ACL tear. Meniscal tears occurred in 21 patients (47%). Meniscal tears requiring surgery occurred in only 10 (40%) of 25 meniscal tears. Seven patients (16%) had medial collateral ligament, posteromedial capsular sprain, or both. Eight patients (18%) had an osteochondral fracture or patellar dislocation associated with an osteochondral fracture. Most knees with a torn meniscus or osteochondral fracture had an ACL tear.

Maffulli et al. (18) performed a prospective arthroscopic study of 106 skeletally mature male athletes who presented with an acute hemarthrosis of the knee caused by sporting activities. They excluded patients with patellar dislocations, radiographic evidence of bone injuries, extraarticular ligamentous lesions, or previous injuries to the same joint. The ACL was injured in 71 patients (67%). In patients with an ACL lesion, associated injuries included meniscal tears (17 patients), cartilaginous loose bodies (6 patients), and minimal osteochondral fractures of the patella (2 patients), the tibial plateau (3 patients), or the femoral condyle (9 patients).

TABLE 20.3. *Chondral changes in ACL-injured knees noted at arthroscopy*

Study	No. of acute ACL patients	Chondral changes (%)	No. of chronic ACL patients	Chondral changes (%)
Noyes (11)	61	20	—	—
DeHaven (10)	—	—	13	69
Indelicato (51)	44	23	56	54
Fowler (50)	—	—	51	22
Daniel (13)	201	18	145	54
Total	306	19	252	47

ACL, anterior cruciate ligament.

The findings on initial work up in isolated (single ligament) acute ACL injury are summarized in Tables 20.2 through 20.4. These studies show the frequency of abnormalities that can accompany an acute ACL injury. These data suggest that in many cases isolated ACL tears (single ligament injuries) are accompanied by acute meniscal tears, chondral injury, or both. This helps us to characterize the newly injured knee as distinct from the knee that presents following reinjury because we can distinguish the symptoms of isolated ACL deficiency from those of articular injury or meniscus tear. The "natural history" of the ACL-deficient knee may be influenced by the presence of occult chondral lesions. Similarly, meniscal tears and/or their treatment may affect the long-term prognosis of ACL-injured knees. An ideal natural history study should document the presence or absence of chondral lesions or meniscal injures in the acute phase so that the specific implications of the additional lesions on an individual patient's prognosis can be determined. The information could be used to counsel patients in whom the presence or absence of acute meniscal tears or articular injury is known from arthroscopy or magnetic resonance imaging (MRI).

Knee Function After Anterior Cruciate Ligament Disruption

Fetto and Marshall (19) published an article in 1980 entitled "The Natural History and Diagnosis of Anterior Cruciate Ligament Insufficiency." Fetto et al. quoted Ivar Palmer who had stated that "the critical study still remained to be done, i.e., a prospective analysis of anterior cruciate insufficiency and its sequelae." Fetto et al.

TABLE 20.4. *Site of chondral damage in chronic ACL-injured knees*

Study	n	Patella (%)	Medial compartment (%)	Lateral compartment (%)
Fowler (50)	51	24	16	7
Daniel (13)	145	24	37	16
Total	196	24	32	14

ACL, anterior cruciate ligament.

concluded that the ACL-deficient knee without surgical treatment "appears to invariably embark upon a course of progressive deterioration and dysfunction." Unfortunately, the study by Fetto et al. did not closely approximate Palmer's ideal "critical study." In the study by Fetto et al. (19), 71% of the patients presented for treatment more than 2 weeks after injury, strongly suggesting potential bias toward symptomatic cases. Of 223 patients with ACL tears, 148 (62%) had additional ligament injuries and an unknown number had sustained meniscal or chondral lesions. Forty-seven patients underwent early ligament surgery and 83 underwent reconstruction at an average of 32 months (range, 6 to 84 months) after injury. The average duration of follow-up on the nonoperative patients was only 22 months (range, 6 to 132 months) after injury. The criteria used to select patients for early or late surgery were not specified.

Nevertheless, it was striking that by 5 years after injury, only 15% of the unoperated knees with isolated or combined ACL ligament injuries rated better than poor on the Hospital for Special Surgery (HSS) knee score especially when the same authors reported 82% with good to excellent results and only 4% with poor results in medial collateral ligament (MCL) injuries (grades I–III). The results of isolated ACL injuries were alleged to be "approximately equal in end-stage total scores" to the results of combined ligament injuries. Details of the follow-up evaluations, however, were scantily reported in this article.

In 1983, Giove et al. (20) reported the results obtained by treating 24 patients with ACL tears by a rehabilitation program emphasizing the hamstrings: "All patients returned to some sports participation, with 14 (59%) returning to their full preinjury level of participation." The patients were selected from a retrospective analysis of hospital records, with follow-up averaging 44 months. The instabilities were apparently mild in comparison to most ACL studies in that only five patients (21%) had a positive pivot shift test. Giove suggested that involuntary guarding augmented by hamstring training might have reduced the percentage with positive pivot shifts. Of the 14 patients who returned to preinjury sports participation, only 3 had no symptoms, whereas 11 had occasional or recurring mild discomfort, swelling, or instability. Eight patients had to reduce sports participation, whereas two returned to only "minimum participation." In this analysis, all sports were treated as a group, but Giove noted that patients who participated in sports such as football, volleyball, basketball, and racquetball did not do nearly as well as those who participated in swimming, golf, bicycling, and running. Thus, a more detailed look at Giove's results shows that ACL tears often caused significant signs and symptoms in patients who play cutting and jumping sports.

Jokl et al. (21) reported on the results of nonoperative treatment of 28 patients with combined severe ACL and MCL injuries. Their study reported better outcomes after the combined injury than most other studies report after isolated ACL injury. The follow-up in this article was particularly short, averaging 3 years, with 13 patients (46%) having follow-up of less than 2 years. Previous articles, such as those of Noyes et al. (22,23), suggest that results may deteriorate with a few years of additional follow-up. Nevertheless, the reported results are striking. Eleven (74%) of 15 patients returned to contact sports, although Jokl et al. did not give details about any signs or symptoms that might accompany participation. Nineteen (68%) of 28 returned to preinjury sports activity. Twenty (71%) were rated as good or excellent on the HSS knee assessment, five (20%) as fair-plus, and three as (4%) fair-minus. Although the authors stated that "our study revealed results much the same as those of McDaniel," McDaniel (48) reported only 21% good to excellent, 45% fair-plus, 30% fair-minus, and 4% poor results. This difference is even more striking because MCL instability can cause a loss of up to 5 points on the 50-point assessment. While McDaniel excluded patients with collateral ligament injuries, all patients in the study by Jokl et al. had acute grade III MCL sprains. Part of the difference in results between the series of Jokl et al. and that of McDaniel may be that all of the patients in the former study were seen on the day of injury, so that there was no bias toward selecting symptomatic patients. In addition, Jokl et al. excluded patients with "mechanical locking of the knee because of torn meniscus" so that the study did not include initial meniscectomies and only 4 (14%) during follow-up, whereas in McDaniel's series, 43 meniscectomies were performed on 53 patients at the index operation and still 8 more (15%) were required during the study.

Walla et al. (24) reported a retrospective study of 38 former athletes who had torn their ACLs at least 2 years before evaluation (mean, 5.6 years). All had positive Lachman and pivot shift tests. None had medial or lateral laxity, and none had undergone ligament reconstruction, although 61% had undergone a meniscectomy. Walla et al. believed that the patients had "progressed quite well," but, as we have previously seen, that is a subjective evaluation. Thirty-one (81%) had sustained a significant reinjury, most within a year of the index injury. Only 12 (32%) could participate in vigorous sports without pain,

swelling, or instability. Moderate or severe radiographic changes were present in 5 (23%) of 23 patients injured less than 5 years before study and in 10 (67%) of 15 injured more than 5 years prior to study. These radiographic changes were reported to be more frequent in patients who had undergone meniscectomy, but data on patients who had not undergone meniscectomy were not provided.

Satku et al. (25) followed up a group of ACL-injured patients for 6 years with the aim of trying to define "patients in whom current and potential disability outweighed the risks of surgery." In these patients, rupture of the ACL was said to be their predominant injury, but other pathology was not specifically excluded. Satku et al. reported that 55 patients (63%) were able to return to preinjury sports after injury, including 4 of the patients with bilateral ACL deficiency. By the time of follow-up (range, 2 to 11 years; average, 6 years), however, only 40 of these 55 were still able to participate in sports. Sixteen (42%) of 38 knees examined less than 5 years after injury had undergone meniscectomy, whereas 40 (68%) of 59 knees examined more than 5 years after injury had undergone meniscectomy. Satku et al. thus implied significant ongoing risks of meniscal injury even several years after ACL injury.

Kannus and Jarvinen (26) reviewed hospital records and identified 98 patients who had been treated conservatively for an acute ACL injury. Enrollment was based on an "unequivocal" examination and the absence of fractures. In addition to clinical examination, 78% had arthrography, 57% underwent examination under anesthesia, 21% underwent arthroscopy, and 78% had arthrotomy as part of the initial workup. Fourteen meniscectomies were performed at the initial procedure. The initial sample included 9% "top-level," 24% competitive, and 38% recreational athletes. Ninety patients were evaluated an average of 8 years after injury. Classification of the ACL injuries according to the standard nomenclature of the American Medical Association (AMA) (27) yielded 41 grade II injuries and 49 grade III tears. Eighty percent of grade III patients reported activity restrictions and 70% showed evidence of degenerative changes on radiographs. Thirty-five percent of grade III patients required ligament reconstruction during the course of the study, and 11 additional patients underwent meniscectomy or removal of loose bodies during that period. None of the group II patients required ligament reconstruction, and only four patients required meniscectomy. Sixty-six percent of grade II patients were still participating in the same activities as before injury. Although grade II patients were considered "partial" injuries in keeping with AMA guidelines, only two of these patients had no evidence of anterior knee laxity on clinical examination, and 78% demonstrated clinical laxity of grade II+ or greater at follow-up. The distinction between complete and partial ACL rupture can be very difficult to make

(28). Given that all patients in this study had an examination that was unequivocal for ACL tear, it is quite possible that many of the group II patients had complete ACL tears (28). Like the earlier study by Chick and Jackson (8), this report strongly indicates that outcomes after ACL injury are related to the degree of knee laxity. These studies offer strong evidence that ACL insufficiency carries a significant risk for progressive knee dysfunction and recurrent injury, particularly among those participating in demanding sports.

Pattee et al. (29) reviewed surgical logs to identify 68 patients who had undergone arthroscopy after a first-time knee injury and been found to have complete ACL rupture. They excluded patients who had undergone ligament reconstruction. The maximum interval from injury to the index procedure was 6 weeks. None of the patients in the study group exhibited a grade III pivot shift. Forty-nine patients (72%) were evaluated an average of 67 months after presentation. Nine patients (18%) required late ACL reconstruction. These patients had an average age of 21 years, which was 7 years younger than the remainder of the sample. In the remaining 40 patients, giving-way was the most common symptom (65%). Pattee et al. observed that few patients considered their instability to be severe, and most coped by modifying their activities. Mild or moderate pain was reported by 61% of patients, usually relating to strenuous or prolonged exercise. Swelling occurred occasionally in 42% of patients. Thirty-three patients (67%) had partial meniscectomy at the index procedure. Only two patients underwent late meniscectomy.

Bonamo et al. (30) reviewed a selected series of 79 patients who had arthroscopy followed by nonoperative treatment for an ACL injury. Sixteen (20%) presented within 1 month of the initial injury, whereas 63 (80%) presented between 1 month and 21 years after the ACL injury. Nine patients had undergone previous meniscectomy. At the index procedure, 27% had debridement of an Outerbridge grade III or IV lesion, and 67% had "significant" meniscal lesions, three of which were reparable. Follow-up ranged from 36 to 102 months after the index procedure. Six patients (8%) had reconstruction during the study period, and ten (13%) were considering reconstruction. At follow-up, most patients had no symptoms with activities of daily living or occupation. With sports, 73% reported "instability," 47% had had at least one episode of giving-way, 30% had postactivity swelling, and 27% had pain. Ninety-five percent of patients had modified their activities, 44% because of the knee and 56% because of lifestyle changes unrelated to the knee. Eighty-nine percent of those not reconstructed were still participating in sports. Twenty-nine (37%) of 79 patients sustained at least one significant reinjury during the study. The risk for reinjury was clearly related to age at presentation. Twelve (80%) of 15 patients between 10 and 19 years old had reinjuries, whereas 41% of patients in their third decade and 10% of patients in their fourth

decade had reinjuries. The authors could not relate poor outcomes to prior meniscectomy or debridement of hyaline cartilage lesions.

In a review of 107 patients with documented ACL tears undergoing arthroscopy for an acute knee injury, Drongowsky et al. (31) evaluated the effect of chondral and meniscus injury on patient function. Seventy-eight percent of the ACL injuries were considered acute at the time of the index procedure. Eighty-five percent of the ACL injuries were considered grade III, and the remainder were grade II using AMA nomenclature (27). Among the 99 patients seen at average follow-up of 51.7 months, there was a significant reduction in sports participation compared with preinjury status. Significant reductions were seen in the number of sports in which subjects participated as well as in the numbers of individuals engaged in sports involving pivoting, cutting, and jumping. The authors noted that injury to the hyaline cartilage was associated with increased symptoms of swelling and pain, and that individuals with these injuries were disabled for lighter activities (e.g., jogging) in addition to more strenuous sports. The authors were unable to demonstrate a similar effect of meniscus injury on the behavior of the ACL-deficient knees in their study. Because this retrospective sample represents a mixed patient population, it is difficult to say that the chondral injuries were in fact acute. If they were not, then clearly these knees were already accumulating damage more rapidly than other knees. Nevertheless, however, this study clearly indicates that chondral damage in an ACL-deficient knee results in disability that does not follow the pattern of most ACL-deficient patients. Because ligament surgery does not directly treat these lesions, ACL reconstruction alone should not be expected to restore these patients to an acceptable level of function. Recent MRI studies have shown bone contusion and cartilage injury to be common in the setting of acute ACL injury (32–37). Further follow-up is needed to ascertain what effect these lesions have on outcomes after ACL rupture.

Prospective Studies of Acute Anterior Cruciate Ligament Tear

There are a handful of prospective studies in the literature that offer the most complete picture of the outcomes to be expected after acute ACL injury (13,38–42). Because prospective studies identify patients at the time of the original injury and account for all patients, including those who recover completely, they minimize selection bias favoring poor outcomes. Although many prospective studies are biased in one way or another, greater documentation of injuries and treatment decisions is available so that the bias tends to be more apparent than in retrospective studies.

Hawkins et al. (41) reported a series of 40 patients with isolated ACL injuries. The mean age at the time of injury was 22 years; 17 of the 40 patients were younger than 20 years old. Follow-up was longer than 2 years for all patients and averaged 4 years. All patients were seen because of the initial injury, not because of continued symptoms, and all were seen within 4 weeks of injury. Twenty-five patients had arthroscopically proven complete ACL tears, whereas 15 were considered to have tears on the basis of Lachman, drawer, and positive pivot shift tests. Four (16%) of the 25 patients who underwent arthroscopy also had meniscal tears and underwent meniscectomy. The ACL injuries were treated with physical therapy and bracing, although most patients did not use their braces.

The follow-up picture was "somewhat grim." Twelve (30%) required late reconstruction because of giving-way. Of the 28 patients who did not undergo ACL reconstruction, 24 (86%) experienced giving-way and restricted their activities to minimize their symptoms. Only four patients (10%) were able to resume the same level of sports without reconstructive surgery. Hawkins et al. developed and described an "arbitrary rating system" incorporating objective and subjective factors. On this scale, there were no excellent ACL injured knees, 5 (12.5%) good knees, 23 (57.5%) fair knees, and 12 (30%) poor knees.

Engebretsen and Tegnander (40) reported on 29 young (mean age, 25 years), active patients followed-up an average of 33 months after presenting within 6 weeks of acute, complete ACL rupture. These patients were unselected because they represented all patients admitted to the hospital with a diagnosis of ACL tear during the enrollment period of the study. Patients were treated with rehabilitation and bracing, although compliance with bracing was inconsistent. Sixteen of 29 patients reported giving-way and only 2 (7%) returned to their preinjury level of activity. Nine of 29 had meniscal tears documented at the initial arthroscopic examination. Of the remaining 20 patients, 7 developed late meniscal tears that required surgery. Thirty-eight percent of patients went on to have late ligament reconstruction. Patients who did not have late reconstruction tended to be lower-demand patients who adjusted their activities to accommodate their knee instability. This study included patients seen up to 6 weeks after the initial injury. Although 6 weeks is probably not enough time to develop a second injury, it is possible that selection of more demanding patients may have occurred during this time. However, within the study sample, more active patients were less likely to tolerate ACL deficiency than patients involved in recreational and less demanding sports, supporting the authors' conclusion that ACL deficiency is not well tolerated in the young athlete.

Clancy et al. (39) performed examination under anesthesia and arthroscopy or open inspection in 99 knees with suspected acute ACL rupture, all of which were confirmed at surgery. Eighty-nine of 99 procedures were performed within 10 days of injury. Sixty-one patients (62%) had a meniscus tear. Twenty-two patients with absent or mild pivot shift were treated conservatively and followed up an average of 48 months later. Nine patients had had partial meniscectomy at the initial procedure. No patient had meniscectomy after the initial procedure. Thirteen patients had good or excellent results, and four were considered failures.

Andersson and colleagues (38,43) followed 59 non–ACL reconstructed patients an average of 58 months after ACL injury. The cohort was part of a consecutive series of 156 patients randomized into three treatment groups: ACL repair, ACL repair plus augmentation, and associated injury repair without ACL repair. Fifteen of the 59 non–ACL reconstructed patients had acute MCL repairs, ten had posterior oblique ligament repairs, and one had an arcuate ligament complex repair. They reported that 23% of the nonreconstructed patients returned to their former level of sports activity.

Meunier et al. (42) recently presented 15-year follow-up of 105 patients randomized after acute ACL injury into conservative (67 patients) versus surgical treatment (38 patients). They reported a higher incidence of subsequent meniscus surgery among the patients initially treated nonoperatively (35%) compared with patients treated with early surgical stabilization (9%). One third of the conservatively treated group underwent late ACL surgery. At follow-up, no difference in activity level or symptoms was detected between the two cohorts. The incidence of degenerative radiographic changes was about 50% in both groups. It is interesting to note how little difference ACL reconstruction made with respect to a number of important outcomes following ACL injury.

Daniel et al. (13) reported on 292 patients followed up for an average of 5.5 years after acute knee injury. Recreational athletes made up a large proportion of the sample, which included no professional or major 4-year collegiate athletes. Fifty-six knees that were stable on KT-1000 testing (injured minus normal difference, ±3 mm at 89 N and manual maximum force) were considered to have normal or partially disrupted ACLs, and were followed up to provide a control group with respect to the ligament injury. Forty-five patients with unstable knees had ACL reconstruction within 90 days of injury. One hundred ninety-one patients with unstable knees underwent a trial of nonoperative treatment. One hundred forty-seven were able to cope with their knee instability sufficiently to avoid ACL reconstruction.

Daniel et al. (44) compared the patients with stable knees (group I) to those with unstable knees (group II) at follow-up to assess the influence of knee instability on outcomes after traumatic hemarthrosis. Prior to injury, more than 85% of patients participated in a level I or II sport at least 50 hours per year. At follow-up, the percentage participating was reduced in both the stable and the unstable groups (Table 20.5), suggesting that much of the activity reduction seen in patients after ACL injury is

TABLE 20.5. *Participation in level I, II, and III sports after traumatic knee hemarthrosis (44)*

	I[a] (h/yr/patient)	II[b] (h/yr/patient)
n	53	139
Before injury	306	322
Follow-up	129	107

[a]Group I, early stable by KT-1000.
[b]Group II, early unstable by KT-1000, coper.

unrelated to knee instability. The mean number of hours of sports participation was reduced in both groups as well. Before injury, 251 patients were participating in a level I or II sport 50 or more hours per year. At follow-up, 127 patients had discontinued participation at this level. Thirty-three patients stated they discontinued a total of 54 level I or II sports activities because of their knee injures. Group I patients had fewer symptoms and impairments than patients in group II. Although 20% of the patients had symptoms of swelling, these complaints were considered mild or infrequent in 97% of all patients with unstable knees who had not been reconstructed.

Functional disability following acute, isolated ACL rupture appears to depend on several factors, including the level of physical activity (1). Participation in higher levels of activity appears to place the ACL-deficient knee at risk for reinjury. In the study by Hawkins et al. (41), only 14% of conservatively treated patients were able to return to unlimited athletic activities. Another 43% returned to sports, but with limitations. Wickiewicz (45) reported that the level of competition within a given sport is very important with the demands on the knee increasing with the level of competition. The study by Daniel et al. (13) included a large proportion of patients performing at lower levels of sports participation than those reported in Wickiewicz's study. In that study, most patients did well with activities of daily living. Furthermore, no patient required a change of occupation as a result of knee instability, although many patients reported functional limitations at demanding, manual jobs (13). In the study by Daniel et al., most ACL-deficient patients were able to participate in low-risk sports activity. They found that the number of preinjury hours of sports participation at levels I and II (46) was an important predictor of the success of conservative treatment (13). Increased participation in the so-called high-risk sports had a strong negative correlation with success of conservative treatment.

As discussed earlier, previous studies have suggested that the degree of knee laxity can be an important determinant of outcomes following ACL rupture (8,26). Subsequently, Eastlack et al. (47) reported no discernible difference in anterior laxity measured with the KT-1000 between "copers" and "noncopers" with ACL deficiency. Daniel and coworkers (13) found that the manual maximum side-to-side injured minus normal (I-N) difference

using the KT-1000 ligament arthrometer (MEDmetric Corporation, San Diego) was predictive of the need for late ligament or meniscus surgery. They performed discriminant analysis of factors known at the time of injury to determine which were predictive of late outcomes. Of the factors evaluated, only the average hours per year of preinjury sports participation, manual maximum side-to-side difference, and age were predictive of late surgery. Because age was not as strong a predictor, it added nothing to the predictive formula if sports participation was considered. Therefore, the authors presented a surgical injury risk factor, or "SURF" for making management decisions in patients presenting with acute ACL rupture (Table 20.6).

Symptomatic Chronic Anterior Cruciate Ligament–Deficient Knee

If it is inappropriate to infer from studies of symptomatic chronically ACL-deficient knees in determining the natural history of the ACL-injured patient, it is equally dubious to assume that the patient presenting with complaints after 2 years of ACL insufficiency will behave as if there were no prior history. These two groups represent different populations; to understand the patient with a symptomatic, chronically unstable knee, it is useful to discuss the literature from that perspective.

In 1980, McDaniel et al. (48) published a report on untreated ruptures of the ACL. McDaniel et al. sought to remedy some of the deficiencies of earlier studies such as short follow-up, inclusion of associated ligament injuries, and extrapolations from animal or cadaver studies. Their data, however, were still based on a retrospective review and therefore subject to unintended case selection and bias. Anterior cruciate lesions were noted at arthrotomy, which was usually performed for meniscectomy. Thus, 43 of the 53 knees studied underwent meniscectomy when the patients entered the study and only patients with symptoms severe enough to warrant arthrotomy could enter the study. Most patients entered the study more than 3 months after the index injury.

One of the main points of the article by McDaniel et al. (48) was that 72% of the patients returned to strenuous sports "at levels ranging from weekend recreational sports to college football and professional baseball." The positive impression this suggests, however, is qualified

TABLE 20.6. *Surgical risk factor (13)*

Side-to-side difference on KT-1000 manual maximum testing	Level I or II sports <50 h/yr	Level I or II sports 50–199 h/yr	Level I or II sports ≥200 h/yr
<5 mm	Low	Low	Moderate
5–7 mm	Low	Moderate	High
>7 mm	Moderate	High	High

by the fact that few details were provided. McDaniel et al. did not give details about which sports the patients played, the level of participation, or the level of symptoms the patients experienced while they played. The average follow-up score on the HSS knee score was 37.8, rating a fair-plus. There was 1 excellent result (2%), 10 good (18%), 24 fair-plus (45%), 16 fair-minus (30%), and 2 poor (4%). Seventy-three percent had a sense of discomfort, 58% had swelling, 56% experienced weakness, 43% had giving-way with unspecified activity, and 68% had radiographic abnormalities, although only 6% had "frank osteoarthritis." This suggests that the results were not as drastically different from those of Fetto and Marshall (19), as the articles' abstracts might suggest.

Many of the patients of McDaniel et al. (48) entered the study at the time of meniscectomy, but eight additional meniscectomies were performed at subsequent surgeries and only eight patients (15%) had both menisci at follow-up. The series clearly reported primarily on the long-term results of ACL-deficient knees that had undergone meniscectomy. In 1983, McDaniel et al. (49) reported further follow-up on all but one of the patients that were presented in the previous study in 1980. The average age of the patients was now 33 years, with follow-up averaging 14 years after injury and 11 years after index arthrotomy. There had been little change in symptoms, sports participation, or function, but radiographic changes had progressed, especially in the compartments that had undergone meniscectomy.

Noyes et al. (23) reported on functional disability in 103 *symptomatic* patients with ACL injuries who were evaluated an average of 5.5 years after injury. Patients with significant collateral ligament injuries were excluded. Most patients had continued to participate in vigorous sports, but none "had proper initial treatment, rehabilitation, or counseling." Noyes et al. pointed out that this group of ACL-injured patients would be expected to have the poorest prognosis. Eighty-five patients (82%) returned to sports after injury, but of these, 53 (62%) sustained a significant reinjury within 1 year of the index injury. Only 36 patients (35% of the total group) were participating in strenuous sports at 5-year follow-up and only 11 had no limitations. These numbers are not much worse than those of Giove et al. (20), despite the fact that Noyes et al. stressed the ominous prognosis, whereas Giove et al. emphasized positive outcomes. This contrast illustrates the importance that the authors' perspectives play in their assessment of their results. As in all areas of science, especially controversial ones, the reader must analyze the data carefully instead of relying entirely on the authors' conclusions.

Thirty-two (31%) of the patients in the study by Noyes et al. (23) reported moderate to severe disability in walking; 45 (44%), in activities of daily living; and 77 (74%), in turning and twisting sports. Of 103 patients, 51 (50%) had undergone meniscectomy, 41 (40%) having had both

medial and lateral menisci removed. These meniscectomized patients had a two- to fourfold increase in symptoms of pain and swelling with activity. Of the patients followed up more than 5 years after injury, 43% showed moderate to severe osteoarthritic changes on radiograph. The authors could not document a statistically significant correlation between radiographic findings and the presence or absence of meniscectomy, although many of the changes "by Fairbank's criteria could be ascribed to meniscectomy." Noyes et al. speculated that some of the patients with pain and swelling might have had meniscal tears that had not been subject to meniscectomy. It is possible, although not substantiated, that meniscal tears themselves may have contributed to Fairbank's changes, making it more difficult to establish a statistically significant effect of meniscectomy.

In the second article of this series, Noyes et al. (22) reported the results of placing 84 patients with symptomatic ACL-deficient knees on a program of rehabilitation, bracing, and activity modification. About one third of these patients improved so that they had minimal or no symptoms with activities of daily living or light recreational activities. Most of these patients still had symptoms, especially during strenuous sports. Only 9% returned to full competitive athletics. About one third of the patients were unchanged despite the program, and one third worsened during the program. Noyes et al. could not predict which patients would improve on their program. They reported that statistical analysis showed that those who experienced giving-way, even only two or three times per year, were at significant risk for developing arthritic changes, although they did not furnish the data that substantiated this assertion. Noyes et al. also enunciated their famous "rule of thirds" for ACL injuries: "that one third of the patients with this injury will compensate adequately and be able to pursue recreational activities, one third will be able to compensate but will have to give up significant activities, and one third will do poorly and will probably require future reconstructive surgery." In their treatment of the patient who presents with a symptomatic ACL-deficient knee, Noyes et al. stressed the importance of counseling the patient with respect to activity modification. A tabulation of articles reporting sports function after nonoperative treatment of ACL tears is presented in Table 20.7; symptoms with activities of daily living are shown in Table 20.8.

Fowler and Regan (50) reported the results of meniscal arthroscopic surgery and rehabilitation in the treatment of patients with symptomatic chronic ACL insufficiency. They stressed that all the patients were symptomatic; thus, this article did not attempt to define the natural history of *all* ACL-injured patients. Fowler and Regan excluded patients with "associated primary collateral or PCL damage." All patients underwent arthroscopic treatment at an average of 4.26 years after injury (range, 6 months to 37 years). They found that 37 (78%) of 51 knees had menis-

TABLE 20.7. *Sports activity in patients with nonoperative treatment of isolated ACL injuries*

Study	Sports participation	Remarks
Chick (8)	83% full athletic activity	Patients with moderate or severe anterior instability excluded
McDaniel (48)	73% in some "strenuous sports"	Little detail on sports functions
	42% no sports restriction	
Giove (20)	59% full preinjury level of participation	Patients involved in "heavy" participation did less well
	13% significant signs or symptoms	
Noyes (22)	35% strenuous sports	Only symptomatic patients included
	11% without limitation	
Walla (24)	42% high-intensity sports with limitations	—
	14% in same sport at same level	
Satku (25)	46% play preinjury sports	Few details about sports
Fowler (50)	22% in pivoting sports with activity modification	All patients symptomatic
	17% uninhibited in pivoting sports	
Daniel (13)	53% play injury sport	No professional or division I college athletes
	31% play the injury sport without hindrance	

ACL, anterior cruciate ligament.

cal damage. Nine patients (17%) had a "full, uninhibited return to pivoting sports, though only five returned to their preinjury level of competition." Eleven (22%) returned to pivoting sports with some modification of activity and awareness of their pathology. Thirteen (25%) returned to athletics, excluding pivoting sports, and 18 (35%) stopped all athletics. Four chose to undergo ACL reconstruction and four others were considering surgery.

Incidence of Meniscus Tears and Chondral Lesions

Woods and Chapman (16) reported in a prospective study of 234 consecutive patients with positive Lachman tests and "either an acute hemarthrosis or continued complaints of pain, effusion, or giving-way following an acute injury" who were examined under anesthesia and by arthroscopy. Patients with collateral ligament injuries were *not* excluded. Meniscus tears were found in 44 (45%) of 99 acute cases, 11 (85%) of 13 subacute cases, and 107 of 122 chronic cases (88%). Table 20.2 presents the results obtained by pooling the series of acute ACL injuries reported by DeHaven (10), Noyes et al. (11), Woods and Chapman (16), and Indelicato and Bittar (51), although the criteria used to select eligible patients were slightly differ-

ent in each study. Of the combined total of 272 patients, 58% had meniscal tears. At the time of the acute arthroscopy, approximately one third of the patients had torn lateral menisci. One ninth of the patients had torn both menisci. Comparing the chronic to the acute knees, we can see that 84% of the chronic cases had meniscal tears, whereas 58% of the acute cases had tears. Sixty-three percent of the chronic cases had torn medial menisci compared with 32% of the acute cases; the percentage with torn lateral menisci was just less than 40% in both chronic and acute cases. All suspected acute ACL tears underwent arthroscopy, but patients with chronic ACL tears underwent arthroscopy only if they were symptomatic. Therefore, we can say that patients with chronic ACL tears *who are symptomatic* appear to have medial meniscal tears much more often than acute cases. These additional meniscal tears could contribute to the degenerative changes seen in some knees with chronic ACL injuries.

Indelicato and Bittar (51) and Woods and Chapman (16) emphasized that many of the meniscal tears in the ACL-injured knees were potentially reparable. Woods and Chapman reported 50% and Indelicato and Bittar reported 65% of meniscal tears in acute ACL-injured knees to be reparable. The incidence of surgically

TABLE 20.8. *Pain, swelling, and "giving way" in chronic ACL patients during activities of daily living*

Study	n	Pain (more than mild or infrequent) (%)	Swelling (more than infrequent) (%)	"Giving way" (%)	Follow-up (yr)	Remarks
McDaniel (48)	49	38	10	Not reported for ADL	14	—
Noyes (22)	103	30	14	21	5.5	Selected population of "worst cases"
Hawkins (41)	40	18	18	11	4	30% who received reconstruction not included
Daniel (13)	34	0	0	9	5	—

ACL, anterior cruciate ligament; ADL, activities of daily living.

TABLE 20.9. *Percentage of meniscus lesions that were judged to be reparable in ACL-injured knees*

Study	No. of acute ACL patients	Reparable meniscal tears (%)	No. of chronic ACL patients	Reparable meniscal tears (%)
Woods (16)	99	50	122	27
Indelicato (51)	44	65	56	57
Daniel (13)	68[a]	17	73[b]	56

ACL, anterior cruciate ligament.
[a]An additional 27 meniscus lesions were "left alone."
[b]An additional 18 meniscus lesions were "left alone."

repaired acute meniscus tears in the San Diego Kaiser series (13) was less than that reported by Woods and Chapman and Indelicato and Bittar, whereas the rate of repair in chronics was higher (Table 20.9). More of the medial meniscus tears were judged reparable than were lateral meniscus tears (Table 20.10).

Chondral changes in the ACL-disrupted knee are presented in Table 20.3. Indelicato and Bittar (51) noted that 10 (23%) of the acute cases demonstrated chondral fractures of the femoral condyles with "free fragments of articular cartilage." Noyes et al. (11) had reported 20%. Indelicato and Bittar noted "significant articular changes" in 30 (54%) of their chronic cases while DeHaven (10) used the same phrase to describe 9 (69%) of the 13 cases of chronic ACL tears with acute hemarthrosis that he arthroscoped. Again it must be noted that only symptomatic chronic ACL cases underwent arthroscopy, so that the numbers we have for the incidence of significant articular changes in chronic ACL cases probably are higher than they would be if all chronic ACL cases were arthroscoped in a prospective, randomized study. The pooled data indicate that the incidence of chondral changes in the chronic population was more than twice the incidence in the acute population. Table 20.4 presents the incidence of chondral lesions by compartment in two studies. Lateral compartment damage was less frequent than damage in the medial and patellofemoral compartments. In examining all the data, however, it is essential to remember that we only have data on those chronic patients whose symptoms were believed to justify arthroscopy or ACL reconstruction.

Late Degenerative Arthritis

Lynch et al. (52) wrote an article in 1983 that had interesting implications regarding the significance of menis-cal injuries in the prognosis of ACL-injured patients. Unfortunately for our purposes, that study group consisted of patients who had undergone successful surgical stabilization of anterior cruciate injuries. Lynch et al. analyzed pain and Fairbank's changes at a mean follow-up of 3.8 years after surgery. Patients were divided into groups consisting of those with no meniscal tear, those with a tear that had been "left alone," those with a tear that had been repaired, and those who had undergone partial or total meniscectomy. In this group of stabilized patients, pain and Fairbank's changes were very infrequent in those who had not injured their menisci. The patients who had undergone meniscal repair did almost as well. Those with tears that had been left alone had a high incidence of pain, but only a moderate incidence of Fairbank's changes, whereas those who had undergone partial or total meniscectomy had much less pain, but a much higher incidence of Fairbank's changes. No similar study of patients with unreconstructed ACLs has been done, although such a study would allow us to differentiate more clearly between the long-term prognosis of an isolated ACL injury without meniscal damage and the isolated ACL injury with meniscal pathology.

Table 20.11 presents data on radiographic changes in chronic ACL patients. Articles with follow-up of 5 years or more report that a high percentage of ACL patients show radiographic changes. Changes judged to be of at least moderate severity are not uncommon. Authors such as Satku et al. (25) and Fowler and Regan (50) reported that radiographic changes correlate with meniscal injury or meniscal surgery, but others such as Giove et al. (20) and Noyes et al. (23) did not corroborate this. Several authors, such as Satku et al. (25) and Walla et al. (24), showed that changes were more severe in those patients who were followed up after longer intervals. No study provided the 30- or 40-year follow-up desirable in study-

TABLE 20.10. *Meniscal tears judged to be reparable in chronic ACL-injured knees*

Study	Medial	Lateral	Total
Woods (16)	31/86 (36%)	6/49 (12%)	37/135 (27%)
Indelicato (51)	31/45 (69%)	6/20 (30%)	37/65 (31%)
Daniel (13)	41/71 (58%)	0/2 (0%)	41/73 (56%)

ACL, anterior cruciate ligament.

TABLE 20.11. *Radiographic changes in patients with nonoperative treatment of isolated ACL injuries*

Study	X-ray changes	Follow-up (yr)	Remarks
Chick (8)	50%, mild changes	2.6	All patients had index meniscectomies
McDaniel (48)	56%, flattening or squaring of femoral condyles 24%, joint space narrowing 10%, "frank osteoarthritis" 14%, normal	14	All had arthrotomies, most had meniscectomies when they entered the study
Giove (20)	59%, "variable degenerative changes" vs 32%, changes in uninvolved knee	3.7	41% had meniscectomy. Meniscectomized knees no worse than others
Noyes (23)	25%, minimum arthritis 21%, moderate or severe arthritis 54%, normal (44% of patients followed up more than five years had moderate or severe changes)	5.5	Only symptomatic patients included. All athletes; 50% had meniscectomies
Walla (24)	39%, moderate or severe arthritis 26%, normal (66% with more than five years' follow-up showed moderate or severe changes)	5.6	All former athletes; 61% had meniscectomies
Hawkins (41)	43%, mild to moderate changes	4	20% had meniscectomies
Satku (25)	44%, mild changes 38%, moderate to severe changes 18%, normal	6	58% had meniscectomies
Daniel (13)	64%, medial compartment 50%, patellofemoral 35%, lateral (predominantly mild x-ray and bone scan changes)	5	Positive correlation between meniscectomy and degenerative changes

ACL, anterior cruciate ligament.

ing potential degenerative changes caused by injuries in young patients.

Satku et al. (25) obtained follow-up radiographs of 49 of the 59 knees they followed up for more than 5 years. Thirty-five of these knees had undergone meniscectomy and five others were said to have clinical signs and symptoms of meniscal injury. Of these 40 knees, 19 (48%) had moderate or severe radiographic "deterioration," whereas none of the nine patients without evidence of meniscal pathology showed such changes. The signs and symptoms said to imply meniscal injury are not specified and could overlap those of posttraumatic arthritis. Nevertheless, there is a strong implication, as in article by Lynch et al. (52), that much of the degenerative effect of ACL injury is mediated by meniscal injury. Lynch et al. correlated degenerative changes in patients who had undergone successful ACL reconstruction with meniscal injury and surgery. Satku et al. suggested a similar correlation in patients whose ligaments had not been reconstructed. In addition, Satku et al. hypothesized that much of the observed deterioration in sports participation could have been due to meniscal injuries and their long-term degenerative effects.

Previous reports have documented that radiographic changes (8,20,23,25,41,48,53) and bone scan changes (13,54,55) occur in the chronic ACL-disrupted knee. The Kaiser study is the first report that presents the results of imaging studies in a large ACL-injured population studied prospectively. Many patients had mild degenerative changes in the index knee. The same was true at 10 years after index injury. Some of the changes on the radiograph and bone scan may be secondary to occult bone lesions sustained at the time of injury (34). In the Kaiser study, meniscus surgery correlated with increased degenerative changes, which supports the findings of previous authors (23,25,56–59). Our earlier report was the first report to correlate degenerative changes with displacement measurements. The manual maximum and quadriceps active tests correlated with an increase in imaging scores ($p < 0.05$).

Partial Anterior Cruciate Ligament Tears

The term "partial" ACL tear has not been clearly defined in the literature; it implies that some of the fibers are torn, but some remain intact. In practice, it generally means that the ligament, while exhibiting signs of injury, still spans the joint without interruption. The extent of ACL tears is difficult to ascertain by arthroscopy. The reported incidence of partial ACL tears is 10% to 28% of all ACL tears (10,11,48,60–62). Umans et al. (63) observed that MRI could not reliably distinguish partial from complete ACL tears. Using strict criteria for describing ACL injury patterns seen on MRI, Roychowdhury et al. (64) compared MRI findings of partial "stable" and "unstable" tears to arthroscopic findings. The investigators could not distinguish partial stable injuries from arthroscopically normal ligaments, nor could they distinguish partial unstable injuries from complete ACL tears. But the observers were able to segregate stable tears (normal ligaments and stable partial tears) from unstable tears (unstable partial tears and complete tears) with 100% sensitivity and 96% specificity. Unfortunately, they did not measure knee stability itself, but only inferred stability based on the continuity of ACL fibers at arthroscopy.

Reports on the outcome of partial ACL tears diagnosed by direct inspection or arthroscopy have been inconsistent (61,65–69). Some authors report that patients with partial ACL tears have no significant instability (68). Others report that the instability and prognosis of patients with partial tears are similar to those of patients with complete tears. A 1-year follow-up evaluation was performed at the San Diego Kaiser Hospital in 30 patients with an acute hemarthrosis who were diagnosed arthroscopically to have a partial ACL tear. Previously reported studies of acute partial ACL tears had not reported stability measurements. Acute KT-1000 measurements in the 30 Kaiser patients revealed that 14 patients had normal stability and 16 had pathologic anterior displacement (KT-1000 injured minus normal difference, ≤3 mm). Follow-up evaluation revealed that 13 of the 14 patients with normal stability acutely had normal stability at follow-up. All 16 of the patients who had pathologic motion acutely had pathologic motion at follow-up. The 1-year evaluation of the patients with pathologic motion was similar to results seen in patients with unrepaired complete ACL disruptions. Function was much better in the patients with partial tears who had normal anterior stability. We currently use the term "partial ACL tear" when a portion of the ACL appears to be intact but damaged, and anterior displacement measurements are normal (KT-1000 anterior manual maximum injured minus normal difference of less than 3 mm). Outcomes among patients in this group appear comparable to outcomes in patients with intact ligaments.

Anterior Cruciate Ligament Injury in Juveniles and Adolescents

ACL injury in the immature athlete poses a particularly difficult problem. A growing number of authors have reported ACL disruptions in patients with open growth plates (70–89). Prior to age 12, most of these disruptions occur by avulsion of the tibial eminence (73–75,82,90). Avulsion of the femoral attachment of the ACL can also occur (86,91). In the adolescent patient, ACL rupture usually represents a midsubstance ACL tear. The mechanism of injury and the incidence of associated collateral ligament injuries and cartilage injuries are similar to those reported in adults (57,92–95).

Mizuta et al. (93) evaluated the results of conservative treatment after complete midsubstance tears of the ACL in 18 skeletally immature patients who presented with an acute hemarthrosis. The average time from initial injury to final evaluation was 51 months, with a minimum of 36 months follow-up. Six patients had an ACL reconstruction during the follow-up period and were assessed immediately before their surgery. All patients had symptoms when reviewed. The modified Lysholm knee score showed one excellent result, one good, eight fair, and eight poor, with a mean score of 64.3. Only one patient had returned to her preinjury level of athletics. Secondary meniscal tears were confirmed in six patients, and three more had the clinical signs of a tear at follow-up. Radiographic evidence of degenerative changes was found in 11 of the 18 patients. The authors noted a positive relationship between prior meniscectomy and degenerative changes at follow-up. They did not evaluate the effect of ACL reconstruction on late degenerative changes. The authors concluded that the results of nonoperative treatment for ACL injuries in this age group are poor and recommended early surgical stabilization.

In skeletally immature patients, the natural history of complete ACL rupture appears to be similar to that in the adult (70,79,81,85). Kannus and Jarvinen (96) reported that in the immature age group, outcomes were strongly influenced by the degree of laxity resulting from the injury (96). As is the case with adults with ACL deficiency, the natural history is believed to be strongly influenced by the degree of exposure to level I activities (97) (Table 20.6). The risk for reinjury may be quite high because of habitually high levels of activity of most persons in this age group. This fact renders conservative treatment problematic (93). The available evidence suggests that it is unlikely young patients will be able to participate in sporting activities after complete ACL tear despite rehabilitation and functional bracing (70,85,93).

Repair of tibial eminence avulsions is associated with good clinical outcomes (91–101), although normal anterior laxity may not be restored (90,102). It seems likely that in many cases a partial midsubstance ACL tear occurs in combination with the fracture. Whether or not a partial midsubstance injury occurs, there is no evidence to suggest that repair of the fractured eminence alone is not sufficient to prevent symptoms and dysfunction.

Because of concerns about physeal injury and growth disturbance with surgical intervention, nonoperative treatment traditionally has been advocated for children with ACL insufficiency. However, the risks of conservative management in the face of a complete ACL rupture must be weighed against the expected risks and benefits of the surgical technique to be used. Extraarticular (nonanatomic) reconstruction and primary repair of the torn ACL have been no more successful in children than in adults (103,104), and cannot be recommended. However, reconstruction by either nonisometric or isometric placement using hamstring tendon grafts can reliably improve knee stability without undue risk for growth disturbance (see Chapter 27) (105–107). In advising the patient and family, the risk for meniscal and joint surface injury secondary to repeated giving-way episodes in the ACL-deficient knee must be balanced against the risk for limb length discrepancy or limb alignment deformity secondary to growth plate arrest resulting from surgery (103).

To date, there has been only one reported case of growth deformity following ACL reconstruction in a skeletally immature patient (108). The report by Koman and Sanders (108) emphasized the importance of observing established surgical principles in avoiding growth complications after intraarticular ACL reconstruction. Bone plugs and hardware such as screws clearly should not cross the growth plate. The position and size of the tunnels relative to the physis also are important. In immature animals, evidence suggests that the risk for physeal disturbance caused by tunnels is determined by the relationship between the cross-sectional area of the tunnel and that of the physis (109,110). In any event, it is prudent to advise the patient's family fully of the risks and goals of both operative and nonoperative treatment at the time the diagnosis is made. If a patient has been fully advised and treated "conservatively," yet nevertheless experiences giving-way episodes with activities, then the prudent course is probably to recommend ligament reconstruction without further delay.

The authors' approach to the ACL-injured patient with open growth plates has been to encourage nonoperative management if possible until less than 1 cm of combined growth remains at the distal femoral and proximal tibial physes, as determined by hand and wrist radiographs (111) and standardized growth charts (112,113). Lo and colleagues (103) and others recommend taking into account family growth history and sexual maturity as well. The patient is advised to avoid activities that involve hard cutting and jumping (International Knee Documentation Committee [IKDC] level I and II sports) (Table 20.12). In the Kaiser study, the risk for a skeletally immature patient sustaining repeated injury to the knee was similar to risk for reinjury among adults. Therefore, we use the SURF table (Table 20.6) in counseling the families of skeletally immature patients presenting with acute

TABLE 20.12. *IKDC sports level*

Level	Activity	Examples
I	Jumping, pivoting, hard cutting	Basketball, football, soccer
II	Lateral motion, less jumping or hard cutting than level I	Baseball, racket sports, skiing
III	Other sports	Jogging, running, swimming

IKDC, International Knee Documentation Committee.

ACL injury. Whatever the course of treatment, the patient and the patient's family must be clearly informed of the options and risks. Patients must be aware that symptoms of instability imply that the knee is at risk for significant reinjury, and that such episodes warrant complete avoidance of the offending activity. If symptomatic knee instability or the patient's goals call for surgery while significant growth remains, a surgical procedure is planned that carries a minimum risk for growth disturbance (83,85,105–107,114,115).

Summary

A review of the data presented reveals several points of consensus. Acute ACL tears are accompanied by meniscal tears in a little more than 50% of cases (Table 20.2). The incidence of lateral tears is slightly greater than medial tears. In chronic ACL-injured patients who have enough symptoms to warrant arthroscopy (and that is a major qualification), four of five patients have meniscal tears and medial tears are much more common than lateral tears. About 40% of surgical meniscus tears are reparable. Studies by Noyes et al. (23), Walla et al. (24), and Satku et al. (25) present information on the number of nonreconstructed ACL-injured patients who came to meniscectomy within 5 years of injury—50%, 61%, and 58%, respectively. Their patients were not specifically preselected because chronic symptoms warranted arthroscopy. Conversely, some meniscal tears were undoubtedly missed in these studies because some patients did not undergo arthrotomy or arthroscopy.

Less information is available regarding chondral changes in ACL-deficient patients (Tables 20.3 and 20.4). Indelicato and Bittar (51) and the Kaiser study both document that chondral changes are more than twice as frequent in chronic patients who come to arthroscopy than in acute patients. In those chronic patients, medial and patellar chondral damage are more common than lateral damage.

McDaniel and Dameron (48,49), Hawkins et al. (41), and the San Diego Kaiser study (13) all point out that most patients with chronic ACL-deficient knees do not have more than mild or infrequent pain with activities of daily living (Table 20.8). These authors also agree that during activities of daily living, few patients have giving-way or more than occasional swelling. Noyes et al. (23), in their study of symptomatic, athletically active patients found more frequent problems during activities of daily living. In the article by Hawkins et al. (41) and in the San Diego Kaiser (13) study, however, some patients left the study group to undergo ACL reconstruction. These were presumably the most symptomatic patients. In the study by Hawkins et al., all patients were initially treated nonoperatively, but 30% subsequently underwent ACL reconstruction. In the San Diego Kaiser study, 20% of the patients underwent acute reconstruction, and 18% of the remainder underwent delayed reconstruction. Although the need for reconstruction is a matter of judgment, these figures are consistent with the famous *rule of thirds* of Noyes et al. according to which one third of patients will need ACL reconstruction. Conversely, it should be emphasized that these two populations were fundamentally different. The Kaiser patients represented all patients presenting with an acute ACL rupture, whereas patients of Noyes et al. were symptomatic patients with chronic ACL insufficiency presenting for treatment.

Each of the studies we have discussed has its specific biases. We have pointed out some of them in the course of this review. Pooling such disparate data represents an interesting but potentially misleading oversimplification. Many of the selection biases (e.g., toward symptomatic patients) are common to most of the articles. Pooling the data does not eliminate such biases and obscures some of the information available to the careful reader of the individual studies.

From the data we now possess, it certainly appears that most patients with ACL injuries do well with activities of daily living even after follow-up in the range of 5 to 15 years. Most can participate in some sports activity if they are inclined to do so, but most will have some limitations in vigorous sports and only a few will be entirely asymptomatic. Approximately half the patients will tear their menisci at the time of ACL rupture. Some of those tears may heal and others will develop. There are more medial meniscus tears in the chronic group than in the acute group. Chondral damage is found in 20% of the patients who undergo acute arthroscopy when their ACL is torn and in more than 40% of those who undergo arthroscopy later. Degenerative changes are seen on radiographs in a substantial number of cases. There is strong evidence linking these changes to meniscal pathology. The Kaiser study (13) documented that patients who undergo partial meniscectomy have more degenerative changes on radiographs at 5 and 10 years follow-up than patients who do not have meniscectomy, regardless of whether or not they have their ACL reconstructed.

Clinicians are frequently presented with the question of whether ACL injury will lead to decreased function and eventual knee arthrosis. Armed with the data currently available regarding the natural history of the ACL-deficient knee, it is possible to outline the possible negative consequences in terms of an injury cascade. Daniel proposed the "ACL injury cascade" as a conceptual framework for understanding the events that may follow ACL injury (Fig. 20.1). In all knees with ACL insufficiency, there is instability that can allow subluxation with certain activities. If sufficient pathologic laxity is present to permit giving-way episodes, sports disability may occur due to joint instability itself. On the other hand, disability may result indirectly from the instability because of a secondary meniscal injury

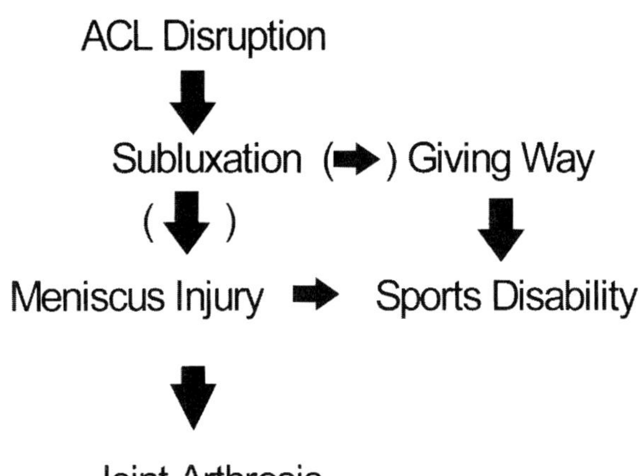

FIGURE 20.1. The anterior cruciate ligament (ACL) injury cascade represents a possible sequence of events that may lead to decreased function, arthrosis, or both. Possible eventualities are demonstrated as arrows with parentheses. (From Daniel DM. Selecting patients for ACL surgery. In: Jackson DW, ed. *The anterior cruciate ligament: current and future concepts.* New York: Raven Press, 1993:255, with permission.)

resulting from joint subluxation. While ACL injury itself may result in only mild degenerative changes on radiographs or bone scans, pathologic joint subluxation can result in meniscal injury. Meniscal injury resulting in meniscectomy is associated with arthrosis, and it is possible that preventing meniscal injury, through either nonoperative or operative means, will decrease the risk for arthrosis.

NONOPERATIVE TREATMENT OF THE ANTERIOR CRUCIATE LIGAMENT–DEFICIENT KNEE

Dye et al. (116) recently explored the broad range of physiologic, anatomic, and kinematic abnormalities that result from ACL disruption. They have proposed the idea of the "envelope of function" (116) to conceptualize the effects of ACL rupture on functional capacity and risk for reinjury. Conservative treatment of the ACL-deficient knee includes activity modification, rehabilitation, and, occasionally, bracing to maximize function and allow the broadest possible range of activities with minimum risk for reinjury or symptoms. It appears that the most important factor in determining the success of conservative treatment is the patient's level of activity (117). In the Kaiser study (13), the single most predictive factor in predicting which patients would need late ACL or meniscal surgery was the patient's level of sports activity prior to the ACL rupture. Probably the most valuable contribution the physician can make in the nonoperative care of these patients is to counsel them fully on the risks associated with high-demand activities in the ACL-deficient knee (22.). The patient must understand the danger of activities that place high functional demands on the knee and must be willing to alter his or her lifestyle and athletic activities.

Rehabilitation of the Anterior Cruciate Ligament–Deficient Knee

Injury to the ACL leads to a number of kinematic and physiologic changes in the knee, including pathologic laxity (118–122), reduced proprioception (123), altered neurosensory reflexes (124–126), changes in muscle function (127–129), and characteristic changes in gait patterns (130–143). Friden et al. (133) compared two groups of ACL-deficient patients; the asymptomatic group demonstrated reduced anterior translation of the knee during gait (dynamic loading) compared with the symptomatic group. The authors postulated that the asymptomatic group compensated for their knee laxity by an unexplained neuromuscular mechanism. In subsequent work by the same group (144,145), the authors reported that proprioceptive deficits in ACL-deficient knees are most pronounced in the nearly extended position and suggested that the abnormalities may interfere with normal joint protective mechanisms. Borsa and coworkers (146) reported similar deficits of threshold detection for joint motion. They recommended a rehabilitation program emphasizing performance-based, weight-bearing, closed kinetic chain exercise for the muscle groups that act on the knee joint "in order to effectively restore reflex stabilization of the lower limb." It has not been established to what extent rehabilitation can correct or compensate for these sensory abnormalities. Nevertheless, rehabilitation of the ACL-deficient knee has focused on enhancing these neuromuscular pathways (1,24,146–148) to reduce the prevalence of functional deficits despite the pathologic laxity that is present in all cases (149).

Tests to evaluate muscle function about the knee have included strength testing (147,150) and the one-leg hop for distance (150,151). Wyatt and Edwardo (152) reported 89% of healthy subjects had a nondominant–dominant quadriceps strength ratio with isokinetic testing at 60° per second of more than 0.8; 90% had a hamstring strength ratio more than 0.8. Daniel et al. (153) reported a left–right one-leg-hop-for-distance ratio of more than 0.9 in 95% of 100 healthy subjects. Barber et al. (154) reported 81% of healthy subjects had a hop ratio of more than 0.9. In the Kaiser follow-up studies (13,155), functional tests were performed in 229 patients at 5 years and in 245 patients at 10 years after index injury. At 10 years after the index injury, the group II patients (unstable, not reconstructed) had a mean injured/noninvolved quadriceps ratio of 0.97 and hamstring ratio of 0.98, greater than the quadriceps ratio of 0.86 and hamstring ratio of 0.90 reported by Kannus (150) in 41 ACL-deficient knees. Prior reports of the involved/noninvolved hop ratio in ACL-deficient patients of 0.9 (156) and 0.82 (154) are less than the mean hop ratio of 0.95 in group II. Group I had better performance than group II on the one-leg-hop-for-distance and quadriceps strength testing at both follow-up intervals ($p < 0.05$) (155).

Much has been written about the importance of interactions between the cruciate ligaments and the quadriceps muscle group (157). Gerber et al. (127) reported that ACL-deficient knees demonstrated significant atrophy of both quadriceps and hamstrings. They noted more severe deficits in the quadriceps than in the hamstring muscle group. It is not clear whether the muscle fiber atrophy is the result of disuse or to alterations of muscle activation patterns (131,133,140,142). The more profound effects seen in the quadriceps group imply that quadriceps strengthening is necessary to restore muscle balance about the knee. However, there is controversy about the best exercise program for achieving the desired level of strength. It has been suggested that so-called open kinetic chain exercises, such as long-arc knee extension, may be harmful to the joint because the loading of both the patellofemoral and tibiofemoral articulations is nonphysiologic (1,158). Arms et al. (158) found that quadriceps activity between full extension and 45° flexion caused significant strain in the ACL. Anterior displacement of the tibia during quadriceps contraction near full extension is due to anterior shear forces generated by the quadriceps (159–163) in terminal extension.

The effects of muscle activity depend not only on the magnitude of the contraction, but also on knee flexion angle and overall body posture during the exercise (164). The term "closed-chain" has been applied to exercises in which the sole of the foot is in contact with the resisting surface, for example the floor or a pedal. Closed-chain exercises have been advocated for two reasons. First, a high joint reaction force, which occurs for example during weight bearing (a classic "closed-chain" configuration), may reduce anterior shear stress at the knee joint (165,166). Second, cocontraction of the hamstrings during these exercises may also reduce anterior shear forces. More et al. (167) suggested that hamstring cocontraction might dynamically stabilize the knee by creating a posteriorly directed force vector at the joint. Greater hamstring muscle strength or alterations in quadriceps activation patterns may reduce the anteriorly directed shear forces that contribute to functional instability in the ACL-deficient knee (168). Walla et al. (24) reported enhanced hamstring reflexes among a group of well-compensated ACL-injured patients as compared with controls and functionally disabled ACL-deficient patients. Furthermore, during high-demand activities, a high net hamstring moment may stabilize knees dynamically against rotational and adduction moments (1,167,169). Hamstring contraction does not appear to restrain anterior translation of the tibia near full extension (170,171). However, the hamstrings are capable of transferring torque from the knee to the hip, and vice versa. As the trunk flexes during weight-bearing exercise, the center of gravity moves forward, reducing the flexion moment at the knee (172). The hamstrings are activated during forward trunk bending to stabilize the hip (172,173). Thus, although the hamstrings may not directly restrain anterior tibial translation in the nearly extended knee, hamstring activity is associated with postural compensation that reduces quadriceps force.

It is an unfortunate development that has allowed the terms "open kinetic chain" and "closed kinetic chain" to assume such a prominent place in our efforts to distinguish "safe" from "unsafe" exercises. In truth, internal forces greatly exceed external forces when the knee joint is loaded (157). Quadriceps forces generated in certain open-chain activities such as kicking a ball are probably much greater than the forces created in most closed-chain rehabilitation activities (165). Therefore, the assertion that closed-chain exercises necessarily create greater joint reaction force is probably not valid. The practical significance of hamstring cocontraction as a direct restraint against anterior tibial translation also is not universally accepted (170,171). It has not been demonstrated that hamstring torque in terminal extension is sufficient to neutralize the very high anterior shear forces that may be produced by quadriceps contraction in this range of flexion (170,171). Theoretically, the crucial factor in distinguishing a safe exercise from an unsafe one is the range of knee flexion where the highest quadriceps forces are generated. In weight-bearing activity, or exercises where the resistance is applied upward against the sole of the foot, the highest quadriceps forces are generated in higher angles of knee flexion, when the moment of knee flexion is greatest. At these angles of flexion, the patellofemoral articulation is more highly congruent, and anterior shear forces accompanying high quadriceps loads are relatively low, even negative (157). As the knee approaches terminal extension, the opposite is true.

From a practical point of view, the Vermont group has studied ACL strain patterns during a wide variety of weight-bearing activities (160,174–176). They have observed a wide range of peak strain values, suggesting that each activity presents a unique pattern of muscle activation. Studies such as these point out the importance of empirically testing different activities to validate their safety in ACL-deficient patients. In general, weight-bearing exercises are capable of exercising the knee extensors and flexors simultaneously, making for an efficient regimen of motor conditioning and promoting muscle balance about the knee. As a general principle in the rehabilitation of the ACL-deficient knee, we prefer exercises that simulate weight-bearing activity.

Bracing

Several types of knee braces are commercially available. The American Academy of Orthopedic Surgery's 1984 *Knee Brace Seminar Report* classified three brace types:

prophylactic, postoperative, and functional. We shall limit this discussion to functional knee braces only, which may be used by patients after ligament rupture to minimize joint impairment and to lower the risk for reinjury. Functional braces have been recommended for patients with pathologic knee motion secondary to ligament disruptions or for patients following knee ligament surgery. The proposed mechanisms of action are a mechanical constraint of joint motion and enhancement of joint position sense and protective neuromuscular reflex pathways.

A number of investigators have demonstrated that functional knee braces decrease anterior joint subluxation in the ACL-disrupted knee at low loads, but do not eliminate joint subluxation (177–185). Mortensen et al. (185) measured anterior displacement with the KT-2000 in ten cadaveric knees with the ligaments intact and the ACL sectioned. They then repeated the measurements after applying a commercial knee brace (Fig. 20.2). Custom braces were made from plaster molds of the limbs. Eleven brace designs were tested on ten knees: Six were custom braces (CTI, Indiana, Lenox Hill, MKS III, Omni TS-7, and Townsend) and five were "off-the-shelf" braces (Don-Joy 4-Point, Ecko, Lerman multiligament, Lorus, and Nuko). One brace design, the Generation II, was tested on five knees. At a 20-lb load, the anterior displacement in the ACL-disrupted knee was reduced 3 mm or more in 10 of 12 braces; at the 40-lb load, a similar reduction occurred in 4 of 12 braces (Fig. 20.3). The pathologic quadriceps displacement was reduced by 50% in 9 of 12 braces (Fig. 20.4). Mortensen et al. (185) also tested the specimens on the Oxford testing rig (157,165). Sectioning the ACL resulted in a small increase in internal tibial rotation in the quadriceps-stabilized knee. Functional knee bracing did not constrain axial rotation. The authors did not observe any significant difference between custom braces and off-the-shelf braces.

Mishra et al. (184) evaluated 42 patients with an ACL-disrupted knee who used a functional knee brace. KT-1000 arthrometer testing was performed as part of the evaluation. When measuring the braced knee, the tibial tubercle sensor was replaced by a hook that fit under the brace to contact the tibial sensor with the skin over the tibial tubercle (Fig. 20.5). In the unbraced state, the 20-lb *I–N* displacement difference was 5 mm. Bracing reduced the displacement but did not restore it to normal (Table 20.13).

Branch et al. (186) investigated the concept that braces may function to enhance joint proprioception. An electromyogram (EMG) study was performed on ACL-injured patients in and out of brace to determine if the use of a brace altered the EMG muscle-firing pattern. There was no significant difference between the braced and unbraced conditions. Beynnon et al. (187) studied the effect that chronic ACL disruption, functional bracing, and a neoprene sleeve have on knee proprioception by measuring the threshold to detection of passive knee

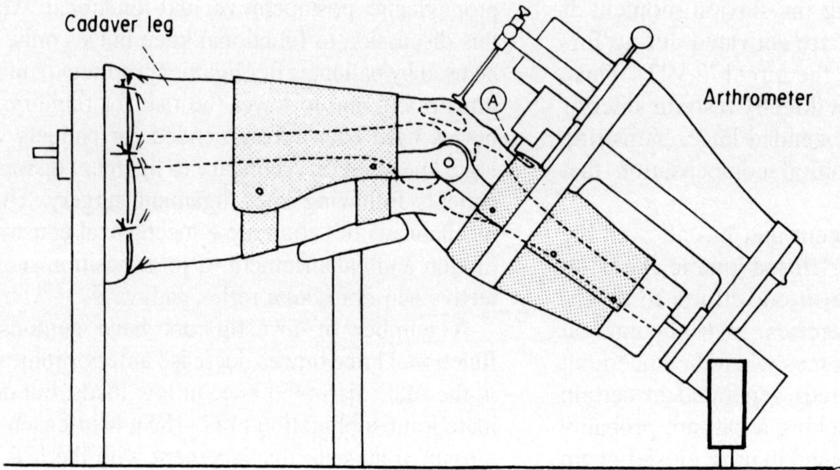

FIGURE 20.2. The KT-1000 arthrometer (MEDmetric, San Diego, CA) was used to test anterior–posterior (A/P) displacement in a cadaver limb. The fresh-frozen limbs were 23 inches in length and were mounted with femoral and tibial intramedullary rods. The thigh soft tissues were sutured to a proximal plate, and a canvas strap was sutured to the patellar tendon to do the quadriceps displacement test. The tibial tubercle pad was replaced with a hook (A) to allow the sensor to be in direct contact with the skin.

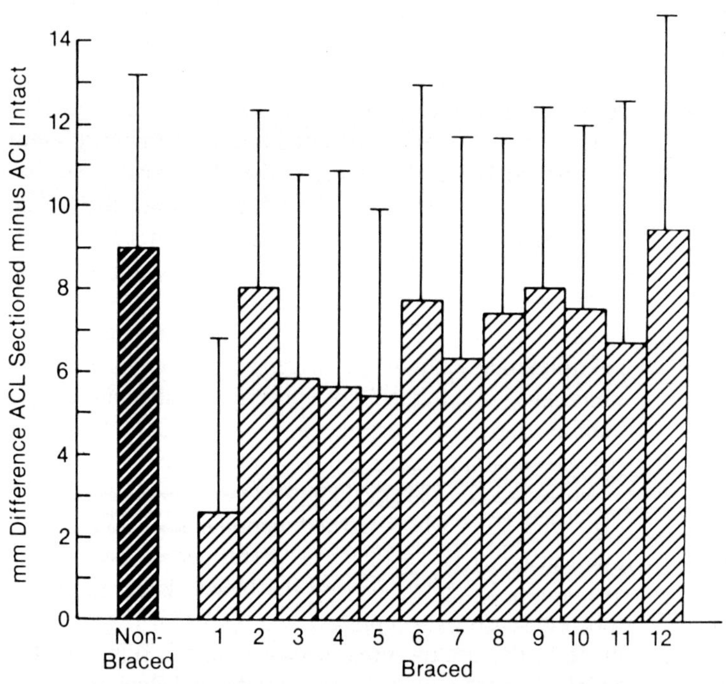

FIGURE 20.3. Anterior displacement tests with the KT-2000 with a 40-lb displacement force. The injured minus intact displacement difference for the unbraced anterior cruciate ligament (ACL)–disrupted knee and the braced ACL-disrupted knees for each brace is given. The results of braces 2 through 12 are similar. The displacement for brace 1 is less than that of the other 11 braces. Brace 1 was a custom-made brace. The brace fit very tightly and caused significant soft tissue deformity that the investigators believed could not be tolerated by a patient.

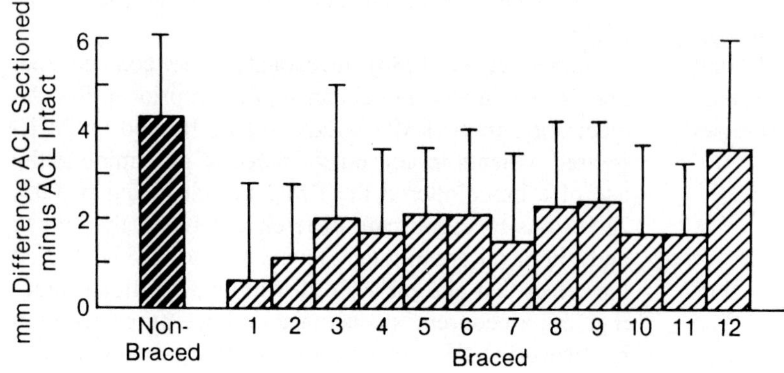

FIGURE 20.4. Quadriceps active displacement was achieved by extending the leg by pulling a strap attached to the quadriceps tendon. The increased displacement after sectioning the anterior cruciate ligament (ACL) is shown for the unbraced and braced conditions.

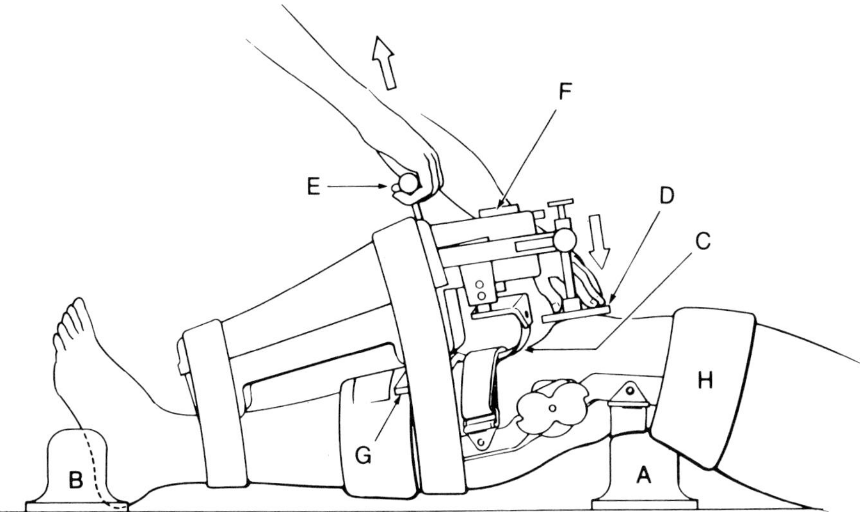

FIGURE 20.5. KT-1000 arthrometer (MEDmetric, San Diego, CA) adapted for knee brace. (*A*) Thigh support, (*B*) foot rest, (*C*) hook adapter for tibial sensor, (*D*) patella sensor, (*E*) force handle, (*F*) displacement dial, (*G*) wooden block adapter for knee brace bulk, (*H*) functional brace.

motion in all three conditions. The threshold to detection of passive knee motion was worse in knees with chronic ACL insufficiency when compared with uninjured knees. This difference was small, and of questionable significance from a clinical and functional perspective. Wearing a functional brace or neoprene sleeve on the ACL-deficient knee did not significantly change the threshold to detection of passive motion in comparison with the same knee without a brace, although improvements were observed. No relationship was detected between the magnitude of AP knee laxity or the grade of

pivot shift and the threshold to detection of passive knee motion.

Investigators have also evaluated brace use by performing functional tests in brace users in and out of their braces. Houston and Goemans (182) performed Cybex strength testing on seven male athletes. Their peak torque was greater at all speeds without the brace. A 15-minute endurance test showed 41% higher blood lactate with brace use. Houston and Goemans concluded that functional knee braces impair muscle performance. Zetterlund et al. (188) studied energy expenditure resulting

TABLE 20.13. *Comparison of mean side-to-side differences in displacement*

Group	n		Anterior drawer (20 lb) at 30 degrees (mm)	Manual maximum at 30 degrees (mm)	Quadriceps active at 30 degrees (mm)
All braces	42	I–N	5.00±2.04	6.45±2.36	4.06±1.71
		B–N	1.41±2.25	2.75±2.32	1.70±1.65
		p^a	<0.001	<0.001	<0.001
Don-Joy 4-point	20	I–N	5.16±1.46	6.29±2.32	4.05±1.94
		B–hN	0.47±1.98	1.97±1.70	1.37±1.58
		p^a	<0.001	<0.001	<0.001
CTI	6	I–N	4.75±4.31	7.42±1.50	5.08±2.06
		B–N	1.17±2.04	2.58±2.29	1.25±1.97
		p^a	<0.05	<0.006	<0.003
Lenox Hill	7	I–N	5.07±1.43	6.79±2.93	4.29±0.95
		B–N	3.00±2.06	4.07±2.32	3.07±1.30
		p^a	0.006	<0.001	<0.043
RKS	9	I–N	4.75±1.56	5.81±2.58	3.13±0.88
		B–N	2.44±2.29	3.56±3.17	1.63±1.53
		p^a	0.001	<0.009	<0.003

I–N, injured minus normal side-to-side difference; B–N, braced injured knee minus normal side-to-side difference.

[a]Matched *t* tests (injured no brace minus normal) versus (injured with brace minus normal).

TABLE 20.14. *Summary of specific task performance, knee pain with sports, knee swelling with sports (number of patients with given response)*

Specific task performance rating				
	Good	Fair	Poor	Unknown	n
Without brace	10	25	7	0	42
With brace	22	16	1	3	42

Knee pain with sports				
	No pain	Mild	Moderate	Severe	Unknown
Without brace	26	11	1	2	2
With brace	35	4	2	0	1

Knee swelling with sports				
	No swelling	With strenuous activity	Moderate	Severe	Unknown
Without brace	26	11	2	1	2
With brace	34	6	1	0	1

from running on a treadmill. A small but significant increase in oxygen consumption and heart rate were noted with brace use. Mishra et al. (184) had brace users perform the 40-yd shuttle run and one-leg hop for distance in and out of the brace. Statistical analysis of the results of the 42 patients tested showed no significant difference with brace use. Some of the more impaired patients did increase their one-leg hop for distance performance with brace use. Warming and Jorgensen (189) studied the effect of functional knee bracing on isokinetic strength in 11 subjects with unilateral ACL insufficiency, using two braces (Donjoy Legend and Bledsoe Brace Force III) and a "placebo brace." The patients were tested on a Biodex Dynamometer at 60° and 180° per second in an isokinetic mode. The experiment used a crossover design with the stable knee as the patient's own control. They observed no statistically significant effect of the two braces compared with the placebo brace and no correlation between knee laxity and the effect of bracing. Kramer et al. (190), in a very thorough and systematic review of the available literature on the effect of bracing on performance in specific dynamic function tests, found insufficient evidence to suggest that functional braces improve functional performance in ACL-deficient patients. There seems to be little evidence to support brace use for improving muscle performance in an ACL-deficient knee.

The following question remains to be answered: **Does the use of a functional brace prevent injury?** The evidence suggests that it does not. Yet, functional braces are commonly used in the unstable knee to prevent further injury and in the reconstructed knee to prevent graft failure. In contrast to the lack of objective documentation that braces are useful, many patients believe they have better function in a brace and, when asked, report that they participate more vigorously in sports activity (Tables 20.14 and 20.15) (184). Mishra et al. (184) reported that patients state that they have fewer giving-way episodes in the brace (Table 20.16). However, there are no published data to support the thesis that braces prevent reinjury or reduce the incidence of giving-way episodes in an ACL-deficient knee, or prevent graft failure after reconstruction.

Authors' Approach to Nonoperative Treatment of the Anterior Cruciate Ligament–Deficient Knee

Our protocol for nonoperative treatment of the ACL-injured patient is shown in (Fig. 20.6). We stress nonimpact, noncompetitive conditioning exercises that will restore strength, stamina, and balance to the quadriceps and other muscle groups of the lower extremity. We agree with Noyes et al. (22,23), Dye et al. (116), Wojtys (1), and others that the most important part of nonoperative management is to understand the patient's objectives and to

TABLE 20.15. *Sport I performance[a] levels: all braces[b] (number of patients with given response)*

	Cannot play	100%	90%	75%	50%	25%	Severe	Unknown
No brace	8	4	1	10	4	3	5	7
With brace	4	1	11	10	7	0	2	7

Sport I class: strenuous = 24, moderate = 18; preinjury hr/yr: mean = 210 (range, 100–1600); postinjury hr/yr: mean = 112 (range, 0–1600).

[a]Preinjury performance established as 100%.

[b]Sport I was the subject's sport of greatest participation prior to injury. A strenuous sport was defined as a sport involving jumping or cutting. A moderate sport was defined as a sport involving running or lateral motion, but not involving jumping or cutting.

TABLE 20.16. *"Giving way" episodes after injury*

"Giving way"	n	Gives way	No giving way	Unknown
No brace (pooled)	42	24	15	3
All braces (pooled)		6	34	2
Without Don-Joy 4-point	20	10	7	3
With Don-Joy 4 point		1	17	2
Without CT	9	4	5	0
With CT		0	9	0
Without Lenox Hill	6	5	1	0
With Lenox Hill		2	4	0
Without RKS	7	5	2	0
With RKS		3	4	0

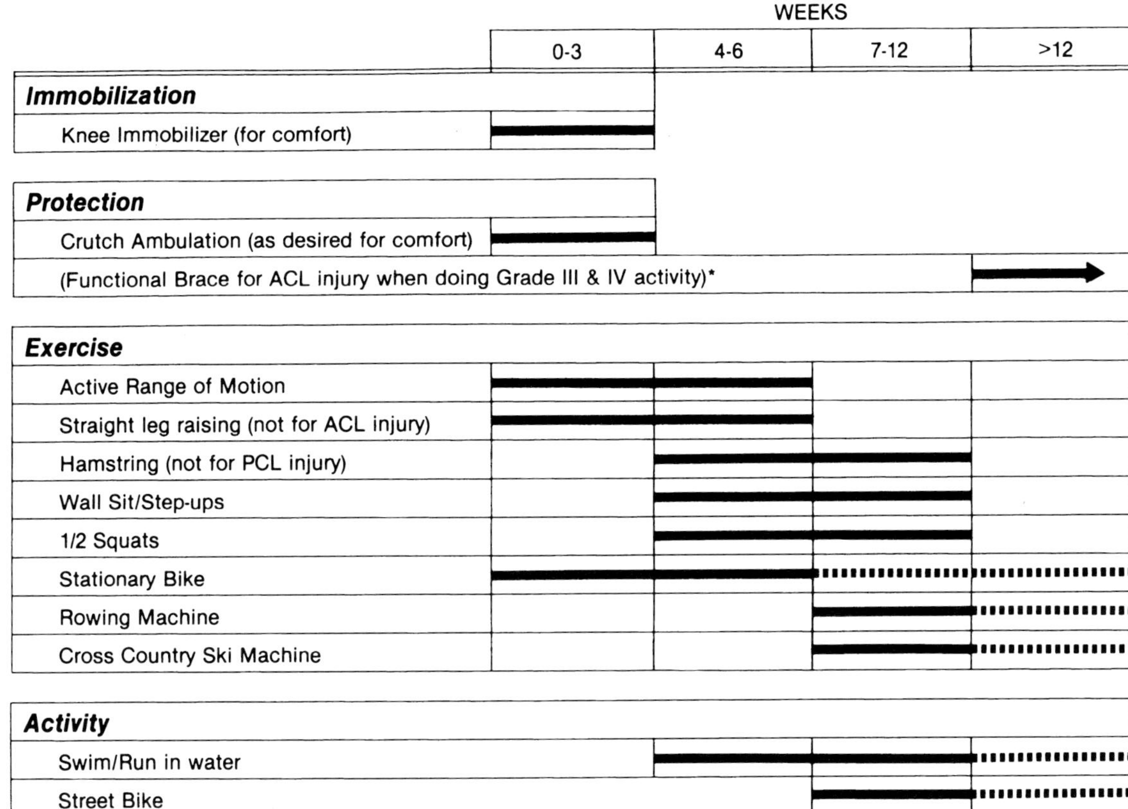

At 12 wks if there is no pain or swelling, full range of motion, and satisfactory strength, activities may progress in this order:

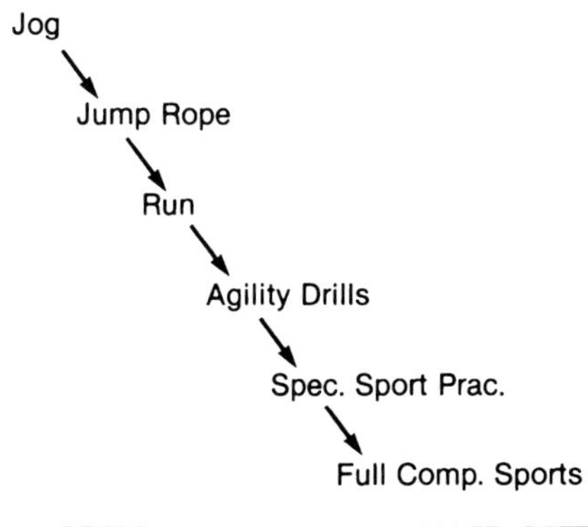

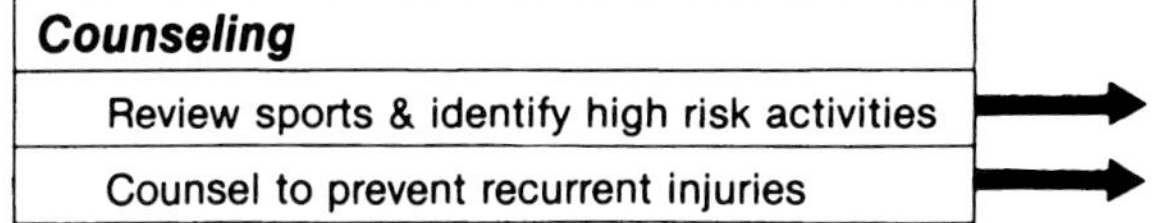

* Efficacy of brace to reduce knee injury has not been documented.

FIGURE 20.6. Nonoperative rehabilitation protocol for single-ligament injury.

communicate the risks presented by the ACL injury (149,191). It is the authors' custom not to recommend functional brace use for patients with ACL disruptions. If an individual patient feels nevertheless that he or she would prefer to use a brace, we recommend a simple, inexpensive knee sleeve, rather than an ACL brace.

REFERENCES

1. Wojtys EM, ed. The ACL deficient knee. *American Academy of Orthopaedic Surgeons Monograph Series* 1994:129.
2. Stark J. Two cases of rupture of the crucial ligaments of the knee-joint. *Edinb Med Surg J* 1850;74:267–271.
3. O'Donoghue DH. An analysis of end results of surgical treatment of major injuries to the ligaments of the knee. *J Bone Joint Surg Am* 1955;37:1–13, 124.
4. Liljedahl SO, Lindvall N, Wetterfors J. Early diagnosis and treatment of acute ruptures of the anterior cruciate ligament: a clinical and arthrographic study of forty-eight cases. *J Bone Joint Surg Am* 1965;47:1503–1513.
5. Jacobsen K. Osteoarthrosis following insufficiency of the cruciate ligaments in man: a clinical study. *Acta Orthop Scand* 1977;48:520–526.
6. Feagin JA Jr, Curl WW. Isolated tear of the anterior cruciate ligament: 5-year follow-up study. *Am J Sports Med* 1976;4:95–100.
7. Youmans WT. The so-called "isolated" anterior cruciate ligament tear or anterior cruciate ligament syndrome: a report of 32 cases with some observation on treatment and its effect on results. *Am J Sports Med* 1978;6:26–30.
8. Chick RR, Jackson DW. Tears of the anterior cruciate ligament in young athletes. *J Bone Joint Surg Am* 1978;60:970–973.
9. Gillquist J, Hagberg G, Oretorp N. Arthroscopy in acute injuries of the knee joint. *Acta Orthop Scand* 1977;48:190–196.
10. DeHaven KE. Diagnosis of acute knee injuries with hemarthrosis. *Am J Sports Med* 1980;8:9–14.
11. Noyes FR, Bassett RW, Grood ES, et al. Arthroscopy in acute traumatic hemarthrosis of the knee: incidence of anterior cruciate tears and other injuries. *J Bone Joint Surg Am* 1980;62:687–695, 757.
12. Hardaker WT Jr, Garrett WE Jr, Bassett FHD. Evaluation of acute traumatic hemarthrosis of the knee joint. *South Med J* 1990;83:640–644.
13. Daniel DM, Stone ML, Dobson BE, et al. Fate of the ACL-injured patient: a prospective outcome study. *Am J Sports Med* 1994;22:632–644.
14. Butler JC, Andrews JR. The role of arthroscopic surgery in the evaluation of acute traumatic hemarthrosis of the knee. *Clin Orthop* 1988;228:150–152.
15. DeHaven KE. Decision-making in acute anterior cruciate ligament injury. *Instr Course Lect* 1987;36:201–203.
16. Woods GW, Chapman DR. Repairable posterior menisco-capsular disruption in anterior cruciate ligament injuries. *Am J Sports Med* 1984;12:381–385.
17. Bomberg BC, McGinty JB. Acute hemarthrosis of the knee: indications for diagnostic arthroscopy. *Arthroscopy* 1990;6:221–225.
18. Maffulli N, Binfield PM, King JB, et al. Acute haemarthrosis of the knee in athletes: a prospective study of 106 cases. *J Bone Joint Surg Br* 1993;75:945–949.
19. Fetto JF, Marshall JL. The natural history and diagnosis of anterior cruciate ligament insufficiency. *Clin Orthop* 1980;147:29–38.
20. Giove TP, Miller SJ 3rd, Kent BE, et al. Non-operative treatment of the torn anterior cruciate ligament. *J Bone Joint Surg Am* 1983;65:184–192.
21. Jokl P, Kaplan N, Stovell P, et al. Non-operative treatment of severe injuries to the medial and anterior cruciate ligaments of the knee. *J Bone Joint Surg Am* 1984;66:714–741.
22. Noyes FR, Matthews DS, Mooar PA, et al. The symptomatic anterior cruciate-deficient knee, II: the results of rehabilitation, activity modification, and counseling on functional disability. *J Bone Joint Surg Am* 1983;65:163–174.
23. Noyes FR, Mooar PA, Matthews DS, et al. The symptomatic anterior cruciate-deficient knee, I: the long-term functional disability in athletically active individuals. *J Bone Joint Surg Am* 1983;65:154–162.
24. Walla DJ, Albright JP, McAuley E, et al. Hamstring control and the unstable anterior cruciate ligament-deficient knee. *Am J Sports Med* 1985;13:34–39.
25. Satku K, Kumar VP, Ngoi SS. Anterior cruciate ligament injuries: to counsel or to operate? *J Bone Joint Surg Br* 1986;68:458–461.
26. Kannus P, Jarvinen M. Conservatively treated tears of the anterior cruciate ligament: long-term results. *J Bone Joint Surg Am* 1987;69:1007–1012.
27. AMA, C.o.t.M.A.o.S.o.t. Standard nomenclature of athletic injuries. Chicago: American Medical Association, 1968;99–100.
28. Hole RL, Lintner DM, Kamaric E, et al. Increased tibial translation after partial sectioning of the anterior cruciate ligament: the posterolateral bundle. *Am J Sports Med* 1996;24:556–560.
29. Pattee GA, Fox JM, Del Pizzo W, et al. Four to ten year followup of unreconstructed anterior cruciate ligament tears. *Am J Sports Med* 1989;17:430–435.
30. Bonamo JJ, Fay C, Firestone T. The conservative treatment of the anterior cruciate deficient knee. *Am J Sports Med* 1990;18:618–623.
31. Drongowski RA, Coran AG, Wojtys EM. Predictive value of meniscal and chondral injuries in conservatively treated anterior cruciate ligament injuries. *Arthroscopy* 1994;10:97–102.
32. Kaplan PA, Walker CW, Kilcoyne RF, et al. Occult fracture patterns of the knee associated with anterior cruciate ligament tears: assessment with MR imaging. *Radiology* 1992;183:835–838.
33. Murphy BJ, Smith RL, Uribe JW, et al. Bone signal abnormalities in the posterolateral tibia and lateral femoral condyle in complete tears of the anterior cruciate ligament: a specific sign? *Radiology* 1992;182:221–224.
34. Rosen MA, Jackson DW, Berger PE. Occult osseous lesions documented by magnetic resonance imaging associated with anterior cruciate ligament ruptures. *Arthroscopy* 1991;7:45–51.
35. Speer KP, Spritzer CE, Bassett FH 3rd, et al. Osseous injury associated with acute tears of the anterior cruciate ligament. *Am J Sports Med* 1992;20:382–389.
36. Vellet AD, Marks PH, Fowler PJ, et al. Occult posttraumatic osteochondral lesions of the knee: prevalence, classification, and short-term sequelae evaluated with MR imaging. *Radiology* 1991;178:271–276.
37. Zeiss J, Paley K, Murray K, et al. Comparison of bone contusion seen by MRI in partial and complete tears of the anterior cruciate ligament. *J Comput Assist Tomogr* 1995;19:773–776.
38. Andersson C, Odensten M, Gillquist J. Knee function after surgical or nonsurgical treatment of acute rupture of the anterior cruciate ligament: a randomized study with a long-term follow-up period. *Clin Orthop* 1991;264:255–263.
39. Clancy WG Jr, Ray JM, Zoltan DJ. Acute tears of the anterior cruciate ligament: surgical versus conservative treatment. *J Bone Joint Surg Am* 1988;70:1483–1488.
40. Engebretsen L, Tegnander A. Short-term results of the nonoperated isolated anterior cruciate ligament tear. *J Orthop Trauma* 1990;4:406–410.
41. Hawkins RJ, Misamore GW, Merritt TR. Follow-up of the acute nonoperated isolated anterior cruciate ligament tear. *Am J Sports Med* 1986;14:205–210.
42. Meunier A, et al. Osteoarthritis after surgical or conservative treatment of the acutely torn anterior cruciate ligament: a randomized study with 15 years follow-up. In: Swedish Orthopedic Society. Skoevde: Acta Orthop Scand 1999;(Suppl 287).
43. Andersson C, Odensten M, Good L, et al. Surgical or non-surgical treatment of acute rupture of the anterior cruciate ligament: a randomized study with long-term follow-up. *J Bone Joint Surg Am* 1989;71:965–974.
44. Daniel DM, Stone ML, Dobson BE, et al. Fate of the ACL-injured patient: a prospective outcome study [see comments]. *Am J Sports Med* 1994;22:632–644.
45. Wickiewicz TL. Meniscal injuries in the cruciate-deficient knee. *Clin Sports Med* 1990;9:681–694.
46. Hefti F, Müller W, Jakob RP, et al. Evaluation of knee ligament injuries with the IKDC form. *Knee Surg Sports Traumatol Arthrosc* 1993;1:226–234.
47. Eastlack ME, Axe MJ, Snyder-Mackler L. Laxity, instability, and functional outcome after ACL injury: copers versus noncopers. *Med Sci Sports Exerc* 1999;31:210–215.
48. McDaniel WJ Jr, Dameron TB Jr. Untreated ruptures of the anterior cruciate ligament: a follow-up study. *J Bone Joint Surg Am* 1980;62:696–705.

49. McDaniel WJ Jr, Dameron TB Jr. The untreated anterior cruciate ligament rupture. *Clin Orthop* 1983;172:158–163.
50. Fowler PJ, Regan WD. The patient with symptomatic chronic anterior cruciate ligament insufficiency: results of minimal arthroscopic surgery and rehabilitation. *Am J Sports Med* 1987;15:321–325.
51. Indelicato PA, Bittar ES. A perspective of lesions associated with ACL insufficiency of the knee: a review of 100 cases. *Clin Orthop* 1985;198:77–80.
52. Lynch MA, Henning CE, Glick RK Jr. Knee joint surface changes: long-term follow-up meniscus tear treatment in stable anterior cruciate ligament reconstructions. *Clin Orthop* 1983;172:148–153.
53. Sommerlath K, Lysholm J, Gillquist J. The long-term course after treatment of acute anterior cruciate ligament ruptures: a 9 to 16 year followup. *Am J Sports Med* 1991;19:156–162.
54. Dye SF, Chew MH. Restoration of osseous homeostasis after anterior cruciate ligament reconstruction. *Am J Sports Med* 1993;21:748–750.
55. Dye SF, Chew MH. The use of scintigraphy to detect increased osseous metabolic activity about the knee. *Instr Course Lect* 1994;43:453–469.
56. Fairbank TJ. Knee joint changes after meniscectomy. *J Bone Joint Surg Br* 1948;30:664–670.
57. Hirshman HP, Daniel DM, Miyasaka K. The fate of unoperated knee ligament injuries. In: Daniel DM, Akeson WH, O'Connor JJ, eds. *Knee ligaments: structure, function, injury, and repair.* New York: Raven Press, 1990:481–503.
58. Johnson RJ, Kettelkamp DB, Clark W, et al. Factors affecting late results after meniscectomy. *J Bone Joint Surg Am* 1974;56:719–729.
59. Tapper EM, Hoover NW. Late results after meniscectomy. *J Bone Joint Surg Am* 1969;51:517–526.
60. Arnoczky SP, Rubin RM, Marshall JL. Microvasculature of the cruciate ligaments and its response to injury: an experimental study in dogs. *J Bone Joint Surg Am* 1979;61:1221–1229.
61. Buckley SL, Barrack RL, Alexander AH. The natural history of conservatively treated partial anterior cruciate ligament tears. *Am J Sports Med* 1989;17:221–225.
62. Feagin JA Jr. Operative treatment of acute and chronic knee problems. *Clin Sports Med* 1985;4:325–331.
63. Umans H, Wimpfheimer O, Haramati N, et al. Diagnosis of partial tears of the anterior cruciate ligament of the knee: value of MR imaging. *AJR Am J Roentgenol* 1995;165:893–897.
64. Roychowdhury S, Fitzgerald SW, Sonin AH, et al. Using MR imaging to diagnose partial tears of the anterior cruciate ligament: value of axial images. *AJR Am J Roentgenol* 1997;168:1487–1491.
65. Farquharson–Roberts MA, Osborne AH. Partial rupture of the anterior cruciate ligament of the knee. *J Bone Joint Surg Br* 1983;65:32–34.
66. McDaniel WJ. Isolated partial tear of the anterior cruciate ligament. *Clin Orthop* 1976;115:209–212.
67. Monaco BR, Noble HB, Bachman DC. Incomplete tears of the anterior cruciate ligament and knee locking. *JAMA* 1982;247:1582–1584.
68. Odensten M, Lysholm J, Gillquist J. The course of partial anterior cruciate ligament ruptures. *Am J Sports Med* 1985;13:183–186.
69. Sandberg R, Balkfors B. Partial rupture of the anterior cruciate ligament: natural course. *Clin Orthop* 1987;220:176–178.
70. Angel KR, Hall DJ. Anterior cruciate ligament injury in children and adolescents. *Arthroscopy* 1989;5:197–200.
71. Angel KR, Hall DJ. The role of arthroscopy in children and adolescents. *Arthroscopy* 1989;5:192–196.
72. Bergstrom R, Gillquist J, Lysholm J, et al. Arthroscopy of the knee in children. *J Pediatr Orthop* 1984;4:542–545.
73. Bradley GW, Shives TC, Samuelson KM. Ligament injuries in the knees of children. *J Bone Joint Surg Am* 1979;61:588–591.
74. DeLee JC. ACL insufficiency in children. In: Feagin J, ed. *The crucial ligaments.* New York: Livingstone, 1988:439–447.
75. DeLee JC, Curtis R. Anterior cruciate ligament insufficiency in children. *Clin Orthop* 1983;172:112–118.
76. Engebretsen L, Svenningsen S, Benum P. Poor results of anterior cruciate ligament repair in adolescence. *Acta Orthop Scand* 1988;59:684–686.
77. Eskjaer S, Larsen ST. Arthroscopy of the knee in children. *Acta Orthop Scand* 1987;58:273–276.
78. Eskjaer S, Larsen ST, Schmidt MB. The significance of hemarthrosis of the knee in children. *Arch Orthop Trauma Surg* 1988;107:96–98.
79. Graf BK, Lange RH, Fujisaki CK, et al. Anterior cruciate ligament tears in skeletally immature patients: meniscal pathology at presentation and after attempted conservative treatment. *Arthroscopy* 1992;8:229–233.
80. Juhl M, Boe S. Arthroscopy in children, with special emphasis on meniscal lesions. *Injury* 1986;17:171–173.
81. Kannus P, Jarvinen M. Knee ligament injuries in adolescents. *J Bone Joint Surg Br* 1988;70:772–776.
82. Kellenberger R, von Laer L. Nonosseous lesions of the anterior cruciate ligaments in childhood and adolescence. *Prog Pediatr Surg* 1990;25:123–131.
83. Lipscomb AB, Anderson AF. Tears of the anterior cruciate ligament in adolescents. *J Bone Joint Surg Am* 1986;68:19–28.
84. Matz SO, Jackson DW. Anterior cruciate ligament injury in children. *Am J Knee Surg* 1988;1:59–65.
85. McCarroll JR, Rettig AC, Shelbourne KD. Anterior cruciate ligament injuries in the young athlete with open physes. *Am J Sports Med* 1988;16:44–47.
86. Robinson SC, Driscoll SE. Simultaneous osteochondral avulsion of the femoral and tibial insertions of the anterior cruciate ligament: report of a case in a thirteen-year-old boy. *J Bone Joint Surg Am* 1981;63:1342–1343.
87. Steiner ME, Grana WA. The young athlete's knee: recent advances. *Clin Sports Med* 1988;7:527–546.
88. Vahasarja V, Kinnuen P, Serlo W. Arthroscopy of the acute traumatic knee in children. Prospective study of 138 cases. *Acta Orthop Scand* 1993;64:580–582.
89. Waldrop JI, Broussard TS. Disruption of the anterior cruciate ligament in a three-year-old child: a case report. *J Bone Joint Surg Am* 1984;66:1113–1114.
90. Bachelin P, Bugmann D. Active subluxation in extension, radiological control in intercondylar eminence fractures in childhood. *Z Kinderchir* 1988;43:180–182.
91. Eady JL, Cardenas CD, Sopa D. Avulsion of the femoral attachment of the anterior cruciate ligament in a seven-year-old child: a case report. *J Bone Joint Surg Am* 1982;64:1376–1378.
92. Lahm A, Erggelet C, Steinwachs M, et al. Articular and osseous lesions in recent ligament tears: arthroscopic changes compared with magnetic resonance imaging findings. *Arthroscopy* 1998;14:597–604.
93. Mizuta H, Kubota K, Shiraishi M, et al. The conservative treatment of complete tears of the anterior cruciate ligament in skeletally immature patients [see comments]. *J Bone Joint Surg Br* 1995;77:890–894.
94. Parker AW, Drez D Jr, Cooper JL. Anterior cruciate ligament injuries in patients with open physes [see comments]. *Am J Sports Med* 1994;22:44–47.
95. Shelbourne KD, Nitz PA. Anterior cruciate ligament injuries in school-aged athletes. In: Reider B, ed. *Sports medicine: the school age athlete.* Philadephia: WB Saunders, 1990.
96. Kannus P, Jarvinen M. Knee ligament injuries in adolescents: eight year follow-up of conservative management. *J Bone Joint Surg Br* 1988;70:772–776.
97. Hefti F, Muller W. Current state of evaluation of knee ligament lesions: the new IKDC knee evaluation form. *Orthopade* 1993;22:351–362.
98. Iborra JP, Mazeau P, Lovahem D, et al. [Fractures of the intercondylar eminence of the tibia in children. Apropos of 25 cases with a 1-20 year follow up]. *Rev Chir Orthop Reparatrice Appar Mot* 1999;85:563–573.
99. Meyers MH, McKeever FM. Fracture of the intercondylar eminence of the tibia. *J Bone Joint Surg Am* 1959;41:209–222.
100. Meyers MH, McKeever FM. Fracture of the intercondylar eminence of the tibia. *J Bone Joint Surg Am* 1970;52:1677–1684.
101. Zaricznyj B. Avulsion fracture of the tibial eminence: treatment by open reduction and pinning. *J Bone Joint Surg Am* 1977;59:1111–1114.
102. Clanton TO, DeLee JC, Sanders B, et al. Knee ligament injuries in children. *J Bone Joint Surg Am* 1979;61:1195–1201.
103. Lo IK, Bell DM, Fowler PJ. Anterior cruciate ligament injuries in the skeletally immature patient. *Instr Course Lect* 1998;47:351–359.
104. Nottage WM, Matsuura PA. Management of complete traumatic anterior cruciate ligament tears in the skeletally immature patient: current concepts and review of the literature. *Arthroscopy* 1994;10:569–573.
105. Bisson LJ, Wickiewicz T, Levinson M, et al. ACL reconstruction in children with open physes [see comments]. *Orthopedics* 1998;21:659–663.
106. Lo IK, Kirkley A, Fowler PJ, et al. The outcome of operatively treated anterior cruciate ligament disruptions in the skeletally immature child. *Arthroscopy* 1997;13:627–634.
107. Matava MJ, Siegel MG. Arthroscopic reconstruction of the ACL with

semitendinosus-gracilis autograft in skeletally immature adolescent patients. *Am J Knee Surg* 1997;10:60–69.

108. Koman JD, Sanders JO. Valgus deformity after reconstruction of the anterior cruciate ligament in a skeletally immature patient: a case report. *J Bone Joint Surg Am* 1999;81:711–715.

109. Guzzanti V, Falciglia F, Gigante A, et al. The effect of intra-articular ACL reconstruction on the growth plates of rabbits. *J Bone Joint Surg Br* 1994;76:960–963.

110. Stadelmaier DM, Arnoczky SP, Dodds J, et al. The effect of drilling and soft tissue grafting across open growth plates: a histologic study. *Am J Sports Med* 1995;23:431–435.

111. Gruelich WW, Pyle SL. *Radiographic atlas of skeletal development of the hand and wrist.* Stanford: Stanford University Press, 1959.

112. Anderson M, Green W, Messner MB. Growth and predictions of growth in the lower extremities. *J Bone Joint Surg Am* 1963;45:7–21.

113. Wester W, Canale ST, Dutkowsky JP, et al. Prediction of angular deformity and leg-length discrepancy after anterior cruciate ligament reconstruction in skeletally immature patients. *J Pediatr Orthop* 1994; 14:516–521.

114. Andrews M, Noyes FR, Barber-Westin SD. Anterior cruciate ligament allograft reconstruction in the skeletally immature athlete. *Am J Sports Med* 1994;22:48–54.

115. McCarroll JR, Shelbourne KD, Porter DA, et al. Patellar tendon graft reconstruction for midsubstance anterior cruciate ligament rupture in junior high school athletes: an algorithm for management. *Am J Sports Med* 1994;22:478–484.

116. Dye SF, Wojtys EM, Fu FH, et al. Factors contributing to function of the knee joint after injury or reconstruction of the anterior cruciate ligament. *Instr Course Lect* 1999;48:185–198.

117. Holden DL, Jackson DW. Treatment selection in acute anterior cruciate ligament tears. *Orthop Clin North Am* 1985;16:99–109.

118. Daniel DM, Stone ML, Sachs R, et al. Instrumented measurement of anterior knee laxity in patients with acute anterior cruciate ligament disruption. *Am J Sports Med* 1985;13:401–407.

119. Karrholm J, Selvik G, Elmqvist LG, et al. Active knee motion after cruciate ligament rupture: stereoradiography. *Acta Orthop Scand* 1988;59:158–164.

120. Marans HJ, Jackson RW, Glossop ND, et al. Anterior cruciate ligament insufficiency: a dynamic three-dimensional motion analysis. *Am J Sports Med* 1989;17:325–332.

121. Markolf KL, Kochan A, Amstutz HC. Measurement of knee stiffness and laxity in patients with documented absence of the anterior cruciate ligament. *J Bone Joint Surg Am* 1984;66:242–252.

122. Shiavi R, Limbird T, Frazer M, et al. Helical motion analysis of the knee, II: kinematics of uninjured and injured knees during walking and pivoting. *J Biomech* 1987;20:653–665.

123. Corrigan JP, Cashman WF, Brady MP. Proprioception in the cruciate deficient knee. *J Bone Joint Surg Br* 1992;74:247–250.

124. Beard DJ, Kyberd PJ, O'Connor JJ, et al. Reflex hamstring contraction latency in anterior cruciate ligament deficiency. *J Orthop Res* 1994; 12:219–228.

125. Krauspe R, Schmidt M, Schaible HG. Sensory innervation of the anterior cruciate ligament: an electrophysiological study of response properties of single identified mechanoreceptors in the cat. *J Bone Joint Surg Am* 1992;74:390–397.

126. Solomonow M, Baratta R, Zhou BH, et al. The synergistic action of the anterior cruciate ligament and thigh muscles in maintaining joint stability. *Am J Sports Med* 1987;15:207–213.

127. Gerber C, Hoppeler H, Claassen H, et al. The lower-extremity musculature in chronic symptomatic instability of the anterior cruciate ligament. *J Bone Joint Surg Am* 1985;67:1034–1043.

128. Snyder-Mackler L, Binder-Macleod SA, Williams PR. Fatiguability of human quadriceps femoris muscle following anterior cruciate ligament reconstruction. *Med Sci Sports Exerc* 1993;25:783–789.

129. Snyder–Mackler L, Delitto A, Stralka SW, et al. Use of electrical stimulation to enhance recovery of quadriceps femoris muscle force production in patients following anterior cruciate ligament reconstruction [see comments]. *Phys Ther* 1994;74:901–907.

130. Andriacchi TP. Dynamics of pathological motion: applied to the anterior cruciate deficient knee. *J Biomech* 1990;23(suppl 1): 99–105.

131. Berchuck M, Andriacchi TP, Bach BR, et al. Gait adaptations by patients who have a deficient anterior cruciate ligament. *J Bone Joint Surg Am* 1990;72:871–877.

132. Co FH, Skinner HB, Cannon WD. Effect of reconstruction of the anterior cruciate ligament on proprioception of the knee and the heel strike transient. *J Orthop Res* 1993;11:696–704.

133. Friden T, Egund N, Lindstrand A. Comparison of symptomatic versus nonsymptomatic patients with chronic anterior cruciate ligament insufficiency: radiographic sagittal displacement during weightbearing [see comments]. *Am J Sports Med* 1993;21:389–393.

134. Goh JC, Bose K, Khoo BC. Gait analysis study on patients with varus osteoarthrosis of the knee. *Clin Orthop* 1993;294:223–231.

135. Jones D, Tanzer T, Mowbray MA, et al. Studies of dynamic ligamentous instability of the knee by electrogoniometric means. *Prosthet Orthot Int* 1983;7:165–173.

136. Kowalk DL, Duncan JA, McCue FC 3rd, et al. Anterior cruciate ligament reconstruction and joint dynamics during stair climbing. *Med Sci Sports Exerc* 1997;29:1406–1413.

137. Maitland ME, Ajemian SV, Suter E. Quadriceps femoris and hamstring muscle function in a person with an unstable knee. *Phys Ther* 1999;79:66–75.

138. Noyes FR, Dunworth LA, Andriacchi TP, et al. Knee hyperextension gait abnormalities in unstable knees: recognition and preoperative gait retraining. *Am J Sports Med* 1996;24:35–45.

139. Noyes FR, Schipplein OD, Andriacchi TP, et al. The anterior cruciate ligament-deficient knee with varus alignment: an analysis of gait adaptations and dynamic joint loadings. *Am J Sports Med* 1992;20: 707–716.

140. Tibone JE, Antich TJ, Fanton GS, et al. Functional analysis of anterior cruciate ligament instability. *Am J Sports Med* 1986;14:276–284.

141. Timoney JM, Inman WS, Quesada PM, et al. Return of normal gait patterns after anterior cruciate ligament reconstruction. *Am J Sports Med* 1993;21:887–889.

142. Vilensky JA, O'Connor BL, Brandt KD, et al. Serial kinematic analysis of the unstable knee after transection of the anterior cruciate ligament: temporal and angular changes in a canine model of osteoarthritis. *J Orthop Res* 1994;12:229–237.

143. Wexler G, Hurwitz DE, Bush–Joseph DA, et al. Functional gait adaptations in patients with anterior cruciate ligament deficiency over time. *Clin Orthop* 1998;348:166–175.

144. Friden T, Roberts D, Zatterstrom R, et al. Proprioception in the nearly extended knee: measurements of position and movement in healthy individuals and in symptomatic anterior cruciate ligament injured patients. *Knee Surg Sports Traumatol Arthrosc* 1996;4:217–224.

145. Friden T, Roberts D, Zatterstrom R, et al. Proprioception after an acute knee ligament injury: a longitudinal study on 16 consecutive patients. *J Orthop Res* 1997;15:637–644.

146. Borsa PA, Lephart SM, Irrgang JJ, et al. The effects of joint position and direction of joint motion on proprioceptive sensibility in anterior cruciate ligament-deficient athletes. *Am J Sports Med* 1997;25:336–340.

147. Friden T, Zatterstrom R, Lindstrand A, et al. Anterior-cruciate-insufficient knees treated with physiotherapy: a three-year follow-up study of patients with late diagnosis. *Clin Orthop* 1991;263:190–199.

148. Ihara H, Nakayama A. Dynamic control joint training for knee ligament injuries. *Am J Sports Med* 1986;14:309–315.

149. Daniel DM, Fithian DC. Indications for ACL surgery. *Arthroscopy* 1994;10:434–441.

150. Kannus P. Ratio of hamstring to quadriceps femoris muscles' strength in the anterior cruciate ligament insufficient knee: relationship to long-term recovery. *Phys Ther* 1988;68:961–965.

151. Harter RA, Osternig LR, Standifer LW. Isokinetic evaluation of quadriceps and hamstrings symmetry following anterior cruciate ligament reconstruction. *Arch Phys Med Rehabil* 1990;71:465–468.

152. Wyatt MP, Edwardo AM. Comparison of quadriceps and hamstring torque values during isokinetic exercise. *J Orthop Sports Phys Ther* 1981;3:48–56.

153. Daniel DM, et al. A measurement of lower limb function. The one-leg-hop-for-distance. *Am J Knee Surg* 1988;1:212–214.

154. Barber SD, Noyes FR, Mangine RE, et al. Quantitative assessment of functional limitations in normal and anterior cruciate ligament-deficient knees. *Clin Orthop* 1990;255:204–214.

155. Daniel DM, et al. A ten-year prospective outcome study of the ACL-injured patient. in Orthopaedic Research Society. 1996. Atlanta, GA: J Bone Jt Surg.

156. Tegner Y, Lysholm J, Lysholm M, et al. A performance test to monitor rehabilitation and evaluate anterior cruciate ligament injuries. *Am J Sports Med* 1986;14:156–159.

157. O'Connor JJ, Biden E, Bradley J, et al. The muscle-stabilized knee. In:

Daniel M, Akeson WA, O'Connor JJ, eds. *Knee ligaments: structure, function, injury, and repair*. New York: Raven Press, 1990:239–277.

158. Arms SW, Pope MH, Johnson RJ, et al. The biomechanics of anterior cruciate ligament rehabilitation and reconstruction. *Am J Sports Med* 1984;12:8–18.

159. Beynnon B, Howe JG, Pope MH, et al. The measurement of anterior cruciate ligament strain *in vivo*. *Int Orthop* 1992;16:1–12.

160. Beynnon BD, Johnson RJ, Fleming BC. The mechanics of anterior cruciate ligament reconstruction. In: Jackson DW, et al., eds. *The anterior cruciate ligament: current and future concepts*. New York: Raven Press, 1993:259–272.

161. Grood ES, Suntay WJ, Noyes FR, et al. Biomechanics of the knee-extension exercise: effect of cutting the anterior cruciate ligament. *J Bone Joint Surg Am* 1984;66:725–734.

162. Huber H, Mattheck CC. The cruciate ligaments and their effect on the kinematics of the human knee. *Med Biol Eng Comput* 1988;26:647–654.

163. Markolf KL, Gorek JF, Kabo JM, et al. Direct measurement of resultant forces in the anterior cruciate ligament: an *in vitro* study performed with a new experimental technique. *J Bone Joint Surg Am* 1990;72:557–567.

164. O'Connor J, Zavatsky A. Anterior cruciate ligament forces in activity. In: Jackson DW, et al., eds. *The anterior cruciate ligament: current and future concepts*. New York: Raven Press, 1993:131–140.

165. Kaufman KR, Daniel DM, Woo SL-Y. Joint kinematics in muscle-stabilized knees, In: Jackson DW, et al., eds. *The anterior cruciate ligament: current and future concepts*. New York: Raven Press, 1993:113–130.

166. Lutz GE, Palmitier RA, An KN. Comparison of tibiofemoral joint forces during open-kinetic-chain and closed-kinetic-chain exercises. *J Bone Joint Surg Am* 1993;75: 732–739.

167. More RC, Karras BT, Neiman R, et al. Hamstrings—an anterior cruciate ligament protagonist: an *in vitro* study. *Am J Sports Med* 1993; 21:231–237.

168. Gauffin H, Tropp H. Altered movement and muscular-activation patterns during the one-legged jump in patients with an old anterior cruciate ligament rupture. *Am J Sports Med* 1992;20:182–192.

169. Andriacchi TP. Functional evaluation of normal and ACL-deficient knee using gait analysis techniques. In: Jackson DW, et al., eds. *The anterior cruciate ligament: current and future concepts*. New York: Raven Press, 1993:153–159.

170. O'Connor JJ. Can muscle co-contraction protect knee ligaments after injury or repair? *J Bone Joint Surg Br* 1993;75:41–48.

171. Wilson D, et al. Effects of hamstrings cocontraction on *in vitro* knee stability. in Orthopaedic Research Society 43rd Annual Meeting. 1997. San Francisco, California: J Bone Joint Surg.

172. Ohkoshi Y, Yasuda K, Kaneda K, et al. Biomechanical analysis of rehabilitation in the standing position. *Am J Sports Med* 1991;19: 605–611.

173. Ohkoshi Y, Yasuda K, Wada T, et al. [Analysis of the shear force exerted on the tibia during standing on bilateral legs with knee flexion]. *Nippon Seikeigeka Gakkai Zasshi* 1990;64:769–778.

174. Beynnon BD, Fleming BC, Johnson RJ, et al. Anterior cruciate ligament strain behavior during rehabilitation exercises *in vivo. Am J Sports Med* 1995;23:24–34.

175. Fleming BC, Beynnon BD, Renstrom PA, et al. The strain behavior of the anterior cruciate ligament during stair climbing: an *in vivo* study. *Arthroscopy* 1999;15:185–191.

176. Fleming BC, Beynnon BD, Renstrom PA, et al., The strain behavior of the anterior cruciate ligament during bicycling: an *in vivo* study. *Am J Sports Med* 1998;26:109–118.

177. Beck C, Drez D Jr, Young J, et al. Instrumented testing of functional knee braces. *Am J Sports Med* 1986; 14:253–256.

178. Beynnon BD, Johnson RJ, Fleming BC, et al. The effect of functional knee bracing on the anterior cruciate ligament in the weightbearing and nonweightbearing knee. *Am J Sports Med* 1997;25:353–359.

179. Beynnon BD, Pope MH, Wertheimer CM, et al. The effect of functional knee-braces on strain on the anterior cruciate ligament *in vivo. J Bone Joint Surg Am* 1992;74:1298–1312.

180. Branch T, Hunter R, Reynolds P. Controlling anterior tibial displacement under static load: a comparison of two braces. *Orthopedics* 1988;11:1249–1252.

181. Colville MR, Lee CL, Ciullo JV. The Lenox Hill brace: an evaluation of effectiveness in treating knee instability. *Am J Sports Med* 1986;14: 257–261.

182. Houston ME, Goemans PH. Leg muscle performance of athletes with and without knee support braces. *Arch Phys Med Rehabil* 1982;63: 431–432.

183. Liggins AB, Bowker P. A quantitative assessment of orthoses for stabilization of the anterior cruciate ligament deficient knee. *Inst Mech Eng [H]* 1991;205:81–87.

184. Mishra DK, Daniel DM, Stone ML. The use of functional knee braces in the control of pathologic anterior knee laxity. *Clin Orthop* 1989;241:213–220.

185. Mortensen W, et al. An *in vitro* study of functional orthoses in the ACL disrupted knee. *Trans Orthop Res Soc* 1988.

186. Branch TP, Hunter R, Donath M. Dynamic EMG analysis of anterior cruciate deficient legs with and without bracing during cutting. *Am J Sports Med* 1989;17:35–41.

187. Beynnon BD, Ryder SH, Konradsen L, et al. The effect of anterior cruciate ligament trauma and bracing on knee proprioception. *Am J Sports Med* 1999;27:150–155.

188. Zetterlund AE, Serfass RC, Hunter RE. The effect of wearing the complete Lenox Hill Derotation Brace on energy expenditure during horizontal treadmill running at 161 meters per minute. *Am J Sports Med* 1986;14:73–76.

189. Warming T, Jorgensen U. The effect of bracing on extension strength in patients with ACL insufficiency. *Scand J Med Sci Sports* 1998;8:14–19.

190. Kramer JF, Dubowitz T, Fowler P, et al. Functional knee braces and dynamic performance: a review. *Clin J Sport Med* 1997;7:32–39.

191. Daniel DM. Selecting patients for ACL surgery. In: Jackson DW, et al., eds. *The anterior cruciate ligament: current and future concepts*. New York: Raven Press, 1993: 251–258.

CHAPTER 21

Principles of Surgery

Part A: Graft Choices and the Biology of Graft Healing

Choll W. Kim and Robert A. Pedowitz

The anterior cruciate ligament (ACL) is one of the most commonly injured structures in the knee. It is estimated that 1 in 3,000 Americans sustains an ACL disruption every year, with approximately 95,000 new injuries each year, and approximately 50,000 reconstructions performed each year (1, and references therein). Consequently, a great deal of effort has been directed at reconstructing this structure. The importance of ACL injury is reflected in the numerous excellent reviews that have been published recently (1–6).

The overall success of ACL reconstruction is a function of multiple factors, including patient selection, the presence of concomitant injuries, mechanical properties of the graft, graft placement and tensioning, the method of graft fixation, the biologic response and remodeling of the graft tissue, and postoperative rehabilitation of the knee. When choosing a graft, the surgeon must consider the initial mechanical properties of the graft, the morbidity of graft harvesting, the remodeling and incorporation of the graft, and ultimate stiffness and strength over time. The biochemical, histologic, neural, and vascular changes that take place in the ACL graft ultimately determine the graft's viability and consequently its ability to act as a functional replacement for the native ACL.

Several general categories of grafts exist (Table 21.1). The autografts, comprised predominantly of the patellar tendon (PT) and hamstrings (HSs), have been the most commonly used ACL grafts. Other autografts include the central quadriceps tendon, Achilles tendon, fascia lata–iliotibial band, plantaris tendon, and reconstituted PT. Allografts are used from cadaveric PTs and HSs, as well as from the ACL, Achilles tendon, and quadriceps tendon. The synthetic grafts constructed from materials such as Gore-Tex, Dacron, carbon, polyester, polylactic acid, and polyprolene have fallen into disfavor due to

their high rate of chronic synovitis and rupture. Various synthetic materials have been used additionally to augment graft reconstruction. Finally, bioengineered grafts using collagen scaffolds and demineralized bone matrix are currently under investigation. They provide additional sources of potential graft material. This section reviews the biology of graft healing as it relates to the various graft choices available.

TABLE 21.1. *Graft choices*

Autografts
 Patellar tendon
 Hamstring tendon
 Semitendinosus
 Gracilis
 Multiple looped
 Central quadriceps
 Achilles tendon
 Fascia lata/iliotibial band
 Meniscus
 Reharvested patellar tendon

Allografts
 Patellar tendon
 Hamstring (semitendinosus/gracilis)
 Fascia lata/iliotibial band
 Achilles tendon
 Anterior cruciate ligament
 Tibialis anterior
 Peroneal tendon

Synthetic grafts
 Gore-Tex
 Dacron
 Carbon filaments
 Polyester

Engineered grafts
 Fabricated collagen bundles
 Demineralized bone matrix

AUTOGRAFTS

Patellar Tendon Autograft

The PT has been one of the most widely used autograft tissues in ACL reconstruction since Jones (7) originally described its use in 1963. This is also the autograft that has been the most extensively studied in experimental models. The PT is a thick fibrous structure on the anterior aspect of the knee joint. Both the central and medial thirds of this structure are commonly used in ACL reconstruction. Histologic, biochemical, and microvascular studies have shown that the PT graft undergoes demonstrable changes in its structure, effectively transforming itself into a ligamentous tissue (8). These changes can be divided into four stages: (a) avascular necrosis, (b) revascularization, (c) cellular proliferation, and (d) remodeling (8–10). Several investigations of PT substitution for the ACL in both human and animal models demonstrate long-term graft viability and suggest that successfully grafted tissue has a histologic appearance like normal ligament, with dense, longitudinally oriented collagen bundles (7,9,11–13).

Morphology

It is known that despite their gross similarities, tendons and ligaments have unique histologic and biochemical characteristics (14). Investigators first noted progressive changes in PT autografts as they heal after implantation. Amiel and coworkers (8,15) performed detailed histologic and biochemical studies in rabbits at 2, 3, 4, 6, and 30 weeks after surgery. They showed that native PT and ACL were similar at gross inspection (Fig. 21.1). Both structures were white, glistening, and firm to palpation. At 2 weeks after surgery, the autografts were noted to be a dull white color, frayed, and necrotic appearing, without adherent synovium. At 4 weeks after surgery, the autografts were swollen to two to three times their original size, glistening, and still without evidence of a synovial sheath. At 6 weeks after

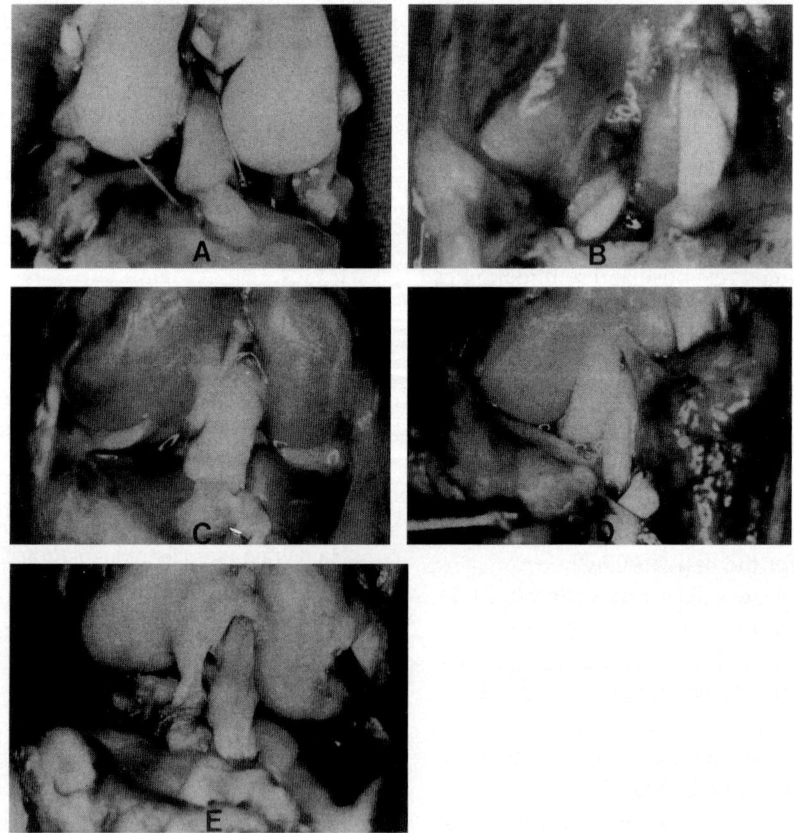

FIGURE 21.1. Gross morphology of femur–anterior cruciate ligament (ACL)–tibia complexes. **A:** Control ACL is white and smooth with compact fibers. **B:** Zero-week patellar tendon autograft is white and flat with compact fibers. **C:** Six-week autograft is white, rounded, and enlarged. **D:** Thirty-week autograft is dull, white, rounded, and small. **E:** Fifty-two-week autograft is dull white, rounded, and small. (From Ballock RT, Woo SL, Lyon RM, et al. Use of patellar tendon autograft for anterior cruciate ligament reconstruction in the rabbit: a long-term histologic and biomechanical study. *J Orthop Res* 1989;7: 474–485, with permission.)

surgery, the autografts showed diminished swelling and a thin synovial envelope emerged. The autografts at 30 weeks were similar to those at 6 weeks. None of the autografts had grossly visible blood vessels. Chiroff (16) reported similar gross morphologic results in the dog model over a 1-year period. Hypertrophy of the intraarticular segment of the PT autograft in the dog model was noted and this continued for up to 1 year after surgery. In addition, development of a covering of synovial membrane occurred by 8 weeks after surgery. In humans, grafts resembled normal ligament tissue when examined 1 year after transplantation (17).

Histology

The four stages of autograft transformation (avascular necrosis, revascularization, cellular proliferation, and remodeling) are evident in histologic studies using rabbits (8,15,18), monkeys (19), and dogs (20). With slight variations in timing, the rabbit model is representative of transformation process.

Avascular Necrosis Stage

The avascular necrosis stage begins as early as 2 days after surgery when there is a relative decrease in tissue cellularity as compared with the tissue of origin (8,21). Seven days after surgery, the cellular population diminished even further, with fibroblasts observed only sporadically in the tissue midsubstance and periphery. By 14 days after surgery, a peripheral rim of round to ovoid cells constituted the entire cellular population, but no fibroblasts were seen centrally (Fig. 21.2). Three weeks after surgery, the tissue's crimp pattern remained similar to that of PT. However, the peritendineum areas showed a marked cellular proliferation, with cells spilling out into the collagenous matrix. The tissue was hypocellular relative to normal PT, but a mixture of cells, some rodlike, others ovoid, were present and oriented longitudinally. By the fourth postoperative week, the number of cells had increased dramatically, approximating the relative cellularity of the normal ACL. Cells were no longer focally concentrated and had spread homogeneously throughout the matrix of the graft. Nuclei present in the 4-week autografts were very similar to those of the ACL. The cells were, for the most part, ovoid, plump, and occasionally rodlike, resembling cells of the ACL. Few spindle-shaped nuclei were seen.

Revascularization Stage

The revascularization stage begins at about 2 weeks and is completed by 8 weeks (19,22), but may require up to 20 weeks (20). Using segmental microangiography techniques in the dog model, Alm and Stromberg (22) showed that revascularization of the paraligamentous and endoligamentous blood supply to the graft was from contributions from the infrapatellar fat pad, the proximal remnant of the excised ACL, and the endosteal vessels at the femoral attachment site. In addition, the posterior synovial fold provides another source of vascular ingrowth (19). From 2 to 6 weeks, the avascular proximal end of the graft was invaded by the endoligamentous vessels from the middle portion of the graft. By the eighth week, the grafts were completely revascularized. From that point, up to the twentieth week, the tissue remodeled to the extent that the collagen bundle arrangement and vascularity resembled the pattern in a normal ligament. The effect this avascular period has on the graft is not completely known. Prior to completion of the revascularization process, the graft is a scaffold on which cells can proliferate and form a new collagenous matrix. Although the early replacement cells are not dependent on the vascular supply for their nutrition, the graft tissue may be vulnerable to stretch, rupture, or alteration in its material properties until the revascularization and subsequent remodeling is complete (21).

Cellular Proliferation Stage

The cellular proliferation stage begins at about 2 to 4 weeks after surgery with a peripheral rim of cells. Kleiner et al. (23) studied the ability of extrinsic cells to repopulate the PT autograft. The intrinsic cells of the native PT autograft were first destroyed by immersion in liquid nitrogen. The PT autograft was then covered in a semipermeable membrane before it was used to reconstruct the ACL (23). Control PT autografts were also treated with liquid nitrogen but were not covered with a semipermeable membrane. Histologic analysis of liquid nitrogen–treated tissue without a membrane cover revealed fibroblastic incorporation of the graft. In contrast, no cells were observed in grafts covered in a semipermeable membrane. These findings suggest that ACL autografts of PT origin are repopulated by cells from an extrinsic origin. The most likely source for these cells is the synovial membrane, which has a combination of macrophagelike cells (type A cells), fibroblastlike cells (type B cells), and undifferentiated cells (type C cells) (24). These cells are adapted for survival in synovial fluid and are present in the joint fluid throughout the postoperative period.

Remodeling Stage

The remodeling stage is a combination of biochemical and ultrastructural events that allows the PT tissue to become more like ACL tissue. The biochemical changes begin as early as 2 weeks, and the structural changes can be seen as early as 6 weeks. To observe the biochemical transformation of PT autografts into a ligamentlike substance, PT autografts were analyzed using three para-

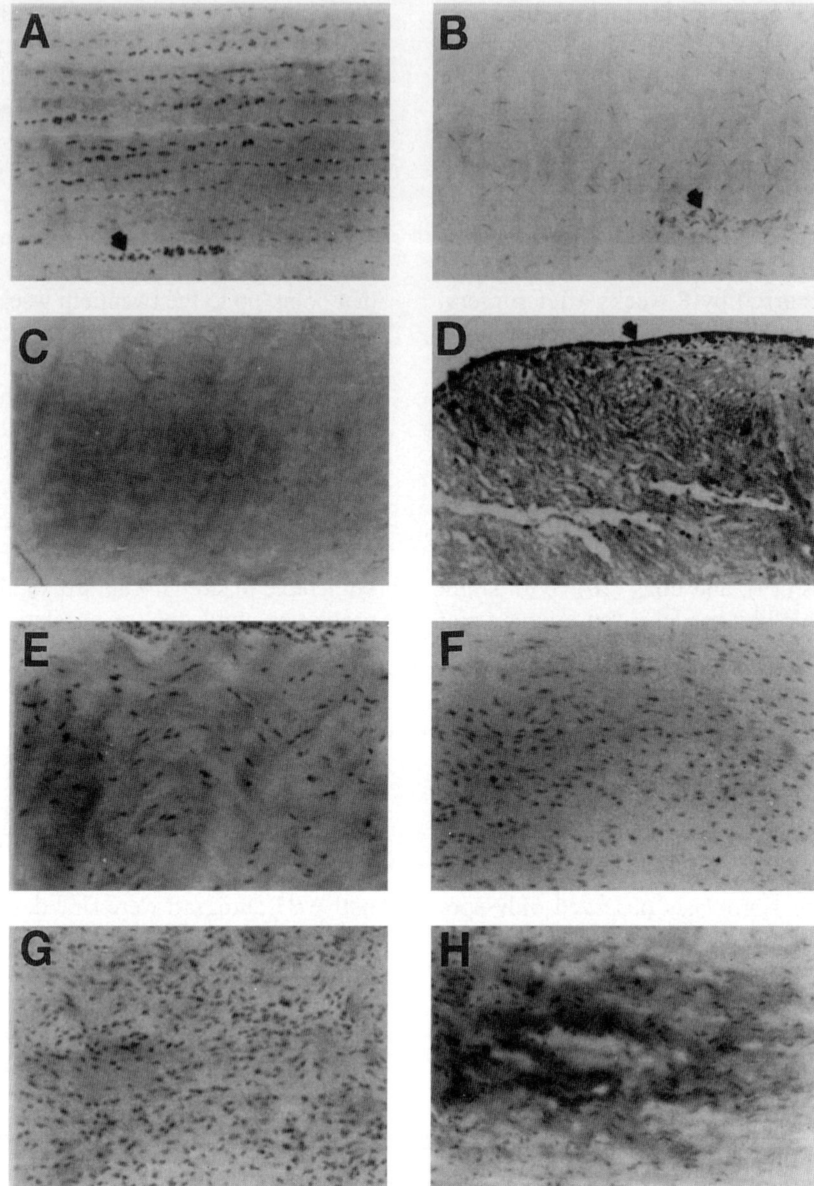

FIGURE 21.2. Histology of normal anterior cruciate ligament (ACL), patellar tendon, and ACL auto-grafts (longitudinal section, coronal plane; hematoxylin and eosin, ×50). **A:** Normal ACL. Note rounded fibroblasts, fine fibrillar crimp, and cluster of potential reserved cells (*arrow*). **B:** Normal patellar tendon. Note spindle-shaped fibroblasts, coarse fibrillar crimp, and peritendineum (*arrow*). **C:** Acellular portion of 2-week autograft. **D:** Rounded fibroblasts inhabit peripheral portion of 2-week autograft (*arrow*). **E:** Focal areas of proliferation are evident in the 3-week autograft, with cells spilling into unoccupied matrix. **F:** Homogeneous distribution of fibroblasts in the 4-week graft. **G:** Relative hypercellularity and rare crimping pattern in 6-week autograft. **H:** Cellular appearance and number in the 30-week autograft are similar to the normal ACL. (From Amiel D, Kleiner JB, Roux RD, et al. The phenomenon of "ligamenti-zation": anterior cruciate ligament reconstruction with autogenous patellar tendon. *J Orthop Res* 1986;4: 162–172, with permission.)

meters with respect to time: collagen cross-linking, collagen typing, and total glycosaminoglycan (GAG) (8). Earlier studies demonstrated measurable differences between tendon and ligament when these tissue were characterized biochemically using these parameters (14). If the autograft actually transforms from a tendinous material to a ligamentous material, one would

expect these biochemical parameters in the autograft to change as well.

Collagen cross-linking characteristics of the ACL autografts changed dramatically as a function of time during the postoperative recovery. As reported previously, normal PT and ACL have distinct reducible cross-link patterns (14). Most notably, the ACL contains a high con-

TABLE 21.2. *Relative amounts of collagen crosslinks in patellar tendon, anterior cruciate ligament, and patellar tendon autografts*

Tissue	DHLNL/HLNL	DHLNL/HHMD
Normal PT	0.23 ± 0.05	0.15 ± 0.03
2-wk graft	0.53 ± 0.07	0.25 ± 0.05
4-wk graft	2.95 ± 0.15	1.60 ± 0.20
6-wk graft	5.23 ± 0.92	2.56 ± 0.87
30-wk graft	4.40 ± 0.80	3.50 ± 0.62
Normal ACL	3.28 ± 0.35	3.65 ± 0.47

PT, patellar tendon; ACL, anterior cruciate ligament; DHLNL, dihydroxylysinonorleucine; HLNL, hydroxylysinonorleucine; HHMD, histidinohydroxymerodesmosine.

From Amiel D, Kleiner JB, Roux RD, et al. The phenomenon of "ligamentization": anterior cruciate ligament reconstruction with autogenous patellar tendon. *J Orthop Res* 1986;4:162–172, with permission.

centration of dihydroxylysinonorleucine (DHLNL) and relatively little histidinohydroxymerodesmosine (HHMD) and hydroxylysinonorleucine (HLNL). The PT exhibits the opposite pattern, with high HHMD and HLNL levels and low DHLNL levels. Because of these differences, collagen cross-linking changes provide an important index of tissue transformation.

Amiel and coworkers (14) noted that a transformation began by 2 weeks after surgery, with an increase in the amount of DHLNL relative to HHMD. By 4 weeks, DHLNL increased dramatically, although HHMD was still high. At 30 weeks, the relative amounts of DHLNL and HHMD appeared to be very similar to those observed for normal ACL and the concentration of HHMD (very high in normal PT) had dropped to levels normally found in ACL. Table 21.2 summarizes the relative amounts of the reducible cross-links found in ACL, PT, and PT autografts at different postoperative time intervals.

In addition to the reducible collagen cross-links, a stable nonreducible cross-link, 3-hydroxypuridinium, was present in those tissue. The concentration of 3-hydroxypyridinium has been found to be four to five times higher in ACL that in PT (14). Autografts at 30 weeks after surgery demonstrated 3-hydroxypyridinium at a concentration that averaged a little more than half that found in normal ACL (Fig. 21.3).

Collagen typing of the tissues provided another valuable parameter for characterizing time-dependent changes in the autograft. PT and ACL have been found to exhibit different collagen-type characteristics (14). Whereas PT had no detectable type III collagen, ACL contained about 10% type III collagen. The predominant

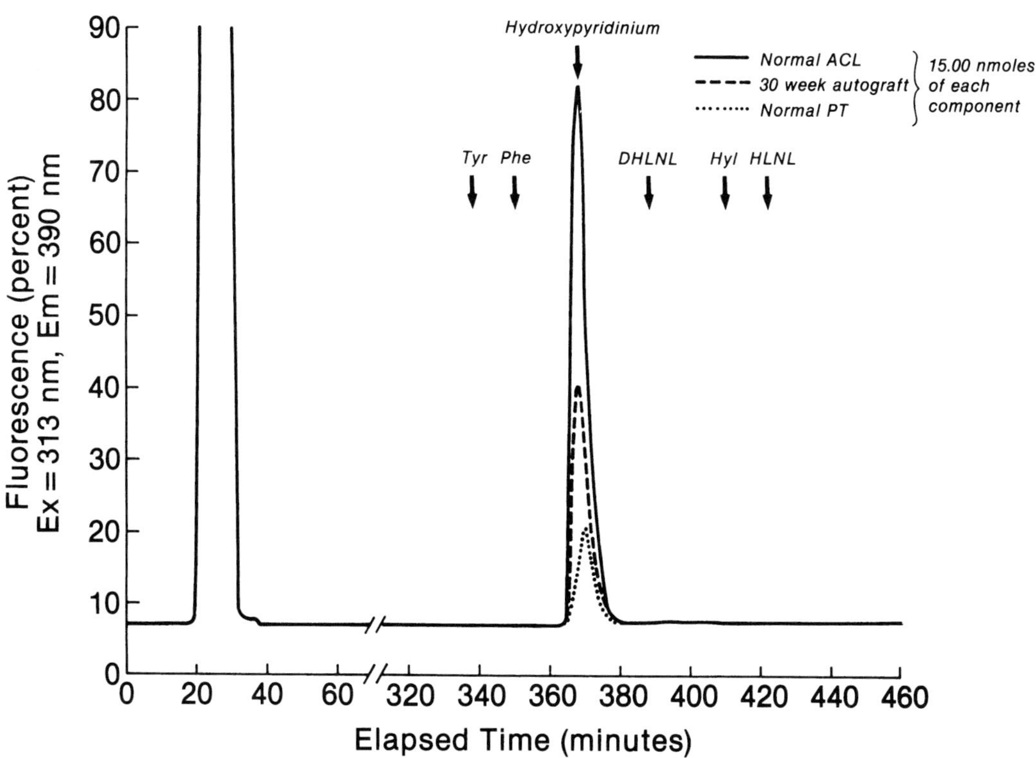

FIGURE 21.3. Isolation of the hydroxypyridinium cross-link by cation-exchange liquid chromatography of the tissue hydrolysates. ACL, anterior cruciate ligament; PT, patellar tendon; DHLNL, dihydroxylysinonorleucine; HLNL, hydroxylysinonorleucine. (From Amiel D, Kleiner JB, Roux RD, et al. The phenomenon of "ligamentization": anterior cruciate ligament reconstruction with autogenous patellar tendon. *J Orthop Res* 1986;4:162–172, with permission.)

TABLE 21.3. *Proportions of type I and type II collagen in patellar tendon, anterior cruciate ligament, and patellar tendon autografts*

Tissue	Type I (%)	Type II (%)
PT	>95	—
2-wk graft	92–95	5–8
4-wk graft	87–90	10–13
6-wk graft	82–85	15–18
30-wk graft	84–88	12–16
ACL	86–89	11–14

PT, patellar tendon; ACL, anterior cruciate ligament.

From Amiel D, Kleiner JB, Roux RD, et al. The phenomenon of "ligamentization": anterior cruciate ligament reconstruction with autogenous patellar tendon. *J Orthop Res* 1986;4:162–172, with permission.

type of collagen in both tissues was Type I. High-pressure liquid chromatography (HPLC) separation of the cyanogen bromide (CNBr) peptides from PT, ACL, and PT autografts at various stages of recovery show that type III collagen was detected in the PT autografts as early as 2 weeks after surgery. The amount of type III collagen reached a maximum at 6 weeks, and it decreased only slightly by 30 weeks. The estimated amount in the PT autograft at 30 weeks was comparable to that found in normal ACL. Table 21.3 summarizes the approximate proportions of type I and III collagens found in the different tissues in the rabbit model.

The normal GAG content of ACL and PT is also different. The ACL contains more than twice the amount of GAG as that contained in PT (14). As early as 2 weeks after surgery, the PT autografts had an increase in the amount of GAG when compared with native PT (Table 21.4). This increased to a maximum at 4 weeks and remained relatively constant up to 30 weeks. During this analogous period, the water content of the graft also

TABLE 21.4. *Total glycosaminoglycan content in patellar tendon, anterior cruciate ligament, and patellar tendon autografts*

Tissue	GAG[a]
PT	3.92 ± 0.16
ACL	9.89 ± 0.56
ACL reconstruction	
2-wk graft	5.62 ± 0.82
4-wk graft	10.72 ± 1.12
6-wk graft	11.71 ± 1.24
30-wk graft	11.42 ± 0.93

GAG, glycosaminoglycan; PT, patellar tendon; ACL, anterior cruciate ligament.

[a]Milligram of hexosamine per gram of dry tissue.

From Amiel D, Frank C, Harwood F, et al. Tendons and ligaments: a morphological and biochemical comparison. *J Orthop Res* 1984;1:257–265; and Amiel D, Kleiner JB, Roux RD, et al. The phenomenon of "ligamentization": anterior cruciate ligament reconstruction with autogenous patellar tendon. *J Orthop Res* 1986;4:162–172, with permission.

seems to increase, corresponding to a decrease in strength (25).

Graft Reinnervation

The importance of the ACL in normal knee kinematics may in part be due to its contribution to proprioception, although the extent of this role has not yet been quantified. Studies in both humans and animals show that native ACL contains mechanoreceptors and free nerve endings (26–31). Patients with ACL disruptions demonstrate deficits in position sense and are slow in recruiting protective muscle reflexes (32–34). Gait analysis studies show there are subtle differences in muscle action such as increased HS activity, decreased net flexion moment, and decreased quadriceps activity termed the "quadriceps avoidance gait" (35–37). This may lead to a syndrome of reflex muscle splinting, repetitive minor injury, and increased laxity (38).

ACL reconstruction using PT and semitendinosus autografts appears to facilitate reinnervation with mechanoreceptors in both humans and animals. When the ACL in humans is torn, the normal mechanoreceptors slowly recede. In untreated ACL lesions, this loss begins 3 months after injury (26). By 9 months after injury, only a few free nerve endings can be found by histology. By 1 year after injury, no free nerve endings can be found. Using a sheep model, Denti et al. (26) showed that Pacini corpuscles and free nerve endings could be found in grafts starting at 3 months and persisting at 9 months (Fig. 21.4). Not surprisingly, artificial grafts did not contain mechanoreceptors. However, PT autografts in the dog showed evidence of reinnervation with mechanoreceptors

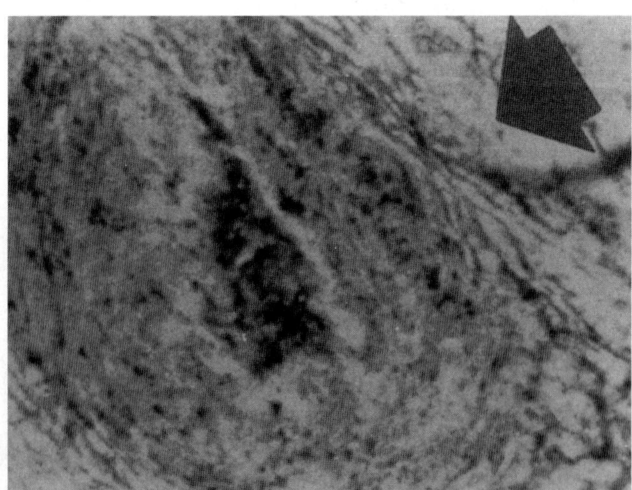

FIGURE 21.4. Bone–patellar bone graft at 6 months shows Pacini corpuscles (*arrow*) in animal models (Ruffini stain; original magnification, ×100). (From Denti M, Monteleone M, Berardi A, et al. Anterior cruciate ligament mechanoreceptors: histologic studies on lesions and reconstruction. *Clin Orthop* 1994;308:29–32, with permission.)

at 6 months (39). Furthermore, two of six cases showed return of somatosensory-evoked potentials, indicating that these neural structures shown on histology may be communicating with the cerebral cortex (39). This reinnervation mimics the neural distribution seen in the native ACL. The native PT contains more free nerve endings (>90%) than mechanoreceptors (<10%). In contrast, the native ACL contains predominantly mechanoreceptors (89%) over free nerve endings (11%). In PT autografts examined at 6 months, mechanoreceptors make up about half of the nerves seen (39). This suggests that the reinnervation process follows the path of ACL development as part of the ligamentization process. The clinical significance of nerve types in ligament versus tendon is not clear in terms of proprioceptive response.

This reinnervation may contribute to the improvement in gait and proprioception following ACL reconstruction. Barrett (40) showed that proprioception after reconstruction was better than in an ACL-deficient knee but still significantly worse than the normal knee at a mean of 3.2 years after reconstruction (range, 1.2 to 6.7 years). Thus, successful ACL reconstruction includes both mechanical restraints to abnormal knee kinematics and neurosensory systems to stabilize the knee during changes in knee position.

Healing in the Bone Tunnel

The bone–ligament junction within the bone tunnel constitutes an important point of fixation in ACL reconstruction, especially during the perioperative period. During the first 1 to 2 months, the main factor affecting the structural strength of graft appears to be the fixation of the graft to the bone (41). After this time, the tensile strength of the interface appears to plateau and the weakest portion of the graft is the midportion of the graft outside the tunnel (41,42). The bone–ligament junction is a highly differentiated functional unit. Four different layers of histologically distinct tissue can be discerned within a 1-mm area. Adjacent to the ligament is a fibrous tissue. The next layer is composed of fibrocartilage, followed by mineralized fibrocartilage and then bone (18,43,44).

Studies in the rabbit model show the onset of cellular proliferation in the graft within the bone tunnel precedes that which occurs in the graft outside the tunnel (18). The process begins with the formation of a loose fibrovascular tissue with a copious cell infiltration. At 1 month, the graft within the tunnel had an abundant number of cells, whereas the graft outside the tunnel was markedly hypocellular. The tissue was more compact with fibers of the transition area aligning in the longitudinal axis of the graft. At 3 months, the graft was adherent to the bone wall and more differentiated than in the sample at 1 month. These cells were oriented in a longitudinal axis and rich in fibrochondrocytelike cells. Penetrating fibers that start from the tendon and cross into bone in an acute

angle (Fig. 21.5) were also visible. These may be similar to the Sharpey's fibers that provide an anchoring system at tendon–bone interfaces. The bone plug was fully incorporated and could no longer be distinguished from surrounding bone. By 6 months, a normal bone–ligament junction could be seen with four differentiated layers composed of fibrous tissue, fibrocartilage, mineralized fibrocartilage, and bone (Fig. 21.6).

Hamstring Autograft

Significant debate continues between proponents of HS and PT autografts for ACL reconstruction. Comparisons of these grafts have concentrated on graft strength, clinical effectiveness, and rates of complications. Graft strength has been measured in several studies that show that the PT and HS autografts have similar ultimate strengths (1,45–47). Both PT and HS autograft reconstructions cause roughly equal degrees of knee flexion weakness (48). It is also hypothesized that patellofemoral disease is likely a consequence of previous disease and/or patellofemoral injury at the time of ACL disruption rather than the type of graft used (1). Although some clinical outcome studies show that both are similarly effective, with only minor variations in knee stability and muscle strength (48,49–55), other prospective comparisons of HS and PT graft reconstructions suggest slightly better stability with PT grafts but with a higher incidence of patellofemoral crepitus (49,55). Currently, most surgeons consider the PT graft to be the gold standard for ACL

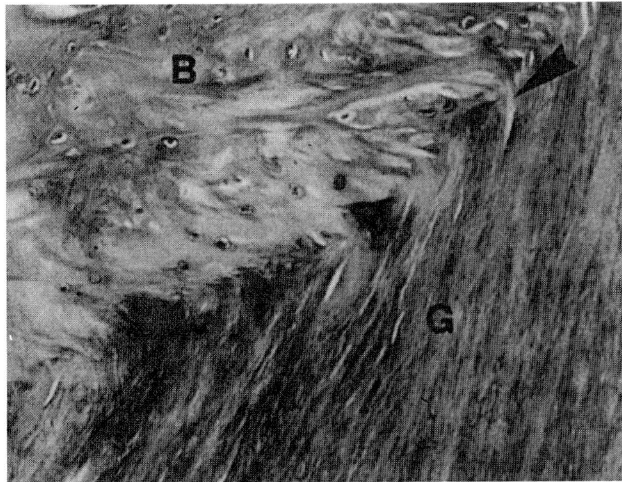

FIGURE 21.5. Longitudinal section of a patellar tendon autograft at 3 months. Inside the femoral tunnel, the graft (*G*) adheres completely to the bone wall (*B*) by a thin transition layer. Some fibers that start from the ligament, cross the transition layer, and enter directly into the bone at an acute angle (*arrow*) can be seen (Gomori–Halmi stain; original magnification, ×20). (From Panni A, Milano G, Lucania L, et al. Graft healing after anterior cruciate ligament reconstruction in rabbits. *Clin Orthop* 1997;343:203–212, with permission.)

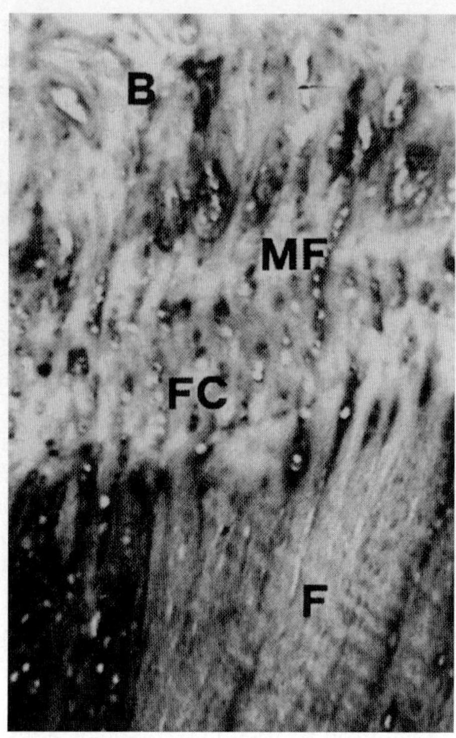

FIGURE 21.6. Longitudinal section of a patellar tendon autograft at 6 months showing four differentiated layers at the bone–ligament interface. A transition from bone (*B*), mineralized fibrocartilage (*MF*), fibrocartilage (*FC*), and fibrous tissue (*F*) can be seen (Gomori–Halmi stain; original magnification, ×10). (From Panni A, Milano G, Lucania L, et al. Graft healing after anterior cruciate ligament reconstruction in rabbits. *Clin Orthop* 1997;343:203–212, with permission.)

reconstruction, but the HS graft provides a nearly comparable alternative for patients with underlying patellofemoral disease and lower activity demands.

Histology

Histologic studies in the rabbit semitendinosus autograft have been performed by Blickenstaff et al. (56). Although the time courses evaluated differ from those of rabbit PT autografts, these studies show that the semitendinosus undergoes a ligamentization process similar to that of the PT (56). At 12 weeks, the intraarticular portion of the HS graft showed interspersed areas of disorganized collagen bundles. Direct comparisons are difficult but it appears 12-week HS grafts resemble PT grafts at 3 to 6 weeks (8). At 26 weeks, the intraarticular portion of the HS grafts demonstrated increased cellularity and dense, longitudinally oriented collagen bundles. This is analogous to the histologic pattern of PT autografts at 30 weeks. Thus, the intraarticular portion of both the HS and PT autografts appears to reach a high level of collagen organization at about 26 to 30 weeks. Prior to this time, the graft material is undergoing revascularization, cellular proliferation, and remodeling. Because no direct com-

parison of HS versus PT autograft healing is available, it is unclear whether there are any significant differences in the temporal sequence of these events.

HS grafts differ from PT grafts in terms of fixation within the bony tunnel. PT grafts are generally harvested with bony blocks and subsequently fixed to the tunnel through a bone-to-bone interface. In contrast, HS grafts tend to be harvested with no bony attachments. Hence, its fixation in the tunnel requires that the HS graft be fixed to the tunnel through a tendon-to-bone interface. It is postulated that bone-to-bone fixation provides greater holding strength and allows a faster rate of healing within the tunnel. Blickenstaff et al. (56) showed that at 12 weeks, the HS graft within the bony tunnel contains bony trabeculae with osteod seams interfacing with a well-organized rim of fibrous tissue. There was a well-demarcated interface between the graft and connective tissue that interdigitated with the bone at acute angles (Fig. 21.7). By this time, the strength of the graft at the tunnel was greater than the intraarticular portion of the graft. This is similar to bio-

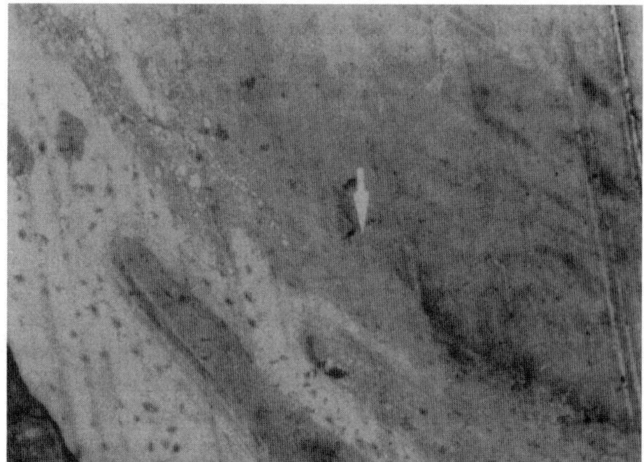

A

B

FIGURE 21.7. A: Twelve-week semitendinosus autograft in bone tunnel. **B:** Twelve-week semitendinosus autograft, intraarticular portion. (From Blickenstaff KR, Grana WA, Egle D. Analysis of a semitendinosus autograft in a rabbit model. *Am J Sports Med* 1997;25:554–559, with permission.)

mechanical studies of tendon healing within a bone tunnel using the dog model of the long digital extensor tendon where failure occurred at the tendon–bone interface at 8 weeks, but at the midsubstance at 12 weeks (41). In the PT model, the strength of the graft within the bone tunnel fixation appears to surpass the strength of the graft in the intraarticular portion at 6 weeks (15). Pinczewski et al. (57) examined the bony attachment of HS tendon autografts in two patients undergoing revision surgery for midsubstance tears. They showed that osteointegration between the HS tendon graft and the bony tunnel occurs by 12 weeks after reconstruction. Thus, 12 weeks appears to be sufficient time for tendon-to-bone integration within the bone tunnel in HS grafts. After this time, the intraarticular portion of the graft becomes the weakest point. Although there is indirect evidence that PT grafts heal within the bone tunnel more rapidly and with greater strength than HS grafts, additional studies are needed to confirm this prevailing belief.

Alternative Autogenous Grafts

As the frequency of ACL reconstruction increases, so have the number of revision cases for graft failures. Current estimates of failures of primary ACL reconstruction range from 0.7% to 8% (58–61). The need for alternative grafts sources becomes evident. This section discusses additional autografts that have been investigated.

Central Quadriceps Tendon

The central quadriceps tendon graft consists of a partial-thickness quadriceps tendon with the prepatellar fascia and PT, which may also include a bone block from the superior patella (4,62–64). A thick graft nearly two times the thickness of the PT can be obtained (62,63).

Biomechanical testing results have been variable. Noyes et al. (65) found that the quadriceps tendon had 14% to 21% of the maximum load of the ACL and 8% to 13% of the maximum load of the central third of the PT. Harris et al. (63) found that the quadriceps tendon had 60% to 200% of the maximum load of a similarly sized PT (63). The reason for this difference is unclear. Clinical results have also been variable. Earlier studies showed that 20% of patients have a positive pivot shift test with only 11 of 45 patients returning to sports without limitation (66). Similarly, Kornblatt et al. (67) found 45% of patients had a positive pivot shift test and that 21% still reported instability symptoms. More recent studies by Howe et al. (59) show better clinical results. In 83 patients with a mean follow-up of 5.5 years, nearly 90% had stable knees on examination. There was also a significant improvement in their ability to return to sports activities (68).

A complication of the quadriceps tendon graft may be extensor mechanism dysfunction. Evaluation of quadri-

ceps strength 3 to 7 years after surgery showed persistent weakness, especially in women (69,70). However, the degree of pain at the bone plug donor site may be less than that for PT grafts (62). No tendon ruptures have been reported thus far.

Achilles Tendon Autograft

The Achilles tendon has also been used to reconstruct the ACL-deficient knee (71). The Achilles tendon autograft is longer than the PT graft and can be taken with a bone plug from the calcaneous. The medial superficial layer is harvested and placed intraarticularly with a calcaneal bone plug fixed to the femoral tunnel and the free end fixed to the tibia with staples. A study of 21 such reconstructions with a follow-up of more than 2 years reported that 85% of patients had a rating of good to excellent. These patients had negative Lachman and pivot shift examinations and tested with less than a 3-mm side-to-side difference with the KT-1000 arthrometer (71). Complications included three cases of Achilles tendinitis, which resolved in 1 year, and one case of graft rupture. There were no Achilles tendon ruptures. However, concern about this complication has resulted in poor acceptance of this technique.

The Achilles tendon appears to remodel in an manner analogous to that of the PT. At 2 weeks after surgery, a thin membranous substance surrounds the graft. Revascularization may start from this membrane. After 1 year, the graft resembles ligament more than tendon, with wavy patterns of collagen fibers aligned along stress lines. Within the bone tunnels, the graft becomes fibrocartilagenous and attached to trabeculae analogous to Sharpey's fibers.

Fascia Lata–Iliotibial Band Autograft

The fascia lata, or fascia of the proximal lateral thigh, forms a condensed fibrous band distally that inserts into the lateral aspect of the proximal tibia. The distal thickened portion is called the *iliotibial tract*. Hey-Groves (72,73) used these grafts for the first ACL reconstructions in the early part of the 1900s. Animal studies in dogs show that iliotibial band grafts are 45% less stiff than control ACL, the yield point was at one third, and the ultimate load was 40% of normal ACL controls (74). Similar to other grafts, the iliotibial band (ITB) also undergoes remodeling and ligamentization, which occurs over a period of 16 weeks in dogs (74).

Clinical studies thus far have shown disappointing results. Insall et al. (75) showed that only about one half of patients claimed their knee was normal. Scott et al. (76) reported that 75% of patients rated their results as excellent, with no limitation of function. More recently, Hooper and Walton (77) performed a comprehensive study of subjective patient outcomes (using a detailed questionnaire) and objective physical examination findings. They found that only 1 of 37 patients was sufficiently happy with the result to rate the knee as normal. The clinical use of the iliotibial band transfer has been limited due to this high rate of ligamentous laxity. Its use with a combined semitendinosus tendon transfer offers improved results (78,79). In this procedure, Zarins and Rowe (79) describe how the free ends of the iliotibial tract and semitendinosus grafts are passed in opposite directions and sutured to each other. In a prospective clinical study of 73 such reconstructions, Billoti et al. (78) show that 92% of patients rated their knees as good to excellent. Complications included pain over the staple that was used to fix the ITB to the tibia, requiring removal in five patients. Fascial hernia at the donor site is another potential complication.

Meniscus Autograft

In situations in which the meniscus is torn and must be otherwise excised, the meniscus itself may be used for ACL reconstruction (80–84). In a study of 100 patients in this category (81), only 10% of patients continued to have a positive Lachman or pivot shift test, and 80% had an overall satisfactory result based on the Zarins and Rowe scale (79). Subjective evaluations showed significant improvement in pain and return to sports (81). Extraarticular augmentation appeared to have no effect on overall results. Results tended to be better in patients younger than 30 years and patients who underwent reconstruction within 1 year of injury. Histologic evaluations in dogs showed that the meniscal graft undergoes metaplasia to ligamentlike tissue (80). In contrast, rabbit and human grafts undergo only mild revascularization but do not undergo ligamentization (85). Rather, the rabbit and human tissues ultimately appeared as hypercellular fibrocartilage (85,86). Tensile testing in the rabbit model show that at 52 weeks, the tensile stress of the graft is 3 kg compared with the normal control ACL, which is 13 kg (85). Complications included adhesions in 11% and graft loosening in 2% of which required PT autograft reconstruction (86). Ferkel et al. (86) suggest that this procedure is indicated only for patients who, in addition to needing reconstruction of the ACL, also have a torn meniscus that would otherwise have to be totally excised. Currently, there is poor acceptance of this procedure because most meniscal fragments large enough to use as a graft tend be repaired.

Reharvested Patellar Tendon Autograft

Recently, a study in dogs evaluated the histologic and mechanical properties of the reharvested PT autograft (87). This study showed that the remaining tissue is thicker and scarlike with collagen fibers oriented longitudinally and more cellular than normal PT. While at 6 months, the collagen fibril size was enlarged and loosely packed, by 12 months the fibrils returned to normal size and degree of packing. Mechanical testing at 6 and 12 months showed decreases in the load to failure to about one half, occurring mainly at midsubstance. Notably, this study did not evaluate the properties of the potential graft after it has been placed intraarticularly and looked instead at properties of the graft at the time of harvest.

Karns et al. (88) described the use of grafts obtained from previously harvested central one-third PT. In that report, no follow-up data were discussed. Kartus et al. (89) have compared the use of reharvested PT autografts from the ipsilateral knee with PT autografts from the contralateral knee for ACL revision surgery in 24 patients. Reharvesting the ipsilateral PT resulted in lower functional scores and a higher rate of complications than revision with the contralateral PT. There were two major complications in the group with revision surgery with the ipsilateral reharvested PT. Based on these results, the authors conclude that the reharvested graft not be used for revision ACL reconstruction until more information is available.

STRENGTH AND BIOMECHANICS OF AUTOGRAFTS

The initial mechanical strength of the various grafts has been studied in detail (65). Testing of ligament strength performed on cadaveric specimens show that the 14-mm-wide PT has the greatest initial strength, having 159% to 168% of the strength of the normal ACL, where the normal ACL has a load to failure of 1,725 N. The semitendinosus and gracilis are less strong, with values about 70% and 49%, respectively (65). However, when the more common 9- to 10-mm-wide PT graft is compared with the multiple-looped HS, the initial strengths are more comparable (45,47,48,90).

There is loss of strength as the grafts remodel over time after transplantation. The nature of this weakness depends on the time after reconstruction. Grafts are weak initially at the fixation points where bone–bone or tendon–bone healing has not yet occurred. After about 6 to 12 weeks, the fixation points heal. At this point, remodeling of the substance of the grafts places the midsubstance of the graft at risk (19,25,74,80,91–96). Exposure of the graft material to excessive tension while it is weak may result in elongation and/or disruption of the graft (97–99). Autograft reconstructions in experimental animals have been performed to quantify changes over time in the biomechanical properties of the graft tissue. Studies have focused on mainly the ultimate load and stiffness of the graft complex at various times after reconstruction.

The PT autograft has been one of the most extensively studied in experimental models. Widely varying biomechanical properties of PT autografts have been reported (Tables 21.5 and 21.6). The general trend, however, is for PT graft remodeling such that stiffness and ultimate load

TABLE 21.5. *Autograft stiffness, experimental/control (%)*

Study	Tissue	Experimental animal	Weeks after surgery				
			0	6–8	12–16	26–30	52–104
Holden (109)	ITT	Goat	2	9	—	—	—
Thorson (93)	ITT	Canine	—	—	10	—	—
van Rens (74)	ITT	Canine	—	—	—	—	45
Butler (102)	ITT/PT	Canine	9	—	23	31	—
Clancy (19)	PT	Primate	—	—	39	—	47
McPherson (100)	PT	Goat	3	—	15	33	35
Yoshiya (95)	PT	Canine	11	—	22	—	—
McFarland (25)	PT	Canine	—	—	15	—	—
Ballock (91)	PT	Rabbit	15	11	—	24	13

ITT, iliotibial tract; PT, patellar tendon.

values reach approximately one third of the control ACL value after as long as 24 months in animal models. Comparable data in human studies are currently lacking. In human and animal studies, most reconstructed joints demonstrated some degree of increased anteroposterior (A/P) translation and articular degeneration.

In a representative study in goats, the ultimate strength and stiffness of PT autografts were low initially but increases to a plateau at about 6 months after surgery (100). Biomechanical evaluation showed that the stiffness of the graft complex was only 7.1 N/mm at the time of surgery, increasing to a maximum of 97 N/mm at 12 months, as compared with 275 N/mm for the controls (Fig. 21.8A). After 24 months, however, the value decreased slightly to 83 N/mm. Ultimate load values followed similar trends. The maximum ultimate load values of the autografts, which occurred at 12 months, were 45% of controls (Fig. 21.8B). McPherson et al. (100) further demonstrated patellofemoral degenerative changes and increased A/P joint laxity in all animals undergoing ACL reconstruction using a central-third PT autograft after 3

to 24 months. Similar results have been shown in the canine (25,95,96,101) and rabbit models (15); slightly better results were found in the Rhesus monkey model (19). Overall, the final stiffness and load values plateau at about 6 months after transplantation and are about 50% of native ACL (19,25,102–104). Based on these data, some treatment protocols for patients undergoing ACL reconstruction allow return to running activities at 6 months (105). No data exist for the time course of graft healing in human models as it relates to graft strength. It would be of interest to delineate these parameters to better coordinate the time course of rehabilitation with the time course of graft healing.

The use of other autograft materials has also yielded similar results. The semitendinosus tendon fails at ultimate loads less than 15% of the normal ACL after 26 weeks of transplantation (92). Various fascia lata–iliotibial tract grafts had strength and stiffness values less than half those of controls in animal models (74,106). The medial meniscus graft failed at 30% of the ultimate load of controls (80,85). This loss in tensile strength, regard-

TABLE 21.6. *Autograft ultimate load, experimental/control (%)*

Study	Tissue	Experimental animal	Weeks afer surgery				
			0	6–8	12–16	26–30	52–104
Holden (109)	ITT	Goat	6	15	—	—	—
O'Donoghue (106)	ITT	Canine	—	—	—	—	23
Thorson (93)	ITT	Canine	—	—	40	—	—
van Rens (74)	ITT	Canine	—	—	—	—	40
Butler (107)	ITT/PT	Canine	14	—	23	28	—
Clancy (19)	PT	Primate	—	—	26	—	52
McPherson (100)	PT	Goat	1	—	15	38	45
Shino (44)	PT	Canine	—	—	—	30	—
Yoshiya (95)	PT	Canine	7	—	20	—	—
Hurley	PT	Canine	—	—	—	—	<32
McFarland (25)	PT	Canine	—	—	23	—	—
Ballock (91)	PT	Rabbit	7	7	—	15	11
Kennedy (92)	ST	Rabbit	—	—	—	13	—
Collins (80)	M	Canine	—	~5	~35	~35	—
Mitsou (85)	M	Rabbit	—	8	—	—	23

ITT, iliotibial tract; PT, patellar tendon; ST, semitendinosus tendon; M, meniscus.

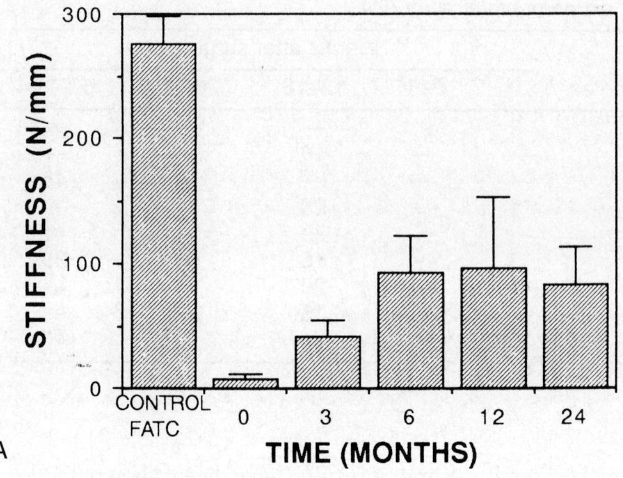

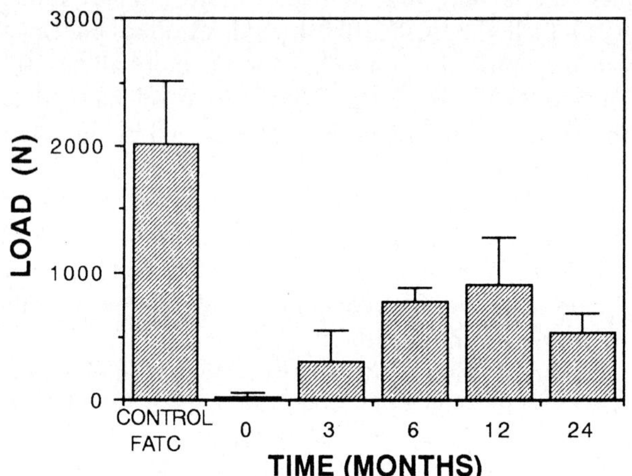

FIGURE 21.8. A: Linear stiffness of control femur–anterior cruciate ligament (ACL)–tibia complex (FATC) and patellar tendon (PT)–reconstructed femur–graft–tibia complex after 0 to 24 months of implantation in a goat model. Linear stiffness of the reconstructed graft–bone complex reach approximately one third of the control ACL value. **B:** Ultimate load of control ACL and PT graft–bone complex. Graft strength improved during the first year of implantation. (From McPherson GK, Mendenhall HV, Gibbons DF, et al. Experimental mechanical and histologic evaluation of the Kennedy ligament augmentation device. *Clin Orthop* 1985;196:186–195, with permission.)

less of the type of graft used, is most likely due to replacement of large collagen fibrils (diameter, >100 nm) with loosely packed small collagen fibrils (diameter, <100 nm) during graft remodeling (19).

It is important to consider that the native ACL is a complex viscoelastic structure. Within the substance of the ligament, different sets of fibers are recruited as the knee joint changes positions (107). This may cause the native ACL to fail at different loads depending on the position of the knee at the time of injury. In addition, normal daily activities impose relatively modest amounts of strain on the ACL, approximately 20% of its failure

capacity (about 445 N) (108,109). The ACL graft must be effective, not only at the extremes, but also at these more common levels of activity. Finally, the ACL must dissipate energy, adjust its lengths, and modulate its internal load distribution as a function of its load history. Thus, a single value for the maximum strength of the ACL graft is not the only mechanical indicator of importance. As the testing of various ACL grafts becomes more sophisticated, such subtle, but important, differences must also be assessed to ultimately determine the best ACL substitute. Currently, the PT and HS autografts continue to be the strongest material for ACL reconstruction.

ALLOGRAFTS

Allograft tissues are useful substitutes to autografts for patients with contraindications to autogenous reconstruction such as a narrow-width PT, an extensor mechanism malalignment (such as patella baja), deficient autogenous tissues, complex multiple ligament reconstructions, or previous failure of an autogenous graft (110–112). Additional advantages of allografts for ACL reconstruction include decreased operative time and no donor site morbidity (111). The disadvantages include limited supply of donor material, potential for disease transmission, possible immune response that may adversely affect graft integrity, and cost. For allografts to be successful, they must be sterile, must be of low immunologic antigenicity, and must provide the biologic scaffold for the graft to attain adequate strength. Several excellent reviews have been published on this topic (110–116).

Allograft Preparation and Storage

Fresh, untreated allogeneic tissues contain immunogenic components, mainly in the form of major histocompatibility antigens expressed on tendon cells. Arnoczky et al. (117) showed that when transplanted in animal models, there is a marked inflammatory response characterized by perivascular cuffing and lymphocyte invasion. Thus, fresh, untreated allografts are rarely used.

Deep freezing or freeze-drying of allografts allows long-term storage of material (118,119). In addition, it greatly reduces graft antigenicity by destroying cells and passenger leukocytes (118–120). Some studies suggest that changes in the material properties of deep-frozen ligaments are not statistically different from those of fresh controls (121,122). Jackson et al. (113) studied the effect of freezing on native ACL using a goat model. By performing the freezing process *in situ*, the native attachment, tension, and orientation of the ligament were maintained throughout the healing process. These studies showed no difference in A/P translation. However, there was a reduction in load to failure (2,274 N in control vs. 1,915 N in frozen ligaments). This suggests that freezing per se has a small but reproducible effect on ultimate graft strength. Histologic evaluation following deep freezing reveals diminished cellularity but maintains the normal fibrous framework of the collagen bundles (Fig. 21.9).

The use of ethylene oxide as a sterilization procedure has been abandoned due to the body's inflammatory response to the degradation products, ethylene chlorhydrin and ethylene glycol, which cause increased incidence of knee effusions (6% to 25%), cyst formation in the bone tunnel (36%), and increased rate of rupture (53%) (110,123–125).

Disease Transmission

An important consideration for allograft ACL reconstruction is the risk for disease transmission. Of the graft choices available, fresh, untreated grafts are the most likely to harbor a virus. In viral recovery studies, cultures from fresh, untreated cadaveric tissue of patients who died of autoimmune deficiency syndrome (AIDS) show that human immunodeficiency virus (HIV) can be cultured from bone in three of five samples and from tendons in two of five samples (126). The process of freezing and freeze-drying decreases the viral load, but does not completely destroy viruses (114).

Gamma irradiation of as little as 2 Mrad has been shown to destroy HIV in some studies (127). In other studies, gamma irradiation of at least 3 to 3.6 Mrad was required to inactivate HIV in tissue culture and ligament–bone tissues (128,129).

When grafts are irradiated, there are associated changes in the structural properties of the graft. Doses of 3 Mrad of radiation on fresh-frozen goat PT allografts cause 27% and 40% reductions in maximum force and strain energy to maximum force, respectively (127,130).

Lower doses of radiation (2 Mrad) show no changes in mechanical properties, but there is a 10% shrinkage in graft length, which requires tensioning to attain original length (110).

As reviewed by DiStephano (110), it seems recipients of bone and relatively avascular soft tissues are unlikely to be infected with HIV. This is in large part due to the implementation of donor screening in 1985 (110). Screening relies on detection of antibodies to HIV-1. Common methods use enzyme-linked immunoassays (EIAs) and rapid latex particle agglutination tests (LAs). Because these screening tests rely on the presence of antibodies to HIV, they will not be useful in screening donors who have recently been infected and have not yet seroconverted, a period ranging from 4 weeks to 6 months. Assessment of HIV risk, taken by medical and social history, attempts to address this gap, but this information is often difficult to obtain in this population of donors. Detection methods directed at the antigens of HIV are available but are not in widespread use due to significant cost. Thus, processed allogeneic tissue, combined with donor screening, provides a relatively safe source of replacement tissue (114). It is estimated that the risk for HIV transmission from allografts is on the order of 1 in 650,000 (131). To date, only one documented case of HIV transmission by a donor is known, which occurred in 1987 (132).

Biology of Allografts

Allografts appear to undergo a maturation process similar to, but slower than, the ligamentization process seen in autografts (44,117,133,134). In postoperative biopsy specimens from humans, grafts were covered with a thick, hypervascular synovial sheath that likely originated from the vascular buds of the infrapatellar fat pad by 6

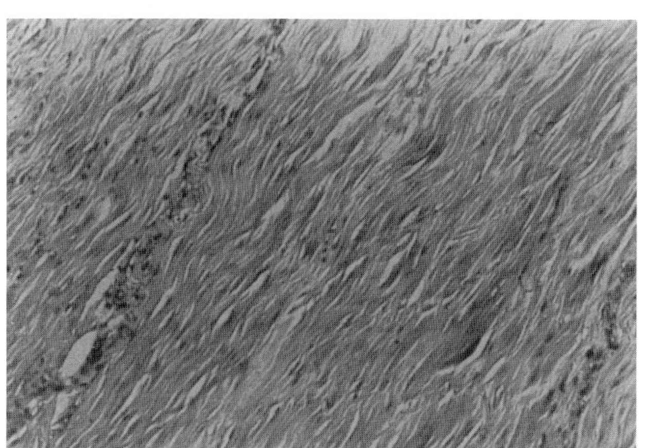
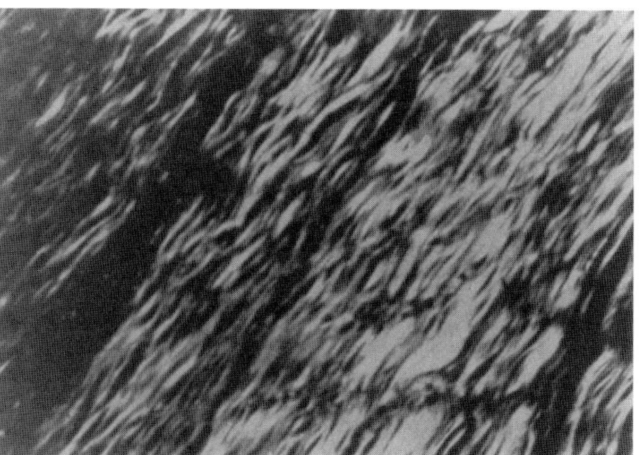

A   B

FIGURE 21.9. A: Photomicrograph of a longitudinal section of deep-frozen patellar tendon allograft 4 months after implantation. **B:** Same specimen viewed under polarized light, showing longitudinal orientation of the collagen bundles (hematoxylin and eosin stain; original magnification, ×100). (From Arnoczky SP, Warren RF, Ashlock MA. Replacement of the anterior cruciate ligament using a patellar tendon allograft: an experimental study. *J Bone Joint Surg Am* 1986;68:376–385, with permission.)

weeks (135,136). By 3 months, the synovial sheath was thinner but remained thicker than normal. Collagen fibers were aligned longitudinally with early hypercellularity present starting at 6 months. Full graft maturity appeared to occur by 18 months. Immunologic rejection was rarely observed in cryopreserved allografts (61).

Histologically, studies show that allografts undergo avascular necrosis, cellular repopulation, revascularization, and collagen remodeling, eventually producing a ligamentlike structure. In a study in goats, comparing similar-sized PT autografts and fresh-frozen PT allografts, Jackson et al. (111,113) showed that the maturation process of allografts lags behind that of autografts. At 6 weeks after transplantation, the allograft sheath showed increased vascularity and a greater inflammatory response than the autograft. At 6 months, electron microscopic ultrastructural analyses showed a greater persis-

tence of large-diameter collagen fibrils and a less robust proliferation of small-diameter collagen fibrils in the allograft group (Fig. 21.10). These findings reflect delayed graft remodeling and consequently a slower time until full graft strength. The autografts showed more robust proliferation of small-diameter collagen fibrils.

Allografts remodel using extrinsic cells to repopulate the graft substance. Using DNA analysis in a goat model, Jackson et al. (113) showed that donor cells are rapidly replaced by host cells. By 4 weeks, no donor DNA is present in any of the grafts. The cells repopulating the allograft tissue are composed of fibroblastic, vascular, and inflammatory cells.

It is intriguing that allografts may be capable of some regeneration of neurologic function. In a dog model, Goertzen et al. (137) showed that deep-frozen bone–ACL–bone allografts display mechanoreceptors

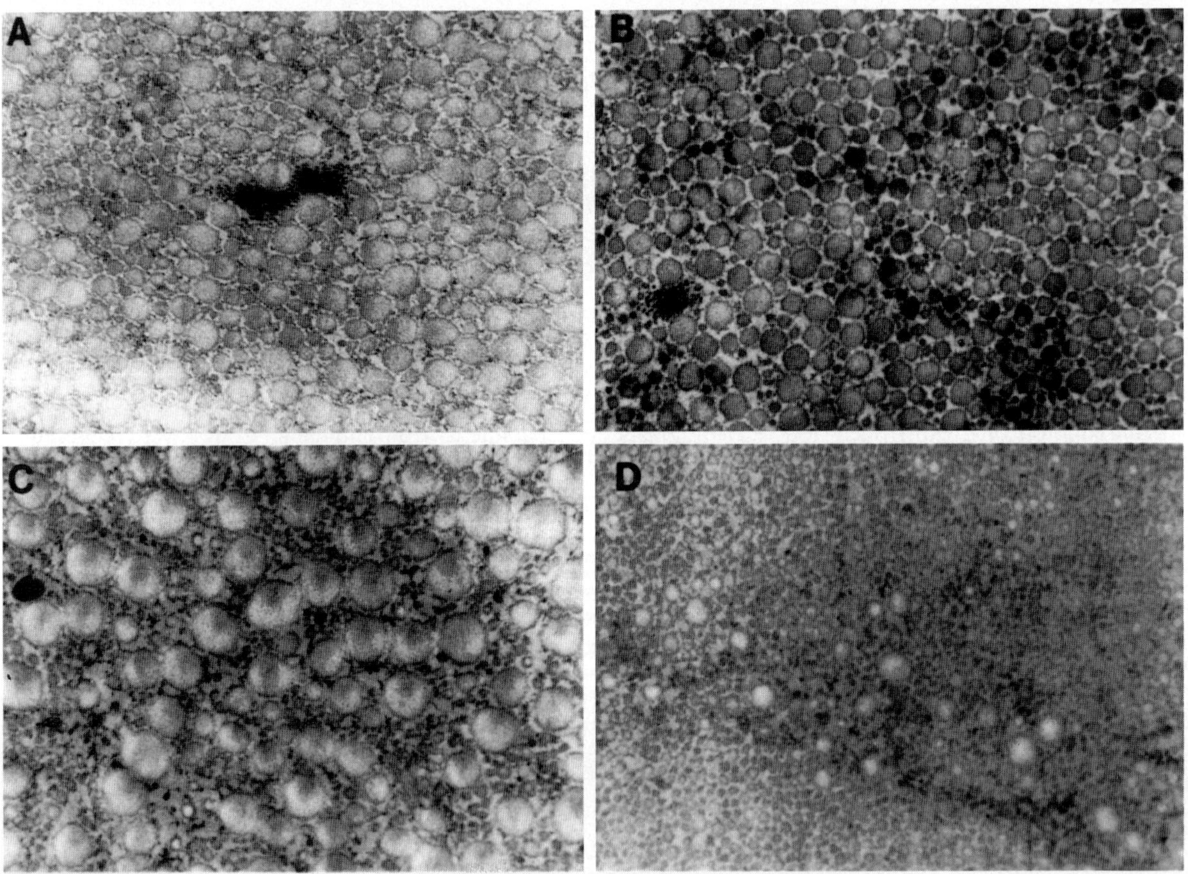

FIGURE 21.10. A: Electron micrograph of normal patellar tendon tissue demonstrating collagen fibrils in the range of 50 to 200 nm in diameter. Most fibrils are in the range of 100 to 150 nm. **B:** Electron micrograph of normal anterior cruciate ligament (ACL) (contralateral knee). Collagen fibrils are in the size range of 50 to 150 nm in diameter. Most fibrils are in the 100-ng range. **C:** Electron micrograph of patellar tendon allograft used for ACL reconstruction, 6 months after transplantation. Collagen fibrils in the range of 200 to 250 ng in diameter are present. **D:** Electron micrograph of patellar tendon autograft used for ACL reconstruction, 6 months after transplantation. Collagen fibrils ranged from 50 to 200 ng in diameter. A marked increase in small-diameter collagen fibrils was observed. Relatively fewer large-diameter fibrils were present. Original magnification, ×52,500. (From Jackson D, Grood E, Goldstein J, et al. A comparison of patellar tendon autograft and allograft used for anterior cruciate ligament reconstruction in the goat model. *Am J Sports Med* 1993;21:176–185, with permission.)

and free nerve endings located mostly near the surface of the allografts and at bony attachments by 6 months after transplantation. Whether this neural ingrowth is capable of providing some return of proprioception as occurs in the native ACL will require further study.

Strength and Biomechanics of Allografts

The biomechanical properties of PT grafts show that graft strength between allografts and autografts differs. Although at 6 weeks the mean maximum loads to failure are comparable, at 6 months the allograft is only about half as strong as the autograft in a goat model (111,113). In addition, A/P translation at 45° of flexion was less in the autograft group at 6 months. In neither group was the normal A/P translation restored to the level of the control group. This is similar to other animal studies that show allografts never attain the strength of the normal ACL (44,120,133,138,139). Direct comparisons of mechanical strength show that the time for allografts to reach maximum strength lags behind that of autografts. Using a dog model, Nikolaou et al. (134) showed that while the breaking strength of autograft PT plateaus at 24 weeks, the breaking strength of allograft PT plateaus later, at 36 weeks (Fig. 21.11). A similar lag has also been shown in augmented PT allografts (140).

Interestingly, human studies have failed to show a clinically significant difference between allografts and autografts. In a retrospective review of 56 autograft and 87 allograft PT ACL reconstructions, Fahey and Indelicato (141) showed that there was no significant difference in symptoms or instrumented laxity between the two groups. Similarly, Shelton et al. (115) compared 30 PT allografts and 30 PT autografts and showed no significant difference in side-to-side arthrometer measurements or Lachman test results. However, there was a greater incidence of glide on pivot-shift testing: 20% in allografts compared with 7% in autografts (115). In a study by Shino et al. (142), clinical comparisons between PT autografts and PT allografts show that thigh muscle extension strength is better in allograft patients than in autograft patients. Differences in A/P laxity were not statistically significant. Additional clinical studies show that allografts are nearly equal in efficacy to autografts when used in the acute ACL injury (135,143,144). In revision cases, allografts fail in one third of knees that have a previously failed reconstruction (145).

Comparing different types of allografts, Noyes and Barber (112) showed that in acute ACL ruptures, the PT allograft is better than the fascia lata allograft. Levitt et al. (146) found no clinical difference between PT and Achilles tendon allografts. Additional studies will be necessary to better identify the best source of allograft tissue. Currently, the PT allograft appears to be the best studied material. Based on limited animal studies on graft maturation, rehabilitation should include a lag of about 3 months compared with the rehabilitation program for autografts, with return to running sports to begin at about 9 months as compared with 6 months for autografts.

XENOGRAFTS

Although the use of grafts from one species to another showed some promise in an animal study, the use of xenografts in humans has shown uniformly poor results (147). Patients encounter persistent synovitis and a high rate of graft rupture (148,149). For these reasons, xenograft transplantation for the treatment of ACL-deficient knees is not widely accepted. As the technology of immune tolerance improves, this alternative source of graft tissue may become more acceptable.

SYNTHETIC AND AUGMENTED GRAFTS

Synthetic materials offer an alternative to biologic tissue for ACL reconstruction (150). When synthetic mate-

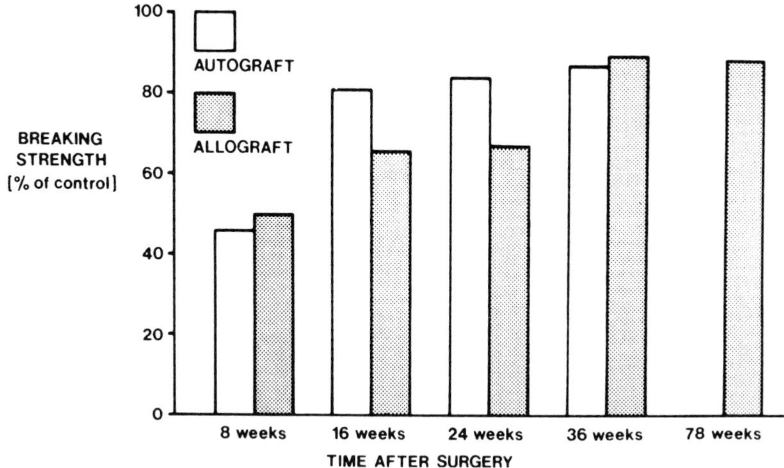

FIGURE 21.11. Comparison of autograft and allograft breaking strength at each time point. (From Nikolaou PK, Seaber AV, Glisson RR, et al. Anterior cruciate ligament allograft transplantation: long-term function, histology, revascularization, and operative technique. *Am J Sports Med* 1986;14:348–360, with permission.)

rials are used, there is no morbidity associated with a donor site and the possibility of transmitting infectious agents through allografts is eliminated (151). The ideal prosthetic ligament should have a high tensile strength, be easily implanted, be durable immediately after surgery to allow aggressive rehabilitation, and have lasting function.

Although numerous types exist, the most popular have been the Gore-Tex braid ligaments, Stryker Dacron ligaments, Kennedy ligament assist devices (LAD), filamentous carbon ligaments, and the Leeds–Keio polyester ligament (151). To date, no synthetic ligament has displayed acceptable function long term. Frank and Jackson (1) showed that 40% to 78% of 855 prosthetic ligaments implanted over a 15-year period compiled from eight different studies fail over time. In addition, synthetic implants are associated with a higher rate of complications, particularly chronic effusions.

Gore-Tex implants, which have been used since 1982, are associated with chronic synovitis with sterile effusions in 5% to 34% of patients (152–154). Ligament failure was noted in 5% to 18% of patients (152–154). Clinically, one third of patients reported buckling at 5 years after reconstruction (154,155). The Dacron prosthesis showed significant synovitis and a rupture rate of 12% by 4 years (156). Clinically, nearly half of patients may have persistent symptoms of instability (157–159). In the longest follow-up to date (9 years), prosthetic ruptures were diagnosed in 44% patients and 14% had acceptable stability and knee function (160). Despite augmentation with autologous tissue, poor results persisted. The Kennedy LAD had a 19.3% failure rate (161). Carbon fibers, which had a failure rate of 24.1% (162), may induce less of an inflammatory response (163). Six-year results of the Leeds–Keio polyester showed only 60% satisfactory results (164).

The pathogenesis of prosthetic ligament–associated chronic synovitis and ligament rupture likely results from small-wear particles as the grafts tenses, bends, and scrapes against bony surfaces (152). Although biologically inert in its original form (165), the small particles activate synovial cells to produce interleukin-1, a powerful modulator of chondrocyte metabolism (166). Interleukin-1 in turn induces an inflammatory response, decreases chondrocyte production of proteoglycans, and induces production of neutral proteinases that can digest the cartilaginous matrix (166). Histologically, there is marked synovial thickening with evidence of acute and chronic inflammation (Fig. 21.12). In some cases, major effusions were indications for graft removal (167).

Although the tensile strength of these prostheses is high initially—for example, the Gore-Tex prosthesis has an initial tensile strength of 4,830 N (168)—long-term complications and an unacceptably high rate of graft failure make the use of prosthetic grafts for ACL reconstruction limited. Further studies to limit small-particle wear

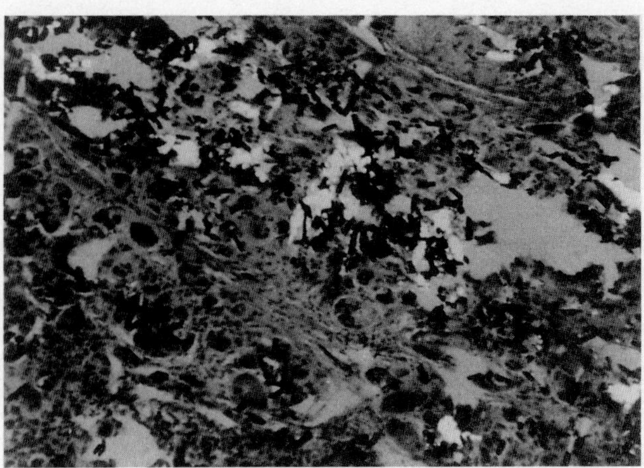

FIGURE 21.12. Histologic view from synovial biopsy a Gortex–anterior cruciate ligament prosthesis. (From Paulos LE, Rosenberg TD, Grewe SR, et al. The Gore-Tex anterior cruciate ligament prosthesis: a long-term follow-up. *Am J Sports Med* 1992;20:246–252, with permission.)

and its consequent inflammatory response must be pursued before this type of reconstruction is recommended.

ENGINEERED GRAFTS

Ligament analogs that allow the graft to remodel by host cellular metabolism have focused on collagen scaffolds composed of either fabricated collagen bundles or demineralized bone matrix (169,170). Collagenous scaffolds promote fibroblast ingrowth and production of extracellular matrix. Compared with tissue culture plates, these scaffolds facilitate continued collagen synthesis about tenfold greater than a tissue culture plate (171). As seeded cells proliferate in the collagen scaffold, they become bipolar and orient themselves along the long of the collagen fibers. Initial studies showed that tensile strength in collagen gels (0.14 MPa) were two orders of magnitude lower than that of ligament tissue (38 MPa) (172). Extruded acid-insoluble collagen fibers have higher tensile strengths of 40 MPa or greater, depending on the cross-linking method (173).

Recently, Jackson et al. (170) used demineralized cortical bone as a biologic matrix. This graft contains collagen and other associated biopolymers, proteoglycans, and glycoproteins (Fig. 21.13). It has the capacity to promote cell growth, differentiation, and remodeling. One-year studies in the goat model show that A/P translation tested at 30 N is 2.1 mm, which is comparable to other ACL reconstruction methods tested in the same animal model. Within the tunnel, there was ingrowth of bone constituents and Sharpey's type fibers at the transition zone but the incorporation process was not complete by 1 year. The intraarticular portion of the graft contained numerous fibrocytes and blood vessels, but ligamentization was incomplete. The time needed to complete the desired remodeling may take several years, making the length of

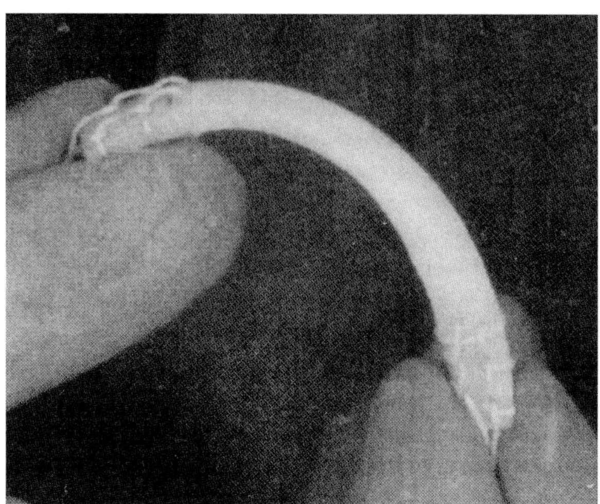

FIGURE 21.13. The appearance of the fully hydrated matrix graft with fixation sutures before implantation. The matrix is firm to the touch but remains relatively pliable. (From Jackson DW, Simon TM, Lowery W, et al. Biologic remodeling after anterior cruciate ligament reconstruction using a collagen matrix derived from demineralized bone: an experimental study in the goat model. *Am J Sports Med* 1996;24:405–414, with permission.)

postoperative protective prohibitive at this time. Continued improvement of this type of graft will be required before it will be of clinical utility. An intriguing possibility is to pretreat graft material with engineered proteins that stimulate fibroblast ingrowth and matrix remodeling.

OVERVIEW

Choosing the best type of graft material for reconstruction of the ACL remains controversial. The most common and best-studied grafts are the PT and HS autografts. As the frequency of ACL reconstruction expands, the need for alternative sources of graft material will also expand. Current efforts to find such alternatives are under intense investigation. Whatever this material may ultimately be, it must possess some important characteristics. The criteria for the optimum ACL graft must include ease of implantation, durability over time, functional similarity to native ACL, low risk for complications, and economic feasibility. A key component of graft durability and function is the appreciation that the ACL is a complex viscoelastic organ. It not only displays inherent strength, but also serves as a proprioceptive device. The native ACL has the ability to modulate itself over various load distributions depending on knee position. Efforts to understanding and ultimately incorporate these complex features into ligament grafts will be the future challenge in ACL reconstruction.

The type of graft does not appear to influence the development of osteoarthritis in patients who have undergone an ACL reconstruction. There continues to be a high incidence of osteoarthritis in patients who undergo ACL reconstruction, particularly in those patients who have concomitant meniscectomy (51,52,174). Currently, the best grafts are those that relieve symptoms of instability. A better understanding of the etiology of osteoarthritis in the ACL-reconstructed knee will be needed to improve this aspect of treatment for the ACL-deficient knee.

The PT autograft continues to be the gold standard by which to compare all other grafts. The current scientific knowledge in the field indicates that there is no clearly superior graft choice for all patients with ACL-deficient knees. The use of allografts is becoming better accepted as screening for viral diseases, graft sterilization techniques, and graft treatment techniques improve. Regardless of the graft choice, all biologic grafts, including autografts and allografts, appear to undergo the ligamentization process. Although the allograft may require more time to complete this process, both graft types must have a period of protection while the graft matures to a ligamentlike structure. Given the variability of results, the surgeon together with patient must explore the advantages and disadvantages of each technique and choose the most appropriate graft for each situation.

REFERENCES

1. Frank CB, Jackson DW. The science of reconstruction of the anterior cruciate ligament. *J Bone Joint Surg Am* 1997;79:1556–1576.
2. Corsetti JR, Jackson DW. Failure of anterior cruciate ligament reconstruction: the biologic basis. *Clin Orthop* 1996;325:42–49.
3. Jaureguito JW, Paulos LE. Why grafts fail. *Clin Orthop* 1996;325:25–41.
4. Marshall JL, Warren RF, Wickiewicz TL, et al. The anterior cruciate ligament: a technique of repair and reconstruction. *Clin Orthop* 1979:97–106.
5. Naranja RJ Jr, Corsetti J, Kuhlman JR, et al. The search for the Holy Grail: a century of anterior cruciate ligament reconstruction. *Am J Orthop* 1997;26:743–752.
6. Paulos LE, Cherf J, Rosenberg TD, et al. Anterior cruciate ligament reconstruction with autografts. *Clin Sports Med* 1991;10:469–485.
7. Jones K. Reconstruction of the anterior cruciate ligament: a technique using the central one-third of the patellar ligament. *J Bone Joint Surg Am* 1963;45:925–932.
8. Amiel D, Kleiner J, Harwood F, et al. The phenomenon of "ligamentization": anterior cruciate ligament reconstruction with autogenous patellar tendon. *J Orthop Res* 1986;4:162–172.
9. Arnoczky SP, Warren RF, Minei JP. Replacement of the anterior cruciate ligament using a synthetic prosthesis: an evaluation of graft biology in the dog. *Am J Sports Med* 1986;14:1–6.
10. Kondo M. An experimental study on reconstructive surgery of the anterior cruciate ligament. *J Jpn Orthop Assoc* 1979;53:521–533.
11. Cabaud HE, Feagin JA, Rodkey WG. Acute anterior cruciate ligament injury and augmented repair: experimental studies. *Am J Sports Med* 1980;8:395–401.
12. Campbell W. Reconstruction of the ligament of the knee. *Am J Surg* 1939;43:473–480.
13. Nimmi M. Collagen: structure, function, and metabolism in normal and fibrotic tissues. *Semin Arthr Rheum* 1983;13:1–85.
14. Amiel D, Frank C, Harwood F, et al. Tendons and ligaments: a morphological and biochemical comparison. *J Orthop Res* 1984;1:257–265.
15. Ballock R, Woo S, Lyon R, et al. Use of patellar tendon autograft for anterior cruciate ligament reconstruction in the rabbit: a long-term histologic and biomechanical study. *J Orthop Res* 1989;7:474–485.
16. Chiroff RT. Experimental replacement of the anterior cruciate ligament: a histological and microradiographic study. *J Bone Joint Surg Am* 1975;57:1124–1127.
17. Alm A, Gillquist J, Streomberg B. The medial third of the patellar lig-

ament in reconstruction of the anterior cruciate ligament: a clinical and histologic study by means of arthroscopy or arthrotomy. *Acta Chir Scand Suppl* 1974;445:5–14.

18. Panni A, Milano G, Lucania L, et al. Graft healing after anterior cruciate ligament reconstruction in rabbits. *Clin Orthop* 1997;343:203–212.

19. Clancy W, Narenchania R, Rosenberg T, et al. Anterior and posterior cruciate ligament reconstruction in rhesus monkeys. *J Bone Joint Surg Am* 1981;63:1270–1284.

20. Arnoczky S, Tarvin G, Marshall J. ACL replacement using patellar tendon. *J Bone Joint Surg Am* 1982;64:217–224.

21. Kleiner J, Amiel D, Harwood F, et al. Early histologic, metabolic, and vascular assessment of anterior cruciate ligament autografts. *J Orthop Res* 1989;7:235–242.

22. Alm A, Stromberg B. Vascular anatomy of the patellar and cruciate ligaments: a microangiographic and histologic investigation in the dog. *Acta Chir Scand Suppl* 1974;445:25–35.

23. Kleiner J, Amiel D, Roux R, et al. Origin of replacement cell for the anterior cruciate ligament autograft. *J Orthop Res* 1986;4:466–474.

24. Dunphy J. *Wound healing.* New York: Medcom Press, 1974.

25. McFarland E, Morrey B, An K, et al. The relationship of vascularity and water content to tensile strength in a patellar tendon replacement of the anterior cruciate in dogs. *Am J Sports Med* 1986;14:436–448.

26. Denti M, Monteleone M, Berardi A, et al. Anterior cruciate ligament mechanoreceptors: histologic studies on lesions and reconstruction. *Clin Orthop* 1994;308:29–32.

27. Krauspe R, Schmidt M, Schaible HG. Sensory innervation of the anterior cruciate ligament: an electrophysiological study of the response properties of single identified mechanoreceptors in the cat. *J Bone Joint Surg Am* 1992;74:390–397.

28. Schultz R, Miller D, Kerr C, et al. Mechanoreceptors in human cruciate ligaments: a histologic study. *J Bone Joint Surg Am* 1984;66:1072.

29. Schutte MJ, Dabezies EJ, Zimny ML, et al. Neural anatomy of the human anterior cruciate ligament. *J Bone Joint Surg Am* 1987;69:243–247.

30. Yahia L, Newman N. Mechanoreceptors in the canine anterior cruciate ligament. *Anat Anz* 1991;173:233–238.

31. Zimny M, Wink C. Neuroreceptors in the tissues of the knee joint. *J Electromyogr Kinesiol* 1991;1:148–157.

32. Barrack R, Skinner H, Buckley S. Proprioception in the anterior cruciate deficient knee. *Am J Sports Med* 1989;17:1–6.

33. Beard D, Kyberd P, Fergusson C, et al. Proprioception after rupture of the anterior cruciate ligament. *J Bone Joint Surg Br* 1993;76:311–315.

34. Wojtys EM, Huston LJ. Neuromuscular performance in normal and anterior cruciate ligament-deficient lower extremities. *Am J Sports Med* 1994;22:89–104.

35. Andriacchi TP, Birac D. Functional testing in the anterior cruciate ligament-deficient knee. *Clin Orthop* 1993;288:40–47.

36. Berchuck M, Andriacchi TP, Bach BR, et al. Gait adaptations by patients who have a deficient anterior cruciate ligament. *J Bone Joint Surg Am* 1990;72:871–877.

37. Solomonow M, Baratta R, Zhou BH, et al. The synergistic action of the anterior cruciate ligament and thigh muscles in maintaining joint stability. *Am J Sports Med* 1987;15:207–213.

38. Kennedy J, Alexander I, Hayes K. Nerve supply of the human knee and its functional importance. *Am J Sports Med* 1982;10:329–335.

39. Barrack R, Lund P, Munn B, et al. Evidence of reinnervation of free patellar tendon autograft used for anterior cruciate ligament reconstruction. *Am J Sports Med* 1997;25:196–202.

40. Barrett DS. Proprioception and function after anterior cruciate reconstruction. *J Bone Joint Surg Br* 1991;73:833–837.

41. Rodeo SA, Arnoczky SP, Torzilli PA, et al. Tendon-healing in a bone tunnel: a biomechanical and histological study in the dog. *J Bone Joint Surg Am* 1993;75:1795–1803.

42. Grana WA, Egle DM, Mahnken R, et al. An analysis of autograft fixation after anterior cruciate ligament reconstruction in a rabbit model. *Am J Sports Med* 1994;22:344–351.

43. Schiavone Panni A, Fabbriciani C, Delcogliano A, et al. Bone-ligament interaction in patellar tendon reconstruction of the ACL. *Knee Surg Sports Traumatol Arthrosc* 1993;1:4–8.

44. Shino K, Kawasaki T, Hirose H, et al. Replacement of the anterior cruciate ligament by an allogeneic tendon graft: an experimental study in the dog. *J Bone Joint Surg Br* 1984;66:672–681.

45. Brown CH Jr., Steiner ME, Carson EW. The use of hamstring tendons

46. Butler DL. Kappa Delta Award paper: anterior cruciate ligament: its normal response and replacement. *J Orthop Res* 1989;7:910–921.

47. O'Neill DB. Arthroscopically assisted reconstruction of the anterior cruciate ligament: a prospective randomized analysis of three techniques. *J Bone Joint Surg Am* 1996;78:803–813.

48. Marder RA, Raskind JR, Carroll M. Prospective evaluation of arthroscopically assisted anterior cruciate ligament reconstruction: patellar tendon versus semitendinosus and gracilis tendons. *Am J Sports Med* 1991;19:478–484.

49. Aglietti P, Buzzi R, Zaccherotti G, et al. Patellar tendon versus doubled semitendinosus and gracilis tendons for anterior cruciate ligament reconstruction. *Am J Sports Med* 1994;22:211–217; discussion, 217–218.

50. Anderson AF, Snyder RB, Lipscomb AB Sr. Anterior cruciate ligament reconstruction using the semitendinosus and gracilis tendons augmented by the Losee iliotibial band tenodesis: a long-term study. *Am J Sports Med* 1994;22:620–626.

51. Daniel DM, Stone ML, Dobson BE, et al. Fate of the ACL-injured patient: a prospective outcome study [see comments]. *Am J Sports Med* 1994;22:632–644.

52. Ferretti A, Conteduca F, De Carli A, et al. Osteoarthritis of the knee after ACL reconstruction. *Int Orthop* 1991;15:367–371.

53. Hillard-Sembell D, Daniel DM, Stone ML, et al. Combined injuries of the anterior cruciate and medial collateral ligaments of the knee: effect of treatment on stability and function of the joint. *J Bone Joint Surg Am* 1996;78:169–176.

54. Karlson JA, Steiner ME, Brown CH, et al. Anterior cruciate ligament reconstruction using gracilis and semitendinosus tendons: comparison of through-the-condyle and over-the-top graft placements. *Am J Sports Med* 1994;22:659–666.

55. Otero AL, Hutcheson L. A comparison of the doubled semitendinosus/gracilis and central third of the patellar tendon autografts in arthroscopic anterior cruciate ligament reconstruction. *Arthroscopy* 1993;9:143–148.

56. Blickenstaff KR, Grana WA, Egle D. Analysis of a semitendinosus autograft in a rabbit model. *Am J Sports Med* 1997;25:554–559.

57. Pinczewski L, Clingeleffer A, Otto D, et al. Integration of hamstring tendon graft with bone in reconstruction of the anterior cruciate ligament. *Arthroscopy* 1997;13:641–643.

58. Holmes PF, James SL, Larson RL, et al. Retrospective direct comparison of three intraarticular anterior cruciate ligament reconstructions. *Am J Sports Med* 1991;19:596–599, discussion 599–600.

59. Howe JG, Johnson RJ, Kaplan MJ, et al. Anterior cruciate ligament reconstruction using quadriceps patellar tendon graft, I: long-term follow-up. *Am J Sports Med* 1991;19:447–457.

60. Shelbourne KD, Mollabashy A, De Carlo M. Acute anterior cruciate ligament injury. *Indiana Med* 1990;83:896–900.

61. Shino K, Inoue M, Horibe S, et al. Reconstruction of the anterior cruciate ligament using allogeneic tendon: long-term follow-up. *Am J Sports Med* 1990;18:457–465.

62. Fulkerson JP, Langeland R. An alternative cruciate reconstruction graft: the central quadriceps tendon. *Arthroscopy* 1995;11:252–254.

63. Harris NL, Smith DA, Lamoreaux L, et al. Central quadriceps tendon for anterior cruciate ligament reconstruction, I: morphometric and biomechanical evaluation. *Am J Sports Med* 1997;25:23–28.

64. Steaubli HU, Jakob RP. Central quadriceps tendon for anterior cruciate ligament reconstruction, I: morphometric and biochemical evaluation [letter]. *Am J Sports Med* 1997;25:725–727.

65. Noyes FR, Butler DL, Grood ES, et al. Biomechanical analysis of human ligament grafts used in knee-ligament repairs and reconstructions. *J Bone Joint Surg Am* 1984;66:344–352.

66. Stanish WD, Kirkpatrick J, Rubinovich RM. Reconstruction of the anterior cruciate ligament with a quadricep patellar tendon graft: preliminary results. *Can J Appl Sport Sci* 1984;9:21–24.

67. Kornblatt I, Warren RF, Wickiewicz TL. Long-term follow-up of anterior cruciate ligament reconstruction using the quadriceps tendon substitution for chronic anterior cruciate ligament insufficiency. *Am J Sports Med* 1988;16:444–448.

68. Kaplan MJ, Howe JG, Fleming B, et al. Anterior cruciate ligament reconstruction using quadriceps patellar tendon graft, II: a specific sport review. *Am J Sports Med* 1991;19:458–462.

69. Yasuda K, Ohkoshi Y, Tanabe Y. Quantitative evaluation of knee insta-

bility and muscle strength after anterior cruciate ligament reconstruction using patellar and quadriceps tendon. *Am J Sports Med* 1992;20: 471–475.

70. Yasuda K, Tomiyama Y, Ohkoshi Y, et al. Arthroscopic observations of autogeneic quadriceps and patellar tendon grafts after anterior cruciate ligament reconstruction of the knee. *Clin Orthop* 1989;246: 217–224.

71. Seo JG, Cho DY, Kim KY. Reconstruction of the anterior cruciate ligament with Achilles tendon autograft. *Orthopedics* 1993;16:719–724.

72. Hey-Groves E. Operation for the repair of the crucial ligaments. *Lancet* 1917;2:674–675.

73. Hey-Groves E. The crucial ligaments of the knee-joint: their function, rupture, and the operative treatment of the same. *Br J Surg* 1920;7: 505–515.

74. van Rens TJ, van den Berg AF, Huiskes R, et al. Substitution of the anterior cruciate ligament: a long-term histologic and biomechanical study with autogenous pedicled grafts of the iliotibial band in dogs. *Arthroscopy* 1986;2:139–154.

75. Insall J, Joseph DM, Aglietti P, et al. Bone-block iliotibial-band transfer for anterior cruciate insufficiency. *J Bone Joint Surg Am* 1981;63: 560–569.

76. Scott W, Ferriter P, Marino M. Intra-articular transfer of the iliotibial tract: two to seven-year follow-up results. *J Bone Joint Surg Am* 1985;67:532–538.

77. Hooper GJ, Walton DI. Reconstruction of the anterior cruciate ligament using the bone-block iliotibial-tract transfer. *J Bone Joint Surg Am* 1987;69:1150–1154.

78. Billoti J, Meese M, Alberta F, et al. A prospective, clinical study evaluating arthroscopic ACL reconstruction using the semitendinosus and iliotibial band: 2- to 5-year follow up. *Orthopedics* 1997;20:125–131.

79. Zarins B, Rowe CR. Combined anterior cruciate-ligament reconstruction using semitendinosus tendon and iliotibial tract. *J Bone Joint Surg Am* 1986;68:160–177.

80. Collins HR, Hughston JC, Dehaven KE, et al. The meniscus as a cruciate ligament substitute. *J Sports Med* 1974;2:11–21.

81. Ferkel RD, Markolf K, Goodfellow D, et al. Treatment of the anterior cruciate ligament-absent knee with associated meniscal tears: instrumented testing and clinical evaluation of two patient groups. *Clin Orthop* 1987;222:239–248.

82. Ivey FM, Blazina ME, Fox JM, et al. Intraarticular substitution for anterior cruciate insufficiency: a clinical comparison between patellar tendon and meniscus. *Am J Sports Med* 1980;8:405–410.

83. Tillberg B. The late repair of torn cruciate ligaments using menisci. *J Bone Joint Surg Br* 1977;59:15–19.

84. Walsh JJ Jr. Meniscal reconstruction of the anterior cruciate ligament. *Clin Orthop* 1972;89:171–177.

85. Mitsou A, Vallianatos P, Piskopakis N, et al. Cruciate ligament replacement using a meniscus. An experimental study. *J Bone Joint Surg Br* 1988;70:784–786.

86. Ferkel RD, Fox JM, Del Pizzo W, et al. Reconstruction of the anterior cruciate ligament using a torn meniscus. *J Bone Joint Surg Am* 1988; 70:715–723.

87. LaPrade RF, Hamilton CD, Montgomery RD, et al. The reharvested central third of the patellar tendon: a histologic and biomechanical analysis. *Am J Sports Med* 1997;25:779–785.

88. Karns DJ, Heidt RS Jr, Holladay BR, et al. Case report: revision anterior cruciate ligament reconstruction [see comments]. *Arthroscopy* 1994;10:148–151, discussion 152–157.

89. Kartus J, Stener S, Lindahl S, et al. Ipsi- or contralateral patellar tendon graft in anterior cruciate ligament revision surgery: a comparison of two methods. *Am J Sports Med* 1998;26:499–504.

90. Steiner ME, Hecker AT, Brown CH Jr, et al. Anterior cruciate ligament graft fixation: comparison of hamstring and patellar tendon grafts. *Am J Sports Med* 1994;22:240–246, discussion 246–247.

91. Ballock RT, Woo SL, Lyon RM, et al. Use of patellar tendon autograft for anterior cruciate ligament reconstruction in the rabbit: a long-term histologic and biomechanical study. *J Orthop Res* 1989;7:474–485.

92. Kennedy JC, Roth JH, Mendenhall HV, et al. Presidential address: intraarticular replacement in the anterior cruciate ligament-deficient knee. *Am J Sports Med* 1980;8:1–8.

93. Thorson E, Rodrigo JJ, Vasseur P, et al. Replacement of the anterior cruciate ligament. A comparison of autografts and allografts in dogs. *Acta Orthop Scan* 1989;60:555–560.

94. Vasseur PB, Rodrigo JJ, Stevenson S, et al. Replacement of the anterior cruciate ligament with a bone-ligament-bone anterior cruciate ligament allograft in dogs. *Clin Orthop* 1987;219:268–277.

95. Yoshiya S, Andrish JT, Manley MTW, et al. Graft tension in anterior cruciate ligament reconstruction: an *in vivo* study in dogs. *Am J Sports Med* 1987;15:464–470.

96. Yoshiya S, Andrish JT, Manley MT, et al. Augmentation of anterior cruciate ligament reconstruction in dogs with prostheses of different stiffnesses. *J Orthop Res* 1986;4:475–485.

97. Beynnon BD, Johnson RJ, Fleming BC, et al. The measurement of elongation of anterior cruciate-ligament grafts *in vivo*. *J Bone Joint Surg Am* 1994;76:520–531.

98. Tohyama H, Beynnon BD, Johnson RJ, et al. The effect of anterior cruciate ligament graft elongation at the time of implantation on the biomechanical behavior of the graft and knee. *Am J Sports Med* 1996; 24:608–614.

99. Yasuda K, Tsujino J, Tanabe Y, et al. Effects of initial graft tension on clinical outcome after anterior cruciate ligament reconstruction: autogenous doubled hamstring tendons connected in series with polyester tapes. *Am J Sports Med* 1997;25:99–106.

100. McPherson GK, Mendenhall HV, Gibbons DF, et al. Experimental mechanical and histologic evaluation of the Kennedy ligament augmentation device. *Clin Orthop* 1985;196:186–195.

101. Figgie HEd, Bahniuk EH, Heiple KG, et al. The effects of tibial-femoral angle on the failure mechanics of the canine anterior cruciate ligament. *J Biomech* 1986;19:89–91.

102. Butler D, Noyes F, Grood E, et al. The effects of vascularity on the mechanical properties of primate anterior cruciate ligament replacements. *Orthop Res Soc Trans* 1983;8:93.

103. Noyes F, Butler D, Paulos L, et al. Intra-articular cruciate reconstruction, I: perspectives on graft strength, vascularization and immediate motion after replacement. *Clin Orthop* 1983;172:71–77.

104. Ryan J, Droupp B. Evaluation of tensile strength of reconstructions of the anterior cruciate ligament using the patellar tendon in dogs. *South Med J* 1966;59:129–134.

105. Shelbourne K, Klootwyk T, DeCarlo M. Update on accelerated rehabilitation after ACL reconstruction. *J Sports Phys Ther* 1992;15:303–308.

106. O'Donoghue DH, Frank GR, Jeter GL, et al. Repair and reconstruction of the anterior cruciate ligament in dogs: factors influencing long-term results. *J Bone Joint Surg Am* 1971;53:710–718.

107. Butler DL, Guan Y, Kay MD, et al. Location-dependent variations in the material properties of the anterior cruciate ligament. *J Biomech* 1992;25:511–518.

108. Beynnon BD, Fleming BC, Johnson RJ, et al. Anterior cruciate ligament strain behavior during rehabilitation exercises *in vivo*. *Am J Sports Med* 1995;23;24–34.

109. Holden JP, Grood ES, Korvick DL, et al. *in vivo* forces in the anterior cruciate ligament: direct measurements during walking and trotting in a quadruped. *J Biomech* 1994;27:517–526.

110. DiStefano V. Anterior cruciate ligament reconstruction: autograft or allograft? *Clin Sports Med* 1993;12:1–11.

111. Jackson DW, Corsetti J, Simon TM. Biologic incorporation of allograft anterior cruciate ligament replacements. *Clin Orthop* 1996;324: 126–133.

112. Noyes F, Barber S. Allograft reconstruction of the anterior and posterior cruciate ligaments: report of ten-year experience and results. *Instr Course Lect* 1993;42:381–396.

113. Jackson D, Grood E, Goldstein J, et al. A comparison of patellar tendon autograft and allograft used for anterior cruciate ligament reconstruction in the goat model. *Am J Sports Med* 1993;21:176–185.

114. Meyers JF. Allograft reconstruction of the anterior cruciate ligament. *Clin Sports Med* 1991;10:487–498.

115. Shelton WR, Papendick L, Dukes AD. Autograft versus allograft anterior cruciate ligament reconstruction. *Arthroscopy* 1997;13:446–449.

116. Shino K. Reconstruction of the anterior cruciate ligament using allogeneic tissues: overview and current practice. *Bull Hosp Joint Dis Orthop Inst* 1991;51:155–174.

117. Arnoczky SP, Warren RF, Ashlock MA. Replacement of the anterior cruciate ligament using a patellar tendon allograft: an experimental study. *J Bone Joint Surg Am* 1986;68:376–385.

118. Cameron RR, Conrad RN, Sell KW, et al. Freeze-dried composite tendon allografts: an experimental study. *Plast Reconstr Surg* 1971;47:39–46.

119. Friedlaender GE, Strong DM, Sell KW. Studies on the antigenicity of bone, I: freeze-dried and deep-frozen bone allografts in rabbits. *J Bone Joint Surg Am* 1976;58:854–858.

120. Jackson DW, Grood ES, Arnoczky SP, et al. Freeze dried anterior cruciate ligament allografts. Preliminary studies in a goat model [published erratum appears in *Am J Sports Med* 1987;15:482]. *Am J Sports Med* 1987;15:295–303.

121. Barad S, Cabaud H, Rodrigo J. The effect of storage at −80 degrees Celsius as compared to 4 degrees Celsius on the strength of rhesus monkey anterior cruciate ligament. *Trans Orthop Res Soc* 1982;7:378.

122. Woo SL, Orlando CA, Camp JF, et al. Effects of postmortem storage by freezing on ligament tensile behavior. *J Biomech* 1986;19:399–404.

123. Jackson DW, Windler GE, Simon TM. Intraarticular reaction associated with the use of freeze-dried, ethylene oxide-sterilized bone-patella tendon-bone allografts in the reconstruction of the anterior cruciate ligament. *Am J Sports Med* 1990;18:1–10, discussion 10–11.

124. Roberts TS, Drez D Jr, McCarthy W, et al. Anterior cruciate ligament reconstruction using freeze-dried, ethylene oxide-sterilized, bone-patellar tendon-bone allografts: two year results in thirty-six patients [published erratum appears in *Am J Sports Med* 1991;19:272]. *Am J Sports Med* 1991;19:35–41.

125. Sterling J, Meyers M, Calvo R. Allograft failure in cruciate ligament reconstruction: Follow-up evaluation in eighteen patients. *Am J Sports Med* 1995;23:173–178.

126. Buck BE, Resnick L, Shah SM, et al. Human immunodeficiency virus cultured from bone. Implications for transplantation. *Clin Orthop* 1990;251:249–253.

127. Spire B, Dormont D, Barrae-Sinoussi F, et al. Inactivation of lymphadenopathy-associated virus by heat, gamma rays, and ultraviolet light. *Lancet* 1985;1:188–189.

128. Conway B, Tomford W, Hirsch M, et al. Effects of gamma irradiation on HIV-1 in a bone allograft model. *Trans Orthop Res Soc* 1990;15:225.

129. Fideler BM, Vangsness CT Jr, Moore T, et al. Effects of gamma irradiation on the human immunodeficiency virus: a study in frozen human bone-patellar ligament-bone grafts obtained from infected cadavera. *J Bone Joint Surg Am* 1994;76:1032–1035.

130. Gibbons MJ, Butler DL, Grood ES, et al. Effects of gamma irradiation on the initial mechanical and material properties of goat bone-patellar tendon-bone allografts. *J Orthop Res* 1991;9:209–218.

131. Allosource, Bone and Tissue Standards. Centennial, CO;1999.

132. American Association of Tissue Banks (AATB). Standards for Tissue Banking. McLean, VA;1999.

133. Jackson DW, Grood ES, Arnoczky SP, et al. Cruciate reconstruction using freeze dried anterior cruciate ligament allograft and a ligament augmentation device LAD: an experimental study in a goat model. *Am J Sports Med* 1987;15:528–538.

134. Nikolaou PK, Seaber AV, Glisson RR, et al. Anterior cruciate ligament allograft transplantation: long-term function, histology, revascularization, and operative technique. *Am J Sports Med* 1986;14:348–360.

135. Shino K, Inoue M, Horibe S, et al. Maturation of allograft tendons transplanted into the knee. An arthroscopic and histological study. *J Bone Joint Surg Br* 1988;70:556–560.

136. Shino K, Inoue M, Horibe S, et al. Surface blood flow and histology of human anterior cruciate ligament allografts. *Arthroscopy* 1991;7:171–176.

137. Goertzen M, Gruber J, Dellmann A, et al. Neurohistological findings after experimental anterior cruciate ligament allograft transplantation. *Arch Orthop Trau Surg* 1992;111:126–129.

138. Curtis RJ, Delee JC, Drez DJ Jr. Reconstruction of the anterior cruciate ligament with freeze dried fascia lata allografts in dogs: a preliminary report. *Am J Sports Med* 1985;13:408–414.

139. Webster DA, Werner FW. Freeze-dried flexor tendons in anterior cruciate ligament reconstruction. *Clin Orthop* 1983;181:238–243.

140. Goertzen M, Dellmann A, Gruber J, et al. Anterior cruciate ligament allograft transplantation for intraarticular ligamentous reconstruction. *Arch Orthop Traum Surg* 1992;111:273–279.

141. Fahey M, Indelicato PA. Bone tunnel enlargement after anterior cruciate ligament replacement. *Am J Sports Med* 1994;22:410–414.

142. Shino K, Nakata K, Horibe S, et al. Quantitative evaluation after arthroscopic anterior cruciate ligament reconstruction: allograft versus autograft. *Am J Sports Med* 1993;21:609–616.

143. Noyes FR, Barber-Westin SD. Reconstruction of the anterior cruciate ligament with human allograft: comparison of early and later results. *J Bone Joint Surg Am* 1996;78:524–537.

144. Shino K, Kimura T, Hirose H, et al. Reconstruction of the anterior cruciate ligament by allogeneic tendon graft: an operation for chronic ligamentous insufficiency. *J Bone Joint Surg Br* 1986;68:739–746.

145. Noyes FR, Barber-Westin SD, Roberts CS. Use of allografts after failed treatment of rupture of the anterior cruciate ligament [see comments]. *J Bone Joint Surg Am* 1994;76:1019–1031.

146. Levitt R, Malinin T, Posada A, et al. Reconstruction of the anterior cruciate ligaments with bone-patellar tendon-bone and Achilles tendon allografts. *Clin Orthop Rel Res* 1994;303:67–78.

147. McMaster WC. A histologic assessment of canine anterior cruciate substitution with bovine xenograft. *Clin Orthop* 1985;196:196–201.

148. Good L, Odensten M, Pettersson L, et al. Failure of a bovine xenograft for reconstruction of the anterior cruciate ligament. *Acta Orthop Scand* 1989;60:8–12.

149. van Steensel CJ, Schreuder O, van den Bosch BF, et al. Failure of anterior cruciate-ligament reconstruction using tendon xenograft. *J Bone Joint Surg Am* 1987;69:860–864.

150. Woods GW. Synthetics in anterior cruciate ligament reconstruction: a review. *Orthop Clin North Am* 1985;16:227–235.

151. Cameron M, Fu F. Prosthetic ligaments in ACL reconstruction. *Bull Rheum Dis* 1994;43:4–6.

152. Glousman R, Shields Jr C, Kerlan R, et al. Gore-Tex prosthetic ligament in anterior cruciate deficient knees. *Am J Sports Med* 1988;16:321–326.

153. Indelicato PA, Pascale MS, Huegel MO. Early experience with the GORE-TEX polytetrafluoroethylene anterior cruciate ligament prosthesis. *Am J Sports Med* 1989;17:55–52.

154. Paulos LE, Rosenberg TD, Grewe SR, et al. The GORE-TEX anterior cruciate ligament prosthesis: a long-term follow-up. *Am J Sports Med* 1992;20:246–252.

155. Ahlfeld SK, Larson RL, Collins HR. Anterior cruciate reconstruction in the chronically unstable knee using an expanded polytetrafluoroethylene PTFE prosthetic ligament. *Am J Sports Med* 1987;15:326–330.

156. Barrett G, Line L, Shelton W, et al. The Dacron ligament prosthesis in anterior cruciate ligament reconstruction: a four-year review. *Am J Sports Med* 1993;21:367–373.

157. Laopex-Vaazquez E, Juan J, Vila E, et al. Reconstruction of the anterior cruciate ligament with a Dacron prosthesis. *J Bone Joint Surg Am* 1991;73:1294–1300.

158. Richmond J, Manseau C, Patz R, et al. Anterior cruciate reconstruction using a Dacron ligament prosthesis: a long-term study. *Am J Sports Med* 1992;20:24–28.

159. Wilk R, Richmond J. Dacron ligament reconstruction for chromic anterior cruciate ligament insufficiency. *Am J Sports Med* 1993;21:374–379.

160. Maletius W, Gillquist J. Long-term results of anterior cruciate ligament reconstruction with a Dacron prosthesis: the frequency of osteoarthritis after seven to eleven years. *Am J Sports Med* 1997;25:288–293.

161. Kdolsky RK, Gibbons DF, Kwasny O, et al. Braided polypropylene augmentation device in reconstructive surgery of the anterior cruciate ligament: long-term clinical performance of 594 patients and short-term arthroscopic results, failure analysis by scanning electron microscopy, and synovial histomorphology. *J Orthop Res* 1997;15:1–10.

162. Meakisalo SE, Visuri T, Viljanen A, et al. Reconstruction of the anterior cruciate ligament with carbon fibres: unsatisfactory results after 8 years. *Knee Surg Sports Traumatol Arthrosc* 1996;4:132–136.

163. Demmer P, Fowler M, Marino A. Use of carbon fibers in the reconstruction of knee ligaments. *Clin Orthop Rel Res* 1991;271:225–232.

164. Dandy D, Gray A. Anterior cruciate ligament reconstruction with the Leeds-Deio prosthesis plus extra-articular tenodesis: results after six years. *J Bone Joint Surg Br* 1994;76:193–197.

165. Salvi M, Velluti C, Misasi M, et al. Ultrastructure of periprosthetic Dacron knee ligament tissue: two cases of ruptured anterior cruciate ligament reconstruction. *Acta Orthop Scand* 1991;62:174–177.

166. Olson E, Kang J, Fu F, et al. The biochemical and histological effects of artificial ligament wear particles: *in vitro* and *in vivo* studies. *Am J Sports Med* 1988;16:558–570.

167. Dahlstedt L, Dalaen N, Jonsson U. Gore-Tex prosthetic ligament vs. Kennedy ligament augmentation device in anterior cruciate ligament reconstruction: a prospective randomized 3-year follow-up of 41 cases. *Acta Orthop Scand* 1990;61:217–224.

168. Bolton C, Bruchman W. The Gore-Tex expanded polytetrafluoroethylene prosthetic ligament: an in vitro and in vivo evaluation. *Clin Orthop Rel Res* 1985;196:202–213.

169. Dunn MG, Tria AJ, Kato YP, et al. Anterior cruciate ligament reconstruction using a composite collagenous prosthesis: a biomechanical and histologic study in rabbits. *Am J Sports Med* 1992;20:507–515.

170. Jackson DW, Simon TM, Lowery W, et al. Biologic remodeling after anterior cruciate ligament reconstruction using a collagen matrix derived from demineralized bone: an experimental study in the goat model. *Am J Sports Med* 1996;24:405–414.
171. Dunn MG, Liesch JB, Tiku ML, et al. Development of fibroblast-seeded ligament analogs for ACL reconstruction. *J Biomed Mat Res* 1995;29:1363–1371.
172. Huang D, Chang TR, Aggarwal A, et al. Mechanisms and dynamics of mechanical strengthening in ligament-equivalent fibroblast-populated collagen matrices. *Ann Biomed Eng* 1993;21:289–305.
173. Dunn MG, Avasarala PN, Zawadsky JP. Optimization of extruded collagen fibers for ACL reconstruction. *J Biomed Mat Res* 1993;27:1545–1552.
174. Aglietti P, Buzzi R, D'Andria S, et al. Long-term study of anterior cruciate ligament reconstruction for chronic instability using the central one-third patellar tendon and a lateral extraarticular tenodesis. *Am J Sports Med* 1992;20:38–45.
175. Amiel D, Kleiner JB, Roux RD, et al. The phenomenon of "ligamentization": anterior cruciate ligament reconstruction with autogenous patellar tendon. *J Orthop Res* 1986;4:162–172.

Part B: Anatomic Placement and Fixation

John W. Miles

ANTERIOR CRUCIATE LIGAMENT TUNNEL PLACEMENT AND FIXATION

Tunnel placement is probably the most important factor in successful ACL surgery. Errors in both femoral and tibial tunnel placement have been blamed for limited postoperative knee range of motion, recurrent effusions, pain, graft elongation, and graft failure.

Tunnel placement not only affects the mechanical properties of the graft but also affects the ligamentization process of graft healing (1).

Anatomy

Normal ACL anatomy forms the basis for our surgical attempts at recreating a ligamentously stable knee and therefore has influenced placement of the femoral and tibial tunnels.

Girgis et al. (2) studied the anatomy of the ACL. The ACL fans out anteriorly as it inserts into a wide depressed area in front of and lateral to the medial intercondylar tubercle. It sends a well-marked slip into the anterior horn of the lateral meniscus. The average distance between the anterior border of the superior articular surface of the tibia and the anterior attachment of the ACL is 15 mm and the average A/P length of the tibial attachment is 30 mm (Fig. 21.14). Girgis et al. also noted that the tibial attachment was wider and stronger than the femoral attachment. The tibial insertion is wider than midsubstance and extends anterior to the notch with the knee in extension. The current ACL grafts are essentially cylindric and cannot recreate this anterior flare.

The ACL is attached to the femur and tibia not as a singular cord but as a collection of individual fibers of different lengths that are not parallel. This has led to a simplistic grouping of fibers as two distinct bands, anteromedial and posterolateral bands (2,3). These bands as distinct bundles do not exist (4).

It also appears that different fibers of the ligament become taut as the knee goes through a range of motion (2,3). The ACL also twists on itself in an outward (lateral) spiral. With the knee extended, the bulk of the ligament (posterolateral portion) is tight and the ACL is flat. As the knee is flexed, the ACL twists 90° on itself (Fig. 21.15). A reconstruction cannot duplicate this arrangement. Because of graft impingement, the anterior fibers of the ACL may not be the fibers the surgeon is trying to reproduce, because of graft impingement. In a cadaveric study, Girgis et al. (2) noted that the ACL was semicircular as it originated from the posteromedial aspect of the lateral femoral condyle (Fig. 21.16).

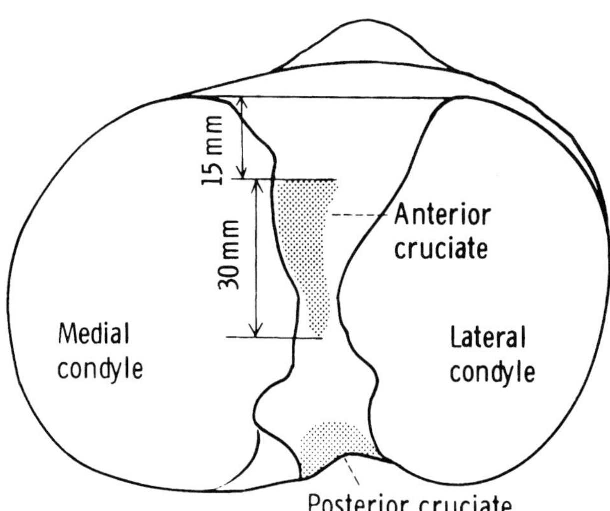

FIGURE 21.14. Anterior cruciate ligament tibial footprint. (From Girgis FG, Marshall JL, Almonajem ARS. The cruciate ligament of the knee joint: anatomical, functional, and experimental analysis. *Clin Orthop* 1975;106:216–231, with permission.)

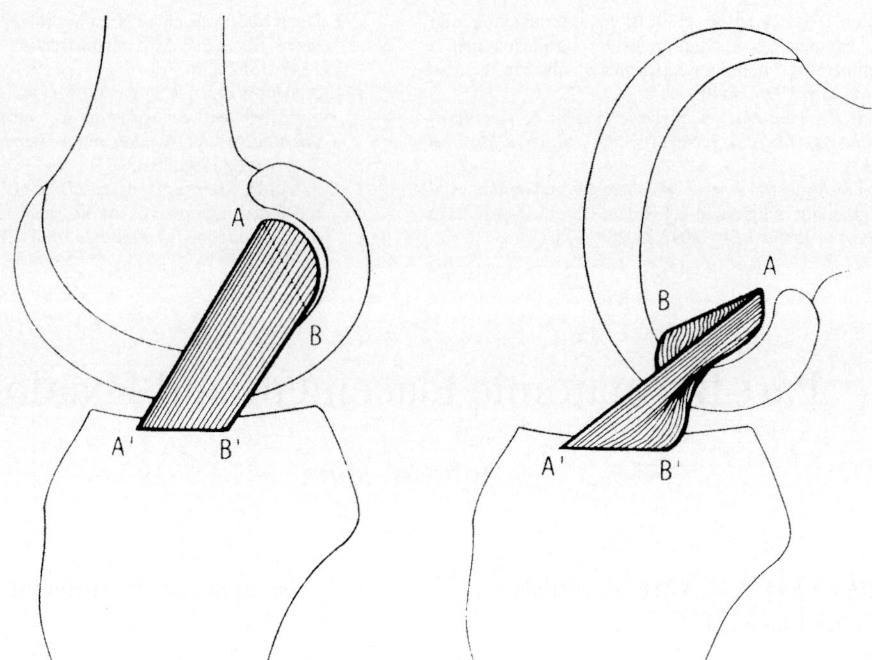

FIGURE 21.15. Schematic drawing representing the changes of the anteromedial and posterolateral portions of the anterior cruciate ligament (ACL) with flexion. (From Girgis FG, Marshall JL, Almonajem ARS. The cruciate ligament of the knee joint: anatomical, functional, and experimental analysis. *Clin Orthop* 1975;106:216–231, with permission.)

Biomechanics

Theoretically, fixation points for an ACL reconstruction should be isometric (i.e., no change in linear separation as the knee is placed through a range of motion). This graft would allow a full range of motion and restoration of nor-mal knee stability. Even in the normal ACL, the existence of truly isometric fibers has been debated (5).

The most ideal or isometric position for a graft based on normal anatomy remains controversial. Studies with different methodologies describe different portions of the ACL as most isometric with anterior, central, or posterior fibers of the ACL having been shown to be most isometric (5–12).

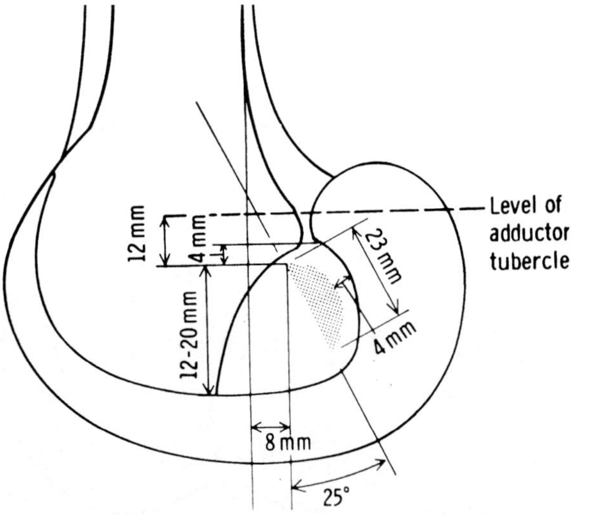

FIGURE 21.16. Drawing of the medial surface of the right lateral femoral condyle showing average measurements and bony relations of the femoral attachment of the anterior cruciate ligament. (From Girgis FG, Marshall JL, Almonajem ARS. The cruciate ligament of the knee joint: anatomical, functional, and experimental analysis. *Clin Orthop* 1975;106: 216–231, with permission.)

Femoral Tunnel

In a widely referenced study, Hefzy et al. (9) demonstrated that altering the femoral attachment of the ACL had a much larger effect than altering the tibial attachment, which helped encourage further evaluation of femoral tunnel placement. In that study, no femoral attachments were completely isometric but there was a zone that was the most isometric as defined by a length change of 2 mm or less. Figure 21.17 shows a contour map for femoral length changes using a central tibial attachment. The shaded areas are those attachments that have a 2 mm or less maximal length change. Line A-A, which runs approximately through the center of the 2-mm region, divides this region into an anterior and posterior portion. The 2-mm zone is wider (i.e., larger) proximally and narrows distally, but along line A-A, there is relative isometry with little change. However, anterior and posterior to this 2-mm zone, small A/P distances lead to much greater length changes as the knee is flexed with points anterior lengthening (i.e., tight in flexion), and points posterior shortening (i.e., lax in flexion).

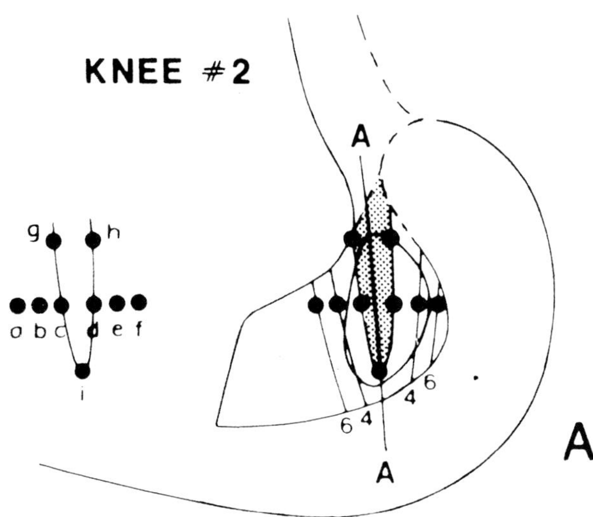

FIGURE 21.17. Contour map line *A-A* is at the center of the 2-mm (isometric) region. By moving to point *A* anteriorly the distance from femur to tibia lengthens by 6 mm as the knee flexes from 0° to 90°. (From Hefzy MS, Grood ES, Noyes FR. Factors affecting the region of most isometric femoral attachments, II: the anterior cruciate ligament. *Am J Sports Med* 1989;17:208–216, with permission.)

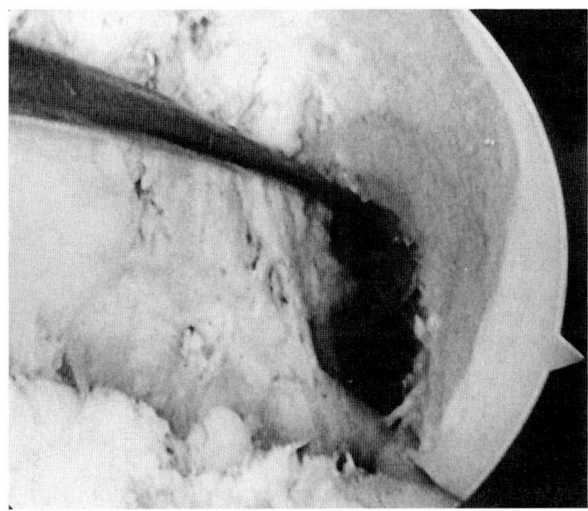

FIGURE 21.18. A probe documents the over-the-top position.

In the past, the most common femoral tunnel error was to place the femoral tunnel too far anteriorly resulting in a graft lax in extension, tight in flexion. This resulted in a knee with limited flexion or if flexion was regained, a nonfunctional graft. Partially as a result of this anterior placement problem, the over-the-top (OTT) position was recommended, which resulted in a graft tight in extension but lax in flexion. The OTT position results in 10 mm of laxity from extension to flexion and, therefore, causes the graft to tighten excessively in knee extension (6).

Femoral Tunnel Technique

Currently, there are three commonly used ways to find the center of the femoral tunnel, which allows placement of a Beath pin or K wire. This location may be selected using direct visualization (freehand), a guide that keys off anatomic landmarks, or a device that measures isometry.

All methods require finding the true OTT position, the most posterior aspect of the intercondylar notch. Once a notchplasty has been performed, this is relatively easy. A shaver is used to remove the proximal portion of the remaining ACL and or fibrous tissue posteriorly. Care is taken not to take a significant amount of bone posteriorly off the femur, because this can change isometry. Clear visualization of the posterior notch is mandatory. There are often small vessels there that require electrocautery. Once clear visualization of the posterior notch has occurred, then a nerve hook can palpate the OTT position superiorly. The nerve hook tip will completely fall behind the notch (Fig. 21.18) in contrast to "residents ridge."

Freehand techniques and the use of an OTT-referenced guide are similar: both pick a specific distance anterior to the OTT position as the entry point for the guidewire. If femoral interference screw fixation is desired, the tunnel site should have 1 to 2 mm of posterior cortex remaining to protect neurovascular structures and provide adequate bone for fixation.

If the surgeon has a 10-mm bone block of patellar–bone–tendon graft, a 10-mm femoral tunnel is selected. A 7-mm offset femoral guide is used; this leaves 2 mm of posterior cortex.

There are many user-friendly femoral guides that use an OTT-referenced system. The "shoe" of the guide slips around the back of the notch with care taken to maintain contact with the posterior cortex with the anterior portion of the shoe (Fig. 21.19).

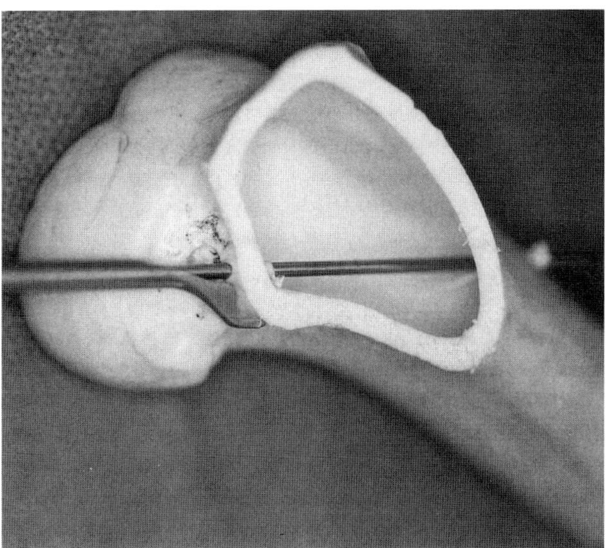

FIGURE 21.19. An over-the-top referenced femoral drill guide.

As described previously, Hefzy et al. (9) noted a larger isometric (2 mm) zone proximally, so most authors are recommending an entry point high in the notch, at the 11- or 1-o'clock position. Because this position puts the K wire and, therefore, the reamer close to the posterior cruciate ligament (PCL), care needs to be taken to not damage the PCL (Fig. 21.20). These guides require use of a more inferior medial portal; however, some guides can be used through the tibial tunnel.

Cooper et al. (13) recently evaluated femoral tunnel placement variables in a cadaveric study. A central tibial tunnel was used. The authors evaluated placing the femoral tunnel at the 12-o'clock (straight up) position or a rotated position at the 10:30- or 1:30-o'clock position. The other variable in the study was in the amount of posterior wall offset using a 5.5- or 7-mm offset guide. A 10-mm femoral tunnel was then reamed. Thus, for the 5.5-mm offset guide, 0.5 mm of posterior wall remained, and for the 7-mm offset guide, 2 mm of posterior wall remained. Therefore, four pin positions were tested with a custom isometer. Excursions of the resulting PT reconstructions were then tested. Isometry was tested and plotted at 15° increments from 0° to 120° of knee flexion. The straight-up, 12-o'clock position using the 7-mm offset guide was the most isometric.

Freehand techniques are similar to that described earlier; however, the surgeon measures the distance with a graduated nerve hook or estimates the distance anterior to the OTT position.

The third commonly used method to find the femoral tunnel involves the use of an isometer. Graf (8) introduced the use of a spring-scale isometer that measures displacement between two points. A small screw or tack is placed at the center of the femoral origin of the ACL after drilling the tibial tunnel. The knee is taken through a range of motion from full extension to the maximum available flexion (usually about 110°) based on patient positioning. An acceptable position is one that allows 1 to 3 mm of elongation (tightening) in the final 20° of extension and 0 to 1 mm of tightening in flexion past 90°. This pattern most closely mimics the native ACL (14).

Based on the known biomechanics of ACL, the tack position can be changed. A commonly used isometer (Acufex, Smith and Nephew Endoscopy, Andover, MA) is described in Figure 21.21. For example, if the tack is moved directly anteriorly, the effect is lengthening of the distance between the tack and the isometer (as the knee is flexed from full extension), which means the graft will tighten in flexion. Some experienced knee surgeons routinely use isometers. Paulos and Rosenberg (14) stated that in their experience, at least 25% of the femoral sites initially selected were changed by the use of an isometer. However, other knee surgeons report no benefit in the routine use of isometers. Barrett et al. (15) compared two groups in which PT ACL reconstructions were performed with the only variable being the use of an isometer. No benefit was found with the use of an isometer.

Sapega et al. (5), in a cadaveric study, noted that in no instance did any portion of the ACL demonstrate truly isometric behavior (a change of 1.0 mm or less). They believed that residual deviation of as much as 3 mm should not be considered nonphysiologic unless it does not follow the shape of the curve of the normal ACL (the shape of the curve of site separation vs. the position of the joint).

Good and Gillquist (16) studied *in vivo* isometer measurements of ACL reconstructions. They found that intraoperative isometry measurements can be used to predict the tension pattern but not the magnitude of that pattern. In other words, a 2-mm deviation from isometry can lead to very different graft tensions in different patients. Fleming et al. (17) evaluated cadaveric specimens with a Kevlar ACL substitute. A spring-scale isometer was used to measure isometry of a selection of femoral and tibial attachment sites. A tensiometer was used to measure tension at different flexion angles. Among other conclusions, the authors reported that "the spring-scale isometer did not accurately predict the tension developed in the ACL substitute during passive range of motion." Colville et al. (18), in a cadaveric study, found that isometry measures do not correlate well with final graft excursion when a bone–PT–bone graft is used. In other words, because of the eccentric nature of a PT autograft, varying graft excursions can be noted depending on where the tendinous portion of the graft is placed in the tunnel.

Morgan et al. (19) compared the current isometers, which have the measuring device at the level of the distal tibial tunnel, to an experimental device measuring isometers proximally at the level of the ACL insertion on the tibia. Significant differences were found between the two methods. The authors report that current isometers do not accurately measure the intraarticular length changes. Johnson et al. (20) report that care must be taken in interpreting isometry data and that clinical judgment and attention to anatomic position of the tunnel is needed.

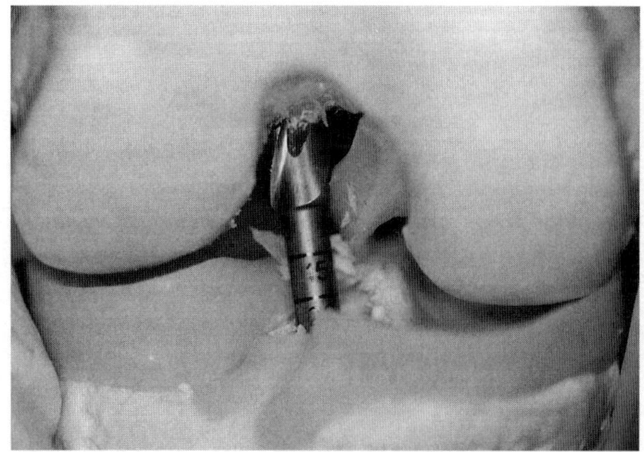

FIGURE 21.20. Care is taken to not damage the posterior cruciate ligament while reaming the femoral tunnel.

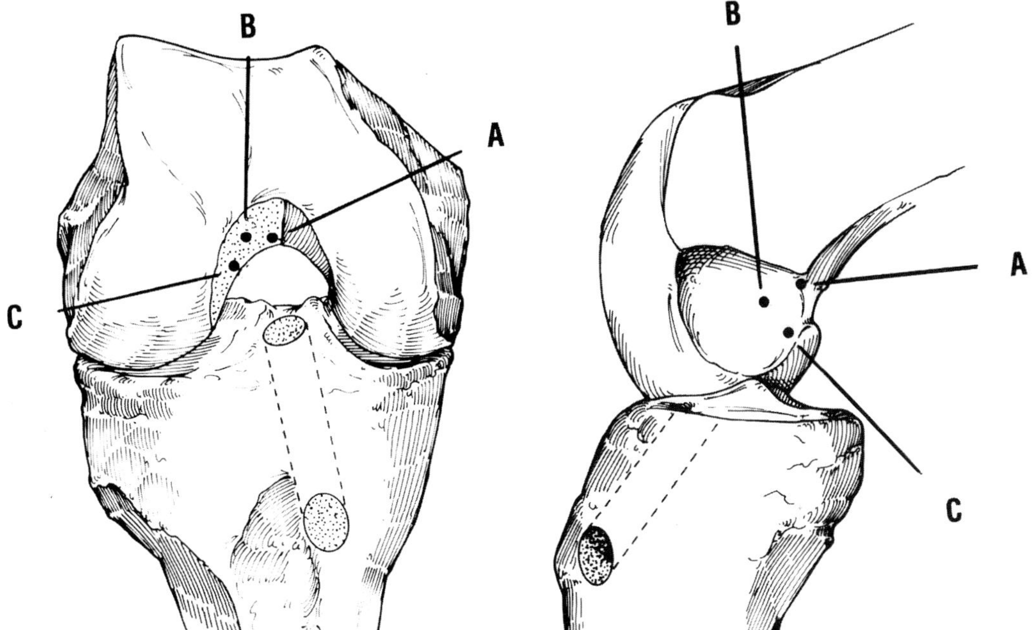

FIGURE 21.21. Point *A* is proximal and high in the notch and typically demonstrates an isometry pattern that mimics normal anterior cruciate ligament. Point *B* is distal (anterior as viewed arthroscopically) and generally demonstrates unacceptable elongation in flexion. Point *C* is lateral and posterior in the notch and generally demonstrates excessive strain in extension. Femoral site behavior will vary slightly depending on the accuracy of the previously selected tibial location. (From Acufex, Smith and Nephew Endoscopy, Andover, MA, with permission.)

A non–spring-scale device, the CA-5000, has been developed. This is a computer-based isometric system that provides a graphic display of relative displacements, according to the angle of flexion. With this device, Fleming et al. (21) noted no significant correlation between isometric measurement and local elongation of the graft measured at the graft mid substance with a Hall-effect transducer.

Graf et al. (22) investigated PT graft abrasion and failure related to diverging tunnels. Their results showed that straight-line tunnels mimicking endoscopic femoral tunnels were significantly less likely to result in a graft failure. Chamfering the tunnels was also found to decrease failure with cyclic loading.

Tibial Tunnel

Over the past decade, femoral graft placement has been emphasized as a source of nonisometric placement. Hefzy et al. (9), as noted earlier, evaluated tibial and femoral attachment sites and noted the greatest effects on isometry by changing the femoral positions. However, smaller changes were noted on the tibial side as well. Moving the tibial insertion point in the A/P plane altered specific geometric variables being measured, altering the location of the most isometric (2-mm zone) femoral zone. Medial lateral changes had a much smaller effect.

Although the tibial side has a smaller effect on isometry, controversy exists regarding placement of the tibial

tunnel. In 1963, Jones (23) described placing a PT graft anteriorly. Many authors describe the anteromedial portion of the ACL as being most isometric (5,8,21,24–26) and an attempt has been made to recreate these fibers. Clancy et al. (24), in an early report of PT ACL reconstructions, recommended placing a Steinman pin 5 mm anterior and medial to the anatomic center of the old stump of the ACL. The reason for the eccentric placement of the tibial tunnel is that when the flat PT is pulled through the tunnel, it will lie posterolaterally in the tunnel, which theoretically places the graft at the anatomic center of the ACL.

O'Brien (25) believed that the most isometric placement of an ACL graft is achieved when the femoral and tibial pivot points are centered on the isometric points for each end of the graft, those being the points "spanning the anterior edge of the ACL." He recommends placing a guidewire at the anterior portion of the ACL anatomic tibial attachment and states that "it is virtually impossible to place the drill hole too far anteriorly as long as the surgeon does not damage the anterior horn attachment of the medial meniscus." O'Brien believed that with this anterior placement, an adequate notchplasty was always necessary. Enlargement of the anterior dimension of the notch by an average of 6.2 mm was necessary.

In 1988, Sidles et al. (12) evaluated potential ligament attachment sites in cadaver knees. These points were digitally recorded and computer-generated isometry maps were generated for both femoral and tibial sites. Posterior tibial insertion sites were "far less isometric than central or anterior sites." Sapega et al. (5) reported that the anteromedial sites were most isometric and should lead the surgeon to recreate these sites.

O'Meara et al. (26), in a study of cadaveric ACL central-third patellar reconstructions, reported that the isometric tibial tunnel should be anterior. The center of the tunnel "lies at the anterior margin of the anatomic attachment of the ACL."

Acker and Drez (6), in a cadaver study using an isometer, found the central anatomic tibial tunnel placement similar to an anterior tibial tunnel placement. However, the posterior tibial tunnel placement was measurably less isometric. Odensten et al. (27) in 1985 in a cadaver study found that the central tibial ACL insertion was isometric and most desirable. Anterior placement was less isometric and posterior placement least isometric.

In a thorough review of the treatment of ACL injuries, Johnson et al. (20) recommended "placement of the graft as closely as possible to the centers of the tibial and femoral attachments of the anterior medial band"; however, anterior graft placement may result in impingement and other problems. The normal ACL has an eccentric anterior flare that cannot be recreated without graft impingement.

Howell et al. (28) evaluated how anterior tibial tunnel placement can result in graft impingement. Estimates were made of how much roofplasty would be needed depending on tibial tunnel placement. The more anterior the tibial tunnel, the more bone would be removed to prevent graft impingement. Howell et al. also showed that it is difficult, if not impossible, to visualize roof impingement as the knee reaches terminal extension.

In 1991, Howell et al. (29) evaluated two sets of patients with HS ACL reconstructions: those that were believed to have impinged grafts and those that were not. The impinged group developed an increased magnetic resonance imaging (MRI) signal in the distal two thirds of the graft. This group also had less knee extension at 1 year and was more likely to have unstable knees.

Howell et al. (30) also studied two groups of PT ACL reconstructions. The roof-impinged group consisted of those knees in which the tibial tunnel was at least partially anterior to the slope of the intercondylar roof on a lateral radiograph of the maximally extended knee, (Fig. 21.22). The unimpinged group differed from the roof-impingement group in that the tibial tunnel was purposely placed more posteriorly on the tibia in the unimpinged group by using a prototype tibial drill guide system. A rigid impingement rod was placed from the tibial tunnel into the notch. A roofplasty was performed until the impingement rod could be freely pistoned with the knee in full extension. No MRI changes were noted in the unimpinged group. However, in the impinged group, by 3 months, the MRI signal increased in the middle and distal portions of the graft. The altered signal did not improve with time. Clinically regaining extension was a problem in the impinged group.

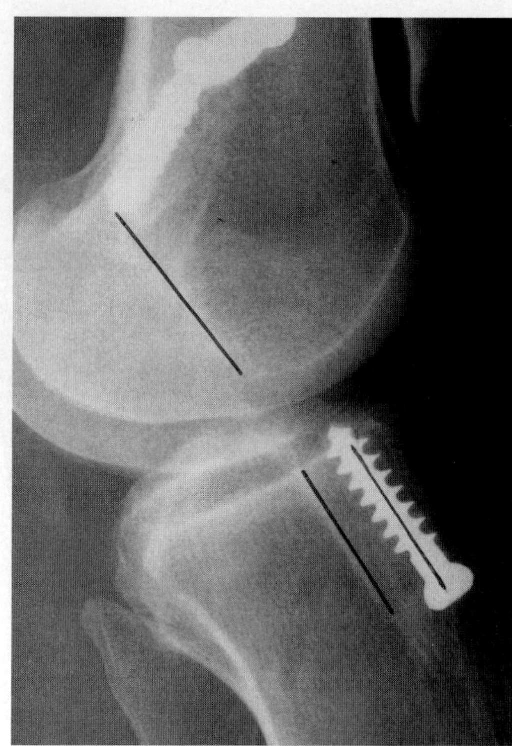

FIGURE 21.22. An impinged graft. Note how most of the tibial tunnel is anterior to the roof with the knee in full extension.

Howell et al. (31) noted poorer results in patients with impinged grafts in terms of extension loss and graft failure. Severity of impingement was again based on radiographic findings from a lateral knee in full extension. In their series severely impinged grafts had a 100% failure rate, the moderate-impingement group had 4 of 14 failures, and the no-impingement group had 3 of 29 failures.

In 1984, Fullerton and Andrews (32) described a calcified nodule as well as a thickened tibial insertion of an ACL reconstruction, which blocked extension. This responded to debridement and additional notchplasty. The authors noted that the tibial graft placement was anterior to the old ACL insertion.

Jackson and Schaefer (33) described a fibrous nodule blocking full extension of ACL-reconstructed knees and described this as a "cyclops" nodule. They report that a component of this problem was related to anterior tibial tunnel placement and inadequate notchplasty.

Marzo et al. (34) described a subgroup of patients with either PT or HS reconstructions that postoperatively demonstrated a clinical syndrome of loss of extension associated with pain at terminal extension, crepitus, and a sensation of a "clunk" near terminal extension. These patients were rearthroscoped and a fibrous nodule in the intercondylar notch was noted. This nodule provided a mechanical block to extension and was responsible for the clunk near extension. Most often, this nodule originated from the anterior portion of the ACL graft and was attached by a pedicle to the tibial insertion site. The authors believed that anterior placement of the graft, particularly on the tibia, contributed to injury to the graft from contact by the intercondylar notch. This injury progressed over time from acute inflammation to disorganized scar formation and eventually to fibrocartilage. This presumably occurs because of the compressive force experienced by the nodule when it is caught between the femur and tibia as the knee is extended. The authors recommended that the tibial tunnel be placed in the posterior one half of the middle third of the tibial ACL insertion.

In a study by Berns and Howell (35), the pressure an ACL graft would be subjected to in full extension by the notch was evaluated as a function of tibial tunnel location. A pressure transducer was used to measure the force transmitted to a graft from the roof in full extension (after a notchplasty). An anterior and a more posterior tunnel were created. The center of the anterior pin was found to lie posteriorly about 25% to 28% from the anterior edge of the tibia. The more posterior pin placement was about 42% posteriorly from the anterior edge of the tibia. Higher roof forces were noted in the anteriorly placed grafts. In addition, the graft contacted the roof (the sensor) much earlier (12.8° of flexion) in the anteriorly placed graft as compared with the more posteriorly placed graft (4.1° of flexion) as the knees were brought in extension.

Romano et al. (36) retrospectively reviewed a group of PT ACL reconstructions to determine if tibial tunnel placement affected final range of motion in the knee. Anterior placement of the tibial tunnel was associated with a loss of both flexion and extension. Although not statistically significant, placement of the tibial tunnel far medially was associated with a trend toward loss of knee flexion.

Mureta et al. (27) evaluated the effects of tibial tunnel placement on a group of quadriceps tendon and HS ACL reconstructions. Radiographic findings were used to evaluate postoperative tunnel position on both A/P and lateral radiographs. Laterally placed tunnels showed a tendency toward less stable knees, more chronic synovitis, and a poorer arthroscopic appearance at the time of relook arthroscopy. One could assume that laterally placed grafts were abraded by the lateral wall of the notch. These authors believed that their results suggested that the tibial drill hole should be positioned around the tip of the medial intercondylar tubercle on the A/P view. The results of Mureta et al. also showed that for anterior placed tibial tunnels, there was a higher incidence of positive Lachman examinations.

In a prospective study, Morgan et al. (37) sought to define constant intra- and extraarticular landmarks for tibial tunnel placement. This tunnel begins 1 cm above the superior margin of the pes anserine insertion and 1.5 cm posteromedial from the medial margin of the tibial tubercle along the superior pes anserine insertion and angles toward the ACL sagittal central insertion point referenced 7 mm anterior to the PCL. This produces a tibial

tunnel parallel with and slightly behind the intercondylar roof in full extension.

Jackson and Gasser (38) described four consistent anatomic landmarks to select the central point of the tunnel: (a) the anterior horn of the lateral meniscus, (b) the medial tibial spine, (c) the PCL, and (d) the ACL stump. They extended an imaginary line from the anterior horn of the lateral meniscus into the stump of the old ACL (Fig. 21.23). This point is consistently located 6 to 7 mm anterior to the anterior border of the PCL, which can be measured with a probe. This tunnel should be in the posterior one half of the ACL footprint. Using their guide system, a 60° tibial angle is selected. By using a calibrated tibial guide system at 55° to 60°, the tibial tunnel will be parallel to the intercondylar roof. They recommended the center of the tunnel medial to lateral be at the base of the midportion of the medial tibial spine.

I use the tibial guide developed by Morgan et al. (37). As described earlier, this is a PCL-referenced ACL guide. The guide pin should be placed so that it nearly touches the PCL (Fig. 21.24), but not so the pin is pushed into the substance of the PCL. The pin should angle toward the normal attachment of the ACL. The guide pin is placed medially in the stump of the old ACL. The tibial tunnel should be placed so that the medial edge of the tunnel is immediately adjacent but does not violate the articular cartilage of the medial tibial plateau.

The ACL graft should contact the lateral aspect of the PCL but should not be significantly deflected around it. A graft placed too laterally will abrade against the wall of the notch. Because this tunnel hugs the PCL, care must be taken in passing the femoral reamer as this can easily damage the PCL.

Morgan et al. (37) believed there was a dynamic interaction between the ACL and PCL, where the PCL may bend around the taut posterior bundle of the ACL in terminal extension, so that this close contact may be important to reproduce.

I use a coring reamer that removes a cylinder of bone to create the tibial tunnel (Figs. 21.25, 21.26). This core of bone is used to make contoured, press-fit, bone grafts for the patellar–tibial tubercle and if necessary, the anterior tibial tunnel bony defects (Fig. 21.27).

The ideal tibial tunnel angle is one that is parallel to the intercondylar roof with the knee in full extension. Based on kinematic principles of a four-bar linkage, Müller (39) noted that the ACL and the intercondylar roof must lie on a line that forms a 40° angle with the long axis of the femur. Good et al. (40) measured this roof angle to be about 35°. If one assumes a femoral intercondylar roof angle of 35°, the tibial guide needs to be set at 55° to the long axis of the tibia to make the tibial tunnel parallel (Fig. 21.28). Most of the current ACL guides can be adjusted, and usually a tibial tunnel angle of about 55° to 60° is fine (Fig. 21.29).

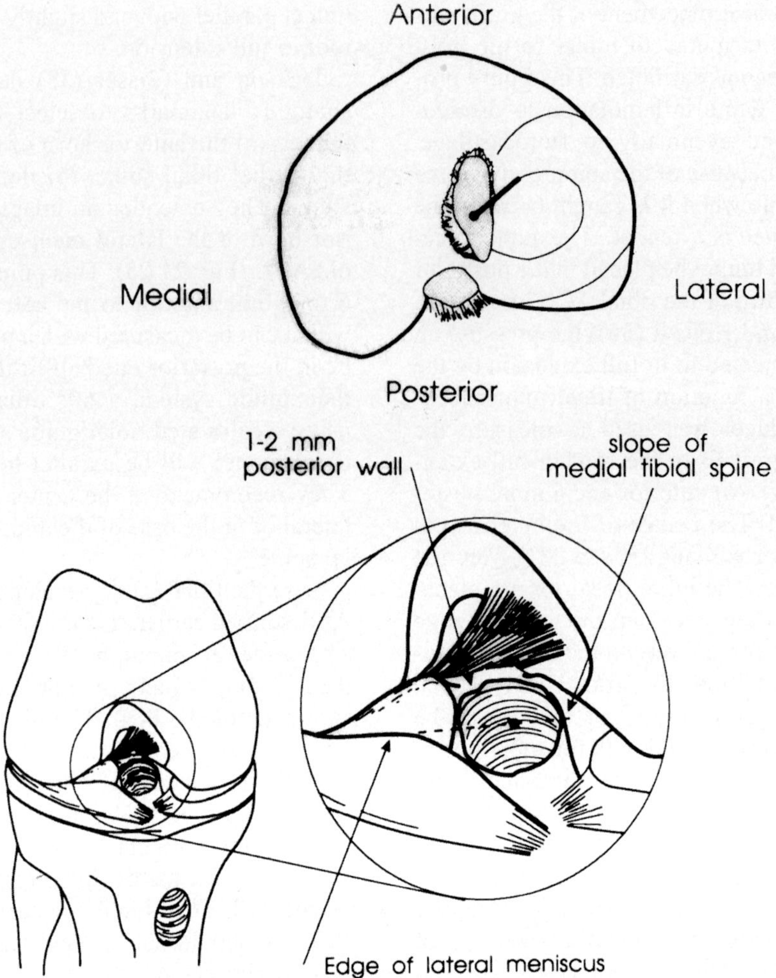

FIGURE 21.23. The anteroposterior center of the tibial tunnel is selected by continuing a line along the inner border of the anterior horn of the lateral meniscus. (From Jackson DW, Gasser SI. Tibial tunnel placement in ACL reconstruction. *Arthroscopy* 1994;10:124–131, with permission.)

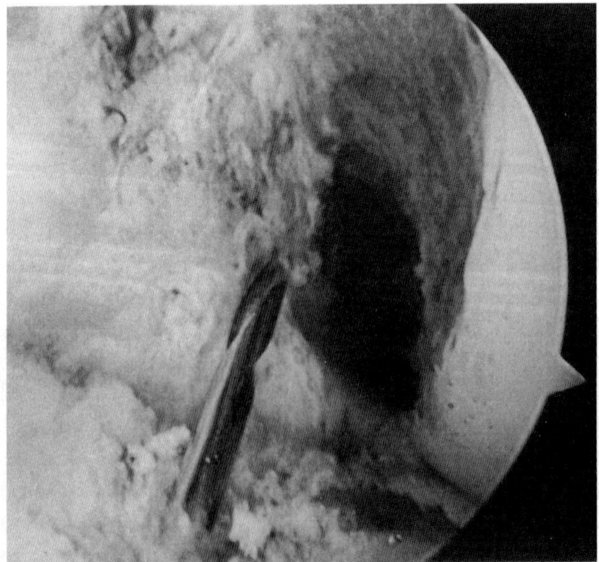

FIGURE 21.24. The tibial guidepin should be closely approximated to the posterior cruciate ligament and medial in the old stump of the anterior cruciate ligament.

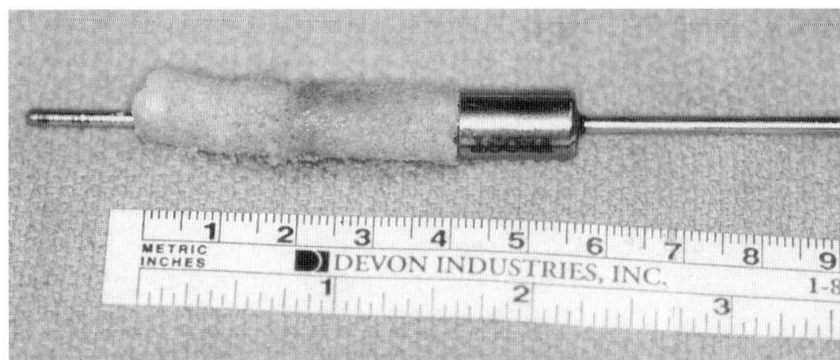

FIGURE 21.25. A core of bone from the coring reamer.

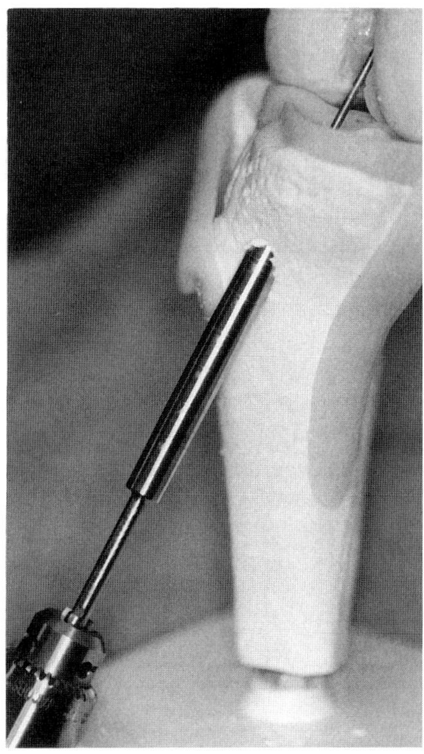

FIGURE 21.26. A coring reamer can be used to drill the tibial tunnel.

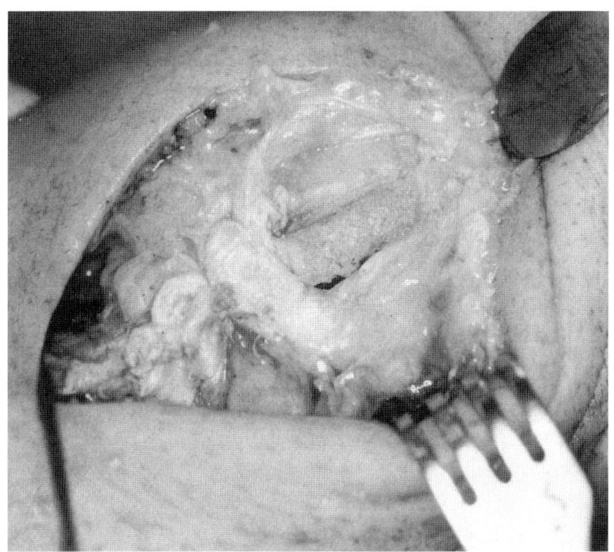

FIGURE 21.27. Bone grafting the patellar defect.

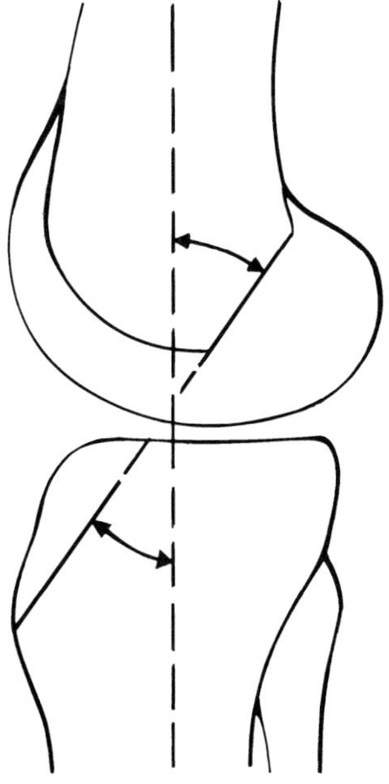

FIGURE 21.28. A roof angle of 35°. To have the tibial tunnel parallel to the roof, a 55° tibial angle is needed.

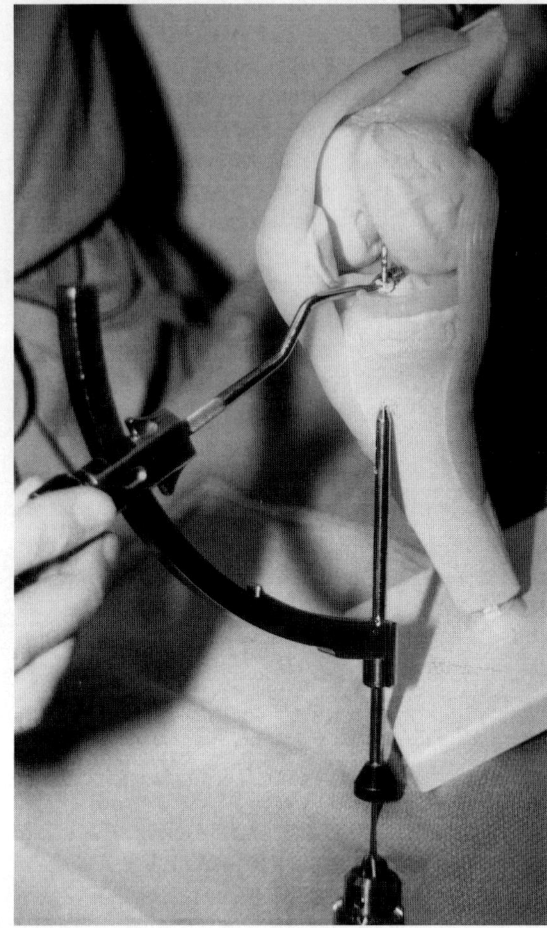

FIGURE 21.29. The adjustable tibial guide should be set at about 55° to 60° to make the tibial tunnel colinear with the femoral notch.

Tibial tunnel length is less important when using two incision techniques. However, when performing endoscopic PT reconstructions, tibial tunnel length becomes more critical. Appropriate tunnel length avoids prominence of the distal bone plug, which can complicate fixation. If the tunnel is too short, the bone plug will protrude and compromise the interference screw fixation. If the tibial tunnel is too long, you may have trouble seeing the tibial bone plug, but that is much less of a problem. Tibial tunnel length is usually slightly shorter and less critical when using HS tendons. There are different methods for calculating tibial tunnel length. I have used a technique, similar to one described by Jackson and Kurzweil, that is simple and easy to use (Fig. 21.30).

I do not currently use an isometer. However, I do test isometry in a basic way. I fix the femoral side and cycle the knee. A gloved finger placed at the tibial tunnel distally estimates any movement of the no. 5 Ethibond and/or the tibial bone plug. Usually, a small tug in the last 15° of terminal knee extension is noted, estimated at less than or equal to 2 mm. If there is more tightening of the graft in terminal extension, then my first thought is roof impingement (especially posterior roof impingement) near terminal extension, which is difficult if not impossible to see. It is possible to remove more bone from the roof without damaging the graft. Also, using a hooded shaver, I will do additional chamfering of the posterior roof, which forms the anterior portion of the femoral tunnel. This usually eliminates the excessive tightening in extension. Another option is to use one of the newer guide systems that use smooth, rigid, cylindric sounds to ascertain if any posterior roof impingement exists prior to passing the graft.

FIXATION

Solid fixation in ACL reconstructions has been the weak link in the postoperative period, which has affected our ability to rehabilitate patients early. Several studies have examined the histology or biomechanics of soft-tissue–healing bone tunnels. VanRens et al. (41) reported on the histologic changes in the bone tunnels of an iliotibial band ACL replacement in a dog model. By 4 weeks, collagen fibers resembling Sharpey's fibers were noted at the interface. At 10 weeks, a tide line marking the border between bone and the graft was seen. This tide line marks the transition between the ligamentous tissue of the normal ACL and bone. By 12 weeks, distinct Sharpey's fibers were noted to continue from the bone into the ligamentous tissue.

Holden et al. (42) investigated fascia lata autografts used to replace the ACL in goats. The mechanical properties were measured at 0, 2, 4, and 8 weeks after surgery. At 0 weeks, failure was related to the types of fixation used. Failure shifted toward graft substance tears at 2, 4, and 8 weeks after surgery with all tears intrasubstance by 8 weeks.

Rodeo et al. (43) evaluated tendon-to-bone healing in a dog model. At 2 weeks, histologically the interface between tendon and bone was composed of vascular, highly cellular fibrous tissue. This layer progressively matured and reorganized, and by 26 weeks continuity between collagen fibers of the tendon and the surrounding bone throughout the length of the tunnel were evident. In this same study, all the 2-, 4-, and 8-week specimens failed biomechanical pullout studies by the tendon pulling out of the bone. All the 12- and 26-week specimens failed by pullout from the clamp or intrasubstance failure. Grana et al. (44), in a rabbit model, noted a faster time course for maturation of the interface between a bone tunnel and a semitendinosus ACL reconstruction. At 2 weeks, all specimens failed biomechanically by the graft pulling out of the femoral tunnel. Grafts tested in the ensuing weeks all failed intrasubstance. Fixation methods can be divided into two basic groups: bone-to-bone and soft tissue to bone.

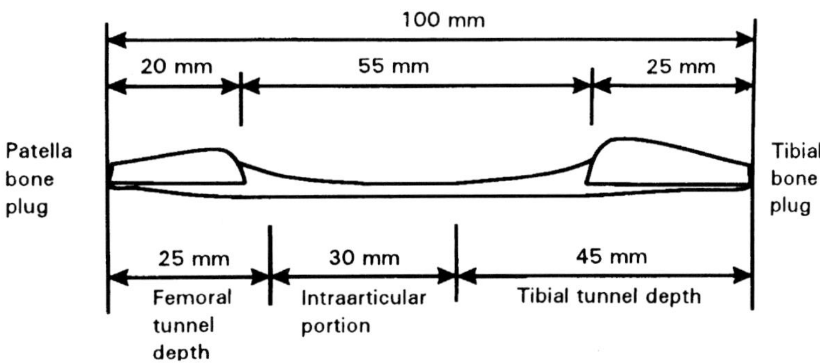

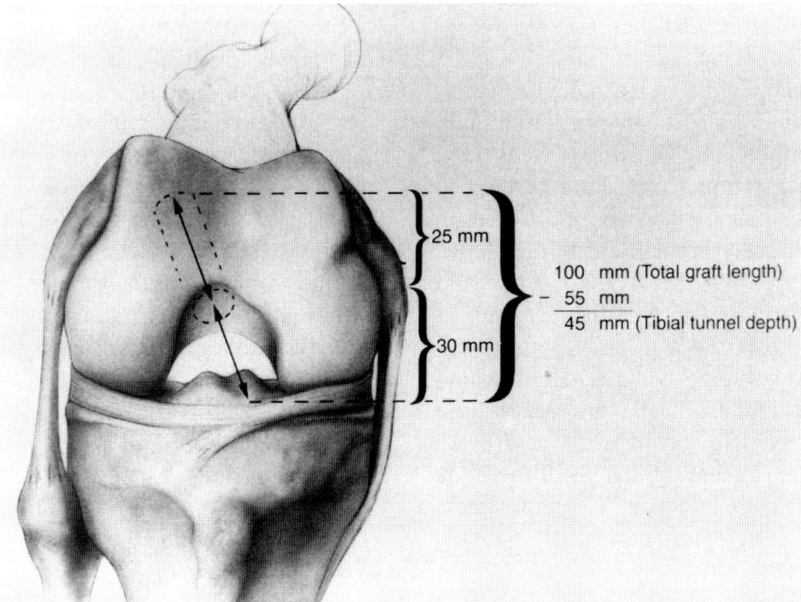

FIGURE 21.30. The calculation of tibial tunnel length. A typical graft has bone plugs of 20 mm and 25 mm, and is 100 mm in length. Assuming a femoral tunnel of 25 mm and an intraarticular distance of 30 mm (the average length of an anterior cruciate ligament), the tibial tunnel must be at least 45 mm in length to accommodate the graft. An additional 5 mm should be added to the calculated length, because drilling a 10- or 11-mm-diameter tibial tunnel effectively shortens the tunnel length by its radius. (From Jackson DW, Kurzweil PR. Anterior cruciate ligament reconstruction. In: Jackson DW, ed. *Master techniques in orthopedic surgery, reconstructive knee surgery.* New York: Raven Press, 1995, with permission.)

Bone-to-Bone Fixation

Lambert (45), in 1983, described interference fixation of a bone–PT–bone ACL graft with a 6.5 mm diameter AO screw. This was refined by Kurosaka et al. (46) in 1987 who described a custom-designed 9.0 screw that substantially increased fixation compared with the 65 AO screw (160 N vs. 436 N pullout strength). They also compared fixing the PT with sutures over buttons (186 N). All graft failures occurred at the fixation site.

Kohn and Rose (47) evaluated the effect of screw size (7- vs. 9-mm Kurosaka screw) and insertion torque on bone–PT fixation. They concluded that a 9-mm screw provided stronger fixation compared with a 7-mm screw in a 10-mm-diameter tunnel. These authors noted that tibial fixation was weaker compared

with femoral fixation and did not recommend 7-mm screws on the tibial side. They also noted that if a 7-mm screw does not provide rigid fixation and the bone plug slips, it can be replaced effectively with a 9-mm screw. The maximum tensile force at failure for 9-mm screws was 727 N on the femoral side and 678 N on the tibial side.

Brown et al. (48) found that the pullout strength of a PT ACL graft placed endoscopically with a 7-mm screw had nearly the strength of a 9-mm screw placed using a two-incision technique (814 vs. 933 N).

In a bovine model, Hulstyn et al. (49) tested fixation strengths of bone–PT reconstructions fixed with different sized screws (5.5, 7.0, and 9.0 mm) in a 10-mm tunnel. The biomechanical parameters were similar for 7- and 9-mm screws. For the 7- and 9-mm screws, there was little difference between 20- and 30-mm length screws.

The effect of bone plug length and Kurosaka screw diameter (7 mm vs. 9 mm) on graft holding strength of cadaver bone–tendon–bone ACL reconstructions was evaluated by Pomeroy et al. (50). Bone plugs of 0.5 cm demonstrated much less pullout strength than 1- or 2-cm bone plugs. Superior pullout strengths for 9-mm screws versus 7-mm screws were also noted.

Matthews et al. (51) evaluated bone–PT–bone fixation in a cadaveric model. They compared a 9×25 Kurosaka interference screw with bone plugs secured using sutures around a screw and post. These two techniques were comparable in terms of failure strength.

Paschal et al. (52) compared biomechanical parameters of two fixation techniques of bone–patellar–tendon autografts in a porcine model. The bone plugs were fixed in tunnels with either a 9-mm Kurosaka interference screw or screw-and-post fixation. Two no. 5 Ticron sutures were passed separately through 2-mm drill holes in the bone block and tied over an AO 6.5 screw and washer. Maximum pullout strength and displacement of the bone graft were compared in a progressive load-to-failure test. Interference screw fixation demonstrated statistically significant higher mean ultimate failure loads at 535 N compared with postfixation at 309 N. There was also less displacement (slippage) of the bone plugs in the tunnels at 110 N of force, 0.32 mm (interference screw) versus 2.21 mm (screw and post). All failures occurred at the fixation site.

Jomha et al. (53), in a pig model, evaluated Kurosaka screw fixation of bone–patellar–tendon ACL reconstructions. These authors realized that potential graft failure may be related to graft–screw divergence. Screws were placed at 0, 10, 20, and 30 degrees of divergence. The pullout strength diminished with increasing divergence (621 N at 0°, 594 N at 10°, 508 N at 20°, 485 N at 30°).

Fanelli et al. (54) retrospectively reviewed 97 patients with an endoscopically performed ACL reconstruction. Based on random differences in surgical technique, one group's postoperative radiographs revealed femoral screw divergence and another group's did not. The authors found no short-term differences in graft failures.

An advantage of interference screw fixation is graft fixation within the bone tunnel closer to the tunnel's articular aperture, thus shortening the length of the graft between the two points of fixation. This was shown in a study of porcine cadaver knees that were "reconstructed" with a bone–PT–bone ACL reconstruction (55). The graft was fixed in one of three positions: the "outside" position (the graft fixed outside the tibial tunnel), the "central" position (the graft fixed at the central point of the tibial tunnel), and the "anatomic" position (the graft fixed at the ACL insertion site). These three reconstructions were compared with the translation of the porcine knee prior to removal of the normal ACL. The level of fixation was statistically significant, with results diminishing as fixation moved away from the joint.

Soft-Tissue Fixation

HS ACL grafts have been used extensively but there has been concern about soft-tissue fixation. Robertson et al. (56) evaluated several options (suture, staple, and two different types of screw and washer or soft-tissue plate). The screw with a washer or soft-tissue plate provided fixation strength between 180 and 238 N.

Steiner et al. (57) in a cadaveric study of ACL fixation techniques, evaluated four fixation techniques for HS reconstructions and four fixation techniques for PT reconstructions compared with the tensile properties of the normal ACL. The strongest fixation technique of both groups was an HS (four-stranded gracilis, semitendinosus) fixed proximally with two screws in a figure-eight pattern and distally with sutures over a screw and post. The PT interference screw fixation supplemented by sutures with a screw and post was a relatively close second. The fixation strength of the groups varied significantly.

Rowden et al. (58) compared interference fixation in a bone–PT–bone reconstruction with a four-stranded HS technique with an endo button proximally and a suture and post distally. One endo button was used for each graft, one for the semitendinosus, one for the gracilis. The HS construct demonstrated failure at 612 versus 416 N for the PT group.

Simonian et al. (59) recently evaluated four-stranded HS fixation with a 9×25-mm bioabsorbable interference screw. To eliminate variations in cadaver bone, a uniform polyurethane foam was used. They compared central screw placement (screw in the middle of the four strands) with eccentric placement. There were no significant differences between pullout strength or graft slippage. All failures occurred at the fixation site. No tendons were cut by the screw in either group. The maximum pullout strength was around 250 N; however, graft slippage (which occurred prior to failure) occurred at much lower loads. For example, 5 mm of graft slippage occurred at between 140 and 160 N.

Pinczewski et al. (60) reported on 2-year follow-up of four-stranded HS ACL endoscopic reconstructions using an interference RCI screw (Smith and Nephew, Carlsbad, CA), 97% of patients had a grade 0 to1 Lachman; 83% of patients had less than 3-mm KT-1000 side-to-side differences.

Recently, there has been increased interest in biodegradable interference screws. Weiler et al. (61) evaluated pullout strengths of bone–tendon–bone interference fixation in calf tibias fixed with six different screws composed of different polymers. All but one of the screws were similar to conventional titanium interference screws in terms of pullout strength.

Weiler et al. (62) compared pullout strengths of a bioabsorbable screw with a round-headed titanium RCI screw for interference fixation of cadaver HSs in bovine tibia. The bioabsorbable screw demonstrated increased pullout strength of 507 N as compared with 419 N for the titanium screw. However, Caborn et al. (63) found no significant differences between an RCI and a bioabsorbable screw for HS fixation.

Another recent option for HS femoral fixation is that of a rigid crosspin at a right angle to the femoral tunnel. The HS tendons loop around this pin or screw in the femoral tunnel. Clark et al. (64) recently reported on the fixation strength of this device in porcine bone and clinical followup on 22 human patients using this fixation for HS ACL reconstructions. The animal fixation strengths ranged from 725 N (35-mm length screw) to 1600 N (70-mm length screw). The clinical results were good with only one late traumatic failure; 18 of the 22 patients had KT-1000 values of less than 3-mm side-to-side differences.

POSTERIOR CRUCIATE LIGAMENT TUNNEL PLACEMENT

The PCL is the primary restraint to posterior translation of the tibia (65). The PCL is narrowest in its midsection (about 13 mm) and fans out superiorly and, to a lesser extent, inferiorly. The width of the femoral origin is broad—approximately 32 mm in an A/P direction. The insertion of the PCL is in a depression on the posterior tibia about 1 cm below the tibia surface (2,66).

The PCL has been divided into a thick anterolateral portion and a smaller posteromedial portion. These portions are inseparable. The anterolateral component is tight in flexion and relatively lax in extension. The posteromedial component is tight in extension and relatively lax in flexion (2) (Fig. 21.31).

Race and Andrew (67) found the anterolateral portion to be four times as large and six times stronger than the posterior portion.

Isometry

In a cadaver study, Grood et al. (68) found the tibial PCL insertion to be much less critical than the femoral origin. No femoral point was totally isometric, although they were able to find a more isometric position, a length change of 2 mm or less with flexion of 0° to 90° (Fig. 21.32). Significant length change occurred as one moved away from this zone. The authors noted that this region averaged 11 mm back from the trochlear articular cartilage. Also, this region extended approximately 1 cm from the roof.

Ogata et al. (69), in another cadaveric study, evaluated changes in length and tension with different femoral posi-

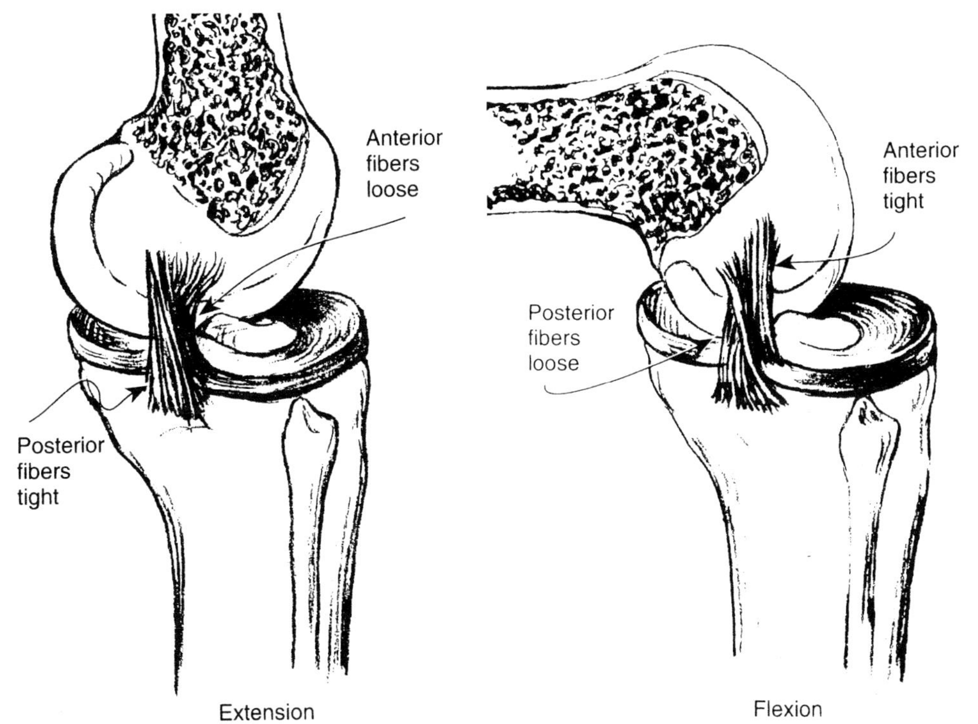

FIGURE 21.31. The two portions of the posterior cruciate ligament. **A:** The smaller posteromedial portion is tight in extension. **B:** The larger anterolateral portion is tight in flexion. (From Miller MD, Harner CD, Koshiwaguchi S. Acute posterior cruciate ligament injuries. In: Fu F, ed. *Knee surgery.* Baltimore, MD: Williams & Wilkins, 1994, with permission.)

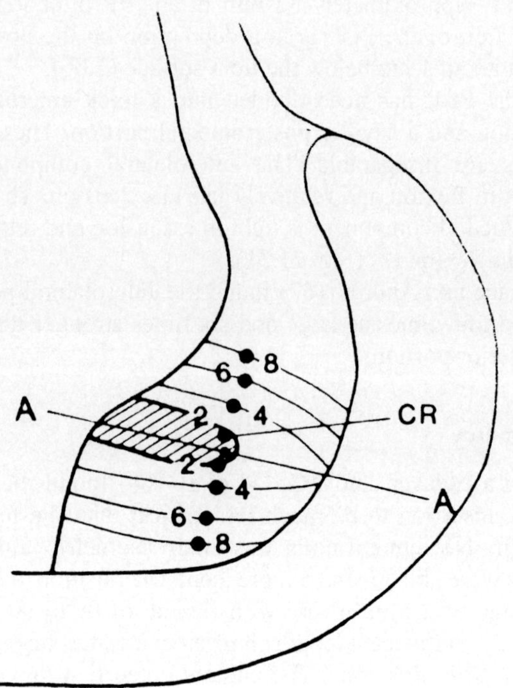

FIGURE 21.32. Line *A-A* represents the most isometric line and is at the center of the 2 mm (most isometric) region. As you move proximal to this area, the tibiofemoral distances became shorter (i.e., a graft would become looser) as the knee is flexed from 0° to 90°. As you move distal (toward the articular cartilage), the tibiofemoral distance became longer (i.e., a graft would tighten) as the knee is flexed from 0° to 90°. (From Race A, Andrew AA. The biomechanical properties of the two bundles of human posterior cruciate ligament. *J Biomech* 1994;27:13–24, with permission.)

tions and a central tibial position. The authors stated that "the fibers attaching to the relatively isometric positions D and E are located within the anterior segment of the posterior fibers of the PCL," (Figs. 21.33, 21.34). They recommended a trial bone tunnel of small diameter be aimed 10 mm proximal (posterior) to the articular edge of the medial femoral condyle at the 10-o'clock position (left knee). Isometry can then be performed and the tunnel can be shifted either toward or away from the articular cartilage. Some authors favor reconstruction of the more isometric fibers of the PCL, others recommend reconstructing the large anterocentral fibers of the PCL that become taut in flexion and will resist posterior tibial translation of a flexed knee.

In a biomechanical study on fresh cadaver knees, Bomberg et al. (70) found that isometric graft placement resulted in a less-satisfactory reconstruction than when the femoral tunnel was located slightly anterior to the center of the femoral PCL attachment zone.

Tibial tunnel placement is not as critical as femoral placement yet is clearly important. Probably placing the tibial tunnel within the main portion of the PCL insertion is adequate.

Tunnel Placement

Drilling and preparing the tibial tunnel is probably the most difficult aspect of PCL reconstructions; however, specific guide systems are available. Thorough, careful

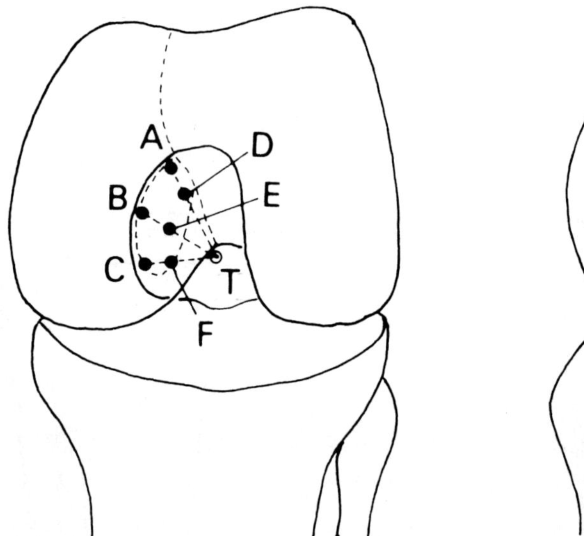
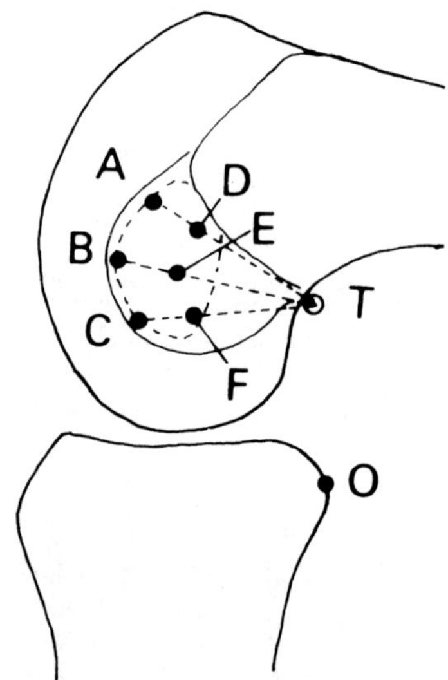

FIGURE 21.33. Anterior and lateral views of the six different posterior cruciate ligament (PCL) femoral attachment sites. Sites *A*, *B*, and *C* were at the very anterior portion of the PCL. Sites *D*, *E*, and *F* were located one third of the distance from each anterior site (*ABC*) to *T*, the most proximal (posterior) portion of the intercondylar notch. Point *O* was a common tibial PCL insertion. (From Grood ES, Hefzy MS, Lindenfield TN. Factors affecting the region of most isometric femoral attachments, II: the posterior cruciate ligament. *Am J Sports Med* 1989;17:197–207, with permission.)

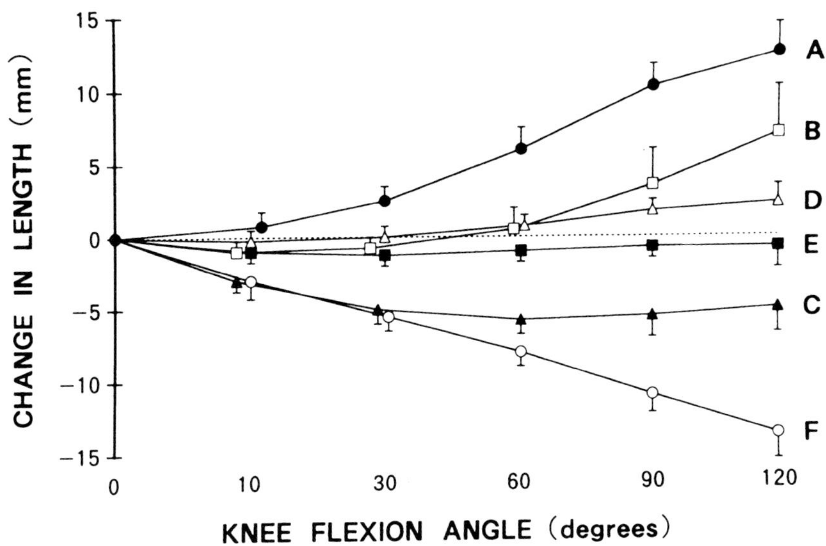

FIGURE 21.34. Changes in length with knee flexion of each point (*A, B, C, D, E, F*). Note that *D* and *E* are nearly isometric. (From Grood ES, Hefzy MS, Lindenfield TN. Factors affecting the region of most isometric femoral attachments, II: the posterior cruciate ligament. *Am J Sports Med* 1989;17:197–207, with permission.)

debridement of the PCL stump is needed. A 70° arthroscope and/or an accessory medial portal may be necessary.

Some practice with the guide is necessary because the guide needs to be placed well around the proximal portion of the posterior tibia. With the tibial guide, the tibial tunnel should be started slightly inferior to the tibial tubercle. Placement of the starting hole too inferior could result in breaking out of the posterior cortex. Placement too superior causes a very acute angle on the graft, which may abrade the graft or make graft passage more difficult (Fig. 21.35). The guide should be placed laterally in the tibial stump of the old PCL.

After the tibial tunnel is completed, the femoral tunnel is drilled. Most techniques use a single tunnel for autograft or allograft tissue; however, a two–femoral-tunnel technique has been described by Paulos using two HS tendons. For a single femoral tunnel an arthroscopic drill guide (Acufex) is placed through the medial portal. The entry point of the pin medially is about halfway between the medial femoral epicondyle and the articular margin of the medial femoral condyle (Fig. 21.36). The entry point of the guidewire is high in the notch, about 1:00 o'clock (right knee) or 11:00 o'clock (left knee). As discussed earlier there is a debate as to whether to recreate the more isometric portion of PCL (this moves the tunnel further back in the notch, i.e., proximal) or to place the graft closer to the articular margin. This placement causes the graft to tighten in flexion, reproducing posterior stability at 90° of knee flexion. Most authors will place the guide pin slightly anterior, about 10 to 12 mm from the articular margin. As noted previously, Bomberg et al. (70) found that femoral tunnels located slightly anteriorly to the femoral isometric point produced the most normal stain pattern. The tunnel can then be drilled to the size of the graft with a cannulated reamer. If you are using an allograft with a bone block (e.g., Achilles), then a nice option is to press-fit the femoral side. The bone block is tapered

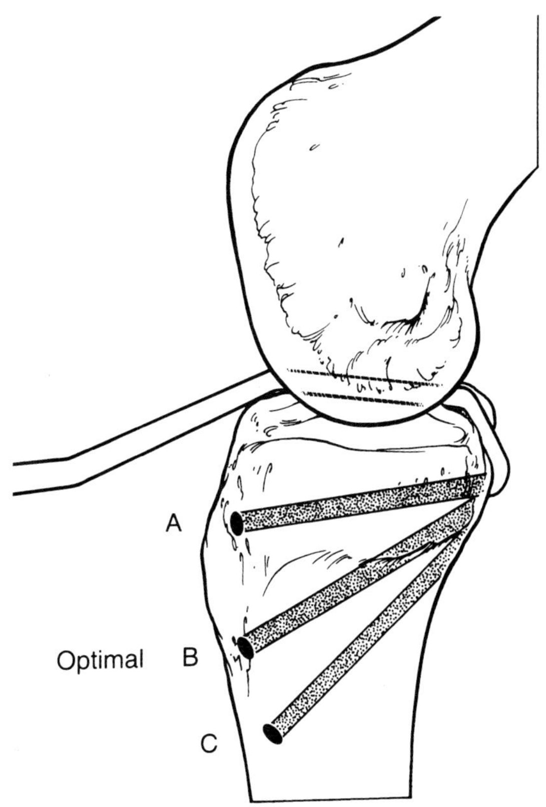

FIGURE 21.35. Entry point *B* is optimal. Point *A* will form a tunnel, which puts excessive stress on the graft posteriorly as it forms a sharp exit angle. Tunnel *C* is too inferior and can cause posterior wall blowout. (From Bullis DW, Fenton PJ, Paulos LE. Arthroscopic reconstruction of the posterior cruciate ligament. In: McGinty JB, ed. *Operative arthroscopy.* Philadelphia: Lippincott–Raven, 1996, with permission.)

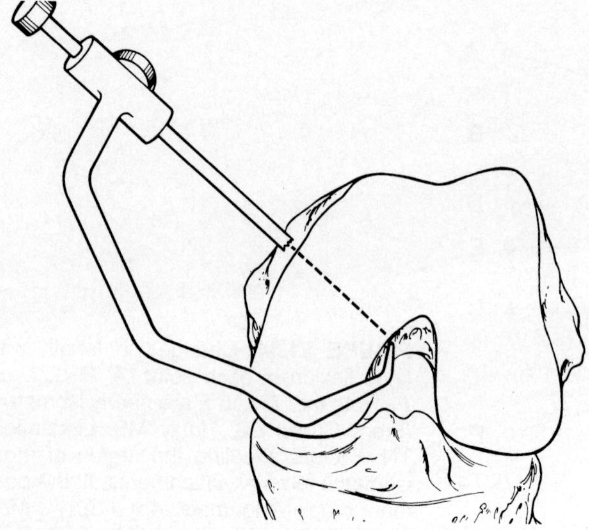

FIGURE 21.36. Posterior cruciate ligament femoral guide placement. (From Bullis DW, Fenton PJ, Paulos LE. Arthroscopic reconstruction of the posterior cruciate ligament. In: McGinty JB, ed. *Operative arthroscopy.* Philadelphia: Lippincott–Raven, 1996, with permission.)

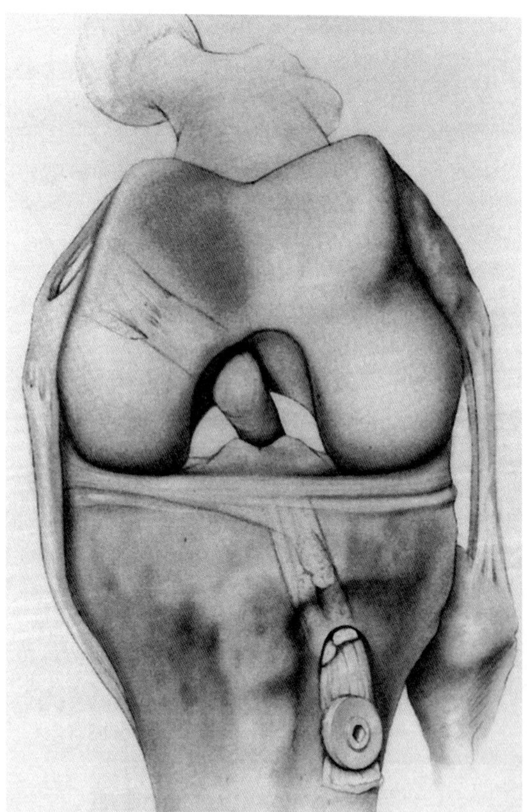

FIGURE 21.37. Completed Achilles tendon allograft posterior cruciate ligament reconstruction. (From Mooney MF, Paulos LE. Arthroscope assisted posterior cruciate ligament repair/reconstruction. In: Jackson DW, ed. *Master techniques in orthopedic surgery, reconstructive knee surgery.* New York: Raven Press, 1995, with permission.)

into a trapezoidal shape. The tunnel is drilled in two stages. The first drill corresponds to the tendinous portion of the graft, usually around 11 or 12 mm, and this is drilled the full length of the tunnel. The second drill corresponds to the midsection of the trapezoidal bone block (usually around 14 mm) and the reaming stops about 15 mm short of the notch. The bone block is wedged in as the graft is pulled into position (Fig. 21.37), but an interference screw can also be added if needed. As with the ACL tunnels the PCL tunnels need to be chamfered, particulately the posterior portion of the femoral tunnel.

REFERENCES

1. Amiel D, Ing D, Kleiner JB, et al. The natural history of the anterior cruciate ligament autograft of patellar tendon origin. *Am J Sports Med* 1986;14:449–462.
2. Girgis FG, Marshall JL, Almonajem ARS. The cruciate ligament of the knee joint: anatomical, functional, and experimental analysis. *Clin Ortho* 1975;106:216–231.
3. Furman W, Marshall JL, Girgis FG. The anterior cruciate ligament: a functional analysis based on postmortem studies. *J Bone Joint Surg Am* 1976;58:179–185.
4. Clark JM, Slides JA. The interrelation of fiber bundles in the anterior cruciate ligament. *J Orthop Res* 1990;8:180–188.
5. Sapega AA, Moyer RA, Schneck C, et al. Testing for isometry during reconstruction of the anterior cruciate ligament: anatomical and biomechanical considerations. *J Bone Joint Surg Am* 1990;72:259–267.
6. Acker JH, Drez D. Analysis of isometric placement of grafts in ACL reconstruction procedures. *Am J Knee Surg* 1989;2:65–70.
7. Bylski-Austrow DI, Grood ES, Hefzy MS, et al. Anterior cruciate ligament replacements: a mechanical study of femoral attachment location, flexion angle at tension g and initial tension. *J Ortho Res* 1990;8:522–531.
8. Graf B. Isometric placement of substitutes for the anterior cruciate ligament. In: Jackson DW, Drez D, eds. *The anterior cruciate deficient knee.* St. Louis: CV Mosby, 1987:102–113.
9. Hefzy MS, Grood ES, Noyes FR. Factors affecting the region of most isometric femoral attachments, II: the anterior cruciate ligament. *Am J Sports Med* 1989;17:208–216.
10. Melhorn JM, Henning CE. The relationship of the femoral attachment site to the isometric tracking of the anterior cruciate ligament graft. *Am J Sports Med* 1987;15:539–542.
11. Odenstein M, Gillquist J. Functional anatomy of the anterior cruciate ligament and a rational for reconstruction. *J Bone Joint Surg Am* 1985;67:257–261.
12. Sidles JA, Larson RV, Garbini JL, et al. Ligament length relationships in the moving knee. *J Ortho Res* 1980;6:593–610.
13. Cooper DE, Urrea L, Small J. Factors affecting isometry of endoscopic anterior cruciate ligament reconstruction: the effect of guide offset and rotation. *Arthroscopy* 1998;14:164–170.
14. Beck CL, Paulos LE, Rosenburg TD. Anterior cruciate ligament reconstruction with the endoscopic technique. *Op Tech Ortho* 1992;2:86–98.
15. Barrett GR, Treacy SH. The effect of intraoperative isometric measurement on the outcome of anterior cruciate ligament reconstruction: a clinical analysis. *Arthroscopy* 1996;12:645–651.
16. Good L, Gillquist J. The value of intraoperative isometry measurements in anterior cruciate ligament reconstruction: an *in vivo* correlation between substitute tension and length change. *J Arthro Rel Surg* 1993;9:525–532.
17. Fleming BC, Beynnon BD, Johnson RJ, et al. Isometric versus tension measurements: a comparison for the reconstruction of the anterior cruciate ligament. *Am J Sports Med* 1993;21:82–88.
18. Colville MR, Bowman RR. The significance of isometer measurements and graft position during anterior cruciate ligament reconstruction. *Am J Sports Med* 1993;21:832–835.
19. Morgan CD, Kalman VR, Grawl DM. Isometry testing for anterior cruciate ligament reconstruction revisited. *Arthroscopy* 1995;11:647–659.
20. Johnson RJ, Beynon BD, Nichols CE, et al. Current concepts review:

the treatment of injuries of the anterior cruciate ligament. *J Bone Joint Surg Am* 1992;74:140–151.

21. Fleming BC, Beynon BD, Nichols CE, et al. An *in vivo* comparison between intraoperative isometric measurements and local elongation of the graft after reconstruction of the anterior cruciate ligament. *J Bone Joint Surg Am* 1994;76:511–519.

22. Graf BK, Herry J, Rothenberg M, et al. Anterior cruciate ligament reconstruction with patellar tendon: an ex vivo study of wear related damage and failure at the femoral tunnel. *Am J Sports Med* 1994;22:131–135.

23. Jones KG. Reconstruction of the anterior cruciate ligament: a technique using the central one-third of the patellar ligament. *J Bone Joint Surg Am* 1963;45:925.

24. Clancy WG, Ray JM, Zohan DJ. Acute tears of the anterior cruciate ligament. Surgical versus conservative treatment. *J Bone Joint Surg Am* 1988;70:1483–1488.

25. O'Brien WR. Isometric placement of anterior cruciate ligament substitutes. *Op Tech Ortho* 1992;2:49–54.

26. O'Meara PM, O'Brien WR, Henning CE. Anterior cruciate ligament reconstruction stability with continuous passive motion: the role of isometric graft placement. *Clin Ortho Rel Res* 1992;277:201–209.

27. Mureta T, Yamamoto H, Ishibashi T, et al. The effects of tibial tunnel placement and roofplasty on reconstructed anterior cruciate ligament knees. *Arthroscopy* 1995;11:57–92.

28. Howell SM, Clark JA, Farley TE. A rationale for predicting anterior cruciate graft impingement by the intercondylar roof. *Am J Sports Med* 1991;19:276–281.

29. Howell SM, Berns GS, Farley EF. Unimpinged and impinged anterior cruciate ligament grafts: MR signal intensity measurements. *Radiology* 1991;179:639–643.

30 Howell SM, Clark JA, Farley TE. Serial magnetic resonance study assessing the effects of impingement on the MR image of the patellar tendon graft. *Arthroscopy* 1992;8:350–358.

31. Howell SM, Taylor MA. Failure of reconstruction of the anterior cruciate ligament due to impingement by the intercondylar roof. *J Bone Joint Surg Am* 1993;75:1044–1055.

32. Fullerton LR, Andrews JR. Mechanical block to extension following augmentation of the anterior cruciate ligament. *Am J Sports Med* 1984;12:166–168.

33. Jackson DW, Schaefer RK. Cyclops syndrome: loss of extension following intra-articular anterior cruciate ligament reconstruction. *Arthroscopy* 1990;6:171–178.

34. Marzo JM, Bowen MK, Warren RF, et al. Intra-articular fibrous nodule as a cause of loss of extension following anterior cruciate ligament reconstruction. *Arthroscopy* 1992;8:10–18.

35. Berns GS, Howell SM. Roofplasty requirements *in vitro* for different tibial hole placements in anterior cruciate ligament reconstruction. *Am J Sports Med* 1993;21:292–298.

36. Romano VM, Graf BK, Keene JS, et al. Anterior cruciate ligament reconstruction: the effect of tibial tunnel placement on range of motion. *Am J Sports Med* 1993;21:415–418.

37. Morgan CD, Kalman VR, Grawl DM. Definitive landmarks for reproducible tibial tunnel placement in anterior cruciate ligament reconstruction. *Arthroscopy* 1995;11:275–288.

38. Jackson DW, Gasser SI. Tibial tunnel placement in ACL reconstruction. *Arthroscopy* 1994;10:124–131.

39. Müller W. *The knee.* Berlin: Springer-Verlag, 1983.

40. Good L, Odenstein M, Gillquist J. Intercondylar notch measurements with special reference to anterior cruciate ligament surgery. *Clin Ortho* 1991;263:185–189.

41. VanRens TJG, Vandenberg AF, Huskes R, et al. Substitution of the anterior cruciate ligament: a long term histologic and biomechanical study with autogenous pedicled grafts of the iliotibial band in dogs. *Arthroscopy* 1986;2:139–154.

42. Holden JP, Grood ES, Butler DL, et al. Biomechanics of fascial lata ligament replacement: early postoperative changes in a goat. *J Orthop Res* 1988;6:639–647.

43. Rodeo SA, Arnoczky SP, Torzilli PA, et al. Tendon healing in a bone tunnel: a biomechanical and histological study in the dog. *J Bone Joint Surg Am* 1993;75:1795–1803.

44. Grana WA, Egle DM, Mahnken R, et al. An analysis of autograft fixation after anterior cruciate ligament reconstruction in a rabbit model. *Am J Sports Med* 1994;22:344–351.

45. Lambert KL. Vascularized patellar tendon graft with rigid internal fixation for anterior cruciate ligament insufficiency. *Clin Orthop Rel Res* 1982;172:85–89.

46. Kurosaka M, Yoshiya S, Andrish JT. A biomechanical comparison of different surgical techniques of graft fixation in anterior cruciate ligament fixation. *Am J Sports Med* 1987;15:225–229.

47. Kohn D, Rose C. Primary stability of interference screw fixation: influence of screw diameter and insertion torque. *Am J Sports Med* 1994;22:334–338.

48. Brown CH, Hecker AT, Hipp JA, et al. The biomechanics of interference screw fixation of patellar tendon anterior cruciate ligament grafts. *Am J Sports Med* 1993;21:880–886.

49. Hulstyn M, Fadale PD, Abate J, et al. Biomechanical evaluation of interference screw fixation in a bovine patellar bone-tendon-bone autograft complex for anterior cruciate ligament reconstruction. *Arthroscopy* 1993;9:417–424.

50. Pomeroy G, Baltz M, Pierz K, et al. The effects of bone plug length and screw diameter on the holding strength of bone-tendon-bone grafts. *Arthroscopy* 1998;14:148–152.

51. Matthews LS, Lawrence SJ, Yahir MA, et al. Fixation strengths of patellar tendon-bone grafts. *Arthroscopy* 1992;9:76–81.

52. Paschal SO, Seeman MD, Ashman RB, et al. Interference fixation vs. post fixation of bone-patellar tendon-bone grafts for anterior cruciate ligament reconstruction. *Clin Orthop Rel Res* 1994;300:281–287.

53. Jomha NM, Raso VJ, Leung P. Effect of varying angles on the pull out strength of interference screw fixation. *Arthroscopy* 1993;9:580–583.

54. Fanelli GC, Desai BM, Cummings PD, et al. Divergent alignment of the femoral interference screw in single incision endoscopic reconstruction of the anterior cruciate ligament. *Contemp Ortho* 1994;28:21–25.

55. Ishibashi Y, Rudy T, Kim HS, et al. The effect of the ACL graft fixation level on knee stability. *Arthroscopy* 1995;11:373.

56. Robertson DB, Daniel DM, Biden E. Soft tissue fixation to bone. *Am J Sports Med* 1986;14:398–403.

57. Steiner ME, Hecker A, Brown CH, et al. Anterior cruciate ligament fixation: comparison of hamstring and patellar tendon grafts. *Am J Sports Med* 1992;22:240–246.

58. Rowden NJ, Sher D, Rogers GJ, et al. Anterior cruciate ligament graft fixation: initial comparison of patellar tendon and semitendinosus autografts in young fresh cadavers. *Am J Sports Med* 1997;25:472–478.

59. Simonian PT, Sussman PS, Baldini TH, et al. Interference screw position and hamstring graft location for anterior cruciate ligament reconstruction. *Arthroscopy* 1998;14:459–464.

60. Pinczewski L, Clingeleffer A. Two year results of endoscopic reconstruction for isolated ACL rupture using quadrupled hamstring tendon autograft and interference screw fixation. Paper presented at: American Academy of Orthopaedic Surgeons 64th Annual Meeting, 1997.

61. Weiler A, Hoffman RFG, Stahelin AC, et al. Hamstring fixation using interference screws: a biomechanical study in calf tibial bone. *Arthroscopy* 1998;14:29–37.

62. Weiler A, Windhagen HJ, Raschke MJ, et al. Biodegradable interference screw fixation exhibits pull-out force and stiffness similar to titanium screws. *Am J Sports Med* 1998;26:119–128.

63. Caborn DNM, Coen M, Neef R, et al. Quadrupled semi-tendinosus-gracilis autograft fixation in the femoral tunnel: a comparison between a metal and a bioabsorbable interference screw. *Arthroscopy* 1998;14:241–245.

64. Clark R, Olsen RE, Larson BJ, et al. Cross-pin femoral fixation: a new technique for hamstring anterior cruciate ligament reconstruction of the knee. *Arthroscopy* 1998;14:258–267.

65. Butler DL, Noyes FR, Grood ES. Ligamentus restraints to anterior-posterior drawer in the human knee: a biomechanical study. *J Bone Joint Surg Am* 1980;62A:259–270.

66. Van Dommelen BA, Fowler PJ. Anatomy of the posterior cruciate ligament: a review. *Am J Sports Med* 1989;17:24–29.

67. Race A, Andrew AA. The biomechanical properties of the two bundles of human posterior cruciate ligament. *J Biomech* 1994;27:13–24.

68. Grood ES, Hefzy MS, Lindenfield TN. Factors affecting the region of most isometric femoral attachments, II: the posterior cruciate ligament. *Am J Sports Med* 1989;17:197–207.

69. Ogata K, McCarthy JA. Measurements of length and tension patterns during reconstruction of the posterior cruciate ligament. *Am J Sports Med* 1992;20:351–355.

70. Bomberg BC, Acker JH, Boyle J, et al. The effect of posterior cruciate ligament loss and reconstruction on the knee. *Am J Knee Surg* 1990;3:85–96.

Part C: Anterior Cruciate Ligament Reconstruction: Techniques Past and Present

Peter D. Laimins and Scott E. Powell

The search for a solution to the problem of ACL insufficiency over the past century has been marked with trials, failures, and partial successes. Attempts at repair, substitution, augmentation, and reconstruction have provided, to varying degrees, short-term stability to the ACL-deficient knee. The 1990s saw the evolution of advances in our understanding of the biology of the reconstructed ligament, the technology of graft fixation, and accelerated rehabilitation protocols that have made ACL reconstruction a successful, reproducible operation with excellent long-term results. A review of techniques once used, modified, and abandoned, sheds light on the evolution of our understanding of ACL reconstruction and provides a foundation for the refinement and development of new techniques in the future.

OPEN PROCEDURES

Repair

Early attempts at primary repair were described as early as 1903 by Robson (1) who reported on suturing the ACL and PCL that were torn "from their upper attachments." Battle (2) reported on the primary repair of ACLs and PCLs torn from the femur. Jones and Smith (3) also described early repair. Pringle (4) reported on three cases of avulsion of the tibial spine repaired with suture. In one case, the patient was injured playing soccer and had lost "any feeling of security in the limb. After open repair, he "hunted, ran to harriers, and danced without any support to the joint."

In 1950, O'Donoghue (5) described a combined injury to the anterior cruciate and medial collateral ligaments with tear of the medial meniscus as the "unhappy triad." He advocated early primary suture repair of the cruciate ligament (Fig. 21.38).

In 1955, O'Donoghue (6) performed an analysis of 80 patients treated with primary repair or reconstruction. Patients with early surgery fared better than those with late surgery. However, of patients with the unhappy triad, repair or reconstruction produced adequate results in only 53% of patients.

In 1965, Liljedahl et al. (7) reported on diagnosis by arthrography and primary repair of the ACL through an arthrotomy incision in 33 patients. Midsubstance tears were repaired by suturing the proximal and distal stumps side-to-side. Proximal ruptures were repaired through drill holes in the lateral femoral condyle. Short-term fol-

low-up of 6 to 18 months in 25 patients found 22 knees with complete stability and full range of motion. Ten of 25 who were active in sports prior to surgery returned to athletic activity.

Marshall et al. (8) described primary repair of the avulsed or, more frequently, the midsubstance tear of the ACL through a medial parapatellar incision. Surgery is performed in the acute setting, ideally within a week of injury. The distal stump of anteromedial fibers and the proximal stump of posterolateral fibers are identified. The synovial sheath is dissected off the ligament and preserved for blood supply to the repaired ligament. Serial sutures are passed anterior to posterior through the ligament beginning near the base and progressing to the torn ends in both the proximal and distal stumps. Anterior and posterior sutures are kept separate. Drill holes are made in the tibia at the anterior and posterior margins of the footprint of the ACL. In the femur, holes are drilled from outside-in using a drill guide. Sutures are brought through either one or, preferably, two drill holes to fan the ligament with the attached sutures (Fig. 21.39).

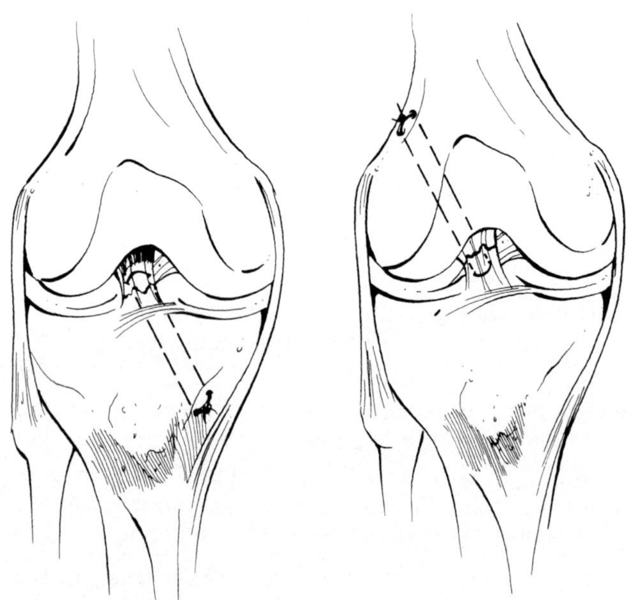

FIGURE 21.38. Repair of anterior cruciate ligament. **Left:** Drill holes through tibia permit passage of suture to secure detached ligament to tibia. **Right:** Similar method to secure proximal end to femur.

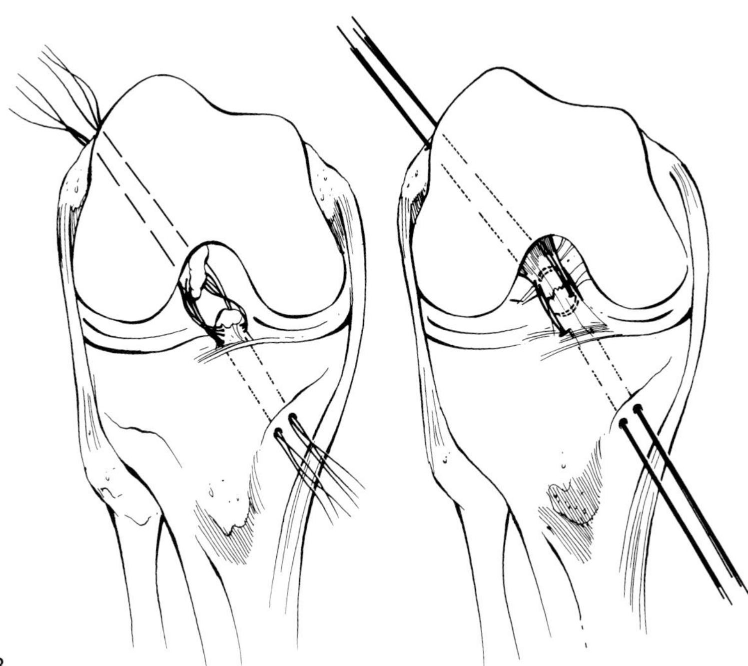

FIGURE 21.39. A: A midportion tear. Looping sutures are placed in the proximal and distal stumps and exit through bone. **B:** When the sutures are drawn tightly, the ligament is reconstituted.

When tissue is inadequate, a strip of fascia lata is used to augment the repair. A 2.5-cm strip of fascia lata is harvested and left attached distally. The graft is tubed and a Bunnell suture placed in the graft. Next, the OTT position is dissected subperiosteally, and a bed of bleeding bone is created with curettes and a curved rasp. The fascia lata graft is passed OTT, through the joint, out through a bony tibial tunnel, and fixed with a staple or heavy sutures on the medial aspect of the tibia. The proximal and distal stumps of the ACL are sutured to the fascia lata strut, and the ligamentum mucosum and synovium are sewn over the graft to enhance blood supply.

In 1989, Jonsson et al. described an augmentation of the repair of the acutely ruptured ACL using a strip of longitudinal patellar retinaculum (9). The band was thought to add strength to the repaired ACL and possibly enhance the healing process through revascularization with anastomotic branches of the medial and inferior geniculate arteries. The graft is harvested from the medial retinaculum and based distally. A 9-mm tibial tunnel is made anterior and medial to the ACL insertion. A lateral femoral incision is made and a femoral tunnel created posterior to the origin of the ACL so that the anterior border of the tunnel is located close to the anatomic center of the origin of the ACL. The graft is passed through the tibial tunnel, out through the femoral tunnel, and tightened over a button or a staple. The midsubstance ACL rupture is repaired using pullout sutures.

Jonsson reported on 28 patients at 5-year follow-up. Only 64% had returned to their preinjury level of activity, and most knees had a slight increase in anterior drawer and Lachman tests.

RECONSTRUCTION

In light of the relatively high failure rates of ACL repair techniques, the search for an adequate substitute for the damaged ACL was begun in the early part of the century and continues to this day. One of the earliest reconstruction techniques was reported in *Lancet* in 1917 (10). Groves (10) reported on "an operation for the substitution of torn crucial ligaments by fascia or tendons." Two years later, he reported on a series of 14 patients treated with open reconstruction of the ACL (11). He wrote, "The War has . . . made the accident comparatively common, and one which can be recognized with considerable certainty even before the knee joint is opened." The procedure begins with a large *U*-shaped incision of the knee and removal of the tibial tubercle with a chip of bone. In an alternative method of open reconstruction, the knee is "merely exposed by vertically splitting the patella." An 8-cm-long strip of the middle third of the iliotibial band is harvested and left attached at the lateral side of the tibia. Drill holes are made in the lateral femoral condyle and anterior tibia. The graft is passed through the femur and knee joint and out through the tibia. "The free end is then passed up to the most prominent point on the inner aspect of the internal condyle, and fixed by sutures and by one ivory nail" (Fig. 21.40). Because his patients were all in the military and were transferred to outposts after recovery, he was unable to report follow-up. He did note that of the 14 cases, "none were made worse by the operation."

Extraarticular procedures were designed to correct the anterolateral rotatory component of instability but did lit-

allow anatomic positioning in the posterior intracondylar notch (12). To increase length, the autograft was modified by including the distal quadriceps tendon and a rolled patellar periosteum attached to the central third of the PT. This construct, however, left the weakest portion of the graft in the intraarticular position. Alternate graft materials included proximally and distally based semitendinosus–gracilis grafts, iliotibial band grafts, prosthetic materials and finally free tendon grafts, allowing adequate length and anatomic intraarticular positioning.

PATELLAR TENDON

In 1963, Jones (12) described a reconstruction technique utilizing a distally based central-third PT autograft with a patellar bone plug (12). Through a medial parapatellar incision, the intercondylar notch is explored and cleared of synovium and periosteum. A modified oscillating saw is used to create a femoral tunnel placed just posterior to the central axis of the femur. The graft is advanced with traction sutures through the PT defect and into the femoral tunnel. A second lateral incision is created to allow suture fixation to the periosteum of the femur (Fig. 21.41).

In 1970, Jones (13) described a modification of his procedure eliminating the need for the second incision. The graft is secured in the femoral tunnel by use of a per-

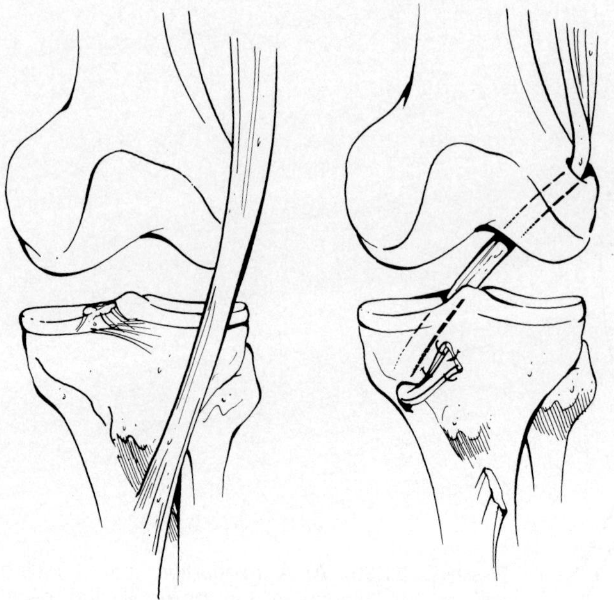

FIGURE 21.40. Formation of a new anterior cruciate ligament from the iliotibial band of fascia.

tle to prevent the more centrally occurring anterior tibial displacement. Thus, procedures with increasing intraarticular anatomic precision were developed. A distally based PT graft with attached patellar bone block was described in the 1960s but frequently lacked sufficient length to

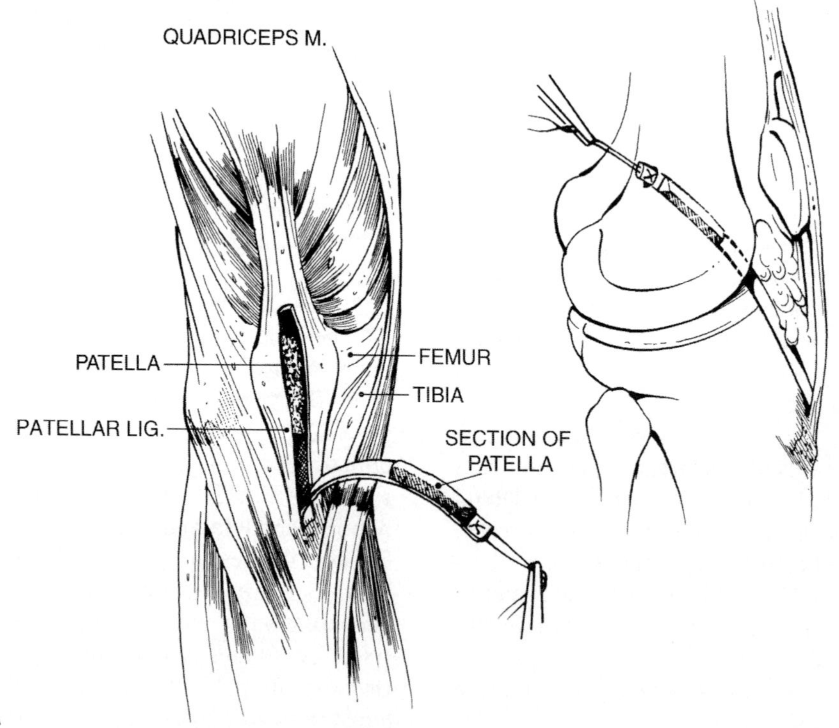

FIGURE 21.41. A: The reflected strip of tendon and attached bone to be used to reconstruct the anterior cruciate ligament. There is a suture in its proximal end. **B:** The new ligament is pulled into the drill hole in the femur so that its proximal portion emerges from the lateral surface of the femur. The ligament is beneath the fat pad. The surgical defects in the quadriceps tendon and the patellar ligament are visualized from behind.

cutaneous pin passed across either the medial or lateral condyle into the patellar bone plug. The pin is cut short and left under the skin.

In 1974, MacIntosh (14) described the use of the lateral third of the PT as an autograft (Fig. 21.42). In this technique, a 1.5-cm strip of distal lateral quadriceps tendon 5 cm in length, lateral patellar retinaculum and patellar aponeurosis, and the lateral PT were harvested as a distally based graft. After drilling a tibial tunnel to the anatomic footprint of the ACL, a lateral incision is made at the distal femur, followed by soft-tissue dissection anterior to the intermuscular septum to the femoral cortex. From within the joint, the OTT position is prepared. The distally based graft is passed through the tibial tunnel. The knee is flexed to 90°, and after application of a posterior tibial drawer, the graft is tensioned and fixed with sutures or staples on the lateral femoral epicondyle.

In 1979, Marshall et al. (15) described a quadriceps tendon substitution procedure for chronic ACL insufficiency (Fig. 21.43). A medial parapatellar incision is made and the joint explored. A notchplasty is performed to eliminate impingement. The graft is composed of the central third of the infrapatellar ligament, the periosteum of the patella, and 6 cm of central quadriceps tendon 2 cm in width. To reinforce the relatively thin pre-PT, the quadriceps tendon is split longitudinally and a segment folded back over the prepatellar periosteum. The patellar periosteum is then tubed with sutures around the piece of quadriceps tendon.

The graft is distally based, remaining attached at the tibial tubercle, and a Bunnell suture is placed through the graft. A bony tunnel is made in the tibia, entering the joint at the midpoint of the insertion of the ACL on the tibia. A lateral incision is made proximal to the lateral femoral condyle. A bony tunnel is created in the lateral femoral condyle, or a subperiosteal tunnel created in the OTT position as described by MacIntosh (14). The graft is passed through the knee and, after application of a posterior drawer, fixed with a staple with the knee flexed at 90° for an OTT placement, or at 30° for a bone tunnel. Ligamentum and synovium are sewn over the graft.

The quadriceps tendon substitution procedure was often performed in conjunction with a medial reconstruction. These included posteromedial reefing, medial collateral ligament (MCL) imbrication, the Bosworth procedure, the O'Donoghue procedure, and distal advancement of the MCL (15). The knee was placed in a cast for 6 weeks and braced with limited motion for another 6 weeks with limitation of full extension until 12 weeks.

In 1988, Kornblatt et al. (16) reported on long-term follow-up of 60 patients treated with the Marshall reconstruction and found the procedure eliminated symptomatic instability in 79% of patients. A residual pivot shift in 45% and symptoms of instability in 21% of patients led the authors to recommend the addition of an extraarticular sling procedure because of the poor strength characteristics of the tissue in the quadriceps tendon substitution.

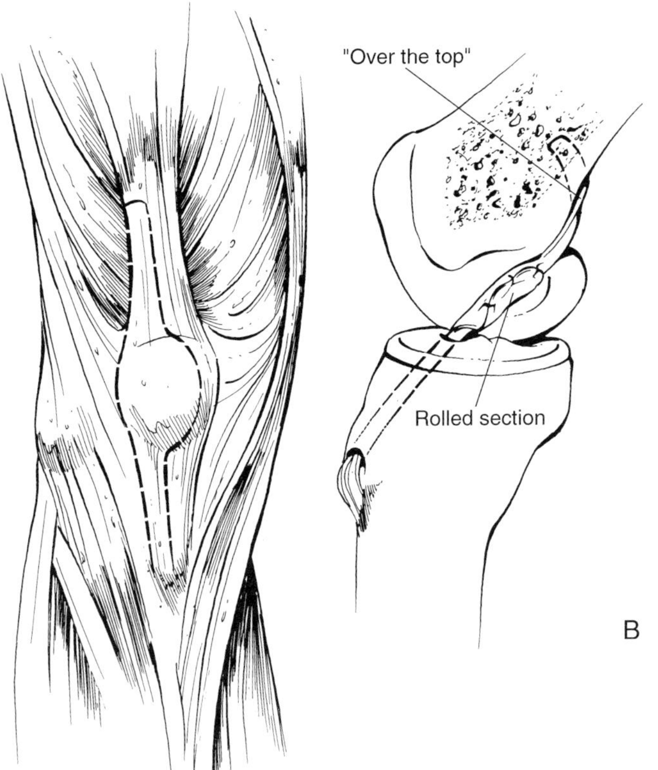

FIGURE 21.42. MacIntosh technique of anterior cruciate ligament reconstruction. **A:** Tendon substitute harvested from lateral portion of patellar tendon and rolled into a tube. **B:** Substitute tendon passed through intercondylar notch and "over-the-top" of lateral femoral condyle.

In 1991, Howe et al. (17) reported on 10-year follow-up of 83 patients who underwent a Marshall reconstruction of the ACL. Ninety-five percent of patients reported no giving-way, and the Lachman maneuver remained negative in 87%. There was no significant difference in postoperative evaluation at 1 and 10 years, demonstrating that results did not deteriorate with time.

In 1976, Eriksson (18) described the use of the medial third of the PT for reconstruction of the ACL (18) (Fig. 21.44). A medial parapatellar incision is made from above the patella to the insertion of the pes tendons. A 1-cm-wide, partial-thickness flap of quadriceps tendon is harvested 4 cm above the superior pole of the patellar. A shallow layer of bone is harvested from the patella. The medial third of the patella tendon is harvested and the distal insertion left attached. A bony tunnel is made through the tibia and enters the joint just medial to the ACL insertion. Sutures are placed through the quadriceps tendon and patellar bone. With the knee flexed, a lateral incision is made. The iliotibial band is incised 2.5 cm from the posterior edge. The knee is maximally flexed and a drill hole made from inside the joint at the origin of the ACL, exiting on the surface of the lateral femoral condyle. The sutures attached to the graft are passed through the tibial and femoral tunnels and through a plastic button. A posterior drawer is placed on the tibia and the sutures tied over the button with the knee at 60° of flexion.

A similar procedure was described by Alm and Gillquist (19) in 1971. The medial third of the PT was dissected from the upper border of the patella down to the

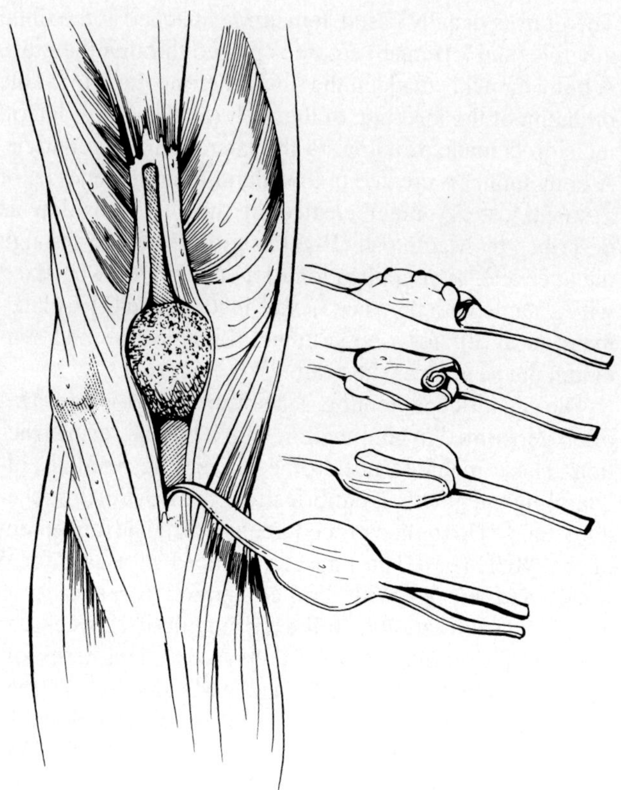

FIGURE 21.43. Harvesting of patelloquadriceps substitution for anterior cruciate ligament.

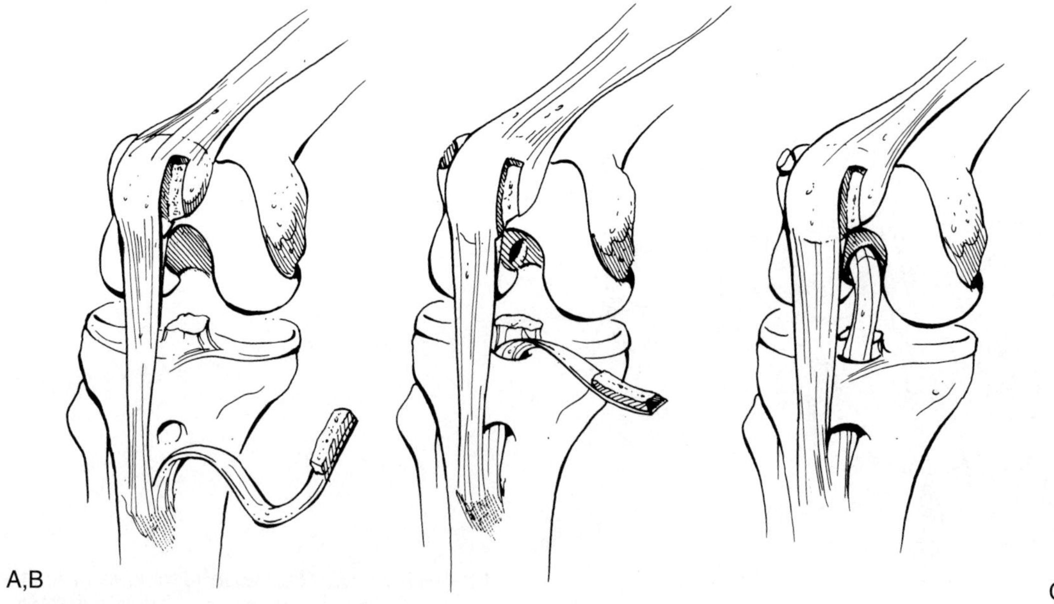

FIGURE 21.44. Eriksson technique of reconstruction of anterior cruciate ligament using split patellar tendon. **A:** Piece of bone dissected off patella and patella tendon split. **B:** Split tendon pulled into knee joint. **C:** Sutures tied and operation completed.

tibial tuberosity, leaving the distal insertion intact. A tibial tunnel was drilled, entering the knee joint at the anatomic insertion tunnel 2 cm deep, which was connected to the lateral femoral cortex with two drill holes. The graft was then advanced through the tunnels with traction sutures and the sutures were tied proximally at the lateral femoral cortex. The knee was immobilized in a cast for 4 weeks, followed by initiation of rehabilitative exercises. At 2-year follow-up, only 66% of 164 patients were able to resume competitive sports.

Drez (20) reported use of a modified Eriksson procedure with a medial pes anserinus transfer and a biceps tendon advancement laterally. Loss of motion was reported in six of ten patients, and no patient returned to preoperative activity level. A report published in 1996 on 6-year follow-up of 29 patients treated with the Eriksson procedure found 21 patients who returned to their preinjury level of activity; the pivot shift was eliminated in 69% of patients (21).

In 1982, Clancy et al. (22) described the use of a free graft of bone–PT–bone for ACL reconstruction. A medial parapatellar incision is made followed by a medial arthrotomy. The vastus medialis is separated from the patella, allowing lateral dislocation of the patella and inspection of the intraarticular structures. Meniscal pathology is addressed, followed by debridement of the notch. Bony tunnels are created in the tibia and femur using drill guides. A free central-third PT graft is harvested with attached tibial and patellar bone blocks and is passed through the tibial and femoral tunnels to its final intraarticular position. The graft is tensioned with the knee at 90° of flexion, with a posterior tibial drawer applied. Fixation is achieved by tying sutures over cortical buttons. Medial and lateral muscle transfers are used on most patients to protect the graft and to reduce anteromedial and anterolateral instability. Medially, a pes anserinus transfer as described by Slocum and Larson (23) and laterally a biceps femoris advancement deep to the fibular collateral ligament are performed. This technique can be performed through an open arthrotomy or through the PT defect. Alternatively, an arthroscopically assisted technique can be used, using arthroscopic drill guides and graft fixation with interference screws.

In 1982, Clancy et al. (22) reviewed 50 patients with a minimum of 2-years of follow-up. They reported good and excellent results in 47 patients, with elimination of the pivot-shift in 41 patients.

SEMITENDINOSUS–GRACILIS

McMaster and colleagues (24) reported in 1974 on use of the gracilis tendon for reconstruction of the torn ACL. The gracilis is harvested through an *S*-shaped medial incision and the muscle belly is sewn to the adjacent semitendinosus through a second proximal incision. The tendon is left attached distally. With the knee in exten-

sion, a guide pin is placed through the tibia and femur to exit the lateral femoral condyle. A tunnel is then drilled through the tibia and femur over the guide pin. The gracilis graft is passed through the joint to exit on the lateral femoral condyle and stapled in place (Fig. 21.45).

In 1975, Cho (25) described a procedure using a distally based semitendinosus graft. Through a medial parapatellar incision, the joint is inspected and the semitendinosus tendon identified and released proximally from surrounding fascial tissue. The musculotendinous junction of the semitendinosus is sutured to the adjacent semimembranosus muscle and tendon. The semitendinosus tendon is left attached distally and routed deep to the remaining pes tendons. Tibial and femoral tunnels are created over guide pins, followed by advancement of the free semitendinosus tendon through the tunnels. The tendon is secured to the lateral femoral epicondyle with staples or sutures. The knee is immobilized at 30° of flexion for 6 weeks, followed by progressive rehabilitation.

Lipscomb et al. (26) used Cho's procedure in 78 patients with ACL-deficient knees. At an average follow-up of 11 months, 86% had significant improvement in stability. They then modified the procedure to include both the semitendinosus and gracilis tendons and reported 84% good results in 342 treated knees at an average of 22 months (27).

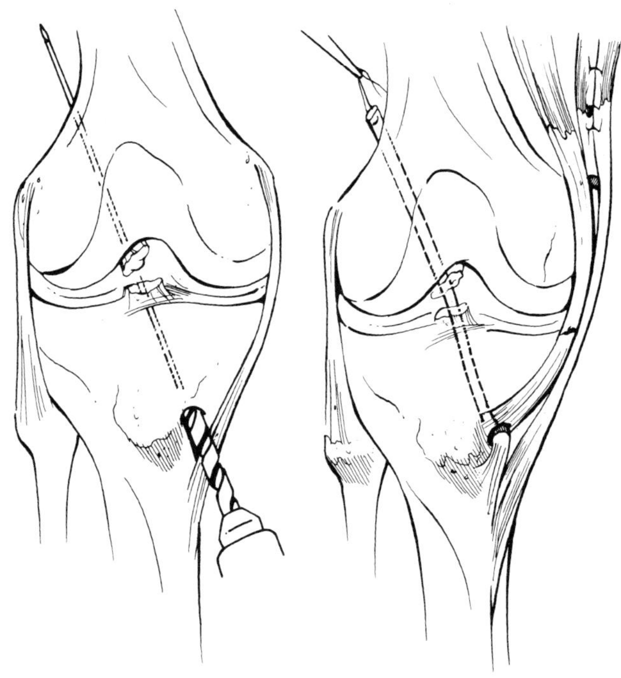

FIGURE 21.45. Left: A drill is passed from the medial tibial metaphysis to exit on the lateral femoral condyle, crossing the joint along the former course of the anterior cruciate ligament. **Right:** The lateral femoral condyle is exposed. The gracilis tendon is passed through the drill hole and stapled to the condyle.

In a technique described in 1983 by Puddu (28), proximally based HS tendons are used as an intraarticular graft. After inspection of the joint through a medial parapatellar arthrotomy, semitendinosus and gracilis tendons are dissected proximally to their musculotendinous junctions. They are detached distally from their tibial insertion with a fleck of bone. A tibial tunnel is drilled through the medial tibial condyle beginning at the anterior edge of the medial collateral ligament approximately 2 to 3 cm below the joint line and enters the joint at the anatomic insertion site of the ACL. The femoral tunnel is created through a lateral incision at the lateral femoral epicondyle. The two-tendon graft is passed through the joint in a distal to proximal fashion and the free end of the graft secured to the iliotibial band.

In 1987, Zaricznyj (29) attempted to recreate the separate anatomic insertions of the anterior and posterior bundles of ACL on the tibia. In this procedure, the knee joint is inspected through a medial arthrotomy. The semitendinosus tendon is identified and dissected proximally to its musculotendinous junction, where it is released and brought into the wound. Two drill holes are created using Steinmann pins, one entering the knee joint anteromedial to the anatomic insertion of the ACL and the other entering posterolateral to the tibial spine. The holes are enlarged to accommodate the graft. A femoral tunnel is drilled 1.3 cm deep at the origin of the ACL. Through a lateral incision over the femoral epicondyle, two drill holes are made to enter the femoral tunnel. The free end of the semitendinosus tendon is then passed through one tibial tunnel, looped over a suture, and pulled distally through the second tibial tunnel. The folded tendon is advanced proximally by pulling sutures through the holes in the femoral tunnel. Sutures are tied proximally and distally to provide graft fixation.

Zaricznyj (29) reviewed 14 patients treated with this procedure at an average follow-up of 3.6 years. The pivot shift test was negative in all patients and all were able to return to their previous occupations. Eight participated in recreational sports, and 12 rated their results as excellent or good.

In 1986, Zarins and Rowe (30) described an open procedure for reconstruction of the ACL-deficient knee combining intra- and extraarticular techniques (Fig. 21.46). The semitendinosus is identified through a medial incision and dissected proximally 20 cm, taking care to maintain its distal attachment. An oblique drill-hole is created in the anteromedial part of the tibia, entering the knee joint at the tibial attachment of the ACL. The iliotibial tract is exposed through the lateral incision with dissection of a 25-cm distally based strip 2 cm wide. Soft-tissue tunnels are created deep to the fibular collateral ligament and over the lateral femoral condyle. An 8-mm groove can be made in the posterior condyle to improve isometry. The free end of the semitendinosus tendon is then passed through the tibial tunnel and knee joint, exiting at the lateral condylar groove anterior to the intermuscular septum, and distally deep to the fibular collateral liga-

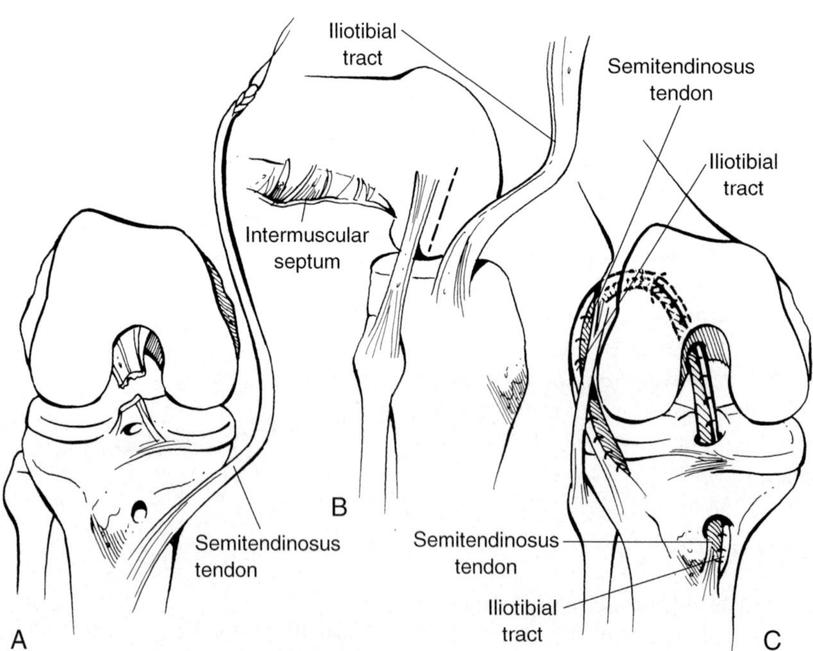

FIGURE 21.46. Zarins and Rowe technique of anterior cruciate ligament reconstruction. **A:** Semitendinosus released at musculotendinous junction, left attached to insertion on anteromedial tibia. **B:** Location of "over-the-top" position, over lateral intermuscular septum. **C:** Final position of composite intraarticular replacement.

ment. The iliotibial tract graft follows the same path in the opposite direction. The grafts are tensioned simultaneously, followed by suturing the grafts to each other and to the posterolateral capsule. After surgery, knee extension is restricted and gradually increased over 9 months with the use of a hinged knee brace.

One hundred patients with chronic instability who were treated with this technique were evaluated at 3 to 7.5 years after surgery, with functional stability achieved in 90%. Anterior drawer was reduced or eliminated in 80 knees, and the pivot shift was eliminated or reduced to 1+ in 91 knees (30).

Initially described as an open procedure, the Zarins–Rowe procedure was later modified by Billotti et al. (31) as an arthroscopic technique. They reported their results in 1997. Femoral and tibial tunnels are prepared using standard ACL drill guides. The semitendinosus graft is fixed to the superior border of the insertion of the iliotibial band, while the iliotibial graft is stapled to the proximal medial tibia. A rehabilitation program is begun on the first postoperative day, including progressive range of motion as tolerated.

Fifty patients were reviewed at 2- to 5-year follow-up, and all showed a statistically significant improvement from preoperative knee scores (31). Ninety-six percent had a negative Lachman test, 92% a negative anterior drawer, and 94% a negative pivot shift test.

In 1991, Brief (32) described a reconstruction to be used in adolescents with open physes, which did not utilize drill holes and, thus, avoided damage to the physes. The semitendinosus and gracilis tendons are harvested through a medial incision, detached from their musculotendinous junctions, and their distal tibial insertions left intact. A lateral incision is made at the distal femur to receive the graft through the OTT position. The tendons are sutured together and passed into the knee joint under the anterior horn of the medial meniscus, through the intercondylar notch and out the knee joint posteriorly. The graft is fixed to the lateral femoral cortex with staples. After surgery, the patient is placed in an adjustable-hinged long leg brace at 25° of flexion. Full range of motion is obtained gradually over 6 weeks.

Brief (32) reviewed a small series of nine patients at 3 to 6 years, and all but one felt improvement in knee stability. None had recurrence of the pivot shift phenomenon. The author pointed out that the graft is not positioned isometrically, tightening somewhat in full extension, and this may have led to stretching of the graft within the first 18 postoperative months as detected by KT-1000 measurements. Overall, six of nine patients were fully satisfied with the results, returning to their preinjury athletic levels.

In 1984, a variation in fixation of HS tendon grafts was described by Gomes et al. (33). Plugs of bone were obtained with a trephine during creation of the tibial and femoral tunnels. A looped semitendinosus free graft was press-fit into bone tunnels using these plugs. The authors reviewed 26 patients treated with this procedure, with good results in 23 cases. Objectively, the pivot shift was negative in all cases, with only one positive Lachman test. Nineteen patients returned to their preinjury sports activity levels.

ILIOTIBIAL BAND

O'Donoghue (34) described the use of a strip of the iliotibial band for reconstruction of the ACL in 1963. A skin incision is made from the midlateral thigh to the fibular head and the fascia lata and the iliotibial band are harvested in a tapering strip. The iliotibial band is dissected off the femur in a continuum with the fascia lata, dissected off of the tibia and left attached distally to the fascia of the calf, creating a strip of tissue about 14 inches in length. The graft is tubed. Through an arthrotomy incision, a tunnel is drilled through the tibia from the lateral side into the footprint of the ACL using specially designed cannulated drills. A tunnel is created in the lateral condyle of the femur at the origin of the ACL. The graft is passed from lateral to medial through the tibia, out through the lateral femoral condyle, and fixed with a staple. The remainder of the graft is stapled from femur to tibia with the knee at 30° of flexion in line with the lateral collateral ligament, folded back proximally, and sutured to the lateral fascia.

In 1981, Insall et al. (35) proposed the use of a proximally based fascia lata graft. Through a lateral incision, the anterior two thirds of the iliotibial band is dissected from Gerdy's tubercle with an attached bone block and fashioned into a tube. A medial parapatellar incision allows a curved clamp to be passed through the intercondylar notch to create an opening in the posterior capsule at the over-the-top position. The bone block and iliotibial band graft are advanced through the capsular opening and intercondylar notch and brought anteriorly. A trough is created in the anteromedial tibial surface to accommodate the bone block, which is fixed in place with a screw. Weight bearing is allowed immediately, with rehabilitative exercises initiated 2 to 3 weeks after the procedure.

Hooper and Walton (36) reviewed 37 patients treated with this technique and found disappointing results. Patients were rarely able to return to their preinjury levels of activity, and most had persistent postoperative objective instability. Because of these results, they discontinued the use of the procedure.

Insall's procedure was modified by Scott et al. (37) in 1985 to include a trough created from the interspinous area to the anterior tibia. They also limited posterior dissection of the iliotibial graft to maintain a firm proximal attachment point to the lateral intermuscular septum. Another modification was described by MacIntosh, who used a distally based strip of the iliotibial band passed deep to the fibular collateral ligament, through the intermuscular septum and OTT position, advanced through the intercondylar notch, and sutured anteriorly at the tibia (38).

EXTRAARTICULAR TECHNIQUES

Numerous extraarticular procedures have been described for recreating stability in the ACL-deficient knee. Early techniques attempted to reestablish stability by reconstructing the medial side of the knee. The Slocum procedure described in 1968 was designed to accentuate the internal rotation function of the pes anserinus on the tibia and thereby improve function in knees with anterior and medial instability (23) (Fig. 21.47). This procedure was used by Slocum as the final step in reconstructing knees for chronic medial ligamentous instability but has also been used in combination with intraarticular and lateral reconstructions for ACL-deficient knees. The pes anserinus is identified through an anteromedial incision. The inferior edge of the semitendinosus tendon is freed from its fascial attachment to the gastrocnemius muscle, followed by sharp dissection of the distal two thirds of the pes insertion on the tibia. The free portion of the pes is reflected anteriorly and medially and sutured to the medial aspect of the patellar and sartorius tendons. The knee is immobilized in a cast at 45° for 3 to 6 weeks, followed by vigorous rehabilitation.

A long-term follow-up study by Freeman et al. (39) in 1982 demonstrated poor results at 10 years. Problems included persistent instability, arthritic changes, and increased anterolateral instability.

Most extraarticular techniques described in the 1970s and 1980s were laterally based procedures using part of the iliotibial band to create a checkrein on anterior tibial displacement relative to the femur. These techniques have been used as the primary procedure for ACL-deficient knees, as well as in combination with intraarticular repairs for acute disruptions and intraarticular reconstructions for chronic instability.

Functional knee instability and the pivot shift phenomenon in ACL-deficient knees occur due to anterolateral rotatory instability of the lateral tibial plateau. The intact iliotibial band subluxes the lateral tibial plateau anteriorly around an intact PCL as the knee is brought into full extension, forcing the tibia to internally rotate relative to the femur. Conversely, an intact ACL produces a relative external rotation of the tibia as full extension is achieved, providing stability in weight-bearing activities. The extraarticular procedures attempt to recreate this function of the ACL by positioning a part of the iliotibial band posterior to the transverse center of knee rotation, thus preventing anterior subluxation of the lateral tibial plateau. The peripheral location of these tenodesis procedures provides a longer moment arm to eliminate rotatory torque forces but at the same time is less effective in preventing the more centrally occurring anterior tibial displacement.

In 1976, MacIntosh and Darby (40) described a procedure in which a 1.5-cm strip of the iliotibial band is harvested from the midportion of the tendon and left attached at Gerdy's tubercle (Fig 21.48). The strip of tendon is passed beneath the fibular collateral ligament, into

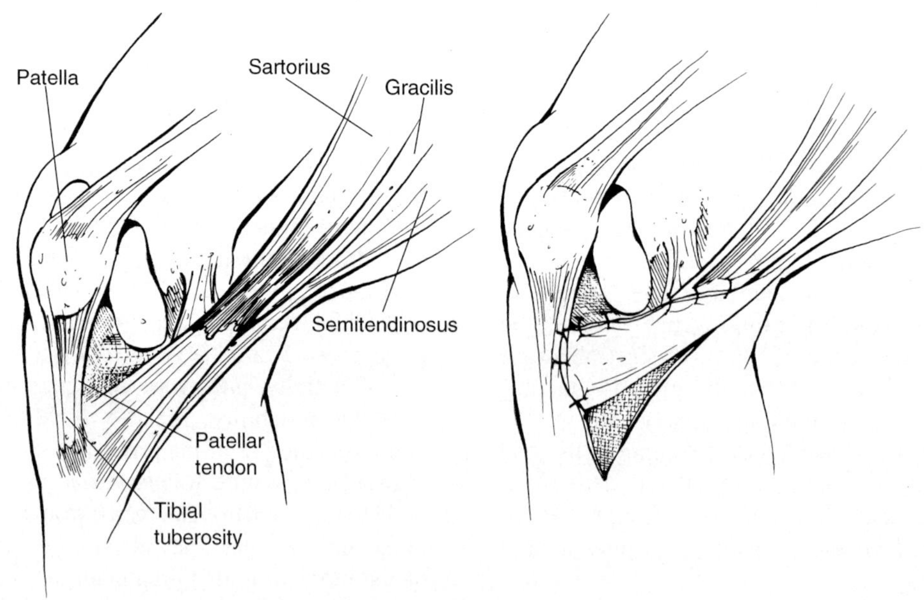

FIGURE 21.47. Slocum transplant of pes anserinus for rotary instability. **A:** Inferior edge of semitendinosus tendon is freed from fascia over calf muscles. Distal two thirds of insertion of pes anserinus is freed from tibia. **B:** Reflected part of pes anserinus is sutured to periosteum over tibial tuberosity, to medial aspect of patellar tendon, to periosteum over proximal tibia, and to sartorius tendon.

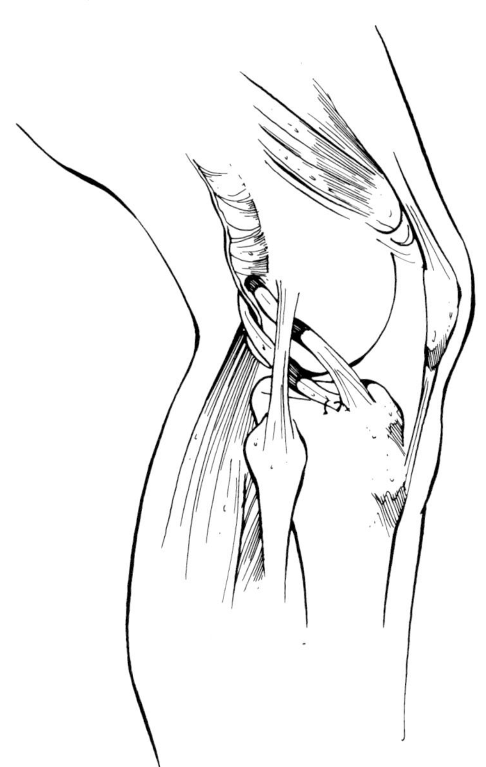

FIGURE 21.48. MacIntosh technique of lateral reconstruction using strip of iliotibial band.

a subperiosteal tunnel on the lateral femoral condyle, through a hiatus created at the distal attachment of the intermuscular septum, and looped back onto itself. With the knee flexed and tibia externally rotated, the strip of tendon is sutured into its attachment at Gerdy's tubercle. A long leg cast is applied for 5 weeks with the knee in 90° of flexion and the foot in external rotation.

A modified MacIntosh technique described by Ireland (41) in 1980 advocated looping the same piece of iliotibial band around the fibular collateral ligament and suturing onto itself rather than reattaching it distally at Gerdy's tubercle. The defect in the iliotibial tract was closed except for the most distal 5 cm.

Another modification of the MacIntosh procedure called for the tendon to be looped back on itself and secured to an area of denuded bone with a staple (42). The iliotibial band is sutured to the fibular collateral ligament. The knee is placed in a brace at 55° of flexion for the first week, then extended to 30° of flexion for the second week. Full extension is reached at week six.

In 1988, Amirault et al. (43) reviewed 27 patients treated with the original MacIntosh procedure and, based on their own classification, found only 52% excellent results. However, 75% of patients were subjectively improved and able to maintain an active lifestyle.

In the same year, Frank and Jackson (44) reviewed 35 patients treated with the MacIntosh procedure and had a

75% satisfactory rating despite a persistent pivot shift in 79% and a positive Lachman test in 80%. They concluded that this technique failed to return most knees to normal when judged by either subjective or objective criteria.

In 1993, Osterman et al. (45) studied the results in 25 patients treated with the lateral substitution procedure and noted subjective postoperative improvement but persistent anteromedial and anterior instability. Anterolateral instability was well controlled.

The Losee procedure described in 1978 used a distally based midsection of the iliotibial tract (46) (Fig. 21.49). The tendon is passed anterior to posterior through a tunnel in the lateral femoral condyle. The exit location of the canal is at the insertion of the lateral head of the gastrocnemius muscle and the posterior capsule. The strip of tendon is woven through the origin of the lateral head of the gastrocnemius 1 cm distal and 5 mm medial to the posterior exit of the tunnel. The tendon is passed horizontally and laterally through the arcuate ligament, beneath the fibular collateral ligament distal to the joint line and fixed to Gerdy's tubercle. As the knee goes into extension, the lateral head of the gastrocnemius tightens, stabilizing the posterolateral corner of the knee. The lateral gastrocnemius and posterior capsule are sutured to the fibular collateral ligament. The knee is placed in a cast at 30° to 45° of flexion for 6 weeks.

The Ellison procedure described in 1979 is a proximally based lateral transfer that routes a central slip of the iliotibial tract with a small piece of attached bone beneath the fibular collateral ligament, which is reattached distal to Gerdy's tubercle to an area of exposed bone (47) (Fig. 21.50). This technique includes a plication of the middle third of the lateral capsular ligament followed by closure of the defect in the iliotibial band to prevent varus instability. If the transfer has been put in the proper position, full extension of the knee is not possible at the time of the procedure. The knee is immobilized for 6 weeks in a long leg cast at 60° with the tibia gently externally rotated. By creating a proximally based band, the transfer provides a dynamic stabilizing component from the tensor fascia.

In 1979, Ellison (47) reviewed 18 patients treated with his technique, with 44% excellent and 39% good results. Durkan et al. (48) performed the Ellison procedure on 104 patients and had 81% subjective and 76% objective excellent or good results. They recommended this procedure for the recreational athlete only. All patients were advised to avoid high-level cutting or jumping activities.

A modification of the Ellison procedure was described by Fox et al. (49) in 1980. The strip of iliotibial band with its attached piece of bone was wrapped around the fibular collateral ligament prior to reattaching it anterior and distal to Gerdy's tubercle. This modification enhanced the tenodesis effect of the procedure. Fox et al. reported their results in 76 patients treated with this modified technique and found fair to excellent results in only 63%; they

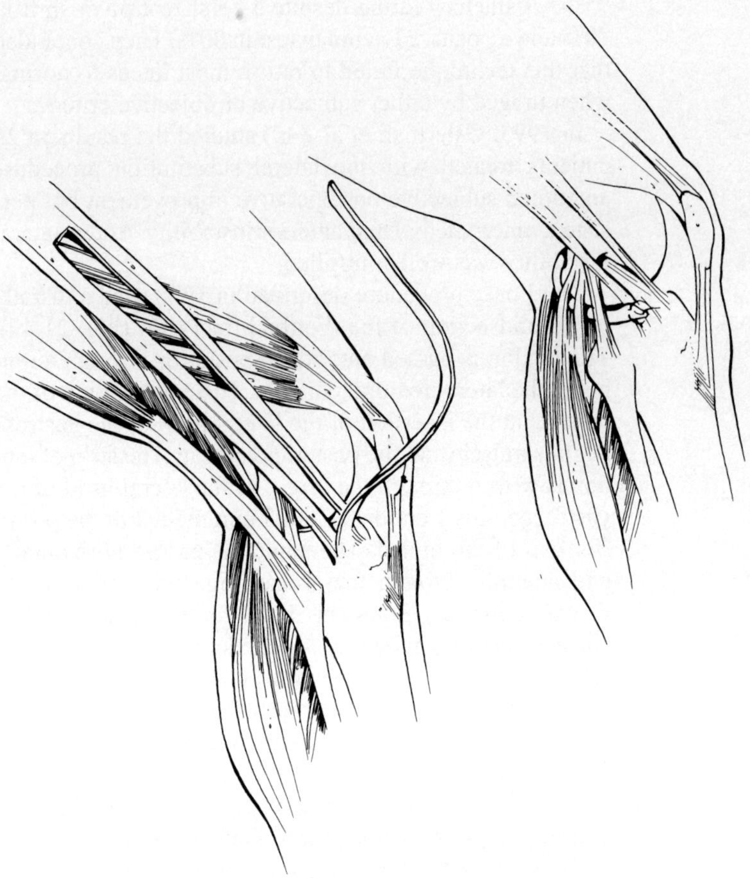

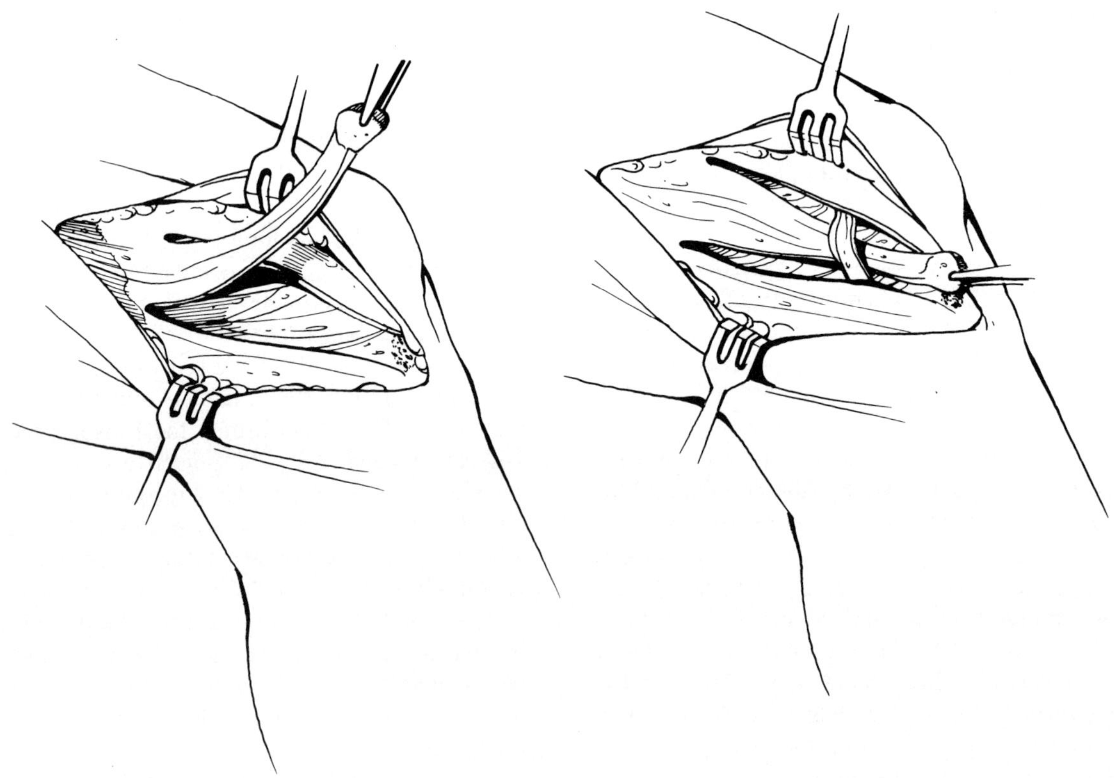

FIGURE 21.49. Losee modification of MacIntosh technique of lateral reconstruction using iliotibial band. **A:** Fascial strip (18 cm long, 1.5 cm wide) of iliotibial tract attached to Gerdy's tubercle. **B:** Imbrication through lateral head of gastrocnemius plus posterolateral corner.

FIGURE 21.50. Ellison technique of lateral reconstruction using strip of iliotibial band.

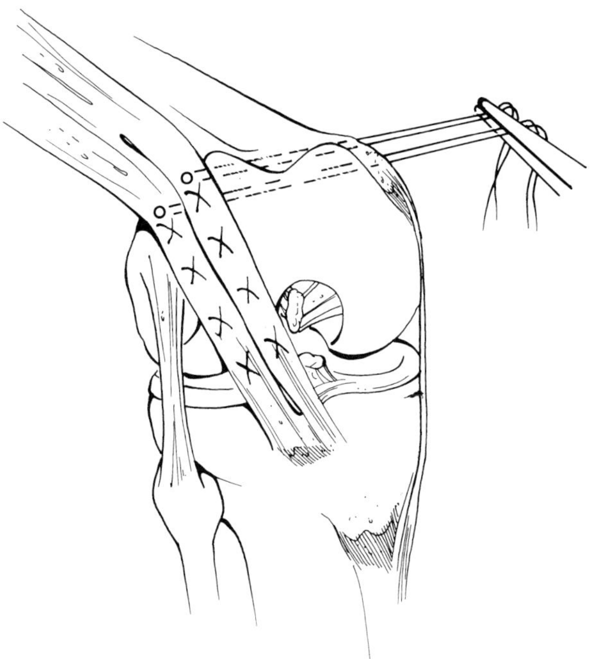

FIGURE 21.51. Attachment of two bundles to lateral femoral condylar area through transosseous drill holes to medial side of femur.

noted disappointing outcomes in patients with 2+ or greater preoperative anterior instability.

In 1983, Andrews and Sanders (50) described an extraarticular procedure in which the iliotibial tract is left intact both proximally and distally and split in line with its fibers 4 cm anterior to its posterior border (Figs. 21.51, 21.52). Two Beath pins are then passed through the distal femur from lateral to medial, exiting the femur through a medial incision and leaving a 1-cm bone bridge over the adductor tubercle. One pin is positioned laterally at the insertion of the intermuscular septum, and the second is placed 5 mm distal and 10 mm anterior to the first at the flare of the lateral femoral condyle. Bunnell-type sutures are placed separately in the two strips of iliotibial tract distal to the pins and pulled through the femur. The sutures are tied medially over the bone bridge with the knee held at 30° of flexion and the tibia externally rotated. The two bundles contribute isometrically to stability, with the posterior bundle tight in extension and the anterior tight in flexion. The knee is placed in a bent-knee cylinder cast for 6 weeks.

In 1985, Andrews reviewed 69 patients treated with his procedure and noted greater than 90% acceptable results both objectively and subjectively.

The lateral tenodesis procedure described by James (51) in 1983 uses a strip of iliotibial band left attached distally at Gerdy's tubercle. The thickest midportion of the tract is harvested in a 2-cm-wide band. A bony tunnel is made through the lateral femoral condyle just proximal and anterior to the origin of the fibular collateral ligament. The tunnel is drilled posterior and medial and exits at the insertion of the lateral gastrocnemius tendon. A tunnel is made in the soft tissue through the arcuate ligament and gastrocnemius tendon and beneath the fibular collateral ligament. The iliotibial graft is passed beneath the fibular collateral ligament, through the tunnel in the arcuate ligament and gastrocnemius tendon, looped anteriorly over these same structures, and passed posteriorly through the same soft-tissue tunnel. The iliotibial tract is brought through the bony tunnel from posterior to ante-

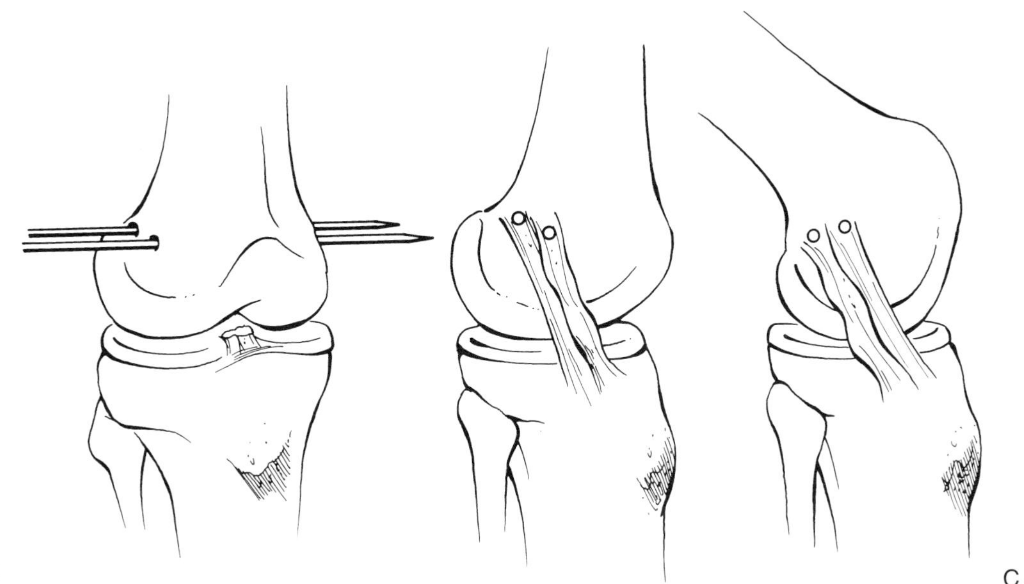

A,B

C

FIGURE 21.52. A: Two points on lateral femoral condyle corresponding to major femoral intraarticular attachments of anterior cruciate ligament. **B:** Posterior band tight in extension. **C:** Anterior band tight in flexion.

rior and beneath the remaining iliotibial band and sutured to the insertion of the fibular collateral ligament. Occasionally a lateral retinacular release is required to prevent maltracking of the patella. The knee is placed in a cast at 30° of flexion.

Jensen et al. (52) reviewed 25 patients treated in this manner, with improvement in 87% of cases. The anterior drawer was eliminated or decreased in 87%, with 100% elimination of the lateral pivot shift. This procedure was indicated for severe chronic anterolateral rotatory instability and was combined with an intraarticular ACL reconstruction.

Hughston (53) described an iliotibial tract tenodesis to the lateral femoral condyle in combination with a plication of the lateral capsular ligament and a biceps femoris advancement. The distal iliotibial band is split in half longitudinally, followed by suturing the posterior band to the intermuscular septum 2 inches proximal to the condyle to prevent anterior subluxation of the lateral tibial plateau. The patient is placed in a long leg cast at 60° of flexion for 6 weeks.

PROSTHETIC LIGAMENTS

Synthetic materials have been used for reconstruction of the ACL since the early part of the century. In 1919, Groves (11) noted that his contemporary, Trethowan, "uses stout strands of twisted silk" to reconstruct the ligament. The 1980s saw a renewed search for synthetic substitutes for the ACL. Although reconstruction of the chronic ACL was usually performed with bone–tendon–bone autograft, the procedure did have problems. The high incidence of patellofemoral pain, up to 30% in some studies, often correlated with a poor result (54–57). Loss of motion remained a problem, despite more aggressive physical therapy protocols (58–60). Moreover, some arthroscopic follow-up studies noted poor quality of the new ligament (61,62). The purpose of prosthetic augmentation devices was to act as an internal strut for protection of the autogenous ACL graft as it undergoes degeneration and revascularization, allow accelerated rehabilitation, and avoid the pitfalls of associated with autogenous PT harvest.

The Leeds–Keio prosthesis was first implanted in patients in 1982 (63). It is an open-weave tube of polyester mesh. It can be fixed to bone at each end with bone plugs. Early reports on its use were encouraging (64). In 1994, Dandy and Gray (65) described 129 patients treated with a Leeds–Keio prosthesis supplemented with an extraarticular MacIntosh lateral substitution reconstruction. Early follow-up showed promise, with recurrent pivot shift in only 4% of patients. These results, however, degenerated with time; at long-term follow-up, 40% of patients had a recurrent pivot shift and nine patients required reoperation.

Another of the prosthetic ligaments introduced in the 1980s was the Stryker–Meadox Dacron ligament pros-

thesis. The graft consisted of a central core of four tightly woven tapes encased by a sheath of loosely woven velour. In 1992, Richmond et al. (66) reported on 35 patients who underwent reconstruction with a Dacron ligament prosthesis for chronic ACL insufficiency. The overall failure rate was 37%, with a failure rate of 78% among patients with associated instability or previous failed ACL reconstruction. In the group of patients with satisfactory results, a subsequent deterioration of clinical stability over time was reported.

In a prospective study published in 1993, Gillquist and Odensten (67) reported on 70 patients with chronic ACL insufficiency who underwent reconstruction with a Dacron prosthesis. At 5-year follow-up, 23% of the prostheses had ruptured, with 55% of patients having good or excellent results. No patient returned to competitive sports. Anterior tibial tunnel placement and associated untreated instabilities contributed to failure of the reconstructions.

The Gore-Tex PTFE graft was a braided configuration of 180 strands of a single continuous fiber of polytetrafluoroethylene (PTFE) with eyelets at either end. Indelicato et al. (68) reported on 41 patients with acute and chronic ACL insufficiency who underwent reconstruction with Gore-Tex PTFE graft. Although 87% of patients had satisfactory results, problems persisted with use of the prosthesis. Four patients had complete rupture of the graft, and nine patients had sterile effusions thought to be due to synovial irritation from the PTFE particles. Tibial tunnel placement, adequate notchplasty, and rasping of tunnel ends had significant impacts on the success of the procedure.

Kennedy and Roth Schmidt (69) originally described the use of a polypropylene braid ligament augmentation device (LAD) in 1980. The LAD was designed to mechanically augment an intraarticular autograft, protect it from disruption during revascularization, and protect it from creep and fatigue failure. The LAD was initially used by Kennedy and Roth Schmidt in conjunction with a modified Marshall reconstruction using quadriceps and PT tubed, passed through the tibial tunnel, and "over the top." In 1985, Roth et al. (70) reviewed 83 patients treated with and without LAD augmentation and found recurrent, symptomatic giving-way in 32% of patients without augmentation and in 11% with augmentation.

In 1996, Grontvedt et al. (71) reported on 100 consecutive patients randomized into two groups using bone–PT–bone autografts with and without LAD augmentation and found no difference between the two groups at 2 years (71). Furthermore, in long-term follow-up of 594 patients treated with bone–tendon–bone autograft with ligament augmentation, 20% of the devices failed. Failures were often accompanied by effusions that resolved when the device was removed. Regardless of failures, good and excellent clinical results were achieved in 83% of patients.

In 1983, a flexible carbon fiber implant was proposed to provide a scaffold for the growth of a new ligament

(73). In many cases, the carbon fibers induced an inflammatory synovial response, a mild foreign-body–giant-cell reaction, and in some cases, skin breakdown over the carbon-fiber knots. Rather than inducing the formation of a "new ligament," the carbon fiber was covered by a thin, fibrous sheath (74). Use of the prosthetic was eventually abandoned.

EXTRAARTICULAR AUGMENTATION OF ANTERIOR CRUCIATE LIGAMENT RECONSTRUCTION

Extraarticular procedures are rarely used today as the primary technique in reestablishing stability in ACL-deficient knees. A number of authors have studied the effects of adding extraarticular procedures to intraarticular ACL reconstruction. In general, no significant benefit was noted in adding a lateral extraarticular procedure to intraarticular reconstruction techniques.

In 1989, Strum et al. (75) compared intraarticular reconstruction to combined intra- and extraarticular techniques. Eighty-four patients underwent intraarticular reconstruction only (central one-third PT graft or torn meniscus graft), and 43 patients were treated with combined intraarticular and lateral extraarticular procedures. No statistical difference was reported between groups. Similar results were noted by Bray et al. (76), who compared 18 patients treated with a MacIntosh lateral substitution alone to 29 with a combined MacIntosh and intraarticular carbon-fiber replacement of the ACL. No statistically significant difference was found between the two groups at 6 years.

O'Brien et al. (77) evaluated 80 open central-third PT autograft reconstructions for chronic ACL-insufficient knees. In 60% of these cases, a simple lateral sling procedure was added with proximal advancement of distally based, iliotibial band strip deep to the fibular collateral ligament. They concluded that the addition of the lateral sling procedure had no effect on overall outcome, and no longer add this procedure. In 1995, Barrett and Richardson (78) studied the effects of adding an iliotibial band tenodesis to arthroscopically assisted intraarticular reconstruction using PT autograft. Thirty-eight patients underwent intraarticular reconstruction alone, whereas in 32 cases an extraarticular augmentation was added. No statistically significant differences were noted either clinically or subjectively between groups.

CLOSED TECHNIQUES

Arthroscopically Assisted Anterior Cruciate Ligament Reconstruction

Open reconstruction techniques for the ACL-deficient knee utilizing a PT or semitendinosus–gracilis autograft have been shown to produce reliable and acceptable results. However, postoperative difficulties with range of motion and patellofemoral pain associated with these open techniques have been noted (54–58). Arthroscopically assisted techniques have been developed in hopes of avoiding these complications and improving ultimate function and return to activity. By performing the intraarticular portion of the surgery arthroscopically, disruption of the knee capsule and synovial membrane is minimized. In addition, arthroscopic instrumentation has been developed to reliably identify intraarticular positions of graft fixation to maximize isometry.

A diagnostic arthroscopy is performed, routinely using inferomedial, inferolateral, and superomedial portals. The menisci are evaluated and treated with arthroscopic repair or debridement. Recent development of intraarticular electrothermal instrumentation has allowed efficient removal of residual ligament and soft tissue from the notch walls by minimizing bleeding and improving visualization. An enlargement of the intercondylar notch is performed with a mechanized burr, removing bone superiorly and laterally to prevent impingement of the graft during movement of the knee.

The arthroscopic equipment is removed and the autograft harvested. If a central-third PT graft is chosen, an anterior longitudinal incision centered over the PT is used. The tendon is identified and measured, the paratenon carefully incised, and the central one third of the PT with attached bone blocks is harvested. Drill holes are placed in each bone block for traction sutures, followed by contouring of the plugs for ease of passage through the bony tunnels, and highlighting the bone–tendon interface with a surgical marker for intraarticular visualization during graft passage. A piece of cancellous bone from the tibia is used to bone-graft the bony defect in the patella.

If a semitendinosus–gracilis autograft is to be used, a vertical incision approximately 4 cm in length is made centered over the tibial insertion of the tendons, which can be estimated by measuring distally three to four fingerbreadths from the joint line. In thin patients with minimal subcutaneous adipose tissue, these tendons can be palpated 2 cm medial to the tibial crest. The fascia overlying the tendons is cleared of soft tissue, followed by an incision along the superior border of the palpable gracilis tendon. A gloved finger is placed inside the fascial incision, allowing palpation of the two tendons. The tibial insertions are sharply dissected, obtaining maximal length. Blunt digital dissection is then used to completely strip soft-tissue attachments from the tendons to the musculotendinous junction. The tendons are harvested using a tendon stripper, taking care to follow their anatomic course in the thigh to avoid premature amputation of the graft. Muscle tissue is removed from the tendons, followed by creation of a triple-stranded graft. Once the graft is harvested, a second longitudinal incision is made on the lateral aspect of the knee. The iliotibial band is incised along its anterior border, followed by elevation of the vastus lateralis from the lateral intermuscular septum. The lateral femur is exposed subperiosteally just proximal to the condylar flare. The arthroscopic instrumentation is reinserted into the knee joint, and the femoral tunnel created with a rear-entry arthroscopic guide at the lateral incision. Next, the tibial tunnel is placed with the use of a drill guide, passing a guide pin from the anteromedial incision into the knee joint. Tunnel edges are smoothed with a rasp to remove sharp edges and prevent graft erosion during knee range of motion. Measuring the maximum diameter of the semitendinosus–gracilis graft or the bone blocks of the PT graft determines tunnel diameter. The graft is then passed through the tunnels into its final intraarticular position. Prior to fixation, the graft is observed intraarticularly during knee motion to ensure lack of impingement superiorly or laterally. If graft impingement is identified, the notch can be enlarged with curettes or a mechanized burr, followed by final fixation.

In 1993, Buss et al. (79) reviewed 68 cases of arthroscopically assisted ACL reconstruction with an autogenous PT graft at a minimum of 2 years after surgery. The authors concluded that an arthroscopically assisted technique produces results comparable to previous open techniques, but with a decreased rate of postoperative patellofemoral pain and need for manipulation of the knee due to loss of motion. In 1995, Ogilvie-Harris and Sekyi-Out (80) reported an interesting complication associated with the lateral incision for the rear-entry guide. In four cases, heterotopic ossification was noted at the femoral incision site, producing pain, clicking, and a palpable mass. This required a second procedure to remove the heterotopic bone formation, which was successfully completed without loss of stability or function.

In 1998, Bach et al. (81) reported the results of 97 patients treated with an arthroscopically assisted two-incision technique, used a central-third PT graft fixed with interference screws (81). At 5 to 9 years, 83% of patients had a negative pivot shift, and less than 2% asymmetry was noted on functional testing. Overall, 97% of patients were satisfied with their outcome and would undergo the procedure again.

Endoscopic Anterior Cruciate Ligament Reconstruction

In an attempt to further decrease postoperative morbidity and to decrease hospital costs by performing the reconstruction on an outpatient basis, purely endoscopic techniques have been developed that eliminate the need for a lateral femoral incision. Endoscopic techniques differ from arthroscopically assisted techniques by creating the femoral tunnel from inside the joint, thus avoiding the lateral femoral dissection and associated morbidity.

As in the arthroscopically assisted technique, an initial diagnostic arthroscopy is performed, followed by graft harvest, notchplasty, and creation of the tibial tunnel. A Beath pin is passed into the knee joint through the tibial tunnel. The pin can be placed freehand at the anatomic femoral origin, or a femoral OTT referencing guide can be used (Fig. 21.53). If interference screw fixation is to be utilized in the femoral tunnel, a 2-mm bony bridge should be left posteriorly to prevent disruption of the tunnel and loss of interference fit. Once the position of the femoral guide pin is determined, the pin is advanced anterolaterally through the cortex and out through the skin. It is important to maintain the knee flexed more than 90° during passage of the guide pin and subsequent reaming of the femoral tunnel to ensure maintenance of an adequate posterior bony bridge. Next, an appropriately sized acorn reamer is advanced manually through the tibial tunnel to prevent inadvertent widening in this tunnel and injury to the PCL. Tunnel depth is determined by graft selection and screw length.

If a central-third PT graft is chosen, the graft is prepared in the same manner as the arthroscopically assisted technique. Preparation of an HS autograft for endoscopic technique uses a quadruple-stranded semitendinosus–gracilis graft, as shorter graft length is required. Both tendons are stripped of their muscular attachments followed by placement of Bunnell-type traction sutures in each of the free ends of the tendons. The two tendons are then placed side-by-side and doubled over a Cottony–Dacron suture at their midpoint. A surgical marker is used to create a line corresponding to the depth of the femoral tunnel. A suture is placed around the neck of the graft to prevent sliding of the

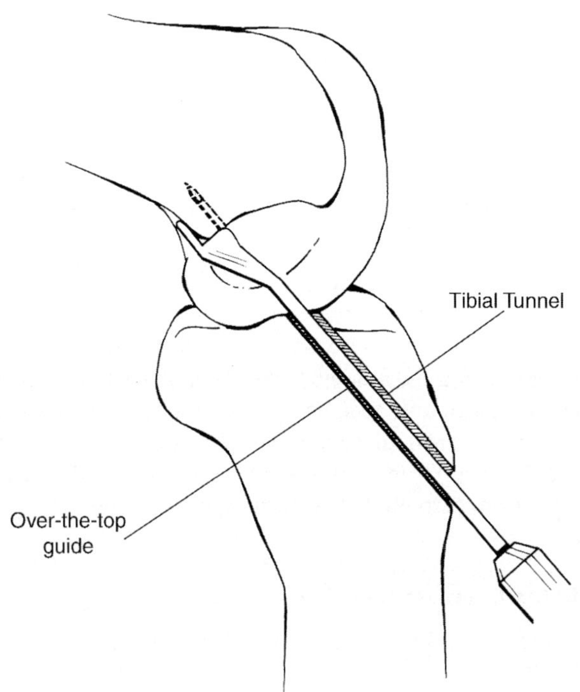

FIGURE 21.53. A Beath pin is passed into the knee joint through the tibial tunnel using a femoral over-the-top referencing guide.

tendons during graft passage. The four legs of the graft are left free to allow equal tensioning of the limbs during final fixation.

The traction suture attached to the femoral side of the graft is passed through the Beath pin. The pin is pulled through the knee joint, bringing the traction suture through the thigh anteriorly. The graft is advanced to its final intraarticular position by pulling on the traction suture and guiding the graft through the tibial tunnel. The mark placed on the graft should be visualized arthroscopically to ensure complete advancement into the femoral tunnel.

Fixation of the PT graft is typically accomplished with interference screws. A variety of fixation devices have been developed for the semitendinosus–gracilis graft, including endoscopically placed buttons at the femoral cortex, bioabsorbable interference screws, transverse pins placed across the femoral tunnel, and interlocking screw devices for fixation of the graft to femoral subchondral or cortical bone. After fixation of the graft, evaluation of range of motion and visualization of the graft is performed to assure lack of impingement and restriction of extension or flexion.

At our institution, we use the endoscopic technique with an autogenous quadruple semitendinosus–gracilis graft. Femoral and tibial tunnel sizes correspond to graft diameter, and fixation is accomplished with bioabsorbable interference screws. To enhance interference fixation, we use screws that are 1 mm in diameter larger than the diameter of the tunnel. We have also developed a low-profile screwdriver (Arthrex, Naples, FL) for use in placement of the femoral interference screw parallel to the femoral tunnel (Fig. 21.54). After insertion of the screw through the inferomedial portal, the screwdriver is advanced through the tibial tunnel anterior to the graft. The screw is placed onto the screwdriver with the use of a hemostat and advanced into the femoral tunnel anterior to the graft. This technique allows parallel placement and advancement of the femoral screw. The four limbs of the graft are tensioned equally through the tibial tunnel while the second interference screw is placed with the knee at 20° of flexion and a posterior drawer applied. We have standardized the depth of screw advancement to leave 5 mm of tunnel for bony ingrowth at both the femoral and tibial insertion sites.

A number of modifications of the endoscopic technique have been described in the literature. Techniques have been developed using a PT graft with press-fit femoral fixation. Malek et al. (82) described creation of a femoral tunnel 1 mm less than the diameter of the bone plug, followed by gentle impaction of the bone plug into the femoral tunnel. By avoiding the use of a screw, potential complications such as loose-screw retrieval and cutting of the graft are avoided. Until bone–interface consolidation occurs, the knee is protected from flexion greater than 100°, because this is the position in which the bone plugs and PT are colinear. Pullout strength has been shown to be

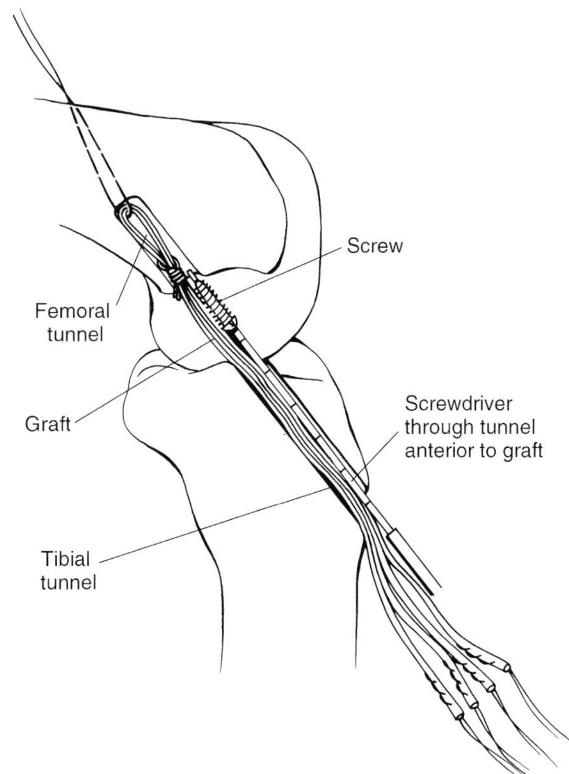

FIGURE 21.54. Low-profile screwdriver (Arthrex, Naples, FL) for use in placement of the femoral interference screw parallel to the femoral tunnel.

similar to strength obtained with an interference screw. Boszotta (83) advocates the use of a circular hollow oscillating saw that allows rapid and standardized harvesting of cylindric bone plugs. This helps to avoid potential patellar fracture due to excessively deep harvest and obviates the need of a femoral interference screw. Placing the knee in 100° of flexion during reaming of the femoral tunnel maximizes femoral pullout strength.

Another modification of the endoscopic technique for PT autograft was described by O'Donnell and Scerpella (84), who suggested the use of an accessory medial parapatellar portal for creation of the femoral tunnel and screw placement. By flexing the knee to 115° and using this relatively distal portal, improvements were noted in screw divergence, tunnel placement, and incidence of graft laceration. Brodie et al. (85) addressed the issue of screw divergence by placing the screwdriver through the tibial tunnel anterior to the graft after introduction of the interference screw through the anteromedial portal, resulting in bone plug–screw divergence angles of less than 5° in nearly 90% of their cases.

In 1998, Bach et al. (86) reviewed 103 patients who had undergone an endoscopic ACL reconstruction with a central-third PT autograft fixed with interference screws. Significant improvement in objective tests of stability was noted, with a negative pivot shift test in 91%, and 4%

to 6% differences in side-to-side functional comparison tests. More than 90% of patients were completely or mostly satisfied with the procedure and indicated that they would undergo the procedure again.

A study published in 1998 by Webb et al. (87) on 82 patients with isolated ACL injuries treated with endoscopic reconstruction with bone–tendon–bone autograft and interference screw fixation demonstrated excellent functional results. Eighty-four percent of patients returned to moderate to strenuous activity. However, graft site pain was present at 24 months in 44% of patients and pain with kneeling was present in 31%.

A rare complication of endoscopic ACL reconstruction was described in a case report by Wiener and Siliski (88). During a revision ACL reconstruction with a PT autograft, at least three passes of the femoral guide pin were made through the anterolateral femoral cortex. At 7 months, the patient suffered a femur stress fracture due to the closely spaced cortical holes. They recommended limiting the number of passes through the femoral cortex by confirming the guide pin position before advancing it through the cortex. If the pin must be repositioned, the angle of knee flexion should be changed to avoid close clustering of cortical holes.

COMPARATIVE STUDIES

Miniarthrotomy Versus Arthroscopically Assisted

Shelbourne et al. (89) studied the effects of arthroscopically assisted techniques in the early postoperative period (<6 months), as most of the anticipated benefits of avoiding open arthrotomy are expected to occur in this time frame. They reported that strength and range of motion improvements and variations occurring at more than 6 months after surgery are most likely due to variables other than the surgical technique. Fifty-two consecutive arthroscopically assisted ACL constructions were matched with 52 miniarthrotomy ACL reconstructions. All knees were reconstructed with autogenous central-third PT grafts. The arthroscopically assisted technique was performed with a lateral femoral approach and a rear-entry drill guide. The open technique was performed through a 6-cm tibial incision followed by a medial arthrotomy. A lateral femoral exposure was created, followed by placement of guide pins. All patients underwent similar postoperative rehabilitative protocols, including immediate full passive extension and early range of motion. No statistical difference was noted between groups in range of motion, KT-1000 measurements, or quadriceps strength scores in the early postoperative period. They concluded that similar successful early clinical results could be achieved with either technique.

In a similar study, Raab et al. (90) hoped to determine whether an arthroscopically assisted technique is less painful, reduces complications, results in more accurate graft placement, and allows rehabilitation to occur more rapidly. One hundred patients were randomly assigned to one of two treatment groups. In the open group, a miniarthrotomy was performed medial to the PT for completion of the notchplasty and determination of graft placement. In the arthroscopically assisted group, these procedures were performed under arthroscopic visualization. A central-third PT autograft was used in all cases, with a rear-entry guide for creation of the femoral tunnel and graft fixation with interference screws. Identical postoperative rehabilitation was followed by both groups, stressing early range of motion followed by strengthening at 6 weeks and running at 8 weeks. No statistically significant difference was identified between the two groups during the first 6 months. Variables measured included thigh atrophy, KT-1000 differences, Lysholm scale, flexion contracture, range of motion, effusion, patellofemoral crepitus, rotational instability, Lachman sign, and complications. Although no differences existed between the two study groups, the authors believe that visualization and femoral tunnel placement are improved in the arthroscopically assisted technique.

Cameron et al. (91) compared an arthroscopically assisted technique with an open procedure using direct visualization of the notchplasty and tunnel placement through a capsulotomy created in the PT defect. The central third of the PT was used as an autograft in both groups. Postoperative rehabilitation was identical, restricting initial range of motion to 10° to 90° of flexion, followed by gradual increase in motion and weight-bearing over 6 months. Results supported the contention that an arthroscopically assisted technique was conducive to better rehabilitation of the quadriceps. The 1-month range of motion, 6-month thigh atrophy, and 6-month quadriceps strength statistically favored the arthroscopically assisted group. Other parameters measured were similar between groups, including postoperative pain, graft placement, and results of Lachman and anterior drawer tests.

Arthroscopically Assisted Versus Endoscopic

Lemos et al. (92) compared femoral interference screw placement in endoscopic and arthroscopically assisted techniques. Fifty patients underwent ACL reconstruction with a PT autograft, equally divided into two groups. In the arthroscopically assisted group, the femoral interference screw was placed under direct visualization through the lateral femoral incision, whereas in the second group the screw was placed endoscopically. Radiographic evaluation revealed no significant divergence in the direct visualization technique, whereas 36% of the endoscopically placed screws showed significant divergence of greater than 5°. The authors raised concern about whether this increased divergence may result in weaker initial fixation strength.

In a study comparing arthroscopically assisted to endoscopic reconstruction techniques, Harner et al. (93) hypothesized that the single incision endoscopic technique would result in equivalent subjective and objective parameters while avoiding the additional incision. Potential benefits would include improved cosmesis, less postoperative pain, and faster rehabilitation. Thirty patients underwent arthroscopically assisted reconstruction with a lateral incision and rear-entry guide; 30 additional knees were reconstructed using a purely endoscopic technique. Central-third PT autografts and allografts were used in all patients. Fifty patients were reviewed at an average of 35 months, and no differences were identified between the groups in the subjective and objective parameters evaluated. A trend was noted in the International Knee Documentation Committee (IKDC) ratings in favor of the endoscopic group. This study concluded that the endoscopic technique is comparable to the traditional two-incision method.

In a similar study, Arciero et al. (94) compared the two procedures using a central-third PT autograft. The decision to use the endoscopic or two-incision technique was based on the length of the autograft. If the total length of the bone–tendon–bone autograft exceeded 10 cm, a two-incision technique was used. Fifty-one patients underwent an arthroscopically assisted reconstruction, whereas 31 patients were reconstructed using an endoscopic technique. Using subjective, objective, and functional criteria, no significant differences were noted between the groups. Trends were identified favoring the endoscopic group in IKDC rating, and the arthroscopically assisted group in increased objective stability. Increased screw divergence was noted radiographically in the endoscopic group. Both techniques provided satisfactory outcomes in most cases.

Reat and Lintner (95) compared the two techniques in an extensive review of subjective and objective parameters. Two groups of 15 patients were evaluated at 15 to 17 months, and no statistically significant difference was identified in operative time, wound complications, early or late postoperative pain and swelling, range of motion, IKDC rating, activity level, function, Lachman test, one-leg hop, isokinetic strength testing, KT-1000 measurements, and increased late laxity. They concluded that the two procedures are essentially identical, both yielding good early results.

In 1997, Sgaglione and Schwartz (96) compared the 2 techniques in 90 consecutive knees reconstructed with either the endoscopic or arthroscopically assisted technique. At approximately 30 to 40 months, no statistically significant differences were noted for complications, including patellofemoral pain, arthrofibrosis, harvest site pathology, or painful hardware. Objective measures of stability were nearly identical in the two groups.

REFERENCES

1. Robson AWM. Ruptured crucial ligaments and their repair by operation. *Ann. Surg* 1903;37:716.
2. Battle WH. A case of suture of the crucial ligaments after open section of the knee-joint for irreducible traumatic dislocation. *Clin Soc Trans* 1900;33:232.
3. Jones R, Smith A. On rupture of the crucial ligaments of the knee, and fractures of the spine of the tibia. *Br J Surg* 1913;1:70.
4. Pringle JH. Avulsion of the spine of the tibia. *Ann Surg* 1907;46;169.
5. O'Donoghue DH. Surgical treatment of fresh injuries to the major ligaments of the knee. *J Bone Joint Surg Am* 1950;32:721–738.
6. O'Donoghue DH. An analysis of end results of surgical treatment of major injuries to the ligaments of the knee. *J Bone Joint Surg Am* 1955;37:1.
7. Liljedahl SO, Lindvall N, Wetterfors J. Early diagnosis and treatment of acute ruptures of the anterior cruciate ligament. *J Bone Joint Surg Am* 1965;47:1503.
8. Marshall JL, Warren RF, Wickiewicz TL, et al. The anterior cruciate ligament: a technique of repair and reconstruction. *Clin Orthop* 1979;143:97–106.
9. Jonsson T, Peterson L, Renstrom P, et al. Augmentation with the longitudinal patellar retinaculum in the repair of an anterior cruciate ligament rupture. *Am J Sports Med* 1989;17:401–408.
10. Groves EWH. Operation for the repair of the crucial ligaments. *Lancet* 1917;11:3.
11. Groves EWH. The crucial ligaments of the knee joint: their function, rupture, and the operative treatment of the same. *Br J Surg* 1919;7:505.
12. Jones KG. Reconstruction of the anterior cruciate ligament: a technique using the central one-third of the patellar ligament. *J Bone Joint Surg Am* 1963;45:925.
13. Jones KG. Reconstruction of the anterior cruciate ligament using the central one-third of the patellar ligament: a follow-up report. *J Bone Joint Surg Am* 1970;52:1302.
14. MacIntosh DL. The anterior cruciate ligament: over-the-top repair. *J Bone Joint Surg Am* 1974;56:1316.
15. Marshall JL, Warren RF, Wickiewicz TL, et al. The anterior cruciate ligament: a technique of repair and reconstruction. *Clin Orthop* 1979;143:97–106.
16. Kornblatt I, Warren RF, Wickiewicz TL. Long-term follow-up of anterior cruciate ligament reconstruction using the quadriceps tendon substitution for chronic anterior cruciate ligament insufficiency. *Am J Sports Med* 1988;16:444.
17. Howe JG, Johnson RJ, Kaplan MJ, et al. Anterior cruciate ligament reconstruction using quadriceps patellar tendon graft, I: long-term follow-up. *Am J Sports Med* 1991;19:447–457.
18. Eriksson E. Reconstruction of the anterior cruciate ligament. *Orthop Clin North Am* 1976;7:167.
19. Alm A, Gillquist J. Reconstruction of the anterior cruciate ligament by using the medial third of the patella ligament. *Acta Chir Scand* 1974;140:289.
20. Drez D. Modified Eriksson procedure for chronic anterior cruciate instability. *Orthopedics* 1978;1:30.
21. Natri A, Jarvinen M, Lehto M, et al. Reconstruction of the chronically insufficient anterior cruciate ligament. *Int Orthop* 1996;20:28.
22. Clancy WG, Nelson DA, Reider B, et al. Anterior cruciate ligament reconstruction using one-third of the patellar ligament, augmented by extra-articular tendon transfers. *J Bone Joint Surg Am* 1982;64:352.
23. Slocum DB, Larson RL. Pes anserinus transplant: a simple surgical procedure for control of rotatory instability of the knee. *J Bone Joint Surg Am* 1968;50:226.
24. McMaster JH, Weinert CR, Scranton P. Diagnosis and management of isolated anterior cruciate ligament tears. *J Trauma* 1974;14:230.
25. Cho KO. Reconstruction of the anterior cruciate ligament by semitendinosus tenodesis. *J Bone Joint Surg Am* 1975;57:608.
26. Lipscomb, AB, Johnston RK, Snyder RB, et al. Secondary reconstruction of anterior cruciate ligament in athletes by using the semitendinosus tendon: preliminary report of 78 cases. *Am J Sports Med* 1979;7:81.
27. Lipscomb AB, Johnston RK, Snyder RB, et al. Evaluation of hamstring strength following use of semitendinosus and gracilis tendons to reconstruct the anterior cruciate ligament. *Am J Sports Med* 1982;10:340.
28. Puddu G. Method for reconstruction of the anterior cruciate ligament using the semitendinosus tendon. *Am J Sports Med* 1983;8:402.
29. Zaricznyj B. Reconstruction of the anterior cruciate ligament of the knee using a doubled tendon graft. *Clin Orth* 1987;220:162.
30. Zarins B, Rowe CR. Combined anterior cruciate ligament reconstruction using semitendinosus tendon and iliotibial tract. *J Bone Joint Surg Am* 1986;68:160.
31. Billotti JD, Meese MA, Alberta F, et al. A prospective, clinical study

evaluating arthroscopic ACL reconstruction using the semitendinosus and iliotibial band: 2- to 5-year follow up. *Orthopedics* 1997;20:125.

32. Brief LP. Anterior cruciate ligament reconstruction without drill holes. *J Arthros Rel Surg* 1991;7:350.

33. Gomes JLE, Marczyk LRS. Anterior cruciate ligament reconstruction with a loop or double thickness of semitendinosus tendon. *Am J Sports Med* 1984;3:199.

34. O'Donoghue DH. Method for replacement of the anterior cruciate ligament of the knee *J Bone Joint Surg Am* 1963;45:905.

35. Insall J, Joseph DM, Aglietti P, et al. Bone-block iliotibial band transfer for anterior cruciate ligament insufficiency. *J Bone Joint Surg Am* 1981;63:560.

36. Hooper GJ, Walton DI. Reconstruction of the anterior cruciate ligament using bone-block iliotibial tract transfer. *J Bone Joint Surg Am* 1987; 69:1150–1154

37. Scott WN, Ferriter P, Marino M. Intra-articular transfer of the iliotibial tract: two- to seven-year follow-up results. *J Bone Joint Surg Am* 1985; 67:532.

38. Bertoia JT, Urovitz EP, Richards RR, et al. Anterior cruciate reconstruction using the MacIntosh lateral-substitution over-the-top repair. *J Bone Joint Surg Am* 1985;67:1183.

39. Freeman BL, Beaty JH, Haynes DB. The pes anserinus transfer: a long-term follow-up. *J Bone Joint Surg Am* 1982;64A:202.

40. MacIntosh DL, Darby TA. Lateral substitution reconstruction. *J Bone Joint Surg Br* 1976;58:142.

41. Ireland J, Trickey EL. MacIntosh tenodesis for anterolateral instability of the knee. *J Bone Joint Surg Br* 1980;62:340.

42. Arnold JA, Coke TP, Heaton LM, et al. Natural history of anterior cruciate tears. *Am J Sports Med* 1979;7:305.

43. Amirault JD, Cameron JC, MacIntosh DL. Chronic anterior cruciate ligament deficiency: long-term results of MacIntosh's lateral substitution reconstruction. *J Bone Joint Surg Br* 1988;70:622.

44. Frank C, Jackson RW. Lateral substitution for chronic isolated anterior cruciate ligament deficiency. *J Bone Joint Surg Br* 1988;70:407.

45. Osterman K, Kujala UM, Kivimaki J, et al. The MacIntosh lateral substitution reconstruction for anterior cruciate deficiency. *Int Orthop (SICOT)* 1993;17:224.

46. Losee RE, Johnson TR, Southwick WD. Anterior subluxation of the lateral tibial plateau. A diagnostic test and operative repair. *J Bone Joint Surg Am* 1978;60:1015.

47. Ellison AE. Distal iliotibial band transfer for anterolateral rotatory instability of the knee. *J Bone Joint Surg Am* 1979;61:330.

48. Durkan JA, Wynne GF, Haggerty JF. Extraarticular reconstruction of the anterior cruciate ligament insufficient knee. *Am J Sports Med* 1989; 17:112.

49. Fox JM, Blazina ME, Del Pizzo W, et al. Extraarticular stabilization of the knee joint for anterior instability. *Clin Orthop* 1980;147:56.

50. Andrews JR, Sanders R. A "mini-reconstruction" technique in treating anterolateral rotatory instability (ALRI). *Clin Orthop* 1983;172:93.

51. James SL. Knee ligament reconstruction. In: Evarts CM, ed. *Surgery of the musculoskeletal system.* New York: Churchill Livingstone, 1983:31–104.

52. Jensen JE, Slocum DB, Larson RL. Reconstruction procedures for anterior cruciate ligament insufficiency: a computer analysis of clinical results. *Am J Sports Med* 1983;11:240.

53. Hughston JC. In: Edmonson AS, Crenshaw AH, eds. *Campbell's operative orthopaedics.* St. Louis: CV Mosby, 1980:972.

54. Halperin N, Hendel D, Fisher S, et al. Anterior cruciate ligament insufficiency syndrome. *Clin Orthop* 1983;179:179–184.

55. Johnson RJ, Eriksson E, Haggmark T, et al. Five- to ten-year follow-up evaluation after reconstruction of the anterior cruciate ligament. *Clin Orthop* 1984;183:122–140.

56. Meyers JF, St. Pierre RK, Sutter JS, et al. Arthroscopic evaluation of anterior cruciate ligament reconstrucitons. *J Arthros Rel Res* 1986;2: 155–161.

57. Roth JH, Kennedy JC, Lockstadt J, et al. Intra-articular reconstruction of the anterior cruciate ligament with or without supplementation by transfer of the biceps femoris tendon. *J Bone Joint Surg Am* 1987;69: 275–278.

58. Graf B, Uhr F. Complications of intraarticular anterior cruciate ligament reconstruction. *Clin Sports Med* 1988;7:835–848.

59. Paulos LE, Rozsenberg TD, Drawbert TJ, et al. Infrapatellar contracture syndrome: an unrecognized cause of knee stiffness with patella entrapment and patella infera. *Am J Sports Med* 1987;15:331–341.

60. Sprague NF. The role of arthroscopic management. *Clin Sports Med* 1987;6:537–549.

61. Kohn D. Arthroscopic evaluation of anterior cruciate ligament reconstruction using a free patellar tendon autograft: a prospective, randomized study. *Clin Orthop* 1990:254:220–224.

62. Meyers JF, St. Pierre RK, Sutter JS. Arthroscopic evaluation of anterior cruciate ligament reconstructions. *J Arthros Rel Surg* 1986;2:155–161.

63. Fujikawa K, Iseki F, Tomatsu T, et al. Microscopic and histological findings after reconstruction of the anterior cruciate ligament reconstruction by the Leeds-Keio artificial ligament. *Knee* 1984;10:35–40.

64. Fujikawa K, Iseki F, Seedhom BB. Arthroscopy after anterior cruciate reconstruction with the Leeds-Keio ligament. *J Bone Joint Surg Br* 1989;71:566–570.

65. Dandy DJ, Gray AJR. Anterior cruciate ligament reconstruction with the Leeds-Keio prosthesis plus extra-articular tenodesis. *J Bone Joint Surg Br* 1994;76:193–197.

66. Richmond JC, Manseau CJ, Patz R, et al. Anterior cruciate reconstruction using a Dacron ligament prosthesis: a long term study. *Am J Sports Med* 1992;20:24–28.

67. Gillquist J, Odensten M. Reconstruction of old anterior cruciate ligament tears with a Dacron prosthesis: a prospective study. *Am J Sports Med* 1993;21:358.

68. Indelicato PA, Pascale MS, Huegel MO. Early experience with the GORE-TEX polytetrafluoroethylene anterior cruciate ligament prosthesis. *Am J Sports Med* 1989;17:55.

69. Kennedy JC, Roth Schmidt AA. The ligament augmentation device (LAD) in the anterior cruciate deficient knee. *Ortho Trans* 1980;4:403.

70. Roth JH, Kennedy JC, Lockstadt H, et al. Polypropylene braid augmented and nonaugmented intraarticular anterior cruciate ligament reconstruction. *Am J Sports Med* 1985;13:321–336.

71. Grontvedt T, Engebretsen L, Bredland T. Arthroscopic reconstruction of the anterior cruciate ligament using bone-patellar tendon-bone grafts with and without augmentation. *J Bone Joint Surg Br* 1996;78: 817–822.

72. Kdolsky RK, Gibbons DF, Kwasny O, et al. Braided polypropylene augmentation device in reconstructive surgery of the anterior cruciate ligament: long term clinical performance of 594 patients and short-term arthroscopic results, failure analysis by scanning electron microscopy, and synovial histomorphology. *J Orthop Res* 1997;1:1–10.

73. Jenkins DHR, Forster IW, McKibbin B, et al. Induction of tendon and ligament formation by carbon implants. *J Bone Joint Surg Br* 1977;59:53.

74. Rushton N, Dandy DJ, Naylor CPE. The clinical, arthroscopic and histologic findings after replacement of the anterior cruciate ligament with carbon-fibre. *J Bone Joint Surg Br* 1983;65:308–309.

75. Strum GM, Fox JM, Ferkel RD, et al. Intraarticular versus intraarticular and extraarticular reconstruction for chronic anterior cruciate ligament instability. *Clin Orthop* 1989;245:188–198.

76. Bray RC, Flanagan JP, Dandy DJ. Reconstruction for chronic anterior cruciate instability. *J Bone Joint Surg Br* 1988;70:100–105.

77. O'Brien SJ, Warren RF, Wickiewicz TL, et al. The iliotibial band lateral sling procedure and its effect on the results of anterior cruciate ligament reconstruction. *Am J Sports Med* 1991;19:21–24, discussion 24–25.

78. Barrett GR, Richardson KJ. The effect of added extra-articular procedure on results of ACL reconstruction. *Am J Knee Surg* 1995;8:1–6.

79. Buss DD, Warren RF, Wickiewicz TL, et al. Arthroscopically assisted reconstruction of the anterior cruciate ligament with use of autogenous patellar-ligament grafts. *J Bone Joint Surg Am* 1993;759:1346–1355.

80. Ogilvie-Harris DJ, Sekyi-Out A. Periarticular heterotopic ossification: a complication of arthroscopic anterior cruciate ligament reconstruction using a two-incision technique. *J Arthrosc Rel Surg* 1995;11: 676–679.

81. Bach BR, Tradonsky S, Bojchuk J, et al. Single-incision endoscopic anterior cruciate reconstruction using patellar tendon autograft. *Am J Sports Med* 1998;26:20–29.

82. Malek MM, DeLuca JV, Verch DL, et al. Arthroscopically assisted ACL reconstruction using central-third patellar tendon autograft with press-fit femoral fixation. *Instr Course Lec* 1996;45:287–295.

83. Boszotta H. Arthroscopic anterior cruciate ligament reconstruction using a patellar tendon graft in press-fit technique: surgical technique and follow-up. *J Arthrosc Rel Surg* 1997;13:332–339.

84. O'Donnell JB, Scerpella T. Endoscopic anterior cruciate ligament reconstruction: modified technique and radiographic review. *J Arthrosc Rel Surg* 1995;11:577–584.

85. Brodie JT, Torpey BM, Donald GD, et al. Femoral interference screw

placement through the tibial tunnel: a radiographic evaluation of inter-ference screw divergence angles after endoscopic anterior cruciate lig-ament reconstruction. *J Arthrosc Rel Surg* 1996;12:435–440.

86. Bach BR, Tradonsky S, Bojchuk J, et al. Arthroscopically assisted ante-rior cruciate ligament reconstruction using patellar tendon autograft. *Am J Sports Med* 1998;26:30–40.

87. Webb JM, Corry IS, Clingeleffer AJ, et al. Endoscopic reconstruction of isolated anterior cruciate ligament rupture. *J Bone Joint Surg Br* 1998;80:288–294.

88. Wiener DF, Siliski JM. Distal femoral shaft fracture: a complication of endoscopic anterior cruciate ligament reconstruction. *Am J Sports Med* 1996;24:244–247.

89. Shelbourne KD, Rettig AC, Hardin G, et al. Miniarthrotomy versus arthroscopic-assisted anterior cruciate ligament reconstruction with autogenous patellar tendon graft. *J Arthrosc Rel Surg* 1993;9:72–75.

90. Raab DJ, Fischer DA, Smith JP, et al. Comparison of arthroscopic and open reconstruction of the anterior cruciate ligament: early results. *Am J Sports Med* 1993;21:680–683, discussion 683–684.

91. Cameron SE, Wilson W, St Pierrre P. A prospective, randomized com-parison of open vs arthroscopically assisted ACL reconstruction. *Orthopedics* 1995;18:249–252.

92. Lemos MJ, Albert J, Simon T, et al. Radiographic analysis of femoral interference screw placement during ACL reconstruction: endoscopic versus open technique. *J Arthrosc Rel Surg* 1993;9:154–158.

93. Harner CD, Marks PH, Fu FH, et al. Anterior cruciate ligament recon-struction: endoscopic versus two-incision technique. *J Arthrosc Rel Surg* 1994;10:502–512.

94. Arciero RA, Scoville CR, Snyder RJ, et al. Single versus two-incision arthroscopic anterior cruciate ligament reconstruction. *J Arthrosc Rel Surg* 1996;12:462–469.

95. Reat J-FP, Lintner DM. One- versus two-incision ACL reconstruction. *Am J Knee Surg* 1997;10:198–208.

96. Sgaglione NA, Schwartz RE. Arthroscopically assisted reconstruction of the anterior cruciate ligament: initial clinical experience and mini-mal 2-year follow-up comparing endoscopic transtibial and two-inci-sion techniques. *J Arthrosc Rel Surg* 1997;13:156–165.

CHAPTER 22

Rehabilitation after Anterior Cruciate Ligament Reconstruction

K. Donald Shelbourne and Thomas E. Klootwyk

The approach to the surgical treatment of knee injuries has changed during the 1990s. In previous years, patients with acute knee injuries had acute surgical repair or reconstruction and then were immobilized for protection. Rehabilitation was initiated later after a period of time to allow graft healing. Rehabilitation now begins preoperatively from the time of the acute injury.

This chapter will describe our approach for a patient who has sustained an anterior cruciate ligament (ACL) injury. We will present the specifics of our ACL rehabilitation program and will emphasize the principles of the program that are applicable to most knee surgeries.

ANTERIOR CRUCIATE LIGAMENT RECONSTRUCTION REHABILITATION

Our ACL rehabilitation program is divided into four phases. The first phase is prescribed preoperatively at the time of the initial diagnosis and continues until the patient has surgery. The second phase begins during surgery when the surgeon ensures that the knee has full range of motion (ROM) after the fixation of the graft. Full ROM is defined as ROM equal to that of the opposite uninjured knee. The phase continues during the first 2 weeks after surgery with emphasis on controlling swelling, regaining ROM (especially full hyperextension), and restoring a normal gait pattern. The third phase usually starts 2 weeks after surgery and involves maintaining full hyperextension and obtaining the final degrees of full flexion. The introduction of simple strengthening and agility activities are added along with stationary biking and stair-stepper workouts. The third phase usually lasts for 2 to 3 weeks. The fourth and final phase begins when the patient has full knee ROM, adequate strength, and confidence in the reconstructed knee. During this phase, leg strength returns to normal and the patient is advanced back into athletic activities.

Phase I: Preoperative

The preoperative rehabilitation phase may be the most important factor in decreasing postoperative rehabilitation problems. The goal of the phase I rehabilitation is to restore full knee ROM and a normal gait and to eliminate knee swelling. The delay in surgery is also used to better prepare the patient mentally for the reconstructive procedure. The combination of avoiding acute surgery and initiating preoperative rehabilitation has done a great deal to advance the recovery and decrease postoperative ROM problems (1,2).

The decision to proceed with the reconstructive surgery is not made on the basis of a certain amount of time from the injury to surgery but is made on the basis of the condition of the knee. Often a 3-week period is stated as the time needed to wait until it is acceptable to proceed with the knee operation. Although, in some cases, 3 weeks will be enough time for the patient to achieve the preoperative goals, some patients may take longer. When the patient has full knee ROM, no knee swelling, a normal gait, and good quadriceps muscle tone, the knee is ready to undergo surgery.

Once the diagnosis of an ACL injury is made, the rehabilitation process is started. The patient sees a physical therapist who will outline the preoperative rehabilitation program for the patient. The patient is shown what exercises to do and how to do them and then is expected to perform the rehabilitation exercises without supervision. The prescribed exercises should be performed three to four times per day and they usually can be done at home or at a health club without the assistance of a physical therapist or athletic trainer.

The first area to be addressed is swelling and pain control. At the initial visit, the patient receives a cold–compression device (Cryo/Cuff; Aircast, Summit, NJ) that can be used throughout the preoperative and postopera-

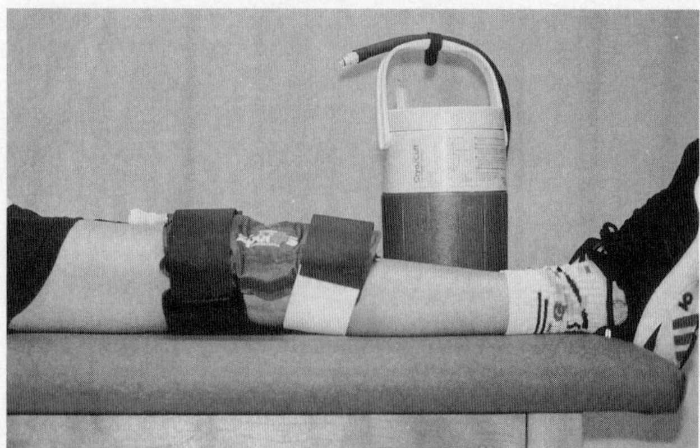

FIGURE 22.1. A Cryo/Cuff provides cold and compression therapy to reduce pain and swelling.

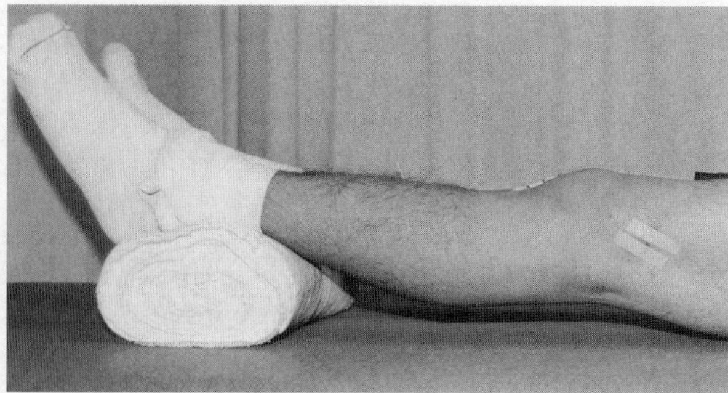

FIGURE 22.2. Heel prop. The heel of the affected leg is propped on a rolled towel so that the thigh is elevated off of the table or floor.

tive rehabilitation process (Fig. 22.1). The device provides not only cold therapy but also compression to reduce pain and swelling. The patient uses the Cryo/Cuff nearly continuously for the first few days after injury. When the knee improves with decreased swelling and less pain, the Cryo/Cuff is used three to four times per day after the rehabilitation exercises are performed.

The second problem to address preoperatively is the lack of full knee ROM. Ninety-seven percent of people have at least some degree of hyperextension in their knees (3). Therefore, when full ROM is to be restored before surgery, the goal is to achieve full hyperextension equal to that of the opposite uninjured knee. The ROM exercises are divided into two areas, extension and flexion. With an acute ACL tear, the patient will hold the knee bent in 10° to 15° of flexion and will complain of pain behind the patella or patellar tendon. This is primarily because the acutely torn ACL becomes impinged as the tibia and femur come into contact with each other when the knee approaches full hyperextension. Secondarily, the pain can be from a bone bruise on the lateral femur and tibia. To be able to restore full knee ROM, two simple exercises are demonstrated: heel props and prone hangs. A heel prop is an exercise where the patient props the heel of the affected leg on a rolled towel (Fig. 22.2). The towel height should be just high enough to elevate the thigh of the affected extremity off the table or floor. With the injured lower extremity in this position, the knee is allowed to relax into extension. In the injured setting, the patient must concentrate on relaxing the hamstring muscles because the muscles will often contract when the knee is placed in this position. The heel prop exercise should be performed three to four times per day for 10 minutes each time.

A second exercise to help regain extension is the prone hang. In this exercise, the patient lies down in a prone position and allows the lower extremities to extend off the end of the table (Fig. 22.3). The distal thigh must be even with the edge of the table to be able to perform the exercise properly. Once again, the patient must concentrate on relaxing the hamstring muscles to allow the knee to achieve full hyperextension. The patient performs this activity three to four times per day for 10 minutes each time. If a table is not available at home, we have found that a set of stairs will work just as well. The patient can lie down at the top of a stairway to extend off the edge of the top step.

When the patient is having difficulty with achieving full hyperextension in spite of compliance with the above exercises, a hyperextension device can be used (Fig. 22.4). This simple device allows the patient to prop the heel on a contoured foam wedge and apply tension on the leg with three Velcro straps. When the leg relaxes, the straps can be adjusted to keep constant pressure toward full hyperextension. The extension board is often loaned to the patient so the exercise can be performed at home.

Exercises to regain full flexion are also performed during the preoperative phase of rehabilitation. The wall slide exercise is performed during the early phases of the rehabilitation when the patient is having difficulty achieving past 90° of flexion. This is a simple exercise done with the patient lying supine and with the foot of the affected extremity on the wall (Fig. 22.5). The patient can easily control the amount of flexion by allowing the foot to slide slowly down the wall.

Once the patient can achieve at least 95° to 100° of flexion, the heel slide exercise is introduced to increase flexion further. The heel slide exercise is performed with the patient's back against the wall. The amount of flexion is increased by pulling the lower leg back toward the buttocks (Fig. 22.6). Surgery will be delayed until the patient has full ROM (full hyperextension and full flexion) equal to that of the opposite uninjured knee.

The third goal of preoperative rehabilitation is to restore a normal gait and to gain leg strength. After the ACL is injured, the patient typically will walk with a bent knee gait pattern. Our goal is to restore the gait to normal as soon as possible after the injury. The patient is instructed how to walk with a normal heel-to-toe gait pattern. The use of crutches for assistance is advised until the patient can walk without a limp. We have found that walking in front of a mirror will greatly assist the patient

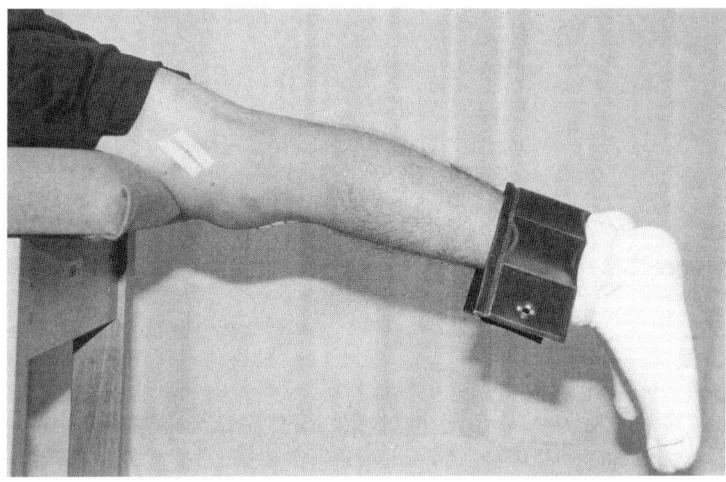

FIGURE 22.3. Prone hang. The patient lies prone so that the distal thighs are at the edge of the table and the lower extremities extend off of the table.

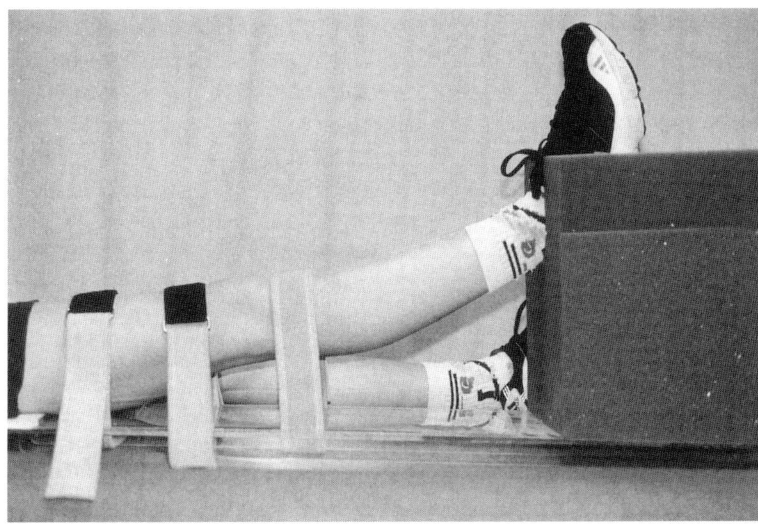

FIGURE 22.4. A hyperextension device is used for patients who are having difficulty achieving full hyperextension equal to the normal contralateral knee.

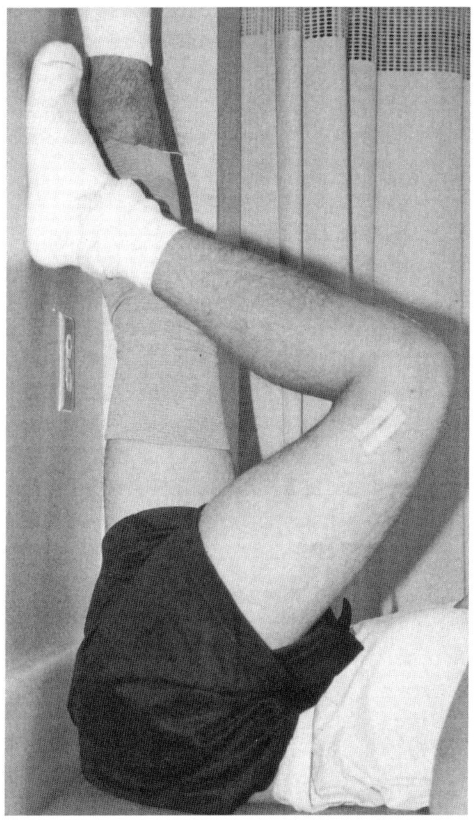

FIGURE 22.5. Wall slide. The foot of the affected leg is placed on the wall and the patient can control the amount of flexion by slowly sliding the foot down the wall.

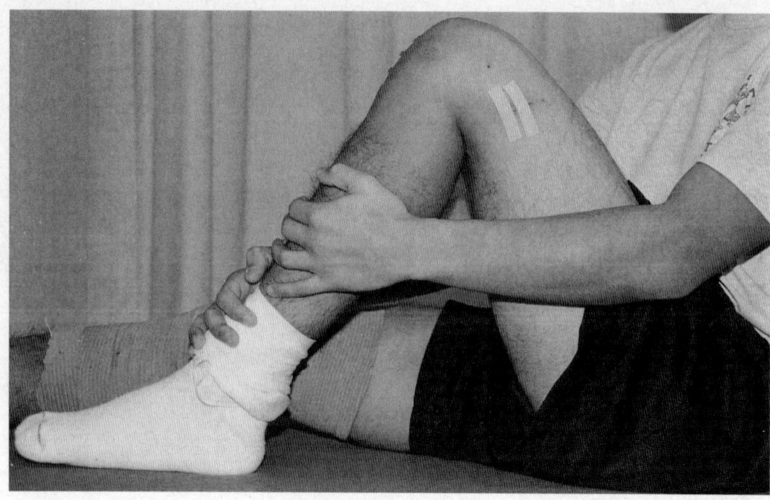

FIGURE 22.6. Heel slides. Once more than 90° of flexion is obtained, heel slides are more useful for gaining flexion.

become aware of how he or she is walking (Fig. 22.7). Walking with a limp can become a habit that is better avoided.

Once swelling has subsided and good ROM and a normal gait have been achieved, leg-strengthening exercises can begin. These exercises are simple and can be performed without the help of a physical therapist. The strengthening activities include quarter knee bends, step-ups at varying degrees of step height, and short-arc quadriceps muscle exercises. The goal of strengthening is to increase strength without increasing knee soreness or swelling.

If the patient wants to undergo surgery as soon as the knee is ready, the strengthening exercises will almost always be limited to the above exercises. If the patient wants to delay the ACL reconstruction until a more convenient time, more aggressive strengthening exercises would include weight-lifting exercises such as leg press, hip sled, and squats.

The last area of the preoperative rehabilitation is patient education and instruction. The mental preparation of the patient is very important to ensure a good clinical result. The more that patients know about the ACL-reconstructive surgery, the less apprehensive they will be with the entire process, and it is our opinion that the patients, therefore, will enjoy a better result.

At the initial visit, we go to great lengths to explain the nature of the ACL tear and the details of the operative reconstruction, the preoperative and postoperative rehabilitation, and the appropriate timing of the surgery. The patient is shown a model of how the reconstruction is performed and a picture booklet of the rehabilitation process (Fig. 22.8). Written details of the surgery and rehabilitation are given to all patients.

Once the patient achieves the preoperative goals, surgery can be performed at any time. If the patient is a student and cannot miss school or tests, the surgery is delayed until a convenient time such as a school vacation. The timing of surgery also applies to someone who is working and has important trips, projects, or meetings scheduled. The surgery is delayed until a convenient time when the patient is able to devote time to knee rehabilitation.

In summary, the preoperative phase of the rehabilitation involves the mental and physical preparation of the patient for surgery. The injured knee should have full

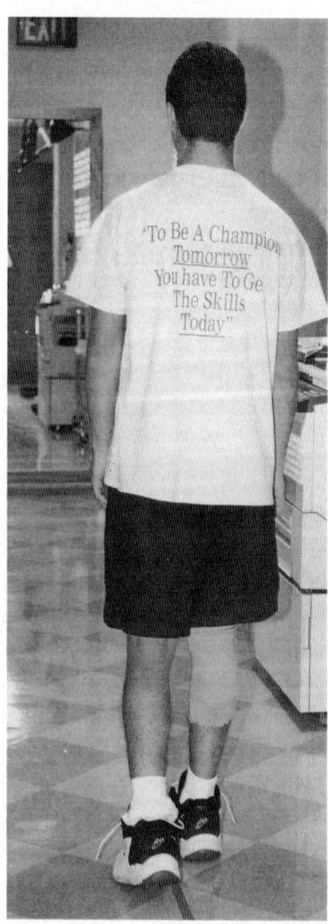

FIGURE 22.7. Walking in front of a mirror gives visual feedback to the patient regarding gait.

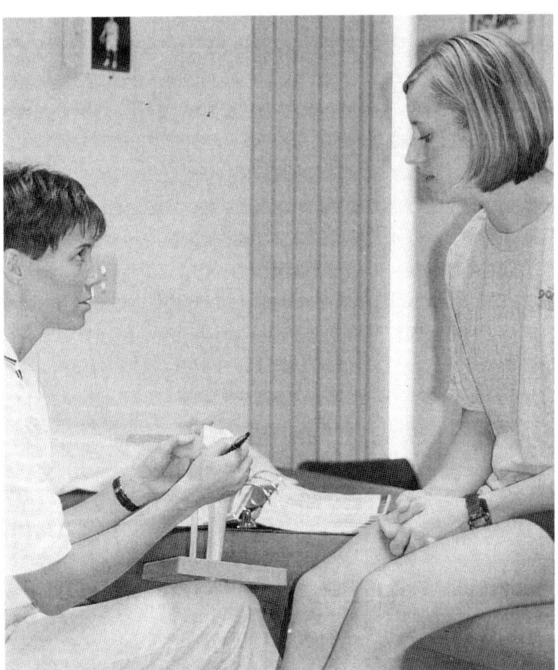

FIGURE 22.8. The surgical procedure and rehabilitation is explained in detail to the patient.

ROM equal to that of the other knee and no knee swelling; the patient should also walk with a normal gait. The patient should fully understand the reconstructive surgery and rehabilitation process. In addition, the surgery should be scheduled at a time that is convenient for school, work, or family schedules.

Phase II: Perioperative

The goals of phase II of the rehabilitation process are to control postoperative swelling, maintain full knee hyperextension, achieve 110° of knee flexion, and start early quadriceps muscle exercises. Phase II begins in the operating room with the fixation of the patellar tendon graft. After the graft is secured into place, the knee is moved through full ROM. We use a suture–button fixation, which is an advantage because the sutures can be retensioned after the knee is moved through full ROM. The suture–button fixation ensures that the fixation of the graft will not capture the knee and limit ROM during the postoperative rehabilitation. After the surgical wounds are closed and the postoperative dressings are applied, the patient is taken to the recovery room for a short stay. Although the rehabilitation has been called "accelerated," the first week after the reconstructive surgery is one of strict bed rest and adherence to the rehabilitation program. After the reconstruction, we admit our patients to the hospital for one night, which gives us several advantages. First, this allows us to begin the patient with the proper rehabilitation program that is to be fol-

lowed for the first week after the reconstruction. Second, it allows the administration of intravenous ketorolac, which provides the patient with excellent postoperative pain relief (4). In addition, our office staff reviews the first-week rehabilitation program with the patient on the morning after the surgery to ensure that the patient is performing the rehabilitation properly.

When the patient arrives to the hospital room after surgery, the reconstructed knee is placed into a continuous passive motion (CPM) machine. The CPM machine is set to move from 0° of extension to 30° of flexion. The patient uses the CPM at all times except when performing specific rehabilitation exercises. We have attempted to discontinue the use of the CPM in the past, but, in office surveys of our patients, the CPM has been rated very highly for providing comfort and decreasing stiffness and important to the recovery from surgery. The CPM provides a predictable means of knee elevation after surgery, and it is used for flexion exercises during the first week.

The maintenance of full knee hyperextension after surgery is an important part of the first week of the rehabilitation program. The patient begins heel prop exercises after being settled into the hospital room. The heel props are performed for 10 minutes each hour from 8 a.m. to 10 p.m. each day for the first week after surgery. In the hospital, the patient uses the end of the bed frame to prop the heel and allow the knee to relax back into full knee hyperextension. A 2-lb (4 to 5 kg) ankle weight can be added to the front of the tibia to assist in the achievement of full hyperextension. As before surgery, full hyperextension is defined as the amount of hyperextension that is present in the opposite normal knee.

The reason for the emphasis on the maintaining full knee hyperextension after surgery is to avoid the symptoms that a postoperative flexion contracture causes, such as activity-related anterior knee pain (5). By maintaining full knee hyperextension after surgery, the newly placed ligament fits perfectly into the notch and prevents this space from potentially filling in with scar tissue, sometimes referred to as a cyclops lesion, and later becoming a block to full hyperextension. The patient continues the hourly hyperextension exercise while at home for the first week after surgery. Instead of a bed frame, a rolled-up towel on the end of the couch can be used.

A second area of emphasis during the first week after surgery is the control of swelling. We use three different methods to accomplish our goal. First, the Cryo/Cuff is placed on the patient's knee in the operating room as part of the postoperative dressings. The patient uses the Cryo/Cuff continually during the first week of recovery except when performing the rehabilitation exercises. Second, the CPM provides a predictable means of knee elevation, which helps control swelling. Third, we emphasize activity modification that restricts the patient to be lying down except to go to the bathroom or to sit at a table to eat meals. We believe that when activities are kept to a minimum for the first week after surgery, patients are not only more comfortable, but they can then proceed with the ROM and strengthening exercises that allow them to return to normal activities of daily living by 2 to 3 weeks after surgery.

A third area of emphasis after the ACL reconstruction is the importance of maintaining leg control through the use of quadriceps muscle exercise. The ability to maintain good leg control in the early postoperative setting assists the patient with ambulation. We recommend three methods to maintain and improve the quadriceps muscle group. First, the patient lifts the reconstructed knee out of the CPM machine at the beginning of each hourly session of extension exercises (Fig. 22.9). Second, the patient performs isometric quadriceps contraction with both legs during the extension session. The isometric contractions are held for 10 seconds, and a set of ten repetitions is performed during each session. Third, the patient does straight leg raises with the opposite normal knee while the patient does the heel prop exercise with the reconstructed knee (Fig. 22.10). This exercise maintains quadriceps muscle leg control in the opposite leg and it automatically "fires" the contralateral quadriceps muscle of the reconstructed leg.

A fourth area of emphasis during the first week after surgery is to increase flexion. Patients begin to work on flexion 4 to 5 hours after the ACL reconstruction. With the Cryo/Cuff removed, the knee is gently flexed up to 110° by increasing the degree of flexion to the highest setting on the CPM machine. The patient controls the speed of the ascent up to 110°. Once the knee is flexed fully in the machine, the machine is placed on pause for 10 minutes. Afterwards, the CPM machine is returned to the normal setting of moving from 0° to 30° of flexion.

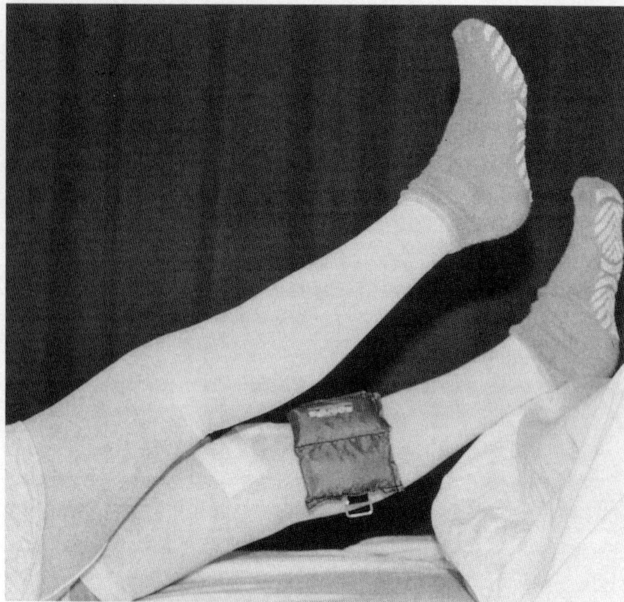

FIGURE 22.10. To maintain quadriceps leg control, the patient can perform straight leg raises with the normal knee while working on extension for the reconstructed knee.

The patient performs the flexion exercise five times per day during the first week after surgery.

Ambulation is the last area of rehabilitation to be addressed with the patients before discharge from the hospital. Although the patients are asked to limit ambulation during the first week after surgery, when they do ambulate, they should attempt to regain a normal gait pattern. Patients are taught to practice a heel-to-toe gait with the assistance of crutches. Patients use crutches until they can ambulate without limping, which usually can be achieved at 1 to 2 weeks after surgery.

Patients are discharged on the morning after the surgery and are instructed to follow the exercise program that was begun in the hospital. For a reminder, a daily exercise chart is given to the patient to complete.

To ensure that the patient is on a correct clinical course, the first follow-up examination is performed by the physician and the physical therapist 1 week after the ACL reconstructive surgery. It is easier to identify and correct problems with ROM, swelling, or poor leg control at 1 week than it is to wait until 2 to 3 weeks after surgery.

During the first visit, the patient is seen by the surgeon to check operative wounds, assess hyperextension and flexion, and evaluate the degree of swelling. The patient is also seen by a physical therapist to advance the rehabilitation program depending on the patient's knee status. At this time, the patient's rehabilitation program changes from the regimented hourly rehabilitation program to a more goal-oriented program.

The goals of the second week of the rehabilitation program are to maintain full knee hyperextension and to con-

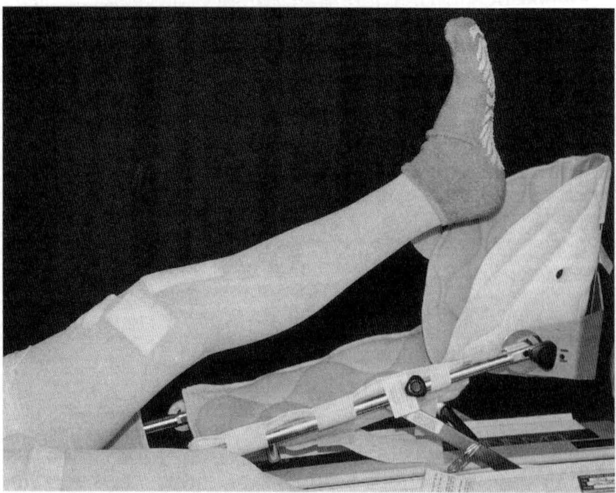

FIGURE 22.9. With his or her own power, the patient should be able to lift the reconstructed leg out of the continuous passive motion machine.

trol swelling by gradually increasing the amount of daily activities. Other goals during the second week of rehabilitation are to resume a normal gait pattern without crutches and to increase knee flexion.

Instead of the hourly extension exercises that the patient did during the first week, the patient is instructed to perform heel props or prone hangs three to four times per day. The number of times the patient does the exercise is not as important as maintaining full knee hyperextension each and every day throughout the week. The patient should perform the hyperextension exercises as much as is needed to maintain full knee hyperextension every day.

To control swelling, patients are encouraged to increase gradually the amount of time walking and doing daily activities. While resting, the leg should be elevated with the Cryo/Cuff on the knee. Usually by 2 weeks after surgery, the patient can tolerate a full day of school activities or a full day of working at a desk.

In addition to extension exercises and an increase in activity the second week after surgery, the patient is guided in the restoration of a normal gait pattern. Patients are reinstructed about a normal gait pattern by watching themselves walk in front of a mirror. Our goal is to have the patients ambulating with a normal gait by the end of the second week after surgery.

The final area of emphasis during the second week after the reconstruction is flexion. At 1 week after surgery, our goal is for the patient to have 90° of knee flexion; at 2 weeks after surgery our goal is 110° to 120° of flexion. This sounds like a large increase, but, if the patient improves flexion by 3° to 4° each day, the flexion goal will be achieved by the end of the second week. The patients can perform and advance these rehabilitation exercises as tolerated. They will be reevaluated at the 2-week postoperative visit by both the surgeon and the physical therapist.

At the 2-week visit, the sutures are removed from the surgical wounds and the patient is advanced further on the rehabilitation program. If the goals of phase II have been met, the patient advances to phase III of the rehabilitation program.

Phase III: Intermediate Postoperative

At the 2-week postoperative visit, the importance of achieving the final degrees of flexion is emphasized. Near the end of this phase of rehabilitation, early functional strengthening exercises and functional sport-specific activities begin.

The final amount of flexion is gained through daily consistent exercise with heel slides. It is important for the patient to understand that at least 130° of flexion must be obtained before intensive strengthening can begin. If aggressive strengthening exercises are attempted before adequate flexion is present, the patient will struggle with obtaining full symmetric flexion and the desired gains in strength will not be realized.

Once 130° of flexion is obtained, aggressive strengthening exercises, such as the stair-stepper and bike workouts, are added to the patient's rehabilitation routine. These activities are not only important for the cardiovascular fitness of the patient but are also an excellent means of early quadriceps and hamstring muscle strengthening. Also, traditional weight-training exercises are added as long as the knee has minimal swelling and the patient has a normal gait. The exercises consist of half-squats, leg press, hip sled, and also some short-arc quadriceps exercises. The time when more formal strength work is started is variable and depends on the status of the patient's knee. We believe that if the rehabilitation goals of 130° of flexion, normal gait, and minimal swelling have been met, there is no reason not to advance the patient back into a more aggressive workout routine. If the patient has not met these goals, aggressive strengthening is not introduced until they are met.

The patient is instructed to perform formal strengthening exercises three times per week. During this early strengthening phase, the patient will feel some tenderness in the area of the patellar tendon. Our instruction to the patient is that some aching in the tendon is desirable because it means that the tendon is being stressed appropriately for gaining strength. If the patient finds that the strengthening exercises lead to an increase in anterior knee pain that persists for 1 to 2 days after the workout, the intensity of the workout needs to be decreased until the symptoms are controlled. Only then can the workout intensity be gradually increased while still controlling for tendon soreness.

An additional area of rehabilitation that is introduced at the beginning of phase III is sport-specific drills. The early agility drills can be the same no matter what sport the athlete plays, but when the general agility activities are mastered, more sport-specific drills are encouraged. For example, if a patient desires to return to basketball, he or she should begin shooting baskets at 3 to 4 weeks after surgery. When confidence and leg strength increase, the activities on the basketball court are advanced. The athlete advances to passing, dribbling, and defensive slide drills, and when those drills are tolerated well, ball-reaction drills are added to the routine. Ball-reaction drills assist the patient with concentrating on the ball and movement of the legs to an unpredictable situation, which allows the athlete to work on reaction time and gaining confidence in the surgically repaired knee. When confidence improves, the patient advances to playing some structured one-on-one, then two-on-two and three-on-three, and finally, full-court basketball.

As you have probably noted, the patient still has not started a formal running program, which is by design. It is our opinion that a formal running program is the last activity that a patient should do. We have observed that when the knee is in the early postoperative phase, the extensor mechanism is still recovering strength. We have also noted that running is an impact activity that the knee does not tolerate well when quadriceps muscle strength is not at least 75% of that of the normal leg. Therefore, we prefer that running be done when the patient does activities that are specific to the desired sport. At or before this time, the patient undergoes the initial postoperative stability and strength testing. The tests are done when the patient has achieved full knee ROM and has had the opportunity to work on strength of the involved extremity. The testing includes a KT-1000 manual maximum test (see Chapter 19C), isokinetic strength testing, leg-press strength testing, and a single-leg hop test. If the patient has a stable knee and adequate strength (isokinetic testing at 180 degrees per second of 60% or greater), he or she is advanced in the rehabilitation program as tolerated.

Phase IV: Final Postoperative

The final phase of the rehabilitation program is the return to full sporting activities. As with the previous three phases of the rehabilitation program, a specific time line is not used; instead the readiness of the knee determines when the patient is ready to return to sports. This phase involves the athlete working with the training and coaching staff on increasing the amount and intensity of the patient's participation in practice. Once again, it is not the time after surgery that is important, but it is the condition of the reconstructed knee and how the athlete is performing in practice and games. We have found that a "functional progression" program provided by the physical therapy staff is of great benefit to the patient at this stage of the rehabilitation process (Table 22.1).

It is important to emphasize that even though the patient has returned to playing sports, the rehabilitation of the knee is not complete. In addition to regular practice, the athlete will still need to do strengthening exercises to regain the final amount of strength and will also need to do additional agility and quickness drills until the feeling of playing normally returns. We have noted that the final aspect of the patient's recovery is the return of the "first step" of quickness. It will often take 2 to 3 months of sport-specific activity before the athlete has completely recovered.

During the recovery phase when the athlete increases the level of activity and practice participation, testing of the knee is done in our physical therapy department. The tests are the same as those performed during phase III of the rehabilitation program, which makes it easy to evaluate progress and guide the patient into areas that still require some rehabilitation.

TABLE 22.1. *Functional progression program*

1. Heel raises on injured leg, 10 times
2. Walk at a fast pace, 50 yd
3. Jumping on both legs, 10 times
4. Jumping on the involved leg, 10 times
5. Jog straight, 50 yd
6. Jog straight and curves, 2 laps
7. Sprint, 40 yd at half speed, ¾-speed, full speed
8. Run figure 8's, 15 yd at half speed, ¾ speed, full speed
9. Cariocas (crossover step), 40 yd, both directions
10. Backward running
11. Cutting to change directions, half speed, ¾ speed, full speed
12. Specific position drills

Finally, all patients are asked to return for research visits at the 1-, 2-, 5-, and 10-year postoperative dates. These visits are used to retest the patient and to evaluate the long-term results of the ACL reconstruction.

SUMMARY

The principles presented in this chapter can be applied to most knee injuries and surgeries. We believe that by taking a perioperative approach to rehabilitation, most of the complications associated with surgery can be prevented. Regardless of the patient's goal for returning to activities, the goal of rehabilitation is to provide a smooth postoperative course that restores the knee to feeling as normal as possible. This goal can be accomplished in most cases with the combination of preoperative and early postoperative modalities and exercises that limit swelling and restore full knee ROM and a normal gait. For patients who followed a perioperative rehabilitation program with ACL reconstruction, the results showed that most patients had good stability, full ROM, a low complication rate, and a predictable return to activities (6).

REFERENCES

1. Mohtadi NGH, Webster-Bogaert S, Fowler PJ. Limitation of motion following anterior cruciate reconstruction: a case control study. *Am J Sports Med* 1991;19:620–624, discussion 624–625.
2. Fisher SE, Shelbourne KD. Arthroscopic treatment of symptomatic extension block complicating anterior cruciate ligament reconstruction. *Am J Sports Med* 1993;21:558–564.
3. DeCarlo MS, Sell K. Normative data for range of motion and single leg hop in high school athletes. *J Sports Rehab* 1997;6:246–255.
4. Shelbourne KD, Liotta FJ, Goodloe SL. Preemptive pain management program for anterior cruciate ligament reconstruction. *Am J Knee Surg* 1998;11:116–119.
5. Shelbourne KD, Trumper RV. Preventing anterior knee pain after anterior cruciate ligament reconstruction. *Am J Sports Med* 1997;25:41–47.
6. Shelbourne KD, Gray T. Anterior cruciate ligament reconstruction with autogenous patellar tendon graft followed by accelerated rehabilitation: a two- to nine-year follow-up. *Am J Sports Med* 1997;25:786–795.

CHAPTER 23

Treatment of Specific Injuries

Part A: Collateral Ligament Injuries

T. Tadashi Funahashi, Diane C. Hillard-Sembell, and Donald C. Fithian

Injuries to the medial collateral ligament (MCL) are the most common ligamentous injuries of the knee, whereas lateral collateral ligament (LCL) injuries are among the least common. In a study of an unselected segment of the general population who presented to a knee injury clinic over a 13-year period, 32% of the injuries in patients with pathologic laxity were isolated injuries to the MCL and 3% represented isolated injuries to the LCL (see Chapter 18). Similarly, Howe and Johnson (1) found isolated LCL injuries accounted for only 4.2% of all knee ligament injuries. The ratio of stable MCL injuries to LCL injuries was 14:1, whereas those with pathologic motion was 11:1. Baseball was the most common sport associated with this injury (18%), followed by soccer, skiing, and vehicular accidents with each at 6%.

Over the past several decades, there have been substantial advances in biomechanical research, resulting in better understanding of the functional anatomy of the knee and improved appreciation for the specific contribution of individual restraints on rotational and translational movement. In-depth analysis of functional biomechanics and clinical outcomes has had an impact on our approach to both diagnosis and treatment of injuries to the collateral ligaments of the knee. In this chapter, we review isolated collateral ligament injuries as well as combined collateral/ACL injury. Isolated and combined injuries involving the posterior cruciate ligament (PCL) are discussed separately in parts B and C. To develop an appropriate treatment plan for ligamentous injuries of the knee, it is important to understand the relevant functional anatomy and biomechanics. We shall then discuss presentation, classification, and treatment.

MEDIAL COLLATERAL LIGAMENT INJURY

Functional Anatomy

The complex anatomy of the medial side of the knee was first appreciated by O'Donoghue (2), who noted that the "medial collateral ligament" consisted of "short thick fibers passing in several directions and in several grouping." Hughston (3) studied the function of individual medial supporting structures, dividing them into "static" and "dynamic" stabilizers. The "static" (or more accurately, "passive") stabilizers are the components of the capsulo-ligamentous complex. The dynamic stabilizers of the medial knee are the pes anserine structures, semimembranosus, and vastus medialis obliques (VMO). The semimembranosus, with its five arms of insertion into the posteromedial aspect of the knee, offers the primary dynamic stabilizing effect (4–6). The pes anserine muscles dynamically stabilize the knee and flex and internally rotate the tibia. The VMO attaches adjacent to the tibial collateral along the adductor tubercle, and the distal extent via the medial retinaculum offers stability to the anterior third of the capsule.

From a surgical point of view, the three-layer description by Warren et al. (7) helps one appreciate the relationship of the various important stabilizing structures. The most superficial layer (layer 1) consists of the deep or sartorial fascia, and encompasses the patellar tendon anteriorly and the popliteal fossa posteriorly. Layer 2 is comprised of the superficial medial collateral ligament. Layer 2 blends anteriorly with layer 1 to form part of the medial patellar retinaculum; and layer 2 blends posteriorly with layer 3, via an oblique group of fibers coursing posteriorly, the posterior oblique ligament (POL) (5). The POL fans out through three arms of attachment: the superficial arm which blends with the pes anserinus sheath, the tibial arm attaching to the peripheral medial meniscus and tibia, and the capsular arm blending with the oblique popliteal ligament. Layer 3 consists of the deep layer of the joint capsule and the medial capsular ligament, which includes the meniscofemoral and meniscotibial portions. At the posterior corner of layer 3 is a confluence of layers 2 and 3 merging also with the semimembranosis tendon sheath, referred to as the oblique popliteal ligament (8,9). The oblique popliteal ligament not only shares fibers with the posterior oblique ligament, but then courses laterally to attach to the lateral femoral condyle and arcuate ligament (10).

Biomechanics

The primary restraint to valgus instability is the superficial MCL (3,11–13). A recent cadaveric study supported earlier findings that the superficial MCL is the primary restraint to valgus stress at any flexion angle (14). The superficial MCL contributes 78% of the restraining force on the medial side of the knee (11). Because of its parallel collagen arrangement, as little as 5 to 8 mm of increased joint space opening indicates a complete failure of the ligament. This is an important point when correlating biomechanical data with physical examination techniques and clinical findings.

The midmedial capsule (deep MCL) primarily functions to limit internal rotation, and does not contribute to significant valgus restraint when the superficial MCL is intact. Therefore, increased tibial rotation results only with a combined sectioning of the superficial *and* deep MCL (12,13,15).

The medial structures also act as major secondary restraints to anterior tibial displacement. Two separate studies (12,15) showed that combined section of the superficial MCL and mid medial capsule led to small changes in anterior translation. However, when the MCL and ACL were both divided, the resulting increase in anterior displacement far exceeded any change seen after individual ligament sectioning. Sectioning the MCL increased the external rotation limit, independent of whether the ACL was intact or sectioned. Subsequent cutting of the posterior oblique ligament and posteromedial capsule further increased the external rotation limit. Clinically, it is also important to remember that increases in external rotation can be caused by posterior subluxation of the lateral tibial plateau instead of the above-described anterior translation of the medial plateau (see section on LCL).

Clinical Evaluation

The mechanism of injury in the majority of MCL injuries involves a valgus force applied laterally about the distal thigh or proximal leg. It is not unusual, however, to find coupled mechanisms such as valgus and rotation, which may inflict damage to both the MCL and the posterior oblique ligament. The most frequent injury is a valgus stress on the joint with the simultaneous internal rotation of the femur on the fixed tibia with the knee in 30° or more of flexion (3,16,17). The athlete will usually experience immediate pain and may report a tearing or popping sensation in the knee.

Clinical examination of the patient with an acute MCL injury reveals medial tenderness, and a variable degree of swelling. It is important to differentiate between localized soft tissue swelling and hemarthrosis. Localized swelling is commonly seen with isolated MCL damage, and hemarthrosis is seen more frequently with associated ACL rupture (17). With combined MCL and ACL injury, extravasation of blood through the tear of the medial capsular structures may reduce the size of the hemarthrosis. Even with an isolated MCL injury the presence or absence of effusion may help the examiner pinpoint the location of the tear. Indelicato (17) has suggested that if there is minimal or no effusion, the capsular tear is interstitial or at the meniscotibial portion of the capsule, which allows extravasation of the fluid from the knee joint. If there is a large effusion, the capsular tear is more likely located at the meniscofemoral portion of capsule, in which case the fluid is less likely to escape the joint. One may postulate several mechanisms by which the location of MCL injury may affect accumulation of fluid within the knee joint. Without reading too much into them, Indelicato's (17) observations are worth bearing in mind from an empirical point of view, as a guide to assessing the location as well as the severity of an MCL injury.

Clinical examination includes valgus stress (abduction) tests at both 30° and full extension. With an MCL injury, examination will demonstrate a positive abduction stress test at 30° of knee flexion. Accurate assessment is possible only if adequate relaxation is achieved, and this is improved by resting the thigh on a bolster (see Fig. 19.42), or on the table edge with the leg off to the side while supporting the foot. The degree of medial joint space opening relative to the contralateral knee is a direct measure of damage and allows classification. The second part of the examination is performed with the knee in full extension. Again, valgus force is applied and the medial opening is compared with the uninjured knee. Full extension loads the posteromedial structures, giving them an important role in restraining valgus and anteriorly directed forces. Research has documented an increase of 7° or more in the abduction limit at full knee extension when the posterior oblique ligament and posteromedial corner were sectioned along with the MCL (11,14). Thus, any medial joint opening in full extension strongly indicates damage to the posterior oblique ligament, or posteromedial capsule, and gross medial opening in full extension strongly indicates damage to the cruciate ligaments (11,14). In both tests, the degree of medial joint opening relative to the uninjured knee provides a measure of damage to the MCL.

In addition, Hughston (3) recommended that the quality of the end point be assessed. He incorporated the quality of the endpoint into his classification of MCL injuries. Medial opening in the amount of 6 to 10 mm with a firm end point was considered a grade 2 MCL injury, and opening of more than 10 mm with no firm end point was considered a grade 3 injury. By definition, a complete MCL tear offers no resistance to valgus stress. Therefore with a complete MCL tear, no firm end point should be encountered. However, despite a complete tear of the MCL an examiner may sense a "soft" end point in the valgus stressed knee in slight flexion as the intact ACL becomes taught. Hughston pointed out that this end point is encountered well beyond the normal medial opening as determined by comparison with the normal contralateral collateral knee. Hughston also recommended performing the anterior drawer test in external rotation to determine whether the MCL injury was proximal or distal to the joint line. When the meniscotibial ligament is torn, the medial meniscus is mobilized allowing the tibia to subluxate anteriorly. If the meniscofemoral ligament is torn, the stabilizing effect of the meniscus is not lost, and hence the drawer is usually normal.

It is extremely important to rule out concomitant damage to other major ligaments, and a thorough knee examination is essential. There is a strong association of ACL injury with complete MCL injury: about 30% of all injuries involving the MCL are combined ACL/MCL tears (see Chapter 18). Therefore a careful and thorough examination should be performed with special attention to the possibility of ACL rupture. Instrumented testing is very helpful because guarding and swelling can render an equivocal "end point" with both anterior and valgus stress. The Pivot shift is particularly difficult to interpret in such cases. PCL or LCL injury must also be excluded via posterior and varus stress tests. Examination of the lateral and posterolateral structures is described later in this chapter.

Injuries to the medial capsular structures may continue into the anterior retinaculum as well, so that a complete examination of the components of the extensor apparatus is important. Patellar dislocation or subluxation may occur occasionally in conjunction with an MCL injury (18). Examination should include palpation to elicit tenderness near the medial border of the patella, at the medial femoral epicondyle, and in the distal fibers of the vastus medialis adjacent to the femoral attachment of the MCL.

Classification

The classification of MCL injury is based primarily on the degree of valgus opening. The commonly used grading system of Hughston (3) describes mild (grade 1)

instability when the absolute opening detected on valgus stressing is 3 to 5 mm and there is a firm end point. Moderate (grade 2) instability represents 6 to 10 mm joint opening and a firm end point, implying that at least some of the MCL fibers still span the join. Severe (grade 3) instability indicates more than 10 mm with no firm end point. It may be more accurate to measure the valgus medial displacement difference in comparison to the opposite side using stress x-ray measurements to determine the amount of medial joint space opening. Using this technique, Daniel (19,20) designated grade 1 injuries as having a side-to-side difference (injured minus noninjured) less than 3 mm, grade 2 as a difference of 3 to 5 mm, and grade 3 for differences greater than 5 mm.

Imaging

Radiographic evaluation should consist of routine anteroposterior, lateral, and sunrise views to document any associated avulsion or osteochrondral fractures. Plain radiographic examination generally adds little to the diagnosis of collateral injuries. Plain radiographs may show the Pelligrini Stieda lesion (calcification near the MCL proximal femoral attachment) in the case of old MCL injury. Stress radiographs help to document the amount of medial opening in response to valgus stress in all patients with more than a trace of valgus instability (grade 2 and 3 MCL injuries). In adults, the radiographs are used to determine the degree of instability (see "Classification" above) (20). Stress views are even more important in the evaluation of skeletally immature patients with increased valgus laxity to exclude distal femoral physeal fracture.

The role of magnetic resonance imaging (MRI) has been studied in the evaluation of medial collateral ligament injury (21–25). Schweitzer (25) described fascial edema and loss of demarcation from adjacent fat, but could not reliably grade the injury on MRI. Rasenberg (23) found a high degree of agreement between clinical grading using instrumented valgus testing and MRI findings, and pointed out that the MRI was valuable in detecting clinically unrecognized additional lesions. Robins (24) found that patients with proximal MCL tears had greater difficulty regaining knee motion than patients with MCL tears at or distal to the joint line. Bone bruises associated with MCL injuries are approximately one-half as common as bone bruises associated with ACL injuries. Miller studied the frequency and natural history of trabecular microfractures noted by MRI, noting complete resolution of symptoms in all cases over 2 to 4 months (22). We do not routinely perform MRI in the setting of acute knee injuries involving the MCL. However, MRI can be useful in specific situations such as multiple ligament injuries where clinical examination is difficult, and in patients who lose motion acutely after injury, to distinguish displaced medial meniscus tears or other intraarticular soft tissue impingement that should be ruled out before "stiffness" is attributed to the MCL injury.

Management

The treatment of isolated MCL injuries has evolved over the past half century (2,26–29). It is generally well accepted that isolated grade 1 and grade 2 injuries will heal satisfactorily and can be treated with a nonoperative aggressive rehabilitation program (30,31). The rehabilitation program should include pain control, early range of motion and weight-bearing, and progress to muscle strengthening and return to functional activity. Protection should be afforded via a hinged knee brace during the early healing, and for protection on return to sporting activity for the first 2 to 6 weeks. Return to sport criteria include resolution of instability and pain, muscle strength at least 80% of the opposite side, and return of motion (30–33). In a study of collegiate football players, players with grade 1 injuries returned to play at an average of 10.6 days, and players with grade 2 injuries returned to play at an average of 19.5 days after injury (30).

Management of grade 3 injuries remains somewhat controversial. Truly isolated grade 3 injuries are rare, and one must carefully evaluate for presence of a associated cruciate, meniscal, or articular cartilage injury. Historically, Palmer (34) recommended surgical treatment, and was dissatisfied with the results of plaster cast treatment of all ligament injuries. O'Donoghue (2) in 1950 advocated immediate repair of all grade 3 tears of the MCL, whether they occurred as an isolated injury or in conjunction with other ligament damage. O'Donoghue popularized this approach to MCL injuries in his review of the surgical treatment of injuries to ligaments of the knee (2). Hughston and Barrett (35) also advocated primary repair of complete MCL disruption. Muller (36) performed primary repair of the MCL and reported good or excellent results in 86%.

Subsequent authors have advocated nonoperative intervention, and in 1974 Ellsasser (28) observed that even severe tears of the MCL in professional football players could be treated nonoperatively with a high degree of success. Ellsasser (28) recommended crutches and physical therapy, but no braces or casts. Ninety-three percent of the players returned to sports within 8 weeks, and 98% ultimately did well without any ligament surgery. Ellsasser (28) stated that "a well-muscled thigh is a prerequisite to the early mobilization program" and that "for the individual with inadequate muscles, use of cylinder cast for 3 or 4 weeks is advisable", but he gave no data to support this suggestion. He also advised that "surgeons who advocate surgical repair for every injury to the knee in which some degree of instability is demonstrable will be operating on many knees that would have an excellent result without operation."

Fetto and Marshal (37) also reported satisfactory results with nonoperative treatment of isolated complete tears of the MCL. Fetto (37) presented a retrospective analysis of 265 grade 2 and 3 MCL injuries, with 6-month follow-up. One hundred fifty patients (57%) underwent surgery at the discretion of the patient and surgeon. Nonoperative treatment of grade 2 injuries yielded 86% good-to-excellent results, as good as operative treatment with respect to valgus instability and total HSS knee score. Isolated grade 3 injuries also did as well nonoperatively as with operative treatment, with 64% good-to-excellent results.

In 1983, Indelicato (17) published his classic article "Non-operative Treatment of Complete Tears of the Medial Collateral Ligament of the Knee." This prospective study compared the results of operative and nonoperative treatment in isolated grade 3 injuries of the MCL. Examination under anesthesia was used to confirm the diagnosis, and arthroscopy ruled out meniscal, chondral, or cruciate ligament associated injuries. "Group 1" patients underwent surgical repair of the MCL and long leg cast with protected weight bearing for 6 weeks. "Group 2" patients were casted, but no surgical intervention performed. After 2 weeks, the group 2 patients were converted to cast brace, motion was allowed from 30° to 80°, and weight bearing was increased as tolerated. At 6 weeks, both groups were placed on the same supervised rehabilitation program, and minimum follow-up was 2.4 years.

Group 1 had 88% good-to-excellent knee scores, and group 2 had 90% good-to-excellent scores. Thus, nonoperative care was as successful as surgical intervention. The group 1 patients regained strength more rapidly than the surgical group. Neither group had completely normal stability of the MCL reestablished when measured against the contralateral knee, but a firm end point was achieved with small degrees of laxity that "appeared to have no functional significance." These findings support Indelicato's (38) most recent recommendations, however his more current rehabilitation program has become more aggressive, with functional progression based on patient comfort and performance rather than on predetermined times.

Jones (39) reported nonoperative treatment of complete isolated MCL tears in high school players. This study looked at nonoperative management only, with the nonoperative protocol being a little more aggressive than the previous study. The patients' knees were immobilized for only 1 week in an off the shelf rehabilitation brace, and then range of motion increased weekly, initially from 36° to 60°, and up to 30° to 110°. Weight bearing was permitted as tolerated, and the brace was removed "when stability was achieved." The mean time in which the knees regained stability in the coronal plane was 29 days, and the athletes returned to competition at a mean of 34 days after injury.

Kannus (32) reported a very poor prognosis for non-operative treatment of grade 3 MCL injuries, but it is critical that in this series, all of the grade 3 MCL patients also had some anterior "instability." Thus few, if any, of the 27 patients in this study represented isolated MCL tears. Treatment of combined injury patterns will be addressed later in this chapter.

The most recent clinical study regarding MCL injury results was reported by Reider (33), and included 5-year follow-up data on 35 athletes with complete MCL sprains. These athletes were treated with early functional rehabilitation and without casting, and 33 patients returned to full preinjury sports participation. Reider (40) also outlined his preferred protocol for early functional rehabilitation in some detail.

Preferred Treatment

Our preferred method for treatment of isolated MCL tears is a nonoperative approach. Based on the literature, it appears that isolated MCL tears can do as well with nonoperative care as with operative repair. Again, it is critical to rule out structural damage to either cruciate ligament, and clinical examination and instrumented testing is generally sufficient. MRI may be helpful to determine coexisting damage. The grade of injury determines initial management and the progression of treatment. In general, incomplete MCL injuries are treated with temporary immobilization using a knee immobilizer or hinged brace, and crutches with weight bearing as pain allows. Range-of-motion exercises as well as isometric and isotonic exercises commence as tolerated. For grade 1 injuries, the athlete may return to play as soon as full range of motion and at least 80% strength is restored. A hinged knee brace is worn for protection for 3 weeks. Athletes with grade 2 injuries may return to sport when full range of motion and strength are restored and the knee has a firm, painless end point on valgus testing. A protective valgus-stabilizing brace is used for the remainder of the season.

An athlete with a grade 3 isolated medial collateral ligament injury is treated initially with a long leg hinged brace to protect against any valgus moment, and depending on the degree of pain, range of motion exercises are begun. If the knee is too painful, the brace is placed in full extension, and as pain subsides, the range of motion is increased. Quadriceps setting and straight leg raises are encouraged immediately, and as range of motion improves, stationary biking is added to the rehabilitation. Crutches are discontinued as pain allows, and pool therapy is also encouraged. Jogging and straight-ahead activities are added as strength improves, and an off-the-shelf hinged brace is worn during this phase and with return to sports. Return to play is allowed once the patient has regained 80% of the strength of the contralateral leg, stability is present, and an agility program has been completed.

COMBINED MEDIAL COLLATERAL LIGAMENT AND ANTERIOR CRUCIATE LIGAMENT INJURY

MCL injury is commonly associated with ACL injury. In a 13-year study of acute knee injuries, 15% of acute knee ligament injuries that resulted in pathologic motion were combined ACL/MCL injuries (see Chapter 18). This represented 30% of all MCL injuries and 24% of all tears involving the ACL. Biomechanical studies have indicated that a total MCL injury seldom occurs without simultaneous involvement of the ACL (11,12,15).

The primary restraint against anterior displacement is the anterior cruciate ligament, and the primary restraint to valgus instability is the medial collateral ligament (3,11,13). Sectioning of the medial ligamentous complex (the superficial medial collateral ligament, medial capsular ligament, and posterior oblique ligament) does not result in an increase in anterior displacement if the anterior cruciate ligament is intact. However, anterior displacement increases if the medial complex is cut when the anterior cruciate ligament has also been sectioned (41). Likewise, because the anterior cruciate ligament acts as a secondary stabilizer against valgus rotation, sectioning of the anterior cruciate ligament exacerbates valgus instability in an MCL-deficient knee.

Combined MCL and ACL injury is usually the result of direct contact, although it can also occur in noncontact situations (42). As previously discussed under isolated MCL injuries, a detailed history and thorough physical examination are imperative. The standard clinical stability tests are performed (see Chapter 19, part A), instrumented testing is carried out (see Chapter 19, part C), and the grade of MCL deficiency is determined (20).

Meniscal injuries may occur in conjunction with combined injuries of the MCL and ACL, with lateral meniscal injuries more common than medial meniscal tears (43). As discussed previously (Isolated MCL section), MRI may be necessary in evaluating patients whose clinical examination is inconclusive.

Management

Although there is general agreement that an isolated injury of the medial collateral ligament heals satisfactorily without operative intervention (17,37,39), there has been more controversy as to the best treatment for combined injuries of the medial collateral and anterior cruciate ligaments (8,9,17,20,32,33,35,37,39,44–55). Traditionally O'Donoghue (2) and Larson (48) advocated acute operative treatment with repair of all damaged structures. But Shelbourne (53) reported an unacceptably high frequency of postoperative stiffness with acute surgical treatment of both components of the combined injury, and many studies have provided a basis for non-surgical treatment of MCL injury.

Jokl (47) reported good or excellent results as determined with the Hospital Sports Special Surgery assessment form on 28 patients who were treated nonoperatively for combined tears of the anterior cruciate and medial collateral ligaments. Less satisfactory results were reported by Kannus (32), who reviewed a series of combined MCL/ACL injuries. In this study the authors reported a very poor prognosis for nonoperative treatment of grade 3 MCL injuries combined with ACL deficiency (32).

In vivo animal studies have suggested that the instability secondary to disruption of the ACL may reduce the quality of healing of the MCL, resulting in more pronounced valgus instability after healing of the MCL (56,57). However, human clinical studies have not detected a deleterious effect on MCL healing with nonsurgical treatment of combined ACL/MCL injuries. Several studies have reported that nonoperative treatment of an MCL injury associated with an acute tear of the ACL has resulted in stable and predictable healing of the MCL (20,58–60).

Crain (59) reviewed serial anterior displacement measurements obtained with the KT-1000 in 55 patients who presented with acute ACL and MCL tears and did not undergo surgery. All ACL injuries were complete, but the degree of MCL injury varied (20% grade 1, 60% grade 2, 20% grade 3). Changes in laxity measurements (manual maximum side-to-side difference) were compared with serial measurements in a sample of isolated ACL-injured patients with respect to changes in their anterior instability over the twelve months following presentation. Among patients with combined injury to the ACL and MCL, anterior laxity decreased from an average of 6.5 mm acutely to 4.5 mm at follow-up. There was no change in anterior laxity over time among patients with isolated ACL ruptures. Grade 3 MCL injuries showed the greatest anterior laxity initially, but had the greatest reduction over the study period (nearly 4 mm). The authors concluded that anterior knee laxity in knees with acute combined ACL/MCL injury will diminish with time, and that the more severe the MCL injury, the greater the reduction that may be anticipated.

Ballmer et al. (61) and Shelbourne and Patel (62) reported good results in combined ACL/MCL injuries with a treatment regimen of reconstruction of the anterior cruciate ligament and nonoperative treatment of the medial collateral ligament. Ballmer documented joint instability with radiographs. Shelbourne and Patel (62) documented the anterior stability with the KT1000 arthrometer testing, but did not document the valgus instability. Hillard-Sembell et al. (20) performed a retrospective study of 66 patients with combined injuries of the ACL and medial collateral ligaments. They compared treatment regimens of combined reconstruction of the anterior cruciate ligament and repair of medial collateral ligament, reconstruction of only the anterior cruciate liga-

ment, and nonoperative management. Roentgenograms were used to document valgus instability. There was no evidence of valgus instability in any of the treatment groups. These clinical studies suggest that there is no benefit to be gained by operative management of the MCL component in the setting of a combined ACL/MCL injury.

Modern treatment approaches to combined ACL/MCL injury focus primarily on the ACL component of the injury or the interaction between the two during healing. Although the quality of healing in dog medial collateral ligaments may be inferior when the "protective" effect of the ACL is lost (56,57), several studies in humans have indicated otherwise (20,61,62). There are at present no convincing studies to suggest that the ACL must be addressed acutely to improve the outcome of the MCL injury, or vice versa. Intermediate-term outcomes in combined ACL/MCL injury appear to be identical to outcomes of isolated ACL injury (20). MCL insufficiency has little if any practical effect on the outcomes of combined ACL/MCL injuries that are treated without surgery (20). Furthermore, reconstruction of the ACL alone in ACL/MCL-deficient knees appears to produce outcomes similar to those reported for isolated ACL deficiency (20,61,62).

Preferred Treatment

Our treatment philosophy is based on three guiding principles. First, a delay of surgical reconstruction of the ACL until the acute inflammatory phase has passed and the full range of motion of the knee has been restored will reduce the prevalence of postoperative complications. Postoperative arthrofibrosis is more common when the ACL reconstruction is done acutely (63,64). Secondly, predictable healing of the MCL can be achieved without surgical intervention, and therefore the initial focus of treatment can be on allowing the MCL to heal with conservative treatment. Finally, immediate surgical intervention is not necessary to address meniscal pathology, because these injuries, if significant, can be addressed at the time of the delayed ACL reconstruction. Although laboratory studies in animals have shown poor healing of the transected MCL in knees with a concomitant torn ACL (56,65), clinical reports in humans with similar injuries has shown predictable healing of the MCL despite the presence of an ACL (60–62).

Initial treatment of the patient with acute combined injuries of the ACL and MCL involves protecting the injured MCL, controlling inflammation and swelling, and restoring normal knee motion. The patient is placed into a protective brace with limited weight bearing. Some authors advocate casting for 2 weeks at 20° of flexion for further protection (66). Robins (24) and Burks (4) have suggested that the location of the MCL rupture is very important among patients with combined ACL and MCL injuries. They describe two distinct groups, each with different prognosis related to return of motion based on the location of the MCL disruption. If the medial collateral ligament injury was proximal, they observed a high rate of stiffness requiring aggressive therapy to restore motion, whereas patients with distal tears achieved motion more easily without needing therapy. Their results suggest that a more sanguine approach to distal injuries may be reasonable, but that proximal injuries must be managed with careful attention to restoring motion. Once full motion is achieved and the knee is rehabilitated, attention can be given to treatment of the ACL.

The decision regarding ACL reconstruction depends entirely on the patient's preinjury activity level and the degree of anterior instability (67). That is to say, the condition of the MCL plays no role in our decision as to whether to reconstruct the ACL. Young athletic patients are best managed with the reconstruction of the ACL, as are older patients who desire to continue in vigorous sporting activities. MCL injury does however play a role in the timing of surgery, whether knee stiffness will need to be addressed, and when the decision can be made to proceed to ACL reconstruction.

ISOLATED LATERAL COLLATERAL LIGAMENT INJURIES

Functional Anatomy

The detailed anatomy of the lateral aspect of the knee is well documented (10,16,68,69). For the purposes of our discussion, the following salient features have impact on the evaluation and treatment of lateral knee injuries. The LCL, popliteus, and the arcuate ligament are considered to be of primary functional significance.

According to Seebacher's (10) description, the LCL lies in the third and deepest layer along with the joint capsule, and runs from the lateral epicondyle of the femur to the proximal lateral aspect of the fibular head. In contrast to the MCL, which is intimately joined with the medial meniscus, the LCL is separated from the lateral meniscus (6). The LCL lies posterior to the axis of rotation, it is tightest in full extension and relaxes in flexion. This relaxation permits the femur to rotate on the tibia (6,70).

As described by Last (69), the popliteus muscle originates from the popliteal surface of the tibia, sloping upward and laterally with half of its tendon inserting just below the epicondyle on the lateral surface of the lateral condyle of the femur. This tendonous portion passes through a plane between the inner capsular laminae and the synovial membrane lining the joint and through a sagittally oriented oval orifice in the capsule (10). The other half of the popliteus muscle ends in a short flat tendon that inserts into the posterior convexity of the lateral meniscus (69).

The joint capsule is divided into two laminae. The superficial lamina encompasses the LCL, and ends pos-

teriorly in the fabellofibular ligament. The inner lamina terminates posteriorly at the Y-shaped arcuate ligament, which spans the junction between the popliteus muscle and its tendon from the fibula to the femur. The arcuate ligament inserts on the apex of the fibular styloid process, and ascends vertically to the lateral head of the gastrocnemius, to the posterior termination of the oblique popliteal ligament. The arcuate ligament adheres firmly to the underlying musculotendinous junction of the popliteus muscle. In addition to its vertical limb, the arcuate ligament fans out medially over the popliteus muscle where it joins the fibers of the oblique popliteal ligament (10).

Biomechanics

Varus Stability

Although the LCL is the primary restraint to varus stresses of the knee, the role of the secondary structures (deep posterolateral structures) appears to be more closely linked to its function than is the case for the medial structures of the knee (12,71,72). Gollehon (73) reported that at all flexion angles, isolated sectioning of either the LCL or the deep posterolateral structures (DPLS; including the arcuate ligament and popliteus) had minimal effect on varus opening, but sectioning both structures resulted in significant increases in varus opening at all flexion angles. Markolf (71), however, reported that LCL sectioning increased varus angulation at all angles, with a tendency towards greater varus opening with increasing flexion. Similarly, Grood (74) reported that increases in varus limits due to isolated LCL sectioning were greatest at 30° of flexion and smallest at full extension. They found that varus angulation further increased when the popliteus and arcuate complex were also sectioned, with the maximum change occurring in full extension (74). Therefore, the presence of an isolated LCL injury is best detected in flexion, whereas the presence of varus instability in full extension indicates incompetence of both the LCL and the DPLS.

Rotational Stability

Kaplan (6) reported that the LCL is relaxed in flexion, permitting rotation of the femur on the tibia. Gollehon (73) reported that when the LCL was left intact and the DPLS was cut, the only significant increase in external rotation was seen at 90° of flexion. However, combined sectioning of the LCL and the DPLS led to increased external rotation of the tibia at both 30° and 90° of knee flexion. The resultant increase in external rotation was greater when both structures were sectioned than the sum of the individual component changes. Interestingly, when the PCL was sectioned along with the LCL and DPLS, a further increase in external rotation was seen at 90°, but not at 30° of flexion (73). Therefore, no individual structure acts as the primary restraint to external rotation, but the posterolateral corner functions in concert as a complex to limit external rotation (73–76).

The LCL and DPLS also appear to work in coupled motion with the ACL (77–79). Wroble (79) demonstrated that ACL deficient knees with simulated posterolateral corner injures have an increased amount of anterior translation in extension, increased adduction, and increased external rotation. He concluded that the lateral structures of the knee are important secondary restraints to anterior translation, and play a role in protecting a reconstructed ACL. LaPrade (78) also demonstrated that sectioning of the LCL increased the forces on the ACL graft under varus loading.

Clinical Evaluation

Lateral Collateral Ligament

As with the medial structures of the knee, knowledge of biomechanical function of the knee ligaments aids the clinician in accurately evaluating an injury. Due to the closely linked functions of the LCL and the deep complex, isolated injuries to either are relatively uncommon. In our experience, approximately 60% of all injuries to the lateral structures occur without associated injury to the cruciate ligaments (see Chapter 18). Isolated injuries to the LCL are relatively benign compared with the more ominous combined injury to the posterolateral corner, and differentiation between the two injuries is critical to appropriate patient care.

The mechanism of injury for most lateral knee injuries involves a varus force applied to the knee. However, similar to the injuries of the medial aspect of the knee, combined injuries to the posterolateral structures may occur as a result of coupled mechanisms such as a varus hyperextension or a combined rotational injury. Depending on the degree of injury, subjective complaints may be limited to pain or discomfort along the lateral aspect of the knee with varus stress. Symptoms may also include pain on weight bearing, with walking on uneven ground, or with lateral cutting movements. Complaints of marked swelling and bruising along the lateral aspect of the leg are generally associated with greater degrees of injury involving the deep posterolateral structures.

Although patients with injury limited to the lateral collateral ligament may present with minimal changes in the external appearance of their knees, patients with greater degrees of injury will frequently have diffuse swelling and ecchymosis along the posterior and lateral aspect of the knee and leg. Swelling of the knee itself may not be dramatic, however, presumably because associated capsular injuries allow extravasation of intracapsular fluid into the surrounding tissues.

The LCL is best palpated with the knee in a figure 4 position. While holding the patient's leg in this position, the LCL is readily palpable as a cord or pencil like structure running from the head of the fibula to the lateral epicondyle of the femur. Attention should be paid to any attenuation of this structure compared with the normal or uninjured side, as well as any tenderness along its path or at the insertion sites. Crepitus at the insertion sites may indicate an avulsion type injury.

Accurate detection of a deficient posterolateral corner may often be difficult, but it is essential for successful treatment of the injured knee. Patients who did not seek appropriate medical attention during the acute phase of their injury may present with more subtle symptoms characteristic of chronic instability. These patients usually have the residuals of a higher grade injury, most commonly that of an unrecognized associated injury to the posterolateral corner. Clinical symptoms may include complaints of "knee giving way backwards," (68) difficulty with stairs, difficulty with higher heels, pain usually at the medial joint line, presumably due to the increased compression forces, and pain along the posterolateral aspect of the knee from stretching of the structures. Noyes (80,81) reported that chronic injuries to the posterolateral structure of the knee may lead to major gait abnormalities characterized by excessive knee hyperextension during the stance phase of gait. Subjective complaints in his series included knee instability, partial or full giving way, medial joint line pain, and pain in the posterolateral soft tissues.

Classification

Based on biomechanical studies, lateral collateral ligament injuries are graded as follows:

Grade 1 = Pain or tenderness without opening to varus stress

Grade 2 = Abnormal joint space opening to varus stress less than 5 mm at 30° of knee flexion, but stable in extension with a firm end point

Grade 3 = Abnormal joint space opening to varus stress greater than or equal to 5 mm at 30° and greater than 3 mm at full extension with a soft end point.

Varus stress testing should be performed both at 30° of knee flexion and in full extension. Laxity on varus testing with the knee at 30° confirms a grade 2 or greater injury to the LCL. For isolated LCL injuries, minimal to no varus instability should be present in full extension, and no increase in external rotation of the knee should be present at 30° or 90° of flexion. Varus laxity in full extension suggests an associated injury to the posterolateral structures. A grade 3 varus instability with the knee at 30° is also highly suspicious for concomitant DPLS and cruciate ligament injury. DeLee (82,83) stated that severe straight lateral instability with >10 mm of joint opening compared with the contralateral knee implied an ACL or PCL injury.

Lateral Collateral Ligament and Posterolateral Corner

As previously mentioned, the likelihood of having a combined injury to the posterolateral corner of the knee with a grade 2 or 3 LCL injury is high. Conversely, however, absence of a LCL injury does not eliminate the possibility of a posterolateral corner injury. LaPrade (84) found that only 23% of knees with a deep posterolateral corner injury had a concomitant fibular collateral ligament injury, and therefore the presence of an intact LCL does not rule out the possibility of a posterolateral corner injury. The External Rotation Dial Test (Fig. 23.1) may assist in delineating these injuries. This test is usually performed with the patient prone with the examiner positioned at the foot of the table. The examiner places an external rotation stress to both legs either through the foot or ankle. The knee is then gently flexed, and the examiner carefully compares the degree of external rotation present in the normal and injured knees (Fig. 23.1). An isolated

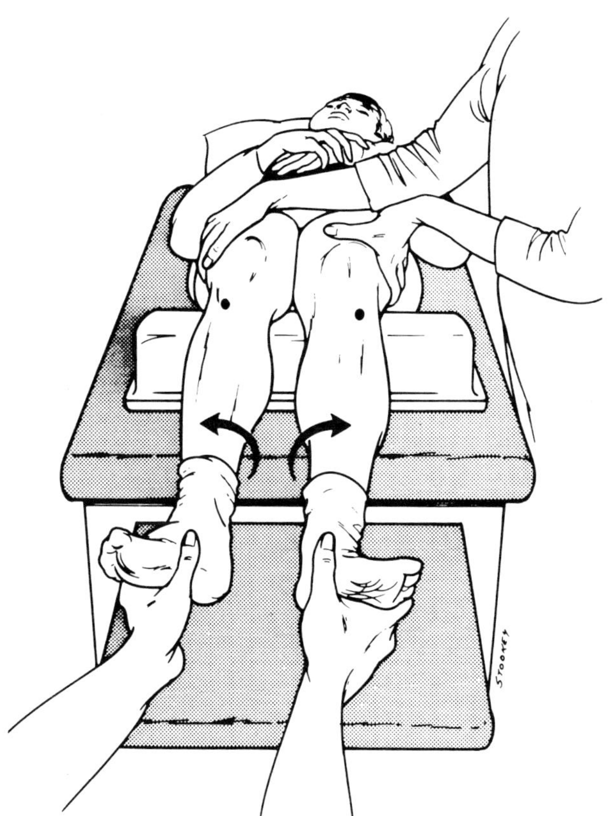

FIGURE 23.1. Evaluation of axial rotation. An assistant stabilizes both femora. The examiner rotates the foot and evaluates tibial rotation by noting the external rotation of the tibial tubercle and the foot. The patient's left leg reveals greater external rotation.

injury to the DPLS (without concomitant injury to the LCL) is confirmed by an increase in external rotation of the tibia at 90° of knee flexion that is not present at 30° of flexion (73). Combined injuries to the LCL and DPLS demonstrate increased external rotation of the tibia at 30° of knee flexion without further increase in external rotation at 90° of flexion. Further increase in tibial external rotation between 30° and 90° of knee flexion suggests an associated PCL injury. The injury to the PCL should be confirmed by the quadriceps active test with or without instrumented measurement as needed (see Chapter 19, part C). Without PCL involvement, no increase in posterior tibial translation should be present at either 30° or 90° of knee flexion when compared with the opposite (uninjured) knee.

Hughston (85) described the External Rotation Recurvatum and the Posterolateral Drawer tests. Briefly, the external rotation recurvatum test is done with the patient supine and relaxed. The lower extremity is then lifted off the examination table by the great toe. For a positive test result, the knee demonstrates both recurvatum and external rotation. One caveat is that this test result is positive only if both the ACL *and* the posterolateral corner are injured. If only the ACL is injured, the knee may go into recurvatum without external rotation, whereas an isolated posterolateral corner injury would not cause recurvatum.

The posterolateral drawer test is done with the patient relaxed in a supine position with the knee flexed at 80° and supported by the examiner. Once complete relaxation is confirmed by palpation of the hamstrings, a posterior drawer force with the knee in neutral rotation is applied. Evidence of a posterolateral corner injury is revealed by the lateral tibial plateau rotating further posteriorly on the femoral condyle. Repeating the test with the knee held in external rotation should accentuate the above, while holding the knee in internal rotation should eliminate the posterior drawer. If the PCL is also injured, the external rotation seen with posterior drawer when the knee is at neutral rotation is eliminated (because the axis of rotation is disrupted), and the posterior drawer remains positive even with the knee held in internal rotation.

Imaging and Other Special Considerations

Although standard radiographic imaging may demonstrate avulsion injuries of the fibular collateral ligament or other capsular structures, plain radiographs provide only limited assistance in delineating these injuries to the lateral ligamentous structures of the knee. However, stress radiography may be helpful if the clinical examination is equivocal, and in measuring the magnitude of instability more objectively.

An accurate evaluation may not be possible given the limitations of a clinical examination in an alert patient with an acutely injured knee. If a high level of suspicion for associated injury is present (e.g., instability on varus stress in full extension), further diagnostic tests are warranted. Though concomitant meniscal pathology appears to be rare, MRI may be helpful in identifying meniscus tears as well as in assessing posterolateral complex injuries (86). LaPrade has noted that MRI can identify injury to the iliotibial band layer, short head of the biceps femoris, meniscotibial ligament, LCL, popliteus origin on the femur, popliteofibular ligament, and the fabellofibular ligament (87). We also have found MRI to be accurate and very useful in preoperative assessment of acute injuries involving the lateral and posterolateral structures. Any question of injury to the deep posterolateral structures of the knee should alert the clinician of the need to proceed with further evaluation, including an examination under anesthesia, a diagnostic arthroscopy, and possible primary repair of the injured structures. Single-photon emission tomography may further assist in differentiating the sites of injury (88).

During arthroscopic evaluation of the knee, if an unexpectedly large amount of lateral compartment laxity is seen in a patient with a major ligamentous injury, one should suspect injury to the DPLS. La Prade (89) described the "drive-through sign" as a positive finding for posterolateral rotatory instability. In a positive drive-through sign, a 4-mm arthroscope can be passed, via a lateral parapatellar tendon portal, under the posterior horn of the lateral meniscus, and be used to view the distal capsular attachment of the coronary ligament without the need to place the knee in a figure 4 position.

Finally, peroneal nerve function should be carefully evaluated. In patients presenting with posterolateral knee injury, La Prade (84) observed a 20% to 27% rate of injury to the peroneal nerve, with 8% of such patients having persistent neuropraxia. The need for nerve conduction studies should be considered in such instances.

Management: Lateral Collateral Ligament and Posterolateral Corner

Perhaps as a result of the rarity of this injury, the literature is sparse regarding the treatment and outcomes of isolated LCL injuries. The consensus appears to be that isolated grade 1 injuries to the LCL do well when treated conservatively. Jones (39) reported 2 cases and Ellsasser (28) reported 10 cases in their series. Both authors implied that LCL injuries had a good prognosis (similar to medial collateral injuries) provided that the cruciate ligaments remained intact. Kannus (90) reported a retrospective study of the long-term nonoperative treatment of grade 2 and 3 LCL injuries. Grade 2 injuries were defined as mild-to-moderate adduction instability at 30° of flexion but normal stability in extension, whereas grade 3 injuries had severe adduction instability at 30° and a mild-to-moderate adduction instability in full extension. All of the patients in his series were treated conservatively with casting for various periods. At an average 8 years follow-up, 82% of those patients with grade 2 injury had returned to their previous level of sports participation. However, 75% of those patients with grade 3 injury were unable to return to preinjury participation levels, and were found to have high frequency of gross laxity, insufficiency of the ACL, muscle weakness, and posttraumatic osteoarthritis. Krukhaug (91) recently reported on 25 patients treated for acute LCL injuries. Seven patients had an isolated LCL injury, whereas the rest of their group had concomitant ligament injuries. Five of five patients who had 1+ laxity initially and had been treated conservatively were stable at follow-up. However, he recommended that patients with grade 3 laxity at initial evaluation be considered for operative repair because they frequently had associated concomitant injuries that required operative intervention.

Preferred Method

There is little controversy that conservative management of isolated LCL injuries results in satisfactory outcomes. We recommend an initial period of diminished activities, while encouraging return of full range of motion, and do not require immobilization or protected weight bearing. For patients with pain on ambulation, a valgus-stressed range-of-motion (ROM) brace is considered along with a period of limited weight bearing, both of which are discontinued once the tenderness is resolved. We allow our patients to return to sports once they have regained full painless range of motion, and pass strength and functional agility testing to minimize the likelihood of a recurrent injury.

Grade 2 injuries should be carefully evaluated to rule out the possibility of an associated posterolateral corner or cruciate ligament injury. True isolated grade 2 injuries are immobilized for a short period (7–10 days) to reduce initial discomfort, and to allow the examiner to reevaluate the knee before initiating definitive treatment. The mechanical axis of the limb is a factor in the rehabilitation of these injuries because of tension generated in the lateral knee ligamentous structures during single-limb stance. For patients with mechanically neutral or valgus knee alignment, after the initial period of rest, we allow early motion and partial weight bearing in a valgus-loaded ROM brace for approximately 6 weeks or until the patient has regained full range of motion and painless weight bearing. However, for patients with mechanically varus knee alignment, we recommend non–weight bearing with a valgus stressed controlled range of motion brace for at least 6 to 8 weeks before allowing weight-bearing activities. We recommend that patients with associated posterolateral corner injuries undergo operative repair of the injured structures within 3 weeks of injury.

In treating grade 2 LCL injuries associated with a cruciate ligament injury, one should maintain a high level of suspicion for a concomitant posterolateral corner involvement. For combined cruciate, LCL, and posterolateral corner injury, we recommend an operative repair of the LCL and posterolateral corner within 2 weeks of the injury, with a concurrent or a staged reconstruction of either or both cruciate ligaments if indicated. However, if the posterolateral corner is not involved, the LCL injury is treated conservatively, and we base our decision for early operative intervention on the need for an ACL reconstruction, using the criteria as delineated by Daniel (SURF Factor) (67).

Grade 3 LCL injuries do poorly when treated nonoperatively, presumably because these injuries are nearly always associated with a posterolateral corner and cruciate ligament injuries. These injuries are treated based on the presence of a posterolateral corner injury similar to the grade 2 LCL injuries.

ANTERIOR CRUCIATE LIGAMENT AND POSTEROLATERAL CORNER

Combined injury to the LCL, posterolateral corner and anterior cruciate ligament requires special consideration. Approximately 30% of all injuries involving the posterolateral structures result also in pathologic ACL laxity (see Chapter 18). Unrecognized posterolateral corner injuries are thought to increase the failure rates of ACL reconstructions (78,79,89,92,93). LaPrade (77) found 11% of ACL injuries had an associated grade 3 posterolateral rotatory instability (PLRI). O'Brien (93) reported that 14% of failures of ACL reconstruction in his series were due to an associated PLRI. Jaureguito (94) reported that grade 1 injuries to the lateral structures do well when treated conservatively, but that in grade 2 injuries and presence of PLRI lead to ACL failures. Johnson et al. (95) reported that missed posterolateral corner injury resulting in rotatory instability could increase the forces on the ACL graft. La Prade (78) measured ACL graft forces before and after sectioning the fibular collateral ligament, the popliteofibular ligament, and the popliteus, and found that forces on the ACL increased dramatically during varus load when the fibular collateral ligament was sectioned. Even greater forces were measured with varus and internal rotation forces, with some further increase on the ACL when the popliteus and popliteofibular ligaments were also sectioned.

Management

For acute injuries within 3 weeks of injury, LaPrade (77) recommends a combined primary repair of the posterolateral corner and an endoscopic ACL reconstruction. Beyond this time he found that the posterolateral structures became ill defined and did not hold sutures well. Before beginning arthroscopy, he first applies repair sutures for the posterolateral structures without tying.

Second, an endoscopic ACL reconstruction is performed, and the graft is fixed with the knee in extension. Finally, the posterolateral repair sutures are tightened with the knee at 60° of flexion and the foot internally rotated (Table 23.1).

For patients who present with a chronic combined ACL and posterolateral corner deficiency, the primary functional disability is first determined by patient history. If both a posterolateral corner and an ACL reconstruction is deemed necessary, a staged procedure is considered, because postoperative rehabilitation for ACL reconstruction requires early full range of motion, whereas repairs and reconstructions of the posterolateral corner require a period of immobilization.

There is no consensus on which reconstructive technique for posterolateral corner insufficiencies provide the best functional outcome. Clancy (96) describes a tenodesis of the long head of the biceps to the lateral femoral epicondyle to reconstruct the fibular collateral ligament. This procedure is effective only when the capsular attachments of the biceps to the posterolateral capsule are not injured, so that the arcuate complex can also be tightened. Albright (97) described a sling procedure for chronic posterolateral corner reconstruction in conjunction with an ACL reconstruction. Using an Achilles tendon or iliotibial band allograft, the graft is passed through a drill hole in the anterior-proximal tibia to the posterior tibia at an exit point immediately medial to the tibiofibular joint. The graft is then passed extra-articularly to a fixation point just proximal to the attachment site of the FCL on the femur. Jakob (98) described a popliteal recession in which the popliteus origin of the femur is osteotomized and countersunk into the lateral femoral condyle through transosseous sutures or a screw and washer. The purpose of his procedure was to restore tension to the entire popliteus complex.

TABLE 23.1. *Tears found in posterolateral knee anatomic structures during surgical exploration for combined grade III ACL-PLRI injuries in 15 patients (77)*

Anatomic structure	Injured	
	n	%
Component of the iliotibial band	15	100
Popliteomeniscal fascicles	14	93
Direct arm short head of biceps femoris	12	80
Capsular arm short head of biceps femoris	11	73
Components of the long head of biceps femoris	10	67
Anterior arm short head of biceps femoris	9	60
Mid-third lateral capsular ligament	9	60
Fabellofibular ligament	8	53
Popliteofibular ligament	7	47
Popliteus origin on femur	4	27
Fibular collateral ligament	4	27
Coronary ligament of the lateral meniscus	4	27
Popliteus musculotendinous junction	0	0

Preferred Treatment

Combined LCL, posterolateral corner, and ACL injuries encountered within 2 to 3 weeks are optimally treated with an operative repair of the LCL and posterolateral structures, and a concomitant ACL reconstruction. Patients who present in the chronic phase with a combined posterolateral corner and ACL deficiency pose a particular challenge. If the posterolateral corner injury is overlooked, the success of the ACL reconstruction may be compromised. Once both injuries have been identified, careful clinical evaluation to determine the primary reason for their knee instability is essential. If clinical indications for an ACL reconstruction are present, we recommend a combined reconstruction of the ACL and posterolateral corner to maximize the likelihood of a successful ACL reconstruction.

However, patients who complain primarily of symptoms associated with their posterolateral rotatory instability are treated for that problem primarily, before ACL reconstruction is considered. If they demonstrate a varus thrust on gait and have a mechanically varus alignment of their knee, we first recommend a realignment osteotomy and a reconstruction of the posterolateral corner. The need for a staged ACL reconstruction should be determined following a period of adequate rehabilitation. For patients with mechanically neutral or valgus aligned knees, realignment osteotomy is not necessary, and the posterolateral corner alone is reconstructed. The ACL may be addressed in the same setting, but we prefer, if possible, a staged procedure. A staged ACL reconstruction offers two main advantages. First, the need for protected immobilization of a posterolateral corner repair and the need for early postoperative mobilization for ACL reconstruction are at odds with one another, so a staged procedure allows the appropriate rehabilitation protocol for the patient following each procedure. Second, the clinical need for an ACL reconstruction can be determined with more certainty after rehabilitation from the posterolateral corner repair, because many patients ultimately choose to alter their activity levels following a major knee injury.

In summary, isolated injuries to the LCL do well when treated conservatively. Concomitant involvement of the posterolateral corner, however, compromises the outcome of ACL reconstruction unless the injury is detected and repaired. The need for early operative intervention is therefore primarily based on the presence of an associated posterolateral corner injury. If surgical intervention is indicated in the acute phase of injury, associated cruciate ligament injuries are also reconstructed. Patients who present with chronic posterolateral corner and/or cruciate ligament pose a challenge because of conflicting surgical and rehabilitation goals. Therefore, when a patient presents with a symptomatic chronic combined ACL and posterolateral corner injury, we prefer to approach the posterolateral reconstruction first, followed later by ACL reconstruction depending on the specific goals of the patient.

REFERENCES

1. Howe J, Johnson RJ. Knee injuries in skiing. *Clin Sports Med* 1982;1: 277–288.
2. O'Donoghue DH. Surgical treatment of fresh injuries to the major ligaments of the knee. *J Bone Joint Surg Am* 1950;32:721–738.
3. Hughston JC, et al. Classification of knee ligament instabilities. Part I. The medial compartment and cruciate ligaments. *J Bone Joint Surg Am* 1976;58:159–172.
4. Burks RT. Gross anatomy. In: Daniel DM, Akeson WH, O'Connor JJ, eds. *Knee ligaments: structure, function, injury, and repair.* New York: Raven Press, 1990:59–76.
5. Hughston JC, Eilers AF. The role of the posterior oblique ligament in repairs of acute medial (collateral) ligament tears of the knee. *J Bone Joint Surg Am* 1973;55:923–940.
6. Kaplan EB. Some aspects of functional anatomy of the human knee joint. *Clin Orthop* 1962;23:18–29.
7. Warren LF, Marshall JL. The supporting structures and layers on the medial side of the knee: an anatomical analysis. *J Bone Joint Surg Am* 1979;61:56–62.
8. Warren RF, Marshall JL. Injuries of the anterior cruciate and medial collateral ligaments of the knee. A long-term follow-up of 86 cases— part II. *Clin Orthop* 1978;136:198–211.
9. Warren RF, Marshall JL. Injuries of the anterior cruciate and medial collateral ligaments of the knee. A retrospective analysis of clinical records—part I. *Clin Orthop* 1978;136:191–197.
10. Seebacher JR, Inglis AE, Marshall JL, et al. The structure of the posterolateral aspect of the knee. *J Bone Joint Surg Am* 1982;64:536–541.
11. Grood ES, Noyes FR, Butler DL, et al. Ligamentous and capsular restraints preventing straight medial and lateral laxity in intact human cadaver knees. *J Bone Joint Surg Am* 1981;63:1257–1269.
12. Markolf KL, Mensch JS, Amstutz HC. Stiffness and laxity of the knee—the contributions of the supporting structures. A quantitative in vitro study. *J Bone Joint Surg Am* 1976;58:583–594.
13. Seering WP, Piziali RL, Nagel DA, et al. The function of the primary ligaments of the knee in varus-valgus and axial rotation. *J Biomech* 1980;13:785–794.
14. Haimes JL, Wroble RR, Grood ES, et al. Role of the medial structures in the intact and anterior cruciate ligament-deficient knee. Limits of motion in the human knee. *Am J Sports Med* 1994;22:402–409.
15. Shoemaker SC, Markolf KL. Effects of joint load on the stiffness and laxity of ligament-deficient knees. An in vitro study of the anterior cruciate and medial collateral ligaments. *J Bone Joint Surg Am* 1985;67:136–146.
16. Hughston JC, et al. Classification of knee ligament instabilities, II. The lateral compartment. *J Bone Joint Surg Am* 1976;58:173–179.
17. Indelicato PA. Non-operative treatment of complete tears of the medial collateral ligament of the knee. *J Bone Joint Surg Am* 1983;65: 323–329.
18. Hunter SC, Marascalco R, Hughston JC. Disruption of the vastus medialis obliquus with medial knee ligament injuries. *Am J Sports Med* 1983;11:427–431.
19. Daniel DM. Diagnosis of a ligament injury. In: Daniel DM, Akeson WA, O'Connor JJ, eds. *Knee ligaments: structure, function, injury, and repair.* New York: Raven Press, 1990:3–10.
20. Hillard-Sembell D, Daniel DM, Stone ML, et al. Combined injuries of the anterior cruciate and medial collateral ligaments of the knee. Effect of treatment on stability and function of the joint. *J Bone Joint Surg Am* 1996;78:169–176.
21. DeMaeseneer M, et al. Normal and abnormal medial meniscocapsular structures. *AJR* 1998;171:969–976.
22. Miller MD, Osborne JR, Gordon WT, et al. The natural history of bone bruises. A prospective study of magnetic resonance imaging-detected trabecular microfractures in patients with isolated medial collateral ligament injuries. *Am J Sports Med* 1998;26:15–19.
23. Rasenberg EI, Lemmens JA, van Kampen A, et al. Grading medial collateral ligament injury: comparison of MR imaging and instru-

mented valgus-varus laxity test-device. A prospective double-blind patient study. *Eur J Radiol* 1995;21:18–24.

24. Robins AJ, Newman AP, Burks RT. Postoperative return of motion in anterior cruciate ligament and medial collateral ligament injuries. The effect of medial collateral ligament rupture location. *Am J Sports Med* 1993;21:20–25.

25. Schweitzer ME, Tran D, Deeley DM, et al. Medial collateral ligament injuries: evaluation of multiple signs, prevalence and location of associated bone bruises, and assessment with MR imaging. *Radiology* 1995;194:825–829.

26. Campbell JD. The evolution and current treatment trends with anterior cruciate, posterior cruciate, and medial collateral ligament injuries. *Am J Knee Surg* 1998;11:128–135.

27. Cox W, Bergfeld J, O'Connor G. Symposium: Functional rehabilitation of isolated medial collateral ligament sprains. *Am J Sports Med* 1979;7: 206–213.

28. Ellsasser JC, Reynolds FC, Omohundro JR. The non-operative treatment of collateral ligament injuries of the knee in professional football players. An analysis of seventy-four injuries treated non-operatively and twenty-four injuries treated surgically. *J Bone Joint Surg Am* 1974;56:1185–1190.

29. McMurray TP. The operative treatment of rupture internal lateral ligament of the knee. *J Bone and Joint Surg* 1918;67:377.

30. Derscheid GL, Garrick JG. Medial collateral ligament injuries in football. Nonoperative management of grade I and grade II sprains. *Am J Sports Med* 1981;9:365–368.

31. Holden DL, Eggert AW, Butler JE. The nonoperative treatment of grade I and II medial collateral ligament injuries to the knee. *Am J Sports Med* 1983;11:340–344.

32. Kannus P. Long-term results of conservatively treated medial collateral ligament injuries of the knee joint. *Clin Orthop* 1988;226:103–112.

33. Reider B, Sathy MR, Talkington J, et al. Treatment of isolated medial collateral ligament injuries in athletes with early functional rehabilitation. A five-year follow-up study. *Am J Sports Med* 1994;22:470–477.

34. Palmer I. On the injuries to the ligaments of the knee joint. *Acta Chir Scand (Suppl)* 1938;81:3–282.

35. Hughston JC, Barrett GR. Acute anteromedial rotatory instability. Long-term results of surgical repair. *J Bone Joint Surg Am* 1983;65: 145–153.

36. Muller W. *The knee: form, function, and ligament reconstruction.* New York: Springer-Verlag, 1983.

37. Fetto JF, Marshall JL. Medial collateral ligament injuries of the knee: a rationale for treatment. *Clin Orthop* 1978;132:206–218.

38. Indelicato PA. Isolated medial collateral ligament injuries in the knee. *J Am Acad Orthop Surg* 1995;3:9–14.

39. Jones RE, Henley MB, Francis P. Nonoperative management of isolated grade III collateral ligament injury in high school football players. *Clin Orthop* 1986;213:137–140.

40. Reider B. Medial collateral ligament injuries in athletes. *Sports Med* 1996;21:147–156.

41. Sullivan D, Levy IM, Sheskier S, et al. Medial restrains to anterior-posterior motion of the knee. *J Bone Joint Surg Am* 1984;66:930–936.

42. Rubenstein RAJ, Shelbourne KD. Management of combined instabilities: anterior cruciate ligament/MCL and anterior cruciate ligament/lateral side. *Oper Tech Sports Med* 1993;1:66–71.

43. Shelbourne KD, Nitz PA. The O'Donoghue triad revisited. Combined knee injuries involving anterior cruciate and medial collateral ligament tears (see comments). *Am J Sports Med* 1991;19:474–477.

44. Aglietti P, et al. Operative treatment of complete lesions of the anterior cruciate and medial collateral ligaments. *Am J Knee Surg* 1991;4: 186–194.

45. Anderson DR, Weiss JA, Takai S. Healing of the medial collateral ligament following a triad injury: a biomechanical and histological study of the knee in rabbits. *J Orthop Res* 1992;10:485–495.

46. Frolke JP, Oskam J, Vierhout PA. Primary reconstruction of the medial collateral ligament in combined injury of the medial collateral and anterior cruciate ligaments. Short-term results. *Knee Surg Sports Traumatol Arthrosc* 1998;6:103–106.

47. Jokl P, Kaplan N, Stovell P, et al. Non-operative treatment of severe injuries to the medial and anterior cruciate ligaments of the knee. *J Bone Joint Surg Am* 1984;66:741–744.

48. Larson RL. Combined instabilities of the knee. *Clin Orthop* 1980;147: 68–75.

49. Noyes FR, Barber-Westin SD. The treatment of acute combined rup-

50. O'Donoghue DH. An analysis of end results of surgical treatment of major injuries to the ligaments of the knee. *J Bone Joint Surg Am* 1955;37:1–13, 124.

51. Petersen W, Laprell H. Combined injuries of the medial collateral ligament and the anterior cruciate ligament. Early ACL reconstruction versus late ACL reconstruction. *Arch Orthop Trauma Surg* 1999; 119(5–6):258–262.

52. Schierl M, Petermann J, Trus P, et al. Anterior cruciate and medial collateral ligament injury. ACL reconstruction and functional treatment of the MCL. *Knee Surg Sports Traumatol Arthrosc* 1994;2:203–206.

53. Shelbourne KD, Baele JR. Treatment of combined anterior cruciate ligament and medial collateral ligament injuries. *Am J Knee Surg* 1988;1:56–58.

54. Shelbourne KD, Porter DA. Anterior cruciate ligament-medial collateral ligament injury: nonoperative management of medial collateral ligament tears with anterior cruciate ligament reconstruction. A preliminary report. *Am J Sports Med* 1992;20:283–286.

55. Woo SL, Inoue M, McGurk–Burleson E, et al. Treatment of the medial collateral ligament injury, II. Structure and function of canine knees in response to differing treatment regimens. *Am J Sports Med* 1987;15: 22–29.

56. Lechner CT, Dahners LE. Healing of the medial collateral ligament in unstable rat knees. *Am J Sports Med* 1991;19:508–512.

57. Woo SL, Peterson RH, Ohland KJ, et al. The effects of strain rate on the properties of the medial collateral ligament in skeletally immature and mature rabbits: a biomechanical and histological study. *J Orthop Res* 1990;8:712–721.

58. Ballmer PM, Jakob RP. The non-operative treatment of isolated complete tears of the medial collateral ligament of the knee. A prospective study. *Arch Orthop Trauma Surg* 1988;107:273–276.

59. Crain EH, Fithian DC, Daniel DM. The change in anterior laxity of combined ACL/MCL injured knees after MCl healing. Presented at the Specialty Day of the American Orthopaedic Society for Sports Medicine, *AAOS Annual Meeting,* Atlanta, GA, 1996.

60. Mok DW, Good C. Non-operative management of acute grade III medial collateral ligament injury of the knee: a prospective study. *Injury* 1989;20:277–280.

61. Ballmer PM, Ballmer FT, Jakob RP. Reconstruction of the anterior cruciate ligament alone in the treatment of a combined instability with complete rupture of the medial collateral ligament. A prospective study. *Arch Orthop Trauma Surg* 1991;110:139–141.

62. Shelbourne KD, Patel DV. Management of combined injuries of the anterior cruciate and medial collateral ligaments. *Instr Course Lect* 1996;45:275–280.

63. Mohtadi NG, Webster-Bogaert S, Fowler PJ. Limitation of motion following anterior cruciate ligament reconstruction. A case-control study. *Am J Sports Med* 1991;19:620–624; discussion 624–625.

64. Shelbourne KD, Wilckens JH, Mollabashy A, et al. Arthrofibrosis in acute anterior cruciate ligament reconstruction. The effect of timing of reconstruction and rehabilitation. *Am J Sports Med* 1991;19:332–336.

65. Woo SL, Hollis JM, Adams DJ, et al. Tensile properties of the human femur-anterior cruciate ligament-tibia complex. The effects of specimen age and orientation. *Am J Sports Med* 1991;19:217–225.

66. Shelbourne KD, Klootwyk TE. Low-velocity knee dislocation with sports injuries. Treatment principles (in process citation). *Clin Sports Med* 2000;19:443–456.

67. Daniel DM, Stone ML, Dobson BE, et al. Fate of the ACL-injured patient. A prospective outcome study (see comments). *Am J Sports Med* 1994;22:632–644.

68. Hughston JC, Jacobson KE. Chronic posterolateral rotatory instability of the knee. *J Bone Joint Surg Am* 1985;67:351–359.

69. Last R. *Anatomy: regional and applied,* 6th ed. New York: Churchill Livingstone, 1978.

70. Brantigan OC, Voshell AF. The mechanics of the ligaments and menisci of the knee joint. *J Bone Joint Surg Am* 1941;23:44–66.

71. Markolf KL, Wascher DC, Finerman GA. Direct in vitro measurement of forces in the cruciate ligaments, II. The effect of section of the posterolateral structures. *J Bone Joint Surg Am* 1993;75:387–394.

72. Wascher DC, Markolf KL, Shapiro MS, et al. Direct in vitro measurement of forces in the cruciate ligaments, I. The effect of multiplane loading in the intact knee. *J Bone Joint Surg Am* 1993;75:377–386.

73. Gollehon DL, Torzilli PA, Warren RF. The role of the posterolateral

and cruciate ligaments in the stability of the human knee. A biomechanical study. *J Bone Joint Surg Am* 1987;69:233–242.

74. Grood ES, Stowers SF, Noyes FR. Limits of movement in the human knee. Effect of sectioning the posterior cruciate ligament and posterolateral structures. *J Bone Joint Surg Am* 1988;70:88–97.

75. Daniel D, Akeson W, O'Connor J. *Knee ligaments: structure, function, injury and repair*. New York: Raven Press, 1990.

76. Veltri DM, Deng XH, Torzilli PA, et al. The role of the cruciate and posterolateral ligaments in stability of the knee. A biomechanical study. *Am J Sports Med* 1995;23:436–443.

77. LaPrade RF, Hamilton CD, Engebretsen L. Treatment of acute and chronic combined anterior ligament and posterolateral knee ligament injuries. *Sports Med Arthrosc Rev* 1997;5:91–99.

78. LaPrade RF, Resig S, Wentorf F, et al. The effects of grade III posterolateral knee complex injuries on anterior cruciate ligament graft force. A biomechanical analysis. *Am J Sports Med* 1999;27:469–475.

79. Wroble RR, Grood ES, Cummings JS, et al. The role of the lateral extraarticular restraints in the anterior cruciate ligament-deficient knee. *Am J Sports Med* 1993;21:257–262, discussion 263.

80. Noyes FR, Barber-Westin SD. Surgical restoration to treat chronic deficiency of the posterolateral complex and cruciate ligaments of the knee joint. *Am J Sports Med* 1996;24:415–426.

81. Noyes FR, Dunworth LA, Andriacchi TP, et al. Knee hyperextension gait abnormalities in unstable knees. Recognition and preoperative gait retraining. *Am J Sports Med* 1996;24:35–45.

82. DeLee JC, Riley MB, Rockwood CA Jr. Acute posterolateral rotatory instability of the knee. *Am J Sports Med* 1983;11:199–207.

83. DeLee JC, Riley MB, Rockwood CA Jr. Acute straight lateral instability of the knee. *Am J Sports Med* 1983;11:404–411.

84. LaPrade RF, Terry GC. Injuries to the posterolateral aspect of the knee. Association of anatomic injury patterns with clinical instability. *Am J Sports Med* 1997;25:433–438.

85. Hughston JC, Norwood LA Jr. The posterolateral drawer test and external rotational recurvatum test for posterolateral rotatory instability of the knee. *Clin Orthop* 1980;147:82–87.

86. Ross G, Chapman AW, Newberg AR, et al. Magnetic resonance imaging for the evaluation of acute posterolateral complex injuries of the knee. *Am J Sports Med* 1997;25:444–448.

87. LaPrade RF, Gilbert TJ, Bollum TS, et al. The magnetic resonance imaging appearance of individual structures of the posterolateral knee. A prospective study of normal knees and knees with surgically verified grade III injuries. *Am J Sports Med* 2000;28:191–199.

88. Cook GJ, Fogelman I. Lateral collateral ligament tear of the knee: appearances on bone scintigraphy with single-photon emission tomography. *Eur J Nucl Med* 1996;23:720–722.

89. LaPrade RF. Arthroscopic evaluation of the lateral compartment of knees with grade 3 posterolateral knee complex injuries. *Am J Sports Med* 1997;25:596–602.

90. Kannus P. Nonoperative treatment of grade II and III sprains of the lateral ligament compartment of the knee. *Am J Sports Med* 1989;17:83–88.

91. Krukhaug Y, Molster A, Rodt A, et al. Lateral ligament injuries of the knee. *Knee Surg Sports Traumatol Arthrosc* 1998;6:21–25.

92. Johnson DL, Coen MJ. Revision ACL surgery. Etiology, indications, techniques, and results. *Am J Knee Surg* 1995;8:155–167.

93. O'Brien SJ, Warren RF, Wickiewicz TL, et al. Reconstruction of the chronically insufficient anterior cruciate ligament with the central third of the patellar ligament. *J Bone Joint Surg Am* 1991;73:278–286.

94. Jaureguito JW, Paulos LE. Why grafts fail. *Clin Orthop* 1996;325:25–41.

95. Johnson DL, Swenson TM, Irrgang JJ, et al. Revision anterior cruciate ligament surgery: experience from Pittsburgh. *Clin Orthop* 1996;325:100–109.

96. Clancy WG. Repair and reconstruction of the posterior cruciate ligament. In: Chapman M, ed. *Operative orthopedics*. Philadelphia: JB Lippincott, 1988.

97. Albright JP. Management of chronic posterolateral instability of the knee: operative technique for the posterolateral corner sling procedure. *Iowa Orthop J* 1994;14:94–100.

98. Jakob RP, Staubli H. Lateral and posterolateral rotatory instability of the knee. In: *Knee and cruciate ligaments*. New York: Spinger-Verlag, 1992.

Part B: Isolated and Combined Posterior Cruciate Ligament and Posterolateral Corner Injuries: Evaluation and Management

Christopher C. Annunziata, J. Robert Giffin, and Christopher D. Harner

The PCL and the posterolateral structures (PLS) serve as important static stabilizers of the knee. The PCL functions as the primary restraint to excessive posterior tibial translation throughout the full range of knee motion and a secondary restraint to posterolateral rotation. The PLS functions predominantly to limit excessive varus opening and external rotation of the knee but also has an important secondary role in posterior tibial translation. Injuries to these structures occur more frequently than once thought. PCL and PLS injuries can occur in isolation but are with increasing frequency becoming recognized as part of a combined ligamentous injury pattern (1–5). Depending on the severity, the disability resulting from these injuries can range from minimal functional alterations to profound limitations in daily activities (6–10).

Although basic science and clinical research on the PCL and PLS has lagged behind that of other ligamentous structures of the knee, recent studies have advanced our understanding of their function, thus improving the ability to diagnose and treat these injuries. Controversy still exists, however, over the natural history of these injuries as well as the indications for surgical intervention, techniques of reconstruction and methods of rehabilitation. Since the basic science, epidemiology and diagnosis of these injuries have been discussed in other chapters, this chapter will only briefly review these topics and will focus on the evaluation and management of isolated and combined PCL and PLS injuries.

BASIC SCIENCE

The PCL consists of three main components: the anterolateral (AL) bundle, the posteromedial (PM) bundle, and the meniscofemoral ligaments (MFL) (11–13). Functionally, the two bundles have different tensioning patterns depending on the degree of knee flexion. The AL bundle is taught with the knee in flexion whereas the PL bundle is taught with the knee in extension (11,14). The precise role of the MFL in knee kinematics has yet to be determined but they do possess significant mechanical strength, suggesting they contribute to knee stability (11,14).

Taken together, the three components of the PCL provide the primary restraint to posterior translation of the tibia and serve as a secondary restraint to excessive external rotation (15–21). Although the PCL functions in this capacity throughout the full range of knee motion, its maximum effect is at 90° of knee flexion where it sustains nearly 100% of a posteriorly directed force (11,15,16,22).

There is a significant functional interaction of the PCL with the PLS (14,23–25). Confusion exists in the literature regarding the PLS because of inconsistent terminology as well as variability in the anatomy of the posterolateral corner structures (6,26–32). The PLS include the popliteus complex, the LCL, and the arcuate ligament. The popliteus complex further consists of the popliteus tendon, the popliteofibular ligament and the popliteal tibial attachments (30,33,34). This complex contributes both statically and dynamically to knee stability. In its static role, it is the primary restraint to excessive external rotation and secondarily assists the PCL with preventing direct posterior translation. Dynamically, with popliteus contraction, there is a significant decrease in the *in situ* forces of the PCL (35,36). No such relationship exists between the LCL and the PCL. The LCL contributes very little to restraining posterior and posterolateral motions. Its primary role is to resist excessive varus rotation. This distinction is very important, as it will directly affect management. A summary of these findings is given in Table 23.2.

Two injury patterns are, therefore, possible with PLS disruptions: posterolateral rotatory instability and varus instability. The interplay of the PCL and the PLS is also important to appreciate. To successfully restore normal posterior laxity it is critical to address the posterior as well as the posterolateral corner structures (3). Despite the increased attention, combined PCL-PLS injury is one of the most complex treatment problems encountered in the management of knee ligament injuries. When there is injury to both of these structures, posterior laxity and

TABLE 23.2. *Kinematic changes in response to isolated and combined injury of the PCL and posterolateral structures under a posterior drawer test*

Injury	PCL	PLS
Isolated		
Posterior translation (90°)	2+	±0
External rotation (30°)	(1+)	1+
Varus	(1+)	1+
Combined (PCL and PLS)		
Posterior translation (90°)	3+	
External rotation (30°)	2+	
Varus	2+	

Values indicate the amount of knee laxity as described by knee classification systems.

PCL, posterior cruciate ligament; PLS, posterolateral structures.

From Harner CD, Höher J. Current concepts: evaluation and treatment of posterior cruciate ligament injuries. *Am J Sports Med* 1998;26:471–482, with permission.

excessive external rotation is more severe than that associated with injury to either in isolation (16,17).

EPIDEMIOLOGY, MECHANISM OF INJURY, AND NATURAL HISTORY

The clinical setting in which the PCL and PLS have been evaluated has implications with regards to incidence, mechanism and extent of injury. The overall incidence of PCL injuries varies from 3% in the general population to 37% of all knee ligament injuries in an emergency department setting (1,2,37,38).

Generally, isolated PCL injuries occur during sporting activities (football, soccer) and result from a noncontact, hyperflexion mechanism (39,40). Combined PCL and PLS injuries, however, result more often from traumatic, contact injuries leading to a direct blow to the tibia (1,2,41). In fact, approximately 95% of the PCL injuries in this setting are associated with other ligamentous injuries in the same knee (2,14). There are many variations of this, but what is important is that the clinician understands there is a distinct difference between the two injury patterns.

Isolated PCL injuries generally have a good prognosis, with the majority of patients returning to their previous level of activity (39,40,42–45). Those with combined PCL and PLS injuries, however, do not do as well and often suffer from both pain and instability (39,40,44–49).

The most common mechanism of PLS injury is a posteriorly directed blow to the tibia with the knee in extension, which forces hyperextension and a varus moment about the knee. Less commonly, severe external rotation is the primary component causing the injury (4). Although these mechanisms can lead to isolated PLS injury, they are more commonly associated with combined injury patterns with the PCL.

EVALUATION

Evaluation of the knee should include an accurate history focusing on the mechanism of injury. The clinical scenario and mechanism of injury may help the clinician in determining the severity and associated injuries. Combined PCL-PLS injuries are commonly associated with damage to bones, vessels, nerves, and other soft tissue structures. Whenever there is a combined injury the possibility of a knee dislocation must be considered. Although popliteal vessel and peroneal nerve integrity should be assessed in any significant knee injury, their function must be particularly scrutinized in this situation since the incidence of injury ranges from 15% to 33% and 9% to 49%, respectively, whether or not the knee is dislocated at the time of evaluation (50–54).

Unlike patients with isolated ACL injuries, those with acute, isolated PCL injuries do not typically report hearing or feeling a "pop." Although many suspect a knee injury, patients do not typically relate a sense of instability (50). They may complain of knee pain, swelling, and stiffness but this is usually only of mild severity. Patients sustaining a combined PCL-PLS injury have pain in the posterolateral knee. They may also note dysesthesias or weakness in the foot due to injury to the peroneal nerve. After the initial swelling from the acute injury has resolved, the patient may note pain and instability of the knee in extension and occasional buckling with weight bearing into hyperextension (5). Chronic injuries to the PCL and PLS can cause disability ranging from almost no functional limitations to severe limitations during activities of daily living (39,40,44,46–49). Those that are symptomatic frequently report pain as their predominant symptom (44–46,48,49,55). In general, chronic, isolated PCL and the more rare, chronic, isolated PLS injuries tend to allow more function whereas the combined pattern with resultant posterolateral instability more often leads to significant functional disability (46). Controversy remains whether the severity corresponds to the degree of abnormal translation (44,46).

A thorough knee examination is essential and should follow the sequence of observation, evaluation of range of motion, palpation, and straight instability followed by specialized testing. Assessment for meniscal damage or other ligamentous injury aside from the PCL and PLS should routinely be performed. Special care must be undertaken when evaluating the ACL in the setting of a PCL-insufficient knee. The noninvolved knee must be examined first to determine the normal relationship of the tibia to the femur since, in the injured knee, the tibia will be subluxed posteriorly. Once this is corrected in the injured knee, standard anterior drawer and Lachman tests can be performed. Significant translation of greater than 10 mm in the sagittal plane suggests injury to both cruciate ligaments (50). Despite increased awareness of PCL

and PLS injuries, they are still frequently not recognized at the initial evaluation.

The most accurate clinical test to assess PCL integrity is the posterior drawer test (37,56). The patient is placed supine and the knee is flexed to 90° while a posteriorly directed force is placed on the proximal tibia. The extent of translation is evaluated by noting the change in the distance of step-off between the medial tibial plateau and the medial femoral condyle. Equally important during this test is to assess the quality of the endpoint. Normally, the plateau is positioned approximately 1 cm anterior to the condyle but can vary, making examination of the contralateral knee essential. PCL injury can be graded with respect to the amount of laxity determined by this test. Grade I is consistent with excessive posterior translation but maintenance of an anterior step-off. Grade II is classified as a 5- to 10-mm translation corresponding to the plateau being displaced flush to the level of, but not posterior to, the condyle. Both of these grades represent partial tears of the PCL. More than 10 mm of translation constitutes a grade III injury, with the plateau displaced posterior to the condyle, and is consistent with a complete tear of the PCL. The degree of sagittal translation should also be assessed with the knee flexed 30°. A slight increase in translation at 30° and not at 90° flexion may indicate a PLS injury; increased sagittal translation at both 30° and 90°, with maximal translation at 90° of knee flexion, is consistent with a PCL injury.

The posterior sag test may provide additional information in evaluating the PCL. The hip and knee are flexed to 90°. With a complete PCL tear, the pull of gravity will displace the tibia posterior to the femur while the examiner supports the weight of the limb by the foot. The quadriceps active test can also aid in the diagnosis of complete ruptures. For this test, the knee is placed at 90° of flexion. While the examiner holds pressure on the foot, the patient is asked to contract the quadriceps. In the presence of a complete tear of the PCL, the patient will achieve dynamic reduction of the posteriorly displaced tibia.

Proper evaluation of the PLS can be difficult with the tibia subluxed posteriorly as in a grade III PCL injury, and so reducing the tibia to neutral is essential before testing for PLS injury (3,56–58). Testing is best performed with the patient positioned prone while an external rotation force is applied to both feet with the knee positioned at 30° and then 90° of flexion. The degree of external rotation is measured by comparing the medial border of the foot to the axis of the femur. Because wide variability of external rotation is possible at these positions, it is essential to compare the results to the contralateral side (59,60). More than a 10-degree difference is considered abnormal (60). The popliteus complex portion of the PLS is the primary restraint to external rotation at all degrees of knee flexion but its effect is maximal at 30°. An increase of 10° or more of external rotation at 30° of knee flexion, but not at 90°, is considered diagnostic of an isolated PLS injury (61). Conversely, the PCL is the secondary restraint to external rotation when the knee is at 90° of flexion (16,17,25). As such, increased external rotation at 30° and 90° of knee flexion suggests a combined PCL-PLS injury (Table 23.2). The recognition of this posterolateral instability component is essential clinically because it may significantly affect the treatment of associated ligamentous instability.

Varus and valgus stress tests are important in assessing the integrity the LCL portion of the PLS. These should be performed with the knee both in full extension and in 30° of flexion. Isolated PCL injury does not significantly affect varus or valgus stability. Increased varus opening at 30° of knee flexion indicates an injury to the LCL and possibly the popliteus complex. Additional slight increased opening also at full extension is consistent with injuries to both of these structures. If there is a large degree of varus opening at full extension, a combined injury of the PLS, PCL and/or the ACL may be present (16,17,19,60,62,63). Other tests such as the reverse pivot shift, external rotation recurvatum, posterolateral drawer and the posterolateral Lachman, can further aid in diagnosing the extent of injury to the PCL and PLS but are more difficult to both reproducibly perform and interpret.

The evaluation of gait and limb alignment is particularly important for those with chronic injury of the PLS. Compared with the medial side of the knee, the articular anatomy of the lateral side is inherently less stable (64). In those with chronic injury to the PLS, the dynamic stabilizers of the lateral knee are not functioning optimally. This may lead to excessive posterolateral rotation and varus opening, commonly known as varus thrust, with heel-strike (64). Therefore, when this gait pattern is seen, it should signify severe instability of the lateral knee. Genu varus is also important to recognize. If this has been present or progressively developed in the setting of PLS injury, it may jeopardize the treatment of the ligamentous injury if not appropriately addressed.

To plan successful treatment for the patient with multiple ligamentous knee injury, it is essential that the examiner determine the extent of injury to all ligaments involved, namely the PCL, popliteus complex, and the LCL.

IMAGING

Standard radiographs are a critical part of the diagnostic evaluation. Adequate anteroposterior and lateral projections should be performed to assess for associated bone injuries. Occasionally bony avulsion from the PCL insertions may be seen. More commonly, in combined PCL-PLS injuries, an avulsion fracture of the fibular head may be seen. These are very subtle findings and the films must be carefully evaluated for these bony injuries

which are typically repairable in the acute setting (33,65). Stress and contralateral views, although not routine, may be helpful in some situations (66). In the setting of a chronic injury, flexion weight-bearing and long cassette radiographs are also essential to assess for arthritis and malalignment, which will potentially affect management.

MRI has become the diagnostic study of choice in evaluating the knee with a presumed PCL injury. This study is 96% to 100% sensitive in detecting tears of the PCL and can also determine the precise location of the tear, with implications for treatment (25,67–69). For example, the femoral "peel-off" injury is particularly amenable to primary repair (70,71). The MRI can be used to assess the menisci, articular surfaces and other ligaments of the knee, which also have relevance to treatment and prognosis. Unfortunately, standard MRI is not routinely helpful in evaluating the PLS (13). The addition of a coronal oblique technique aligned along the axis of the popliteus tendon may prove to be of further assistance in evaluating this region (64).

A bone scan may prove helpful in the evaluation and management of the PCL injured knee. Patients with long-standing PCL injuries are predisposed to early medial and patellofemoral compartment chondrosis (37,42,72). In the setting of an isolated PCL-deficient knee with medial and/or patellofemoral compartment pain and normal radiographs, a bone scan to assess these compartments may be helpful. If there is increased uptake, then surgical intervention may be beneficial (73). If there is no increased uptake, then a continued nonoperative approach is our treatment of choice.

CLASSIFICATION

PCL and PLS injuries can each be classified according to associated injuries (isolated or combined), severity (partial vs. complete), and timing (acute vs. chronic) (10,14,74). Each of these variables affects treatment and outcome.

Combined injuries are those in which there is injury to other significant structures in the knee aside from the PCL, most notably including the PLS. Distinguishing between the isolated and the more common, combined complete PCL tear is more difficult, as noted previously (3), but is critical because the treatment and prognosis is different. Isolated injuries, in general, may be treated nonoperatively and have an excellent prognosis (10,39,40,42,43). Combined injuries have a more guarded prognosis. Better results may be possible in this group with early surgical intervention rather than with conservative treatment (14).

PLS injuries can occur in isolation, involving any component of the PLS, the LCL, popliteus complex, or the arcuate ligament, to varying degrees although this is rare. PLS injuries are more commonly associated with injury to the cruciate ligaments, particularly the PCL (1–3). This can be conceptualized as part of a posterolateral instability pattern with the severity of injury occasionally progressing from partial PLS injury to complete and then to combined PCL-PLS injury (33).

Severity is measured clinically and corresponds to the degree of laxity in the PCL, being either partial (grades I or II) or complete (grade III). Grade III injuries involve disruption of both the AL and PM bundles. Complete tears occasionally occur in isolation but frequently result in a combined injury pattern. The severity of damage to the PLS can be determined during the physical examination by the degree of abnormal laxity in varus opening or external rotation, respectively.

A classification has been proposed that takes into account the varying degrees of posterior and posterolateral instability resulting from combined PCL-PLS injury (75). This scheme stresses the importance of recognizing the individual components, the PCL, LCL, popliteus complex and the arcuate ligament, and the role of each in the instability pattern. The primary determinant of the level of injury is the degree of laxity in full extension because this is thought to correlate well with the degree of associated, combined ligament injury (75). As mentioned, it is imperative to recognize all the structures that are injured to optimize the chance of functional recovery.

Acute versus chronic injury distinction for both the PCL and PLS is somewhat arbitrary. An injury that has occurred within 3 weeks is considered acute. A chronic injury is one that has been present greater than 3 weeks and in fact is usually months old. The importance of making this distinction lies in the benefit of early surgical intervention particularly for isolated PLS and combined PCL-PLS injuries, which will be discussed later. In the acute setting, early surgery facilitates primary repair of the PLS. After 3 weeks, significant scar formation limits the success of primary repair, and typically commits the surgeon to waiting 3 months to allow completion of the healing response before surgical reconstruction can be implemented. Chronic injuries may become associated with significant pericapsular stretching leading to a more extensive rotational instability pattern or the development of arthrosis. This could lead to substantial difficulty in determining the extent of the injury as well as the optimal treatment plan. The categorization of isolated PCL injuries into acute or chronic, however, is not as important as in the combined injury pattern. Injuries of this structure alone do not lead to significant scar formation and therefore adequate surgical treatment for the majority of isolated PCL injuries is not as significantly affected by timing.

TREATMENT

The treatment protocol for these injuries depends on many factors. The timing, severity, and extent of associated injuries are all important prognostic factors that

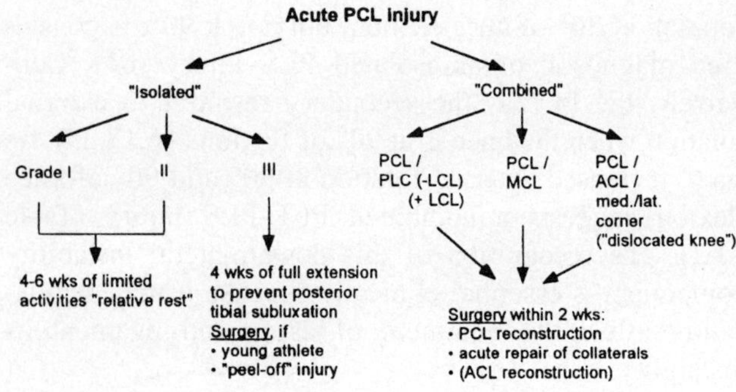

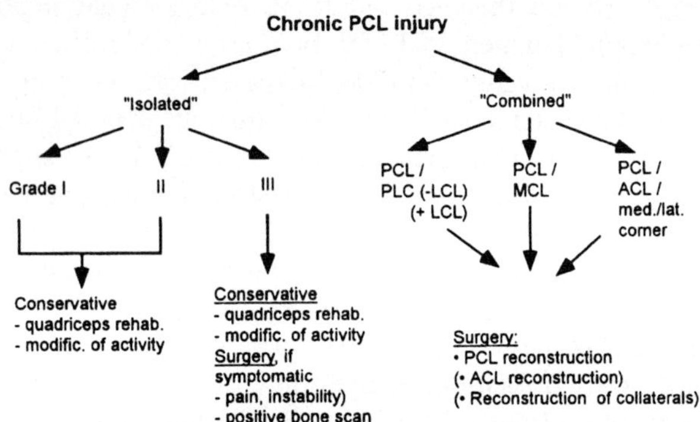

FIGURE 23.2. Treatment algorithm for acute and chronic posterior cruciate ligament (PCL) injuries. LCL, lateral collateral ligament; MCL, medial collateral ligament; ACL, anterior cruciate ligament. (From Harner CD, Höher J. Current concepts: evaluation and treatment of posterior cruciate ligament injuries. *Am J Sports Med* 1998;26:471–482, with permission.)

must be considered prior to intervention. Algorithms have been developed to aid the physician in treating these difficult problems but it is important to consider the individuality of each patient before pursuing a specific treatment (Fig. 23.2).

Nonoperative

Most acute, isolated grade I and II PCL injuries do not require surgical intervention (3,39,40,42,43). The likely benign course is related to the remaining integrity both of the secondary restraints and of various portions of the PCL. Treatment is focused on protected weight-bearing and quadriceps rehabilitation. In our experience, most patients recover rapidly and return to sports within 2-4 weeks of the injury. In acute grade III injuries, the rehabilitative course is not as predictable and frequently requires a longer time. Because of the possibility of occult PLS injury, we recommend 2 to 4 weeks of immobilization in full extension. This will minimize the posterior displacing effect of both gravity and the hamstrings on the tibia and will allow the PLS injury, if present, to heal with less stress (76,77). After the period of immobilization, the mainstay of rehabilitation is quadriceps strengthening to counteract posterior tibial subluxation (76,77). Quadriceps sets, straight leg raises, and partial weight bearing with crutches is initiated. At the end of 4 weeks, active-assisted ROM exercises are implemented and weight bearing is progressed to tolerance. Functional exercises such as biking and stair climbing, as well as leg presses and knee extensions follow this. After grade III injuries, it is usually at least 3 months before the athlete is able to return to sport. Unfortunately, some do not heal well with nonoperative therapy, and the athlete is unable to return to sport without some type of intervention. PCL functional braces may be used, but have not been effective in our experience; these patients may ultimately require surgery.

Similar to those with acute injuries, patients with chronic, isolated, grades I and II PCL injuries usually respond well with physical therapy while braces provide little benefit. Occasionally, some with chronic, grade II injuries will develop recurrent swelling and pain. In these situations, radiographs or a bone scan may be helpful to assess the status of the joint compartments. If the bone scan is notable for increased uptake, activity modification and physical therapy are recommended. Surgical intervention is usually avoided in these patients because current techniques have not been consistent in restoring the knee to normal function.

This is not the case in patients with chronic, grade III deficiencies. Surgery is recommended in these patients if they become symptomatic despite maximizing physical therapy intervention. In these cases, surgery can potentially provide enough stability to minimize the medial and/or patellofemoral compartment pain. We have found that in most of these injuries, there is some deficiency in the PLS. We, therefore, would recommend a PLS reconstruction in conjunction with the PCL reconstruction, as described in the next section.

Recommended treatment for an isolated, partial PLS injury, although rare, is almost universally nonoperative (64). Most patients do well with a protocol of knee immobilization in full extension for approximately 3 weeks followed by progressive functional rehabilitation exercises. Those who do not respond to this protocol should be carefully evaluated to determine if there is an abnormal gait pattern, evidence of limb malalignment or symptomatic increase in instability. If these are present, the patient may benefit from surgical intervention. Patients with isolated, complete PLS tears or combined injuries do poorly with nonsurgical treatment (64). Treatment for these injuries is focused on individual repair of all the involved structures.

Operative

Recent advances in the study of PCL and PLS injuries have led to a better understanding of the function and disability associated with these injuries. Although contro-versy still exists, this has led to more acceptable indications for surgical intervention. The issues of timing and type of reconstruction remain unresolved because there currently are no long-term studies that specifically address these issues.

Surgical intervention starts with a thorough preoperative assessment to determine the extent of the injury. These cases should be performed in a semi-elective setting with a skilled operating room staff. In addition, because of the proximity of the vessels to the tibial tunnel placement in certain reconstruction techniques, a vascular surgeon may be immediately required should injury to these structures occur. Any operative procedure should start with a complete examination under anesthesia. This is valuable not only for confirming the PCL injury but, more importantly, to assess the other potentially injured structures, particularly the PLS. Arthroscopy is also uniformly performed to confirm the extent of the injury and to assist with the repair or reconstructive procedure. The surgeon must be familiar with and capable to perform the repair or reconstruction options for the PCL as well as those of the collateral and capsular structures to ensure the optimal surgical outcome.

Several different methods have been developed for PCL and PLS reconstruction, emphasizing the fact that no current technique has met with reproducibly excellent results. Most surgeons now agree that restoration of normal anatomy yields the best potential for consistent results after PCL reconstruction (14,57,62,74). Numerous variables exist, including graft choice, graft placement, type of fixation, and postoperative rehabilitation.

A variety of tissues have been used for reconstruction. Autologous tissues include ipsilateral or contralateral bone-patellar tendon-bone, hamstrings, iliotibial band, or central quadriceps tendon. Bone-patellar tendon-bone and Achilles tendon are the most commonly used allograft tissues. We currently favor Achilles tendon allograft because of its high tensile strength, ease of passage and lack of donor site morbidity. Additional benefits of this graft include its exceptional size and length making it quite versatile when compared with other graft options. Multiple methods of fixation also exist, including interference fixation (metal or bioabsorbable) and remote fixation (Endobutton [Smith & Nephew Endoscopy, Andover, MA]), plastic buttons, cortical screws and washers, or staples. No single technique is universally accepted. The treating surgeon should be familiar with several of these options so that the final choice can depend on the surgical situation.

Posterior Cruciate Ligament

True isolated PCL injuries rarely require surgical intervention. Occasionally, those who have sustained grade III injuries and continue to be symptomatic despite extensive nonoperative treatment may benefit from surgical intervention, as mentioned earlier. Currently, most surgery in which the PCL is reconstructed involves combined ligament injury patterns (44–46,78), since many of the symptomatic, isolated, grade III injuries are likely associated with occult concomitant ligamentous injury, particularly involving the PLS (16,46,60,79). When a coexistent PLS injury is overlooked, surgical treatment of the PCL may have a higher risk for failure (23).

Surgical intervention for PCL injuries can be divided into primary repair and reconstruction. Unfortunately, as with ACL injuries, primary repair of midsubstance PCL tears has not been consistently successful. With avulsion injuries, however, primary repair typically results in a favorable outcome (65,80,81). Avulsion most commonly occurs on the femoral side of the ligament, but can also occur on the tibial side where it is usually associated with a large bone fragment. Surgical repair of these avulsions should be performed within 2 weeks of the injury. The femoral and tibial avulsions are approached through an anteromedial arthrotomy and a standard or modified posterior knee approach, respectively (82). They can then be fixed with either screws or sutures through drill holes depending on the presence and size of the bone fragment (33).

Current reconstructive options include single-bundle, double-bundle, tibial inlay or a combination of these techniques (79). None of these options, however, can effectively reproduce all the components of the PCL complex. The single-bundle technique was developed to reconstruct the AL bundle because of its larger size and greater biomechanical properties (11,13,83,84). In an attempt to place the graft in the anatomic position of the native AL bundle, a single tibial and femoral tunnel is utilized. An arthroscopic-assisted technique using the Achilles tendon is recommended (85). Because of recent biomechanical data suggesting that the addition of a second bundle significantly decreases posterior tibial translation, the double-bundle technique has become our preferred procedure, instead of the traditional single-bundle technique (86).

In performing the double-bundle reconstruction, the patient is positioned supine and a tourniquet is placed over the thigh (87). A detailed examination under anesthesia is performed followed by a systematic diagnostic arthroscopy. After confirmation of the PCL tear, the remnants are debrided using a posteromedial and standard anterior portals. Care is taken to avoid injury to the closely situated neurovascular structures. A tibial tunnel is then created from the anteromedial tibia and directed posteriorly to the native PCL tibial insertion (Fig. 23.3). The correct position is critical and should be checked with intraoperative radiographs after the guide wire is placed and before final drilling. After the tibial tunnel is completed, attention is then focused to creating the femoral tunnels. The lateral portal is enlarged and then utilized to create two tunnels, one corresponding to the AL and the other to the PM bundle insertion sites on the

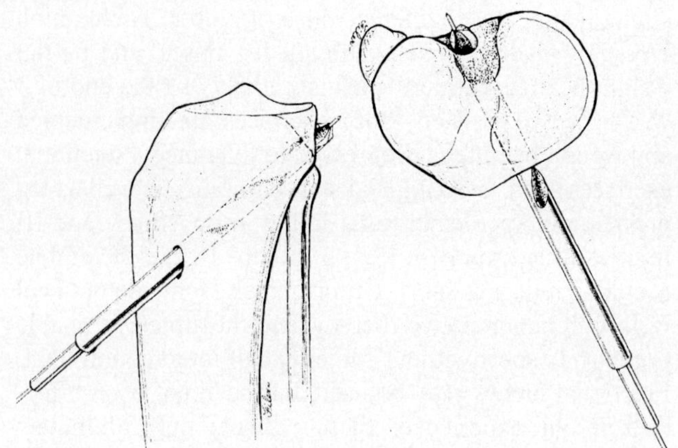

FIGURE 23.3. Posterior cruciate ligament tibial tunnel drilling. The angle of the proximal tibiofibular joint frequently serves as an adequate preliminary guide to correct tunnel placement. (From Miller MD, Harner CD, Kashiwaguchi SL. Acute posterior cruciate ligament injuries. In: Fu FH, Harner CD, Vince KG, eds. *Knee surgery, vol. 1.* Philadelphia: Lippincott Williams & Wilkins, 1994, with permission.)

medial femoral condyle (Fig. 23.4). The semitendinosus (or gracilis) is then harvested while an Achilles tendon allograft is prepared. Both of these grafts are then passed anterograde through the tibial tunnel, and, subsequently, retrograde into the femur with the Achilles tendon passed into the AL tunnel and the hamstring tendon passed into the PM tunnel (Fig. 23.5). The grafts are first fixed on the femoral side and then cycled. The Achilles graft, representing the reconstructed AL bundle, is tensioned at 90° and then fixed with a screw and pegged washer on the tibia. Subsequently, the hamstring tendon, or reconstructed PM bundle, is tensioned at 30° of flexion and then secured in a similar fashion or tied over a post (Fig. 23.6).

The rehabilitation protocol is, in general, slower than that for isolated ACL reconstruction. A hinged knee brace is placed and locked in extension for 4 weeks. During the ensuing 4 weeks, range of motion exercises are initiated while weight-bearing and strengthening exercises are progressed. The patient is expected to achieve full motion and a normal gait at approximately 3 months after surgery after which time more intensive therapy programs are initiated.

The tibial inlay technique recently has regained popularity (83,88–90). For this technique, a posterior approach to the knee is performed, and the graft is secured directly into a trough in the posterior tibia. The graft can then be directed straight to the femoral tunnel (90). This obviates the need for the excessive bend around the tibia and is followed by a standard single or double-bundle technique into the femur. This approach is technically demanding and requires a prone or lateral decubitus position, adding operative time and becoming particularly burdensome when attempting repair of a combined ligament injury. At this time, tibial fixation variation has not been shown to

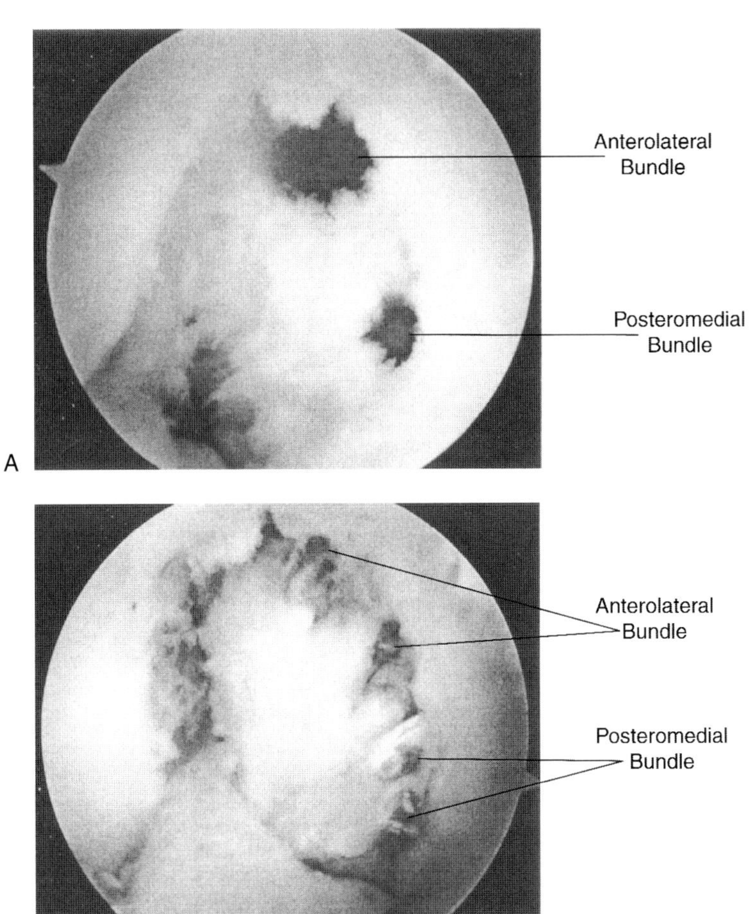

FIGURE 23.4. Positioning of femoral tunnels. **A:** The superior and inferior tunnels are positioned at the respective attachment sites of the anterolateral and posteromedial bundles. **B:** The same femoral condyle with the Achilles tendon allograft and semitendinosus autograft in place.

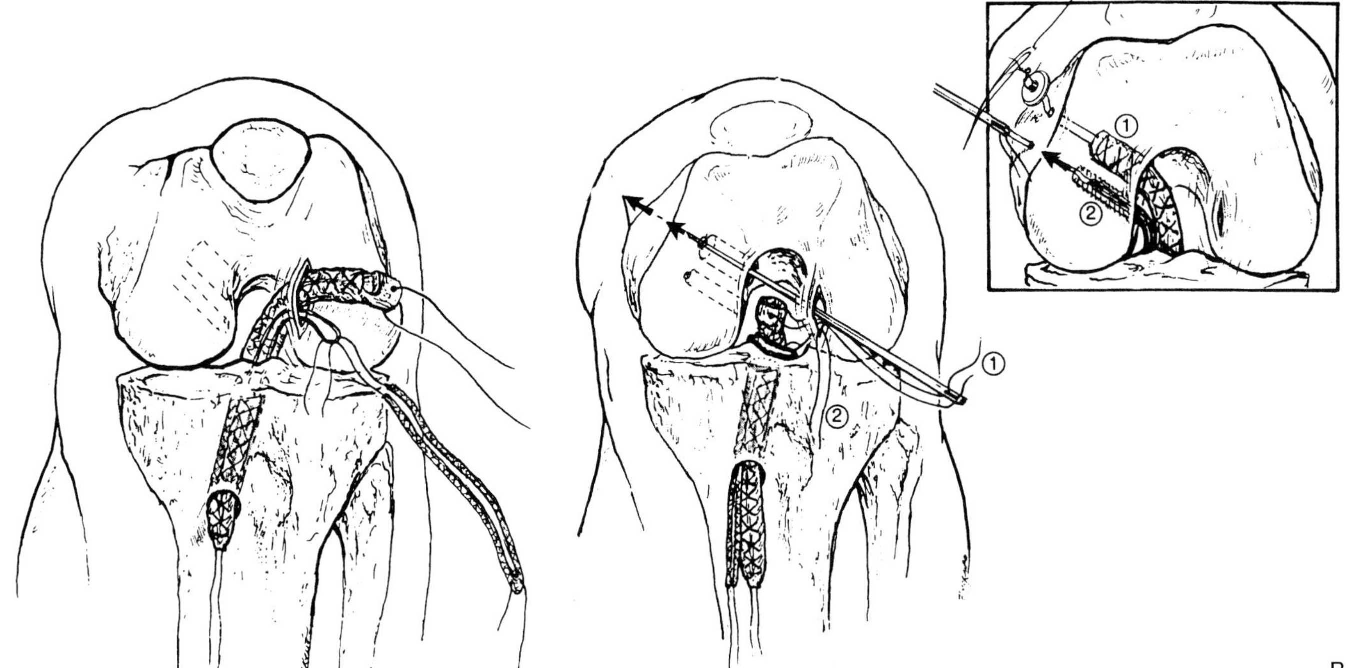

FIGURE 23.5. Graft placement. **A:** Achilles tendon allograft and semitendinosis autograft passed in anterograde fashion through the tibial tunnel. **B:** Grafts are then fixed into corresponding femoral tunnels. (From Petrie RS, Harner CD. Double bundle posterior cruciate ligament reconstruction technique: University of Pittsburgh approach. *Oper Tech Sports Med* 1999;7:118–126, with permission.)

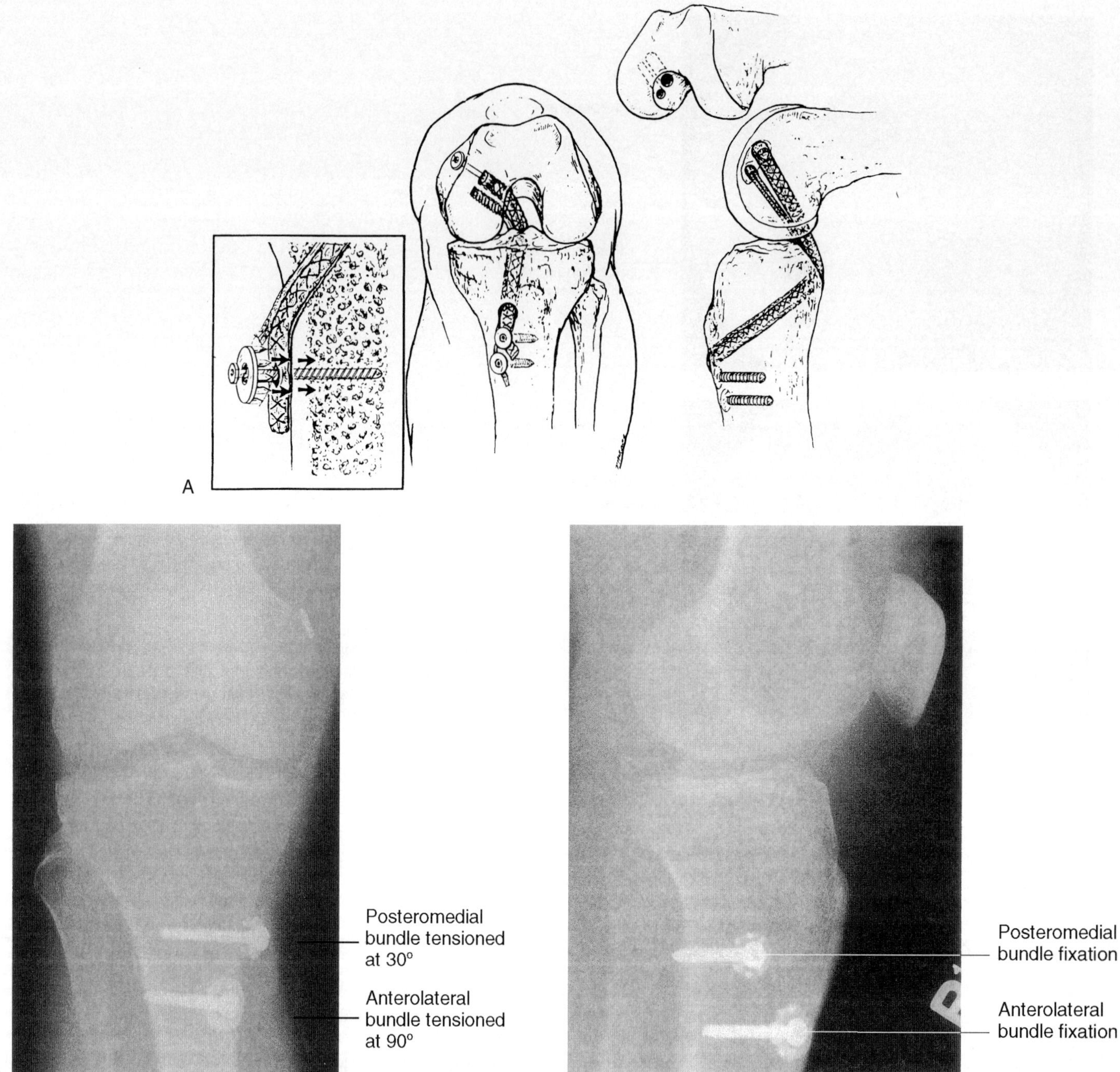

FIGURE 23.6. Tibial fixation of the posterior cruciate ligament graft. **A:** Illustration of individual graft fixation. **B:** Postoperative radiograph with fixation in place. (From Petrie RS, Harner CD. Double bundle posterior cruciate ligament reconstruction technique: University of Pittsburgh approach. *Oper Tech Sports Med* 1999;7:118–126, with permission.)

significantly affect the behavior of the graft, and so the theoretical benefits may not outweigh the technical demands of this technique (88–91).

Posterolateral Structures

Aside from the few cases of isolated, partial injuries, most tears of the PLS require surgical intervention. The combined PCL-PLS injury must be appropriately identified since, if mistaken for an isolated PCL injury and treated nonsurgically, posterior and posterolateral instability will invariably persist (1,2,14,33,34,50). Treatment of the acute PLS injury is generally more successful than that for the chronic injury, and therefore, acute reconstruction is recommended for both acute, isolated, complete PLS and combined PCL-PLS injury (3–5,46,60,79).

The timing for surgical treatment of the injured PLS is critical, with acute repairs consistently giving more favorable results than reconstruction of chronic injuries (46,60,64,79). Two reasons are proposed for this discrepancy. First, injuries to this region, unlike PCL ruptures, are associated with significant scar formation within the first 2 weeks, as previously mentioned. Attempts at surgical repair beyond this time frame are frequently disappointing both in localizing discrete anatomic structures and in finding any sturdy tissue to repair. Accordingly, surgical options for chronic injuries are reconstructions rather than repairs. Many reconstructive techniques have been described but none has consistently shown better results than acute repair.

Treatment of PLS injuries therefore is centered on recognizing the acute injury and following with the immediate, direct anatomic repair of all ligamentous injuries, preferably within the first 2 weeks. Depending on the quality of the tissue or type of injury, repair or reconstructive techniques may be utilized. Our approach begins with a lateral "hockey-stick" incision paralleling the posterior edge of the iliotibial band, which is then split, exposing the deep structures of the LCL anteriorly, and the lateral head of the gastrocnemius muscle and underlying popliteus complex more posteriorly. Special attention is given in identifying the injured structures. In cases where the posterolateral capsular structures are avulsed off their femoral attachments with preservation of the popliteus tendon, direct repair of these structures utilizing suture anchors is recommended. The LCL should also be assessed and, if present, an avulsion injury should similarly be repaired with suture anchors. Occasionally there is interstitial tearing of this structure, mandating concomitant reconstruction (92) (Fig. 23.7). For this, an Achilles tendon allograft is used. The LCL can be detached and elevated from its distal insertion and the allograft bone block is then fixed vertically into the fibular head using interference screw fixation. The native LCL can then be tensioned proximal and distal to the graft. Suture anchors are then placed into the lateral epicondyle, with passage of the suture arms through the Achilles tendon and proximal LCL to reinforce the repair.

The extent of injury to the popliteus and more importantly its attachments to the fibula through the popliteofibular ligament must then be visualized. The popliteofibular ligament has become recognized as a significant component of the popliteus complex, particularly as a static stabilizer (60). We, therefore, believe that this step is the most crucial to the overall success or failure of the procedure. In cases where this tendon is avulsed off of its tibial or femoral insertion, tension and anatomic restoration of this structure is created through the use of sutures in combination with femoral or fibular fixation by means of a blind tunnel and one of several possible fixation devices. Tension is applied with the knee in 20° to 30° of flexion during the final fixation. If the popliteus tendon

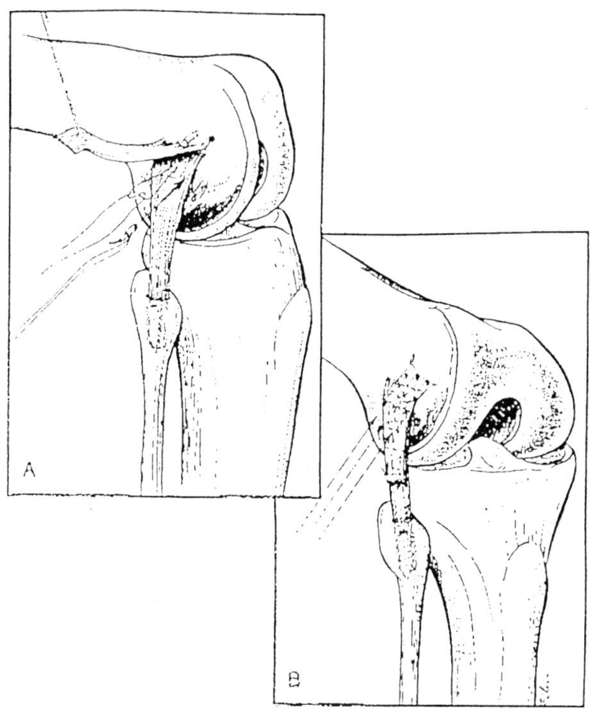

FIGURE 23.7. LCL reconstruction with Achilles tendon allograft. **A:** The torn or stretched LCL is elevated from its fibular insertion, and the allograft bone block is fixed in a tunnel in the proximal fibula using an interference screw. The tensioned graft is then fixed to the lateral epicondyle using multiple suture anchors. **B:** The native LCL is tensioned and sutured to the graft. (From Cole BJ, Harner CD. The multiple ligament injured knee. *Clin Sports Med* 1999;18:241–262, with permission.)

tissue cannot be repaired by this approach, reconstruction is indicated as described later for the chronic injury.

Chronic injuries still present a therapeutic challenge. Attempts at primary repair in this setting often lose stability over time (64). To improve long-term results, other techniques have been recommended, including arcuate ligament advancement, biceps tenodesis and popliteofibular ligament reconstruction with allograft or autograft tissue, but no consensus exists on which is the best procedure (6,55,62,93–98).

The initial evaluation of limb alignment and gait is essential for those with chronic injuries. If varus malalignment or a lateral thrust exists, a proximal tibial osteotomy may be necessary to correct the alignment. If unrecognized or ignored, ligamentous repair or reconstruction in this setting will have a significant risk for failure due to chronic repetitive stretching of the reconstruction with time (46,60,64). The osteotomy may be performed in conjunction with PLS reconstruction but we favor performing a staged operation, since the osteotomy alone may alleviate the patients symptoms, avoiding further surgical intervention (60). Otherwise, delayed reconstruction can be performed.

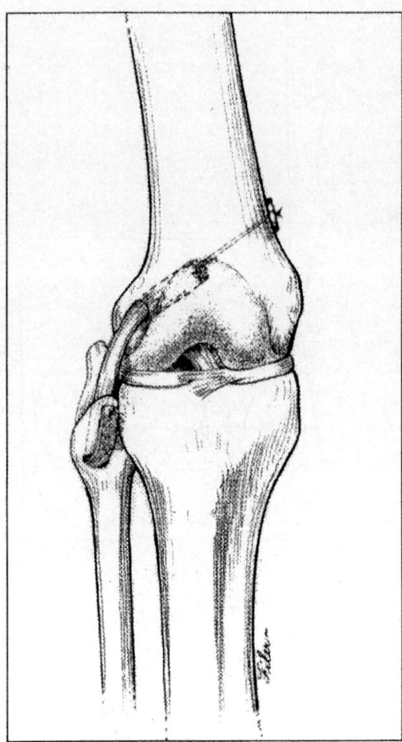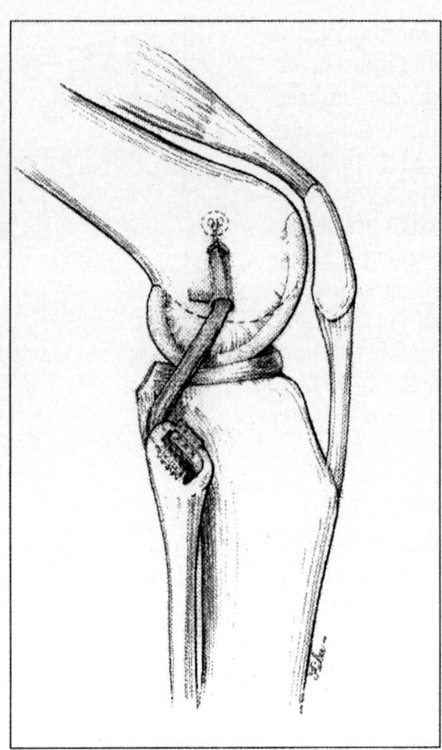

FIGURE 23.8. Popliteofibular ligament reconstruction using an interference screw for fibular fixation and a Hewson button for femoral fixation.

Chronic cases of posterolateral instability demonstrate tissue redundancy and excessive scarring posterior to the LCL, and identification of the particular structures of the popliteus complex is difficult, as mentioned previously. In this situation, we currently recommend anatomic reconstruction of the popliteofibular ligament. Utilizing the same approach to the lateral knee, the LCL is identified and if part of the injury pattern, reconstructed as described earlier. An oblique tunnel oriented similarly to the course of the ligament is then created in the proximal fibula. A proximal, blind femoral tunnel is then created at the anatomic insertion site of the popliteus tendon along the epicondylar axis of the femur. An Achilles tendon allograft is then passed under the LCL into the proximal and distal tunnels. Fixation at the fibular tunnel can be performed with soft tissue or conventional interference screws while the femoral side is stabilized with either a soft tissue interference screw, a button tied over the medial cortex through a separate skin incision, or a combination of these fixation methods (Fig. 23.8). The knee is maintained in 20° to 30° of flexion with neutral to slight internal rotation of the foot as the graft is tensioned and secured.

Combined Posterior Cruciate Ligament–Posterolateral Structures

Combined PCL-PLS is one of the most complex treatment problems encountered in managing knee ligament injuries. When both the PCL and PLS are ruptured, substantial posterior translation, external rotation and varus opening can all be present at differing angles of knee flexion (46). This combination creates a complex surgical puzzle (62). With several patterns of injury possible, it is difficult to have one surgical plan. It is essential to determine which and to what extent structures are injured. Ideally, combined PCL-PLS injuries should also be treated within the first 1 to 2 weeks. In the chronic setting, the surgeon must determine the need for an initial osteotomy, as described for the isolated PLS injury. Subsequently, all the injured soft tissue structures should be appropriately repaired or reconstructed to achieve the best chance for successful treatment.

In these cases, we recommend the simultaneous reconstruction of the PCL and PLS. The PCL is reconstructed first using the double-bundle technique to the point of femoral side fixation. Attention is then focused on the acute repair or reconstruction of the popliteofibular ligament and, if necessary, the LCL. Both can be reconstructed with a double-armed technique, but we favor approaching the reconstruction of the popliteofibular ligament and LCL individually with the approach outlined earlier (62). Subsequent to preparing the posterolateral aspect of the knee, the PCL graft is secured into the tibia. The knee is then placed in 30° of flexion where final posterolateral stabilization is performed. After surgery the patients follow a similar protocol as for PCL reconstruction.

SUMMARY

Recent studies have significantly advanced the understanding of the structure and function of both the PCL and PLS. Injuries to these structures are increasingly being recognized through improvements in examination techniques and diagnostic imaging studies. Despite this, treatment remains controversial. In general, most PCL injuries can be successfully treated nonoperatively while injuries to the PLS frequently require surgical intervention. Treatment of the combined PCL-PLS injuries continues to be one of the most challenging in ligamentous surgery of the knee. Although several surgical techniques have been developed, the most important factors associated with successful return of knee function are the early diagnosis and acute surgical treatment of this injury pattern.

REFERENCES

1. Fanelli GC. Posterior cruciate ligament injuries in trauma patients. *Arthroscopy* 1993;9:291–294.
2. Fanelli GC, Edson CJ. Posterior cruciate ligament injuries in trauma patients: Part II. *Arthroscopy* 1995;11:526–529.
3. Baker CL Jr, Norwood LA, Hughston JC. Acute posterolateral instability of the knee. *J Bone Joint Surg Am* 1983;65:614–618.
4. DeLee JC, Riley MB, Rockwood CA Jr. Acute posterolateral rotatory instability of the knee. *Am J Sports Med* 1983;11:199–207.
5. Hughston JC, Jacobson KE. Chronic posterolateral rotatory instability of the knee. *J Bone Joint Surg Am* 1985;67:351–359.
6. Watanabe Y, Moriya H, Takahashi K, et al. Functional anatomy of the posterolateral structures of the knee. *Arthroscopy* 1993;9:57–62.
7. Terry GC, LaPrade RF. The posterolateral aspect of the knee: anatomy and surgical approach. *Am J Sports Med* 1996;24:732–739.
8. Marshall JL, Girgis FG, Zelko RR. The biceps femoris tendon and its functional significance. *J Bone Joint Surg Am* 1972;54:1444–1450.
9. Terry GC, LaPrade RF. The biceps femoris muscle complex at the knee: its anatomy and injury patterns associated with acute anterolateral-anteromedial rotatory instability. *Am J Sports Med* 1996;24:2–8.
10. Markolf KL, Wascher DC, Finerman GA. Direct in vitro measurement of forces in the cruciate ligaments, Part II: the effect of section of the posterolateral structures. *J Bone Joint Surg Am* 1993;75:387–394.
11. Harner CD, Xerogeanes JW, Livesay GA, et al. The human posterior cruciate ligament complex: an interdisciplinary study. Ligament morphology and biomechanical evaluation. *Am J Sports Med* 1995;23:736–745.
12. Harner CD, Baek GH, Vogrin TM, et al. Quantitative analysis of human cruciate ligament insertions. *Arthroscopy* 1999;15:741–749.
13. Race A, Amis AA. The mechanical properties of the two bundles of the human posterior cruciate ligament. *J Biomech* 1994;27:13–24.
14. Harner CD, Höher J. Current concepts: evaluation and treatment of posterior cruciate ligament injuries. *Am J Sports Med* 1998;26:471–482.
15. Butler DL, Noyes FR, Grood ES. Ligamentous restraints to anterior-posterior drawer in the human knee. A biomechanical study. *J Bone Joint Surg Am* 1980;62:259–270.
16. Gollehon DL, Torzilli PA, Warren RF. The role of the posterolateral and cruciate ligaments in the stability of the human knee. A biomechanical study. *J Bone Joint Surg Am* 1987;69:233–242.
17. Grood ES, Stowers SF, Noyes FR. Limits of movement in the human knee. Effect of sectioning the posterior cruciate ligament and posterolateral structures. *J Bone Joint Surg Am* 1988;70:88–97.
18. Pearsall AW, Pyevich M, Draganich LF, et al. In vitro study of knee stability after posterior cruciate ligament reconstruction. *Clin Orthop* 1996;327:264–271.
19. Veltri D, Deng X-H, Torzilli PA, et al. The role of the popliteofibular ligament in the stability of the human knee. A biomechanical study. *Am J Sports Med* 1996;24:19–27.
20. Van Dommelen BA, Fowler PJ. Anatomy of the posterior cruciate ligament: a review. *Am J Sports Med* 1989;17:24–29.
21. Warren R, Arnoczky SP, Wickiewicz TL. Anatomy of the knee. In: Nicholas JA, Hershman EB, eds. *The lower extremity and spine in sports medicine*. St. Louis: CV Mosby, 1986:657–694.
22. Fox RJ, Harner CD, Sakane M, et al. Determination of in situ forces in the human posterior cruciate ligament using robotic technology: a cadaveric study. *Am J Sports Med* 1998;26:395–401.
23. Harner CD, Höher J, Vogrin TM, et al. The effect of sectioning of the posterolateral structures on in situ forces in the human posterior cruciate ligament. *Trans Orthop Res Soc* 1998;23:47.
24. Harner CD, Vogrin TM, Höher J, et al. The effects of loading the popliteus muscle on the intact and PCL deficient knee. *Trans Orthop Res Soc* 1997;43:863.
25. Veltri DM, Deng X-H, Torzilli PA, et al. The role of the cruciate and posterolateral ligaments in stability of the knee. A biomechanical study. *Am J Sports Med* 1995;23:436–443.
26. Kaplan EB. The fabellofibular and short lateral ligaments of the knee joint. *J Bone Joint Surg Am* 1961;43:169–179.
27. Last RJ. The popliteus muscle and the lateral meniscus with a note on the attachment of the medial meniscus. *J Bone Joint Surg Br* 1950;32:93–99.
28. Lovejoy JF Jr, Harden TP. Popliteus muscle in man. *Anat Rec* 1971;169:727–730.
29. Seebacher JR, Inglis AE, Marshall JL, et al. The structure of the posterolateral aspect of the knee. *J Bone Joint Surg Am* 1982;64:536–541.
30. Staubli HU, Birrer S. The popliteus tendon and its fascicles at the popliteal hiatus: gross anatomy and functional arthroscopic evaluation with and without anterior cruciate ligament deficiency. *Arthroscopy* 1990;6:209–220.
31. Staubli HU, Rauschning W. Popliteus tendon and lateral meniscus. *Am J Knee Surg* 1991;4:110–121.
32. Sudasna S, Harnsiriwattanagit K. The ligamentous structures of the posterolateral aspect of the knee. *Bull Hosp Joint Dis Orthop Inst* 1990;50:35–40.
33. Müller W. *The knee: form, function and ligament reconstruction*. Berlin: Springer-Verlag, 1983.
34. Staubli HU. Posteromedial and posterolateral capsular injuries associated with posterior cruciate ligament insufficiency. *Sports Med Arthrosc Rev* 1994;2:146–164.
35. Harner CD, Höher J, Vogrin TM, et al. The effects of a popliteus load on in situ forces in the posterior cruciate ligament on knee kinematics. *Am J Sports Med* 1998;26:669–673.
36. Höher J, Harner CD, Vogrin TM, et al. In situ forces in the posterolateral structures in the knee under posterior tibial loading in the intact and posterior cruciate ligament-deficient knee. *J Orthop Res* 1998;16:675–681.
37. Clancy WG Jr, Shelbourne KD, Zoellner GB, et al. Treatment of knee joint instability secondary to rupture of the posterior cruciate ligament. Report of a new procedure. *J Bone Joint Surg Am* 1983;65:310–322.
38. Miyasaka KC, Daniel DM. The incidence of knee ligament injuries in the general population. *Am J Knee Surg* 1991;4:3–8.
39. Fowler PJ, Messiah SS. Isolated posterior cruciate ligament injuries in athletes. *Am J Sports Med* 1987;15:553–557.
40. Parolie JM, Bergfeld JA. Long-term results of nonoperative treatment of isolated posterior cruciate ligament injuries in the athlete. *Am J Sports Med* 1986;14:35–38.
41. Kennedy JC, Grainger RW. The posterior cruciate ligament. *J Trauma* 1967;7:367–377.
42. Keller PM, Shelbourne KD, McCarroll JR, et al. Non-operatively treated isolated posterior cruciate ligament injuries. *Am J Sports Med* 1993;21:132–136.
43. Shelbourne KD, Davis TJ, Patel DV. The natural history of acute, isolated, non-operatively treated posterior cruciate ligament injuries: a prospective study. *Am J Sports Med* 1999;27:276–283.
44. Satku K, Chew CN, Seow H. Posterior cruciate ligament injuries. *Acta Orthop Scand* 1984;55:26–29.
45. Torg JS, Barton TM, Pavlov H, et al. Natural history of the posterior cruciate ligament-deficient knee. *Clin Orthop* 1989;246:208–216.
46. Cooper DE, Warren RF, Warner JJP. The posterior cruciate ligament and posterolateral structures of the knee: anatomy, function and patterns of injury. In: Tullos HS, ed. *Instructional Course Lecture, vol 40*. Park Ridge: American Academy Orthopaedic Surgeons, 1991:249–270.
47. Cain TE, Schwab GH. Performance of an athlete with straight posterior knee stability. *Am J Sports Med* 1981;9:203–208.
48. Cross MJ, Powell JF. Long-term follow-up of posterior cruciate ligament rupture: a study of 116 cases. *Am J Sports Med* 1984;12:292–297.
49. Dandy DJ, Pusey RJ. The long-term results of unrepaired tears of the posterior cruciate ligament. *J Bone Joint Surg Br* 1982;64:92–94.

50. Harner CD, Bennett CG. Posterior cruciate ligament injuries. In: Arendt EA, ed. *Orthopaedic knowledge update: sports medicine 2*. Rosemont, IL: American Academy of Orthopaedic Surgeons, 1999:317–326.

51. Green NE, Allen BL. Vascular injuries associated with dislocation of the knee. *J Bone Joint Surg* 1977;59:236–239.

52. Wascher DC, Dvimak PC, DeCoster TA. Knee dislocation: initial assessment and implications for treatment. *J Orthop Trauma* 1997;11: 525–529.

53. Shields L, Mital M, Cave E. Complete dislocation of the knee: experience at the Massachusetts General Hospital. *J Trauma* 1969;9:192–215.

54. Taft T, Almekinders L. The dislocated knee. In: Fu F, Harner CD, Vince K, eds. *Knee surgery*. Baltimore: Williams and Wilkins, 1994:837–858.

55. Hughston JC, Degenhardt TC. Reconstruction of the posterior cruciate ligament. *Clin Orthop* 1982;164:59–77.

56. Covey DC, Sapega AA. Injuries to the posterior cruciate ligament. *J Bone Joint Surg Am* 1993;75:1376–1386.

57. Noyes FR, Barber-Westin SD. Treatment of complex injuries involving the posterior cruciate and posterolateral ligaments of the knee. *Am J Knee Surg* 1996;9:200–214.

58. Noyes FR, Stowers SF, Grood ES, et al. Posterior subluxations of the medial and lateral tibiofemoral compartments. An in vivo ligament sectioning study in cadaveric knees. *Am J Sports Med* 1993;21:407–414.

59. Cooper DE. Tests for posterolateral instability of the knee in normal subjects: results of examination under anesthesia. *J Bone Joint Surg Am* 1991;73:30–36.

60. Veltri DM, Warren RF. Posterolateral instability of the knee. In: Jackson DW, ed. *Instructional Course Lectures, vol. 44*. Rosemont, IL: American Academy of Orthopaedic Surgeons, 1995:441–453.

61. Albright JP, Brown AW. Management of chronic posterolateral rotatory instability of the knee: surgical technique for the posterolateral sling procedure. In: Zuckerman JD, ed. *Instructional Course Lectures, vol 48*. Rosemont, IL: American Academy Orthopaedic Surgeons, 1999: 369–378.

62. Cooper DE. Treatment of combined posterior cruciate ligament and posterolateral injuries of the knee. *Oper Tech Sports Med* 1999;7: 135–142.

63. Veltri DM, Deng XH, Torzilli PA, et al. The role of the cruciate and posterolateral ligaments in stability of the knee: a biomechanical study. *Am J Sports Med* 1995;23:436–443.

64. LaPrade RF. The medial collateral ligament complex and the posterolateral aspect of the knee. In: Arendt EA, ed. *Orthopaedic knowledge update: sports medicine 2*. Rosemont, IL: American Academy of Orthopaedic Surgeons, 1999:317–326.

65. Meyers MH. Isolated avulsion of the tibial attachment of the posterior cruciate ligament of the knee. *J Bone Joint Surg Am* 1975;57: 669–672.

66. Hewett TE, Noyes FR, Lee MD. Diagnosis of complete and partial posterior cruciate ligament ruptures: stress radiography compared with KT-1000 arthrometer and posterior drawer testing. *Am J Sports Med* 1997;25:648–655.

67. Grover JS, Bassett LW, Gross ML, et al. Posterior cruciate ligament: MR imaging. *Radiology* 1990;174:527–530.

68. Polly DW, Callaghan JJ, Sikes RA, et al. The accuracy of selective magnetic resonance imaging compared with the findings of arthroscopy of the knee. *J Bone Joint Surg Am* 1988;70:192–198.

69. Turner DA, Prodromos CC, Petasnick JP, et al. Acute injuries of the ligaments of the knee: magnetic resonance evaluation. *Radiology* 1985; 154:717–722.

70. Pouranas J, Symeonides P. The results of surgical repairs of acute tears of the posterior cruciate ligament. *Clin Orthop* 1991;267:103–107.

71. Barrett G, Savoie F. Operative management of acute PCL injuries with associated long term results. *Orthopaedics* 1991;14:687–692.

72. Dejour H, Walch G, Peyrot J, et al. The natural history of rupture of the posterior cruciate ligament. *Fr J Orthop Surg* 1988;2:112–120.

73. Torg J, Barton T, Pavlov H, et al. Natural history of posterior cruciate deficient knee. *Clin Orthop* 1982;164:59–77.

74. Petrie RS, Harner CD. Evaluation and management of the posterior cruciate injured knee. *Oper Tech Sports Med* 1999;7:93–103.

75. Cooper DE. Classification of posterior cruciate ligament injury patterns. Presented at the International PCL Study Group Meeting, Dijon, France, 1995.

76. Höher J, Harner CD, Vogrin TM, et al. Hamstring loading increases in situ forces in the PCL. *Trans Orthop Res Soc* 1998;23:48.

77. Renstrom P, Arms SW, Stanwyk TS, et al. Strain within the anterior cruciate ligament during hamstring and quadriceps activity. *Am J Sports Med* 1986;14:83–87.

78. O'Donoghue DH. An analysis of end results of surgical treatment of major injuries of the ligaments of the knee. *J Bone Joint Surg Am* 1955; 37:1–13.

79. Miller MD, Bergfeld JA, Fowler PJ, et al. The posterior cruciate ligament injured knee: principles of evaluation and treatment. In: Zuckerman JD, ed. *Instructional Course Lectures, vol. 48*. Rosemont, IL: American Academy of Orthopaedic Surgeons, 1999:199–207.

80. Gross M, Glover JS, Bassett LW, et al. Magnetic resonance imaging of the PCL: clinical use to improve diagnostic accuracy. *Am J Sports Med* 1992;20:732—737.

81. Richter M, Kiefer H, Hehl G, et al. Primary repair for posterior cruciate ligament injuries: an eight-year follow up of fifty-three patients. *Am J Sports Med* 1996;24:298–305.

82. Burks RT, Schaffer JJ. A simplified approach to the tibial attachment of the posterior cruciate ligament. *Clin Orthop* 1990;254:216–219.

83. Benedetto KP, Hackl W, Fink C. Mittelfristige Ergebnisse der hinteren Kreuzbandrekonstrúktion mit dern LAD-augmentierten Lig. Patellae. *Arthroskopie* 1995;8:95–99.

84. Race A, Amis AA. Are anatomic PCL reconstructions superior to isometric? An in-vitro biomechanical analysis. *Trans Orthop Res Soc* 1997;43:874.

85. Klimkiewicz JJ, Harner CD, Fu FH. Single bundle posterior cruciate ligament reconstruction: University of Pittsburgh approach. *Oper Tech Sports Med* 1999;7:105–109.

86. Harner CD, Janaushek MA, Kanamori A, et al. Biomechanical analysis of a double bundle posterior cruciate ligament reconstruction. *Am J Sports Med* 2000;28:144–151.

87. Petrie RS, Harner CD. Double bundle posterior cruciate ligament reconstruction technique: University of Pittsburgh approach. *Oper Tech Sports Med* 1999;7:118–126.

88. Berg EE. Posterior cruciate ligament tibial inlay reconstruction. *Arthroscopy* 1995;8:95–99.

89. Jacob RP, Edwards JC. Posterior cruciate ligament reconstruction: anterior-posterior two stage technique. *Sports Med Arthrosc Rev* 1994;2: 137–145.

90. Miller MD, Olszewski AD. Posterior cruciate ligament injuries: new treatment options. *Am J Knee Surg* 1995;8:351–355.

91. Bach BR Jr, Daluga DJ, Mikosz R, et al. Force displacement characteristics of the posterior cruciate ligament. *Am J Sports Med* 1992;20: 67–72.

92. Cole BJ, Harner CD. The multiple ligament injured knee. *Clin Sports Med* 1999;18:241–262.

93. Clancy WG. Repair and reconstruction of the posterior cruciate ligament. In: Chapman M, ed. *Operative orthopaedics*. Philadelphia: JB Lippincott, 1981:1651–1655.

94. Fanelli GC, Giannotti BF, Edson CJ. Arthroscopically assisted combined posterior cruciate ligament/posterolateral complex reconstruction. *Arthroscopy* 1996;12:521–529.

95. Fleming RE, Blatz DJ, McCarroll JR. Posterior problems in the knee: posterior cruciate insufficiency and posterolateral rotatory insufficiency. *Am J Sports Med* 1981;9:107–113.

96. Maynard MJ, Deng X, Wickiewicz TL, et al. The popliteofibular ligament. Rediscovery of a key element in posterolateral instability. *Am J Sports Med* 1996;24:311–316.

97. Noyes FR, Barber-Westin SD. Surgical reconstruction of severe chronic posterolateral complex injuries of the knee using allograft tissues. *Am J Sports Med* 1995;23:2–12.

98. Noyes FR, Barber-Westin SD. Surgical restoration to treat chronic deficiency of the posterolateral complex and cruciate ligaments of the knee joint. *Am J Sports Med* 1996;24:415–426.

Part C: Evaluation and Treatment of the Multiple Ligament Injured Knee

Christopher C. Annunziata, J. Robert Giffin, and Christopher D. Harner

The purpose of this section is to present our current approach to the multiple ligament-injured knee. Although the potential combinations that exist under this topic seem endless, we will simplify this and focus on combined ligament-injured knees that involve both cruciate ligaments. Basically, we will be discussing the evaluation and management of the dislocated knee. Combinations that will be focused on are the ACL/PCL, ACL/PCL medial side, and ACL/PCL lateral side injuries. This section will be organized into epidemiology and mechanism of injury, associated injuries, classification, evaluation and management.

EPIDEMIOLOGY AND MECHANISM OF INJURY

The vast majority of knee dislocations result in both the ACL and PCL being ruptured (1–6). Complete bicruciate knee ligament injuries will, therefore, be considered synonymous to knee dislocations for the purpose of this discussion (7–11). The reported incidence of knee dislocations has ranged from 0.001% to 0.013% of patients evaluated for orthopedic injuries (12–17). The actual incidence, however, may be higher since many dislocations can be missed either due to the frequent occurrence of spontaneous reduction (20% to 56%) or because of attention drawn to other significant injuries (5,7,14–22). In the future, the reported incidence of knee dislocations may rise with the faster average speed of vehicles, the increased number of people participating in sports and the better recognition of this injury (23).

Knee dislocations typically occur as a result of extreme forces on the knee (23,24). Although they can occur with trivial mechanisms such as slipping off a curb, more than 50% are caused by high- or low-energy trauma such as in motor vehicle accidents or contact sports (3,17,25, 27–29). The injurious force may occur directly, as in the typical "dashboard" mechanism with a posteriorly directed force to the anterior tibia, or indirectly as with sudden hyperextension of the knee (7,28,29). High-energy accidents may also result in pure varus or valgus rotation leading to dislocation (24).

ASSOCIATED INJURIES

The devastating nature of knee dislocations is related predominantly to the high incidence of injury to structures other than the supporting ligaments. It is essential that the treating physician be aware of these potentially limb-threatening injuries.

Injuries to the popliteal artery—from intimal tears to complete disruption—occur in approximately 33% of knee dislocations (12,14,17,24,25,29–40). Despite this high risk, some go undetected in this setting, predominantly due to the difficulty in assessing the integrity of the vasculature. Although the absence of adequate capillary refill or palpable pulses is highly suggestive of arterial compromise, their presence does not completely exclude the possibility of injury to the circulation (7,31, 33,37,38,41–43). Thus, the liberal use of arteriography in the evaluation of knee dislocations may be indicated (11,28,31,32,38,40,44). Poor collateral flow around the knee that is not adequately restored within 6 to 8 hours has led to reported amputation rates as high as 86% (31).

Besides the vasculature, both the tibial and peroneal nerves can be injured in the setting of a knee dislocation. The peroneal nerve is involved in 9% to 49% of cases (12, 13,15,17,24,29,34,37,45,46). Nerve injury commonly occurs with disruption of the lateral ligamentous structures (7,11). Most cases result in a neuropraxic pattern of injury although complete transection can occur. Regardless, functional return is generally poor, with more than 50% achieving only limited recovery (14,17,29,34,45).

Avulsion injuries are commonly seen with knee dislocations, with avulsions of the cruciate ligaments involved in 50% to 80% of the cases (30,34). Avulsions should not be mistaken for more severe fractures involving the condyles or tibial plateau (14,15,34,46). Although no reliable estimate exists, it is generally felt that these severe fracture-dislocations are underreported (1). With associated soft tissue complications and pronounced joint instability, early bony fixation is mandatory, as is soft tissue repair or reconstruction. Such associated injuries generally result in worse outcomes when compared with fracture alone (1,7,34). Open injuries have been reported with 19% to 35% of the dislocations, as have injuries to the extensor mechanism and other tendons around the knee (14,15,17,47).

CLASSIFICATION

A classification system is helpful only if it provides assistance in developing a treatment plan, comparing results and predicting prognosis. In light of this, no classification system for knee dislocations is perfect. Dislocations of joints can be discussed in terms of degree, timing, and direction. Those involving the knee can be partial, associated with spontaneous reduction, or complete at initial presentation. The distinction between acute and chronic is somewhat arbitrary, but may have implications for treatment: as with PCL/PLS injuries, treatment in the acute setting usually involves some aspects of primary repair, whereas treatment after 3 weeks typically warrants reconstruction of the involved structures.

Classically, knee dislocations have been discussed in terms of the tibial position relative to the femur (48). Anterior and posterior dislocations are most common, whereas medial, lateral, and rotatory dislocations occur less frequently. The least common displacement, posterolateral, has been well described because of the difficulty with closed reduction. This is due to the "button-hole" effect of the medial femoral condyle through the capsule, which can lead to a high incidence of peroneal nerve palsy and skin necrosis (16,49,50). Although the positional system of classification is helpful in determining the method of reduction and in predicting associated injuries, it has limitations. Under this classification, both cruciate ligaments are assumed torn, but isolated injuries to these structures have been reported in some knee dislocations (3,4). The system also fails to address the spontaneously reduced dislocation or to delineate the status of the collateral ligaments or potential patterns of ligament damage (1,7,11).

We have found the classification presented by Schenck's group to be most helpful (9) (Table 23.3). This system is purely anatomic; distinguishing between structures involved and patterns of injury (7,18,31,36). Four classes of injury are presented, with five basic patterns, further sub-classified by associated injuries (7,18,31,36). One significant omission from each of these classification systems is the lack of attention to articular cartilage and meniscal damage; such associated injuries may

TABLE 23.3. *Classification of knee dislocations*

Class	Injury
KDI	PCL—intact knee dislocation, usually ACL and LCL torn, also includes ACL—intact knee dislocation with complete PCL tear
KDII	ACL and PCL torn, collaterals intact
KDIII—M	ACL, PCL, MCL—corner torn; lateral side intact
KDIII—L	ACL, PCL, LCL—corner torn; medial side intact
KDIV	All 4 ligaments torn

PCL, posterior cruciate ligament; ACL, anterior cruciate ligament; LCL, lateral collateral ligament; MCL, medial collateral ligament.

From Schenck RC Jr, Hunter RE, Ostrum RF, et al. Knee dislocations. In: Zuckerman JD, ed. *Instructional course lectures, vol. 48.* Rosemont, IL: American Academy of Orthopaedic Surgeons, 1999:515–522, with permission.

impact significantly on the ultimate functional outcome. For the best possible guide to diagnosis, treatment and prognosis, all these systems should be taken into consideration (23).

TREATMENT

The goals of treatment are to restore knee stability, reestablish a normal ROM, and return the patients to their preinjury level of function, while attempting to guard against late posttraumatic arthritis. Each patient must be treated individually, taking age, occupation, lifestyle, and expectations into consideration. Before surgical intervention, several factors must be addressed. These include adequately delineating the extent of injury, defining the appropriate timing of surgery, and determining what type of repair or reconstruction and graft sources will be necessary.

Initial Evaluation

The evaluation of the knee in the acute trauma setting must include a history emphasizing the mechanism of injury and a thorough neurovascular examination of the entire lower extremity. This is essential since some patients with multiple trauma may have a knee dislocation that is unrecognized because the focus of attention may have been directed toward other life-threatening injuries. Special attention is given to peroneal and tibial nerve function as well as the skin of the lower extremity. Popliteal and pedal pulses, capillary refill and compartment swelling are evaluated by comparison to the contralateral side. Attention then is directed to the supporting structures of the knee itself. Eliciting gross instability of two or more ligaments should give rise to a high clinical suspicion for a knee dislocation even if it is not obvious on radiographic images (1). An algorithm of our initial approach to the multiple ligament-injured knee is presented in Figure 23.9.

If the knee is dislocated on presentation, closed reduction should be attempted immediately after obtaining radiographs. The reduction maneuver is based on the mechanism of injury and direction of dislocation and should be performed expeditiously to avoid persistent compression or stretching of the neurovascular structures. Once accomplished, joint congruence and circulatory status must immediately be reevaluated. Depending on the results, emergent surgery may be required.

Once the knee is reduced and the neurovascular examination is complete, a ligamentous evaluation can be performed. Many different patterns of multiligamentous injury can occur. These can vary from the infrequent cases of only one of the cruciate ligaments being ruptured or no collateral ligament involvement to the more common bicruciate injury combined with lateral or medial-sided injury (15,17,24,28,34). Injuries to other structures may also be underestimated. Extensive capsular, articular

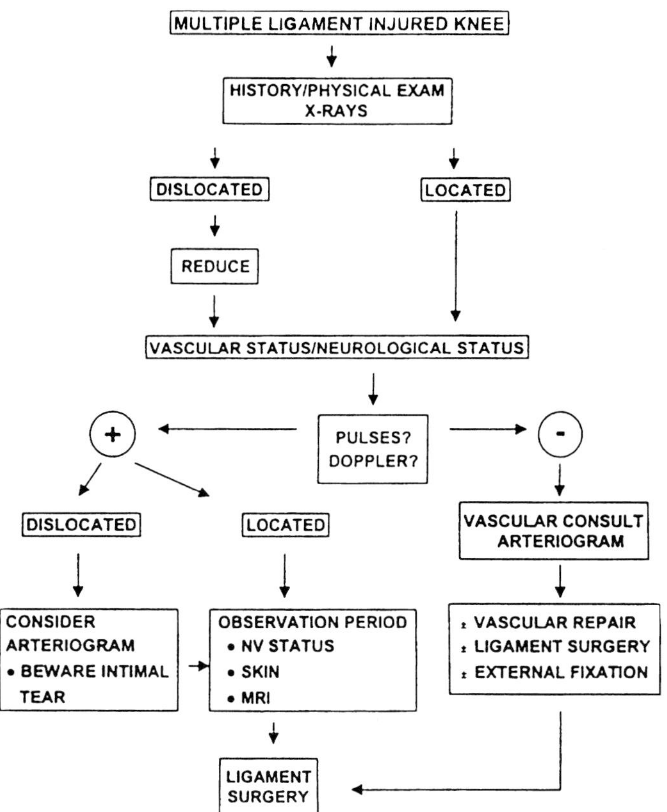

FIGURE 23.9. Treatment algorithm for the multiple-ligament injured knee. (Marks P, Harner CD. The ACL in the multiple ligament injured knee. *Clin Sports Med* 1993;12:825–838, with permission.)

cartilage, and meniscal damage can occur as well as tears to the muscles or tendons around the knee. Due to the significant pain, swelling, and gross instability commonly associated with these injuries, the best evaluation will come from an examination under anesthesia. Despite the extent of injury, however, a flexion arc of 0° to 30° is usually obtainable in the acute setting. Applying varus or valgus stress at 30° may reveal significant opening, suggesting injury to a collateral ligament, while opening at full extension indicates additional PCL and/or ACL damage (1,51–56). The integrity of the ACL can also be assessed with a gentle Lachman's test at 30°. Special care should be taken to avoid accidental hyperextension or redislocation of the knee. In the knee that can be flexed to 90°, testing of the PCL and PLS can be performed but this is usually impossible in the acute setting.

If emergent surgery is not required, imaging studies can be exceedingly helpful. Standard radiographs will provide information as to the mechanism of injury and allow some prediction of the possible extent of ligamentous injury. They will also demonstrate associated avulsion or significant periarticular fractures of the tibia, femur or patella. In addition to plain radiographs, stress radiographs in certain cases have been suggested to determine the degree of ligamentous laxity (7,23). In cases of chronic injury, a bone scan may be helpful to distinguish whether persistent pain is from instability or posttraumatic arthritis (57,58).

In the setting of the multiple ligament-injured knee, MRI has proven to be invaluable (Fig. 23.10). Not only is it the best study to evaluate the integrity of the ligaments,

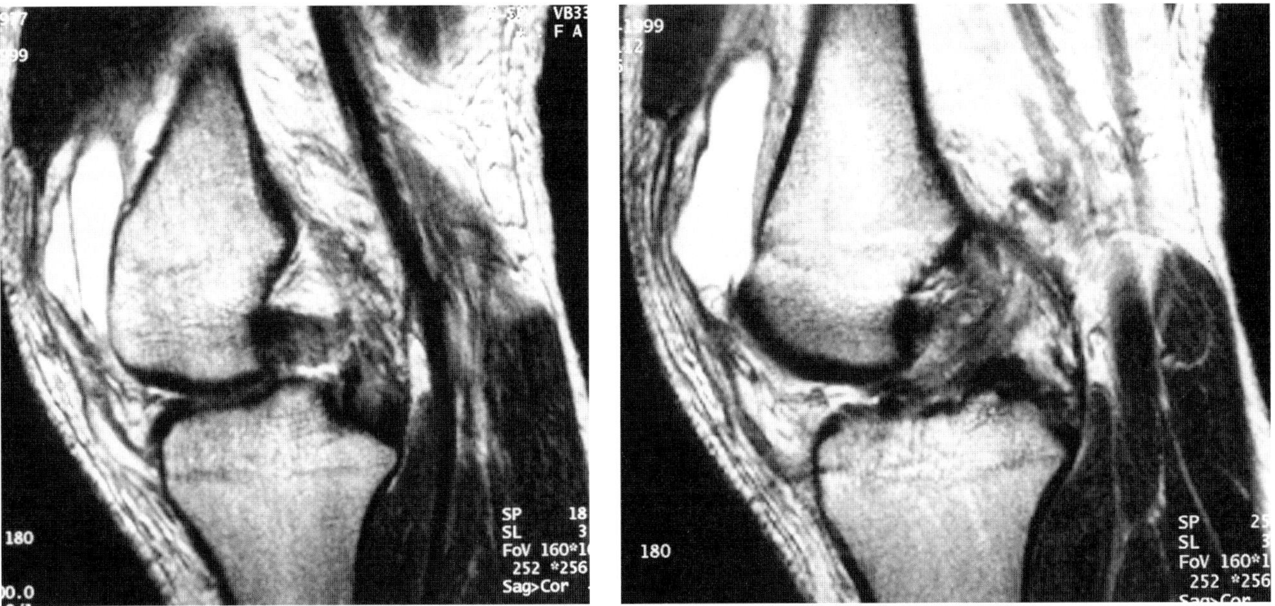

FIGURE 23.10. Magnetic resonance image of a multiple-ligament injured knee. Sequential T2-weighted sagittal images notable for **(A)** a torn posterior cruciate ligament and **(B)** a torn anterior cruciate ligament.

but it will also provide information about other structures such as the menisci, articular cartilage, extensor mechanism and bone, which if injured can lead to a poor outcome. MRI provides information necessary for identifying which structures will need to be addressed surgically and what resources will be required (7,9,10,19,20,59,60). Perhaps most importantly, preoperative counseling becomes possible regarding prognosis. Although these studies are helpful, the final assessment and treatment decisions stem from the examination under anesthesia.

Timing

Although the definitive treatment remains controversial, some surgical indications are well accepted. Emergent surgical intervention is necessary when adequate blood flow has not been restored after proper reduction or when a reduction can not be obtained in a closed manner. Impending or true compartment syndrome and open injury are also situations requiring immediate treatment including fasciotomy and irrigation and debridement respectively.

Some injuries may not require immediate intervention but are best treated in an urgent manner, within the first 24 to 48 hours from the injury. These include significant lower extremity fractures, such as those of the distal femur or tibial plateau, as well as disruption of the extensor mechanism. Treatment of these injuries is essential to achieve adequate periarticular stabilization and active joint mobility prior to ligamentous reconstruction.

Treatment should be delayed in the setting of multiligament injury or nerve disruption. Although controversial, most authors would recommend operative treatment of the multiple ligament-injured knee with the possible exception of older, sedentary individuals and those few that are stable after reduction (1,6,7,11,14–17,23,24,26, 28–30,34,37,44–46,50,61–75).

Operative Treatment

The treatment of the multiple ligament-injured knee remains controversial. Many opinions exist regarding the appropriate care of the damaged ligamentous structures and other associated injuries. We will present our approach to the management of the significant associated injuries but will focus predominantly on the treatment of the combined ligament injuries.

Vascular Injuries

Our treatment of vascular injuries is based on the examination. The pedal pulses are evaluated before and after reduction. If they are not restored or if there is any evidence of ischemia, we obtain an immediate vascular surgery consultation and prepare for urgent surgical exploration. At this point limb salvage takes priority over knee stability. A "one-shot" arteriogram in the operating room followed by exploration and repair is preferred in our institution. Communication is essential between the orthopedic and vascular surgeons when planning the timing of repair, placement of incisions and postoperative immobilization. Arterial repair typically involves resection of the injured segment and reanastomosis with an interposition graft. If possible the popliteal vein is also reconstructed to potentially limit the development of late venous insufficiency or thrombosis, and to optimize arterial patency after reconstruction (13,37,42,43,76). Prophylactic fasciotomies are uniformly performed after revascularization. We will also repair bony avulsions or collateral ligament tears only if encountered in the approach for the vascular procedure. Most vascular surgeons prefer to keep the knee in slight flexion after surgery to take tension off the repair. Although it is of primary importance to maintain a well functioning vascular graft, knee flexion may prolong tibial subluxation until the time of ligamentous reconstruction, and thus may later prohibit successful reduction. Generally the knee can safely be placed in an immobilizer, but if there is any concern of significant instability or subluxation that could compromise the repair, we have a low threshold for placing an external fixator across the joint until ligamentous reconstruction can be performed.

Although immediate treatment is straightforward in the setting of absent pulses, detection of strong palpable pulses does not exclude the possibility of an arterial injury (7,31,33,37,38,41–43). Vascular injury may not develop immediately. In fact, undetected intimal tears can lead to vascular compromise several days after the injury (30,33,38,42,47,77). Therefore, many different approaches to treatment in this setting have been discussed in the literature, including observation, serial examination with ankle-brachial index evaluation, Doppler pressure measurements and definitive arteriography (5,23,26,30–35,38,77). It remains the responsibility of the treating physician to diagnose and treat any arterial injury promptly. One should never assume that vascular compromise is caused by self-limited arterial spasm. We recommend the liberal use of arteriography if there is any asymmetry of pulses and even when pulses return to normal after reduction.

These patients are at high risk for the development of deep venous thrombosis during the period before definitive surgical reconstruction due to potential popliteal vein injury and relative immobility. Because of this, appropriate prophylaxis should be considered.

Nerve Injuries

The initial assessment of sensory and motor function is crucial. The immediate treatment of a neurologic deficit should be aimed at relieving ischemia or impending compartment syndrome rather than primarily repairing the nerve injury. Prevention of contracture is a high priority, but the outcome of direct nerve injury in this setting remains unknown. Injuries can range from complete disruption to mild traction. If the nerve is intact, at least 3 months of observation is warranted to assess for spontaneous recovery (78). Functional return may take up to 1 year, whereas neurolysis has been suggested to potentially expedite this (15). If the nerve is intact but a deficit exists at the time of surgery, we will perform a release of the fascial bands where the peroneal nerve enters the anterior and lateral compartments to prevent postoperative edema from potentially causing compression. Although immediate microsurgical repair of sharply transected nerves has generally proven to be practical, we think that it is best, in this setting, to tag the cut ends for later identification and cable grafting (1,79).

Ligament Injuries

As previously stated, if immediate surgery is required for vascular, open, or irreducible injury, we will attempt primary repair of collateral ligament tears and significant bony avulsions through the incisions created, when deemed feasible (e.g., if the wound is not contaminated and the vascular repair is secure) (1,23). Definitive surgery for the remaining ligamentous and other intraarticular injuries is performed later.

If immediate surgery is not required for associated injuries, the operation to repair the multiple ligament-injured knee should be delayed for 1 to 2 weeks but not longer than 3 weeks. This offers several advantages. It will allow for a period of vascular monitoring during the resolution of acute inflammation. Range of motion and quadriceps tone will partially return, potentially reducing the risk for postoperative arthrofibrosis (26). Various degrees of healing will also take place. Capsular healing occurs quickly and will allow an arthroscopic-assisted approach to surgery thus minimizing the extent of tissue dissection. Fortunately, healing of other complete tears, such as the collaterals or PLS, is not full in the short term. Scarring of these structures will therefore be minimal, allowing for their identification and repair. Significantly more scarring will occur in the chronic setting, leading to poorer results with attempted primary repair. If surgery must be delayed beyond 3 weeks, it may be prudent to wait until full range of motion is established and consider late reconstruction if the patient develops residual laxity leading to functional instability (1).

As with other orthopedic injuries, preferences in treating the multiple ligament-injured knee have cycled throughout the years and optimal treatment remains ill-defined. Before the mid-1970s, most pertinent literature focused on nonsurgical approaches consisting of closed reduction followed by immobilization (14,24,29,40,46). Results tended to vary with the duration of closed treatment: longer periods of immobilization resulted in stable but stiff knees whereas brief periods led to excellent motion but frequently unacceptable instability (7,11,29, 80). With recent advances in knee ligament surgery, many now feel comfortable recommending operative treatment of this injury with the goal of improving stability while retaining motion (1,6,7,11,14–17,23,24,26,28–30,34,37, 44–46,50,61–75).

The literature pertaining to the multiple ligament–injured knee is sparse, and no single treatment approach has been accepted by all. Several reasons for this exist. First, the relative infrequency of the injury presents few subjects for study. Second, the reports tend to vary with respect to the combined ligament-injury patterns included. Third, the methods of treatment and tools for subsequent evaluation have been inconsistent. The current opinion is that surgical intervention will result in superior stability and range of motion while nonoperative treatment will lead to unacceptable stiffness or instability, but this belief has not yet been proven with a reliable clinical study. Unfortunately, no prospective study currently exists to compare surgical to nonsurgical treatments of this injury, since this would subject some patients to the documented ill effects of immobilization not typically encountered with surgical intervention (7,23,81).

In our experience, these patients are at high risk for persistent and progressive functional instability, and surgical treatment has given a more predictable outcome without the complications of immobilization. The concern for postoperative arthrofibrosis with subsequent restricted motion is well appreciated in this setting (26, 28,34,65,67). Some authors have proposed that staging the reconstruction of cruciate injuries decreases the risk for postoperative arthrofibrosis (26,82). In fact, it is not known whether it is the concomitant repair or reconstruction of all the injured ligaments, or the lack of early mobilization that puts the knee at greatest risk for limited functional mobility (23). Others have not found that simultaneous reconstruction increases this risk (61,67, 71,83). Since the ACL and PCL serve different stabilizing functions, we believe the best reproduction of knee kinematics must involve reconstruction of both cruciate ligaments. In addition, we believe associated ligament injuries resulting in grade III laxity have a limited ability to heal in a functional position without excess laxity. Therefore, we recommend the simultaneous repair or reconstruction of all, complete, ligamentous tears in the multiple ligament–injured knee followed by early motion once significant nerve, vessel, and skin injuries, if present, have been addressed. This subjects the patient to fewer operations, decreases concern for late instability, and limits the possibility of arthrofibrosis.

Repair Versus Reconstruction

Repair or reconstruction of the ligamentous injuries depends on the structure involved. In the setting of a knee dislocation, the vast majority of cruciate injuries are midsubstance tears. Primary repair of a midsubstance tear in a cruciate ligament has not been successful (84). We therefore reconstruct this type of injury. In the case of bony avulsion injuries of the cruciate ligaments, however, primary repairs have been successful (85,86). This is either performed using nonabsorbable sutures passed through small drill holes tied over a cortical bridge of bone or screw fixation depending on the size of the associated bone fragment (84).

With respect to the medial and lateral structures, primary repair has met with better results. Avulsions or intrasubstance tears of the MCL may be directly repaired. Similar injuries to the LCL can also be repaired, but we tend to supplement the repair of intrasubstance tears with a graft reconstruction. This is done because of less consistent healing as well as the limited success in treating chronic insufficiency of the LCL if it were to occur. If peripheral meniscal tears or capsular avulsions are encountered, they are also repaired primarily. Beyond 3 weeks, however, scar formation and soft tissue contracture limits the success of primary ligamentous repair thus reconstructive procedures often become necessary.

Several different grafts may be utilized for reconstruction. Depending on the extent of injury, autografts may be obtained from the ipsilateral or contralateral patellar, hamstring, or quadriceps tendons. In our hands, however, allograft tissue is used predominantly over autograft in the multiple ligament–injured knee. The use of allograft eliminates graft site morbidity, decreases dissection time and reduces the number and extent of incisions in an already substantially traumatized knee (5,61,65,71). It also decreases intraoperative tourniquet time as well as postoperative pain and stiffness (87). The risk for disease transmission with the use of allograft tissue has been exceedingly low (88). Additional factors influencing graft selection include the mechanical characteristics, type of fixation, and the morbidity of tissue loss. We prefer allograft bone–patellar tendon–bone to reconstruct the ACL and allograft Achilles tendon to reconstruct the LCL. For PCL reconstruction, we perform a single-bundle technique in the acute setting and more recently a double-bundle technique for chronic injuries. Achilles tendon allograft is utilized for both reconstructive techniques with the addition of an ipsilateral hamstring tendon for the double-bundle technique. We also use one of the ipsilateral hamstring tendons as an autograft to reconstruct the PLS. This can be harvested without an additional incision, using the approach described later.

Operative Technique

The patient is positioned supine on the operative table. A tourniquet is placed high on the leg but not inflated unless needed. The surgical prep should allow for wide exposure of the entire lower extremity. Due to the proximity of the popliteal vasculature to the surgical approach, a doppler probe is placed on the field to confirm the presence of pedal pulses at the start and finish of the case.

An examination under anesthesia is performed to more completely define the extent of ligamentous insufficiency. Special attention is focused on the collateral ligaments. Injuries to these structures will guide the decision of where and when to make the necessary incisions. If capsular healing is adequate and the injury pattern permits, we begin with arthroscopy to first define the pathology not readily appreciated by examination or imaging studies. Arthroscopic techniques are then used throughout as much of the procedure as possible to limit the extent of dissection. In the setting of MCL insufficiency and significant valgus laxity, however, we will typically begin with a medial-based incision.

Medial Side Injury (Anterior Cruciate Ligament/Posterior Cruciate Ligament/Medial Collateral Ligament)

A medial incision is begun at the level of the vastus medialis and continues anteriorly over the femoral epicondyle and extends to the anteromedial tibia just medial to the patellar tendon (89) (Fig. 23.11). The sartorial fascia is then split and reflected allowing exposure and subsequent evaluation of the MCL and capsule. Continuing with a short medial parapatellar arthrotomy, access to the knee joint for cruciate, meniscus and articular cartilage evaluation and treatment can be obtained. At this point, attention is then focused on cruciate reconstruction. This is performed with a combination of graft material including ipsilateral HT autograft, which can easily be harvested through this medial incision. Following this, the meniscus is repaired with 2–0 nonabsorbable sutures, whereas capsular and MCL avulsions are repaired

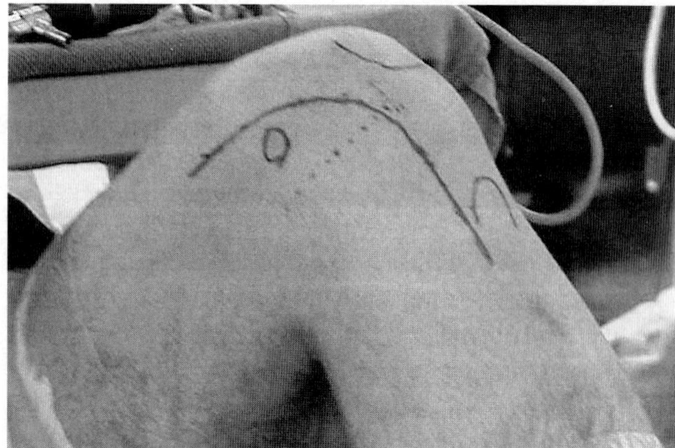

FIGURE 23.11. Approach for anterior cruciate ligament–posterior cruciate ligament medial side injury. Not seen is a sterile Doppler probe present at the foot of the bed.

anatomically with suture anchors. Intrasubstance MCL tears are repaired primarily using number 2 nonabsorbable sutures with a modified-Kessler stitch.

Lateral Side Injury (Anterior Cruciate Ligament/Posterior Cruciate Ligament/Lateral Collateral Ligament/Posterior Ligament Complex)

In contrast to the medial side, if the lateral structures are torn, an arthroscopic approach is advocated initially to obviate the need for both medial and lateral incisions, which could potentially cause skin necrosis. Following this, a curvilinear incision beginning midway between the fibular head and Gerdy's tubercle is created which will continue proximally to the lateral epicondyle, paralleling the posterior border of the iliotibial band (ITB). The peroneal nerve is identified proximally, posterior to the biceps femoris (BF), and traced distally to the point of entrance into the anterior compartment of the leg. Following release of the nerve from the fascial bands as it enters the lateral compartment, gentle neurolysis is performed to release any gross hematoma. The interval between the posterior edge of the ITB and the BF is developed and the ITB insertion is partially released in subperiosteal fashion from Gerdy's tubercle and reflected anteriorly. Repair is routinely performed with suture anchors during the closure. A vertical incision is then made at the posterior border of the LCL while making sure to protect or coagulate the inferior geniculate vessel located in the interval between the LCL and capsule. This window allows visualization of the lateral meniscus and popliteal tendon.

A thorough, systematic inspection of the posterolateral aspect of the knee is performed. The lateral meniscus, capsule, BF tendon, ITB and the arcuate complex of the PLS are repaired using the same techniques as on the medial side, employing free sutures as well as suture anchors. Avulsions of the LCL and popliteal tendon are directly repaired, but more commonly, interstitial tears of these structures require concomitant reconstruction (see Chapter 22). The LCL is usually reconstructed utilizing AT allograft and reinforced with the native LCL. If the popliteal tendon is significantly injured, the popliteofibular ligament is reconstructed anatomically with a semitendinosus autograft. It is first fixed into the native attachment site on the lateral condyle then passed deep to the LCL, tensioned and sutured back to itself after passing through a tunnel created in the fibular head.

Cruciate Ligament Reconstruction

Because the principles of cruciate reconstruction are discussed elsewhere, this section will focus on the unique technical aspects and order of simultaneous cruciate reconstruction (Table 23.4). The tibial tunnels are created first with the PCL followed by the ACL (89). This is then

TABLE 23.4. *Steps in ligament reconstruction*

Step	Action
1	*Begin tibial tunnels:* Place guide wire for the single PCL tunnel followed by guide wire for the single ACL tunnel
2	*Confirm radiographically:* Obtain intraoperative lateral knee radiograph to confirm correct wire placement
3	*Begin femoral tunnels:* Create single ACL followed by double PCL tunnels while waiting for radiograph
4	*Complete tibial tunnels:* Once radiographically confirmed, drill PCL tunnel first, followed by ACL tunnel
5	*Position grafts:* a. Pass both PCL grafts retrograde through tibial tunnel then anterograde through each femoral tunnel b. Pass ACL anterograde through tibial then femoral tunnels
6	*Fix grafts at femur:* Fix PCL grafts then ACL graft with screw and/or distant fixation techniques
7	*Prepare medial and/or lateral structure(s):* Performmedial and/or lateral side repairs or reconstructions but do not definitively secure
8	*Fix PCL graft at tibia:* While recreating the anteromedial tibial step-off, fix the anterolateral bundle at 90°, then the posteromedial bundle at 30°
9	*Fix ACL graft at tibia:* Fix ACL graft at full extension
10	*Secure medial and/or lateral structure(s):* Complete fixation of medial and/or lateral side repairs or reconstructions

PCL, posterior cruciate ligament; ACL, anterior cruciate ligament.

From Cole BJ, Harner CD. The multiple ligament injured knee. *Clin Sports Med* 1999;18:241–262, with permission.

followed by the creation of the femoral tunnels in opposite order. The tunnels for ACL reconstruction should be placed at the anatomic attachment sites on the femur and tibia. Since the PCL is also absent, the posterior edge of the anterior horn of the lateral meniscus is utilized as a guide to the center of the tibial footprint. The guide pin is then inserted usually at an angle of 47.5° but may be increased to allow for a longer tibial tunnel. The femoral tunnel is placed at the 11 o'clock position for the right knee and the 1 o'clock position for the left knee while leaving an 1- to 2-mm cortical bridge on the posterior aspect of the lateral femoral condyle.

A single or double-bundle technique is utilized for the reconstruction of the PCL depending on the timing of treatment. The double-bundle technique will be described briefly while further details of this procedure can be reviewed in Chapter 22. The PCL tibial tunnel is also drilled through the anteromedial tibia distal enough from the usual site of the ACL tibial tunnel so as to leave at least a 2-cm cortical bridge. The tunnel is angled such

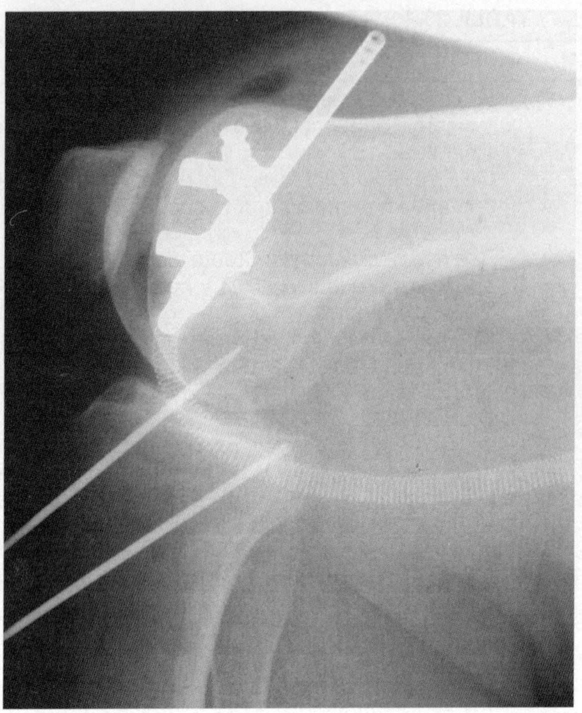

FIGURE 23.12. Intraoperative lateral radiograph of the knee taken after placement of anterior cruciate ligament and posterior cruciate ligament tibial tunnel guide wires. Appropriate placement should be confirmed before proceeding with final drilling.

that it parallels the proximal tibiofibular joint. A 70-degree arthroscope placed through the notch or through an accessory posteromedial portal is frequently used to visualize and prepare the tibial footprint. The guide pin should exit at the distal and lateral aspect of the native PCL tibial footprint and its position (as well as that of the ACL tibial tunnel) should be confirmed by an intraoperative lateral radiograph (Fig. 23.12). Two femoral tunnels are created through the anterolateral portal corresponding to the attachment sites of the anterolateral and posteromedial bundles.

After all the tunnels are created, the grafts are passed and then initially fixed in the femoral tunnels. The PCL grafts are passed first. They are placed through an enlarged anterolateral portal, passed through the tibial tunnel and then placed into the femoral tunnels with the use of a Beath pin. The ACL graft is then passed in the traditional manner, retrograde from the tibial to femoral tunnel. The PCL grafts are also fixed first with interference and/or distant fixation techniques. Interference screw fixation of the ACL graft then follows.

Prior to graft fixation on the femur, the medial or lateral repairs are performed as described previously but not definitively secured. Tightening and subsequent fixation of the PCL in the tibial tunnel is then performed while reproducing the normal tibial step-off of the medial tibial plateau in relation to the femoral condyle.

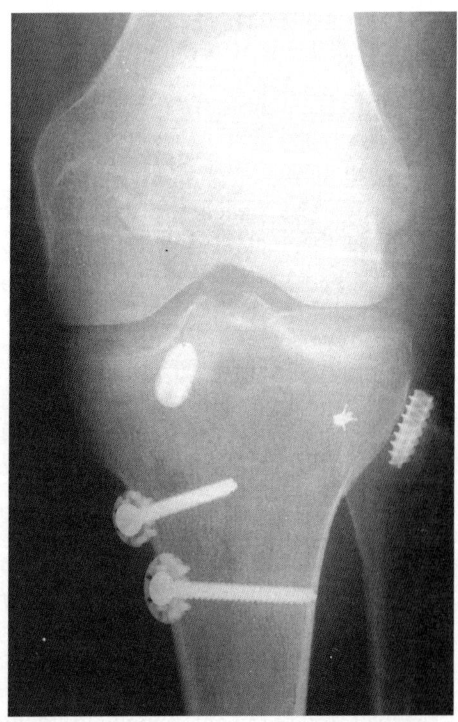
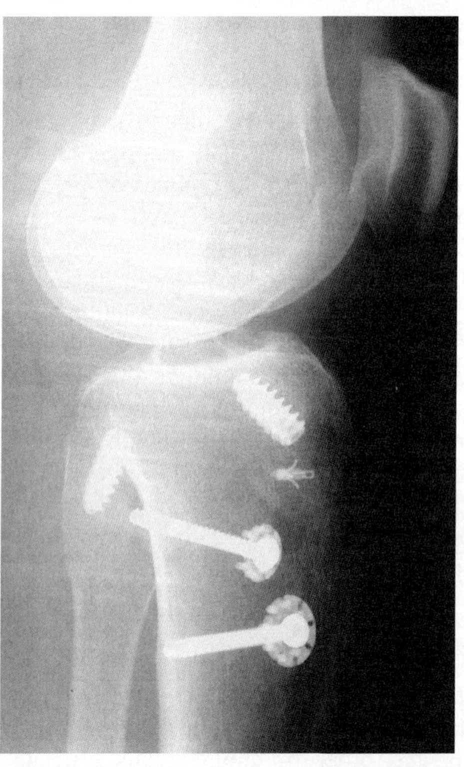

FIGURE 23.13. Postoperative **(A)** anterior and **(B)** lateral radiographs following anterior cruciate ligament, posterior cruciate ligament, and lateral collateral ligament reconstruction and primary repair of the popliteofibular ligament.

The AT is tightened and fixed with a bicortical screw and soft tissue washer at 90° while the HT is secured with a similar device or tied over a screw and washer at 30°. This will recreate the anterolateral and posteromedial bundles of the PCL and, therefore, reestablish the "central-pivot" of the knee (27). The ACL graft is then secured in full extension using a standard interference screw. Cyclical loading should be performed to pretension all of the grafts before final tibial fixation. Following the fixation of the cruciate grafts in the tibia, the remaining extraarticular repairs or reconstructions are completed. Adequate range of motion is confirmed and drains are placed in the medial or lateral wounds if needed. The knee is then placed in a hinged knee brace locked in full extension. Radiographs should be obtained after surgery to confirm appropriate tibiofemoral reduction and graft fixation (Fig. 23.13).

Postoperative Rehabilitation

Although no study currently exists to clarify how aggressive rehabilitation can be, we focus on early, controlled motion to limit the possibility of arthrofibrosis. This is very important because stiffness can be a greater problem than instability after surgical treatment. For the first 4 weeks the knee is maximally protected. Full extension is maintained in the brace while non–weight-bearing ambulation with crutches is recommended. Quadriceps isometric exercises are begun immediately, but active hamstring exercises are avoided for 3 months to avoid undue posterior stress on the reconstruction. Passive ROM exercises with the assistance of a therapist are begun within the first week in the prone position or with support of the posterior proximal tibia to prevent posterior subluxation. After 4 weeks the brace may be unlocked for ambulation and sleeping. Weight bearing is advanced as tolerated unless a PLS repair or reconstruction was performed, in which case ambulation remains partial for 3 months. ROM frequently returns slowly and may take up to 6 months for return of full flexion.

SUMMARY

Appropriate management of the multiple ligament–injured knee remains controversial. The clinician must have a high index of suspicion for a knee dislocation and the inherent associated risk for limb-threatening injuries. Once stabilized, consideration should be given to ligamentous repair or reconstruction of all grade III ligament injuries within the first 3 weeks of injury. Although these cases are some of the most technically challenging in knee surgery, adequate knee stability and range of motion can be reproduced after anatomic reconstruction and appropriate rehabilitation.

REFERENCES

1. Cole BJ, Harner CD. The multiple ligament injured knee. *Clin Sports Med* 1999;18:241–262.
2. Bellabarba C, Bush-Joseph C, Bach BJ. Knee dislocation without anterior cruciate ligament disruption. A report of three cases. *Am J Knee Surg* 1996;9:167–170.
3. Cooper D, Speer K, Wickiewicz T, et al. Complete dislocation of the knee without posterior cruciate ligament disruption. *Clin Orthop* 1992;284:228–233.
4. Shelbourne KD, Pritchard J, Rettig A, et al. Knee dislocations with intact PCL. *Orthop Rev* 1992;21:607–611.
5. Wascher DC, Dvirnak PC, DeCoster TA. Knee dislocation: initial assessment and implications for treatment. *J Orthop Trauma* 1997;11:525–529.
6. Bratt HD, Newman AP. Complete dislocation of the knee without disruption of both cruciate ligaments. *J Trauma* 1993;34:383–389.
7. Schenck RC Jr. The dislocated knee. In: Schafer M, ed. *Instructional Course Lectures, vol. 43.* Rosemont, IL: American Academy of Orthopaedic Surgeons, 1994:127–136.
8. Schenck RC, Burke RL. The dislocated knee. *Perspect Orthop Surg* 1991;2:119–134.
9. Schenck RC, Burke R, Walker D. The dislocated knee: a new classification system [abstract]. *South Med J* 1992;85:35–S1.
10. Schenck RC Jr, Nonweiler D, DeLee JC. The incomplete bicruciate ligament pattern: a report of two cases. *Orthop Rev* 1993;22:1249–1252.
11. Schenck RC Jr, Hunter RE, Ostrum RF, et al. Knee dislocations. In: Zuckerman JD, ed. *Instructional Course Lectures, vol. 48.* Rosemont, IL: American Academy of Orthopaedic Surgeons, 1999:515–522.
12. Hoover NW. Injuries of the popliteal artery associated with fractures and dislocations. *Surg Clin North Am* 1961;41:1099–1112.
13. Welling R, Kakkasseril J, Cranley J. Complete dislocations of the knee with popliteal vascular injury. *J Trauma* 1981;21:450–453.
14. Meyers MH, Harvey JP Jr. Traumatic dislocation of the knee joint, a study of eighteen cases. *J Bone Joint Surg Am* 1971;53:16–29.
15. Meyers MH, Moore TM, Harvey JP Jr. Follow-up notes on articles previously published in the journal: traumatic dislocation of the knee joint. *J Bone Joint Surg Am* 1975;57:430–433.
16. Quinlan AG, Sharrard WJW. Postero-lateral dislocation of the knee with capsular interposition. *J Bone Joint Surg Br* 1958;40:660–663.
17. Shields L, Mital M, Cave EF. Complete dislocation of the knee: experience at the Massachusetts General hospital. *J Trauma* 1969;9:192–215.
18. Walker DN, Hardison R, Schenck RC Jr. A baker's dozen of knee dislocations. *Am J Knee Surg* 1994;7:117–124.
19. Reddy PK, Posteraro RH, Schenck RC Jr. The role of MRI in evaluation of the cruciate ligaments in knee dislocations. *Orthopedics* 1996;19:155–169.
20. Schenck RC Jr. Management of PCL injuries in knee dislocations. *Oper Tech Sports Med* 1993;1:143–147.
21. Kremchek TE, Welling RE, Kremchek EJ. Traumatic dislocation of the knee. *Orthop Rev* 1989;18:1051–1057.
22. Siliski JM. Evaluation and treatment of dislocation of the knee. *Mediguide Orthop* 1992;10:1–7.
23. Good L, Johnson RJ. The dislocated knee. *J Am Acad Orthop Surg* 1995;3:284–292.
24. Kennedy JC. Complete dislocation of the knee joint. *J Bone Joint Surg Am* 1963;45:889–904.
25. Bunt TS, Malone JM, Moody M, et al. Frequency of vascular injury with blunt trauma-induced extremity injury. *Am J Surg* 1990;160:226–228.
26. Shelbourne KD, Porter DA, Clingman JA, et al. Low-velocity knee dislocation. *Orthop Rev* 1991;20:995–1004.
27. Hughston JC, Bowden JA, Andrews JR, et al. Acute tears of the posterior cruciate ligament: results of operative treatment. *J Bone Joint Surg Am* 1980;62:438–450.
28. Roman PD, Hopson CN, Zenni EJ Jr. Traumatic dislocation of the knee: a report of 30 cases and literature review. *Orthop Rev* 1987;16:917–924.
29. Taylor AR, Arden GP, Rainey HA. Traumatic dislocation of the knee: a report of forty-three cases with special reference to conservative treatment. *J Bone Joint Surg Br* 1972;54:96–102.
30. Frassica F, Sim F, Staeheli J, et al. Dislocation of the knee. *Clin Orthop* 1992;263:200–205.

31. Green N, Allen B. Vascular injuries associated with dislocation of the knee. *J Bone Joint Surg Am* 1977;59:236–239.

32. Kendall R, Taylor D, Salvian A, et al. The role of arteriography in assessing vascular injuries associated with dislocations of the knee. *J Trauma* 1993;35:875–878.

33. Ottolenghi C. Vascular complications in injuries about the knee joint. *Clin Orthop* 1982;165:148–156.

34. Sisto D, Warren R. Complete knee dislocation: a follow-up of operative treatment. *Clin Orthop* 1985;198:94–101.

35. Treiman G, Yellin A, Weaver F, et al. Examination of the patient with knee dislocation. The case for selective arteriography. *Arch Surg* 1992;127:1056–1063.

36. DeBakey ME, Simeone FA. Battle injuries of the arteries in world war II: an analysis of 2,471 cases. *Ann Surg* 1946;123:534–579.

37. Jones RE, Smith EC, Bone GE. Vascular and orthopedic complications of knee dislocation. *Surg Gynecol Obstet* 1979;149:554–558.

38. McCoy GF, Hannon DG, Barr RJ, et al. Vascular injury associated with low-velocity dislocations of the knee. *J Bone Joint Surg Br* 1987;69:285–287.

39. McCutchen JD, Gilham NR. Injury to the popliteal artery associated with dislocation of the knee: palpable distal pulses do not negate the requirement for arteriography. *Injury* 1989;20:307–310.

40. Reckling FW, Peltier LF. Acute knee dislocations and their complications. *J Trauma* 1969;9:181–191.

41. Grimley RP, Ashton F, Slaney G, et al. Popliteal artery injuries associated with civilian knee trauma. *Injury* 1981;13:1–6.

42. O'Donnell TF Jr, Brewster DC, Darling RC, et al. Arterial injuries associated with fractures and/or dislocations of the knee. *J Trauma* 1977;17:775–784.

43. Savage R. Popliteal injury associated with dislocation of the knee. *J Bone Joint Surg Am* 1977;59:236–239.

44. Walker DN, Rogers W, Schenck RC Jr. Immediate vascular and ligamentous repair in a closed knee dislocation: case report. *J Trauma* 1994;35:898–900.

45. Taft T, Almekinders L. The dislocated knee. In: Fu F, Harner CD, Vince K, eds. *Knee surgery.* Baltimore: Williams & Wilkins, 1994:837–858.

46. Thomsen PB, Rud B, Jensen UH. Stability and motion after traumatic dislocation of the knee. *Acta Orthop Scand* 1984;55:278–283.

47. O'Donoghue D. An analysis of end results of surgical treatment of major injuries to the ligaments of the knee. *J Bone Joint Surg Am* 1955;37:1–13.

48. Harner CD, Miller M. Graft tensioning in PCL surgery. *Oper Tech Sports Med* 1993;1:115–120.

49. Quinlan A. Irreducible posterolateral dislocation of the knee with button-holing of the medial femoral condyle. *J Bone Joint Surg Am* 1966;48:1619–1621.

50. Hill JA, Rana NA. Complications of posterolateral dislocations of the knee: case report and literature review. *Clin Orthop* 1981;154:212–215.

51. Gollehon DL, Torzilli PA, Warren RF. The role of the posterolateral and cruciate ligaments in the stability of the human knee. A biomechanical study. *J Bone Joint Surg Am* 1987;69:233–242.

52. Grood ES, Stowers SF, Noyes FR. Limits of movement in the human knee. Effect of sectioning the posterior cruciate ligament and posterolateral structures. *J Bone Joint Surg Am* 1988;70:88–97.

53. Veltri D, Deng X-H, Torzilli PA, et al. The role of the popliteofibular ligament in the stability of the knee: a biomechanical study. *Am J Sports Med* 1996;24:19–27.

54. Veltri D, Warren RF. Posterolateral instability of the knee. In: Jackson DW, ed. *Instructional Course Lectures, vol. 44.* Rosemont, IL: American Academy of Orthopaedic Surgeons, 1995:441–453.

55. Cooper DE. Treatment of combined posterior cruciate ligament and posterolateral injuries of the knee. *Oper Tech Sports Med* 1999;7:135–142.

56. Veltri D, Deng X-H, Torzilli PA, et al. The role of the cruciate and posterolateral ligaments in stability of the knee: a biomechanical study. *Am J Sports Med* 1995;23:436–443.

57. Clancy WG. Repair and reconstruction of the posterior cruciate ligament. In: Chapman M, ed. *Operative orthopaedics.* Philadelphia: Lippincott, 1988:1651–1665.

58. Skyhar MJ, Warren RF, Oritz GJ, et al. The effects of sectioning the posterior cruciate ligament and the posterolateral complex on the articular contact pressure within the knee. *J Bone Joint Surg Am* 1993;75:694–699.

59. Fowler PJ. Imaging of the posterior cruciate ligament. In: Fanelli GC, ed. *Posterior cruciate ligament injuries. A practical guide to management.* New York: Springer-Verlag, 2001.

60. Harner CD, Hoher J. Current concepts: evaluation and treatment of posterior cruciate ligament injuries. *Am J Sports Med* 1998;26:471–482.

61. Fanelli G, Giannotti B, Edson C. Arthroscopically assisted combined anterior and posterior cruciate reconstruction. *Arthroscopy* 1996;12:5–14.

62. Malizos K, Xenakis T, Mavrodontidis A, et al. Knee dislocations and their management. *Acta Orthop Scand Suppl* 1997;275:80–83.

63. Marks P, Harner CD. The ACL in the multiple ligament injured knee. *Clin Sports Med* 1993;12:825–838.

64. Montgomery J. Dislocation of the knee. *Orthop Clin North Am* 1987;18:149–156.

65. Shapiro M, Freedman E. Allograft reconstruction of the anterior and posterior cruciate ligaments after traumatic knee dislocation. *Am J Sports Med* 1995;23:580–587.

66. Veltri D, Warren RF. Isolated and combined posterior cruciate injuries. *J Am Acad Orthop Surg* 1993;1:67–75.

67. Burger RS, Larson RL. Acute dislocations. In: Larson RL, Grana WA, eds. *The knee: form, function, pathology, and treatment.* Philadelphia: WB Saunders, 1993:501–512.

68. Fanelli GC, Feldman DD. Management of combined anterior cruciate ligament/posterior cruciate ligament/posterolateral complex injuries of the knee. *Oper Tech Sports Med* 1999;7:143–149.

69. Fanelli G, Giannotti B, Edson C. Current concepts review. The posterior cruciate ligament arthroscopic evaluation and treatment. *Arthroscopy* 1994;10:673–688.

70. Fanelli GC, Giannotti BF, Edson CJ. Arthroscopically assisted combined posterior cruciate ligament/posterolateral complex reconstruction. *Arthroscopy* 1996;12:521–530.

71. Noyes FR, Barber-Westin SD. Reconstruction of the anterior and posterior cruciate ligaments after knee dislocation. Use of early protected postoperative motion to decrease arthrofibrosis. *Am J Sports Med* 1997;25:769–778.

72. Leffers D. Dislocations and soft tissue injuries of the knee. In: Browner BD, Jupiter JB, Levine AM, et al, eds. *Skeletal trauma: fractures, dislocations, ligamentous injury.* Philadelphia: WB Saunders, 1992:1724–1729.

73. Maynard MJ, Warren RF. Surgical and reconstructive technique for knee dislocations. In: Jackson DW, ed. *Reconstructive knee surgery: master techniques in orthopaedic surgery.* New York: Raven Press, 1995:161–183.

74. Moore TM. Fracture-dislocation of the knee. *Clin Orthop* 1981;156:128–140.

75. Lipscomb AB, Anderson AF. Surgical reconstruction of both the anterior and posterior cruciate ligaments. *Am J Knee Surg* 1990;3:29–40.

76. Bishara R, Pasch A, Lim L, et al. Improved results in the treatment of vascular injuries with fracture and dislocations. *J Vasc Surg* 1986;3:707–711.

77. Chapman J. Popliteal artery damage in closed injuries of the knee. *J Bone Joint Surg Br* 1985;67:420–423.

78. White K. The results of traction injury to the common peroneal nerve. *J Bone Joint Surg Br* 1968;50:346–350.

79. Lundborg G, Rydevik B, Manthorpe M, et al. Peripheral nerve: the physiology of soft tissue repair. In: Woo SL-Y, Buckwalter JA, eds. *Injury and repair of the musculoskeletal soft tissues.* Park Ridge: American Academy of Orthopaedic Surgeons, 1988:297–352.

80. Almekinders L, Logan T. Results following treatment of traumatic dislocations of the knee joint. *Clin Orthop* 1992;284:203–207.

81. Montgomery TJ, White J, Roberts TS, et al. Orthopedic management of dislocations of the knee: a comparison of surgical reconstruction and immobilization. *Orthop Trans* 1992;16:225.

82. Yeh W-L, Tu Y-K, Su J-Y, et al. Knee dislocation: treatment of high-velocity knee dislocation. *J Trauma* 1999;46:693–701.

83. L'Insalata J, Irrgang J, Allen A, et al. Multiple ligament reconstruction for knee dislocation: results at a minimum two years follow-up. Presented at American Orthopaedic Society for Sports Medicine Specialty Day, San Francisco, CA, February 16, 1997.

84. Marshall J, Warren R, Wickiewicz T, et al. The anterior cruciate ligament: a technique for repair and reconstruction. *Clin Orthop* 1979;143:97.

85. Meyers MH. Isolated avulsion of the tibial attachment of the posterior cruciate ligament of the knee. *J Bone Joint Surg Am* 1975;57: 669–672.
86. Richter M, Kiefer H, Hehl G, et al. Primary repair for posterior cruciate ligament injuries: an eight-year follow up of fifty-three patients. *Am J Sports Med* 1996;24:298–305.
87. Harner C, Olson E, Fu F, et al. The use of fresh frozen allograft tissue in knee ligament reconstruction: indications, techniques, results and controversies. In: *The ACL-deficient knee*. Washington DC: American Academy of Orthopaedic Surgeons, 1992:28–46.
88. Buck R, Malinin T, Brown M. Bone transplantation and human immunodeficiency virus: an estimate of risk acquired immunodeficiency syndrome (AIDS). *Clin Orthop* 1989;240:129.
89. Klimkiewicz JJ, Petrie RS, Harner CD. ACL/PCL/MCL reconstruction: University of Pittsburgh arthroscopically assisted technique. *Oper Tech Sports Med* 1999;7:150–153.

CHAPTER 24

Clinical Outcome Studies for Knee Ligament Injuries

Marc F. Swiontkowski and Elizabeth A. Arendt

Accurate assessment of clinical outcomes is essential in orthopedic surgery for several reasons: to document the natural history of untreated orthopedic conditions, to determine the effectiveness of individual treatments, and to compare efficacy of different treatments. Despite this essential need, individual practitioners as well as organizations rarely perform routine analysis of their treatment of musculoskeletal disease and injury, surgical and nonsurgical.

This chapter will discuss the assessment of knee ligament injuries and their treatments, provide a historical review, and describe current outcome assessment tools.

Webster's Dictionary definition of outcome is "something that follows as a result or consequence." Following this definition, outcomes research, or outcome analysis, can take on a variety of aspects. Donabedian, in his classic work, first used the word in describing the continuum of diagnosis, process of care, and outcome (1). Currently, outcomes assessment of medical and surgical practice habits has emerged as the valued tool to help shape medical policy and practice habits as we approach the twenty-first century.

One can divide research in medical practice into two general domains. The first is efficacy research, which is primarily the technical side of medicine. This is research done to determine if a procedure works at all. It is generally conducted in the hands of the developer of the treatment or in a high volume practice environment. The second type of research is effectiveness research, and this is the domain in which outcomes research is placed. Effectiveness research is done to find out whether the procedure works well when applied to the general population, and what are the patient-oriented results of that particular procedure.

Liang and Jette (2), in a critical review of functional assessment, listed five criteria necessary for an accurate assessment of a clinical outcome:

1. The outcome measure (assessment instrument) should permit quantification.
2. Data collection procedures should be standardized.
3. The instrument should accurately measure what it purports to measure (validity).
4. The measure should be reliable.
5. The instrument should distinguish changes that are adequate for its intended purpose.

Outcomes research, then, is a compilation of end result measures. These outcome measures can vary from measurements of technical success to measurements of patient-oriented or functional outcomes. Current research emphasis is placed on the latter, patient-oriented outcomes, to address the deficiencies in previous clinical research methods. Clinical practice of medicine, including surgery, is dependent on the knowledge base created by those who carry out research, develop new ideas and technologies, and teach and report on this information (3). Thus, if research and literature are deficient in a disease recognition and treatment, so too will there be deficiencies in the clinical practice designed to care for that disease state.

Meta-analysis is a relatively new concept of structured literature review. The technique of meta-analysis was designed as a way to aggregate reports of randomized clinical trials. What is required in any meta-analysis is high-quality data which have consistent definition of terms, patient groups, and outcomes data. Meta-analysis then groups these individual research/clinical trials together, to report a clinical finding or overall effect. The strength of a meta-analysis is the pooling of numbers, increasing statistical power and providing a more stratified and comprehensive picture of disease states and treatment impact. Attempts at meta-analysis have resulted in structured literature reviews that demonstrate that there are a variety of common orthopedic conditions for which there are serious deficiencies in the quality of the literature (3). A paucity of orthopedic conditions have enough studies conforming to the high-quality guidelines of a meta-analysis to permit such critical review.

In addition to the deficiencies in clinical research methods and tools, other factors have stimulated the emergence of outcomes research. These include the rapidly rising costs of health care. However, beyond economic incentives, outcomes research should be the essential element to aid the practitioner in the assessment of the quality and appropriateness of medical care.

The emergence of knowledge concerning variations in practice patterns is another factor that is stimulating more quality outcome research. The technical ability to investigate variation in practice patterns in a given area has emerged as a tool that is important to medical practice. Small-area analysis involves a calculation of population-based rates of medical care utilization by hospitals, patients, and health care providers. This concept of small-area variations was developed by Wennberg and Gittelsohn (4). They discovered that the rates of utilization of almost all kinds of medical care were strikingly different. Moreover the variations appeared to be almost exclusively the result of differences in beliefs among physicians about the best way to treat various conditions. From a perspective of not only cost but also quality, the resolution of variations in practice patterns deserves prompt attention by both the individual practitioner and medical organizations. It is this apparent inefficiency for the medical profession to understand the appropriateness and the effectiveness of medical and surgical practice that provides the biggest impetus to the medical profession to invest in outcomes research.

OUTCOME MEASUREMENTS

Outcome research uses measurement. The techniques of measurement can focus on the process of care, or clinical results (radiographic results, range of motion, muscle strength, knee stability). Instruments can also focus on patient-oriented outcomes (functional activities of daily living, quality of life). In the past decade, methods to assess physical function by self-administered questionnaires have improved tremendously, and have become the cornerstone in outcomes assessment. Other measures that could be performed include work status, pain, and patient satisfaction with the process of care. Though relief of the pain is one of the primary reasons for the performance of most orthopedic procedures, pain is a subjective state; there is no gold standard by which to measure its state. However, valid and reliable measurements of chronic pain have been developed (5–7). Graphic representation of a subjective experience was first described by Freyd (8), where he described the graphic rating scale and outlined the advantages of such a system. A visual analog

scale was introduced by Labib (9) to analyze pain and function after total joint arthroplasty. Visual analog scales have shown high test–retest reliability, and their effectiveness in demonstrating measurements of sensory stimulus in a functional capacity have been well delineated (8–13). A visual analog scale to analyze subjective knee complaints has been described (14). Visual analog or graphic rating scales are felt to be more sensitive than traditional descriptive pain scales (9,15).

The measurement properties research instruments should include are validity (the ability to measure what the instrument is supposed to measure), reliability (reproducibility from one administration to another), and sensitivity (the ability to measure change over time).

Numerical scoring systems (rating scales) has been the most popular orthopedic outcome measure in the last 25 years. These rating scales specifically address the first two of Liang and Jette's requirements for an accurate assessment of clinical outcome. The Iowa hip scale (16), introduced in 1963, was perhaps the first widely used rating scale. More than 100 cumulative numerical scoring systems have since been developed in orthopedics to address joint and musculoskeletal issues. These have allowed for quantification of assessment, as well as a standardization of data collection. This allows the potential advantage to include the use of statistical methods to analyze the effects of treatment and the possible establishment of quantitative guidelines for instituting different treatment regimens. The rationale for using numerical scales has been to facilitate comparisons between different groups. Most of these have a final score consisting of the reduction of all assessment data into a single numerical value. One of the main concerns with many of the existing rating scales, is that few have examined the data analysis associated with their use. A review by this author of the orthopedic literature from 1969 to 1991 revealed 63 different rating scales in the area of adult reconstructive orthopedics (17). These were developed for the following areas of orthopedic surgery: total joint arthroplasty, osteotomy, arthrodesis, excisional procedures of the wrist, and soft tissue stabilization and realignment procedures. Of these 63 scales identified, as originally described, 33 (52%) were used for postoperative and preoperative comparison, whereas only 3 (5%) did so with statistical analysis. Only two (4%) of the studies compared the rating scale to the patient's overall subjective satisfaction. In no study did investigators adequately subject their assessment scales to well-adopted measures of validity (2,18,19). Finally, these rating scales mixed clinical outcomes (objective measures) with functional outcomes.

The major potential advantage of numerical rating scales is that they allow quantitative assessment and standardization of data collection. The greatest drawback of rating scales is data loss. This data loss occurs on multiple levels. During the construction of a rating scale, important qualitative information is often omitted, or qualitative information is reduced to a quantitative measurement. The methodology used to construct rating scales often weights the variables comprised in the final score arbitrarily. The weighting is typically loosely based on the researchers' (usually an orthopedic surgeon) perception of what is most important to the patient. Weighting can only be adequately determined by direct patient input, as well as with the use of regression analysis techniques (19). Historically, most rating scales do not consider the importance of the patient's perspective in determining the relative weight of the scores, and the techniques used to assess pain have typically been inadequate. Additional data are lost when one compares preoperative and postoperative values for individual variables. Frequently the score preoperatively is combined into one number as well as one number for the postoperative result, and these are compared. Therefore, individual areas, such as instability, function, and pain, are reduced to one score. This greatly reduces the amount of information, and much valuable information is lost to the reader/evaluator of the published study. This limits the usefulness of the study for the individual reader, and markedly limits the ability to compare studies across different groups. Some authors have tried to get away from quantitative groupings and have tried to convert their cumulative scores into qualitative groupings (excellent, good, fair, poor). Although this improves categorizations by not quantifying qualitative terms, this form of rating can also be viewed as arbitrary, secondary to values and perceptions designated by the researcher/author of the grading scale.

Validity is another major area in which orthopedic rating scales must be critically examined. Few authors attempt to compare their rating scales to the patients' overall subjective assessment of their treatment; this would serve as the simplest attempt to validate a scoring system. Validation and formulation of new clinical assessment tools involve a complex process (18). Typically, this work involves investigators from social sciences who specialize in outcome assessment and statistical methods. The creation of a valid instrument by which to measure assessment is an arduous task. Examples of early validated assessment measurements are the arthritis impact measurement scale (20), the sickness impact profile, and the health assessment questionnaire (21).

A final issue to address is how cost should be measured in outcome measurements. Certainly the cost of health care is an increasingly important factor in modern medical practice and should be considered in the evaluation of effectiveness. This is frequently done in two ways. A cost benefit analysis compares expenditures for different programs or interventions and expresses all outcomes, including morbidity and death, in an economic term. This kind of cost benefit model is a challenge methodically and raises major ethical concerns when the model tries to measure lives saved or the quality of life in monetary terms.

A cost effectiveness model allows costs to be subtracted from benefits and express the net benefit for each intervention or program evaluated. This requires that all health outcomes be measured in some quantitative way and this is expressed in commensurate units. An example of a commensurate unit of cost effectiveness is a quality-adjusted life year (QALY). This is an improvement over the cost analysis model. However, it is difficult to always measure variables in commensurate units.

Therefore, a perfect outcome assessment tool should use sophisticated psychometric techniques to derive the scale and the scale should be validated. A pain scale typically using visual analog techniques should be added. These elements will allow use of statistical techniques to analyze all aspects of the outcome. The scales should be used in clinical series that are comparable, with large enough numbers to minimize error. The group should be studied long enough for faults or positive and negative variables to have emerged. Only factors that are quantifiable should be quantified. The answers that are produced should provide conclusions that are constructive to the question that is being asked. This is the ideal of which there are few examples in the knee ligament literature.

HISTORICAL PERSPECTIVE

The surgical treatment of injured ligaments to the knee was first detailed in the English literature by Hey Grove in 1919 (22). However, it is perhaps O'Donoghue in the 1950s that can be credited with advancing the surgical treatment of ligamentous knee injuries (23). In addition to this advancement, O'Donoghue published an analysis of the end results of surgical treatments of major ligaments knee injuries (24). In this article, he thought that the best outcome could be obtained by early, meticulous, surgical repair of the damaged ligaments. The author thought that by itemizing the torn structures and what was repaired at the time of surgery, and examining the patient after surgery, one could learn much in regards to effective treatment for various injuries. In addition to an objective examination, O'Donoghue used a questionnaire format in which he asked four questions–Question A: "does your knee bother you?" with yes and no as possible answers; Question B: "is it as good as your other knee?"; Question C: "are you completely happy with the results of your operation" (this question is least valuable because it may reflect loyalty to the surgeon); Question D: "has your knee kept you from participating in athletics?". O'Donoghue thought that this was the most significant question of all.

O'Donoghue thus reported the results of surgical repairs and knee ligament injuries employing postoperative personal examination and patient questionnaires as a mechanism of data collection on which conclusions were based. His original article centered the bulk of the "outcome assessment" on a questionnaire that largely involving the patient's perspective of the end results. In later articles, O'Donoghue expanded his reported parameters to include a greater number of concrete observations, including increasing numbers of objective tests of the knee. In 1973 (25), he outlined a comprehensive diagnostic protocol for examination of the injured knee. As interest increased in knee ligament injuries, so did the number of parameters investigators recognized as being significant. Jones (26) and Slocum (27) incorporated the preoperative examination in addition to the postoperative examination. This preoperative examination included rotatory instability. In addition to increasing the complexity and number of parameters in the objective examination, investigators began to add another dimension to the injury profile and postoperative evaluation by including functional tests such as running, jumping, and squatting to their evaluation methods (28).

As an appreciation of the myriad of factors that surgeons thought important in postoperative evaluations grew, attempts to formulate standardized systems of evaluation emerged. During this time, comprehensive approaches to other joints in surgical procedures in orthopedic literature began to appear (29). In 1975, Kettlecamp developed a scoring scale for evaluation of the arthritic knee (19). He conformed to rigid criteria in developing this scoring scale, including the following:

1. The scale must measure an important characteristic of the knee.
2. The clinical variables must be those that can be quantified by an orthopedic surgeon in his office.
3. Total points derived from the scoring scales should be related to the clinical results.

During this time, organized methods of evaluations for knee ligaments injuries became more numerous and more sophisticated. Early leaders in this field were Marshall (30) and Palmar (31). Marshall's score had a place for the patient's own evaluation, which was divided into four qualitative descriptors (normal, severe, improved, worse). Marshall claimed that stability was highly important for successful rehabilitation and return to function, therefore, Marshall's rating system covered symptoms, activity grading, and results of simple functional tests. Many of the items were graded in a binary fashion (binary having to do with yes or no answers) as opposed to a numerical grading system. Palmar (31) understood that symptoms, while shown to correlate with overall status of the knee, may be disguised or hidden by a change in lifestyle or activity. His evaluation was divided into four gross categorizations that correlated well with the patient's own evaluation of his or her condition and the physicians clinical assessment of the status of the knee.

In 1982, Lysholm (32) introduced a scoring scale that he felt correlated better with the classification that the patients gave themselves. They used a numerical scale that they found preferable to the binary questions that were largely used in Marshall's rating system. Lysholm (33), and later Tegner thought that a more differentiated picture of disability can be obtained with a scoring (numerical) scale. They can be credited with recognizing that limitations in knee function may be masked by an involuntary low activity level. Lysholm's scale (Table 24.1) placed increased emphasis on knee instability. They thought that this was justified by previous work demonstrating a high correlation between the feeling of instability and the inability to return to a sport. Tegner improved on Lysholm's functional questionnaire by proposing an activity score as an adjunct, which numerically graded functional status depending on work and sport performance (Table 24.2).

TABLE 24.1. *Lysholm knee scoring scale*

Parameter	Score
Limp (5 points)	
None	5
Slight or periodical	3
Severe and constant	0
Support (5 points)	
None	5
Cane or crutch	2
Weight-bearing impossible	0
Locking (15 points)	
No locking or catching sensations	15
Catching sensation but no locking	10
Locking occasionally	6
Locking frequently	0
Instability (25 points)	
Never giving way	25
Rarely during sports or severe exertion	20
Frequently during sports or severe exertion (or incapable of participation)	15
Occasionally in daily living activities	10
Often in daily living activities	5
Every step	0
Pain (25 points)	
None	25
Inconstant and slight during severe exertion	20
Marked during severe exertion	15
Marked on or after walking >2 km	10
Marked on or after walking <2 km	5
Constant	0
Swelling (10 points)	
None	25
On severe exertion	6
On ordinary exertion	2
Constant	0
Stair climbing (10 points)	
No problems	10
Slightly impaired	6
One step at a time	2
Impossible	0
Squatting (5 points)	
No problems	5
Slightly impaired	4
Not beyond 90E	2
Impossible	0

Noyes and coworkers (34) developed a knee rating scale that represented a move back toward a more comprehensive evaluation system originally reported by Marshall and coworkers. Their system was not binary. Noyes recorded activity levels using a self-assessment of one's

TABLE 24.2. *Tegner activity score*

10. Competitive sports
    Soccer-national and international elite
9. Competitive sports
    Soccer, lower divisions
    Ice hockey
    Wrestling
    Gymnastics
8. Competitive sports
    Bandy
    Squash or badminton
    Athletics (jumping etc.)
    Downhill skiing
7. Competitive sports
    Tennis
    Athletics (running)
    Motocross, speedway
    Handball
    Basketball
    Recreational sports
    Bandy and ice hockey
    Squash
    Athletics (jumping)
    Cross country (track) both recreational and
    competitive
6. Recreational sports
    Tennis and badminton
    Handball
    Basketball
    Downhill skiing
    Jogging (at least 5 times per week)
5. Work
    Heavy labor
    Competitive sports
    Cycling
    Cross-country skiing
    Recreational sports
    Jogging on uneven ground at least 2 times per week
4. Work
    Moderately heavy labor (e.g., truck driving, heavy
    domestic work)
    Recreational sports
    Cycling
    Cross-country skiing
    Jogging on even ground at least 2 times per week
3. Work
    Light labor (e.g., nursing)
    Competitive and recreational sports
    Swimming
    Walking in forest possible
2. Work
    Light labor
    Walking on uneven ground possible but impossible to
    walk in forest
1. Work
    Sedentary work
    Walking on even ground possible
0. Sick leave or disability pension because of knee
    problems

ability to perform three sport levels; this was a numerical scale from 0 to 100. He thought that one needed to check the consistency of the patient's answers; therefore, every patient was interviewed before recording the results in the computer for data analysis. This represented a more complex system. He thought, however, that his system improved on the previous potential sources of errors by not combining many variables into an overall point score. He also thought that this system could adequately assess alterations in lifestyle and the intensity of athletic activities before and after treatment. Noyes and coworkers (35–38) emphasized the assessment of function before and after surgical intervention. Their numerical scale, called the Cincinnati knee ligament rating system (38), includes a physical examination, instrumented testing, as well as a four-part evaluation format to assess symptoms and functions (Table 24.3). This four-part evaluation includes:

1. A symptom rating scale assessing pain, swelling, and partial and full giving way depending on six specifically defined activity levels.
2. An objective assessment of function in a series of activities including walking, stair climbing, squats, running, jumping, and pivoting.
3. A sports activity rating scale that stratifies functions depending on four levels of sport type and level and frequency of participation.
4. A final rating system that provides an overall grade defined by the lowest score in any individual category.

Another popular knee rating system, much represented in past literature on knee ligament injuries and their treatment results, is the Hospital for Special Surgery (HSS) rating system first was published in 1988 (30). This rating system integrated a composite subjective assessment as well as subjective and objective functional testing, and an objective assessment (physical examination). Specific sports were categorized according to how potentially demanding participation could be. One major difference with the HSS score was of the 45 points on the objective examination of the knee, only 16 specifically addressed the anterior cruciate ligament. Twenty of the remaining points assess collateral ligaments, posterior cruciate ligaments, and posterolateral corner.

A group of knee surgeons from Europe and America met in 1987 and founded the International Knee Documentation Committee (IKDC) (39). The Knee Documentation Committee was formed because the members of this group felt that none of the previously stated forms had found worldwide acceptance, and they had a strong concern that a scoring system that attributed numerical factors to qualitative factors was arbitrary and not comparable with each other when factors were added together in a single score (40). Common terminology and an evaluation form was created by this group. This form was suggested to be the standard form

TABLE 24.3. *Cincinnati knee ligament rating scale*

Parameter	Points
Normal knee with strenuous work or pivoting sports	100
Able to do moderate work or pivoting sports	80
Able to do light work or light pivoting sports	60
Able to do ADL alone	40
Moderate symptoms with ADL	20
Severe symptoms with ADL	0

Assessment of ADL function: ADL and sports

ADL rating	Points
Walking	
Normal	40
Some limits	30
3–4 blocks	20
<1 block, cane	0
Stair climbing	
Normal	40
Some limits	30
11–30 steps	20
1–10 steps	0
Squatting/kneeling	
Normal	40
Some limits	30
6–10 squats	20
0–5 squats	0

Sports rating	Points
Straight running	100
Fully competitive	80
Some limits	60
Half speed	40
Unable	0
Jumping/landing	100
Fully competitive	80
Some limits	60
Half speed	40
Hard twisting/cutting/pivoting	
Fully competitive	100
Some limits	80
Half speed	60
Unable	40

Sports activity rating scale

Levels	Points
I. Participates 4–7 days/week	
A. Jumping, cutting, pivoting (e.g., soccer)	100
B. Twisting, turning (e.g., raquet sports)	95
C. Running (e.g., cycling, swimming)	90
II. Participates 1–3 days/week	
A. Jumping, cutting, pivoting	85
B. Twisting, turning	80
C. Running	75
III. Participates 1–3 times/month	
A. Jumping, cutting, pivoting	65
B. Twisting, turning	60
C. Running	55
IV. No sports	
A. No problems with ADL	40
B. Moderate problems with ADL	20
C. Severe problems with ADL	0

ADL, activities of daily living.

for use in all publications on the results of the treatment of knee ligament injuries. It was formulated by consensus and is a concise one-page form (Table 24.4) including a documentation section, a qualification section, and an evaluation section. For evaluation there are four problem areas: subjective assessment, symptoms, range of motion, and ligament examination. These are supplemented by four additional areas that are documented but not included in the evaluation: compartment findings, pathology, radiology findings, and a single functional test. The form can be used before and after surgery. Each parameter is qualified as normal, nearly normal, abnormal, and severely abnormal. The members felt that this qualification was less subjective and emotional than "very good, good, fair, and poor." Each problem area within the evaluation section is qualified for the group qualification. The worst qualification within the group is taken as the section qualification; the worst group qualification is taken as the final evaluation. If the knee is abnormal in any of the problem areas, it can not be entered as a normal knee. The hope was that this new form would enable a better comparison between treatment methods among different examinations and different study groups.

SUMMARY OF HISTORIC SCORING SYSTEMS

The Lysholm score is a subjective assessment of function: it does not emphasize an investigative physical examination, but rather a patient assessment. With the evolving trends in outcome study toward patient, rather than investigator interpretation of the results, this scoring system is a better reflection of outcome as we are currently defining it. The HSS rating is weighted more toward the objective assessment (45 points). However, in a comparison of Lysholm and HSS scores, these two scores were found to be highly correlative with each other (41), but not correlative with the Cincinnati knee rating final scores. The Cincinnati knee ligament rating system is clearly the most elaborate and detailed assessment of activity-related symptoms and function of the ligamentously reconstructed knee. When comparing the same patients between the Lysholm, HSS scores, and the Cincinnati knee ligament questionnaires, the patient score is consistently higher on Lysholm and HSS than on the Cincinnati knee score. The Cincinnati knee score, however, was able to better stratify patients that were in stressful pivotal type sports versus more recreational type sports. This means that the Cincinnati Knee Score is less likely to have inflated results due to symptoms masked by low activity levels. It is for this reason that Tegner added an activity rating scale; this can be a useful supplement to any numerical scale, including HSS or Lysholm. This need for stratification in regards to activity levels is important, demonstrating the need for large study samples.

TABLE 24.4. *The 2000 International Knee Documentation Committee (IKDC) knee examination form*

2000
IKDC KNEE EXAMINATION FORM

Patient Name:___________________________   Date of Birth:______/______/______
                                                                                 Day   Month   Year

Gender: □F   □M   Age:___________   Date of Examination:______/______/______
                                                                                 Day   Month   Year

Generalized Laxity: □tight   □normal   □lax

Alignment: □obvious varus   □normal   □obvious valgus

Patella Position: □obvious baja   □normal   □obvious alta

Patella Subluxation/Dislocation: □centered   □subluxable   □subluxed   □dislocated

Range of Motion (Ext/Flex):   Index Side: passive______/______/______   active______/______/______
                              Opposite Side: passive______/______/______   active______/______/______

SEVEN GROUPS	FOUR GRADES				*Group Grade			
	A Normal	B Nearly Normal	C Abnormal	D Severely Abnormal	A	B	C	D
1. Effusion	□ None	□ Mild	□ Moderate	□ Severe	□	□	□	□
2. Passive Motion Deficit								
ΔLack of extension	□ <3°	□ 3 to 5°	□ 6 to 10°	□ >10°				
ΔLack of flexion	□ 0 to 5°	□ 6 to 15°	□ 16 to 25°	□ >25°	□	□	□	□
3. Ligament Examination (manual, instrumented, x-ray)								
ΔLachman (25° flex) (134N)	□ -1 to 2mm	□ 3 to 5mm(1$^+$)	□ 6 to 10mm(2$^+$)	□ >10mm(3$^+$)				
		□ <-1 to −3	□ <-3 stiff					
ΔLachman (25° flex) manual max	□ -1 to 2mm	□ 3 to 5mm	□ 6 to 10mm	□ >10mm				
Anterior endpoint:	□ firm		□ soft					
ΔTotal AP Translation (25° flex)	□ 0 to 2mm	□ 3 to 5mm	□ 6 to 10mm	□ >10mm				
ΔTotal AP Translation (70° flex)	□ 0 to 2mm	□ 3 to 5mm	□ 6 to 10mm	□ >10mm				
ΔPosterior Drawer Test (70° flex)	□ 0 to 2mm	□ 3 to 5mm	□ 6 to 10mm	□ >10mm				
ΔMed Joint Opening (20° flex/valgus rot)	□ 0 to 2mm	□ 3 to 5mm	□ 6 to 10mm	□ >10mm				
ΔLat Joint Opening (20° flex/varus rot)	□ 0 to 2mm	□ 3 to 5mm	□ 6 to 10mm	□ >10mm				
ΔExternal Rotation Test (30° flex prone)	□ <5°	□ 6 to 10°	□ 11 to 19°	□ >20°				
ΔExternal Rotation Test (90° flex prone)	□ <5°	□ 6 to 10°	□ 11 to 19°	□ >20°				
ΔPivot Shift	□ equal	□ +glide	□ ++(clunk)	□ +++(gross)				
ΔReverse Pivot Shift	□ equal	□ glide	□ gross	□ marked	□	□	□	□
4. Compartment Findings			crepitation with					
ΔCrepitus Ant. Compartment	□ none	□ moderate	□ mild pain	□ >mild pain				
ΔCrepitus Med. Compartment	□ none	□ moderate	□ mild pain	□ >mild pain				
ΔCrepitus Lat. Compartment	□ none	□ moderate	□ mild pain	□ >mild pain				
5. Harvest Site Pathology	□ none	□ mild	□ moderate	□ severe				
6. X-ray Findings								
Med. Joint Space	□ none	□ mild	□ moderate	□ severe				
Lat. Joint Space	□ none	□ mild	□ moderate	□ severe				
Patellofemoral	□ none	□ mild	□ moderate	□ severe				
Ant. Joint Space (sagittal)	□ none	□ mild	□ moderate	□ severe				
Post. Joint Space (sagittal)	□ none	□ mild	□ moderate	□ severe				
7. Functional Test								
One Leg Hop (% of opposite side)	□ ≥90%	□ 89 to 76%	□ 75 to 50%	□ <50%				
****Final Evaluation**					□	□	□	□

*   Group grade: The lowest grade within a group determines the group grade
** Final evaluation: the worst group grade determines the final evaluation for acute and subacute patients. For chronic patients compare preoperative and postoperative evaluations. In a final evaluation only the first 3 groups are evaluated but all groups must be documented. Δ Difference in involved knee compared to normal or what is assumed to be normal.

The tendency to combine a raw data score into one categoric score data is thought to be a primary source of error. The Cincinnati knee ligament rating system avoids raw score combinations and separately lists 20 factors deriving the final overall grade by incorporating the lowest common result of each factor. This is similar to the International Knee Society evaluation, which has the worst qualification within the group taken as a group qualification. The worst group qualification is then taken as a final evaluation. This is an improvement, with less data loss and better overall assessment of end results.

In the recent past, quantitative assessments of function have been popularized with function tests being performed, comparing the uninjured and injured/postoperative limb. The HSS, IKDC, and the Cincinnati Knee scoring systems incorporate one or more functional tests in their end result measure. However, there have been numerous studies looking at functional tests that demonstrate that one can score well on a functional test and still have objective laxity on physical examination as well as subjective reports of giving way (35,41). The lack of a functional test correlating with a measurement of ACL function is consistent with Noyes and coworkers (35,42). Noyes looked at four hop tests and showed that there was a low sensitivity rate in any of the hop tests. Fifty percent of the patients who had anterior cruciate–deficient knees scored satisfactorily on a single-leg hop test. If one would do two hop tests together, 62% of the population performed abnormally, increasing the sensitivity. No statistically significant relationship was found between the KT-1000 arthrometer results and any one of the five functional test results (35). Noyes thought that the hop tests used in the study were not sensitive enough to detect functional limitations in ACL-deficient knees. They concluded that functional tests must be used in conjunction with other clinical assessment tools.

GENERIC HEALTH MEASURES

Generic measures of health status have been developed to assess the outcomes of treatment. Few of these have been used to evaluate the results of orthopedic treatments in sports or ligaments knee injuries. The Short-Form Health Survey (SF-36), developed by John Ware and colleagues, is a generic health status measure that is patient-based, and obtains the patient's assessment of his or her behavioral function, subjective well being, and perceptions of health. The reliability of SF-36 in populations including general and chronic disease states in the orthopedic treatment of arthritis have been well documented. In 1996, Shapiro looked at 113 patients divided into groups who underwent ACL reconstructive surgery versus those who were treated without surgery (43). They found that SF-36 scales that were less based on physical health (general health, vitality, social functioning, motion, and mental health) had no correlations at any period of time between the patient groups. However, the three SF-36 parameters that were based more on physical health (physical functioning role, role physical, and bodily pain) had a statistically different change in one parameter (role physical) from baseline to 6 months in the surgically treated group. There were trends toward significance in the other two physical health–based parameters (physical functioning role and bodily pain). They concluded that the SF-36 health status assessment could not be used as a discriminate index to classify ACL-injured

patients into groups for various treatments. The three physical health based scales of the SF-36 did correlate with the final IKDC score; they did not correlate with the objective measurement of stability.

This study again points out the disparity between the generic subjective measurements of outcome as provided by the SF-36 and the objective measurement of laxity. This suggests that there are issues beyond laxity that contribute to the primary function of the patient after ACL surgery. It also suggests that the SF-36 lacks sensitivity or was unable to detect subtle changes in functioning resulting from differences in laxity. This continues to be a problem in knee laxity index scores. There likely needs to be a more sophisticated test to detect subtle changes in function. Minor differences in laxity is likely masked by the patient's change in lifestyle or habits based on the qualitative state of their knee (43). The patients' rating of their own knee function is independent of the results of static and dynamic tests commonly used to assess knee stability and function. There is an assumption that an independent relationship exists between knee joint function and knee stability. Knee function and knee stability, however, may be mutually exclusive entities in the ACL reconstructed knee (44,45). A recent study that looked at patients 5 years after an ACL reconstruction compared objective instability and functional activity scores (46). They found that there was no correlation between objective instability and a functional activity score. The assumption that the severity of joint laxity after ACL injury is directly related to the degree of instability is widely held (47–50). Changes in joint laxity measurements continue to be a major criterion by which successful outcomes are documented after ACL reconstruction. In addition, there have been a paucity of studies that have looked at joint laxity measurements and functional outcomes after conservative treatment of the ACL-injured patient (50–52). The relationship between the clinical (objective) sign of joint laxity, the subjective feeling of instability, and functional activities as currently measured by functional outcome studies, fail to show a strong correlation between objective signs and functional instability (53).

CURRENT OUTCOME ASSESSMENT TOOLS

Conventional research techniques for clinical management have generally focused on process based (clinical) outcomes. These include fracture union, ROM, infection, etc. In orthopedic research these clinical outcome measures have dominated the published literature and with very few exceptions have not used health related outcomes that are patient derived, standardized, and validated. As Wennberg recently stated "We need a way to assure the American people that the needed evaluations of clinical theory are done in a timely way, before plausible but wrong ideas get institutionalized into the everyday practice of medicine" (54). This will require the use of clinical trial method wherever possible, and standardized outcome assessment (preferably multicenter) wherever practical (55,56). Outcome assessment herein defined must include patient-derived, health-oriented outcomes combined with traditional clinical outcomes, and given the evolving competitive marketplace, patient satisfaction data.

Large databases in existence have great utility for studying the process of care but have little, if any, patient-oriented functional data (57–62). The only outcomes commonly available are mortality, complications, length of stay, and charges (63). We would need to begin to routinely collect patient-oriented functional outcome data to enhance the use of such large data sets.

Several well-validated general health status instruments have been widely used in medical research (Table 24.5).

TABLE 24.5. *Health-related questionnaire instruments and scoring resources*

Instrument	Method of administration	Training time required	Length of time to complete	Population	Conditions used for	Where and how to obtain instrument
SF-36	Self or interviewer	2 hr	5–10 min	All	General health status/quality of life measures	Medical Outcomes Trust 20 Park Plaza Suite (1014) Boston, MA 02116-4313
SIP	Self or interviewer	1 wk	30 min	All	General health status/quality of life measures	Ann Skinner 624 N. Broadway Rm 647 Baltimore, MD 21205
WOMAC	Self	1 wk	10 min	Arthritis patients	Arthritis	Jane Campbell, London Health Science Center (Suite 303) South Campus 375 South Street, London, Ontario N6A-4G5 Canada
Nottingham Health Profile	Self	1 wk	10 min	All	General health status/quality of life measures	Jim McEwan, Department of Public Health, University of Glasgow, Glasgow G12 8QQ United Kingdom
QWB	Trained interviewer	2 wk	12 min	All	General health status/quality of life measures	Holly Teetzel, Dept. Family and Preventive Med., Box 0622, University of California, San Diego, 9500 Gilman Drive, La Jolla, CA 92093
AAOS Instruments UE, LE, Spine and Pediatrics	Self or interviewer	1 wk	Variable (module dependent) 10–40 min	Patients of specific age or regions of disease/ injury	Quality of life measure applied to regional (or specific age group) musculoskeletal populations	Director research and Scientific Affairs, American Academy of Orthopaedic Surgeons, 6300 North River Road, Rosemont, IL 60018
MFA	Self or interviewer	2 hr	15min		Quality of life measure applied to musculoskeletal disease	Department of Orthopaedics, Box 35979825 Ninth Avenue, Seattle, WA 98104

SF-36, Short Form-36; SIP, sickness impact profile; WOMAC, Western Ontario and McMaster University Osteoarthritis Index; QWB, Quality of Well-Being Scale; AAOS, American Academy of Orthopaedic Surgeons; MFA, musculoskeletal function.

These instruments or scales attempt to assess all aspects of an individual's function including physical, social, and mental well-being. A partial list would include the SF-36 (Short Form-36 developed by John Ware, Ph.D. and the Rand Corporation Medical Outcomes Study), the SIP (sickness impact profile developed by Marilyn Bergner, Ph.D. and coworkers at the University of Washington), the quality of well-being scale (QWB; widely used in the United Kingdom to develop QALY), and the Nottingham Health Profile (63). The latter has been used in an important study on the functional outcomes of patients undergoing amputation versus limb salvage for severe open tibial fractures (64). All of these scales share certain characteristics that make their use appealing for the orthopedic community. They are health-related, address the individual instead of a disease or organ, are from the patients' perspective, and were scientifically validated. They share the characteristics of being internally consistent, reproducible, are responsive to clinical change over time, and have the ability to discriminate between severity of conditions. Disease-specific functional outcomes questionnaires can be developed but must undergo the same type of vigorous validation to assure users that the instrument measures what it proposes to measure (65). A brief discussion of each of the three most widely used general health status instruments, the SF-36, the SIP, and the QWB seems useful.

The SF-36 is perhaps the most broadly studied, refined, and widely applied of the general health status instruments (66,67). Its 36 questions relate to 6 different functional subscales: bodily pain, role function (physical and mental health), social function, physical function, energy/fatigue, and general health perceptions. These scales are scored separately without an aggregate scale. This may represent a small limitation of this tool. It has been validated as a broadly reliable and reproducible questionnaire that has been applied to numerous health conditions. It is also validated to be reliable as a questionnaire delivered by interviewer, by mail, or by telephone and takes 5 to 7 minutes to complete. These are major advantages as it is practical for use in the busy clinic or office. It has not been widely applied to orthopedic conditions. This is rapidly changing, as one of the authors noted nearly 10% of the papers presented from the podium at the 1994 annual meeting of an orthopedic subspecialty society included SF-36 data. It is generally considered to have a "floor" effect for musculoskeletal conditions. This implies that patients with clinically relevant functional disability are not adequately characterized by the questions in the physical function section. This is especially true for high functional demand athletes. Of the general health status instruments available, the authors generally recommend this tool.

The SIP is a 136 endorsable item questionnaire that ideally is interviewer administered and takes 25 to 35 minutes to complete (68,69). Less information exists on self and mail administration. It was developed to provide a measure of the effects or outcomes of health care that can be used for evaluation, program planning and policy formation. It has 12 different domains addressed by the endorsable statements (the patient simply affirms that a statement of disability applies to them) which are scored independently, aggregated into a physical and psychosocial subscale, and pooled to give a single score. The scale is 0 to 100 (no disability is 0), however, scores in excess of 35 or so bring worthwhile quality of life into serious question. A rough approximation of a relevant difference is 2 points (statistically). The SIP has been widely used in multiple health conditions and has been used in musculoskeletal injury where it has proven to be useful (70,71). It requires training to administer, however, so it is best recommended for well funded outcome studies or controlled trials where interviewers can be trained and employed. It too suffers from a floor effect, and low sensitivity for the lesser degrees of musculoskeletal disability.

The QWB scale forms the foundation for the cost effectiveness tool termed the QALY (72). It was designed to be a commonly used effectiveness measure for policy analysis and resource allocation. Patients are classified by their responses to the questionnaire on their level of physical activity (three levels), mobility (three levels), social activity (five levels), and according to the one symptom or problem that bothered them the most on the day of assessment (choice of 22 symptom complexes). The QWB is then calculated by combining preference weights. The preference weights were derived from responses to a household survey that asked respondents to rate their preference for various health states on a 1 to 10 scale, ranging from death to perfect health. Multiple QWB scores are calculated separately for each of 6 days preceding interview, and the final score is taken as the average over the 6 days. The scale ranges from 0 to 1 with 1 being a state of perfect health and 0 equivalent to death. The QWB takes 20 to 25 minutes to administer and cannot be self-administered. Using values generated on the scale from large populations and multiplying that value times a year and the cost of the intervention gives the QALY. The QALY is therefore defined as the well-life expectancy; the product of QWB scores and the expected duration of life in each functional level defined by the QWB. QALYs provide a way to estimate trade-offs between costs and benefits of health interventions. The physical dimension of the QWB scale very likely has a moderate-to-severe floor effect for relevant musculoskeletal disability. Generally speaking, when orthopedic interventions have been studied using the QALY methodology, they have fared well. This is especially true for hip arthroplasty and operative management of hip fracture.

The lack of a well-validated general health status tool to assess musculoskeletal disability, which does not demonstrate the floor effects discussed above is apparent.

Because musculoskeletal injury and disease is responsible for more loss of productive years of life than any other disease process, the need to develop such a scale is apparent. For 5 years, a National Institutes of Health–sponsored effort was conducted to develop and validate a general health status instrument that emphasizes musculoskeletal function. Beginning with open-ended interviews of patients with musculoskeletal injury and disease, a pool of items was developed that was supplemented by interviews with practitioners who treat these diseases (orthopedists, rehabilitation physicians, physical therapists, occupational therapists, and trainers) and a review of all validated published questionnaires. The patients who were interviewed consisted of individuals with injury (bone and soft tissue-ligamentous) involving the upper and lower extremity. Patients with arthritis (rheumatoid and osteoarthritis), and a diffuse group of "overuse" syndromes (including carpal tunnel syndrome, lateral epicondylitis, and rotator cuff disease in the upper extremity and anterior knee pain and plantar fasciitis in the lower extremity) were enrolled. The pool of items for the Musculoskeletal Functional Assessment Instrument (MFAI) was narrowed to 177 by the frequency of complaint, clinical importance, and patient perceived significance of the functional disability. This scale was subjected to reproducibility testing and 119 patients took the questionnaire besides several objective measures. These included ROM, self-selected walking speed, timed stair climbing, and isokinetic testing in the lower extremity, and ROM, grip dynamometer, the Jebsen-Taylor functional test, and isokinetic testing in the upper extremity. These data and correlation matrices were used to further reduce the MFAI to 100 items. Scaling exercises to rank the items of functional disability were conducted with a group of 50 patients with musculoskeletal disease and injury. The long form MFA takes 13 to 15 minutes for an individual with an eighth grade reading level to complete. Its development, responsiveness, reproducibility and validation testing have been published. It is best used for funded efficacy studies although it can be self-administered.

These data were used to develop a short MFAI of 46 items using the same psychometric techniques. The 36-item function scale and the 12-item "bother" have a scaled format to increase the sensitivity. The "bother" scale is a patient utility scale where patients can relate how much their functional difficulties impede or "bother" them. This aspect of the tool may be useful for managing individual patients, although this theory has not been tested. The short form will be useful for office based outcomes and multicenter effectiveness assessments which are necessary to study the majority of entities within the field of musculoskeletal injury because of the low incidence of many types of injury that we are required to treat. It is hoped that the American Academy of Orthopaedic Surgeons, and the subspecialty societies will play key roles in facilitating these types of investigations.

The American Academy of Orthopaedic Surgeons has developed a series of validated functional questionnaires that are made available to the orthopedic community for office based assessments. The general module uses the SF-36 for general health status measurement. The spine, pediatric (age under 18), upper and lower extremity modules provide greater sensitivity for their respective functional domains. Both the upper and lower extremity modules have sections for high functional demand athletes. These instruments may be most useful for funded outcomes programs that are attempting to document efficacy of a treatment method.

Most recently, two measurement scales have been developed and designed specifically for knee conditions. The Quality of Life Outcome Measure is a patient-based, subjective outcome measure for chronic anterior cruciate ligament deficiency (73) that was developed, pretested, and validated.

The Activities of Daily Living Scale of the Knee Outcome Survey is a patient-reported measure of functional limitations imposed by pathological disorders and impairments of the knee during activities of daily living (74).

We will likely see the emergence of new outcome tools for specific knee conditions. As these tools emerge, specific clinical applications and reports on their use will result in a more refined understanding of knee conditions and out treatment of specific disorders.

CONCLUSION

The ideal study of the natural history of knee ligament injury or a rehabilitative–surgical intervention should use:

1. Clinical (objective) outcomes measures (laxity, ROM, strength testing, etc.)
2. A patient self-reported functional measure (ideally stratified to include varying levels of sport and work)
3. A measure of patient satisfaction with the process of care
4. Cost

The study should include pre- and postobservation or intervention assessment points, and the use of active follow-up (scheduled for all subjects at the same intervals). The next decade should bring to the practicing knee surgeon an abundance of well-done outcome studies that will enhance the physician and patient decision-making process and improve the results of care.

REFERENCES

1. Donabedian A. Evaluating the product of medical care. *Milbank Quest* 1966;44:166–203.
2. Liang MH, Jette AM. Measuring functional ability in chronic arthritis. *Arthritis Rheum* 1981;24:80–86.

3. Keller RB, Rudicel SA, Liang MH. Outcomes research in orthopaedics. Instructional course lectures. *Am Acad Orthop Surg* 1994;43:599–611.

4. Wennberg A, Gittelsohn J. Variations in medical care among small areas. *Sci Am* 1982;246:120–134.

5. Melzack R. The McGill pain questionnaire: major properties and scoring methods. *Pain* 1975;1:277–299.

6. Scott J, Huskisson EC. Graphic representation of pain. *Pain* 1976;2:76–184.

7. Williams RC. Toward a set of reliable and valid measurements for chronic pain assessment and outcome research. *Pain* 1988;35:239–251.

8. Freyd M. The graphic rating scale. *J Educ Psychol* 1923;14:83–102.

9. Labib S, Fisher W, Laurin CA. The use of visual analog scales (VAS) in assessment of pain and function in arthroplasty patients [abstract]. *Orthop Trans* 1986;10:598.

10. Bond A, Lader M. The use of analogue scales in rating subjective feelings. *Br J Med Psychol* 1974;47:211–218.

11. Cella DF, Perry SW. Reliability and concurrent validity of three visual analogue mood scales. *Psychol Rep* 1986;59:827–833.

12. Harms–Ringdahl K, Carlsson AM, Ekholm J, et al. Pain assessment with different intensity scales in response to loading of joint structures. *Pain* 1986;27:401–411.

13. Huskisson EC, Jones J, Scott PJ. Application of visual-analogue scales to the measurement of functional capacity. *Rheum Rehab* 1976;15:185–187.

14. Flandry F, Hunt JP, Terry GC, et al. Analysis of subjective knee complaints using visual analog scales. *Am J Sports Med* 1991:112–118.

15. Carlsson AM. Assessment of chronic pain. Aspects of the reliability and validity of the visual analogue scale. *Pain* 1983;16:87–101.

16. Larson CB. Rating scale for hip dislocations. *Clin Orthop* 1963;31:85.

17. Swiontkowski MF. Outcomes measurement in orthopaedic trauma surgery. *Injury* 1995;26:653–657.

18. Tugwell P, Bombardier C. A methodologic framework for developing and selecting endpoints in clinical trials. *J Rheumatol* 1982;9:758–762.

19. Kettlecamp D, Thompson C. Development of a knee scoring scale. *Clin Orthop Relat Res* 1975;107:93–99.

20. Meenan RF, Gertman PM, Mason JH, et al. The arthritis impact measurement scales: further investigation of a health status measure. *Arthritis Rheum* 1982;25:1048–1053.

21. Fries JF, Spitz PW, Young DY. The dimensions of health outcomes: the health assessment questionnaire, disability and pain scales. *J Rheum* 1982;9:789–793.

22. Groves H. The crucial ligaments of the knee joint. Their function, rupture, and the operative treatment of the same. *Br J Surg* 1919;7:505–515.

23. O'Donoghue DH. Surgical treatment of fresh injuries to the major ligaments of the knee. *J Bone Joint Surg Am* 1950;50:211–225.

24. O'Donoghue DH. An analysis of end results of surgical treatment of major injuries to the ligaments of the knee. *J Bone Joint Surg Am* 1955;37:1–13.

25. O'Donoghue DH. Treatment of acute ligamentous injuries of the knee. *Orthop Clin North Am* 1973;40:617.

26. Jones KG. Reconstruction of the anterior ligament. *J Bone Joint Surg Am* 1963;45:925.

27. Slocum DB, Larson RL. Pes anserinus transplantation. *J Bone Joint Surg Am* 1963;45:925.

28. Smillie IS, ed. *Diseases of the knee joint*. London: Churchill-Livingston, 1974:29.

29. Harris WH. Traumatic arthritis of the hip after dislocation and acetabular fractures; treatment by mold arthroplasty. *J Bone Joint Surg Am* 1969;51:737.

30. Marshall JL, Fetto JF, Botero PM. Knee ligament injuries: a standard evaluation method. *Clin Orthop* 1977;123:115–129.

31. Palmar I. Injuries to the ligaments of the knee joint. *Suppl Acta Orthop Scand* 1938;170–173.

32. Lysholm J, Gillquist J. Evaluation of knee ligament surgery results with special emphasis on use of a scoring scale. *Am J Sports Med* 1982;10:150–154.

33. Tegner Y, Lysholm J. Rating systems in the evaluation of knee ligament injuries. *Clin Orthop* 1985;198:43–49.

34. Noyes FR, Barber SD, Mooar LA. A rationale for assessing sports activity levels and limitations in knee disorders. *Clin Orthop* 1989;246:238–249.

35. Barber SD, Noyes FR, Mangine RE, et al. Quantitative assessment of functional limitations in normal and anterior cruciate ligament-deficient knees. *Clin Orthop* 1990;255:204–214.

36. Noyes FR, Barber SD, Mangine RE. Bone-patellar ligament-bone and fascia lata allografts for reconstruction of the anterior cruciate ligament. *J Bone Joint Surg Am* 1990;72:1125–1136.

37. Noyes FR, McGinnis GH, Mooar LA. Functional disability in the anterior cruciate insufficient knee syndrome. Review of the knee rating systems and projected risk factors in determining treatment. *Sports Med* 1984;1:278–302.

38. Noyes FR, ed. *The Noyes knee rating system: an assessment of subjective, objective, ligamentous, and functional parameters*. Cincinnati: Cincinnati Sports Medicine Research and Educational Foundation, 1993.

39. Hefti F, Muller M, Jakob RP, et al. Evaluation of knee ligament injuries with the IKDC form. *Knee Surg Sports Traumatol Arthrosc* 1993;1:226–234.

40. Hefti F, Muller M. Current state of evaluation of knee ligament injuries with the IKDC knee evaluation form. *Orthopaedics* 1993;22:351–362.

41. Sgaglione NA, Del Pizzo W, Fox JM, et al. Critical analysis of knee ligament rating systems. *Am J Sports Med* 1995;23:660–667.

42. Noyes FR, Barber SD, Mangine RE. Abnormal lower limb symmetry determined by function hop tests after anterior cruciate ligament rupture. *Am J Sports Med* 1991;19:513–518.

43. Shapiro ET, Richmond JC, Rockett SE, et al. The use of a generic, patient-based health assessment (SF-36) for evaluation of patients with anterior cruciate ligament injuries. *Am J Sports Med* 1995;23:660–667.

44. Sekiya I, Muneta T, Ogiuchi T, et al. Significance of the single-legged hop test to the anterior cruciate ligament-reconstructed knee in relation to muscle strength and anterior laxity. *Am J Sports Med* 1998;26:384–388.

45. Wilk KE, Romaniello WT, Soscia SM, et al. The relationship between subjective knee scores, isokinetic testing, and functional testing in the ACL reconstructed knee. *J Orthop Phys Ther* 1994;20:60–73.

46. Seto JL, Drofino AS, Morissey MC, et al. Assessment of quadriceps/hamstring strength, knee ligament stability, functional and sports activity levels five years after anterior cruciate ligament reconstruction. *Am J Sports Med* 1988;16:170–180.

47. Fetto JF, Marshall JL. The natural history and diagnosis of anterior cruciate ligament insufficiency. *Clin Orthop* 1980;147:29–38.

48. Johnson RJ, Ericksson E, Haggamark T, et al. Five- to ten-year follow-up evaluation after reconstruction of the anterior cruciate ligament. *Clin Orthop* 1984;183:122–140.

49. Lysholm J, Gillquist J. Evaluation of knee ligament surgery results with special emphasis on the use of a scoring scale. *Am J Sports Med* 1982;10:150–154.

50. Noyes FR, Mooar PA, Matthews DS, et al. The symptomatic anterior cruciate-deficient knee, Part 1: the long-term functional disability in athletically active individuals. *J Bone Joint Surg Am* 1983;65:154–162.

51. Anderson KC. Knee laxity and function after conservative treatment of anterior cruciate ligament injuries: a prospective study. *Int J Sports Med* 1993;14:150–153.

52. Lephart SM, Perrin DH, Fu FH, et al. Relationship between selected physical characteristics and functional capacity in the anterior cruciate ligament-insufficient athlete. *J Orthop Sports Phys Ther* 1992;16:174–181.

53. Snyder-Mackler L, Fitzgerald GK, Bartolozzi AR, et al. The relationship between passive joint laxity and functional outcome after anterior cruciate ligament injury. *Am J Sports Med* 1997;25:191–195.

54. Wennberg JE. Letter to the editor. *N Engl J Med* 1994;331:815.

55. Deyo RA, Inui TS, Leninger JD, et al. Measuring functional outcomes in chronic disease; a comparison of traditional scales and a self-administered health status questionnaire in patients with rheumatoid arthritis. *Med Care* 1983;21:180–192.

56. Schroeder SA. Outcome assessment 70 years later: are we ready? *N Engl J Med* 1987;316:160–162.

57. Cutler SJ, Latourette HB. A national cooperative program for the evaluation of end results in cancer. *JNCI* 1959;22:633–646.

58. Pollock DA, McClain PW. Trauma registries: current status and future prospects. *JAMA* 1989;262:2280–2283.

59. Schwartz RJ, Jacobs LM, Yaezel D. Impact of pre-hospital center care on length of stay and hospital charges. *J Trauma* 1989;29:1611–1615.

60. Sniezek JE, Finklea JF, Graciter PL. Injury coding and hospital discharge data. *JAMA* 1989;262:2270–2272.

61. Vestrup JA, Phang T, Veresi L, et al. The utility of a multi center trauma registry. *J Trauma* 1994;37:375–378.

62. Weddell JM. Registers and registries: a review. *Int J Epidemiol* 1973;2:221–228.

63. McEwen J. The Nottingham Health Profile: a measure of perceived health. In: Teeling-Smith G, ed. *Measuring the social benefits of medicine*. London Office of Health Economics, 1983:75–84.

64. Georgiadis GM, Behrens FF, Joyce MJ, et al. Open tibial fractures with severe soft tissue loss, limb salvage compared with below knee amputation. *J Bone Joint Surg Am* 1993;75:1431–1441.

65. Levine DW, Simmons BP, Koris MJ, et al. A self-administered questionnaire for the assessment of severity of symptoms and functional status in carpal tunnel syndrome. *J Bone Surg Am* 1993;75:1585–1592.

66. Stewart AL, Hayes RD, Ware JE. The MOS short form general health survey; reliability and validity in a patient population. *Med Care* 1988;26:724–735.

67. Tarlov AR, Ware JE, Greenfield S, et al. The medical outcomes study: an application of methods for monitoring the results of medical care. *JAMA* 1989;262:925–930.

68. Bergner M, Bobbitt RA, Carter WB, et al. The sickness impact profile: development and final revision of a health status measure. *Med Care* 1981;19:757–805.

69. Bergner M, Bobbitt RA, Pollaro WE, et al. The sickness impact profile: validation of a health status measure. *Med Care* 1976;14:57–67.

70. MacKenzie EJ, Burgess AR, McAndrew MP, et al. Patient-oriented functional outcome after unilateral lower extremity fracture. *J Orthop Trauma* 1993;7:393–401.

71. MacKenzie EJ, Cushing BM, Jurkovich GJ, et al. Physical impairment and functional outcomes six months after severe lower extremity fractures. *J Trauma* 1993;34:528–538.

72. McDowell I, Newell C. *Measuring health: a guide to rating scales and questionnaires*, New York: Oxford University Press, 1987:125-133.

73. Mohtadi N. Development and validation of the quality of life outcome measure (questionnaire) for chronic anterior cruciate ligament deficiency. *Am J Sports Med* 1998;26:350–359.

74. Irrgang JJ, Snyder-Mackler L, Wainner RS, et al. Development of a patient-reported measure of function of the knee. *J Bone Joint Surg Am* 1998;80:1132–1145.

CHAPTER 25

Outcomes Following Anterior Cruciate Ligament Surgery

Edmond P. Young and Donald C. Fithian

The frequency with which the anterior cruciate ligament (ACL) is reconstructed and the convergence of techniques of reconstruction and rehabilitation imply a high level of confidence in the success of the operation (1). There is now a vast amount of literature on the function, biology, and biomechanics of the ACL, as well as on techniques of ACL reconstruction and rehabilitation (1,2). Yet, although knee ligament reconstruction surgery has undergone considerable evolution over the past 25 years, the criteria by which we judge success and failure are not yet clearly defined (3). There are few studies that clearly document the natural history of the ACL-deficient knee and the risk factors associated with a poor outcome (4–6). Without this as a foundation, the vast literature on surgical results has limited practical value, because the benefits of treatment cannot be measured directly.

The patient with an ACL-disrupted knee is at risk for functional impairment, secondary meniscus tear, and the development of joint arthrosis. The cascade of events from ACL disruption to secondary injuries with meniscus tears to joint arthrosis has been documented (7–11). What is the effect of ACL reconstructive surgery on this process? It is clear that some patients are able to cope with their ACL-disrupted knee without sustaining secondary injuries (8,10,12–15). Some cope without modifying their lifestyle, others modify their athletic participation, and others cope by discontinuing athletic participation.

The purpose of ACL reconstruction is to restore normal function by reestablishing the restraints to anterior tibiofemoral motion, yet it has only recently been established that the degree of objective instability is related to the function in the postoperative knee (16–19). Rather than reporting results solely in terms of physical impairments, outcomes research has begun to refocus our attention on the patient's overall function and satisfaction. Several clinical outcomes instruments have been used to assess function of the injured knee (20–24). Shapiro et al. (25) have assessed the validity of a generic instrument (the SF-36) in evaluating patients following ACL injury and treatment. Mohtadi (26) has developed a quality-of-life outcome measure for the chronically ACL-deficient knee. The fundamental purpose of the development of such outcomes measures is to not only assess the objective results of surgery, but also in a rigorous and scientific manner to determine the effectiveness of the surgery in the broader sense of its effects on the patient's overall function (27).

PROBLEMS WITH EXISTING LITERATURE

Prospectively collected data on outcomes of injury and treatment are essential because the data allow us to apply an informed decision process in advising the patient who has sustained a knee injury. It further allows greater participation of the patient in decisions regarding his or her knee. The worst we can do, as surgeons, is to create a situation that is in fact worse for the patient than the one with which we were first presented. In surgery, as in all things, wisdom requires understanding one's limitations. The decision whether to reconstruct the ligament should be guided by realistic goals and expectations. The goals of ACL reconstruction are determined by the symptoms, disabilities, and other undesirable clinical outcomes of ACL injury. The expectations must be guided by specific evidence that surgery will—or will not—prevent or ameliorate those untoward outcomes.

The ideal outcome study would be designed as a prospective, blinded, randomized study with a matched control group. The groups being compared must be similar in composition and risk for adverse or favorable outcomes to minimize *susceptibility bias*. The groups would be evaluated before and after treatment by the same tester, separate from the treating physician, to eliminate *detection bias*

(28). If a study is designed to compare two surgical procedures, it is essential that surgeons for procedure A are equally as skilled as the surgeons for procedure B to eliminate *performance bias*. Most of the existing literature regarding results of anterior cruciate ligament surgery consists of retrospective studies or chart reviews, which are susceptible to all the previous forms of bias.

Length of follow-up is also important when considering the results of any ligament surgery. Reports of knee surgery, except in rare instances, require a 2-year follow-up. We have found that most graft failures are revealed by 6 months after surgery (29). However, vigorous return to sporting activity does not usually occur until the second year after injury. A 2-year follow-up provides evaluation of the motion limits and patient function. A 5-year follow-up is probably needed to evaluate the success of the ligament reconstruction in preventing late meniscus tears. Although intercondylar radiographic changes may be seen as early as 6 months after an ACL injury (30), a follow-up of 10 years is probably required to evaluate the efficacy of ligament surgery in reducing the incidence of degenerative arthritis.

EVALUATING THE RESULTS OF KNEE LIGAMENT SURGERY

Motion Limits

The KT arthrometer has been used to measure anterior–posterior displacement and to diagnose an ACL disruption (31–38). We have found the manual maximum test to be the most accurate clinical test for diagnosing complete ACL rupture (5,6,39). Compared with arthroscopy, the manual maximum test was 97% specific and 96% sensitive in diagnosing complete ACL rupture (6). Therefore, in the Kaiser studies, the term "KT unstable" is used essentially synonymously with "ACL deficient."

The primary goal of ACL reconstruction is to restore the normal restraints to anterior tibiofemoral motion. Therefore, anterior displacement measurements are an important indication of surgical success. A successful operation should try to return patients to their preinjury state. Buss et al. (40), Bach et al. (16), Faustgen et al. (41) and others have reported results of instrumented testing in follow-up studies on current techniques of autograft bone–patellar tendon–bone ACL reconstruction. The available data for manual maximum KT testing are presented in Table 25.1. It is clear from these studies that ACL reconstruction using currently accepted graft sources is effective in reducing the pathologic anterior tibiofemoral motion associated with ACL deficiency. However, many patients have some degree of residual anterior instability on instrumented testing (16–18). It is not clear from the literature the point at which postreconstruction anterior laxity will allow symptomatic subluxation and increased risk for reinjury.

In contrast to the well-established criteria for documenting insufficiency of the native ACL, the definition of

TABLE 25.1. *Manual maximum KT arthrometer data, injured minus normal difference (I - N)*

Reference	Year	Cases (n)	Procedure	Mos f/u	I-N difference
Buss (12)	1993	68	Two-incision PT	32	91% 0–3 mm
Harner (40)	1994	30	Arthroscopic PT	29	1.6 ± 2.0 mm
		30	Two-incision PT	30	1.8 ± 3.4 mm
Faustgen (30)	1994	201	Arthroscopic PT	36	3.8 mm
			Two-incision PT		(3.4 mm w/ early mobilization)
			Two-incision PT/LAD		
O'Neill (64)	1996	40	Two-incision ST-G	42	83% 0–3 mm
		40	Two-incision PT		93% 0–3 mm
		45	Arthroscopic PT		87% 0–3 mm
Daniel (18)	1996	71	ACL repair	121	3.0 mm acute
			ITB		3.4 mm late
			Arthroscopic ST-G		
			Two-incision PT		
			Arthroscopic PT		
Stringham (80)	1996	66	Autograft PT	34	80% 0–3 mm
		47	Allograft PT		70% 0–3 mm
Sgaglione (72)	1997	45	Arthroscopic PT	30	75% 0–3 mm
		45	Two-incision PT	41	78% 0–3 mm
Feagin (34)	1997	68	Two-incision ST-G	58	83% 0–5 mm
		69	Two-incision PT		89% 0–5 mm
Bach (9)	1998	97	Arthroscopic PT	79	1.0 ± 3.0 mm
Plancher (67)	1998	75	Two-incision PT	55	1.4 ± 3.3 mm
Howell (45)	1999	67	Arthroscopic ST-G	25	93% 0–3 mm
		41	Two-incision ST-G	26	82% 0–3 mm
Patel (65)	2000	32	Arthroscopic PT	70	87% 0–3 mm

TABLE 25.2. *Arthrometer measurements, millimeters of injured minus normal difference (I - N)*

Group	I: Early stable		II: Coper		III: Early reconstruction		IV: Late reconstruction+	
Displacement force	89 N	MM[a]	89 N	MM	89 N	MM	89 N	MM
Acute injury								
Clinic	−0.0	0.2	3.4	6.0	4.1	6.5	3.7	6.1
Anesthesia	−1.1	0.2	3.9	6.6	4.8	7.2	3.6	5.7
12 mo after injury								
	n = 20		*n = 105*		*n = 33*		*n = 34*	
Clinic	0.6	0.7	3.6	5.2	2.2	3.0	5.3	7.5

[a]Manual maximum + measurements before ligament surgery.

postreconstruction graft failure is not firmly established in the literature. Graft failure has been defined arbitrarily as a displacement difference of greater than 5 mm (17,33,40,41,51). Barber et al. (17) have pointed out that postoperative instability measurements should include not only mean values, but also the distribution of measured values. Bach (33) and Faustgen (18) both reported a greater frequency of symptoms, impairment, and sports disability in patients with manual maximum differences greater than 5 mm after ACL reconstruction.

In the Kaiser 10-year follow-up study (5), both early and follow-up laxity and motion measurements were reported if the patient had not had ligament surgery in the preceding 24 months and had normal contralateral knees. Table 25.2 presents mean side-to-side differences for the 89 N and manual maximum tests at the initial clinical examination, under anesthesia, and at 12-month follow-up for the stable hemarthrosis population (group I), patients with ACL insufficiency who did not undergo ligament reconstruction (group II), the early ACL reconstructed patients (group III), and the patients reconstructed late (group IV). Initial clinical measurements were highly predictive of later test results in patients who had not undergone reconstruction before repeat testing (groups I, II, and IV). Instrumented testing is well tolerated by the conscious patient with an acutely injured knee; therefore, the accuracy of the manual maximum

test was not improved by performing it under anesthesia. Table 25.3 presents the results of instrumented testing at 5-year follow-up. In comparing the surgical groups to nonsurgically treated patients, Table 25.3 presents the distribution of side-to-side differences using 3 mm as the threshold. A significant injured-minus-normal difference (I-N) was noted between group I and other groups ($p < 0.01$) on all tests. There was a difference between group II versus groups III and IV on the manual maximum test ($p < 0.05$). Anterior displacement measurements for both the early and late reconstructed populations increased slightly over time after ligament surgery, but at follow-up was clearly less than the prereconstruction condition ($p < 0.0001$).

Symptoms and Impairment

Previous studies of ACL-injured patients have used a variety of reporting systems combining symptoms, impairments, range of motion, radiologic findings, and patient activity (21,52–57). This requires assigning a relative importance to each item to allow a final score to be calculated. To permit the greatest opportunity to compare the outcome of the patients in our study with other studies, the results of each measurement parameter are presented and no total score or grade was assigned to the patient outcome.

TABLE 25.3. *KT-1000 displacement measurements, millimeters of injured minus normal difference (I - N) follow-up evaluation*

Group	I: Early stable	II: Coper	III: Early reconstruction	IV: Late reconstruction
Patient number	53	134	43	33
Quadriceps active				
Mean	0.4	3.0	2.4	2.4
<3 mm	89%	44%	49%	55%
89 N				
Mean	0.5	2.3	1.7	2.5
<3 mm	93%	55%	63%	61%
134 N				
Mean	0.6	3.1	2.3	2.8
<3 mm	92%	39%	49%	45%
Manual maximum				
Mean	0.7	5.0	3.7	4.3
<3 mm	91%	16%	33%	30%

TABLE 25.4. *Symptoms and impairments final evaluation*

Group	I: Early stable	II: Coper	III: Early reconstruction	IV: Late reconstruction
n	53	139	45	33
Symptoms (%)				
Pain (> mild and infrequent)	11	21	27	24
Swelling	6	18	36	33
Giving way with sports	4	18	20	3
Giving way with ADL	0	9	16	3
Impairments (%)				
Walk	8	6	11	11
Climb	10	24	36	24
Stairs	13	22	24	24
Kneel	21	37	64	64
Squat	19	40	40	55
Run	15	37	33	39
Jump	13	34	33	36
Cut	13	56	42	52

ADL, activities of daily living.

Group I patients had fewer symptoms and impairments than the group II, III, and IV patients (Table 25.4). Late pain and swelling are fairly common among patients who have suffered an ACL injury, and the Kaiser study *did not* indicate that these complaints are less frequent after ligament reconstruction. In addition, low levels of giving way with sports are reported with *similar* frequency in groups II, III, and IV. Swelling and difficulty kneeling were more common in patients who had undergone reconstruction ($p < 0.05$). Eighty-three percent of the patients who had late ligament surgery said they were better after the ligament surgery, none said they were worse.

To put this in perspective, it should be pointed out that while many patients reported pain, for most it was mild and infrequent. Symptoms of pain and swelling were less in group II patients ("copers") than previously reported in chronic ACL patients (14,58–60). Symptoms of giving way were also less than previously reported (14,58,61).

Occupation and Sports

Disability for sports after ACL injury is the principle reason that patients request ligament surgery. Therefore, documenting pre- and postinjury sports activity is an important part of the patient evaluation. A number of systems have been used to document sports activity (24,37,52,54,57,62). The essential elements are sport level, participation level, performance, symptoms during or after participation, and frequency of play or exposure. The International Knee Documentation Committee has divided sports into three levels based on the committee's perception of the risk for injury to the knee when participating in that sport.

In the Kaiser study, sports were documented as hours per year of participation in sports by sports level (Table 25.5). Before injury, 92% of patients played a sport at least 50 hours a year; at follow-up the number was 50%. The average hours of sports participation had decreased from 322 hours a year to 223 hours a year. The patients had discontinued 33 level I or II sports because of the knee injury. Before injury, groups III and IV reported the most hours of sports participation, and group I patients the least (Table 25.5). The hours per year of participation in preinjury sports was reduced in all groups at follow-up. The greatest reductions were among patients who had ligament reconstruction. Much of the sports activity change over the follow-up period was due to changes in lifestyle not related to the knee injury. Brace use for sports by group was I, 2%; II, 14%; III, 11%; and IV, 18%.

In the Hawkins study (58), 90% of the patients with a nonreconstructed knee were still playing sports, but 75% were playing at a decreased level. Andersson (4) reported that 23% of the nonreconstructed patients returned to their former level of sports activity.

TABLE 25.5. *Participation in level I, II, and III sports (hours/year/patient)*

Group	I: Early stable	II: Coper	III: Early reconstruction	IV: Late reconstruction
Age (y)	25	29	24	22
n	53	139	45	33
Preinjury sports				
Pre-injury	306	322	459	523
Follow-up	129	107	110	122
Follow-up (total sports)	217	223	268	281

The return to occupational activity has also been examined. Larkin (63) found no difference in return to work between acute and chronically reconstructed patients, with all patients returning to their previous occupations, including those requiring heavy or very heavy occupational activities. Wexler (64) studied a subset of 22 patients who underwent ACL reconstruction with an associated Workers' Compensation claim and found that outcomes were no different than those for their historical controls. Scores using the Noyes Occupational Factor increased from 48 before surgery to 60 after surgery, although no score was reported for preinjury occupational level. All but two patients were able to return to at least their previous level of work. SF-36 scores were similar to those of the general population, although mental health scores were lower. Noyes (65) compared the results of a cohort of 20 patients undergoing work-related ACL reconstruction with a matched, nonrandomized group of 19 non–work-related patients. No significant difference was found with respect to ligament function, subjective analysis, or overall Cincinnati Knee Rating System score. No significant difference was found between anteroposterior displacements, although no manual maximum data were presented. There was, however, a significant difference with respect to the number of days of lost employment, both before and after surgery. Industrial patients returned to work an average of 222 days after surgery, compared with 37 days for nonindustrial patients. In the Kaiser study, no patient stated that they had changed work because of the knee injury.

Function Testing

Tests used to evaluate knee function have included strength testing (66,67) and the one leg hop-for-distance (66,67). In terms of strength testing, Wyatt (68) reported 89% of normal subjects had a nondominant/dominant quadriceps strength ratio with isokinetic testing at 60° per second of 0.8 and 90% had a hamstring strength ratio of 0.8. The nonreconstructed patients (group II) in the Kaiser study had a mean injured/noninvolved quadriceps ratio of 0.97 and hamstring ratio of 0.98. This was greater than the quadriceps ratio of 0.86 and hamstring ratio of 0.90 reported by Kannus in 41 ACL-deficient knees (67). The group III and IV reconstructed/noninvolved quadriceps ratio of 0.90 and hamstring ratio of 0.93 may be compared with the quadriceps ratio of 0.90 and hamstring ratio of 0.97 previously reported in 24 ACL-reconstructed patients (66).

The one leg hop-for-distance test is a measure of agility, strength, and confidence in the lower extremity. Daniel et al. (69) reported a left/right one-leg-hop-for-distance ratio of 0.9 in 95% of 100 healthy subjects. Barber (17) reported 81% of normal subjects had a hop ratio of 0.9. The 10-year Kaiser study revealed a 0.95 ratio for the group II copers, comparable to 1.0 for group I, 0.92 for group III, and 0.91 for group IV. Prior reports of the involved/noninvolved hop ratio in ACL-deficient patients of 0.9 (55) and 0.82 (17) are less than the mean hop ratio of 0.95 in group II.

Incidence of Late Arthrosis

Previous reports have documented radiographic changes (10,13,14,58,60,70,71) and bone scan changes (72). The Kaiser 10-year fate study was the first to document the results of imaging studies in a large, ACL-injured population prospectively studied. Many patients had mild degenerative changes by radiography and moderate changes by bone scan in the index knee. Some of the changes on radiography and bone scan may be secondary to occult bone lesions sustained at the time of the injury that are diagnosed by MRI in most ACL-injured patients (73). Meniscus surgery correlated with increased degenerative changes, supporting the findings of previous authors (10,11,13,14,37,58,60). The relationship between meniscectomy and osteoarthrosis has been previously documented (74–76).

The Kaiser study was also the first to describe an increased incidence of degenerative joint disease in ACL-reconstructed patients. This may be explained in part by a higher incidence of meniscus surgery in the reconstructed patients. However, a comparison of bone scan scores for patients who did not have meniscus surgery also revealed a greater incidence of arthrosis in the reconstructed patients. Five possible explanations were proposed: (i) greater injury in the reconstructed knees before surgery than in the patients who did not choose reconstruction, (ii) joint injury occurring at the time of surgery, (iii) the joint's response to stress deprivation after surgery (77), (iv) prolonged joint inflammation after surgery (78,79), and (v) abnormal joint mechanics after surgery (79). Casteleyn has proposed that the increased incidence in arthrosis postreconstruction may be related to the increased activity level permitted by the ACL reconstruction. As proposed by Dye (80), activity levels outside the "envelope of function" of the reconstructed knee may lead to loss of joint homeostasis, and ultimately irreversible degenerative changes.

Secondary (Late) Surgery

Surgery performed after the patient has recovered from the index injury is termed late surgery. In the Kaiser study, all surgery more than 90 days after the index injury is termed late surgery. Late surgery may include repeat arthroscopy, debridement, meniscectomy, meniscal repair, or revision ACL reconstruction. Plancher et al. (48) reported on 72 subjects (75 knees) older than 40 years with an average of 55 months follow-up. Thirteen patients (17%) required late surgery, five because of reinjury. The previously reported incidence of late meniscectomy in the ACL-injured knee/years of follow-up are as follows: 16%/12 years (71), 10%/4 years (58), 24%/5 years (81). The incidence in the Kaiser study was 20%/5 years. The reported incidence of late reconstruction in the ACL-injured knee ranges from 25% to 38% (58,81,82). In the Kaiser study, 44 of the 191 KT unstable knees were reconstructed late (23%). Table 25.6 shows that patients who need late surgery generally do so within 24 months of the initial injury (5). Over the 10-year period following ACL rupture, patients with unstable knees who did not have early ligament reconstruction were nearly three and one-half times *more* likely to require late surgery for meniscus injury, ligament stabilization, or salvage than patients who were reconstructed within 90 days of injury (5). In the Kaiser study, seven of the patients had a post-surgical manipulation under anesthesia to restore motion, five of these patients had been reconstructed early and two reconstructed late. A total of 25 surgical procedures were performed after ligament surgery. These procedures included treatment of infection (77), metal removal (83), arthroscopy (70), and a second ACL reconstruction (31). Seven of the patients sustained meniscus tears after an ACL reconstruction. One meniscus tear was repaired and six were excised. Twenty-one patients had a meniscus repair with an ACL reconstruction. There has been no further surgery in 18 patients. One patient had a second meniscus repair with a second reconstruction, and two had the meniscus subsequently excised.

In the Kaiser study a number of factors were associated with the risk for undergoing late surgery had for a meniscus tear or an ACL reconstruction ($p < 0.05$). Stepwise discriminant analysis revealed that the two important variables for predicting late meniscus, ligament, or salvage surgery were: (i) the total preinjury hours per year of sport level I and II participation and (ii) the manual maximum displacement difference at within 3 months after injury. No additional variables improved the ability to predict which patient would have late meniscus or ligament surgery. A guide to the patient's surgical risk factor (SURF) has been proposed based on these two variables, and is outlined in Chapter 20. We currently recommend early reconstruction for patients in the "high" SURF risk category and nonoperative treatment of patients at "low" risk. A prospective, randomized study is now underway to determine the most appropriate treatment of "moderate" risk patients.

PROSPECTIVE COMPARISON STUDIES

Most of the literature on the unoperated, ACL-injured knee and the "natural history" of the ACL-injured knee is retrospective and has analyzed patients with chronic ACL disruptions presenting with knee symptoms (14,84), mixed patient populations presenting with acute or chronic injuries (7), patients with failed ACL repairs (52), and patient populations gleaned from surgical logs (60,61,83) or hospital records (59). The ideal study of patient outcomes would be designed prospectively to identify all patients who sustained their injury within the clinical population considered to be at risk. It would document definitively the presence of the injury and exclude or subcategorize patients with regard to additional injuries (e.g., other ligament injuries, fractures, chondral injuries, and meniscal injuries). Treatments would be randomized within groups at similar levels of risk for poor outcomes, and patients would be followed at regular intervals for a sufficient time until they reached a steady state with respect to late outcomes. No such study has yet been done. Outcomes research in orthopedic surgery remains highly developmental, and clinical instruments are still being evaluated for use in evaluating specific conditions of the knee (25,26).

Four prospective studies of acute ACL rupture have been published with at least 4 years follow-up. Clancy (85) reported a 48-month follow up of 92 patients, Hawkins a 45-month follow-up of 40 patients, and Andersson (4,81) a 58-month follow-up of 59 patients. At the Kaiser Hospital in San Diego, Daniel et al. have pub-

TABLE 25.6. *Review of type and timing of surgery in KT stable and unstable knees*

After injury (mo)	KT grade stable (early phase) n = 56			KT grade unstable (early phase) n = 236		
	Surgical examination	ACL reconstruction	Meniscus surgery	Surgical examination	ACL reconstruction	Meniscus surgery
0–3	18	0	5	190	45	54
9–12	2	0	0	25	15	13
13–24	1	1[a]	1	26	17	14
25–36	0	0	0	12	5	9
37–48	2	0	2	9	3	5
49–60	1	1[b]	1	4	2	2
61–72	1	0	0	6	3	5
73–84	0	0	0	1	1	1

[a]ACL disruption with second injury.
[b]ACL disruption with index injury.

lished a 5-year follow-up study of 292 patients presenting to us with their first acute traumatic hemarthrosis (6), and 266 of these patients were subsequently reevaluated 10 years after the index injury (5). All of these studies fall short of the standards described previously. Nevertheless, there is much they can teach us in predicting patient outcomes, counseling patients, and identifying areas in need of further study.

All of the patients in the Clancy and Andersson studies were surgically evaluated. Clancy treated 92 patients with an acute ACL disruption. He reconstructed 70 patients (those with a "moderate or severe" pivot shift), and treated nonoperatively 22 patients (those with an "absent, trace or mild" pivot shift). Andersson randomized 156 patients into three treatment groups: ACL repair, ACL repair plus augmentation, and associated injury repair without ACL repair, which is the ACL nonoperative population. Fifteen of the non-ACL surgery patients in Andersson's study had acute medial collateral ligament repairs, ten had posterior oblique ligament repairs, and one had an arcuate ligament complex repair. Hawkins did not report on what basis it was decided to treat the 40 ACL-injured patients in his study without ACL reconstructive surgery or what percentage of his ACL-injured patients the nonoperative group represented. Twenty-five of the Hawkins patients were evaluated surgically (58).

The remainder of the patients were not examined surgically as "examination without anesthesia was sufficient for diagnosis in 15 of the patients, all of whom had a positive Lachman test, anterior drawer and pivot shift maneuver."

In the Kaiser study, Daniel et al. identified all patients presenting with an acute posttraumatic knee hemarthrosis who met strict study entry criteria. The incidence of ACL disruption in a patient with an acute traumatic hemarthrosis has been previously reported to range from 62% to 77% (62,86–88). In the Kaiser study, 81% of acute hemarthroses were KT unstable. All patients were examined clinically with the KT-1000 Knee Ligament Arthrometer (MEDMetric, San Diego), and many had diagnostic arthroscopy (6). Patients were grouped according to early phase (within 90 days of knee injury) knee stability measurements and whether they underwent knee ligament reconstruction (Fig. 25.1). The patients with a stable knee and hemarthrosis were presumed to have a normal ACL or partial tear of the ACL. This population was included because follow-up studies had not previously been reported for this population and they served as a comparison group to the unstable ACL-injured knees.

The Kaiser Study, like those of Clancy and Hawkins, was not randomized. The study was designed prospec-

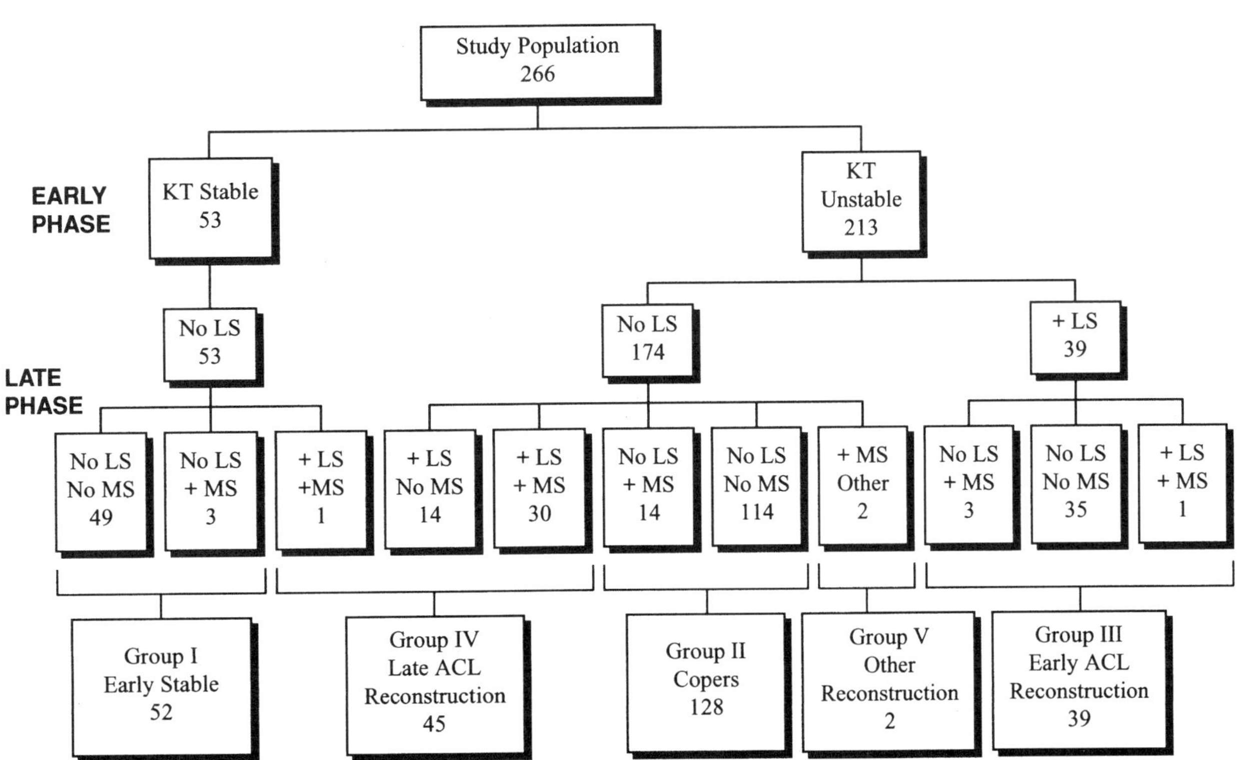

FIGURE 25.1. Flow chart depicting the makeup of study groups in the Kaiser study.

tively as an observational study to document outcomes rather than to specifically test hypotheses comparing different methods of treatment. The patients were not randomized into treatment groups, but selected their own treatment program. The treatment groups therefore were undoubtedly different in a number of ways, which may lead to bias against favorable outcomes in some of the groups, or for more favorable outcomes in others. Surgical technique and postoperative rehabilitation have changed markedly in the past 10 years. All this must be borne in mind as the results are interpreted. Despite these limitations, it is instructive to compare the outcomes of the stable hemarthrosis population (group I), patients with ACL insufficiency who did not undergo ligament reconstruction (group II), the early ACL reconstructed patients (group III), and the patients reconstructed late (group IV).

The only prospective studies that compare the outcome of a reconstructed group of patients with a nonoperative group of patients are those by Andersson (4), Clancy (85), and the Kaiser study (6). In the Andersson study, the level of activity was higher in the reconstructed patients, although the mean knee score was not significantly different. In the Clancy study, 44% of the nonreconstructed patients had a good or excellent result versus 97% with an ACL reconstruction. In the Kaiser study, 83% of the patients who had late ACL reconstructive surgery stated they were improved by the ligament surgery, and in most their hours of sports participation increased over their ACL-disrupted condition. The follow-up evaluation in the Kaiser study revealed the symptoms of giving way, swelling, and pain were *not* different between the nonreconstructed and reconstructed groups. The impairment inventory was *not* different between the two groups with the exception that the reconstructed patients had more trouble kneeling. The postinjury sports participation was *similar* for the two groups of patients at 10 years average follow-up.

The Kaiser 5-year study was the first published report examining the direct effects of ligament surgery on degenerative arthritis. The follow-up evaluation included radiographs (30° standing posteroanterior, 30° lateral, and tunnel views) and bone scans of both knees. A disturbing finding in the Kaiser study was a small but increased incidence of degenerative joint disease in the reconstructed patients, compared with the patient treated without ACL surgery, which could not be entirely explained by a higher incidence of meniscus injury in the ACL-reconstructed patients before their reconstruction. Figure 25.2 demonstrates the 5- and 10-year radiographic scores by groups. As documented by the Kaiser study, the level of arthrosis is mild if the menisci remain intact. ACL surgery does indeed protect the meniscus and thereby spares the knee from the arthritis that develops after meniscectomy. DeHaven has reported the incidence of meniscus tears after meniscus repair is higher in the ACL-disrupted knee than the ACL-reconstructed knee (89). However, at this time there is no evidence to support the thesis that ACL reconstructive surgery prevents arthritis in the ACL-injured knee that has undergone meniscectomy.

The Kaiser study documented that ACL surgery decreased the measured joint instability. Both the Andersson and the Kaiser study showed a higher incidence of late meniscus tears in the ACL-disrupted knee versus the ACL-reconstructed knee. Because it has proven useful for assessing a patient's risk for late meniscal or ligament surgery, we strongly recommend routine use of instrumented testing in the evaluation and management of patients with acutely injured knees. Determination of an individual's SURF risk level provides valuable information for the physician counseling a patient following knee injury. For the patient presenting with a primary knee injury and ACL insufficiency as determined by the KT-1000 manual maximum test, we view ACL reconstruction as a prophylactic measure in patients who are considered at risk for reinjury and subsequent meniscus or ligament surgery.

Other prospective comparative studies have been done to compare the results of different operative techniques

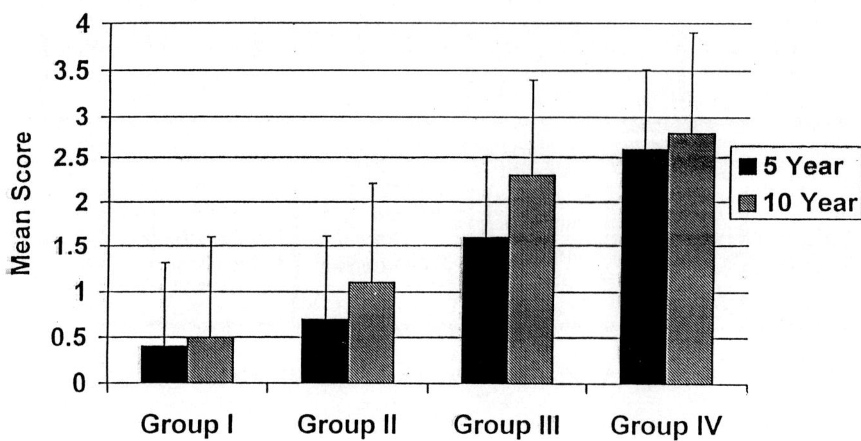

FIGURE 25.2. Radiographic scores at 5- and 10-year follow-up.

without comparing those results to nonoperated controls. Marder et al. (90) performed a prospective, randomized study comparing two-incision hamstring and patellar tendon techniques. A total of 72 patients was evaluated at a mean 29-month follow-up. No significant difference was found between groups with respect to Zarins-Rowe score, return to activity, or manual or instrumented laxity testing. KT-1000 results were only reported at 20-pound load, however. Isokinetic testing did reveal a difference with hamstring peak torque approximately 10% greater in the patellar tendon group. Two revision cases were included in the study, both in the patellar tendon group.

O'Neill et al. (43) studied 125 patients in a prospective, randomized study with mean 42-month follow-up. The authors compared the results of ACL reconstruction using two-incision hamstring (group I), two-incision patella tendon (group II), and endoscopic patella tendon (group III). Evaluation of patient outcomes included comparisons of return to athletic activity, graft failure, KT-2000 arthrometry, muscle strength testing, and single leg hop. Lysholm and Gillquist and International Knee Documentation Committee (IKDC) scores were also reported. A Lysholm score of at least 90 was achieved by roughly 90% of patients in each group, with no statistical difference among groups. Similarly, IKDC ratings were nearly 90% A or B in groups I and II, and 96% in group III, again not statistically significant. Single leg hop was also at least 90% of the uninvolved contralateral limb in approximately 90% of patients in all groups with no statistical difference noted. Group II showed the least laxity by KT-2000, with manual maximum difference of 3 mm or less in 93% of patients, compared with 83% and 87% in groups I and III, respectively. The mean follow-up was 42 months. Revision ACL cases were not excluded, although the authors did not state the distribution of revision cases among the three groups.

Harner et al. (42) reported on 50 patients studied prospectively, 24 of whom underwent two-incision patellar tendon reconstruction and 26 of whom underwent endoscopic reconstruction. They were evaluated at 35- and 29-month follow-up, respectively. The groups were not randomized, but rather comprised two consecutive series of patients. Only patients with chronic, isolated ACL tears were studied, with both allograft and autograft cases included. Sixty-seven percent of the two-incision group and 60% of the endoscopic group were able to return to the same or higher level of sports activity. Ninety-six percent of the two-incision group and 97% of the endoscopic group showed a KT-1000 manual-maximum difference of five or less. IKDC ratings were normal or nearly normal in 58% of patients in the two-incision group and 81% of patients in the endoscopic group.

Victor et al. (91) studied 73 patients in a prospective study with 2-year follow-up to compare the results of ACL reconstruction using patellar tendon autograft versus allograft. The study was not randomized; choice of technique was based on availability of allograft donor tissue. No statistically significant difference was found with respect to KT-1000 arthrometry, but only 20-pound force data were reported, and no side-to-side data were provided. Autograft patients had a mean Lysholm score of 92.6, and a Tegner score of 4.75, whereas allograft patients scored 85.4 and 4.41, respectively. No statistical difference was found.

AREAS FOR FUTURE RESEARCH

A great deal of literature exists examining the outcomes following ACL surgery, but the results on which we base our recommendations for surgery remain fragmented. Although reported results are quite good overall, the absence of a uniform standard for the reporting of results makes comparisons difficult, and the number of available long-term, prospective, randomized studies remains lacking. Variables such as surgical technique, graft choice, and rehabilitation protocols must also be accounted for when evaluating study data. All of these factors make it difficult to formulate a treatment plan for the patient with ACL insufficiency that is based on rigorous, scientific evidence. Further research will be necessary before we are able to demonstrate clearly to what degree ACL surgery improves on the natural history of the injury, and to identify in advance those patients who are most likely to benefit from surgical intervention.

REFERENCES

1. Wojtys EM. The ACL deficient knee. In: *American Academy of Orthopaedic Surgeons monograph series*. Rosemont, IL: AAOS, 1994.
2. Daniel DM, Teitge RA, Grand WA, et al. Knee and leg: soft-tissue trauma. In: Frumoyer JW, ed. *Orthopaedic knowledge update*. Rosemont, IL: AAOS, 1990:55–59.
3. Mohtadi N. Quality of life assessment as an outcome on anterior cruciate ligament reconstructive surgery. In: Jackson DW, ed. *The anterior cruciate ligament. Current and future concepts*. New York: Raven Press, 1993:439–444.
4. Andersson C, Odensten M., Gillquist J. Knee function after surgical or nonsurgical treatment of acute rupture of the anterior cruciate ligament: a randomized study with a long-term follow-up period. *Clin Orthop* 1991;264:255–263.
5. Daniel DM, Fithian DC, Stone ML, et al. A ten-year prospective outcome study of the ACL-injured patient. In: *63rd annual meeting, AAOS*. Atlanta, 1996.
6. Daniel DM, Stone ML, Dobson BE, et al. Fate of the ACL-injured patient. A prospective outcome study [see comments]. *Am J Sports Med* 1994;22:632–644.
7. Butler DL, Noyes FR, Grood ES. Ligamentous restraints to anterior-posterior drawer in the human knee. A biomechanical study. *J Bone Joint Surg Am* 1980;62:259–270.
8. Hirshman HP, Daniel DM, Miyasaka K. The fate of unoperated knee ligament injuries. In: Daniel DM, Akeson WH, O'Connor JJ, eds. *Knee ligaments: structure, function, injury and repair*. New York: Raven Press, 1991:481–503.
9. Jacobsen K. Osteoarthrosis following insufficiency of the cruciate ligaments in man: a clinical study. *Acta Orthop Scand* 1977;48:520–526.
10. Satku K, Kumar VP, Ngoi SS. Anterior cruciate ligament injuries. To counsel or to operate? *J Bone Joint Surg Br* 1986;68:458–461.
11. Sherman MF, Warren RF, Marshall JL, et al. A clinical and radiographical analysis of 127 anterior cruciate insufficient knees. *Clin Orthop* 1988;227:229–237.

12. Fowler PJ, Regan WD. The patient with symptomatic chronic anterior cruciate ligament insufficiency. Results of minimal arthroscopic surgery and rehabilitation. *Am J Sports Med* 1987;15:321–325.

13. Miller SJ, Kent BE, Sanford TL, et al. Non-operative treatment of the torn anterior cruciate ligament. *J Bone Joint Surg Am* 1983;65:184–192.

14. Noyes FR, Mooar PA, Matthews DS, et al. The symptomatic anterior cruciate-deficient knee, Part I: the long-term functional disability in athletically active individuals. *J Bone Joint Surg Am* 1983;65:154–162.

15. Wallace MP, Howell SM, Hull ML. In vivo tensile behavior of a four-bundle hamstring graft as a replacement for the anterior cruciate ligament. *J Orthop Res* 1997;15:539–545.

16. Bach BR Jr, Jones GT, Sweet FA, et al. Arthroscopy-assisted anterior cruciate ligament reconstruction using patellar tendon substitution. Two- to four-year follow-up results. *Am J Sports Med* 1994;22:758–767.

17. Barber-Westin SD, Noyes FR. The effect of rehabilitation and return to activity on anterior-posterior knee displacements after anterior cruciate ligament reconstruction. *Am J Sports Med* 1993;21:264–270.

18. Faustgen J, Lane J, Stone ML, et al. Functional recovery after patella tendon ACL surgery: the effect of early mobilization. In: *62nd annual meeting, AAOS*, Orlando, 1994.

19. Sgaglione NA, Warren RF, Wickiewicz TL, et al. Primary repair with semitendinosus tendon augmentation of acute anterior cruciate ligament injuries. *Am J Sports Med* 1990;18:64–73.

20. Hefti F, Muller W. [Current state of evaluation of knee ligament lesions. The new IKDC knee evaluation form]. *Orthopade* 1993;22:351–362.

21. Lysholm J, Gillquist J. Evaluation of knee ligament surgery results with special emphasis on use of a scoring scale. *Am J Sports Med* 1982;10:150–154.

22. Marshall JL, Fetto JF, Botero PM. Knee ligament injuries: a standardized evaluation method. *Clin Orthop* 1977;123:115–129.

23. Noyes FR, McGinniss GH, Mooar LA. Functional disability in the anterior cruciate insufficient knee syndrome. Review of knee rating systems and projected risk factors in determining treatment. *Sports Med* 1984;1:278–302.

24. Tegner Y, Lysholm J. Rating systems in the evaluation of knee ligament injuries. *Clin Orthop* 1985;198:43–49.

25. Shapiro ET, Richmond JC, Rockett SE, et al. The use of a generic, patient-based health assessment (SF-36) for evaluation of patients with anterior cruciate ligament injuries. *Am J Sports Med* 1996;24:196–200.

26. Mohtadi N. Development and validation of the quality of life outcome measure (questionnaire) for chronic anterior cruciate ligament deficiency. *Am J Sports Med* 1998;26:350–359.

27. Keller RB, Hoover H. Quality improvement foundations. A professional challenge instructional course lecture. In: *Outcomes and effectiveness in musculoskeletal research and practice*. San Diego: AAOS, 1995.

28. Rudicel S. Sports injury research. How to avoid bias. *Am J Sports Med* 1988;16(suppl 1):S48–S52.

29. Daniel DM, Woodward EP, Losse GM, et al. The Marshall/Macintosh anterior cruciate ligament reconstruction with the Kennedy ligament augmentation device: report of the United States clinical trials. In: Friedman MJ, Ferkel RD, eds. *Prosthetic ligament reconstruction of the knee*. Philadelphia: WB Saunders, 1988:71–78.

30. Feagin JA Jr, Cabaud HE, Curl WW. The anterior cruciate ligament: radiographic and clinical signs of successful and unsuccessful repairs. *Clin Orthop* 1982;164:54–58.

31. Anderson AF, Lipscomb AB. Preoperative instrumented testing of anterior and posterior knee laxity. *Am J Sports Med* 1989;17:387–392.

32. Bach BR Jr, Jones GT, Hager CA, et al. Arthrometric results of arthroscopically assisted anterior cruciate ligament reconstruction using autograft patellar tendon substitution. *Am J Sports Med* 1995;23:179–185.

33. Bach BR Jr, Warren RF, Flynn WM, et al. Arthrometric evaluation of knees that have a torn anterior cruciate ligament. *J Bone Joint Surg Am* 1990;72:1299–1306.

34. Dahlstedt LJ, Dalen N. Knee laxity in cruciate ligament injury. Value of examination under anesthesia. *Acta Orthop Scand* 1989;60:181–184.

35. Franklin JL, Rosenberg TD, Paulos LE, et al. Radiographic assessment of instability of the knee due to rupture of the anterior cruciate ligament. A quadriceps-contraction technique [see comments]. *J Bone Joint Surg Am* 1991;73:365–372.

36. Sommerlath K. Instrumented testing of sagittal knee laxity in stable and unstable knees. *Am J Knee Surg* 1991;4:70–78.

37. Steiner ME, Brown C, Zarins B, et al. Measurement of anterior-posterior displacement of the knee. A comparison of the results with instrumented devices and with clinical examination. *J Bone Joint Surg Am* 1990;72:1307–1315.

38. Wroble RR, Van Ginkel LA, Grood ES, et al. Repeatability of the KT-1000 arthrometer in a normal population. *Am J Sports Med* 1990;18:396–399.

39. Daniel DM, Stone ML. KT-1000 anterior-posterior displacement measurements. In: Daniel DM, Akeson WH, O'Connor JJ, eds. *Knee ligaments: structure, function, injury, and repair*. New York: Raven Press, 1990:427–444.

40. Buss DD, Warren RF, Wickiewicz TL, et al. Arthroscopically assisted reconstruction of the anterior cruciate ligament with use of autogenous patellar-ligament grafts. Results after twenty-four to forty-two months. *J Bone Joint Surg Am* 1993;75:1346–1355.

41. Faustgen JP, Daniel DM, Stone ML, et al. Impairment in post ACL reconstructed patients versus measured postoperative laxity. In: *62nd annual meeting, AAOS*. Orlando, 1994.

42. Harner CD, Marks PH, Fu FH, et al. Anterior cruciate ligament reconstruction: endoscopic versus two-incision technique [see comments]. *Arthroscopy* 1994;10:502–512.

43. O'Neill DB. Arthroscopically assisted reconstruction of the anterior cruciate ligament. A prospective randomized analysis of three techniques. *J Bone Joint Surg Am* 1996;78:803–813.

44. Stringham DR, Pelmas CJ, Burks RT, et al. Comparison of anterior cruciate ligament reconstructions using patellar tendon autograft or allograft. *Arthroscopy* 1996;12:414–421.

45. Sgaglione NA, Schwartz RE. Arthroscopically assisted reconstruction of the anterior cruciate ligament: initial clinical experience and minimal 2-year follow-up comparing endoscopic transtibial and two-incision techniques. *Arthroscopy* 1997;13:156–165.

46. Feagin JA Jr, Wills RP, Lambert KL, et al. Anterior cruciate ligament reconstruction. Bone-patella tendon-bone versus semitendinosus anatomic reconstruction. *Clin Orthop* 1997;(341):69–72.

47. Bach BR Jr, Tradonsky S, Bojchuk J, et al. Arthroscopically assisted anterior cruciate ligament reconstruction using patellar tendon autograft. Five- to nine-year follow-up evaluation. *Am J Sports Med* 1998;26:20–29.

48. Plancher KD, Steadman JR, Briggs KK, et al. Reconstruction of the anterior cruciate ligament in patients who are at least forty years old. A long-term follow-up and outcome study. *J Bone Joint Surg Am* 1998;80:184–197.

49. Howell SM, Deutsch ML. Comparison of endoscopic and two-incision techniques for reconstructing a torn anterior cruciate ligament using hamstring tendons. *Arthroscopy* 1999;15:594–606.

50. Patel JV, Church JS, Hall AJ. Central third bone-patellar tendon-bone anterior cruciate ligament reconstruction: a 5-year follow-up. *Arthroscopy* 2000;16:67–70.

51. O'Brien SJ, Warren RF, Pavlov H, et al. Reconstruction of the chronically insufficient anterior cruciate ligament with the central third of the patellar ligament. *J Bone Joint Surg Am* 1991;73:278–286.

52. Feagin JA Jr, Blake WP. Postoperative evaluation and result recording in the anterior cruciate ligament reconstructed knee. *Clin Orthop* 1983;172:143–147.

53. Noyes FR, Barber SD. The effect of an extra-articular procedure on allograft reconstructions for chronic ruptures of the anterior cruciate ligament. *J Bone Joint Surg Am* 1991;73:882–892.

54. Straub T, Hunter RE. Acute anterior cruciate ligament repair. *Clin Orthop* 1988;227:238–250.

55. Tegner Y, Lysholm J, Lysholm M, et al. A performance test to monitor rehabilitation and evaluate anterior cruciate ligament injuries. *Am J Sports Med* 1986;14:156–159.

56. Windsor R, Insall J, Warren RF, et al. The hospital for special surgery knee ligament rating form. *Am J Knee Surg* 1988;1:140–145.

57. Zarins B, Rowe CR. Combined anterior cruciate-ligament reconstruction using semitendinosus tendon and iliotibial tract. *J Bone Joint Surg Am* 1986;68:160–177.

58. Hawkins RJ, Misamore GW, Merritt TR. Followup of the acute nonoperated isolated anterior cruciate ligament tear. *Am J Sports Med* 1986;14:205–210.

59. Kannus P, Jarvinen M. Conservatively treated tears of the anterior cruciate ligament. Long-term results. *J Bone Joint Surg Am* 1987;69:1007–1012.

60. McDaniel WJ Jr, Dameron TB Jr. Untreated ruptures of the anterior

cruciate ligament. A follow-up study. *J Bone Joint Surg Am* 1980;62: 696–705.

61. Pattee GA, Fox JM, Del Pizzo W, et al. Four to ten year followup of unreconstructed anterior cruciate ligament tears. *Am J Sports Med* 1989;17:430–435.

62. Noyes FR, Barber SD, Mooar LA. A rationale for assessing sports activity levels and limitations in knee disorders. *Clin Orthop* 1989;246: 238–249.

63. Larkin JJ, Barber-Westin SD. The effect of injury chronicity and progressive rehabilitation on single-incision arthroscopic anterior cruciate ligament reconstruction. *Arthroscopy* 1998;14:15–22.

64. Wexler G, Bach BR Jr, Bush-Joseph CA, et al. Outcomes of anterior cruciate ligament reconstruction in patients with workers' compensation claims. *Arthroscopy* 2000;16:49–58.

65. Noyes FR, Barber-Westin SD. A comparison of results of arthroscopic-assisted anterior cruciate ligament reconstruction between workers' compensation and noncompensation patients. *Arthroscopy* 1997;13: 474–484.

66. Harter RA, Osternig LR, Standifer LW. Isokinetic evaluation of quadriceps and hamstrings symmetry following anterior cruciate ligament reconstruction [see comments]. *Arch Phys Med Rehabil* 1990;71: 465–468.

67. Kannus P. Ratio of hamstring to quadriceps femoris muscles' strength in the anterior cruciate ligament insufficient knee. Relationship to long-term recovery. *Phys Ther* 1988;68:961–965.

68. Wyatt M, Edwardo A. Comparison of quadriceps and hamstring torque values during isokinetic exercise. *J Orthop Sports Phys Ther* 1981;3: 48–56.

69. Daniel DM, Stone ML, Riehl B, et al. A measurement of lower limb function. The one-leg-hop-for-distance. *Am J Knee Surg* 1988;1: 212–214.

70. Chick RR, Jackson DW. Tears of the anterior cruciate ligament in young athletes. *J Bone Joint Surg Am* 1978;60:970–973.

71. Sommerlath K, Lysholm J, Gillquist J. The long-term course after treatment of acute anterior cruciate ligament ruptures. A 9 to 16 year followup. *Am J Sports Med* 1991;19:56–62.

72. Dorchak JD, Barrack RL, Alexander AH, et al. Radionuclide imaging of the knee with chronic anterior cruciate ligament tear. *Orthop Rev* 1993;22:1233–1241.

73. Rosen MA, Jackson DW, Berger PE. Occult osseous lesions documented by magnetic resonance imaging associated with anterior cruciate ligament ruptures. *Arthroscopy* 1991;7:45–51.

74. Fairbank TJ. Knee joint changes after meniscectomy. *J Bone Joint Surg Br* 1948;30:664–670.

75. Johnson RJ, Kettelkamp DB, Clark W, et al. Factors effecting late results after meniscectomy. *J Bone Joint Surg Am* 1974;56:719–729.

76. Tapper EM, Hoover NW. Late results after meniscectomy. *J Bone Joint Surg Am* 1969;51:517–526.

77. Akeson WH. The response of ligaments to stress modulation and overview of the ligament healing response. In: Daniel DM, Akeson WH, O'Connor JJ, eds. *Knee ligaments: structure, function, injury and repair.* New York: Raven Press, 1990:315–327.

78. Amiel D, Kuiper S. Experimental studies on anterior cruciate ligament grafts: histology and biochemistry. In: Daniel DM, Akeson WH, O'Connor JJ, eds. *Knee ligaments: structure, function, injury and repair.* New York: Raven Press, 1990:379–388.

79. Sachs RA, Reznik A, Daniel DM, et al. Complications of knee ligament surgery. In: Daniel DM, Akeson WH, O'Connor JJ, eds. *Knee ligaments: structure, function, injury and repair.* New York: Raven Press, 1990:505–520.

80. Dye SF. The knee as a biologic transmission with an envelope of function: a theory. *Clin Orthop* 1996;(325):10–18.

81. Andersson C, Odensten M, Good L, et al. Surgical or non-surgical treatment of acute rupture of the anterior cruciate ligament. A randomized study with long-term follow-up. *J Bone Joint Surg Am* 1989;71: 965–974.

82. Engebretsen L, Tegnander A. Short-term results of the nonoperated isolated anterior cruciate ligament tear. *J Orthop Trauma* 1990;4:406–410.

83. Arnold JA, Coker TP, Heaton LM, et al. Natural history of anterior cruciate tears. *Am J Sports Med* 1979;7:305–313.

84. Funk FJ Jr. Osteoarthritis of the knee following ligamentous injury. *Clin Orthop* 1983;172:154–157.

85. Clancy WG Jr, Ray JM, Zoltan DJ. Acute tears of the anterior cruciate ligament. Surgical versus conservative treatment. *J Bone Joint Surg Am* 1988;70:1483–1488.

86. Butler JC, Andrews JR. The role of arthroscopic surgery in the evaluation of acute traumatic hemarthrosis of the knee. *Clin Orthop* 1988; 228:150–152.

87. DeHaven KE. Decision-making in acute anterior cruciate ligament injury. *Instr Course Lect* 1987;36:201–203.

88. Hardaker WT Jr, Garrett WE Jr, Bassett FH. Evaluation of acute traumatic hemarthrosis of the knee joint. *South Med J* 1990;83: 640–644.

89. DeHaven KE. Meniscus repair in the athlete. *Clin Orthop* 1985;198: 31–35.

90. Marder RA, Raskind JR, Carroll M. Prospective evaluation of arthroscopically assisted anterior cruciate ligament reconstruction. Patellar tendon versus semitendinosus and gracilis tendons. *Am J Sports Med* 1991;19:478–484.

91. Victor J, Bellemans J, Witvrouw E, et al. Graft selection in anterior cruciate ligament reconstruction—prospective analysis of patellar tendon autografts compared with allografts. *Int Orthop* 1997;21:93–97.

Special Clinical Issues

CHAPTER 26

Surgical Decisions and Treatment Alternatives

Meniscal Tears, Malalignment, Chondral Injury, and Chronic Arthrosis

James P. Tasto, Steven Tradonsky, Brad S. Cohen, and Timothy J. Hunt

In this chapter, we describe the current treatment modalities for meniscal and chondral injuries and provide a comprehensive review of the literature, treatment regimens, indications, and contraindications for the treatment of chronic arthrosis. Specifics of newer methods of chondrocyte and osteochondral transplantation are addressed, and we have included a section on the role of alignment in the treatment of ligamentous and chondral injuries of the knee.

MENISCAL TEARS

History

The first documented meniscal repair was performed in 1883 by Thomas Annandale (1). The treatment of meniscal tears in the late 1800s consisted of closed manipulation followed by cast immobilization. If this treatment method failed, meniscal excision was performed. In 1909, Jones (2) advocated complete meniscectomy if painful episodes recurred after an attempt at reduction of the meniscal tear. In 1936, King (3) performed canine experiments addressing the natural history of a torn meniscus. He performed various degrees of partial and total meniscectomies and found that articular cartilage degeneration was in direct proportion to the amount of meniscus excised. In a subsequent experiment, he found that tears that communicated with the peripheral synovium were likely to heal, whereas those within the substance of the meniscus were unlikely to heal (4).

Because total meniscectomy was the treatment of choice, there was a paucity of long-term data to support

this method. Most reports focused on short-term results, which were satisfactory in most cases. In 1948, Fairbank compared the preoperative and postoperative radiographs of patients between 7 months and 14 years after meniscectomy (5). It was in this report that the classic changes of osteoarthritis were described. Changes included osteophyte formation, joint space narrowing, and flattening of the femoral condyle in the involved compartment. In 1975, Cox et al. (6) reported that partial meniscectomy resulted in less severe degenerative changes than total excision of the meniscus. As a result of these investigations, it was determined that total meniscectomy was not a benign procedure and that orthopedic surgeons should concentrate on meniscal preservation when possible.

Biomechanics

The meniscus serves several important functions within the knee joint, including load transmission, shock absorption, stability, joint lubrication, and possibly proprioception. The menisci also improve the congruity of the articulating surfaces and increase the surface area of joint contact, aiding in load transmission (7).

The knee bends 2 to 4 million times per year, and the forces across the femoral-tibial articulation are two to four times body weight. Between 50% and 100% of the load transmitted through the knee is transmitted through the menisci, depending on the position of the knee. With the knee in extension, 50% of the compressive load is transmitted through the menisci, and 85% of the load is transmitted through the menisci with the knee in 90° of flexion (8). Analyses of compressive loads across the menisci show that the medial meniscus transmits 40% to 50% of the load in the medial compartment, whereas the lateral meniscus may transmit as much as 65% to 75% of the load on the lateral side (9). Several studies have shown that the ability of the joint to transmit load is reduced by removal of all or part of the menisci. Medial meniscectomy reduces the contact area by 50% to 70%, which significantly increases load per unit area and results in articular cartilage damage and degeneration (8). Contact stress, which is a function of force per unit area, has been shown to increase by a factor of two- to fourfold (10).

Johnson and Pope (11) demonstrated that the menisci absorb energy by undergoing elongation as load is placed on the knee joint. As the joint compresses, the menisci extrude peripherally, and the circumferentially oriented collagen fibers elongate. The menisci absorb the greatest amount of energy at low loading rates, but even at more rapid rates, the shock-absorption characteristics probably contribute significantly (10). The shock-absorption capacity of the normal knee is reduced 20% by a meniscectomy (12).

Levy et al. (13) compared the stabilizing effects of the medial and lateral menisci in the intact knee and in the anterior cruciate ligament (ACL)–deficient knee. A significant increase in anteroposterior translation occurred in the ACL-deficient knee after excising the medial meniscus. They concluded that the medial meniscus is a secondary stabilizer of the knee and that it is therefore subjected to shear forces in the ACL-deficient knee (14). The lateral meniscus has been shown to be much more mobile, and it is less likely to sustain shear forces than the medial meniscus.

The menisci contribute to joint lubrication by spreading a film of nutrient synovial fluid over the articular surfaces and reducing the space available in which fluid can pool (15). After meniscectomy, the coefficient of friction increases by 20% (16).

Structure

The mean composition of the adult meniscus is 75% collagen, 8% to 13% noncollagenous protein, and 1% hexosamine (17). Ninety percent of meniscal cartilage is type I, distinguishing it from articular cartilage, which is predominantly type II (18). The collagen fibers are primarily oriented circumferentially, allowing the menisci to resist elongation as hoops resist expansion of a barrel (11). These stresses within the meniscus have been called *hoop stresses*. Some fibers are oriented radially and act as ties within the meniscus, preventing longitudinal splitting from compression forces (15). The arrangement of collagen fibers allows the translation of vertical compressive loads in the knee joint to circumferential stresses (19).

Meniscal Circulation and Biology of Healing

The blood supply to the menisci originates from the superior and inferior branches of the medial and lateral geniculate arteries. Branches from these vessels form a perimeniscal capillary plexus in the capsular and synovial attachments of the meniscus. Arnoczky and Warren (20) demonstrated that the perimeniscal capillary plexus penetrates the peripheral 10% to 30% of the medial meniscus and 10% to 25% of the lateral meniscus (Fig. 26.1). King showed that tears in the peripheral portion of the meniscus healed, whereas more central tears had little healing potential. Arnoczky and Warren (21) characterized the healing response of the meniscus in a dog model.

Two pathways, extrinsic and intrinsic, may result in meniscal healing. The extrinsic mechanism is activated when the meniscus is injured. Injury to the meniscus results in formation of a fibrin clot that acts as a scaffold for vascular ingrowth and the attraction of undifferentiated mesenchymal cells and nutrients that are necessary to accomplish healing. A fibrovascular scar is formed by 10 weeks, and remodeling of the region will occur over the ensuing several months. In the free margin of the meniscus, where the vascular supply is limited, the healing response is limited.

The intrinsic pathway requires unlocking of the meniscal fibrochondrocytes to produce a healing response. If the cells are provided with the appropriate environment, they can proliferate and synthesize the matrix required to produce a reparative response (22). It is thought that fibrin clot acts as a scaffold in addition to providing the mitogenic and chemotactic factors necessary to provide a healing response.

The more centrally a tear is located within the meniscus, the less likely it is to heal. In these central tears, stimulation of the healing process is required (Fig. 26.2). Red-red lesions (i.e., vascular tissue on both sides of the

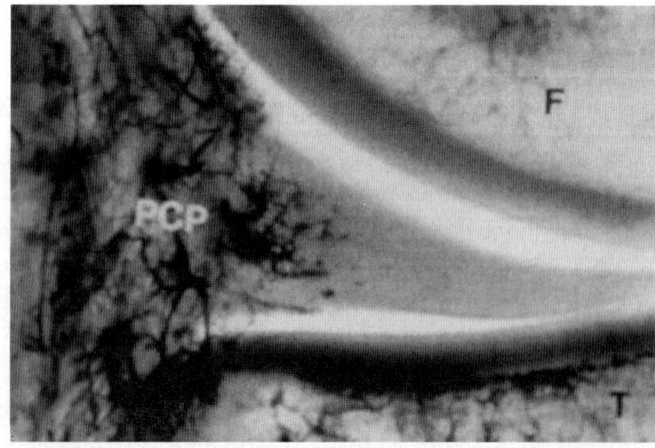

FIGURE 26.1. The perimeniscal capillary plexus *(PCP)* penetrates the peripheral 10% to 30% of the meniscus. F, femur; T, tibia. (From Arnoczky SP, Warren RF. Microvasculature of the human meniscus. *Am J Sports Med* 1982;10:90–95, with permission.)

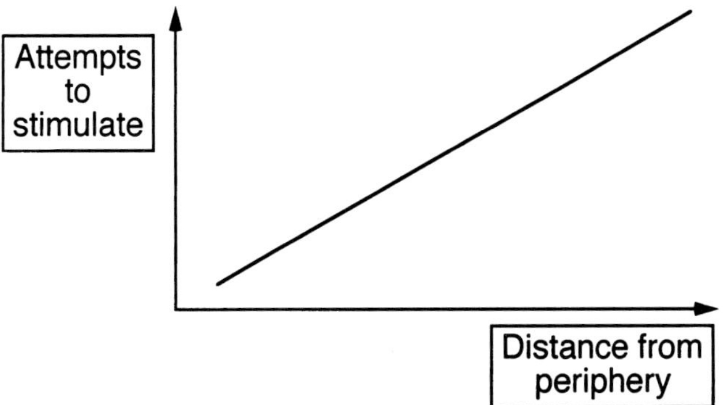

FIGURE 26.2. The farther a tear is from the vascular periphery, the more must be added to the system (e.g., synovial abrasion, fibrin clot) to stimulate the healing process.

repair) and red-white lesions (i.e., vascular tissue on the capsular side and avascular tissue on the free margin side) tend to heal more readily when adequate stabilization is obtained. White-white lesions (i.e., avascular tissue on both sides) are much less likely to heal without stimulation such as synovial abrasion or the addition of a fibrin clot.

Classification of Meniscal Tears

Meniscal tears are described by appearance and location. Cooper et al. (23) devised a classification system for the location of meniscal tears. The menisci have been divided into three radial zones and four circumferential zones (Fig. 26.3). Tears are also described according to the plane of the tear relative to the tibial plateau (Fig.

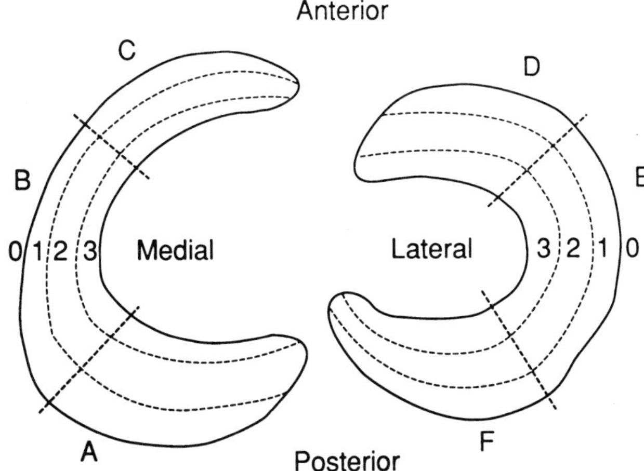

FIGURE 26.3. Zone classification of the meniscus. The most anterior zone of the lateral meniscus is *D*. Zero is the meniscosynovial junction, 1 is the outer third, 2 is the middle third, and 3 is the inner third of each meniscus. (Adapted from Cooper DE, Arnoczky SP, Warren RF. Arthroscopic meniscal repair. *Clin Sports Med* 1990;9:589–607, with permission.)

26.4). Vertical tears are perpendicular to the plateau, and horizontal tears are parallel to the plateau. Radial tears are vertical tears that travel from the free edge of the meniscus toward the meniscosynovial junction. Longitudinal tears propagate in a circumferential manner in an anteroposterior direction. Vertical tears may be partial or full thickness. Complex tears comprise two or more tear patterns and are described as such. Certain tear patterns have been given descriptive terms such as bucket-handle or parrot-beak tears.

Repair

Indications for Repair or Excision

The decision to repair or excise a specific meniscal lesion is simplified by separation of lesions into those that are reparable and those that may be reparable. Reparable tears tend to be traumatic in nature, are within the vascular zone, and have no damage to the meniscal body. Tears longer than 1 cm that are oriented in a vertical-longitudinal direction and located in the periphery of the meniscus fall into the reparable category (24). Meniscal tears in the avascular region have a lower potential for healing and require enhancement to stimulate healing. These techniques include rasping the femoral and tibial surfaces of the synovium and possible placement of a fibrin clot. Damage to the meniscal body is a contraindication to repair because there is no evidence for return of the normal biomechanical properties to the meniscal tissue (24).

The average age of the patient undergoing meniscal repair is 21 years (range, 12 to 42 years) (25). Eighty percent of patients with reparable menisci have a concurrent acute or chronic ACL tear. Patient age is relevant only because older patients are more willing to adjust their lifestyle. However, patients younger than 50 years of age should be considered candidates for repair. Cannon and Vittori (26) showed that meniscal repairs in patients older than 30 have higher healing rates than in those younger than 30 years.

Tears in the red-red and red-white zones have excellent healing potential (26). It can sometimes be difficult, however, to determine the vascularity of the tear. If bleeding is not seen, a tear located within 3 mm of the periphery can be presumed to lie within the vascular region of the meniscus. Tears more than 5 mm from the periphery are in the avascular zone and have poor healing potential. The 3- to 5-mm range has a variable vascular pattern, and tears in this region have an intermediate prognosis (27).

Regardless of ACL status, vertical-longitudinal tears measuring less than 1 cm that cannot be displaced more than 3 mm, radial tears less than 5 mm, and simple horizontal cleavage tears are stable and do not require repair. All vertical-longitudinal and displaced bucket-handle tears in an ACL-deficient knee should be repaired, as

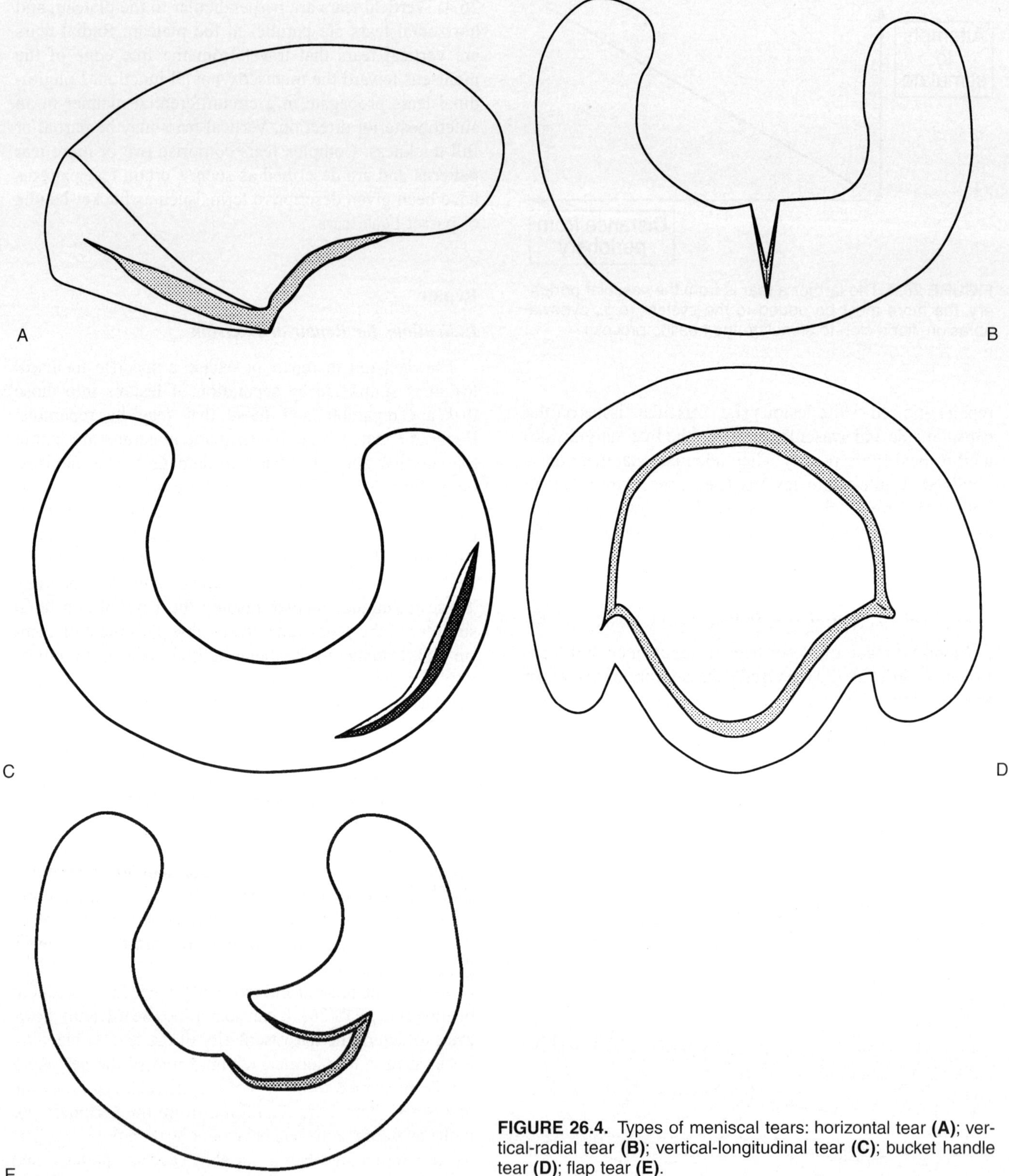

FIGURE 26.4. Types of meniscal tears: horizontal tear **(A)**; vertical-radial tear **(B)**; vertical-longitudinal tear **(C)**; bucket handle tear **(D)**; flap tear **(E)**.

long as the repair is performed in conjunction with an ACL reconstruction. The combined meniscal repair and ACL reconstruction improves healing rates of the meniscal tear and increases the longevity of the articular surface of the knee (28).

If a meniscal tear is unlikely to heal, taking into account the previously outlined considerations, a partial meniscectomy should be performed. Degenerative tears, complex tears, flap tears, and unstable radial tears should be considered for partial meniscectomy.

Repair Principles

The conditions necessary to promote healing are similar to other repairs within the musculoskeletal system. Healing potential must be stimulated, and the defect must be stabilized. Stimulation is accomplished by synovial abrasion or the addition of a fibrin clot. Stability is inherent to the tear pattern, as described earlier, or stability must be introduced to the tear by suture reapproximation or immobilization (29).

The most common methods used to achieve stability in meniscal repair are performed arthroscopically. The arthroscopic surgical morbidity rate is lower, suture placement is very accurate, and tears not amenable to open repair can be reached using modern arthroscopic techniques. Arthroscopic techniques can be divided into inside-out, outside-in, and all-inside methods. The inside-out technique was initially performed percutaneously but is currently combined with a posteromedial or posterolateral incision to avoid neurovascular injury.

Common to all of these procedures is placement of horizontal or vertical mattress sutures that approximate both surfaces of the torn meniscus. There are two schools of thought about suture type. Many surgeons use nonabsorbable sutures thinking that the meniscus is not very vascular and requires a long period of healing. Users of absorbable sutures believe that the nonabsorbable suture puckers the meniscus and causes permanent deformation (29). In one study, Barrett et al. (30) found that nonabsorbable sutures (2–0 Ethibond) had a much lower failure rate than absorbable sutures (00 PDS). It was therefore recommended that permanent sutures be used to allow for longer and more stable fixation and to permit more complete maturation and remodeling. Kohn et al. (31) demonstrated that vertical mattress suturing has strength that is superior to horizontal mattress suturing, because vertical mattress suturing captures more collagen fibers.

Tears of the medial meniscus should be performed in a position of relative extension. This approach allows the saphenous nerve to be pulled anterior to the posteromedial corner, protecting the nerve from injury. This position also prevents plication and obliteration of the posterior capsular recess, averting a flexion contracture. Repairs of the lateral meniscus should be repaired with the knee in 50° to 70° of flexion, allowing the peroneal nerve to drop posteriorly (32).

In the inside-out technique, single- and double-barrel, zone-specific cannulas can be used to place horizontal or vertical mattress sutures through the meniscus. The advantage of the inside-out technique is that it enhances the surgeon's ability to place sutures accurately, producing excellent coaptation of the meniscus. The most difficult aspect is retrieval of the 6-cm needles through the posterior incisions. The Henning technique uses a 2–0 Ethibond (Ethicon, Somerville, NJ) suture with double-armed, taper-ended Keith needles. After a reparable meniscal tear is identified, the meniscal edges are débrided arthroscopically using a rasp or a full-radius cutter. A separate posteromedial or posterolateral incision is then made. The incision is made to expose the capsule, allowing direct visualization for suture retrieval. The arthroscope is placed in the ipsilateral portal, and a single- or double-armed cannula is placed through the contralateral portal. This allows the sutures to be aimed away from the popliteal structures and toward the accessory incision. The tip of the suture needle may be advanced beyond the end of the cannula and used to reduce the meniscus. The needle is then advanced across the tear and through the capsule. Most surgeons advocate placing sutures on both the femoral and tibial sides of the meniscus. Vertical sutures allow space for more sutures, but horizontal sutures are easier to place. Sutures are then pulled taut to assess the coaptation of the edges and are tied over the capsule (33).

The posteromedial approach to the knee is performed through a 4-cm incision centered at the joint just posterior to the medial collateral ligament. The knee is flexed to 90° to protect the saphenous vein and nerve. The subcutaneous tissues are bluntly dissected, exposing the sartorial fascia. This fascia is divided in line with the skin incision. A retractor is placed deep to this layer but anterior to the medial head of the gastrocnemius to protect the posterior neurovascular structures. The posteromedial joint line should be palpable at this point, and the repair can be performed (32,33).

The posterolateral approach is made through a 4-cm incision just posterior to the lateral collateral ligament at the level of the joint line. Dissection is done between the anterior border of the biceps and the posterior border of the iliotibial band. Blunt dissection is performed between the arcuate complex and the lateral head of the gastrocnemius. A retractor is introduced to protect the neurovascular structures, and repair can proceed. The peroneal nerve lies medial to the biceps and is not protected by retraction of the biceps alone. It is the retracted gastrocnemius that protects the peroneal nerve (32,33).

The outside-in repair technique was developed in the 1980s by Warren. The technique was developed to avoid the neurovascular injuries that had been reported with the inside-out technique. This procedure allows very rapid suture placement and is excellent to reach tears in the anterior and middle third of the meniscus. This method delivers suture (0 PDS) through the lumen of an 18-gauge spinal needle, directed from a known safe zone through the capsule and through the meniscal tissue under arthroscopic control. The arthroscope is in the contralateral portal. The suture is then retrieved through an ipsilateral portal, and an interference knot is tied in the end of the retrieved suture. The spinal needle is removed, and the free suture end is used to retrogradely move the knot to reduce the meniscal tear. This procedure is repeated several times until the tear is stable. After stability has been achieved, the sutures are tunneled subcutaneously and tied over the capsule (34).

In 1991, Morgan (35) described the all-inside technique of meniscal repair. The technique was developed to safely and effectively suture meniscal tears in the posterocentral, peripheral portions of the posterior horns of the menisci. He felt that these tears were difficult to approach by the inside-out or outside-in techniques. The all-inside technique ties the sutures over the meniscus and does not include the capsule. This approach prevents the possibility of a flexion contracture. The disadvantages of the technique are that it is technically very demanding and requires visualization in the posterior compartment with a 70-degree scope placed through the intercondylar notch, which requires special training for the surgeon. It also requires a posterior operative cannula, which carries some potential risk for neurovascular complications. Because this technique is very difficult to perform, newer devices have become available to make the all-inside method technically achievable. The T-Fix device (Acufex Microsurgical, Inc., Mansfield, MA) has a short, rigid Delrin T attached to a braided, nonabsorbable suture that is preloaded inside and deployed through a delivery needle. The T grabs inside the tissue and provides an anchor for the suture. These anchors are placed side by side, and arthroscopic knots are tied. Bionx Implants (Blue Bell, PA) has developed a polylactic acid tack, the Meniscal Arrow, and the system allows placement of several tacks with a relatively easy insertion technique (Fig. 26.5). This technique requires no arthroscopic knot tying, which makes it quite appealing. Strength testing of the Meniscal Arrow has shown that it has a pull-out strength equivalent to a horizontal Maxon stitch in a bovine meniscal model (36).

In performing the arrow technique, meniscal width should be determined to choose appropriate arrow length. If the repair is to be done in conjunction with an ACL reconstruction, the meniscus should be repaired first. The meniscal edges should be débrided to generate bleeding using a rasp, trephine needle, or mechanical shaver. However, care should be taken not to alter the architecture of the meniscal body.

Planning arrow placement aids in reduction and maintaining the reduction during the repair. For posterior

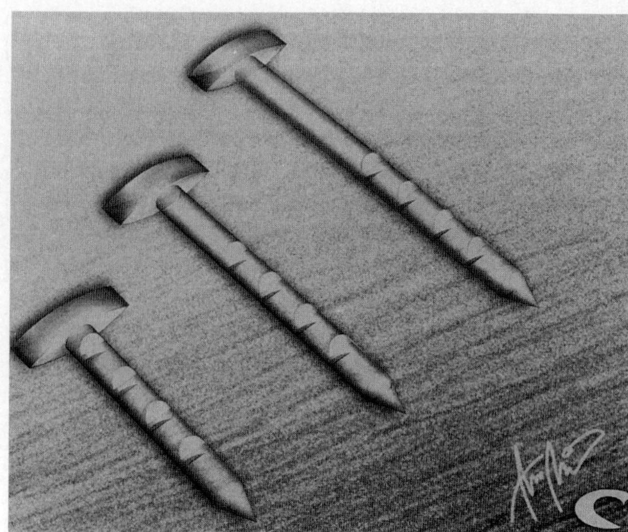

FIGURE 26.5. Meniscal Arrow (Bionx Implants, Inc., Blue Bell, PA).

tears, the first arrow should be placed in the most posterior position. The next arrow should be placed in the center of the tear. Subsequent arrows should be placed by alternating anterior and posterior to the center arrow. In more medial tears, the middle of the tear is fixed first, and subsequent arrows are placed anterior and posterior to the center arrow.

The appropriate cannula should be chosen to allow an approach to the tear as perpendicular as possible to ensure maximum fixation in the circumferential fibers of the meniscus. Standard portals are usually adequate to obtain a perpendicular position. However, if they are not adequate, additional portals should be made. The selected cannula is inserted with the obturator in place to avoid grabbing soft tissue on insertion. This also helps to prevent damage to the articular surface on introduction into

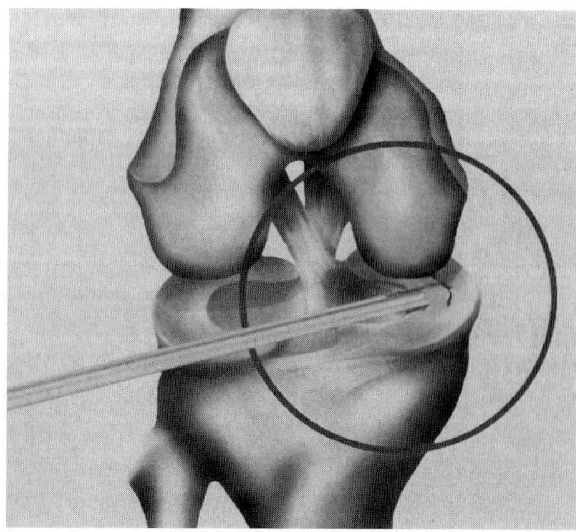

FIGURE 26.6. Cannula shown reducing meniscal tear with a stylet in place to aid reduction.

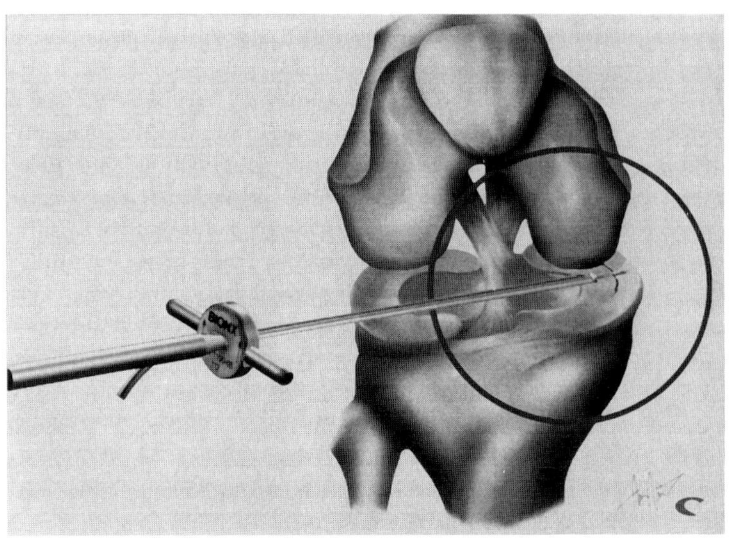

FIGURE 26.7. The Meniscal Arrow (Bionx Implants, Inc., Blue Bell, PA) is seated on the meniscal surface after channel preparation. A stylet holds the reduction.

the joint. The cannula should then be used to reduce the meniscal tear. The obturator is removed, and the reduction is maintained using the sharp tip of the cannula. When using the straight cannula, a stylet can be used to maintain the reduction while placing the arrow (Fig. 26.6).

The channel being prepared for the arrow should include 3 to 5 mm of the central portion of the meniscus to ensure that enough tissue is available to accommodate the T-head of the arrow. Fixation can be maximized by keeping the cannula and the T-head as parallel as possible to the joint line. While maintaining firm pressure on the cannula, the surgeon inserts the cutting needle into the cannula and the meniscus. The needle protrudes 13 mm from the end of the cannula and can be used as a gauge for the selection of the appropriate-length arrow. To prevent postoperative pain from the sharp tip of the arrow, no more than 1 mm should protrude beyond the capsule.

Deploying the 13 mm of the sharp needle seats it against the head of the cannula.

The inflow irrigation should be turned off, and the needle should be removed. The arrow is placed into the cannula, which allows only the proper orientation. The blunt obturator is used to seat the arrow to the meniscal surface (Fig. 26.7). A change in pressure is required when the arrow contacts the meniscal surface. The arrow is driven into the meniscus using a mallet.

A recently developed pneumatic-powered gun appears to have simplified this delivery system (Fig. 26.8). Preliminary clinical evaluations seem to validate ease of use and better reproducibility. Pull-out strengths have also been enhanced.

The arrow must be completely driven into the meniscal surface, or "countersunk." The obturator must be fully seated against the cannula to ensure that the arrow is fully

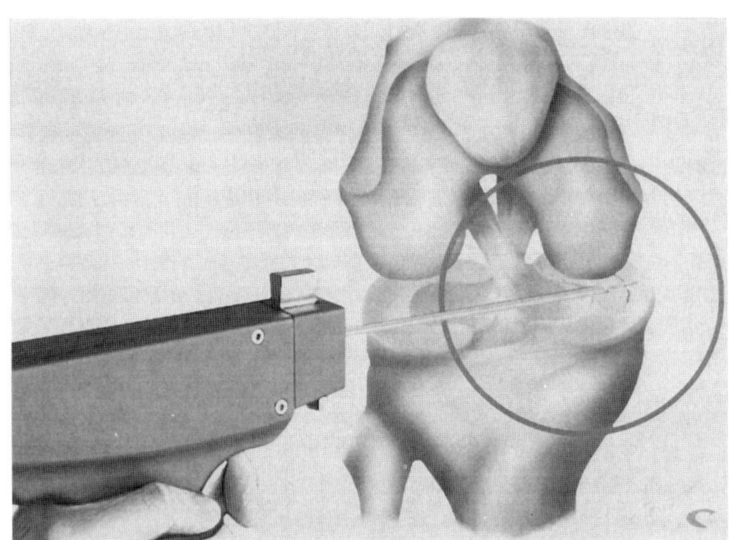

FIGURE 26.8. Alternative delivery system. Automated Meniscal Arrow (Bionx Implants, Inc., Blue Bell, PA) gun is used for insertion. More than one arrow can be delivered with this system.

implanted. If the T-head can be palpated, the cannula should be replaced, and the arrow should be tapped in farther. If the arrow needs to be extracted, it should be rotated 90° before removal.

The cannula can be shifted to a new position to insert another arrow. A distance of 5 mm should be maintained between the shafts of the arrows, not the T-heads.

Results of Meniscal Surgery

The success rate of meniscal repair reported in the literature is 78% to 100% (23). Using second-look arthroscopy or arthrography, 75% to 80% show complete healing, 15% show partial healing, and 5% to 10% show failure of healing (7). Rodeo and Warren (37) reported a series of patients who underwent an outside-in meniscal repair with 2-year follow-up and who had an 86% success rate. Sixty-seven percent were asymptomatic with evidence of complete healing, and 19% were minimally symptomatic with evidence of partial healing. A 14% failure rate was attributed to patients with significant symptoms or objective evidence of failure to heal. Patients with stable knees had a higher propensity for the meniscal repair to heal (85%) than patients with unstable knees (62%). The failure rate was only 5% for patients undergoing concomitant ACL reconstruction. The hemarthrosis related to ACL reconstruction is thought to provide serum factors necessary for meniscal healing (37).

Cannon reported his results of inside-out meniscal repairs. He followed 117 of 160 repairs with arthrography or second-look arthroscopy. Seventy-nine percent of repairs were done in conjunction with ACL reconstruction. Twenty-five were in cruciate-stable knees. Seventy-five percent of tears were healed or incompletely healed. Eighty-two percent of repairs done in conjunction with ACL reconstruction healed, whereas only 48% of isolated meniscal repairs had successful outcomes. Tears with an increased rim width larger than 4 to 5 mm and tears longer than 2 cm had higher failure rates. Tears longer than 4 to 5 cm had a 60% failure rate. In general, lateral meniscal repairs did better than medial meniscal repairs (84% vs. 70%) (34).

Reigle et al. (38) had no failures among 87 patients (69 with concomitant ACL reconstruction) using the all-inside technique. Eighteen patients had isolated lateral meniscal tears. Barrett et al. (39) reported preliminary results using the T-Fix suture anchor in 21 meniscal repairs. All patients had associated ACL reconstructions. At follow-up, four patients were symptomatic and underwent second look-arthroscopy. Three of the tears had healed, and one had failed. No studies have reported results using Bionx Meniscal Arrows, but preliminary results are promising.

Complications in Meniscal Surgery

The overall complication rate in meniscal repair surgery is reported as 2.8% to 29%. Complications have included saphenous neuropathy, arthrofibrosis, popliteal artery laceration, peroneal neuropathy, deep infection, deep venous thrombosis, pulmonary embolus, meniscal cysts, and reflex sympathetic dystrophy. Saphenous neuropathy is the most common complication, and most patients describe it as a minor nuisance. Arthrofibrosis occurs in 7% to 10% of cases. This is complicated by the fact that most meniscal repairs are performed in conjunction with ACL reconstruction (also associated with a significant rate of arthrofibrosis). Most complications are transient and resolve spontaneously or with appropriate treatment. However, it is important to be aware of the potential complications of this otherwise extremely beneficial procedure (40).

Postoperative Rehabilitation after Meniscal Repair

Two schools of thought exist with regard to the appropriate rehabilitation program after meniscal repair. Most surgeons use a restrictive rehabilitation program, advocating immobilization and partial weight bearing in the first 4 to 6 weeks after a repair (34,41). The rationale, as reported by DeHaven et al. (25), was to protect the repair site and to allow maturation of a fibrovascular scar. Because no reports were available on the use of a more aggressive rehabilitation protocol, Shelbourne (42) performed a series of isolated meniscal repairs and changed only the postoperative motion and weight-bearing status to compare outcomes. The accelerated group was encouraged to bear weight and move their knees as tolerated. The protocol emphasized prevention of swelling and effusions. The patients in the accelerated program gained motion 4 weeks earlier and returned to full activity approximately 10 weeks earlier, with no overall difference in success rates between the two groups. For patients undergoing ACL reconstruction concomitantly, the rehabilitation protocol should follow the surgeon's normal routine, encouraging range of motion along with weight bearing as tolerated. The risks of jeopardizing the meniscal repair are far less than the risks of losing motion in an ACL reconstruction. Restrictive and accelerated rehabilitation protocols have led to successful results in meniscal repair surgery, and the accelerated protocol does not seem to compromise the results in isolated repairs or those in combination with ACL reconstruction.

Enhancement Techniques

To increase healing rates of meniscal repairs in the relatively avascular (red-white) zones and in the avascular (white-white) zones, efforts have been made to enhance the vascularity of these areas and to provide a better healing environment. Débridement of devitalized tissue should be performed to expose a bleeding surface on at least one side of the tear. However, débridement should be limited to the superficial tissue covering the meniscal edges. This is typically done with a full-radius resector blade or meniscal rasp. Vascular access channels have been made with large-bore needles to allow fibrovascular ingrowth into the avascular region of the meniscus. The problem with the vascular access channels is that they cut across the circumferentially oriented collagen fibers and disturb the normal architecture (43). Trephination therefore has become more of a standard approach. This technique uses an 18-gauge needle to create multiple puncture sites to allow vascular ingrowth. The channels produced are smaller in diameter than the vascular access channels and cause minimal damage to normal architecture (44). Synovial abrasion of the femoral and tibial surfaces can be performed to stimulate a proliferative vascular response to increase the success rate of repair within the red-white zone (45). Increased hemarthrosis associated with ACL reconstruction is thought to provide various growth factors necessary for healing of the meniscus. By providing the factors and a scaffold necessary for healing to occur, the fibrin clot has been used to support and induce a healing response in the avascular portion of the meniscus (22). These techniques can be used to enhance healing rates of tears within the red-white zone but have not been shown to improve healing in the white-white zone.

Meniscectomy

When a meniscal tear is unable to be repaired, partial meniscectomy should be performed. Two types of partial meniscectomies have been described. Segmental meniscectomy involves removing the entire width of the meniscus out to the meniscocapsular junction, and circumferential meniscectomy involves removing some length of the central portion of the meniscus. After segmental meniscectomy, menisci retain no load-transmitting properties, whereas menisci after a circumferential meniscectomy retain load-transmission capabilities proportional to the amount of meniscus remaining (46).

The goal of partial meniscectomy is to preserve as much normal tissue as possible while removing damaged, unstable, or abnormal tissue. *Balancing* of the meniscal remnant should be performed by removing some normal tissue to prevent stress concentration at an edge that could lead to tearing of the residual meniscus (47). In performing a partial meniscectomy, all mobile fragments should be removed. A sequence of cutting and probing should be performed to assess remnant stability. A smooth, contoured residual rim with no sudden changes in shape should be left behind. The meniscosynovial junction should be protected, and when in doubt, the surgeon should always leave more meniscus than less (48).

Balancing a radial tear requires removing enough tissue on both sides of the tear to create a smooth C-shaped central edge. This should be done to prevent propagation of the tear anteriorly or posteriorly, which will result in a flap tear. Treatment of a vertical–longitudinal tear requires removal of the central fragment, followed by

tapering of the anterior and posterior edges to create a smooth inner margin of meniscus. Flap tears are treated by principles similar to those previously described. While treating a horizontal cleavage tear, the sequence of cutting and probing should be performed. This may require resection of the tibial and femoral lamina or only the unstable lamina. Because the meniscal remnants may still participate in load transmission, only the unstable fragments should be excised (29).

Meniscal surgery is quite complex and requires the surgeon to be experienced with many different techniques. The goal of meniscal surgery is to retain as much of the normal biomechanics within the knee as possible.

ACUTE CHONDRAL INJURY AND CHRONIC ARTHROSIS

Anterior Cruciate Ligament Injury

In an acute ACL injury, there is an anterior subluxation of the lateral tibia on the lateral femoral condyle. There are several proposed mechanisms for the subchondral fracture or "bone bruise" that is seen on magnetic resonance imaging (MRI) (49). These include the pivot-shift phenomenon, the reduction of the pivot-shift phenomenon, and a hyperextension injury of the knee. Bone bruises are seen on roughly 80% of knee MRI scans after acute ACL injuries. Most common sites of the subchondral fractures are the terminal sulcus of the lateral femoral condyle and the posterolateral surface of the tibial plateau. Free water shifts, acute edema, and inflammation are best seen on T2-weighted images.

Follow-up MRI studies have been done after initial MRI scans to evaluate the outcomes of these bone lesions. In one series in which the follow-up period was 6 to 12 months, there were apparent sequelae in 67% of cases (50), including overt cartilage loss or deficit in 48% and an osteochondral defect in 14%. There is still no consensus on whether these bone bruises result in degenerative arthrosis, but single-impact loads can produce a subsequent osteoarthritic picture. In a canine model, a single impact of 2,170 N was applied through the skin to the patellofemoral joint (51). At 6 months, the histologic picture of the patellofemoral joint included fibrillation, subchondral bone formation, and loss of safranin-O staining; these are hallmarks of osteoarthritis.

Overt cartilage damage or fracture was detected in 20% to 46% of knees undergoing arthroscopy after an acute ACL injury (52–54). Twenty percent of the patients had injury to the lateral femoral condyle, 13% to the lateral tibial plateau, 20% to the medial femoral condyle, and 6% to the medial tibial plateau. Some patients had multiple areas of involvement.

The arthroscopic incidence of chondral defect after a chronic ACL injury reported in the literature has ranged from 42% to 69% (52,55,56). Most of these lesions are in the lateral femoral condyle or lateral tibial plateau. Ongoing studies are attempting to define the clinical outcomes, especially in regard to degenerative changes after an acute chondral injury.

Posterior Cruciate Ligament Injury

The incidence of chondral injuries as a result of an acute posterior cruciate ligament (PCL) injury varies in the literature. No injuries were encountered in some series, but in others, the incidence was as high as 25% (57–59). Acute chondral injuries tend to occur in the lateral and patellofemoral compartments.

Additional injuries to the posterolateral corner (generally defined as the popliteus muscle and tendon, lateral collateral ligament, and posterolateral capsule) have been found to increase the instability caused by a PCL injury (60). A cadaveric sectioning study found that there was a significant increase in the pressure in the medial and patellofemoral joints after sectioning the posterolateral corner in a PCL injury model (60). The investigators referred to this as a "reverse Maquet effect." In general, degenerative changes from a chronic PCL injury tend to occur in the medial and patellofemoral compartments. These series have included radiographic, arthroscopic, and arthrotomy studies. The incidence of degenerative changes ranged from 36% to 50% in the medial compartment and 16% to 31% in the patellofemoral area (57,59,61). One study did find, however, that the distribution was roughly equal between the medial and lateral compartments for degenerative changes (62). It also found that there is a much higher incidence of degenerative changes with a combined injury to the PCL and posterolateral corner.

Arthroscopic Classifications

There have been many classification systems proposed over the years for articular cartilage injury. Historically, one of the more popular has been the Outerbridge classification (63). That system, as well as others, is not comprehensive in its ability to describe with a simple grading system the essential details of the injury to the cartilage surface. Conversely, some systems are so elaborate as to be cumbersome. In the past 12 years, there has been advancement in classification as arthroscopy has become more commonplace. Four systems during that time have been published (64–67). Each of the classification systems attempts to use size, depth, and location of the lesion. In some, specific proposed etiologic mechanisms are included for different types of lesions. Others have offered scoring systems that have been difficult to use. Their advantage, however, is a more comprehensive analysis of the spectrum of chondral injuries in an attempt to make comparison possible in clinical research. The fact that there have been many systems without one being used universally indicates how difficult it is to be comprehensive without being burdensome. However, the classification system of Bauer and Jackson (65) is a system in which the types are readily recognizable and that offers a probable mechanism of injury (Fig. 26.9), including acute injuries and chronic degenerative changes.

Arthroscopic Treatments

Increasing attention has been paid to chondral injuries in the literature since the mid-1980s. An early article entitled "Chondral Fractures—Cause for Confusion" focused on West Point cadets who were thought to have meniscal injuries (68). At the time of arthroscopy, however, chondral fractures were encountered. Three of the eight cadets had ACL injuries. Treatment was standardized. This included excision of the loose cartilage down to bone and curetting to bleeding bone if the lesions were larger than 5 mm in diameter. The investigators found that the chondral fractures seemed to have roughly three times the recovery length compared with a corresponding meniscal injury. They concluded that chondral fractures usually manifested in a skeletally mature patient and offered a poor prognosis compared with osteochondral fractures, which tended to occur in adolescents, have a bloody effusion, and have a more rapid healing rate. Other series subsequently published had higher numbers of patients but tended to offer poor long-term follow-up. The short-term outcomes were thought to be very good.

Biopsy after cartilage shaving was performed and compared with no treatment (69). Biopsies were performed from 3 months to 2.5 years later. In the patients who underwent shaving, no new superficial zone was formed, and the cartilage was fibrillated. There appeared to be increased metabolism in the radial zone and increased cell necrosis near the surface. In the group that had no shaving, the superficial fibers were tangential to the articular surface. There were increased chondrocytes in the superficial zone, increased metabolism in the radial zone, and a "significantly smaller" rate of cell necrosis. In general, the study's authors believed that shaving was detrimental.

Chondral injury that occurs in a stable knee was also studied. A mechanism was proposed for injury to the medial femoral condyle where the tibial spine abuts the medial femoral condyle with flexion and internal rotation (70). Abutment was demonstrated in this series through direct observation with arthroscopy.

Surgeons have attempted to identify prognostic factors found at the time of arthroscopy and correlate these with long-term outcomes. In one series, complete vertical excision of the loose cartilage was performed with drilling of the subchondral bone. Several factors were consistent with a good prognosis, and many other factors were consistent with a poor prognosis (64). Patients were not allowed to bear weight for 8 weeks. Results were based on the presence or absence of locking, effusion,

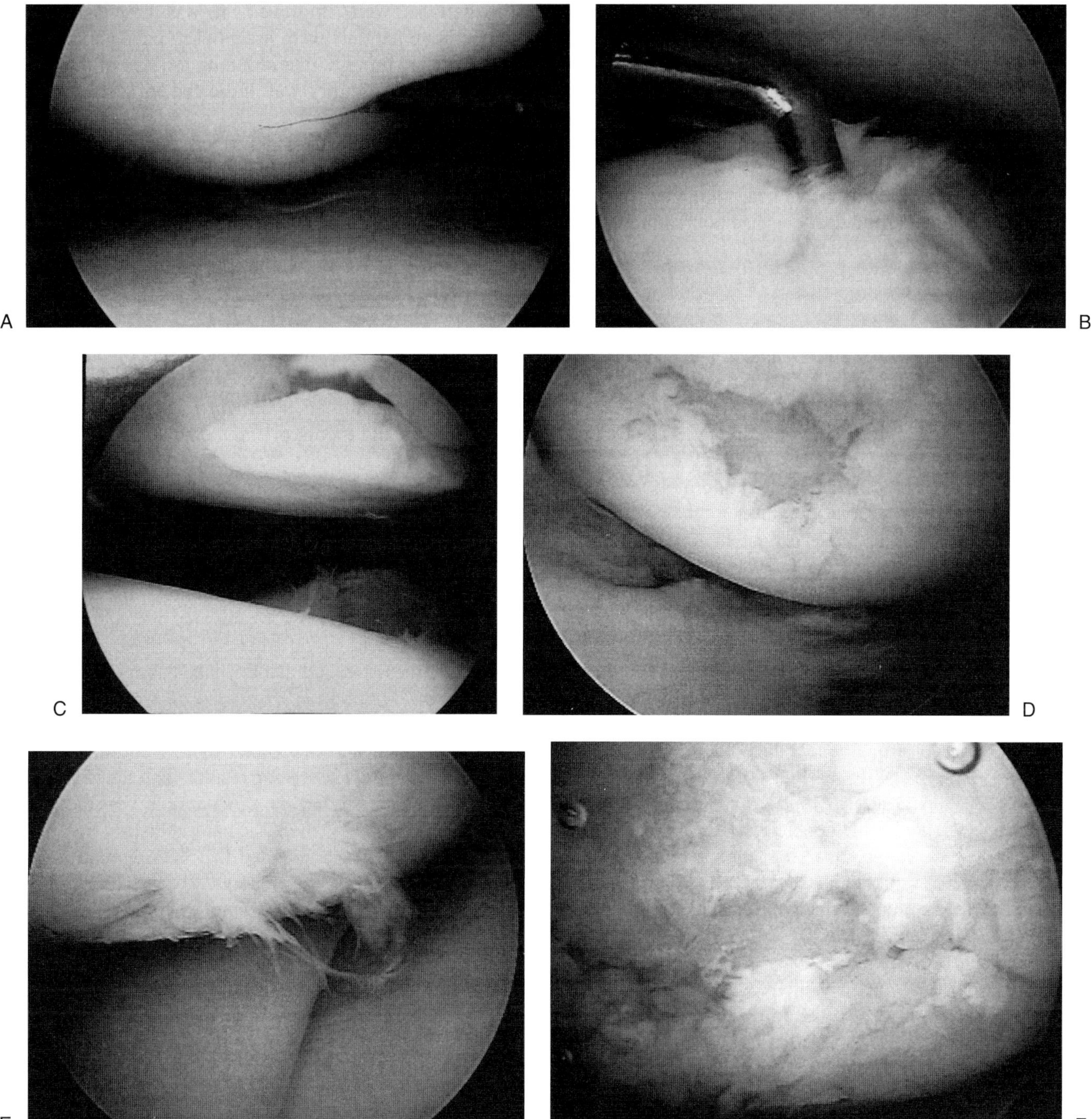

FIGURE 26.9. Classification of chondral lesions: type I, linear crack type **(A)**; type II, stellate fracture **(B)**; type III, flap type **(C)**; type IV, crater type **(D)**; type V, fibrillation type **(E)**; type VI, degrading type **(F)**. (From Bauer M, Jackson RW. Chondral lesions of the femoral condyles: a system of arthroscopic classification. *Arthroscopy* 1988;4:97–102, with permission.)

pain, and range of motion. In general, the best prognoses were found with acute, small- to medium-sized lesions and partial-thickness lesions. Preservation of the tidemark in the partial-thickness lesions was believed to offer some protection. Worse prognoses were found for larger lesions, full-thickness injuries, chronic degenerative arthrosis, and eburnated bone in the submeniscal, weight-

bearing surface and for older patients in poor health. In that same series, arthroscopy was repeated in 71% of the patients at 12 to 15 months after the initial arthroscopy. Fifty-seven percent of the patients underwent biopsy. The biopsy revealed, in the best situations, a cauliflower-like, bumpy surface with good staining for glycosaminoglycans. In the worst situations, there appeared to be a carpet of fibrous tissue overlying a depression, with no staining for glycosaminoglycans and no chondrocytes evident.

Other investigators have attempted to determine the long-term outcome of isolated defects to the femoral and tibial weight-bearing surfaces. In one series, 28 young athletes with grade II to III Outerbridge injuries with a minimum diameter of 1 cm were studied with arthroscopy (71). Three of the 28 had fragments removed with drilling, and 25 of the patients had no treatment. The patients were followed clinically and with radiographs at 12 to 15 years. At the follow-up evaluation, the average Lysholm score (72) was 92; 10 had excellent results, 12 had good results, and 6 had limited activities of daily living. During the interval follow-up, five had additional arthroscopic procedures, including three for removal of loose bodies and two for diagnosing the source of pain. Radiographs were graded using combined Ahlback and Fairbanks systems (5,73). There was no radiographic arthrosis in 12, no joint space obliteration in 4, less than 50% joint space reduction in 11, and more than 50% joint space reduction in 1. The investigators felt the results were strikingly good. There was, however, twice the amount of joint space narrowing on average compared with similar partial meniscectomy series (74).

One study attempted to compare their standardized treatment protocol with that for autologous cartilage transplantation techniques (75). The lesions were débrided to a stable border, and the calcified cartilage was débrided to bleeding bone with a curette or shaver. A grading system from the cartilage transplant literature was used (49). At 1 year, Ahlback's treatment protocol yielded six excellent, nine good, zero fair, and zero poor results. These results compared favorably with autologous cartilage transplantation techniques. MRI was also used to determine preoperatively the cartilage injuries but had an accuracy rate of only 21%.

One group (76) attempted to repair avulsed pieces of cartilage from the femoral condyle with a fibrin sealant and polydioxanone. It was determined on second-look arthroscopy at 14 to 16 weeks after initial fixation that the cartilage could best be reapproximated if there was a small piece of bone attached to the fragment. The investigators believed that the fixation was questionable, and no long-term results have been presented regarding the quality of the cartilage.

Chronic Arthrosis of the Knee

In the early 1940s, two series were presented before the advent of arthroscopy in which housekeeping-type procedures were done for chronic degenerative arthritis (77,78). The researchers thought that these rough surfaces resulted from repeated microtrauma and caused irritation and symptoms. They believed that, by removing the irritated surface, they would be reducing the patient's symptoms. In these series, more than 95% of the patients were improved. It was emphasized that cooperative patients were essential to have good results. Haggart (78) thought that reducing the size of the patella or excising it entirely was indicated in severe patellofemoral disease.

Insall and Pirdie (79) described the operation made popular by Pridie that included drilling of the subchondral bone in an attempt to encourage fibrocartilage repair. Sixty patients were studied. Pain relief was better in 40, the same in 16, and worse in 4. Function improved in 30, remained unchanged in 22, and was worse in 8.

In 1974, Jackson (80) reported the early use of arthroscopy in the degenerative knee. He believed that arthroscopy was indicated for early detection, appropriate treatment preparation, avoidance of unnecessary intraarticular surgery, limited treatment of simple excision of loose bodies and meniscal fragments, and for follow-up and research. Since that time, there have been several studies published about arthroscopic débridement of meniscal and chondral injuries. A few of these series have included débridement of the osteophytes as well.

Two series that used the same outcome scale, which was based on patient satisfaction, function, and comfort, had a combined 131 knees and an average follow-up period of more 13 months (81,82). In these series, there was no drilling or abrasion. The average age of the patients was about 55 years. The results were fairly consistent. In one series, there were 74% good, 10% fair, and 16% poor results. In the other, there were 72.1% good, 16.3% fair, and 11.6% poor results. The latter group of investigators stated that the procedure is best thought of as a palliative one in which the natural history may not be affected (82). They concluded that débridement was not indicated in severely degenerative knees. The number of lesions, not the type, was found to correlate with outcome.

The specific effect of chondral débridement versus meniscal débridement and lavage was also studied (83). A series of 207 patients were followed for an average of 24 months after the index procedure. The groups were subdivided into those having cartilage procedures, meniscus procedures, combined procedures, or lavage only. In general, the best results were reported for the group receiving chondral débridement alone. The investigators commented that subsequent lavage yielded equally favorable results compared with initial lavage, a finding that contradicted those of another series in which subsequent arthroscopies had less favorable results with each repeat treatment (84).

The specific population of elderly patients with decreased activity levels was also studied (85). The average age of the patients was 63 years. Sixty percent of them had tri-compartmental involvement. The early failures were associated with longer symptoms, severe radiographic changes, and malalignment. The best results correlated with short-term symptoms, mild-to-moderate degenerative change on radiographs, and the presence of crystalline deposits. Age, weight, compartment location, and preoperative range of motion were shown to have no effect.

Other researchers have echoed the effect of severe osteoarthrosis on successive débridement. One series found a reoperation rate of 67%, defined as failure, within 36 months because of severe osteoarthrosis. This compares with only a 32% failure rate over the same time interval for all degrees of osteoarthrosis. There appeared to be no correlation with the patients' demographics, physical findings, arthroscopic findings, or specific procedure performed (86).

Patient satisfaction with arthroscopic débridement was studied (87). The patient population in this series averaged 58.1 years, and the average follow-up period was 50.6 months; 74% of patients felt they would repeat the procedure, and 26% would not (87). The favorable results tended to deteriorate with time. The study's authors stressed there was a very low complication rate despite the mediocre results, and they felt no bridges were burned by the use of arthroscopic débridement.

The effect of alignment on outcome was studied by Salisbury et al. (88). In this series, débridement of 52 patients was performed with Outerbridge-like grade III or IV changes. The patients were divided into groups based on alignment: varus, normal, and valgus. The patients were evaluated for pain and function. A score of 10 on the pain scale was considered to be the same or worse pain than before the procedure. The patients were seen at final follow-up at an average of 27.5 months. Patients with varus deformities showed 32% fair to good results, with a pain rating of 8.5. Those with normal alignment showed 94% fair to good results, with a pain rating of only 3.4. Those with valgus alignment, although smaller in number, had generally poor results.

The technique of abrasion arthroplasty evolved in an attempt to create reparative fibrocartilage. This procedure is generally attributed to Johnson (89). The subchondral bone is débrided with a motorized burr to approximately 1 to 2 mm deep (Fig. 26.10). In his clinical series, Johnson treated 99 knees in 95 patients with an average age of 60 years. The minimal follow-up was 2 years. Seventy-four percent of the knees were improved, 7% were the same, 15% were worse, and 3% provided no answer. Repeat radiographs were obtained for 64 of the patients at 2 years. Fifty percent of the knees had a wider joint space. This was believed by the investigator to be caused by reparative fibrocartilage. He chose abrasion arthroplasty because he noticed no cartilage coalescence on second-look arthroscopy after drilling. Johnson stressed that débridement is intracortical and not cancellous. If "red" bone is exposed, the débridement was believed to be too deep. Tourniquet release and pressure reduction to allow assessment of bleeding is emphasized to check for the proper depth of burring.

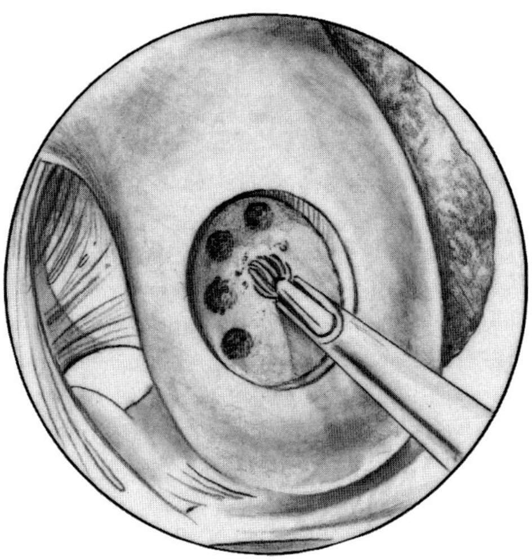

FIGURE 26.10. Abrasion chondroplasty. (From Miller MD. Atlas of chondral injury treatment. *Oper Tech Orthop* 1987; 7:289–293, with permission.)

The healing response was studied, and nonvascular, fibrous, spindle-cell tissue was seen at about 8 weeks. By 4 to 6 months, there appeared to be some cartilaginous tissue in the same area, and by 9 months, a reparative fibrocartilage was attached to the subchondral bone and adjacent hyaline cartilage. One biopsy was performed 4 years after the index procedure, and the tissue was found to be fibrocartilage after appropriate staining and histologic analysis. The tidemark was restored. The author compared the histology of drilling with that of abrasion (89). It was proposed that abrasion provided a viable and cellular ingrowth. The drilling was said to provide an acellular myxomatous central area. It was felt that contraindications to abrasion alone were severe malalignment, mechanical instability, and a patient who is likely to be uncooperative with the postoperative protocol. There were, however, no contraindications based on the size and location of these lesions.

Two other series in the literature presented favorable results for abrasion arthroplasty after similar techniques (90,91). In one study, the abrasion arthroplasty was compared with débridement alone (92). With abrasion, 53% of patients were improved, 37% were unchanged, and 10% were worse. With débridement alone, 32% were improved, 50% were unchanged, and 11% were worse. Another series studied 55 patients with an average age of 62 years. All had severe arthritis. At follow-up, 47% had excellent, 33% had good, 4% had fair, and 16% had poor results, based on the scale used for total-knee arthroplasties (91,93).

In 1989, the first of two studies appeared in which abrasion arthroplasty was found to be not as favorable as débridement alone (94). In 1991, another published series had similarly discouraging results (95). In general, abrasion arthroplasty has fallen out of favor, but there are still several advocates of the procedure.

Only one publication in the literature deals with arthroscopic drilling as a treatment for degenerative arthrosis (96). There were 22 patients who had follow-up examinations at an average of 25.1 months. Ninety percent of the patients had grade II or IV Outerbridge changes. The results showed that 80% of the patients had decreased pain or were totally relieved of their pain. The investigators theorized that this decrease in pain correlated with a reduction in intraosseous pressure. However, this point was not investigated. No increase in joint space was seen at 6 to 8 months. No correlation was proposed between the extent of arthritis and the final results.

A microfracture technique using an awl was developed in which multiple holes were created 3 to 4 mm apart (Fig. 26.11). This is done to avoid thermal injury (97). The desired result is the same as that of an abrasion arthroplasty: ingrowth of fibrocartilage. The researchers (97) reported 77 patients with full-thickness defects. The initial treatment was a perpendicular débridement. Forty-six patients used continuous passive motion (CPM) after surgery, and 31 patients did not. The patients underwent second-look arthroscopy at an average interval of 64 weeks for the CPM group and 73 weeks for the non-CPM group. Cartilage assessment was based on its appearance, with a score of 1 being normal and 5 indicating chronic changes consistent with "bare bone." Interval improvement was 2.67 with CPM and 1.67 without. Rodrigo et al. (97) thought that the improvement was unrelated to the size of the lesion or age of the patient.

Steadman et al. (98) reported more than 1,200 patients who had undergone the microfracture procedure. Further technical issues were emphasized in the article. At follow-up, which was as long as 5 years after surgery, the overall results showed that 75% of the patients were improved, 20% were unchanged, and 5% were worse.

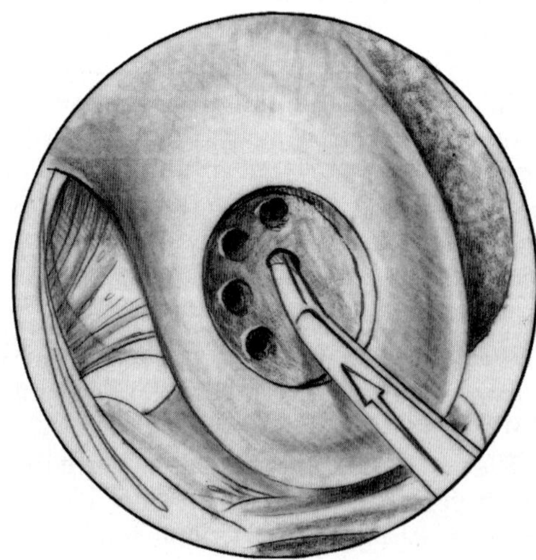

FIGURE 26.11. Microfracture with an awl. (From Miller MD. Atlas of chondral injury treatment. *Oper Tech Orthop* 1987; 7:289–293, with permission.)

In 1934, Burman (99) observed that in using arthroscopy, "It was in the group of arthritic cases that we had the pleasant surprise of seeing marked improvement in the joint following arthroscopy." Arthroscopy in 1934 was limited in its treatment options. Lavage was thought to be the effective treatment modality.

Since that time, there have been several reports attempting to document the contribution of lavage to patients' improvement after arthroscopy. In one series (100), a group of patients with osteoarthrosis underwent lavage and physical therapy. A control group consisted of those who had undergone physical therapy alone. The results indicated that the relief was better in the lavage group at 1 year. Another series (101) presented as a treatment simple irrigation with 3 L normal saline. The results at 1 year showed that 25 of the 29 patients had good or excellent results. At 2 years, 17 of the 21 available patients had good or excellent results.

A recent development in the treatment of chondral injury is the use of radiofrequency and laser chondroplasties. There are no long-term studies published on the use of these modalities in regard to patient outcomes or residual effects on cartilage. Short-term results with radiofrequency are promising, but there have been some reported adverse effects with laser.

Cartilage transplantation must be considered in the treatment of these acute and chronic cartilage injuries. The methods include chondrocyte, autologous osteochondral, and allograft transplantation. These specific treatment modalities are presented in Chapter 14.

ALIGNMENT

Role of Alignment in Treatment of Ligamentous and Chondral Injuries

Assessment of limb alignment is an important component of the decision-making process when evaluating a patient with a ligamentous injury. Tibiofemoral alignment in the coronal plane can be described relative to the weight-bearing axis (i.e., mechanical axis) or relative to the axis formed between the tibia and femur (i.e., anatomic axis) (Fig. 26.12).

In the normal knee, the mechanical axis (i.e., weight-bearing axis) is depicted diagrammatically as a line drawn from the center of the femoral head to the center of the ankle joint. This is most accurately measured on a double-stance, weight-bearing, anteroposterior radiograph that includes the hips, knees, and ankles on a single, 3-ft film (Fig. 26.12). In the normal knee, the mechanical axis is in 1.2° of varus (102). If the mechanical axis passes medial to the knee center, the limb is in varus alignment. Conversely, if it passes lateral to the knee center, the limb is in valgus. The exact degree of varus or valgus is reflected by the angle formed between the mechanical axis and the tibial shaft axis.

Importance of Alignment in Ligamentous Deficiency

Malalignment in the absence of ligamentous deficiency causes increased joint contact pressure, ultimately resulting in premature chondral wear and arthrosis. Clinically, valgus alignment occurs less frequently and is seldom a cause of significant dysfunction in the younger individual, although it may be associated with premature lateral arthritis in the middle-aged patient. The remainder of this discussion focuses on the association between varus alignment and ligament deficiencies.

Varus angulation at the knee can have several causes. In the so-called physiologic varus, the mechanical axis passes medial to the center of the knee in the absence of any other injury. The incidence of physiologic varus among patients with an acute ACL injury has not been defined. Medial meniscal loss or medial joint space arthrosis, both of which result in joint space narrowing, may aggravate primary varus or physiologic varus.

There is good evidence that the lateral collateral ligament is the primary restraint to varus angulation and that superimposition of a lateral collateral ligament injury on a preexisting physiologic varus results in two potential causes of varus angulation; this is called *double varus* (103,104). Lateral ligament deficiency may develop in the absence of a lateral ligament injury if the lateral ligaments become attenuated (105,106). This may occur if the patient with primary varus sustains an ACL injury. Because the ACL is a secondary restraint to varus angulation, the combination of primary varus and ACL disruption may in time result in stretching of the lateral ligaments with resultant double varus.

Numerous investigators have described an increase in varus angulation, posterior translation, external rotation, and coupled external rotation after sectioning of the posterolateral complex (104–107). When a posterolateral ligament injury occurs in the presence of primary varus angulation, the knee demonstrates varus angulation and varus recurvatum while standing or walking. This is seen clinically as knee hyperextension during stance or during the stance phase of gait. Varus recurvatum is accentuated in the presence of a PCL injury, with or without posterolateral corner laxity. This condition has been called *triple varus*.

Cartilage wear is determined ultimately by the joint reaction forces, which are a combination of the static and dynamic forces across the knee. The surgeon needs to evaluate each component separately and to determine which of these can be, or should be, corrected. These components include, but are not limited to, bony alignment, ligament deficiencies, muscle forces, and gait adaptations. Gait analysis is a means of assessing all these components functionally.

Clinical Findings

The goal of the clinical evaluation is to determine whether the symptoms described by the patient can be

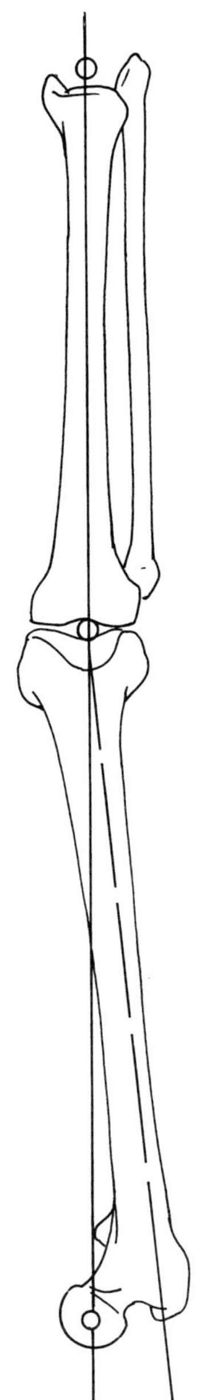

FIGURE 26.12. The mechanical axis system.

Limb alignment can also be described by the angle formed between the tibia and the femur (i.e., anatomic axis). The anatomic axis has a wide range of normal values, with an average of 5° of valgus (102). Although easier to measure clinically and radiographically, it does not represent the forces across the knee and should not be the sole determinant in planning surgical procedures.

Although ligament deficiencies can be addressed by ligament repair or reconstruction, malalignment can only be corrected by bony realignment (i.e., osteotomy), and the challenge in clinical practice is to determine which patients with ligament deficiencies and associated alignment abnormalities require or would benefit from either or both of these procedures.

attributed to malalignment, ligament deficiency, meniscal or chondral lesions, or any combination of these conditions. Each patient needs to be carefully evaluated so that all components of the pathologic process are identified. Poor surgical outcomes are often related to a failure to identify and address the various components of the problem. Most clinicians believe that failure to address the bony varus when performing an ACL or a lateral complex reconstruction results in a high surgical failure rate.

In the assessment of the injured knee, it is important to assess tibiofemoral alignment clinically, and if there is concern regarding alignment, full-length, weight-bearing radiographs should be obtained to make accurate measurements. Clinical examination must also determine the full extent of ligamentous injury by evaluating each ligament or ligament complex as discussed in previous chapters.

Varus alignment alone results in medial-sided symptoms, which are often activity related and relieved by rest. Meniscal injuries or early arthrosis usually cause clicking or locking, which may be reproduced by varus loading during clinical evaluation.

ACL deficiency causes subluxation episodes usually in association with rotational or pivoting maneuvers. Lateral ligament insufficiency can also result in instability during walking and is often more apparent during pivoting movements. A lateral thrust may occur during normal walking and can be accentuated by running. Patients with mild lateral ligament injuries may not demonstrate a lateral thrust and may only complain of lateral pain with activities. Injuries to the posterolateral complex may result in varus recurvatum, which in severe cases can be seen during stance, but in less severe cases, it may be apparent only during gait.

Gait Analysis

Gait analysis has been used to scientifically determine the forces about the normal knee and compare them with the knee with abnormal alignment or ligament deficiency. Gait analysis allows accurate determination of the adduction moment about the knee. This information is useful in predicting the results of surgical procedures performed in cases of varus alignment. The degree of radiographically measured varus is not the sole determinant of the adduction moment about the knee, which is influenced by a number of other factors, including lower limb rotational alignment (i.e., toe-in results in greater adduction than toe-out) and gait adaptations.

Adduction moment is an important indicator of the success of high tibial osteotomy. Prodromos (108) demonstrated that patients with a high adduction moment are more likely to develop recurrent varus after a high tibial osteotomy and suggested that knees with a high adduction moment should be overcorrected at the time of surgery. This has not been proved clinically.

Noyes et al. (105,109) demonstrated that patients with ACL injures and varus alignment have markedly increased tensile forces in the lateral ligaments with gait, suggesting that these patients may be at risk for stretching of the lateral ligaments if the varus is not addressed. However, there are no long-term follow-up clinical studies of this effect.

Treatment of Malalignment

Management of Varus Malalignment in Anterior Cruciate Ligament Injuries

Although the decision-making process about treatment of patients with primary varus or with isolated ligament injuries has been fairly well defined, the management of patients with varus alignment and associated ligament injuries is more difficult and not as well supported scientifically. The physician needs to decide whether the patient requires ligament reconstruction, osteotomy, or both and decide in which sequence to perform the various procedures.

Patients with ligamentous injuries in the absence of bony malalignment should be managed as discussed in previous chapters. When bony malalignment exists, the surgeon should consider bony realignment in association with or in place of ligament reconstruction.

Although many clinicians believe that physiologic varus in the presence of an acute ACL injury increases the risk for ligament reconstruction failure, there are no data to support corrective osteotomy in this situation. Patients should, however, be cautioned that without surgery they are at increased risk for stretching the lateral ligament structures, with resulting double varus and lateral thrust, which may be more difficult to treat. There are no reports on the results of ACL reconstruction performed for acute ACL injuries in the presence of varus malalignment. The large series of ACL reconstructions do not discuss the increased failure rate in varus knees that has been reported anecdotally.

For the varus-aligned, chronically ACL deficient–knee, careful evaluation of the exact symptoms should guide the surgeon's decision about correction of the appropriate abnormality. Symptoms of instability warrant a ligament reconstruction, whereas symptoms of medial compartment arthrosis or medial meniscal tears should be treated with arthroscopy followed by realignment.

There are many reports of surgery for the treatment of malalignment and associated ligament injuries. The literature, however, is confusing, and the clinician needs to separate those undergoing osteotomy only, ligament reconstruction only, or combinations of these patients. Patents undergoing combined or sequential procedures should also be differentiated.

Noyes et al. (105) reported 41 patients who underwent high tibial osteotomy for varus malalignment in the presence of chronic ACL deficiency. Thirty patients also underwent stabilization procedures for instability (14 extraarticular and 16 ACL reconstructions). At a mean follow-up of 58 months, improvements were observed for pain with daily activities in 50% of patients.

Dejour et al. (110) reported results of combined ACL reconstruction and high tibial osteotomy in 44 patients at an average of 3.5 years after surgery. All patients had symptomatic ACL-deficient knees and varus malalignment, and 26 patients were able to return to low-level but not competitive sports.

Boss et al. (43) described 27 of 34 patients who underwent combined ACL reconstruction and high tibial osteotomy. They reported no perioperative complications, but only 25% of patients regained their preinjury level of sporting activity; however, 50% of patients were able to participate in a higher level of sporting activity after surgery. Only two thirds of patients had less than 3 mm of anterior translation compared with the normal knee.

Latterman and Jakob (111) reported 27 of 30 patients who underwent surgical procedures for varus malalignment in the presence of ACL instability. Three groups of patients were described. Group 1 only underwent osteotomy, group 2 underwent an osteotomy with simultaneous ACL reconstruction, and group 3 underwent osteotomy followed at 6 to 12 months by ACL reconstruction. None of the patients was completely free of pain at follow-up, with 8 of 28 patients reporting pain even with light activities. No patient had less than 3 mm of side-to-side difference on the Lachman test, and 9 of the 27 patients had a positive pivot-shift test. The International Knee Documentation Committee score did improve for 23 of the 27 patients. However, on radiographic examination, progression of osteoarthritis was demonstrated in all patients. The investigators reported a very high rate of complications, with 4 of 11 patients undergoing only osteotomy having some complication, 3 of the 8 patients undergoing staged procedures, and 5 of the 8 patients undergoing simultaneous procedures demonstrating significant complications.

Neuschwander and Drez (112) reported results for five patients who underwent combined ACL reconstruction and high tibial osteotomy because of symptoms of instability and medial arthrosis. They reported no complications and average side-to-side differences of 3.1 mm. All patients had instability eliminated with an improvement in functional levels. They recommend the procedure be reserved only as a salvage procedure.

Many surgeons have stated that combined high tibial osteotomy and ACL reconstruction should be considered a salvage procedure only, and the consensus seems to be that this procedure should be recommended to patients with severe symptoms who are too young for other reconstructive procedures (105,111–114). Patients should be cautioned that the goal of surgery is to decrease pain and instability and that expectations of return to high-level athletic activity are unrealistic.

There has been much discussion regarding the order in which combined procedures should be done and whether they should be performed at a single operative session or as staged procedures. Careful review of the literature does not reveal a definite conclusion, but some guidelines can be suggested. Combined surgical procedures seem to be associated with an increased rate of complications and should be avoided if possible. Many patients appear to respond well to an initial osteotomy, obviating the need for ligament reconstruction even in the presence of preoperative instability symptoms. In the chronic situation in which patients already have some attenuation of the lateral ligaments, many surgeons suggest realignment of the limb (by high tibial osteotomy) before ligament reconstruction. In the case of lateral or posterolateral ligament reconstruction, this approach is almost certainly beneficial because reconstruction of these ligaments in the presence of varus alignment has been shown to have a high failure rate.

No reports discuss acute PCL or posterolateral injuries in the presence of primary varus. Veltri and Warren (115) recommend osteotomy and ligament reconstruction to correct varus alignment in association with chronic posterolateral ligament injuries. They also point out that, when the osteotomy is performed initially, the patients' symptoms often abate enough that ligament reconstruction can be avoided.

Complications of Surgery for Correction of Malalignment

Data for results of osteotomy are obtained primarily for patients undergoing osteotomy for malalignment, not for patients undergoing osteotomy in the presence of ligamentous deficiency. In the setting of pure malalignment, complications as high as 30% have been demonstrated (116):

Inadequate valgus: 20%
Recurrent varus: 5% to 30%
Nonunion: 1% to 3%
Infection: 1% to 8%
Fracture: 2% to 3%
Neurologic: 1% to 10%
Vascular: less than 1%

Although very high complication rates for combined osteotomy and ligament reconstruction could be expected, they have not been reported in the previously described series.

Surgical Procedures

Numerous techniques of high tibial osteotomy have been described, and a discussion of the merits of each of these is beyond the scope of this chapter. The exact surgical technique is probably not as important as the degree of correction obtained. Most modern techniques involve resection of a wedge of bone in the tibial metaphysis to convert the varus to a mild valgus alignment. Several guides have been marketed to simplify this resection, and numerous surgeons suggest that overcorrection to 9° to 10° of anatomic valgus is necessary to optimize long-term results (92,117,118). Another technique has been to aim to obtain a mechanical axis that passes through the medial one third of the lateral tibial plateau. Although static measurement of the varus alignment on full-length radiographs has its limitations, it remains the most practical means of calculating the degree of correction necessary.

Valgus producing high tibial osteotomy has been shown experimentally to decrease the medial joint forces (92) and demonstrated clinically to limit the progression of medial arthrosis (92,117,118). Prodromos (108) suggested that the results of surgery might be influenced by other factors (e.g., high or low adduction moment), but this idea has not been proved in any scientific fashion.

REFERENCES

1. Annandale T. An operation for displaced semilunar cartilage: the classic. *Clin Orthop* 1990;260:3–5.
2. Jones R. *Notes on derangements of the knee.* : AGT Fisher, 1909:969.
3. King D. The function of semilunar cartilages. *J Bone Joint Surg Am* 1936;18:1069.
4. King D. The healing of semilunar cartilages. *J Bone Joint Surg Am* 1936;18:333.
5. Fairbank TJ. Knee Joint changes after meniscectomy. *J Bone Joint Surg Br* 1948;30:664–670.
6. Cox JS, Nye CE, Shaeffer WW, et al. The degenerative effect of partial and total resection of the medial meniscus in dogs' knees. *Clin Orthop* 1975;109:178–183.
7. Rodeo S, Warren R. Meniscal repair using the outside-to-inside technique. *Clin Sports Med* 1996;15:469–481.
8. Ahmed AM, Burke D. *In vivo* measurement of static pressure distribution in synovial joint. Part I: Tibial surface of the knee. *J Biomech Eng* 1983;105:201–209.
9. Shrive N. The weight-bearing role of the menisci of the knee. *J Bone Joint Surg Br* 1974;15:381.
10. Krause WR, Pope MH, Johnson RJ, et al. Mechanical changes in the knee after meniscectomy. *J Bone Joint Surg Am* 1976;58:599–604.
11. Johnson RJ, Pope MH. *Functional anatomy of the meniscus. AAOS symposium on reconstruction of the knee.* St. Louis: CV Mosby, 1978:3–13.
12. Voloshin AS, Wosk J. Shock absorption of meniscectomized and painful knees. A comparative *in vivo* study. *J Biomed Eng* 1983:5:157–161.
13. Levy IM, Torzilli PA, Warren RF. The effect of medial meniscectomy on anterior-posterior motion of the knee. *J Bone Joint Surg Am* 1982;64:883–888.
14. Levy IM, Torzilli PA, Warren RF. The effect of lateral meniscectomy on motion of the knee. *J Bone Joint Surg Am* 1989;71:401–406.
15. Renstrom P, Johson R. Anatomy and biomechanics of the menisci. *Clin Sports Med* 1990;9:523–533.
16. MacConail MA. The movements of bones and joints. Part III: The synovial fluid and its assistants. *J Bone Joint Surg Br* 1950;32:244.
17. Ingman AM, Ghosh P, Taylor TKF. Variation of collagenous and non-collagenous proteins of human knee joint menisci with age and degeneration. *Generentologia* 1974;20:212–233.
18. Eyre DR, Koob TJ, Chun LE. Biochemistry of the meniscus: unique profile of collagen types and site dependent variations in composition. *Trans Orthop Res Soc* 1983;8:56.
19. Ghosh P, Taylor T, Phil D. The knee joint meniscus: a fibrocartilage of some distinction. *Clin Orthop* 1987;224:52–63.
20. Arnoczky SP, Warren RF. Microvasculature of the human meniscus. *Am J Sports Med* 1982;10:90–95.
21. Arnoczky SP, Warren RF. The microvasculature of the meniscus and its response to injury—an experimental study in the dog. *Am J Sports Med* 1983;11:131–141.
22. Arnoczky SP, Warren RF, Spivak JM. Meniscal repair using an exogenous fibrin clot: an experimental study in dogs. *J Bone Joint Surg Am* 1988;70:1209–1217.
23. Cooper DE, Arnoczky SP, Warren RF. Arthroscopic meniscal repair. *Clin Sports Med* 1990;9:589–607.
24. DeHaven KE, Arnoczky SP. Meniscal repair. Part I: Basic science, indications for repair, and open repair. *J Bone Joint Surg Am* 1994;76:140–152.
25. DeHaven KE, Black KP, Griffiths JH. Open meniscus repair: technique and two to nine year results. *Am J Sports Med* 1989;17:788–795.
26. Cannon WD, Vittori JM. The incidence of healing in arthroscopic meniscal repairs in anterior cruciate ligament–reconstructed knees versus stable knees. *Am J Sports Med* 1992;20:176–181.
27. Dehaven KE. Decision-making factors in the treatment of meniscal lesions. *Clin Orthop* 1990;252:49–54.
28. Belzer JP, Cannon WD. Meniscal tears: treatment in the stable and unstable knee. *J Am Acad Orthop Surg* 1993;1:41–47.
29. Newman AP, Daniels AU, Burks RT. Principles and decision making in meniscal surgery. *Arthroscopy* 1993;9:33–41.
30. Barrett GR, Richardson K, Ruff CG, et al. The effect of suture type on meniscal repair. *Am J Knee Surg* 1997;10:2–9.
31. Kohn D, Plitz W, Reiss G, et al. Meniscus replacement using a tendon autograft—an experimental study. Paper presented at the meeting of the American Academy of Orthopaedic Surgeons, Anaheim, California, 1991.
32. Mooney MF, Rosenberg TD. Meniscus repair: the inside-out technique. In: *Master techniques in orthopaedic surgery: reconstructive knee surgery.* New York: Raven Press, 1995:69–86.
33. Schulte K, Fu F. Meniscal repair using the inside-to-outside technique. *Clin Sports Med* 1996;15:455–467.
34. Cannon WD, Morgan CD. Meniscal repair. Part II: Arthroscopic repair techniques. *J Bone Joint Surg Am* 1994;76:294–311.
35. Morgan CD. The "all-inside" meniscal repair. *Arthroscopy* 1991;7:120–125.
36. Albrecht-Olsen P, Lind T, Kristensen G, et al. Failure strength of a new meniscus arrow repair technique: biomechanical comparison with horizontal suture. *Arthroscopy* 1997;13:183–187.
37. Rodeo SA, Warren RF. Meniscal repair using the outside-to-inside technique. *Clin Sports Med.* 1996;15:469–481.
38. Reigle CA, Mulhollan JS, Morgan CD. Arthroscopic all-inside meniscus repair. *Clin Sports Med* 1996;15:483–498.
39. Barrett GR, Treacy S, Ruff CG. Preliminary results of the T-fix endoscopic meniscus repair technique in an anterior cruciate ligament reconstruction population. *Arthroscopy* 1997;13:218–223.
40. Austin KS. Complications of arthroscopic meniscal repair. *Clin Sports Med* 1996;15:613–619.
41. DeHaven KE. Meniscus repair in the athlete. *Clin Orthop* 1985;198:31–35.
42. Shelbourne KD, Patel DV, Adsit WS, et al. Rehabilitation after meniscal repair. *Clin Sports Med* 1996;15:595–612.
43. Boss A, Stutz G, Oursin C, et al. Anterior cruciate ligament reconstruction combined with valgus tibial osteotomy (combined procedure). *Knee Surg Sports Traumatol Arthrosc* 1995;3:187–191.
44. Arnoczky SP, Adams ME, DeHaven KE, et al. The meniscus. In: Woo SL-Y, Buckwalter J, eds. *NIAMSAAOS workshop on the injury and repair of the musculoskeletal soft tissues.* Park Ridge, IL: American Academy of Orthopaedic Surgeons, 1988:487–537.
45. Henning CE. Arthroscopic repair of meniscus tears. *Orthopedics* 1983;6:1130–1132.
46. Grood ES. Meniscal function. *Adv Orthop Surg* 1984:193–197.
47. Whipple TL. Arthroscopic surgery: the meniscus rim after operative arthroscopy. *Contemp Orthop* 1984;9:25–32.

48. Metcalf RW. The torn medial meniscus. In: Parisien JS, ed. *Arthroscopic surgery*. New York: McGraw-Hill, 1988:93–110.

49. Ahlback S. Osteoarthritis of the knee: a radiographic investigation. *Acta Radiol* 1968;(suppl 277):5–72.

50. Vellet AD, Marks PH, Fowler PJ, et al. Occult post-traumatic osteochondral lesions of the knee: prevalence, classification and short-term sequelae evaluated with MR imaging. *Radiology* 1991;187:271–276.

51. Thompson RC, Oegema TR, Lewis JL, et al. Osteoarthrotic changes after acute transarticular load. *J Bone Joint Surg Am* 1991;73:990–991,101.

52. Indelicato PA, Bittar ES. A perspective of lesions associated with ACL insufficiency of the knee. *Clin Orthop* 1985;198:77–80.

53. Spindler KP, Schils JP, Bergfeld JA, et al. Perspective study of osseous, articular, and meniscal lesions in recent anterior cruciate ligament rears by magnetic resonance imaging and arthroscopy. *Am J Sports Med* 1993;21:551–557.

54. Noyes FR, Bassett, RW, Groodes ES, et al. Arthroscopy in acute traumatic hemarthrosis of the knee. *J Bone Joint Surg Am* 1980;62:687–757.

55. Dehaven KE. Diagnosis of acute knee injuries with hemarthrosis. *Am J Sports Med* 1980;8:9–14.

56. Fowler PJ, Regan WD. The patient with symptomatic chronic anterior cruciate ligament insufficiency. *Am J Sports Med* 1987;15:321–325.

57. Clancy WG, Shelbourne KD, Zoellner GB, et al. Treatment of knee joint instability secondary to rupture of the posterior cruciate ligament. *J Bone Joint Surg Am* 1983;65:310–322.

58. Fowler PJ, Messieh SS. Isolated posterior cruciate ligament injury in athletes. *Am J Sports Med* 1987;15:553–557.

59. Geissler WB, Whipple TL. Intra-articular abnormalities in association with posterior cruciate ligament injuries. *Am J Sports Med* 1993;21:846–849.

60. Skyhar MJ, Warren RF, Ortiz GJ, et al. The effects of sectioning of the posterior cruciate ligament and the posterolateral complex on the articular contact pressures within the knee. *J Bone Joint Surg Am* 1993;74:694–699.

61. Parolie JM, Bergfeld JA. Long-term results of nonoperative treatment of isolated posterior cruciate ligament injuries in the athlete. *Am J Sports Med* 1986;14:35–38.

62. Torg JS, Barton TM, Pavlov H. Natural history of posterior cruciate ligament–deficient knee. *Clin Orthop* 1989;246:208–216.

63. Outerbridge RE. The etiology of chondromalacia patellae. *J Bone Joint Surg Br* 1961;43:752–757.

64. Dzioba RB. The classification and treatment of acute articular cartilage lesions. *Arthroscopy* 1988;4:72–80.

65. Bauer M, Jackson RW. Chondral lesions of the femoral condyles: a system of arthroscopic classification. *Arthroscopy* 1988;4:97–102.

66. Noyes FR, Stabler CL. A system for grading articular cartilage lesions at arthroscopy. *Am J Sports Med* 1989;17:505–513.

67. Dougados M, Ayral X, Listrat V, et al. The SFA system for assessing articular cartilage lesions at arthroscopy of the knee. *Arthroscopy* 1994;10:69–77.

68. Hopkinson WJ, Mitchell WA, Curl WW. Chondral fractures of the knee: cause for confusion. *Am J Sports Med* 1985;13:309–312.

69. Schmid A, Schmid F. Results after cartilage shaving studied by electron microscopy. Proceedings. *Am J Sports Med* 1987;15:386–387.

70. Terry GC, Flandry F, Van Manen JW, et al. Isolated chondral fractures of the knee. *Clin Orthop* 1988;234:170–177.

71. Messner K, Maletius W. The long term prognosis for severe damage to the weight-bearing cartilage in the knee. *Acta Orthop Scand* 1996;67:165–168.

72. Lysholm J, Gillquist J. Evaluation of knee ligament surgery results with special emphasis on use of a scoring scale. *Am J Sports Med* 1982;10:150–154.

73. Tapper EM, Hoover NW. Results after meniscectomy. *J Bone Joint Surg Am* 1969;51:517–526.

74. Rockborn P, Gillquist J. Outcome of the arthroscopic meniscectomy. *Acta Orthop Scand* 995;66:113–117.

75. Levy AS, Lohnes J, Sculley S, et al. Chondral delamination of the knee in soccer players. *Am J Sports Med* 1996;24:364–369.

76. Maletius W, Lundberg M. Refixation of large chondral fragments on the weight-bearing area of the knee joint: a report of two cases. *Arthroscopy* 1994;10:630–633.

77. Magnuson PB. Joint debridement surgical treatment of degenerative arthritis. *Surg Gynecol Obstet* 1941;73:1–9.

78. Haggart GE. The surgical treatment of degenerative arthritis of the knee joint. *J Bone Joint Surg* 1940;22:717–729.

79. Insall J, Pirdie A. Debridement operation for osteoarthritis of the knee. *Clin Orthop* 1974;101:61–67.

80. Jackson RW. The role of arthroscopy in the management of the arthritic knee. *Clin Orthop* 1974;101:28–35.

81. Sprague NF. Arthroscopic debridement for degenerative joint disease. *Clin Orthop* 1981;160:118–123.

82. Gross DE, Brenner SL, Esformes I, et al. Arthroscopic treatment of degenerative joint disease of the knee. *Orthopedics* 1991;14:1317–1321.

83. Jackson RW, Silver R, Marans H. Arthroscopic treatment of degenerative joint disease [abstract]. *Arthroscopy* 1986;2:114.

84. Ogilvie-Harris DJ, Fitsialos DP. Arthroscopic management of the degenerative knee. *Arthroscopy* 1991;7:151–157.

85. Baumgaertner MR, Cannon WD, Vittori JM, et al. Arthroscopic debridement of the arthritic knee. *Clin Orthop* 1990;253:197–202.

86. Davis PF, Bocell JR, Tullols HS. Arthroscopic treatment in the presence of osteoarthritis of the knee. *Trans Am Acad Orthop Surg* 1990:568. Abstract presented at the *AAOS* Annual Meeting, New Orleans, LA, 1990.

87. Timoney JM, Kneisl JS, Barrack RL, et al. Arthroscopy in the osteoarthritic knee long term follow-up. *Orthop Rev* 1990;19:371–379.

88. Salisbury RB, Nottage WM, Gardner B. The effect of alignment on results in arthroscopic debridement of the degenerative knee. *Clin Orthop* 1985;198:268–272.

89. Johnson L. Arthroscopic abrasion arthroplasty historical and pathological perspective: present status. *Arthroscopy* 1986;2:54–69.

90. Friedman MJ, Berasi CC, Fox JM. Preliminary results with abrasion arthroplasty in the osteoarthritic knee. *Clin Orthop* 1984;182:200–205.

91. Chandler EJ. Abrasion arthroplasty of the knee. *Contemp Orthop* 1985;11:21–29.

92. Fujisawa Y, Masuhara K, Shiomi S. The effect of high tibial osteotomy on osteoarthritis of the knee: an arthroscopic study of 54 knee joints. *Orthop Clin North Am* 1979;10:585–608.

93. Brittberg M, Lidahl A, Nilson A, et al. Treatment of deep cartilage defects of the knee with autologous chondrocyte transplantation. *N Engl J Med* 1994;331:889–895.

94. Bert JM, Maschka K. The arthroscopic treatment of unicompartmental arthrosis: a five year follow-up study of abrasion arthroplasty plus arthroscopic debridement and arthroscopic debridement alone. *Arthroscopy* 1989;5:25–32.

95. Rand J. Role of arthroscopy in osteoarthritis of the knee. *Arthroscopy* 1991;7:358–363.

96. Richards RN, Lonergan RP. Arthroscopic surgery for relief of pain in the osteoarthritic knee. *Orthopedics* 1984;7:1705–1707.

97. Rodrigo JJ, Steadman JR, Silliman JF, et al. Improvement of full thickness chondral defect healing in the human knee after debridement and microfracture using continuous passive motion. *Am J Knee Surg* 1994;7:109–116.

98. Steadman JR, Rodkey WG, Singleton SB, et al. Microfracture techniques for full thickness chondral defects: technique and clinical results. *Oper Tech Orthop* 1997;7:300–304.

99. Burman MS, Finklestein H, Mayer L. Arthroscopy of the knee joint. *J Bone Joint Surg* 1934;16:255–268.

100. Livesley PJ, Doagherty M, Needoff M, et al. Arthroscopic lavage of osteoarthritic knees. *J Bone Joint Surg Br* 1991;73:922–926.

101. Edelson R, Burks RT, Bloebaum RD. Short-term effects of knee washout for osteoarthritis. *Am J Sports Med* 1995;23:345–349.

102. Hsu RW, Himeno S, Coventry MB, et al. Normal axial alignment of the lower extremity and load bearing distribution at the knee. *Clin Orthop* 1990;255:215–223.

103. Galehon DI, Torzilli PA, Warren RF. The role of the posterolateral and cruciate ligaments in the stability of the human knee: a biomechanical study. *J Bone Joint Surg Am* 1987;69:233–242.

104. Grood ES, Stowers SF, Noyes FR. Limits of movement in the human knee: effects of sectioning the posterior cruciate ligament and posterolateral structures. *J Bone Joint Surg Am* 1988;70:88–97.

105. Noyes FR, Barber-Westin SD, Simon R. High tibial osteotomy and lig-

ament reconstruction in varus angulated, anterior ligament cruciate-ligament deficient knees: a two to seven year follow up study. *Am J Sports Med* 1993;21:2–12.

106. Markolf KL, Wascher DC, Finnerman GA. Direct *in vitro* measurements of forces in the cruciate ligaments. Part II: The effect of sectioning the posterolateral structures. *J Bone Joint Surg Am* 1993;75:387–394.

107. Nielsen S, Helmig P. The static stabilizing function of the popliteal tendon in the knee: an experimental study. *Arch Orthop Trauma Surg* 1986;104:357–362.

108. Prodromos CC, Andriachi TP, Galante JO. A relationship between gait and clinical changed following high tibial osteotomy. *J Bone Joint Surg Am* 1985;67:1188–1195.

109. Noyes FR, Barber-Westin SD. Surgical restoration to treat chronic deficiency of the posterolateral complex and cruciate ligaments of the knee joint. *Am J Sports Med* 1996;24:415–426.

110. Dejour H, Neyret P, Boileau P, et al. Anterior cruciate ligament reconstruction combined with valgus tibial osteotomy. *Clin Orthop* 1994;299:220–228.

111. Latterman C, Jakob RP. High tibial osteotomy alone or combined with ligament reconstruction in anterior cruciate ligament-deficient knees. *Knee Surg Sports Traumatol Arthrosc* 1996;4:32–38.

112. Neuschwander DC, Drez D Jr, Paine RM. Simultaneous high tibial osteotomy and ACL reconstruction for combined genu varum and symptomatic ACL tear. *Orthopedics* 1993;16:679–684.

113. O'Neill DF, James SL. Valgus osteotomy with anterior cruciate ligament laxity. *Clin Orthop* 1992;278:153–159.

114. Miller MD, Fu FH. The role of osteotomy in the anterior cruciate ligament-deficient knee. *Clin Sports Med* 1993;12:697–708.

115. Veltri DM, Warren RF. Posterolateral instability of the knee. *Instr Course Lect* 1995;44:441–453.

116. Shives TC, Morrey BF. Alternative reconstructive procedures. In: Morrey BF, ed. *Joint replacement arthroplasty.* New York: Churchill Livingstone, 1991.

117. Coventry MB, Bowman PW. Long term results of upper tibial osteotomy for degenerative arthritis of the knee. *Acta Orthop Belg* 1982;48:139–146.

118. Koshino T, Tsuchiya K. The effect of high tibial osteotomy on osteoarthritis of the knee. Clinical and histological observations. *Orthopedics* 1979;3:37–45.

CHAPTER 27

Ligament Injuries in Children and Adolescents

Henry G. Chambers

Although rare in children and adolescents, ligament injuries about the knee present significant diagnostic and therapeutic challenges. The incidence and severity of the injury depends on the size of the child, their sport, and as the adolescent approaches maturity, possibly even the sex of the child. In this chapter, the epidemiology of knee ligament injuries in children, unique physical examination findings, imaging challenges, and therapeutic approaches to the various ligament injuries are explored.

EPIDEMIOLOGY

There seems to be a spectrum of injuries to the knee in children. Younger children sustain metaphyseal fractures. Teenagers with low-energy trauma may experience anterior cruciate ligament (ACL) rupture, whereas those who have high-energy trauma may have physeal injuries (1). Fractures in the young child may be a representation of their small size and the relatively lower energy imparted in sports. It had been postulated that increased ligamentous laxity (especially in children) would predispose to a greater injury rate. However, Grana and Moretz (2) found no correlation between ligamentous laxity and the occurrence or type of injury.

Alpine or downhill skiing is one of the most dangerous sports for children (3–5). Blitzer et al. (6) found that one fifth of skiing injuries were knee injuries. Deibert et al. (7) performed a large (>3 million skier visits), long-term (12 years) study of skiing injuries in children, adolescents, and adults. The medial collateral ligament injury rate in children from 1981 to 1987 was 20% (51 of 255), decreasing to 7% (19 of 273) for the period from 1987 to 1994. For adolescents, the rate was 9.6% (78 of 813) in the first period and 8.8% (58 of 660) in the second period. One ACL injury occurred between 1981 and 1987 and two occurred between 1987 and 1994. The adolescent age group had a 3.9% incidence of ACL tears in the first period and 4.7% in the second period. These findings compared with a 15.2% to 19% incidence for adults. The investigators felt that the overall 58% decrease in children's accidents was related to the use of properly functioning modern equipment (7). Although most of those who sustain snowboarding injuries are children and adolescents, the incidence of knee injury is significantly lower than for alpine skiing (8–11).

The quick stopping and direction changing in basketball predisposes the knee to ligamentous injuries. Several studies have documented the increased incidence of knee injuries among women who play basketball (12,13). Gray et al. (14) reported a total of 19 ACL ruptures in female players compared with only 4 ACL injuries in male basketball players during the same period. Possible causative factors for this increase in ACL in women may be extrinsic (i.e., body movement, muscular strength, shoe-surface interface, and skill level) or intrinsic (i.e., joint laxity, limb alignment, notch dimensions, and ligament size) (15,16). Loudon et al. (17) found a significant correlation between ACL injuries and knee recurvatum, "navicular drop," and extrinsic subtalar pronation.

Football represents the leading cause of ACL tears in adolescents (18–21). In a survey of coaches from Kentucky, Stocker et al. (22) found an incidence of 0.055 knee injuries per player (257 knee injuries in 4,690 players). Volleyball also has a significant rate of ACL and medial collateral ligament injuries, with the most injuries caused by landing from a jump in the attack zone (23). Soccer is relatively safe, with a rate of 3.7 to 5.6 injuries per 1,000 hours (only one ACL tear) (23,24).

PHYSICAL EXAMINATION

A high index of suspicion must be entertained when evaluating children or adolescents with knee injuries. Many children present late with ligamentous or meniscal injuries because the initial examining physician underestimated the significance of the physical examination findings and a hemarthrosis. The differential diagnosis for a child with an acute hemarthrosis includes ACL tears, tibial spine avulsion fractures, patellar dislocations, osteochondral fractures, meniscal tears, physeal fractures of the distal femur, and medial collateral ligament tears (25). A posterior cruciate ligament (PCL) tear may not demonstrate a large hemarthrosis.

Anterior Cruciate Ligament Injury

The standard physical examination techniques (e.g., Lachman, anterior drawer, pivot shift) used in evaluating adults have the same validity in children (26–28). Although children do have greater ligamentous laxity than adults, a side-to-side comparison usually aids in the diagnosis. Children are often more apprehensive than adults, and it can be difficult to perform these tests, particularly the pivot-shift test. Physical examination of the child under general anesthesia increases its accuracy. Donaldson et al. (29) found that the pivot-shift test was initially positive in only 35% of knees, increasing to 98% under anesthesia. The Lachman test was equally sensitive to examination under anesthesia. The anterior drawer test was positive in 70% of the knees, increasing to 91% under anesthesia. Instrumented analysis (e.g., KT-1000) has a great advantage in the documentation and reproducibility of side-to-side differences. Newer testing equipment designed for children has been introduced and may further aid in the evaluation of children with ACL injuries.

Tibial Spine Avulsion Injuries

Tibial spine avulsion injuries manifest with a large hemarthrosis and with the signs of an ACL injury (e.g., positive Lachman test, positive anterior drawer test). The meniscus (usually medial) may be entrapped in the fracture site. The diagnosis is usually made by the anteroposterior and lateral radiograph results. Radiographs should be obtained as part of the examination of any knee in a child or adolescent with a hemarthrosis. A severe medial ligamentous injury also may be associated with a tibial spine fracture (30).

Patellar Dislocation

Often, the medical history of children is difficult to elicit. Even with ACL injuries, they say that their "knees dislocated." Patellar dislocations are frequently associated with a large hemarthrosis. Tenderness is experienced in the medial peripatellar region, and there is an occasional defect in the retinaculum. There may also be tenderness at the adductor tubercle, indicating a patellofemoral ligament tear.

Osteochondral Fractures

A twisting knee injury or a patellar dislocation can lead to a chondral or osteochondral fracture. A tense hemarthrosis with tenderness over either femoral condyle of a flexed knee may signify an osteochondral fracture. Radiographs, computed tomography (CT), or magnetic resonance imaging (MRI) can be used to help define the lesion and its extent. Chondral lesions are more common in children because the cartilage is thicker and therefore more prone to shear injury. Frequently, the diagnosis is made only at the time of arthroscopy.

Physeal Fractures

Physeal fractures are rare injuries of the distal femur. They must be distinguished from medial collateral ligament or lateral complex injuries in the child. There is usually a tense hemarthrosis with tenderness along the entire distal femur at the physis (i.e., adjacent to the upper pole of the patella or 2 to 3 cm above the joint line). If the fracture is limited to one condyle, tenderness will be greater at the involved physis. Laxity may be identified on varus or valgus stress testing. A diagnosis is usually made on the basis of plain radiographs. Occasionally, stress radiographs may be necessary to distinguish collateral ligament injury from physeal fractures. This is especially true in children and adolescents who have severe soft tissue edema and ecchymosis.

The examiner must also be aware of the relationship between Salter Harris III fractures of the medial femoral condyle and midsubstance ACL tears. Brone and Wroble (31) reported three cases of ACL tears associated with Salter Harris III fractures and found four other cases in the literature (Fig. 27.1).

Meniscal Tears

Meniscal tears are often associated with ACL tears, medial collateral ligament tears, or both, and can lead to a significant hemarthrosis. Popping and especially locking of the knee in slight flexion are important symptoms. Joint line tenderness is very helpful if present, but its absence does not exclude a diagnosis of a meniscal tear. The McMurray test is nonspecific, but a positive result may suggest further investigation. In the very young child, clunking and increased "laxity" on the Lachman test may indicate a discoid meniscus.

Medial Collateral Ligament Injuries

Tenderness of the medial knee at the origin, midsubstance, or insertion of the medial collateral ligament aids in the diagnosis of a ligament strain (grade I). With valgus stress applied to the knee in slight flexion, there may be opening of the joint with a good end point (grade II). If the knee opens medially without an end point, there is a grade III tear with a possibility of a concomitant ACL tear.

Tibial Tubercle Avulsion Injury

A large hemarthrosis occurs when there is an avulsion of the tibial tubercle with the patellar tendon. There is tender-

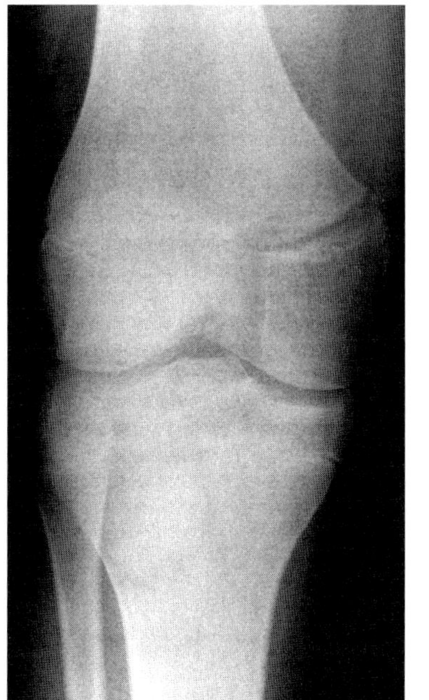
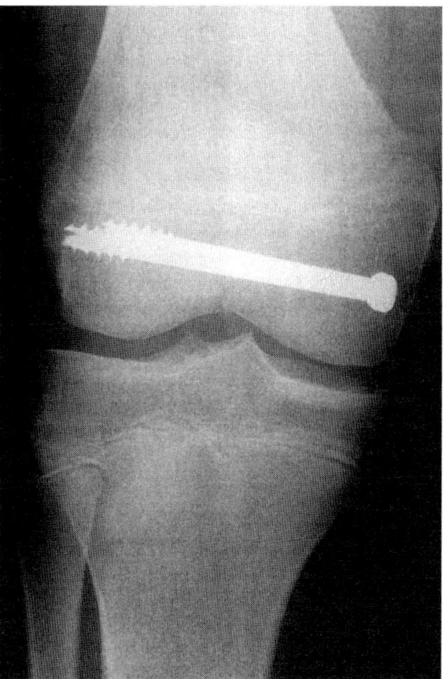

FIGURE 27.1. **A:** Salter Harris III fracture. **B:** After open reduction and internal fixation.

ness and edema over the entire anterior surface of the knee, and crepitus may be present over the tibial tubercle. The patella is often high riding. This injury may be missed on a cursory examination because the finding of patella alta on the lateral radiograph is often subtle. In more extensive fractures, the fracture line may extend posteriorly into the knee joint and include the ACL (Fig. 27.2).

Posterior Cruciate Ligament and Posterolateral Complex Injuries

PCL tears are rare in children. The physical findings are the same as for adults. However, because of their rarity, the injury is often missed at first examination. It is usually diagnosed when the child or adolescent begins

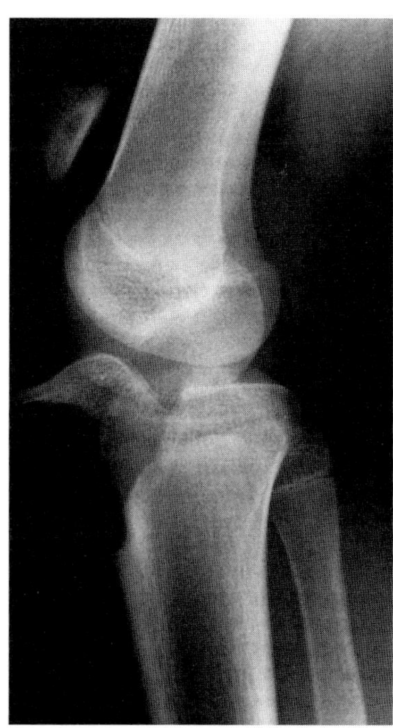
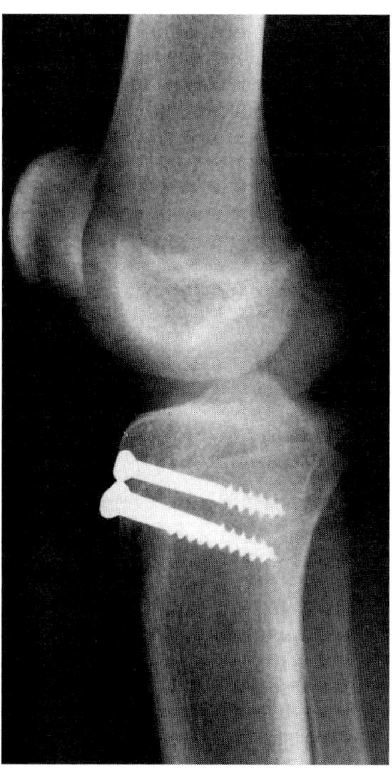

FIGURE 27.2. **A:** Tibial tubercle avulsion injury. **B:** After open reduction and internal fixation.

complaining of pain in the knee and medial joint line symptoms. Children have a higher incidence of bony avulsion fractures from the posterior tibia than adults. These fractures are amenable to open reduction and internal fixation.

IMAGING

Although the history and clinical examination suggest the diagnosis in most cases, imaging studies are often needed. Because of the high incidence of fractures in this age group, at least anteroposterior and lateral radiographs of the knee should be obtained. It is also recommended that a Merchant or sunrise view be obtained to evaluate the patellofemoral joint, looking for osteochondral fractures from the patella or distal femur. A tunnel view should be obtained to evaluate the intercondylar notch and a possible osteochondral fracture. Occasionally, oblique radiographs of the knee are necessary to identify avulsion fractures at the medial and lateral margins of the proximal tibia.

Magnetic resonance imaging can be used to confirm the clinical diagnosis or to make the diagnosis if the clinical diagnosis is in question. Gelb et al. (32), however, found (in adult patients), that MRI was only 95% sensitive and 88% specific for the diagnosis of ACL tears relative to a 100% specificity and sensitivity for clinical examination. The results were even poorer for evaluation of meniscal injuries (82% and 87%) and worse in articular surface damage (33%). They concluded that MRI is unnecessary in most knee disorders and not a cost-effective test (32). It does not appear to be helpful in the grading of medial collateral ligament tears (33). Others have found that MRI is a helpful adjunct in the evaluation of knee injuries (34,35). In studies in which the MRI was used to evaluate knee injuries in children, it was found that, although the MRI might aid in the diagnosis of meniscal injuries, there was still a problem identifying the ACL because of its small size (36,37) or poor sensitivity in finding an ACL tear (64%) (38). Rangger et al. (39) suggested that MRI should be done in all cases in which the clinical diagnosis has been reduced to a suspected meniscal injury. MRI has also been effective in the diagnosis of posterolateral complex injuries of the knee (40), and it is the only way to diagnosis bone bruises or contusions (41,42).

The diagnosis of collateral ligament injuries can be very difficult. There is an inherent laxity in many children, and differentiation between ligamentous and physeal injuries is critical. The use of stress radiographs can be helpful. The best method of performing a radiographic stress test, especially if trying to distinguish between a medial collateral ligament injury and a Salter Harris I fracture of the distal femur, is to place the child supine and tie a belt or strap around the distal thighs with the knees slightly flexed (approximately 20%) over a pillow. The feet are then abducted as the radiograph is taken (Fig. 27.3). This simple test differentiates medial collateral ligament tears, which open at the joint, from a Salter Harris I fracture, which opens at the physis. Other than its use in differentiating physeal fractures from medial collateral ligament tears, stress radiography seems to have little role in the evaluation of acute knee injuries in children. Although it is sensitive in the diagnosis of PCL tears, clinical examination or MRI provides sufficient information (43,44).

My approach to the use of imaging in children's knee injuries is to obtain anteroposterior, lateral, tunnel, and Merchant views of all injured knees. Comparison views may be necessary but are not ordered routinely. Knee pain in children may be referred from hip pathology such as Legg-Calvé-Perthes syndrome or slipped capital

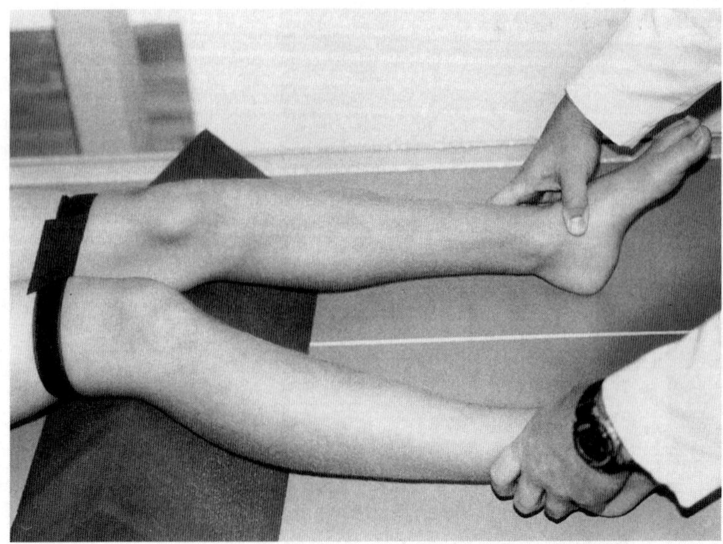

FIGURE 27.3. Technique for performing a stress radiograph to discriminate a medial collateral ligament tear from a physeal injury.

femoral epiphysis, and if there is any doubt, anteroposterior and frog lateral pelvis radiographs should be obtained. Occasionally, the child is uncooperative or too uncomfortable to examine. An examination can be performed 7 to 10 days later. If there is still a question of a ligamentous laxity injury or meniscal tear, an MRI scan can be ordered, with the realization that it may not be the definitive test. Rarely, when it is difficult to distinguish between physeal fractures and a medial collateral ligament tear, stress radiographs can be performed.

ROLE OF ARTHROSCOPY IN CHILDREN

After a complete clinical examination and appropriate injury studies, the diagnosis may still be in doubt. Several studies have addressed this problem in children with hemarthroses. Ure et al. (45) performed arthroscopy in 104 patients younger than 18 years who had hemarthroses. They found that the most frequent diagnosis was patellar dislocation (45% of children and 29% of adolescents). The preoperative diagnosis was shown to be wrong or incomplete in 41% of the children and 24% of the adolescents and in only 36% of the children were meniscal tears suspected before surgery. They concluded that every child with a hemarthrosis of the knee should have arthroscopy (45). Matelic et al. (46) reported similar findings for 21 children, with osteochondral fractures found in 14 (67%) of the patients. Preoperative radiographs failed to identify the fracture in 36% of the patients. The highest incidence of unsuspected pathologic findings from clinical evaluation and standard imaging, coupled with findings of additional pathology (i.e., meniscal tears, osteochondral and chondral fractures, and partial ACL tears), warrants considering diagnostic arthroscopy in all children who have an acute hemarthrosis (47–52).

TREATMENT OF LIGAMENT INJURIES IN CHILDREN

Collateral Ligament Injuries

Medial collateral ligament injuries often occur in conjunction with other ligamentous injuries (e.g., ACL), osteochondral fractures, or meniscal injuries (53). It was once thought that medial collateral ligament injuries could not occur before physeal closure. However, it is clear that medial collateral ligament tears do occur at the origin, midsubstance, or insertion of the ligament (54).

Earlier studies suggested that the injured medial collateral ligament needed to be repaired or at least immobilized, especially in the presence of an ACL tear (54,55). However, later studies suggest that treatment with a cast brace or prefabricated brace with free range of motion can lead to good or excellent results (56–60).

Isolated tears of the medial collateral ligament should be treated by placing the knee in a range of motion brace set from 0° to 90°. After 10 to 14 days, the range of motion can be increased to full flexion. The brace is left in place for 4 to 6 weeks. The knee should be tested for laxity before allowing the child or adolescent to return to cutting activities.

Lateral collateral injuries may have associated bony avulsions or even fibular physeal injuries. These physeal injuries are usually nondisplaced or minimally displaced but should be treated with immobilization in a knee immobilizer or cylinder cast. An ACL tear may be associated with a lateral collateral ligament tear. Associated posterolateral complex injuries must be completely excluded because they often require operative repair, even in children and adolescents.

Posterior Cruciate Ligament Injury

PCL injuries are rare injuries in children and are therefore often missed at the initial evaluation of a knee injury (61). It can be helpful to know the mechanism of injury, which is usually a fall onto a flexed knee, a dashboard injury in a motor vehicle accident, or severe hyperextension (62,63). A PCL injury has been found in a 10-year-old child after a femur fracture (64). The degree of joint effusion is usually less than with an ACL tear, and evaluation of posterior laxity can be difficult in a child (65). Whereas ACL injuries give the patient instability, PCL injuries may be associated with disability from degenerative disease of the medial joint compartment (66,67).

Children have a higher incidence of bony avulsion injuries from the tibial insertion but may also have a bony avulsion of the femur. Anteroposterior, lateral, and oblique radiographs of the knee usually demonstrate the avulsion. Midsubstance tears can be identified with MRI (Fig. 27.4).

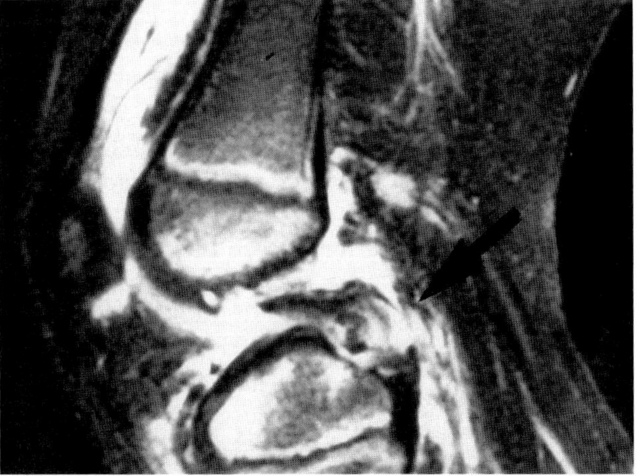

FIGURE 27.4. Magnetic resonance imaging of a 7-year-old child with a midsubstance posterior cruciate ligament tear.

The bony avulsion should be repaired with interepiphyseal sutures or screw fixation (68). Arthroscopies should be performed before prone positioning of the patient because of the high incidence of associated injuries (69). Because the repair of PCL injuries is controversial in adults, it may be prudent to treat the knee with physical therapy (range of motion) and strengthening combined with a PCL brace (keeping the knee in slight flexion) until the child is skeletally mature (70–74).

Combined PCL and posterolateral complex injuries are extremely difficult to treat in adults and in children. There are no natural history studies of children with this injury combination, and the most prudent approach is to perform any surgery (e.g., posterolateral repair, proximal advancement) that does not violate the physis of the femur, tibia, or fibula (75–77). Bracing until skeletal maturity with a reassessment of the functional laxity at that time should be the conservative approach.

Midsubstance Anterior Cruciate Ligament Tears

Although once thought to be rare in children and adolescents, the incidence of ACL tears seems to be rising because of increased awareness or increased sports participation (78,79). It has been found in children as young as 3 years (80–82). It was once thought that most children would sustain a physeal injury rather than an ACL injury. Skak et al. (1) found that low-energy trauma was associated with ligamentous injuries and that high-energy trauma was associated with a physeal injury.

The natural history of ACL tears is not entirely predictable. Some children do well without an ACL, but others are unable to do even simple activities. Many early studies report that this can be a benign injury. However, longer follow-up demonstrates that there was a preponderance of fair to poor results (83–86). Clancy et al. (76) reported the significance of the pivot-shift test as a predictor of the need for ACL reconstruction. When the pivot-shift test was not strongly positive, one half of the patients did well after treatment with a nonoperative program of functional rehabilitation. Patients with unstable knees (i.e., strongly positive pivot-shift test result) had better results after reconstruction.

Several articles have evaluated the effect of ACL injuries in skeletally immature patients. Angel and Hall (47) reviewed 27 patients who had ACL tears. Forty-one percent of the patients had associated pathology, and another 41% had or were recommended to have ACL reconstruction. Mizuta et al. (87) evaluated 18 patients who were skeletally immature and treated conservatively for a mean of 51 months. The modified Lysholm knee score showed one excellent, one good, eight fair, and eight poor results. Only one patient returned to her preinjury level of athletics. Fifty percent had meniscal tears, and radiographic evidence of ligamentous changes were found in 11 of 18 patients. Janarv et al. (88) reported

similar findings, with 68% of their patients requiring ACL reconstruction because of the failure of conservative care (88). Pressman et al. (89) performed a long-term (5-year) retrospective review of 42 children and evaluated the efficacy of treatment and the clinical results of operative and nonoperative management. They found that intraarticular reconstruction provided the best outcome, confirmed by clinical examination and patient satisfaction outcome reports.

Besides the knee instability and inability to participate in sporting activities, there is an increased risk for meniscal tears. Williams et al. (90) found 56% (13 of 24) of their patients had coexistent meniscal tears. Graf et al. (91) reviewed 12 patients with midsubstance tears of the ACL and found that 6 patients had 8 meniscal tears (4 medial and 4 lateral). These young patients were braced, and all developed "giving way" episodes (91).

The primary concern in treating ACL injuries in children is that the most successful reconstructions are intraarticular and require drill holes to be placed in the proximal tibia and distal femur. In children who are not skeletally mature, these drill holes must cross the growth plate or physis. If a bony bridge crosses the physis, a longitudinal or angular growth arrest may occur (92). This concern has provided the backdrop for the controversy surrounding the treatment of ACL injuries in children and adolescents.

There are four primary treatment options for the skeletally immature child or adolescent with an ACL tear: nonoperative; repair of the ligament tear; nonoperative treatment until the child is near or at skeletal maturity, at which time the ACL reconstruction is performed; or ACL reconstruction close to the time of the injury, regardless of age.

Nonoperative treatment does not have a good predictable outcome and carries the possibility of long-term instability, meniscal tears, and degenerative joint disease (85,91,93–99). Another concern with nonoperative treatment is that this population of young athletes is often the most noncompliant group of patients.

Repair of the Anterior Cruciate Ligament

As in adults, it does not appear that repair of the ACL in children leads to a stable knee. DeLee and Curtis (100) compared ACL repair in three children and found that there was a significant degree of ACL laxity at follow-up examination in two of the three patients (100). Engebretsen et al. (101) found that the knees were unstable in five of eight children after 3 to 8 years of follow-up after ACL repair and that all of the children had lower activity levels.

ANTERIOR CRUCIATE LIGAMENT RECONSTRUCTION

The decision to perform an ACL reconstruction must take several factors into account: the goals of the child, the ability to comply with possible preoperative and postoperative activity limitations, the ability to cooperate with the postoperative rehabilitation, their degree of skeletal maturity, the presence of an associated meniscal injury, and the extent to which the ACL instability is affecting their activities of daily living and sporting activities.

Skeletal maturity can be assessed in several ways. In girls, age at menarche provides an important clue to their growth. Girls usually grow for approximately 18 months after menarche. An anteroposterior radiograph of the left hand can be taken to correlate with skeletal maturity using the Greulich and Pyle atlas (102). However, there is a large range of "normal" bone ages at the teenage years using this method. Plain radiographs of the knee can be used to subjectively rate the physis as "wide open" or "approaching maturity." The Tanner scale can be used to stage the sexual maturity of adolescents based on pubic hair and breast development in girls and pubic hair and penis or testes development in boys (Table 27.1).This is often an embarrassing examination for teenagers, and even parents challenge its necessity. Assessment of a recent growth spurt or proximity in height to their parents or siblings can also be used to help assess skeletal maturity.

Patients can be considered skeletally immature if they meet the following criteria: anteroposterior and lateral radiographs of the knee with "wide open" physes, no adolescent growth spurt, patient significantly shorter than older siblings or parents (10 to 15 cm), and the Tanner stage of 1 or 2. The child can be considered mature if he or she has radiographs demonstrating closing physes, had undergone an adolescent growth spurt, is of similar height to siblings and parents (within 2.5 to 5 cm), and the Tanner stage is 4 or 5 (98).

When faced with a child with an ACL-deficient knee, many factors must be considered—not only if and when a reconstruction should be performed, but also what type and technique. McCarroll et al. (98) recommend waiting until the child is almost skeletally mature and then performing the standard patellar tendon graft. Using this technique, they found that 55 of 60 patients were able to return to their previous sport, and 5 were active in less strenuous sports. They had no abnormal growth related to the intraarticular reconstruction (98).

Lo et al. (103) evaluated five patients who had radiographically open physes. Three had reconstructions using hamstring tendons, and two had patellar tendon grafts. They used a 6-mm tibial drill hole and over-the-top positioning of the femur. After a mean of 7.4 years, they had no evidence of limb-length discrepancy and less than 3 mm of anterior–posterior displacement on clinical examination of the knee.

Because of the possibility that bone graft (from the bone–tendon–bone construct of the patellar tendon graft) would cause a growth arrest, many centers have been performing hamstring tendon ACL reconstructions. There is controversy about the best graft material (104,105), and there is much bias in the current literature. Studies have used traditional drill holes through the physes with semitendinosus, gracilis, or both tendons (78,106), drill holes through the tibial physis and a femoral over-the-top position (107), or a technique in which the hamstring graft is placed under the medial meniscus on the tibia and then over-the-top on the femur (108,109). Andrews et al. (110) had good results using a 7-mm, centrally placed allograft (fascia lata or Achilles tendon) combined with an over-the-top femoral placement (Fig. 27.5). My algorithm incorporates both techniques and depends on the age, skeletal maturity, and activity level of the child (Fig. 27.6).

TABLE 27.1. Maturation in adolescence

Stage	Pubic hair	Genitalia	Breasts
Boys			
1	None	Prepubertal penis, testis, and scrotum	
2	Sparse, straight	Enlargement of testes and scrotum, no change in the size of the penis	
3	Darker, curling extends laterally	Enlargement of penis, testes and scrotum	
4	Coarse, curly, does not extend to the thigh	Further growth of testes and scrotum. Increased breadth of penis	
5	Adult Type	Adult size and shape	
Girls			
1	None		Prepubertal, no breast tissue
2	Sparse, straight		Breast bud
3	Darker, curling		Breast mound and areola enlarge
4	Coarse, abundant		Breast enlarged, areola forms mound
5	Adult type, extends to medial thigh		Adult type, areola part of breast contour

Adapted from Tanner JM. Growth at adolescence, Second Ed. Oxford, UK: Blackwell, 1960.

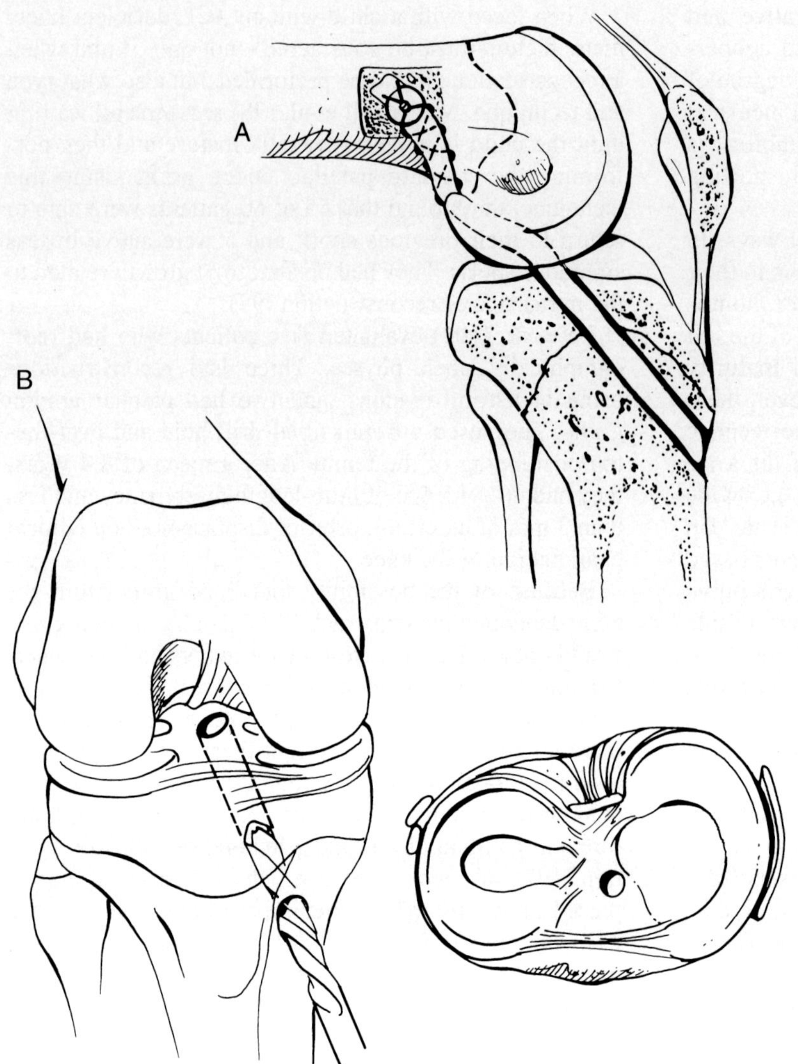

FIGURE 27.5. A: Over-the-top position in the lateral femoral condyle with elevation of the periosteal H flaps and roughening of the femoral cortical trough. **B:** A 7-mm drill hole is made through the anteromedial aspect of the tibia (approximately 3 cm), passing proximal to the epiphyseal plate in the center of the growth plate in a perpendicular fashion and slightly posterior to the anatomic anterior cruciate ligament insertion. (From Andrews M, Noyes FR, Barber-Westin SD. Anterior cruciate ligament allograft reconstruction in the skeletally immature athlete. *Am J Sports Med* 1994;22:48–54, with permission.)

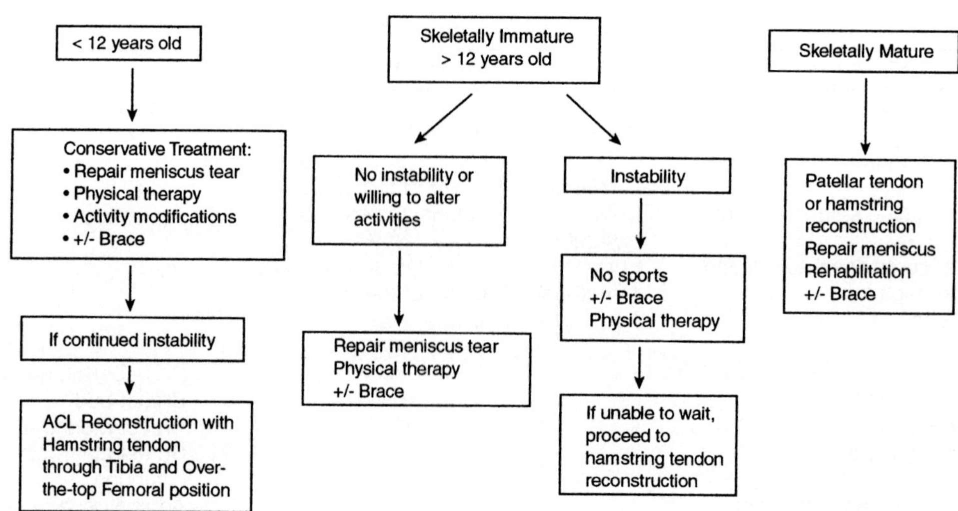

FIGURE 27.6. Treatment of a child with an anterior cruciate ligament (ACL) injury.

TIBIAL SPINE INJURIES

The ACL is attached to the medial tibial spine, which is part of the tibial eminence. With stress, the incompletely ossified tibial eminence fails before the ligament through the cancellous bone of the subchondral plate (111). With this injury, the ACL is often stretched. The fracture may extend into the weight-bearing portion of the tibia (112), and the meniscus may be entrapped under the bony fragment (18,113).

Meyers and McKeever (114) classify these fractures as three basic types: type I is nondisplaced, type II is hinged or partially displaced, and type III is completely displaced. Zaricznyj (115) added type IV to include fractures with comminution of the fragment (Fig. 27.7).

The traditional teaching is that type I and type II fractures can be treated conservatively in slight flexion (20°) (114,116,117), but McClennan (118,119) demonstrated that this position does not reduce the fracture fragment. Most surgeons agree that reduction should be performed in cases of type III or type IV fractures.

However, the method and outcome of reduction is controversial. Treatment of type III and type IV fractures has included open or arthroscopically placed sutures or wire through the epiphysis and the ligament to hold the fragment in place (120–124), percutaneous Kirschner wire placement (118,119,125), or screw fixation (126,127). I prefer performing arthroscopy to evaluate the meniscus, evaluating the ability to reduce the fragment in a closed manner and then performing a mini-open arthrotomy to anatomically repair the fracture to the bed with a nonabsorbable suture through the epiphysis (Fig. 27.8).

Outcome studies have demonstrated that, even with anatomic reduction and regardless of the technique of fixation, there is often residual laxity. Most of the patients are asymptomatic, however. Willis et al. (128) found a 75% incidence of laxity as measured by the KT-1000 arthrometer. Smith (129) evaluated 12 patients who had open reduction and internal fixation and found that all had laxity. Others (88,111,130,131) found similar laxity. Molander et al. (132) did not find any laxity

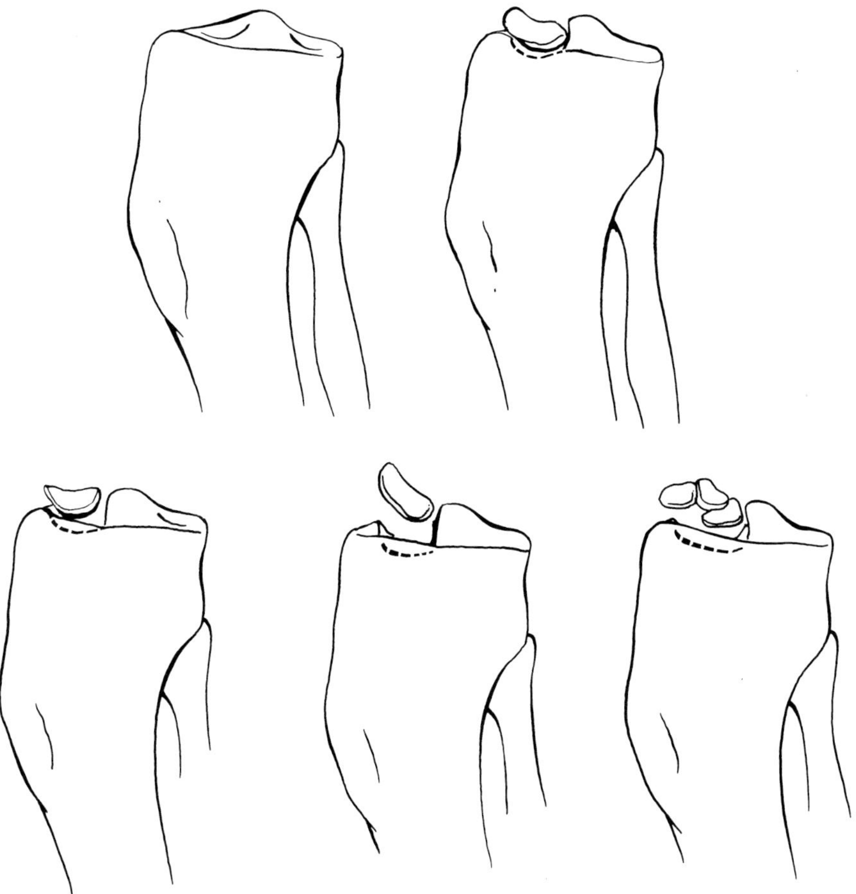

FIGURE 27.7. Classification of intercondylar eminence fractures. (From Zaricznyj B. Avulsion fracture of the tibial eminence: treatment by open reduction and pinning. *J Bone Joint Surg Am* 1977;59:1111–1114, with permission.)

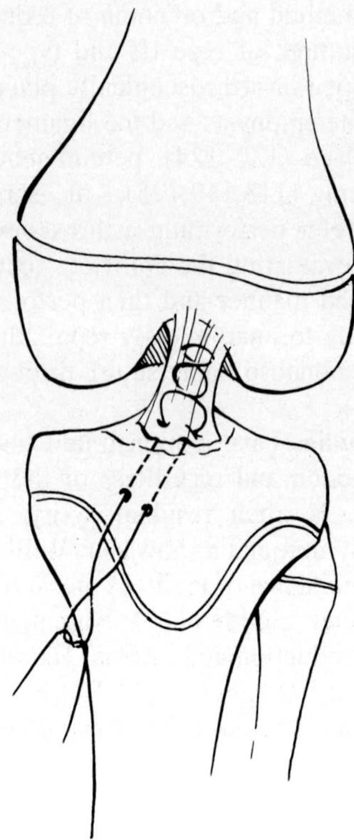

FIGURE 27.8. Method of fixation for an intercondylar eminence fracture.

but did not use instrumented testing. McClennan arthroscopically evaluated type III fractures after they had healed and found that there were often large (>3 mm) displacements. He concluded that, in his patients, there could be long-term morbidity with extension loss, chondromalacia, quadriceps weakness, and ligamentous instability; that the loss of reduction was common after closed reduction; that tibial spine fractures were not reduced by the femoral condyles; and that type III fractures should have open reduction, ACL tensioning, internal fixation, and aggressive rehabilitation (118, 119). In the rare case in which the bone block is so large that there is loss of full extension, a femoral notchplasty (Leuger) or an excision of a wedge of tibial bone can be performed (133).

CONCLUSIONS

The diagnosis and treatment of children's knee ligament injuries are challenging. Open physes, thick articular cartilage, and the developmental issues of childhood and adolescents combine to complicate the care of the injured knee. A careful history and physical examination, judicious use of the appropriate imaging technique, and knowledge of the pathoanatomy can lead the practitioner to the correct diagnosis and treatment.

REFERENCES

1. Skak SV, Jensen TT, Poulsen TD, et al. Epidemiology of knee injuries in children. *Acta Orthop Scand* 1987;58:78–81.
2. Grana WA, Moretz JA. Ligamentous laxity in secondary school athletes. *JAMA* 1978;240:1975–1976.
3. Garrick JG, Requa RK. Injury patterns in children and adolescent skiers. *Am J Sports Med* 1979;7:245–248.
4. Shorter NA, Jensen PE, Harmon BJ, et al. Skiing injuries in children and adolescents. *J Trauma* 1996;40:997–1001.
5. Ungerholm S, Engkvist O, Gierup J, et al. Skiing injuries in children and adults: a comparative study from an 8-year period. *Int J Sports Med* 1983;4:236–240.
6. Blitzer CM, Johnson RJ, Ettlinger CF, et al. Downhill skiing injuries in children. *Am J Sports Med* 1984;12:142–147.
7. Deibert MC, Aronsson DD, Johnson RJ, et al. Skiing injuries in children, adolescents, and adults. *J Bone Joint Surg Am* 1998;80:25–32.
8. Chow TK, Corbett SW, Farstad DJ. Spectrum of injuries from snowboarding. *J Trauma* 1996;41:321–325.
9. Davidson TM, Laliotis AT. Snowboarding injuries, a four-year study with comparison with alpine ski injuries. *West J Med* 1996;164:231–237.
10. Pigozzi F, Santori N, DiSalvo V, et al. Snowboard traumatology: an epidemiologic study. *Orthopedics* 1997;20:505–509.
11. Sutherland AG, Holmes JD, Myers S. Differing injury patterns in snowboarding and alpine skiing. *Injury* 1996;27:423–425.
12. Baker MM. Anterior cruciate ligament injuries in the female athlete. *J Womens Health* 1998;7:343–349.
13. Gomez E, DeLee JC, Farney WC. Incidence of injury in Texas girls' high school basketball. *Am J Sports Med* 1996;24:684–687.
14. Gray J, Taunton JE, McKenzie DC, et al. A survey of injuries to the anterior cruciate ligament of the knee in female basketball players. *Int J Sports Med* 1985;6:314–316.
15. Arendt E, Dick R. Knee injury patterns among men and women in collegiate basketball and soccer. NCAA data and review of literature. *Am J Sports Med* 1995;23:694–701.
16. Hewett TE, Stroupe AL, Nance TA, et al. Plyometric training in female athletes. Decreased impact forces and increased hamstring torques. *Am J Sports Med* 1996;24:765–773.
17. Loudon JK, Jenkins W, Loudon KL. The relationship between static posture and ACL injury in female athletes. *J Orthop Sports Phys Ther* 1996;24:91–97.
18. Chandler JT, Miller TK. Tibial eminence fracture with meniscal entrapment. *Arthroscopy* 1995;11:499–502.
19. DeLee JC, Farney WC. Incidence of injury in Texas high school football. *Am J Sports Med* 1992;20:575–580.
20. Halpern B, Thompson N, Curl WW, et al. High school football injuries: identifying the risk factors. *Am J Sports Med* 1988;16(Suppl 1):S113–S117.
21. Pritchett JW. A claims-made study of knee injuries due to football in high school athletes. *J Pediatr Orthop* 1988;8:551–553.
22. Stocker BD, Nyland JA, Caborn DN, et al. Results of the Kentucky high school football knee injury survey. *J Ky Med Assoc* 1997;95:458–464.
23. Ferretti A, Papandrea P, Conteduca F, et al. Knee ligament injuries in volleyball players. *Am J Sports Med* 1992;20:203–207.
24. Schmidt-Olsen S, Jorgensen U, Kaalund S, et al. Injuries among young soccer players. *Am J Sports Med* 1991;19:273–275.
25. Eiskjaer S, Larsen ST, Schmidt MB. The significance of hemarthrosis of the knee in children. *Arch Orthop Trauma Surg* 1988;107:96–98.
26. Clanton T, Delee JC, Sanders B, et al. Knee ligament injuries in children. *J Bone Joint Surg Am* 1979;61:1195–1201.
27. Jensen JE, Conn RR, Hazelrigg G, et al. Systematic evaluation of acute knee injuries. *Clin Sports Med* 1985;4:295–312.
28. Sandberg R, Balkfors B, Henricson A, et al. Stability tests in knee ligament injuries. *Arch Orthop Trauma Surg* 1986;106:5–7.
29. Donaldson WFD, Warren RF, Wickiewicz T. A comparison of acute anterior cruciate ligament examinations. Initial versus examination under anesthesia. *Am J Sports Med* 1985;13:5–10.
30. Hayes JM, Masear VR. Avulsion fracture of the tibial eminence associated with severe medial ligamentous injury in an adolescent. A case report and literature review. *Am J Sports Med* 1984;12:330–333.
31. Brone LA, Wroble RR. Salter Harris type III fracture of the medial femoral condyle associated with an anterior cruciate ligament tear.

Report of three cases and review of the literature. *Am J Sports Med* 1998;26:581–586.

32. Gelb HJ, Glasgow SG, Sapega AA, et al. Magnetic resonance imaging of knee disorders. Clinical value and cost-effectiveness in a sports medicine practice. *Am J Sports Med* 1996;24:99–103.

33. Schweitzer ME, Tran D, Deely DM, et al. Medial collateral ligament injuries: evaluation of multiple signs, prevalence and location of associated bone bruises, and assessment with MR imaging. *Radiology* 1995;194:825–829.

34. Le Vot J, Solacroup JC, Leonetti P, et al. Correlations between clinical examination/MRI/arthroscopy in the acute traumatic knee [in French]. *J Chir (Paris)* 1994;131:144–153.

35. Ng J, Baron M, Ng AC, et al. Traumatic knee injuries: the accuracy of MRI compared with arthroscopy. *Indiana Med* 1989;82:886–890.

36. King SJ. Magnetic resonance imaging of knee injuries in children. *Eur Radiol* 1997;7:1245–1251.

37. King SJ, Carty HM, Brady O. Magnetic resonance imaging of knee injuries in children. *Pediatr Radiol* 1996;26:287–290.

38. Zobel MS, Borrell JA, Liegel MJ, et al. Pediatric knee MR imaging: pattern of injuries in the immature skeleton. *Radiology* 1994;190:397–401.

39. Rangger C, Klestil T, Kathrein A, et al. Influence of magnetic resonance imaging on indications for arthroscopy of the knee. *Clin Orthop* 1996;330:133–142.

40. Ross G, Chapman AW, Newberg AR, et al. Magnetic resonance imaging for the evaluation of acute posterolateral complex injuries of the knee. *Am J Sports Med* 1997;25:444–448.

41. Engebretsen L, Arendt E, Fritts HM. Osteochondral lesions and cruciate ligament injuries. MRI in 18 knees. *Acta Orthop Scand* 1993;64:434–436.

42. Snearly WN, Kaplan PA, Dussault RG. Lateral-compartment bone contusions in adolescents with intact anterior cruciate ligaments. *Radiology* 1996;198:205–208.

43. Harilainen A, Myllynen P, Rauste J, et al. Diagnosis of acute knee ligament injuries: the value of stress radiography compared with clinical examination, stability under anaesthesia and arthroscopic or operative findings. *Ann Chir Gynaecol* 1986;75:37–43.

44. McPhee IB, Fraser JG. Stress radiography in acute ligamentous injuries of the knee. *Injury* 1981;12:383–388.

45. Ure BM, Tiling T, Roddecker K, et al. Arthroscopy of the knee in children and adolescents. *Eur J Pediatr Surg* 1992;2:102–105.

46. Matelic TM, Aronsson DD, Boyd DW Jr, et al. Acute hemarthrosis of the knee in children. *Am J Sports Med* 1995;23:668–671.

47. Angel KR, Hall DJ. Anterior cruciate ligament injury in children and adolescents. *Arthroscopy* 1989;5:197–200.

48. Harvell JC Jr, Fu FH, Stanitski CL. Diagnostic arthroscopy of the knee in children and adolescents. *Orthopedics* 1989;12:1555–1560.

49. Haus J, Refior HJ. The importance of arthroscopy in sports injuries in children and adolescents. *Knee Surg Sports Traumatol Arthrosc* 1993;1:34–38.

50. Kloeppel-Wirth S, Koltai JL, Dittmer H. Significance of arthroscopy in children with knee joint injuries. *Eur J Pediatr Surg* 1992;2:169–172.

51. Stanitski CL, Harvell JC, Fu F. Observations on acute knee hemarthrosis in children and adolescents. *J Pediatr Orthop* 1993;13:506–510.

52. Vahasarja V, Kinnuen P, Serlo W. Arthroscopy of the acute traumatic knee in children. Prospective study of 138 cases. *Acta Orthop Scand* 1993;64:580–582.

53. Garvin GJ, Munk PL, Vellet AD. Tears of the medial collateral ligament: magnetic resonance imaging findings and associated injuries. *Can Assoc Radiol J* 1993;44:199–204.

54. Bradley GW, Shives TC, Samuelson KM. Ligament injuries in the knees of children. *J Bone Joint Surg Am* 1979;61:588–591.

55. Hastings DE. The non-operative management of collateral ligament injuries of the knee joint. *Clin Orthop* 1980;147:22–28.

56. Lundberg M, Messner K. Long-term prognosis of isolated partial medial collateral ligament ruptures. A ten-year clinical and radiographic evaluation of a prospectively observed group of patients. *Am J Sports Med* 1996;24:160–163.

57. Mok DW, Good C. Non-operative management of acute grade III medial collateral ligament injury of the knee: a prospective study. *Injury* 1989;20:277–280.

58. Petermann J, von Garrel T, Gotzen L. Non-operative treatment of acute medial collateral ligament lesions of the knee joint. *Knee Surg Sports Traumatol Arthrosc* 1993;1:93–96.

59. Reider B. Medial collateral ligament injuries in athletes. *Sports Med* 1996;21:147–156.

60. Reider B, Sathy MR, Talkington J, et al. Treatment of isolated medial collateral ligament injuries in athletes with early functional rehabilitation. A five-year follow-up study. *Am J Sports Med* 1994;22:470–477.

61. Moyer RA, Marchetto PA. Injuries of the posterior cruciate ligament. *Clin Sports Med* 1993;12:307–315.

62. Mayer PJ, Micheli LJ. Avulsion of the femoral attachment of the posterior cruciate ligament in an eleven-year-old boy. *J Bone Joint Surg Am* 1979;61:431–432.

63. Sanders W, Wilkins K, Neidre A. Acute insufficiency of the posterior cruciate ligament in children. *J Bone Joint Surg Am* 1980;62:129–131.

64. Goodrich A, Ballard A. Posterior cruciate ligament avulsion associated with ipsilateral femur fracture in a 10-year-old child. *J Trauma* 1988;28:1393–1396.

65. Rubenstein RA, Shelboursneck A, McCarroll JR, et al. The accuracy of the clinical examination in the setting of posterior cruciate ligament injuries. *Am J Sports Med* 1994;4:550–557.

66. Bickerstaff DR. Posterior cruciate ligament injuries. *Br J Hosp Med* 1997;58:129–133.

67. Boynton MD, Tietjens BR. Long-term followup of the untreated isolated posterior cruciate ligament-deficient knee. *Am J Sports Med* 1996;24:306–310.

68. Satku K, Chew CN, Seow H. Posterior cruciate ligament injuries. *Acta Orthop Scand* 1984;55:26–29.

69. Loos WC, Fox JM, Blazina ME, et al. Acute posterior cruciate ligament injuries. *Am J Sports Med* 1981;9:86–92.

70. Fowler PJ, Messieh SS. Isolated posterior cruciate ligament injuries in athletes. *Am J Sports Med* 1987;15:553–557.

71. Hughston JC, Bowden JA, Andrews JR, et al. Acute tears of the posterior cruciate ligament. Results of operative treatment. *J Bone Joint Surg Am* 1980;62:438–450.

72. Moore HA, Larson RL. Posterior cruciate ligament injuries. Results of early surgical repair. *Am J Sports Med* 1980;8:68–78.

73. Richter M, Kiefer H, Hehl G, et al. Primary repair for posterior cruciate ligament injuries. An eight year follow-up of fifty-three patients. *Am J Sports Med* 1996;24:298–305.

74. Strand T, Molster AO, Engesaeter LB, et al. Primary repair in posterior cruciate ligament injuries. *Acta Orthop Scand* 1984;55:545–547.

75. Baker CL, Norwood LA, Hughston JC. Acute combined posterior cruciate and posterolateral instability of the knee. *Am J Sports Med* 1984;12:204–208.

76. Clancy WG Jr, Ray JM, Zoltan DJ. Acute tears of the anterior cruciate ligament. Surgical versus conservative treatment. *J Bone Joint Surg Am* 1988;70:1483–1488.

77. Noyes FR, Barber-Westin SD. Surgical restoration to treat chronic deficiency of the posterolateral complex and cruciate ligaments of the knee joint. *Am J Sports Med* 1996;24:415–426.

78. Nottage WM, Matsuura PA. Management of complete traumatic anterior cruciate ligament tears in the skeletally immature patient: current concepts and review of the literature. *Arthroscopy* 1994;10:569–573.

79. Sullivan JA. Ligament injury of the knee in children. *Clin Orthop* 1990;255:44–50.

80. Corso SJ, Whipple TL. Avulsion of the femoral attachment of the anterior cruciate ligament in a 3-year-old boy. *Arthroscopy* 1996;12:95–98.

81. Eady JL, Cardenas CD, Sopa D. Avulsion of the femoral attachment of the anterior cruciate ligament in a seven-year-old child. A case report. *J Bone Joint Surg Am* 1982;64:1376–1378.

82. Schaefer RA, Eilert RE, Gillogly SD. Disruption of the anterior cruciate ligament in a 4-year-old child. *Orthop Rev* 1993;22:725–727.

83. Engstrom B, Gornitzka J, Johansson C, et al. Knee function after anterior cruciate ligament ruptures treated conservatively. *Int Orthop* 1993;17:208–213.

84. Fetto JF, Marshall JL. The natural history and diagnosis of anterior cruciate ligament insufficiency. *Clin Orthop* 1980;147:29–36.

85. Kannus P, Jaervinen M. Knee ligament injuries in adolescents: 8 year follow-up of conservative management. *J Bone Joint Surg Br* 1988;70:772–776.

86. Sandberg R, Balkfors B, Nilsson B, et al. Operative versus non-operative treatment of recent injuries to the ligaments of the knee. A prospective randomized study. *J Bone Joint Surg Am* 1987;69:1120–1126.

87. Mizuta H, Kubota K, Shiraishi M, et al. The conservative treatment of complete tears of the anterior cruciate ligament in skeletally immature patients. *J Bone Joint Surg Br* 1995;77:890–894.

88. Janarv PM, Nystrom A, Werner S, et al. Anterior cruciate ligament injuries in skeletally immature patients. *J Pediatr Orthop* 1996;16:673–677.

89. Pressman AE, Letts RM, Jarvis JG. Anterior cruciate ligament tears in children: an analysis of operative versus nonoperative treatment. *J Pediatr Orthop* 1997;17:505–511.

90. Williams JS Jr, Abate JA, Fadale PD, et al. Meniscal and nonosseous ACL injuries in children and adolescents. *Am J Knee Surg* 1996;9:22–26.

91. Graf BK, Lange RH, Fujisaki CK, et al. Anterior cruciate ligament tears in skeletally immature patients: meniscal pathology at presentation and after attempted conservative treatment. *Arthroscopy* 1992;8:229–233.

92. Guzzanti V, Falciglia F, Gigante A, et al. The effect of intra-articular ACL reconstruction on the growth plates of rabbits. *J Bone Joint Surg Br* 1994;76:960–963.

93. Barrack RL, Buckley SL, Bruckner JD, et al. Partial versus complete acute anterior cruciate ligament tears. The results of nonoperative treatment. *J Bone Joint Surg Br* 1990;72:622–624.

94. Kannus P, Jarvinen M. Conservatively treated tears of the anterior cruciate ligament. Long-term results. *J Bone Joint Surg Am* 1987;69:1007–1012.

95. Lehnert M, Eisenschenk A, Zellner A. Results of conservative treatment of partial tears of the anterior cruciate ligament. *Int Orthop* 1993;17:219–223.

96. Lipcomb AB, Anderson AF. Tears of the anterior cruciate ligament in adolescents. *J Bone Joint Surg Am* 1986;68:19–28.

97. McCarroll JR, Rettig AC, Shelbourne KD. Anterior cruciate ligament injuries in the young athlete with open physes. *Am J Sports Med* 1988;16:44–47.

98. McCarroll JR, Shelbourne KD, Porter DA, et al. Patellar tendon graft reconstruction for midsubstance anterior cruciate ligament rupture in junior high school athletes. An algorithm for management. *Am J Sports Med* 1994;22:478–484.

99. Shelbourne KD, Patel DV, McCarroll JR. Management of anterior cruciate ligament injuries in skeletally immature adolescents. *Knee Surg Sports Traumatol Arthrosc* 1996;4:68–74.

100. DeLee JC, Curtis R. Anterior cruciate ligament insufficiency in children. *Clin Orthop* 1983;172:112–118.

101. Engebretsen L, Svenningseen S, Beaum P. Poor results of anterior cruciate ligament repair in adolescence. *Acta Orthop Scand* 1988;59:684–686.

102. Greulich W, Pyle S. *Radiographic atlas of skeletal development of the hand and wrist.* Stanford, CA: Standford Press, 1959.

103. Lo IK, Kirkley A, Fowler PJ, et al. The outcome of operatively treated anterior cruciate ligament disruptions in the skeletally immature child. *Arthroscopy* 1997;13:627–634.

104. Aglietti P, Buzzi R, Zaccherotti G, et al. Patellar tendon versus double semitendinosus and gracilis tendons for anterior cruciate ligament reconstruction. *Am J Sports Med* 1994;22:211–217.

105. Steiner ME, Hecker AT, Brown CH Jr, et al. Anterior cruciate ligament graft fixation. Comparison of hamstring and patellar tendon grafts. *Am J Sports Med* 1994;22:240–246.

106. Matava MJ, Siegel MG. Arthroscopic reconstruction of the ACL with semitendinosus-gracilis autograft in skeletally immature adolescent patients. *Am J Knee Surg* 1997;10:60–69.

107. Karlson JA, Steiner ME, Brown CH, et al. Anterior cruciate ligament reconstruction using gracilis and semitendinosus tendons. Comparison of through-the-condyle and over-the-top graft placements. *Am J Sports Med* 1994;22:659–666.

108. Brief LP. Anterior cruciate ligament reconstruction without drill holes. *Arthroscopy* 1991;7:350–357.

109. Parker AW, Drez D Jr. Anterior cruciate ligament injuries in patients with open physes. *Am J Sports Med* 1994;22:44–47.

110. Andrews M, Noyes FR, Barber-Westin SD. Anterior cruciate ligament allograft reconstruction in the skeletally immature athlete. *Am J Sports Med* 1994;22:48–54.

111. Wiley JJ, Baxter MP. Tibial spine fractures in children. *Clin Orthop* 1990;255:54–60.

112. Pellacci F, Mignani G, Valdiserri L. Fractures of the intercondylar eminence of the tibia in children. *Ital J Orthop Traumatol* 1986;12:441–446.

113. Bursten DB, Viola A, Fulkerson JP. Entrapment of the medial meniscus in a fracture of the tibial eminence. *Arthroscopy* 1988;4:47–50.

114. Meyers MH, McKeever FM. Fracture of the intercondylar eminence of the tibia. *J Bone Joint Surg Am* 1970;52:1677–1684.

115. Zaricznyj B. Avulsion fracture of the tibial eminence: treatment by open reduction and pinning. *J Bone Joint Surg Am* 1977;59:1111–1114.

116. Driessen MJ, Winkelman PA. Fractures of the intercondylar eminence of the tibia in childhood. *Neth J Surg* 1984;36:69–72.

117. Oostvogel HJ, Klasen HJ, Reddingius RE. Fractures of the intercondylar eminence in children and adolescents. *Arch Orthop Trauma Surg* 1988;107:242–247.

118. McLennan JG. Lessons learned after second-look arthroscopy in type III fractures of the tibial spine. *J Pediatr Orthop* 1995;15:59–62.

119. McLennan JG. The role of arthroscopic surgery in the treatment of fractures of the intercondylar eminence of the tibia. *J Bone Joint Surg Br* 1982;64:477–480.

120. Brunelli G. Fractures of the intercondylar tibial eminence. *Ital J Orthop Traumatol* 1978;4:5–12.

121. Kogan MG, Marks P, Amendola A. Technique for arthroscopic suture fixation of displaced tibial intercondylar eminence fractures. *Arthroscopy* 1997;13:301–306.

122. Matthews DE, Geissler WB. Arthroscopic suture fixation of displaced tibial eminence fractures. *Arthroscopy* 1994;10:418–423.

123. Perez CL, Garcia SG, Gomez CF. The arthroscopic knot technique for fracture of the tibia in children. *Arthroscopy* 1994;10:698–699.

124. Prince AR, Moyer RA. Arthroscopic treatment of an avulsion fracture of the intercondylar eminence of the tibia. Case report. *Am J Knee Surg* 1995;8:114–116.

125. Bale RS, Banks AJ. Arthroscopically guided Kirschner wire fixation for fractures of the intercondylar eminence of the tibia. *J R Coll Surg Edinb* 1995;40:260–262.

126. Lubowitz JH, Grauer JD. Arthroscopic treatment of anterior cruciate ligament avulsion. *Clin Orthop* 1993;294:242–246.

127. Mirbey J, Besancenot J, Chambers RT, et al. Avulsion fractures of the tibial tuberosity in the adolescent athlete. Risk factors, mechanism of injury, and treatment. *Am J Sports Med* 1988;16:336–340.

128. Willis RB, Blokker C, Stoll TM, et al. Long-term follow-up of anterior tibial eminence fractures. *J Pediatr Orthop* 1993;13:361–364.

129. Smith JB. Knee instability after fractures of the intercondylar eminence of the tibia. *J Pediatr Orthop* 1984;4:462–464.

130. Bachelin P, Bugmann P. Active subluxation in extension, radiological control in intercondylar eminence fractures in childhood. *Z Kinderchir* 1988;43:180–182.

131. Baxter MP, Wiley JJ. Fractures of the tibial spine in children. An evaluation of knee stability. *J Bone Joint Surg Br* 1988;70:228–230.

132. Molander ML, Wallin G, Wikstad I. Fracture of the intercondylar eminence of the tibia: a review of 35 patients. *J Bone Joint Surg Br* 1981;63:89–91.

133. Fyfe IS, Jackson JP. Tibial intercondylar fractures in children: a review of the classification and the treatment of mal-union. *Injury* 1981;13:165–169.

CHAPTER 28

Complications of Knee Ligament Surgery

Raymond A. Sachs, Alan M. Reznik, Dale M. Daniel, and Mary Lou Stone

Knee ligament surgery has many risks. However, for the athlete participating in high-risk sports, joint instability commonly results in repeated injury, progressive impairment, and joint damage, and knee ligament surgery is often indicated. Table 28.1 presents the incidence of complications associated with knee ligament surgery using two sources of information: a review of all complications

TABLE 28.1. *Complications of knee ligament surgery*

Complication	Incidence		
	Literature	SD1	SD2
Anesthetic mortality	0.01%	0%	0%
Vascular injury	0.01%	0%	0%
Cutaneous nerve injury	50%	NS	NS
Major nerve injury	0%	0%	0.005%
Tourniquet palsy	22–100%[a]	NS	NS
DVT and PE (clinical)	3.5%	0.75%	0.25%
Skin necrosis	2%	0.75%	0%
Superficial infection	4%	NS	2.5%
Deep infection	1.6%	1.5%	0.1%
Reflex sympathetic dystrophy	0%	0%	0%
Secondary procedure for stiffness	4%	7%	0.8%
Graft impingement	NS	3%	1%
Flexion contracture	32%	20%[b]	1%
Patella femoral pain	32%	19%	NS
Quadriceps weakness	47%	62%[c]	NS
Effusion	13%	12%	NS
Knee pain	15–65%[d]	NS	NS
Extensor disruption	1%	0%	0.2%
Growth plate disturbance	8%	0%	0%
Secondary procedure within 6 mo	NS	10%	2.5%

NS, not studied or insufficient data.

[a]Estimates based on reports in patients undergoing arthrotomy for nonligamentous surgery.

[b]Prone heel height difference = 5 cm.

[c]Quadriceps strength <80% of contralateral normal knee.

[d]Represents knee pain from all sources combined.

from knee ligament surgery reported in the orthopedic literature before the year 2000 and the clinic records and follow-up evaluations of ligament surgery performed at the San Diego Kaiser Hospital between 1983 and 2000. The San Diego patients were divided into two groups for the purpose of this presentation. The SD1 group consists of 390 patients with a mixture of open and arthroscopically assisted anterior cruciate ligament (ACL) and multiple ligament reconstructions performed between 1983 and 1988 and using multiple graft sources. Most patients were immobilized in flexion and instructed to avoid bearing weight on the limb after surgery. The SD2 group consists of 1,354 patients with arthroscopic ACL reconstructions performed between 1990 and 2000 and using bone–patellar tendon–bone (BPTB) as the graft source. These patients were immobilized in full extension and allowed weight bearing as tolerated with range of motion outside the brace four times per day.

ANESTHETIC MORTALITY

Anesthetic mortality in knee ligament surgery has been reported in the literature (1–7). Lunn et al. (1) reviewed anesthetic complications in all types of surgery in Cardiff, Wales, between 1972 and 1977 (n = 108,878). Lunn et al. (1) constructed five overall risk categories based on the subjective assessment of the patient's degree of overall illness. The categories were nearly identical to the American Society of Anesthesiologists (ASA) classification (2). There were 197 deaths. The results of this study can be summarized as follows:

Anesthesia believed causative of death: 1 case per 10,000 patients

Anesthesia partly or totally causative of death: 2 case per 10,000 patients

Deaths related at all to anesthesia: 5 cases per 10,000 patients

These figures are probably applicable to a general orthopedic surgery practice. However, patients undergoing knee ligament surgery are the youngest and healthiest segment of the population (ASA class I or II). ASA class I and II patients make up more than 80% of all patients (1–3) but suffer less than 40% of anesthetic deaths (4). In this special subgroup, the mortality due to anesthesia is no greater than 0.5 deaths per 10,000 patients. There were no major anesthetic complications in SD1 or SD2.

VASCULAR INJURIES

There were no cases of vascular injuries in SD1 or SD2. Hohf's (8) 1960 survey of vascular injuries in orthopedic operations identified 352 cases in 1,163 responses. Sixty-one were associated with knee injury. Knee surgery vascular injuries resulted in 21 amputations, which represented 34% of reported vascular injuries to the knee. Arthrotomy represented more than one half of the cases (32 patients), and tourniquet-induced thrombosis was responsible for 2 cases. The popliteal artery was injured in 85% of the cases. The remaining 15% of the injuries around the knee were divided among the anterior tibial, posterior tibial, genicular, and recurring collateral arteries.

There are several reports of vascular injury associated with knee dislocation (9,10). McCoy (10) reported four cases of low-velocity knee dislocations with vascular injuries, only one of which had overt signs of vascular disruption. Three of the four cases were sports injuries. This study points out that intimal tears may be present with distal pulses intact. The investigators recommend an arteriogram in all cases of knee dislocation, regardless of the presence of peripheral pulses. The possibility of a knee dislocation should be considered when dealing with multiple ligament injuries.

Green (9) evaluated 245 knee dislocations and found a 32% incidence of popliteal artery injury. In knees with a straight anterior or posterior dislocation, 40% were associated with a vascular lesion. When the artery was not explored (19 cases), 89% of the injuries resulted in amputation. There were uniformly poor results and an 85% amputation rate if exploration and repair was performed after 8 hours. When repair was done within 8 hours, there was an 87% limb-salvage rate. They attributed these findings to irreversible changes occurring after 6 to 8 hours of ischemia. They recommended early exploration and repair along with prophylactic fasciotomy in all cases of vascular injury after dislocation.

There are several reports of vascular injury after arthroscopic surgery. DeLee's survey (11) of 118,590 cases revealed 9 cases of vascular injury, representing approximately 1% of all complications (11). Four of the nine cases resulted in amputations. Jeffries (12) reported two cases of popliteal artery injury after partial lateral meniscectomy. He cautions against the cavalier use of power suction shavers in the posterior lateral compartment of the knee. Popliteal artery aneurysm has been reported after meniscectomy (13). Meniscal repairs are also associated with vascular injury when the posterior lateral meniscus is involved (10).

Roth and Bray (14) reported a vascular complication from placing an artificial ligament in the over-the-top position. An arteriogram revealed a sharp cutoff of the popliteal artery. The artery was found trapped between the ligament graft and bone when the popliteal fossa was explored. The limb's vascularity was restored by bypassing the entrapment with a saphenous vein graft.

FLUID EXTRAVASATION AND COMPARTMENT SYNDROME

Fruensguaard and Holm (15) reported compartment syndrome as a complication of arthroscopy. Noyes and Spievak (16) studied fluid dissection that can occur with flexion of a knee distended for the purpose of arthroscopy. In 300 clinical cases, they saw this on four occasions with rapid resolution after tourniquet release. They reported that fluid could dissect by the path of the semimembranous bursa, beneath the pes anserinus, and into the calf muscles, even with an intact knee capsule. In cadaveric specimens, they demonstrated that extravasation of fluid can cause an elevation of pressure in the calf compartments high enough to initiate a compartment syndrome. Cadaveric studies by Peek and Haynes (17) revealed that the presence of a capsular defect elevated compartment pressures 80 mm above normal. In swine hind limbs, the pressure elevation caused by saline extravasation had returned to normal within 15 minutes after the tourniquet was released in the side without a capsular defect. In the swine model with a capsular defect, the pressure remained greater than 40 mm Hg for at least 8 hours after the tourniquet was released. Histologic studies of the limbs tested 8 days after pressurization revealed fibrous replacement of intracompartmental muscles on the capsular defect side, but no changes in the limb without a capsular defect. The results imply that extravasation with a capsular tear can cause compartment syndrome and tissue death. This experimental result is analogous to compartment syndrome in humans, because pressures within a compartment greater than 30 to 40 mm Hg are considered diagnostic of compartment syndrome in the clinical setting (18–20).

Compartment syndrome has not been reported as a result of ligament reconstruction in the literature. However, in SD2, one case of ACL reconstruction was aborted because of intraoperative compartment syndrome caused by fluid extravasation into the calf. The clinician should be aware of this possible complication and monitor the size, swelling, and circulatory status of the limb intraoperatively and postoperatively. When the diagnosis is entertained, prompt compartment pressure measurements should be made and fasciotomy performed when indicated.

NEUROLOGIC INJURY IN KNEE LIGAMENT SURGERY

Incision Nerve Injury

Probably no aspect of knee ligament surgery receives less attention than the simple act of making a skin incision, but the occurrence of postoperative numbness, dysesthesia, or painful neuromas after a median parapatellar incision is common. In the words of Kummel (21), "The current management of the infrapatellar branch of the saphenous nerve in knee surgery resembles the old saying about the weather: Everybody talks about it but nobody does anything."

The saphenous nerve becomes subcutaneous above the medial side of the knee, where it emerges behind the tendon of the sartorius muscle. It gives off one or more infrapatellar branches that curve forward to supply the anteromedial part of the leg below the knee and run downward with the great saphenous vein to give off a series of medial cutaneous branches (22). The infrapatellar nerve is rarely a single nerve and usually consists of a plexus or multiple rami, which extend above and below the joint line on the medial aspect of the knee, frequently crossing over extensively into the lateral side of the knee. No incision on the medial side of the knee can be assured of avoiding the nerve (21,23). Swanson (24) reported that 63% of 87 patients undergoing open medial meniscectomy showed immediate dysesthesia after the operation and that dysesthesia persisted in 44.4% at 6 months. Johnson and Kettlecamp (25) reported 76 patients who had medial arthrotomies and 18 patients who had lateral arthrotomies. Of the patients with medial incisions, 54% had sensory loss, which in 30% was irritating and disabling to some extent. Of the patients with lateral incisions, 33% had sensory loss, but only 11% complained of irritation or hypersensitivity. The problem of damage to the infrapatellar branch of the saphenous nerve may extend beyond numbness or dysesthesia. Poehling et al. (26), in an examination of 35 patients with clinically significant reflex sympathetic dystrophy of the knee, found evidence of insult to the infrapatellar branch of the saphenous nerve in all patients. They suggested that patients with persistent, nonmechanical pain syndromes of the knee often have had trauma to the infrapatellar branch of the saphenous nerve, and in a high percentage of these patients, vasomotor abnormalities can be demonstrated.

Damage to superficial nervous structures is most likely to occur at two points during knee ligament surgery. First, damage to the infrapatellar branch of the saphenous nerve may occur during a medial arthrotomy incision or midline prepatellar incision, particularly if no attempt is made to isolate rami during the superficial dissection. Second, cutaneous branches of the saphenous nerve proceeding distally in the leg may be damaged during repair of the tibial insertion of the medial collateral ligament or during harvesting of the semitendinosus or gracilis tendons or during medial meniscus repair. It is likely that a certain incidence of damage to superficial nerves on the medial side of the knee is unavoidable during complex knee ligament surgery. However, use of laterally based skin incisions whenever possible and careful dissection in the region of the sartorius tendon and muscle can limit morbidity.

Nerve Injury in Arthroscopic Procedures

In a nationwide review commissioned by the Arthroscopy Association of North America, DeLee (11) reported 63 neurologic injuries in 118,590 arthroscopies. In a review of 2,640 arthroscopic procedures done by a large, experienced group of arthroscopists, neurologic injury was reported in 0.7% of patients (27). Reports of injury to the saphenous nerve during arthroscopically assisted meniscus repair vary from 1% to 22% of cases (28–30). Injury to the peroneal nerve has been reported less often but was damaged in 1 of 96 meniscal repairs performed by Miller (29). Avoidance of neurologic injury during arthroscopic meniscus repair may be accomplished by adopting a "semi-open" technique, always inserting a retractor in a posterolateral or posteromedial incision of the knee so as to protect the respective neurovascular structures at risk (31).

Nerve Injury from Tourniquet Use

Cushing (32) described the pneumatic tourniquet in 1904. Its use in knee ligament surgery is now taken for granted. The sparsity of reports on adverse effects from tourniquet use has no doubt fostered the impression that it is without risk. However, it is likely that large numbers of patients incur transient nerve injury during knee ligament surgery, but complete recovery occurs within a few days to a few weeks.

Ochoa et al. (33) reported the delayed recovery of peripheral nerves after surgery is the result of a slowly resolving axonal compression syndrome caused by the pneumatic tourniquet. Their studies revealed a conduction block or reduced conduction velocity at the site of the tourniquet, with normal conduction velocities being maintained in nerve fibers distal to the tourniquet. Histologic studies showed local demyelination under the tourniquet with preservation of axonal continuity. They concluded that the nerve lesion associated with tourniquet use occurs at the edge of the cuff and consists of longitudinal shearing of the axon in relation to the Schwann cell as a result of the pressure gradient caused by the tourniquet. In most cases, this lesion is reversible.

Fowler et al. (34) produced confirmatory data. By maintaining a cuff pressure of 1,000 mm Hg in baboons for 1 to 3 hours, he produced a consistent paralysis of distal muscles lasting up to 3 months. There was a significant correlation between the duration of compression and subsequent conduction block. When cuff pressure was reduced to 500 mm Hg, similar but lesser changes occurred. Rorabeck and Kennedy (35) performed an experimental study in dogs, varying pneumatic tourniquet pressure from 250 to 500 mm Hg and varying the time of application from 1 to 2 hours. Impairment of sciatic nerve conduction velocity occurred with *every* tourniquet application, regardless of pressure and duration of application. In all cases, recovery occurred after release of the tourniquet. The rate of recovery was related to pressure and time.

Dobner and Nitz (36) prospectively studies 24 patients undergoing meniscectomy with the use of a tourniquet and compared them with 24 patients undergoing meniscectomy without the use of a tourniquet. Their results showed that 71% of patients in the tourniquet group had electromyographic (EMG) evidence of denervation and a functional capacity of 39% of the normal leg when tested 6 weeks after surgery. No patient in the control group had evidence of denervation, and at 6 weeks, the average functional capacity was 79%. In a similar study, Saunders et al. (37) observed 48 patients after meniscectomy. Thirty patients (38) demonstrated EMG abnormalities after arthrotomy. Eighty-five percent of the patients with tourniquet times longer than 60 minutes had abnormal EMG patterns. Seventy-one percent had abnormalities with times of 30 to 60 minutes, 58% with times of 15 to 30 minutes, and 22% with times of less than 15 minutes.

There are few reports of tourniquet problems associated with ACL reconstruction in the literature. Guanche (39) reported an isolated case of tourniquet-induced tibial nerve palsy during an unremarkable ACL reconstruction. No other such cases have been reported nor observed in our own series. Hooper et al. (40) randomized 30 ACL reconstructions to 2 groups. One group was operated with a tourniquet, and the second group had reconstructions done without a tourniquet. They reported no difference in the duration of surgery or postoperative pain as measured by opioid consumption. Daniel et al. (41) retrospectively evaluated 94 patients in 2 groups; one group had ACL reconstruction under tourniquet control, and the second group had reconstruction without a tourniquet. Quadriceps strength recovery was delayed in the tourniquet group at the 6- and 12-week examinations. However, there was no difference between the two groups at the 1-year evaluation.

Early postoperative weakness of quadriceps function after knee ligament surgery has often been attributed to pain inhibition or lack of motivation. Delayed recovery may be the result of an axonal compression syndrome caused by the pneumatic tourniquet or may be caused by direct muscle injury induced by muscle compression (37,42,43). Clinical studies have shown that the degree of conduction block is related to increased pressure and increased duration of tourniquet application. Surgeons therefore should minimize the tourniquet pressure and the time that the tourniquet is used. The use of wider tourniquets may allow lower cuff inflation pressures and decrease muscle and nerve injury (44).

DEEP VEIN THROMBOSIS

Venous thromboembolic disease is the leading cause of death among patients who survive at least 7 days after trauma (45). Although the incidence of venous thromboembolic disease has been studied after meniscectomy and after total-knee replacement, there are few studies of the incidence of thrombotic or embolic complications after knee ligament surgery. Cullison et al. (46) prospectively studied 67 patients after ACL reconstruction using compression ultrasonography 2 to 3 days after surgery. Patients were studied from the popliteal vein to the inguinal ligament. Only one patient had a thrombosis in the femoral vein, and the thrombus was absent at repeat examination on postoperative day 10.

Clinical risk factors for the development of venous thrombosis may include advanced age, previous venous thromboembolism, malignant disease, cardiac failure, prolonged immobilization, obesity, and varicose veins (47). However, the subject of risk factors remains controversial. Stulberg et al. (48), in a review of 638 total-knee replacements, found no high-risk population. Cohen et al. (49) found no significant differences in venous thrombosis with patient age, sex, corticosteroid therapy, spinal versus general anesthesia, or tourniquet time. Only previous venous thromboembolic disease was predictive of increased risk. McKenna et al. (50) found that patients who had taken preoperative aspirin or other nonsteroidal antiinflammatory medications had a significantly lower incidence of thromboembolism after total-knee arthroplasty than their unmedicated counterparts. They found no other significant differences between the two groups.

An overview of the literature indicates that the incidence of deep vein thrombosis (DVT) increases with increasing complexity of the operation and with increasing age. Reports of DVT after arthroscopic surgery range from 0.1% to 1.6% (11,51,52). With knee arthrotomy, an incidence as low as 8% was reported by Nilsen et al. (53) in their study of patients 20 to 35 years old, whereas an incidence of 57% was reported by Cohen et al. (49) for older patients undergoing knee arthrotomy for degenerative disease. For patients undergoing total-knee arthroplasty, there is general agreement that the incidence of DVT is high, with rates of 46% to 72% reported (48,50,54,55).

Patients undergoing knee ligament surgery are usually young, athletic, and healthy. They have none of the risk factors identified by Kakkar et al. (47) and by Hull and Raskob (56), except for the possible adverse effect of postoperative immobilization. It is not surprising that thromboembolic disease after knee ligament surgery is rarely reported. However, the preponderance of research indicates that, even in this most favored population, some patients develop silent, postoperative DVT. It is likely that most thrombi are small and localized in the calf. Although rare, a sudden, fatal, pulmonary embolus originating from the lower extremity and occurring without premonitory clinical signs may be the most common cause of mortality after knee ligament surgery.

One case of clinically evident DVT was observed in SD1, as well as one case of nonfatal pulmonary embolus. In SD2, there were two clinical cases of DVT and one nonfatal pulmonary embolus.

KNEE INFECTION

Deep sepsis can be a devastating complication of ACL reconstruction. McAllister et al. (57) reported a series of 831 ACL reconstructions. Four (0.48%) of the 831 developed deep sepsis. Risk factors associated with sepsis were thought to be previous knee surgery and associated meniscal repair. Williams and Warren (58) reported their series of 2,500 arthroscopically assisted ACL reconstructions at the Hospital for Special Surgery. Seven (0.3%) of their patients had postoperative sepsis. Six of seven had concomitant open procedures such as meniscal repair, medial collateral ligament, or posterolateral corner reconstruction

In SD1, there were six infections (1.5%). Three infections were superficial. All superficial infections centered on a screw with spiked washer used to attach a hamstring graft to the proximal tibia. Two infections manifested as failures to heal the distal end of the tibial wound. The infection resolved with the use of oral antibiotics and removal of the fixation device, which was performed 7 and 12 weeks after the initial surgery. One knee remained stable, and instability recurred in the other. The third superficial infection followed a blow to the anterior aspect of the knee 6 months after surgery, with wound breakdown over the screw and soft tissue washer. After the fixation device was removed and the patient was placed on oral antibiotics, the infection resolved, and the knee remained stable. Three infections were deep. None occurred within 8 weeks of ligament surgery. All occurred after a secondary arthrotomy procedure.

In one case, the infection followed an open procedure, with lateral release performed to gain joint motion 2 months after an acute patellar tendon–ACL reconstruction. Two weeks after the secondary open procedure, the patient presented with chills, fever, and pyarthrosis, a sample of which was cultured and grew *Staphylococcus aureus*. The patient was treated with open débridement, intravenous antibiotics, a rotation flap for secondary wound closure, and a split-thickness skin graft to the donor site. The patient's infection resolved, and she regained good knee function.

A second case developed after an arthroscopic procedure to gain range of motion was performed 7 months after an acute medial collateral ligament repair and hamstring graft–ACL reconstruction. This was the patient's fourth secondary procedure performed to gain joint motion,

including an arthrotomy 6 months after the ligament surgery. Three days after the arthroscopy, the patient presented with a pyarthrosis, a cultured sample of which grew *Bacteroides fragilis* and *S. aureus*. Open wound débridement was performed, and antibiotics were administered intravenously. The infection resolved, but the patient developed a painful arthrofibrosis in 20° of flexion.

The third deep infection developed after a procedure to retension an over-the-top, 8-mm, polypropylene-patellar tendon composite graft 6 months after the index procedure. Two weeks after the secondary procedure, the patient presented with chills and fever. Joint aspiration was cultured and grew *Staphylococcus epidermidis*. The composite graft was removed. An iliotibial band procedure was performed (59) at the time of the graft removal. The patient was placed on intravenous antibiotics, and the infection resolved.

In SD2, 34 patients (2.5%) were placed on oral antibiotics for wound "cellulitis." One additional patient had infection around the tibial screw, necessitating removal. Only one patient (0.1%) had pyarthrosis. This patient ultimately required metal and graft excision to bring his infection under control.

REFLEX SYMPATHETIC DYSTROPHY OF THE KNEE

Reflex sympathetic dystrophy (RSD) is an accepted term for a disorder that includes a constellation of symptoms with a wide array of causes (60–62). Classically, it manifests in any extremity as hypersensitivity to painful stimuli associated with cool, mottled skin; limb atrophy; osteoporosis; increased vascularity of the limb; and restricted range of motion. Clinical situations associated with RSD include injuries involving soft tissues, fractures, treatment of fractures (particularly cast immobilization), surgical procedures of any type, and nerve trauma. The incidence of classic RSD after trauma to the hand or foot is 0.9% (62). An examination of 3,000 knee injuries (most without surgical pathology) yielded 14 cases of RSD, a 0.5% incidence rate (63). Our review of knee ligament reconstruction literature did not discover reports of RSD. There were no cases diagnosed in SD1 or SD2.

GRAFT COMPLICATIONS

Graft Donor Site Complications

The most common autograft tissues used for ACL are the hamstring tendons and the middle one third of the patellar tendon. Donor graft site morbidity should be considered when planning ligament graft surgery.

Complications of bone patellar tendon bone reconstruction have been reported. There are 13 cases of patella fracture in the literature, with approximately one half occurring in the immediate postoperative period and the other one half occurring up to 1 year after surgery (64). There are

10 reported cases of patellar tendon rupture after ACL reconstruction using BPTB autograft. All cases occurred within 10 months of surgery (65). Three cases of tibial fracture at the site of graft harvest are also reported in the literature (66–68), as well as two cases of femoral fracture at the site of femoral graft fixation (69,70).

Cabaud et al. (71) evaluated the patellar tendon in dogs after using the middle one third for ACL reconstruction. They reported no loss of strength at 4 months and increased strength at 8 months after reconstruction. However, in a similar study using dogs (n = 22), Burks et al. (72) reported the patellar tendon strength after harvesting the middle one third to be 70% of the control side at 3 months and 60% at 6 months. The cross-sectional area of the tendon was larger than the control side at 3 and 6 months, and histologic examination revealed poor collagen organization. Burks et al. (72) harvested the middle third of the patellar tendon and closed the prepatellar fascia, but not the defect. At 3 and 6 months, the mean tendon length was 10% shorter than the control side. Paulos et al. (73) reported symptomatic patella baja resulting from patella tendon graft harvest for ACL surgery.

The effect of harvesting the patellar tendon on patellofemoral morbidity was discussed by Huegel and Indelicato (74) in a 6-month comparison of allograft versus autograft. In the allograft group, 68% (15 of 22) were asymptomatic and had 80% quadriceps strength. Only 20% (5 of 25) in the autograft group had 80% quadriceps strength, and 60% had donor site or patellofemoral discomfort. A different view was offered by Rubinstein et al. (75) and by Shelbourne and Trumper (76). They studied 20 patients who had a BPTB graft harvested from the contralateral knee. All had full range of motion at 3 weeks. None demonstrated contractures or patella baja. Quadriceps strength averaged 69% by 6 weeks, 93% at 1 year, and 95% at the 2-year follow-up assessment. No anterior knee pain or soreness was experienced by any patient at the 1-year examination. The investigators concluded that harvesting BPTB autograft, by itself, was the source of only minimal morbidity.

Patellar tendon and hamstring tendons were the most common graft sources in SD1. Table 28.2 provides the data 1 year after surgery on 180 patients who were sorted

TABLE 28.2. *Evaluation 1 year after ACL reconstruction (n = 180)*

| | Graft source | | | |
| | Patella tendon | | Hamstring tendon(s) | |
Postoperative flexion (degrees)	30[b]	0[a]	30[b]	0[a]
Number	60	56	45	19
Age (mean)	25	26	23	26
Surgery within 6 wk of injury	7 (12%)	15 (27%)	21 (47%)	5 (26%)
Flexion contracture[c]				
Mean	4	2	4	1
5°	19 (32%)	6 (6%)	11 (24%)	0
Flexion loss >10°	4 (7%)	0	4 (9%)	0
Patellar irritability >1[d]	5 (8%)	0	3 (7%)	0
Quadriceps index[e]				
Mean	61	74	75	81
<80	49 (82%)	30 (54%)	25 (49%)	7 (37%)
Flexion index[e]				
Mean	75	97	88	88
<90	27 (45%)	15 (27%)	22 (49%)	10 (53%)
Hop index[e]				
Mean	75	81	83	84
<90	45 (45%)	36 (64%)	28 (62%)	7 (37%)
KT-1000 30°				
20-lb anterior				
Mean	1.5	1.8	2.7	2.2
>2.5	20 (33%)	17 (30%)	23 (51%)	10 (53%)
Manual maximum				
Mean	2.9	3.2	2.8	3.6
>2.5	29 (48%)	35 (63%)	25 (56%)	12 (63%)
>5.0	8 (13%)	8 (14%)	9 (20%)	3 (16%)

[a]Postoperative immobilization in 0° of flexion and postoperative program.
[b]Postoperative immobilization in 20–30° of flexion for 3 wk followed with a range of motion brace or hinged cast for an additional 3 to 4 wk with a range of motion of 20–100°.
[c]Flexion contracture measured as prone heel height difference, 1 cm = 1 degree.
[d]There were no contralateral knees with patella irritability >1.
[e]Quadriceps, flexion, and hop index are expressed in relation to the contralateral normal knee (injured/normal × 100).

into four groups based on the graft source and postoperative rehabilitation program. The graft source used in surgery was selected by the surgeon. The hamstring was often selected as the graft source in the less athletic patient having an ACL reconstruction in association with a meniscus repair. The patellar tendon was usually selected for patients involved in high-risk sports or for patients with greater joint instability. Despite the fact that the patient groups are dissimilar, the data are of interest. In the patellar tendon group, a higher percentage of patients had flexion contracture, quadriceps weakness, and poor hop function. Using a hamstring tendon graft source did result in decreased knee flexion strength, but overall, it appeared to result in less morbidity. However, by KT-1000 measurements, better stability was obtained with the patellar tendon graft.

BPTB was the graft source in SD2. We had two patella fractures. One occurred during graft harvest and was immediately fixed, and the second fracture occurred 6 weeks after surgery and required secondary surgery.

Allograft Reconstruction

Allograft reconstruction has gained a measure of popularity, mainly because of ease of reconstruction and ease of postoperative rehabilitation. Bone, tendon, and ligament tissue appear to provoke only a minimal immune response, allowing their transplantation without the need for preoperative tissue typing or postoperative immune suppression. However, allograft implantation is not without problems. Several basic science studies have shown that allograft is not as rapidly remodeled or incorporated into host tissue as comparable allograft (77–81). The use of allograft raises other issues and potential disadvantages such as scarcity, potential for disease transmission, and cost-effectiveness (78).

Allograft sterilization and preservation constitute a complex issue. Previously, it was common for freeze-dried allograft to be preserved in ethylene oxide. Unfortunately, after transplantation, a high failure rate ensued, along with a characteristic persistent synovial reaction and chronic inflammatory response. Ethylene chlorhydrin, a toxic reaction product of ethylene oxide, could be found within the allograft and within the synovium for up to 14 months (82,83).

It is common for fresh-frozen allografts to be sterilized using gamma irradiation. High doses of gamma irradiation (4 mrad) have been effective in eradicating the human immunodeficiency virus. Unfortunately, the dose level required for 100% eradication of the virus causes degradation of the biomechanical properties of the graft such that it becomes unsuitable for ACL reconstruction. Lower levels of gamma irradiation (1.5 to 2.5 mrad) are now commonly used. At these levels, the graft loses approximately 15% of its biomechanical strength, but it is still in the acceptable range for implantation (84).

Many studies comparing the results of allografts with those of autografts have been published (85–89). Shelton et al. (85) randomized 60 patients with patella tendon grafts. They examined patients at 3, 6, 12, and 24 months and found no difference in patellofemoral pain, swelling, range of motion, or KT-1000 measurements at any time. There was no difference in patellofemoral crepitus or thigh circumference at 12 and 24 months. Twenty percent of the allograft group was found to have a pivot shift at 24 months, compared with 7% of the autograft group. Victor et al. (86) compared 48 autografts with 25 allografts and found no difference in any measurement at 24 months. However, there were three repeat ruptures in the allograft group and none in the autograft group. Stringham et al. (87) re-examined 47 autografts and 31 allografts at an average of 3 years after surgery. There had been four repeat ruptures in the allograft group, but no other substantial differences were observed between the groups.

Allograft ligament reconstruction is an acceptable substitute for autograft in most patients. However, because allograft incorporates more slowly into the host than autograft and because allograft loses some of its mechanical strength during the sterilization process, allograft ACL reconstruction has a somewhat higher rate of failure than comparable autograft surgery. On the positive side, allograft does appear to result in less loss of quadriceps function within the first 3 months of surgery, but this is balanced by the slight chance of infectious disease transmission and the significantly greater expense involved with these grafts.

POSTOPERATIVE GRAFT IMPINGEMENT

Postoperative impingement of the ACL graft in the intercondylar notch may block full extension or may produce a chafing of the graft that can weaken it with resulting disruption. Graft impingement is predominantly affected by placement of the tibial tunnel. Anterior or lateral placement of the tibial tunnel may result in graft impingement unless a notchplasty is performed (see Chapter 21B). Yaru et al. (90) observed that anterior tibial translation produced by active extension of the knee caused graft impingement in a greater flexion arc than could be produced with passive knee extension. They recommended that with passive motion there should be a 2-mm clearance between the anterior portion of the intercondylar notch and the ligament graft to avoid impingement when the patient actively extends.

Lane et al. (91) reported 12 cases (3%) that postoperatively demonstrated an audible and palpable "thunk" as the patient extended his or her knee. The thunk was rarely painful, but in the more severe cases, it was annoying. In no patient could the thunk be produced by passively extending the leg. In six cases, the thunk was annoying enough that the patients consented to arthroscopic surgery. Arthroscopy was performed under local anesthesia so the knee could be actively extended to produce the thunk. In all six patients, arthroscopy revealed impingement of the graft on the anterior, lateral, or both walls of the intercondylar notch, and the condition was reduced or eliminated by excising bone to open the anterior portal of the intercondylar notch.

At the 6-month follow-up assessment, 12 cases (1%) of thunking were identified in SD2. For 11 of these patients, the problem resolved after arthroscopic notchplasty. The 12th patient changed insurance providers and was lost to follow-up.

JOINT STIFFNESS

The goal of ligament reconstruction is to restore normal knee kinematics. A knee with a 10° flexion contracture is probably a greater impairment than the usual knee with an ACL disruption. The past decade has seen a dramatic change from prolonged postoperative rehabilitation in flexion to immobilization in complete extension and aggressive resumption of range of motion. As a result, the incidence of postoperative joint stiffness has been markedly diminished (92,93). Cosgarea et al. (94) retrospectively analyzed 188 ACL reconstructions. The postoperative protocol changed over 4 years from immobilization in 45° of flexion for 1 week, to immobilization in 45° of flexion but with motion started at 48 hours, and to bracing in full extension with motion started at 24 hours after surgery. The incidence of arthrofibrosis diminished from 23% to 3% as rehabilitation became more aggressive. The investigators also found a diminished incidence of arthrofibrosis when surgery was delayed more than 3 weeks from the time of injury. Dandy and Edwards (95) reported their series of 194 patients. Diminished postoperative knee extension was directly correlated with the position of postoperative immobilization. In their series, 59% of patients immobilized in flexion had a postoperative flexion contracture, whereas only 2.5% of patients immobilized in extension lacked full extension. All persistent cases of flexion contracture eventually came to arthroscopy. In every case, the surgeons found soft tissue in the intercondylar notch (i.e., cyclops lesion) blocking full extension, and removal solved the patient's problem. The study's authors postulate that most blocks to full extension are mechanical in nature and that true arthrofibrosis is rare.

Paulos et al. (73) reported stiffness of the knee after surgery caused by fibrous hyperplasia of the anterior soft tissues of the knee, including the anterior fat pad, and shortening of the patellar tendon. Paulos et al. (73) emphasized the importance of early patella mobilization to prevent development of the condition.

After properly performed ligament surgery followed by short periods of bracing in extension, mobilization of the limb with passive stretching and active range of motion usually restore joint motion. Occasionally, manip-

ulation under anesthesia, arthroscopic release of adhesions (96,97), and open surgery are necessary (73,98). We have found the Exercycle to be a useful range of motion device.

Mohtadi et al. (99) reviewed 527 ACL reconstructions and reported that 37 patients (7%) were manipulated because they failed to gain a satisfactory range of motion. A satisfactory range of motion was defined as 10° to 120° by 3 months after surgery. In a comparison between the manipulated and nonmanipulated patients, researchers reported no statistically significant differences between the two groups in relation to age, sex, knee, meniscal repair, or performance of a concomitant medial collateral ligament repair. They reported that manipulation was needed by 11% (25 of 228 cases) if surgery was done less than 6 weeks after injury, compared with 4% (12 of 299 cases) if the surgery was done 6 or more weeks after injury.

Our experience was similar (Table 28.3). In SD1, a range of motion procedure under anesthesia was performed on 27 patients (7%) within 12 months of the ligament surgery. There were 329 patients in SD1 who had single-ligament ACL reconstruction surgery only. Sixteen (5%) of those patients had postoperative manipulation under anesthesia. There were 61 patients in SD1 with multiple-ligament repairs, and 11 (18%) of those patients had manipulation, a significantly higher rate than for the single-ligament surgery group ($p < 0.005$). Nine percent of patients (12 of 132) who had ACL reconstruction within 6 weeks of injury had manipulation, but only 2% (4 of 197) who had ACL reconstruction greater than 6 weeks after injury had manipulation ($p < 0.005$).

In SD2, only 10 patients (0.8%) required secondary surgery for stiffness, perhaps reflecting the positive effects of many current advances in surgery and rehabilitation.

CYCLOPS LESION

In 1990, Dandy and Edwards (95) published results of their study of a series of 13 patients with loss of extension after BPTB reconstruction. They described the consistent arthroscopic finding of a soft tissue nodule in the intercondylar notch, which they called a *cyclops lesion*. Since then, Dandy's findings have been confirmed by others. Marzo et al. (100) reported 21 patients with restricted knee extension at an average of 4 months after surgery. All had fibrous nodules occupying the intercondylar notch. Removal of the cyclops lesion resulted in resolution of the flexion contracture in all cases. Histologic evaluation of the cyclops lesion revealed dense fibroconnective tissue with occasional fibrocartilage elements.

In SD2, three patients (0.2%) were found to have a cyclops lesion. Arthroscopic resection led to successful resolution of flexion contracture in all cases.

FLEXION CONTRACTURE, PATELLOFEMORAL PAIN, AND QUADRICEPS WEAKNESS

Flexion contracture, patellofemoral pain, and quadriceps weakness are the three most common complications of knee ligament surgery. They are implicated in suboptimal results after ACL reconstruction and are causes for patient dissatisfaction.

Flexion Contracture

Before 1986, patients in SD1 were immobilized in 30° of flexion for 3 weeks after surgery and then placed in a hinged cast or brace with a 30-degree extension stop for another 3 to 5 weeks. Evaluation 1 year after surgery revealed that 30 (29%) of 105 patients had a flexion contracture of more than 5°, measured as a prone heel height difference of more than 5 cm. (Referenced to 0° of extension, 16 patients [15%] had a flexion contracture of more than 5°.) There was a positive correlation between flexion contracture, patellar irritability, quadriceps weakness, and impairment on the same one-leg hop for distance (Fig. 28.1). There was a positive correlation between flexion contracture and age (107).

Since 1986, the operated knee has been braced in extension. The incidence of flexion contracture in SD1 patients with patellar tendon grafts dropped from 32% to 11% ($p < 0.005$) and, in hamstring graft patients, from 24% to 0% ($p < 0.01$) (Table 28.2). In SD2, the incidence of flexion contracture dropped markedly to less than 1% (10 of 1,354), again reflecting the favorable marriage of arthroscopic technique, bracing in extension, early weight bearing, and passive range of motion.

Patellofemoral Pain

A 1982 San Diego Kaiser retrospective review of 36 patients with normal patellofemoral joints at the time of surgery revealed that only one third had normal patellofemoral clinical examination results 1 year after surgery. Of the remaining patients, one third had anterior knee crepitus but no pain, and the other third had anterior knee crepitus and anterior knee pain. A later review of 126 postoperative patients found a 19% incidence of patellofemoral pain (101). Correlations between patellar symptoms and other factors are presented in Figure 28.1. The effects of patellar irritability and knee flexion contracture were found to be additive in their effect on quadriceps strength. One year after surgery, 17 (94%) of 18 patients with a flexion contracture of more than 5° and an irritable patella had quadriceps strength of less than 80% of the contralateral knee, compared with 18 (54%) of 33 patients with a flexion contracture of less than 6° and no patella irritability. As shown in Table 28.2, 8% of knees immobilized after surgery in 30° of flexion had moderate to severe patellar irritability (i.e., discomfort

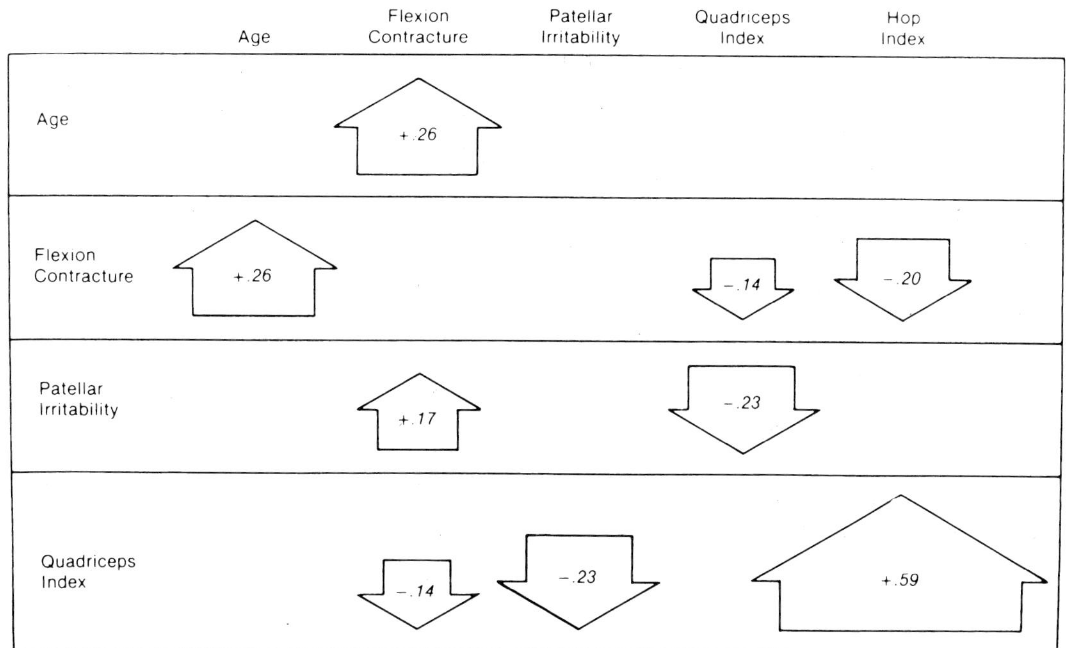

FIGURE 28.1. Evaluation of 126 patients 1 year after anterior cruciate ligament reconstruction. Patients were treated by postoperative cast immobilization in 30° of flexion for 3 weeks, followed by a range of motion brace with a 30° extension stop for 3 to 5 weeks. *Arrows* indicate statistically significant ($p < 0.01$) correlations. The value within each arrow states the extent of the correlation. Positive correlations are indicated as arrows pointing up, and negative correlations are indicated by arrows pointing down. Flexion contracture is defined as a prone heel height difference of more than 5 cm.

TABLE 28.3. *Secondary procedures within 12 months of ligament surgery*

Indication	Patients	Manipulation closed	Arthroscopy	Other operative procedures
Single-ligament ACL surgery (n = 329)				
Limited range of motion	16	20	2	2
Fixation failure	3			3
Chronic effusion	4		4	1
Metal removal	2			2
Graft impingement	3		3	
Skin graft	2			2
Infection	2		1	1
Total	32 (10%)	20	10	11
Multiple-ligament surgery (n = 61)				
Limited range of motion	11	11	5	2
Infection				1
Total	11 (18%)			

with patellar manipulation), but none of the 75 patients immobilized in 0° of flexion had moderate or severe patellar irritability. In no patient did the contralateral knee have moderate or severe patellar irritability.

Quadriceps Weakness

Quadriceps weakness is the single most common problem reported after ACL reconstruction. It was reported by 47% of patients in our literature review. In 180 of the patients in SD1, peak extension torque at 60 degrees/second was measured 1 year after surgery and compared with the normal, contralateral knee. One hundred eleven patients (62%) had quadriceps strength of less than 80% of the contralateral normal knee. An additional test used to compare limb function was the one-leg hop for distance. This test evaluates strength and confidence in the tested leg (see Chapter 26). The hop for distance on the operated knee by 116 patients (64%) was less than 90% of that on the contralateral normal knee. As demonstrated in Figure 28.1, there is a positive correlation between quadriceps weakness and a flexion contracture. Patients immobilized postoperatively at 0° of flexion had less flexion contracture and greater quadriceps strength 1 year after surgery than those immobilized at 30° of flexion (Table 28.2).

Effusion

Joint effusion occurs after all knee ligament surgery. Many patients have persistent effusions for 3 to 9 months (Table 28.4). Like many observations, the reported incidence of effusion depends largely on the evaluation system of the examiner (see Chapter 26). The incidence of joint surface injury in the acute ACL-injured knee is about 20%, and the incidence in the chronic ACL-injured knee is about 50%. It is therefore likely that many patients will have an effusion detected on follow-up examination that results from the joint surface pathology.

The reported incidence of chronic effusion after ligament surgery in the literature is 13% (Table 28.1). In SD1, 12% of patients had an effusion 1 year after ACL surgery. Four of the five patients with the largest effusions had their autogenous graft augmented with a 3M Kennedy ligament augmentation device (LAD). The incidence of effusion may increase when synthetic ligaments are used. Olsen et al. (102) reported that synthetic ligament wear particles induced elevated levels of neutral proteinases in tissue culture. *In vivo* studies revealed that wear particles accumulated in the synovial and subsynovial tissue, resulting in a mild to moderate synovial hypertrophy. Effusions have been associated with a number of synthetic ligaments: carbon fiber, Dacron, LAD, and Gore-Tex (103,104).

Young et al. (105) reviewed studies of nerve pathways and quadriceps function, which reflected changes that occurred as a response to effusion. They observed that, when saline is injected into the normal knees, the amount of quadriceps inhibition was related to the amount of fluid injected. As little as 40 mm of saline may inhibit more than 50% of the nerve activity in the quadriceps. Based on these studies and the work of others, the investigators suggested a network of factors that contribute to quadriceps inhibition and flexion contracture.

Review of the SD1 1-year postoperative data suggests a relationship between effusion and a decrease in quadriceps strength. The quadriceps index for the 25 patients with an effusion was 60%, and it was 71% for the 180 patients without an effusion.

Ogilvie-Harris et al. (106) examined the effect of prostaglandin inhibition and the subsequent decrease in periarticular inflammation on the rate of recovery after arthroscopic meniscectomy. This double-blind study of 139 patients showed that the use of a prostaglandin inhibitor (i.e., naproxen sodium) resulted in significantly less pain, less synovitis, and less effusion. There was a significantly more rapid return of quadriceps function,

TABLE 28.4. *Recovery after ligament surgery*

Parameter	Postoperative week			
	2	6	12	24
Effusion				
0	0	0	8%	57%
1	36%	62%	80%	38%
2	64%	28%	12%	5%
3	0	0	0	0
Knee circumference (I − N)				
<1 cm	8%	12%	13%	30%
1–3 cm	69%	84%	83%	69%
>3 cm	22%	4%	4%	1%
Mean cm	2.9	1.8	1.4	1.0
Thigh circumference (N − I)				
<1 cm	8%	3%	3%	21%
1–3 cm	70%	28%	57%	67%
>3 cm	22%	68%	40%	12%
Mean cm	2.3	4.2	3.3	1.6
Flexion contracture[a]				
<1 cm	30%	11%	35%	57%
1–5 cm	42%	39%	45%	39%
6–10 cm	22%	41%	16%	4%
>10 cm	5%	10%	4%	0%
Mean cm	3.9	5.9	3.3	1.3
Flexion (degrees)				
0–40	26%	2%	0%	0%
41–90	70%	32%	4%	0%
91–120	4%	53%	35%	12%
>120	0%	13%	62%	88%
Mean	4	101	123	130
KT-1000 (I − N)				
20 lb				
>2.5 mm		13%	31%	37%
Mean mm		−0.05	1.9	1.9
Manual max.				
>2.5 mm			41%	51%
>5 mm			9%	13%
Mean			2.2	2.7
Quad active				
<2.5 mm		16%	24%	40%
Mean		−0.02	1.0	2.0
Pivot shift				
0				89%
1				10%
2				1%
3				0%

[a]Measured as a prone heel height difference (1 cm = 1 degree).

range of motion, sports participation, and gainful employment with the use of nonsteroidal antiinflammatory drugs compared with the patients who were not given that drug.

GROWTH PLATE DISTURBANCES

Growth disturbance, angular deformity, and loss of joint congruity are sequelae of injury (fractures) of the growth plate and are therefore concerns of surgeons attempting to reconstruct the ACL in patients with significant growth potential (107,108). Studies on growth and leg-length discrepancy have yielded some data with which to assess the risk to patients of paraphyseal or transphyseal surgery. If 1 cm is an acceptable leg-length discrepancy, after the age of 15.5 years for the average boy and the age of 14 years for the average girl (using the 50th percentile of growth as a guide), growth plate disturbance is not an issue (109). It is our approach to calculate the bone age from wrist radiographs and estimate the remaining distal femoral and proximal tibial growth in any patient with open growth plates considered for ACL reconstruction surgery. There were nine patients younger than 15 in the San Diego Kaiser Review of 500 ACL-injured patients. Ligament surgery was not performed immediately in any of the nine youths.

In the only large series of ACL reconstructions in adolescent athletes, Lipscomb and Anderson (110) addressed the possibility of growth arrest. They examined knee stability and complications in 24 patients seen after reconstructions using semitendinosus and gracilis tendons intraarticularly and Ellison or Losse extraarticular supplementation. Their study population consisted of 11 patients with completely open physes and 13 with partially open physes. In this series, an 8-mm drill hole was placed in the femoral epiphysis (avoiding the femoral physis), and a 6.4-mm drill hole was placed across the tibial physis. Preoperative measurements of leg-length discrepancies were not made. Postoperative measurements after skeletal maturity revealed less than 5-mm difference in 17 patients. For the five patients with 6- to 10-mm differences, the injured limb was shorter in two and longer in three. The two remaining reconstructions resulted in one limb 2 cm shorter and one limb 1.3 cm longer than the uninjured side. The 2-cm difference was attributed to the use of staples for ligament fixation, which spanned the epiphysis. No explanation for the 1.3-cm leg lengthening was given.

Stadelmaier et al. (111) examined growth plate inhibition in immature dogs. Tunnels were drilled across the femoral and tibial physes. In drill holes that were left empty, a bony bridge spanning the growth plate developed in all dogs as early as 2 weeks after surgery. However, when the drill holes were filled with fascia lata autograft, none developed a bony bridge, and all maintained normal growth plate anatomy for the duration of the study. This finding provides basic scientific support to explain the relatively small number of growth abnormalities reported after ACL reconstruction in children and adolescents.

REOPERATION

Review of SD2 showed three (0.2%) reoperations within 1 week for retensioning of a loose tibial bone plug. There were four (0.3%) late operations for removal of painful screws. Ten operations (0.8%) were performed for stiffness, and one operation was performed for possible early graft failure. Eleven operations were done for graft impingement and two for sepsis. One operation was performed for open reduction and internal fixation of a patellar fracture. In total, 33 patients (2.5%) required secondary surgery within 6 months of the index procedure.

SUMMARY

During the past 17 years that we have been collecting data, the incidence of complications associated with ligament reconstruction has markedly diminished. Arthroscopy, improved implantation technique, postoperative immobilization in extension rather than flexion, early weight bearing, early range of motion, early muscle rehabilitation, and improved pain control may have all had a part in the diminution of joint stiffness, weakness, and pain.

Unfortunately, a small incidence of infection and thromboembolic disease may be unavoidable. Transient nerve and muscle injury, however, may be on the decline because of the trend toward lower tourniquet pressures and shorter operating times for ACL reconstruction. Many surgeons now avoid use of the tourniquet altogether.

Short- and long-term graft source complications and failures remain an unsolved problem. Artificial ligaments have been a disappointment, and allografts, although promising, still have a small risk of disastrous infection, slightly inferior overall results, and increased costs. Lack of a perfect graft source perhaps remains the single largest unsolved problem in ligament reconstruction surgery.

REFERENCES

1. Lunn JN, Hunter AR, Scott DB. Anaesthesia-related surgical mortality. *Anaesthesia* 1983;38:1090–1096.
2. Miller DB. *Anesthesia*, 2nd ed, vol 16. New York: Churchill Livingston, 1988:315–320.
3. Vacanti CJ, VanHouten RJ, Hill RC. A statistical analysis of the relationship of physical status to postoperative mortality in 68,388 cases. *Anesth Analg* 1970;49:564–566.
4. Goldstein A Jr, Keats AS. The risk of anesthesia. *Anesthesiology* 1970;33:130–143.
5. Cooper JB, Newbower RS, Kitz RJ. An analysis of major errors and equipment failures in anesthesia management: considerations for prevention and detection. *Anesthesiology* 1984;60:34–42.
6. Tinker JH. In: Rogers MD, ed. *Current practice in anesthesiology.* Toronto: BC Decker, 1988:1–5.
7. Keats AS. In: Orkin FK, Cooperman LH, eds. *Complications in anesthesiology.* Philadelphia: JB Lippincott, 1983:3–13.
8. Hohf RP. Arterial injuries occurring during orthopaedic operations. *Clin Orthop* 1963;28:21–37.
9. Green NE, Allen BL. Vascular injuries associated with dislocation of the knee. *J Bone Joint Surg Am* 1977;59:236–239.
10. McCoy GF, Hannon DG, Barr RJ, et al Vascular injury associated with low-velocity dislocations of the knee. *J Bone Joint Surg Br* 1987;69:285–287.
11. DeLee JC. Complications of arthroscopy and arthroscopic surgery: results of a national survey. *Arthroscopy* 1985;1:214–220.
12. Jeffries JT, Gainor BJ, Allen WC, et al. Injury to the popliteal artery as a complication of arthroscopic surgery. A report of two cases. *J Bone Joint Surg Am* 1987;69:783–785.
13. Jimenez F, Utrilla A, Cuesta C, et al. Popliteal artery and venous aneurysm as a complication of arthroscopic meniscectomy. *J Trauma* 1988;28:1404–1405.
14. Roth JH, Bray RC. Popliteal artery injury during anterior cruciate ligament reconstruction: brief report. *J Bone Joint Surg Br* 1988;70:840.
15. Fruensgaard S, Holm A. Compartment syndrome complicating arthroscopic surgery: brief report. *J Bone Joint Surg Br* 1988;70:146–147.
16. Noyes FR, Spievack ES. Extraarticular fluid dissection in tissues during arthroscopy. A report of clinical cases and a study of intraarticular and thigh pressures in cadavers. *Am J Sports Med* 1982;10:346–351.
17. Peek RD, Haynes DW. Compartment syndrome as a complication of arthroscopy. A case report and a study of interstitial pressures. *Am J Sports Med* 1984;12:464–468.
18. Matsen FAD. Compartment syndrome. A unified concept. *Clin Orthop* 1975;113:8–14.
19. Mubarak SJ. A practical approach to compartmental syndromes. Part II. Diagnosis. *Instr Course Lect* 1983;32:92–102.
20. Whitesides TE, Haney TC, Morimoto K, et al. Tissue pressure measurements as a determinant for the need of fasciotomy. *Clin Orthop* 1975;113:43—51.

21. Kummell BM. Preservation of infrapatellar branch of saphenous nerve during knee surgery. *Orthop Rev* 1974:43–45.

22. Hollinshead WH. *Anatomy for surgeons,* 2nd ed. New York: Harper & Row, 1969.

23. Chambers GH. The prepatellar nerve. A cause of suboptimal results in knee arthrotomy. *Clin Orthop* 1972;82:157–159.

24. Swanson AJ. The incidence of prepatellar neuropathy following medial meniscectomy. *Clin Orthop* 1983;181:151–153.

25. Johnson RJ, Kettlekamp DB, Clark W, et al. Factors affecting late results after meniscectomy. *J Bone Joint Surg Am* 1974;56:719–729.

26. Poehling GG, Pollock FE Jr, Koman LA. Reflex sympathetic dystrophy of the knee after sensory nerve injury. *Arthroscopy* 1988;4:31–35.

27. Sherman OH, Fox JM, Snyder SJ, et al. Arthroscopy—"'no-problem surgery." An analysis of complications in two thousand six hundred and forty cases. *J Bone Joint Surg Am* 1986;68:256–265.

28. Barber FA, Stone RG. Meniscal repair. An arthroscopic technique. *J Bone Joint Surg Br* 1985;67:39–41.

29. Miller DB Jr. Arthroscopic meniscus repair. *Am J Sports Med* 1988;16:315–320.

30. Morgan CD, Casscells SW. Arthroscopic meniscus repair: a safe approach to the posterior horns. *Arthroscopy* 1986;2:3–12.

31. Scott GA, Jolly BL, Henning DE. Combined posterior incision and arthroscopic intra-articular repair of the meniscus. An examination of factors affecting healing. *J Bone Joint Surg Am* 1986;68:847–861.

32. Cushing H. Pneumatic tourniquets: with especial reference to their use in craniotomies. *Med News N Y* 1904;84:269–277.

33. Ochoa J, Danta G, Fowler TJ, et al. Nature of the nerve lesion caused by a pneumatic tourniquet. *Nature* 1971;233:265–266.

34. Fowler TJ, Danta G, Gilliatt RW. Recovery of nerve conduction after a pneumatic tourniquet: observations on the hind-limb of the baboon. *J Neurol Neurosurg Psychiatry* 1972;35:638–647.

35. Rorabeck CH, Kennedy JC. Tourniquet-induced nerve ischemia complicating knee ligament surgery. *Am J Sports Med* 1980;8:98–102.

36. Dobner JJ, Nitz AJ. Postmeniscectomy tourniquet palsy and functional sequelae. *Am J Sports Med* 1982;10:211–214.

37. Saunders KC, Louis DL, Weingarden SI, et al. Effect of tourniquet time on postoperative quadriceps function. *Clin Orthop* 1979;143:194–199.

38. Livingston LA. The quadriceps angle: a review of the literature. *J Orthop Sports Phys Ther* 1998;28:105–109.

39. Guanche CA. Tourniquet-induced tibial nerve palsy complicating anterior cruciate ligament reconstruction. *Arthroscopy* 1995;11:620–622.

40. Hooper J, Rosaeg OP, Krepski B, et al. Tourniquet inflation during arthroscopic knee ligament surgery does not increase postoperative pain. *Can J Anaesth* 1999;46:925–929.

41. Daniel DM, Lumkong G, Stone ML, et al. Effects of tourniquet use in anterior cruciate ligament reconstruction. *Arthroscopy* 1995;11:307–311.

42. Patterson S, Klenerman L. The effect of pneumatic tourniquets on the ultrastructure of skeletal muscle. *J Bone Joint Surg Br* 1979;61:178–183.

43. Pedowitz RA, Gershuni DH, Schmidt AH, et al. Muscle injury induced beneath and distal to a pneumatic tourniquet: a quantitative animal study of effects of tourniquet pressure and duration. *J Hand Surg Am* 1991;16:610–621.

44. Moore MR, Garfin SR, Hargens AR. Wide tourniquets eliminate blood flow at low inflation pressures. *J Hand Surg Am* 1987;12:1006–1011.

45. Fitts WT Jr. Thromboembolism: the clinical picture. *J Trauma* 1969;9:661–667.

46. Cullison TR, Muldoon MP, Gorman JD, et al. The incidence of deep venous thrombosis in anterior cruciate ligament reconstruction. *Arthroscopy* 1996;12:657–659.

47. Kakkar VV, Howe CT, Nicolaides AN, et al. Deep vein thrombosis of the leg. Is there a "high risk" group? *Am J Surg* 1970;120:527–530.

48. Stulberg BN, Insall JN, Williams GW, et al. Deep-vein thrombosis following total knee replacement. An analysis of six hundred and thirty-eight arthroplasties. *J Bone Joint Surg Am* 1984;66:194–201.

49. Cohen SH, Ehrlich GE, Kauffman MS, et al. Thrombophlebitis following knee surgery. *J Bone Joint Surg Am* 1973;55:106–112.

50. McKenna R, Bachmann F, Kaushal SP, et al. Thromboembolic disease in patients undergoing total knee replacement. *J Bone Joint Surg Am* 1976;58:928–932.

51. Orbon RJ, Poehling GG. Arthroscopic meniscectomy. *South Med J* 1981;74:1238–1242.

52. Walker RH, Dillingham M. Thrombophlebitis following arthroscopic surgery of the knee. *Contemp Orthop* 1983 :29–33.

53. Nilsen DW, Westre B, Jaer O, et al. A clinical and phlebographic study of postoperative deep vein thrombosis following knee meniscus extirpation. *Thromb Haemost* 1982;47:291–292.

54. Kaushal SP, Galante JO, McKenna R, et al. Complications following total knee replacement. *Clin Orthop* 1976;121:181–187.

55. Lotke PA, Ecker ML, Alavi A, et al. Indications for the treatment of deep venous thrombosis following total knee replacement. *J Bone Joint Surg Am* 1984;66:202–208.

56. Hull RD, Raskob GE. Prophylaxis of venous thromboembolic disease following hip and knee surgery. *J Bone Joint Surg Am* 1986;68:146–150.

57. McAllister DR, Parker RD, Cooper AE, et al. Outcomes of postoperative septic arthritis after anterior cruciate ligament reconstruction. *Am J Sports Med* 1999;27:562–570.

58. Williams RJ 3rd, Laurencin CT, Warren RF, et al. Septic arthritis after arthroscopic anterior cruciate ligament reconstruction. Diagnosis and management. *Am J Sports Med* 1997;25:261–267.

59. Arnold JA. A lateral extra-articular tenodesis for anterior cruciate ligament deficiency of the knee. *Orthop Clin North Am* 1985;16:213–222.

60. Ficat RP. *Reflex sympathetic dystrophy*. Baltimore: Williams & Wilkins, 1977:149–169.

61. Livingston WK. *Pain mechanisms: a physiologic interpretation of causalgia and its related states,* 1st ed. New York: McMillan, 1943.

62. Poplawski ZJ, Wiley AM, Murray JF. Post-traumatic dystrophy of the extremities. *J Bone Joint Surg Am* 1983;65:642–655.

63. Tietjen R. Reflex sympathetic dystrophy of the knee. *Clin Orthop* 1986;209:234–243.

64. Benson ER, Barnett PR. A delayed transverse avulsion fracture of the superior pole of the patella after anterior cruciate ligament reconstruction. *Arthroscopy* 1998;14:85–88.

65. Marumoto JM, Mitsunaga MM, Richardson AB, et al. Late patellar tendon ruptures after removal of the central third for anterior cruciate ligament reconstruction. A report of two cases. *Am J Sports Med* 1996;24:698–701.

66. Moen KY, Boynton MD, Raasch WG. Fracture of the proximal tibia after anterior cruciate ligament reconstruction: a case report [See comments]. *Am J Orthop* 1998;27:629–630.

67. Morgan E, Steensen RN. Traumatic proximal tibial fracture following anterior cruciate ligament reconstruction. *Am J Knee Surg* 1998;11:193–194.

68. el-Hage ZM, Mohammed A, Griffiths D, et al. Tibial plateau fracture following allograft anterior cruciate ligament (ACL) reconstruction. *Injury* 1998;29:73–74.

69. Johnson DL. Distal femoral fracture: a complication of endoscopic anterior cruciate ligament reconstruction—a case report [Letter; comment]. *Am J Sports Med* 1998;26:603.

70. Noah J, Sherman OH, Roberts C. Fracture of the supracondylar femur after anterior cruciate ligament reconstruction using patellar tendon and iliotibial band tenodesis. A case report. *Am J Sports Med* 1992;20:615–618.

71. Cabaud HE, Feagin JA, Rodkey WG. Acute anterior cruciate ligament injury and augmented repair. Experimental studies. *Am J Sports Med* 1980;8:395–401.

72. Burks RT, Haut RC, Lancaster RL. Biomechanical and histological observations of the dog patellar tendon after removal of its central one-third. *Am J Sports Med* 1990;18:146–153.

73. Paulos LE, Rosenberg TD, Drawbert J, et al. Infrapatellar contracture syndrome. An unrecognized cause of knee stiffness with patella entrapment and patella infera. *Am J Sports Med* 1987;15:331–341.

74. Huegel M, Indelicato PA. Trends in rehabilitation following anterior cruciate ligament reconstruction. *Clin Sports Med* 1988;7:801–811.

75. Rubinstein RA Jr, Shelbourne KD, VanMeter CD, et al. Isolated autogenous bone-patellar tendon-bone graft site morbidity. *Am J Sports Med* 1994;22:324–327.

76. Shelbourne KD, Trumper RV. Preventing anterior knee pain after anterior cruciate ligament reconstruction. *Am J Sports Med* 1997;25:41–47.

77. Goertzen MJ, Buitkamp J, Clahasen H, et al. Cell survival following bone-anterior cruciate ligament-bone allograft transplantation: DNA fingerprints, segregation, and collagen morphological analysis of multiple markers in the canine model. *Arch Orthop Trauma Surg* 1998;117:208–214.

78. Jackson DW, Corsetti J, Simon TM. Biologic incorporation of allograft anterior cruciate ligament replacements. *Clin Orthop* 1996;324: 126–133.
79. Kirkpatrick JS, Seaber AV, Glisson RR, et al. Cryopreserved anterior cruciate ligament allografts in a canine model. *J South Orthop Assoc* 1996;5:20–29.
80. Jackson DW, Grood ES, Goldstein JD, et al. A comparison of patellar tendon autograft and allograft used for anterior cruciate ligament reconstruction in the goat model. *Am J Sports Med* 1993;21:176–185.
81. Jackson DW, Simon TM, Kurzweil PR, et al. Survival of cells after intra-articular transplantation of fresh allografts of the patellar and anterior cruciate ligaments. DNA-probe analysis in a goat model. *J Bone Joint Surg Am* 1992;74:112–118.
82. Roberts TS, Drez D Jr, McCarthy W, et al. Anterior cruciate ligament reconstruction using freeze-dried, ethylene oxide-sterilized, bone-patellar tendon–bone allografts. Two year results in thirty-six patients [Published erratum appears in *Am J Sports Med* 1991;19:272]. *Am J Sports Med* 1991;19:35–41.
83. Jackson DW, Windler GE, Simon TM. Intraarticular reaction associated with the use of freeze-dried, ethylene oxide-sterilized bone-patella tendon-bone allografts in the reconstruction of the anterior cruciate ligament. *Am J Sports Med* 1990;18:1–10; discussion 10–11.
84. Fideler BM, Vangsness CT Jr, Lu B, et al. Gamma irradiation: effects on biomechanical properties of human bone-patellar tendon-bone allografts. *Am J Sports Med* 1995;23:643–646.
85. Shelton WR, Papendick L, Dukes AD. Autograft versus allograft anterior cruciate ligament reconstruction. *Arthroscopy* 1997;13:446–449.
86. Victor J, Bellemans J, Witvrouw E, et al. Graft selection in anterior cruciate ligament reconstruction–prospective analysis of patellar tendon autografts compared with allografts. *Int Orthop* 1997;21:93–97.
87. Stringham DR, Peomas CJ, Burks RT, et al. Comparison of anterior cruciate ligament reconstructions using patellar tendon autograft or allograft. *Arthroscopy* 1996;12:414–421.
88. Lephart SM, Kocher MS, Harner CD, et al. Quadriceps strength and functional capacity after anterior cruciate ligament reconstruction. Patellar tendon autograft versus allograft. *Am J Sports Med* 1993;21: 738–743.
89. Saddemi SR, Frogameini AD, Fenton PJ, et al. Comparison of perioperative morbidity of anterior cruciate ligament autografts versus allografts. *Arthroscopy* 1993;9:519–524.
90. Yaru NC, Daniel DM, Penner D, et al. The effect of tibial attachment site on graft impingement in an anterior cruciate ligament reconstruction. *Am J Sports Med* 1992;20:217–220.
91. Lane JG, Daniel DM, Stone ML. Graft impingement after anterior cruciate ligament reconstruction. Presentation as an active extension "thunk." *Am J Sports Med* 1994;22:415–417.
92. Epstein RM. Morbidity and mortality from anesthesia: a continuing problem. *Anesthesiology* 1978;49:388–389.
93. Noyes FR, Mangine RE, Barber S. Early knee motion after open and arthroscopic anterior cruciate ligament reconstruction. *Am J Sports Med* 1987;15:149–160.
94. Cosgarea AJ, Sebastianelli WJ, DeHaven KE. Prevention of arthrofibrosis after anterior cruciate ligament reconstruction using the central third patellar tendon autograft. *Am J Sports Med* 1995;23:87–92.
95. Dandy DJ, Edwards DJ. Problems in regaining full extension of the knee after anterior cruciate ligament reconstruction: does arthrofibrosis exist? [See comments]. *Knee Surg Sports Traumatol Arthrosc* 1994;2:76–79.
96. Parisien JS. The role of arthroscopy in the treatment of postoperative fibroarthrosis of the knee joint. *Clin Orthop* 1988;229:185–192.
97. Sprague NF 3rd, O'Connor RL, Fox JM. Arthroscopic treatment of postoperative knee fibroarthrosis. *Clin Orthop* 1982;166:165–172.
98. Nicoll EA. Quadricepsplasty. *J Bone Joint Surg Br* 1963;45:483–490.
99. Mohtadi NG, Webster-Bogaert S, Fowler PJ. Limitation of motion following anterior cruciate ligament reconstruction. A case-control study. *Am J Sports Med* 1991;19:620–624; discussion 624–625.
100. Marzo JM, Bowen MK, Warren RF, et al. Intraarticular fibrous nodule as a cause of loss of extension following anterior cruciate ligament reconstruction. *Arthroscopy* 1992;8:10–18.
101. Sachs RA, Daniel DM, Stone ML, et al. Patellofemoral problems after anterior cruciate ligament reconstruction. *Am J Sports Med* 1989;17: 760–765.
102. Olson EJ, Kang JD, Fu FH, et al. The biochemical and histological effects of artificial ligament wear particles: in vitro and in vivo studies. *Am J Sports Med* 1988;16:558–570.
103. Rusch RM. In: Freidman MJ, Ferkel RD, eds. *Prosthetic reconstruction of the knee*. Philadelphia: WB Saunders, 1988:52–58.
104. Indelicato PA, Pascale MS, Huegel MO. Early experience with the Gore-Tex polytetrafluoroethylene anterior cruciate ligament prosthesis. *Am J Sports Med* 1989;17:52–55.
105. Young A, Stokes M, Iles JF. Effects of joint pathology on muscle. *Clin Orthop* 1987;219:21–27.
106. Ogilvie-Harris DJ, Bauer M, Corey P. Prostaglandin inhibition and the rate of recovery after arthroscopic meniscectomy. A randomised double-blind prospective study. *J Bone Joint Surg Br* 1985;67:567–571.
107. Clanton TO, DeLee JC, Sanders B, et al. Knee ligament injuries in children. *J Bone Joint Surg Am* 1979;61:1195–1201.
108. Czitrom AA, Salter RB, Willis RB. Fractures involving the distal epiphyseal plate of the femur. *Int Orthop* 1981;4:269–277.
109. Moseley CF. A straight line graph for leg length discrepancies. *Clin Orthop* 1978;136:33–40.
110. Lipscomb AB, Anderson AF. Tears of the anterior cruciate ligament in adolescents. *J Bone Joint Surg Am* 1986;68:19–28.
111. Stadelmaier DM, Arnoczky SP, Dodds J, et al. The effect of drilling and soft tissue grafting across open growth plates. A histologic study. *Am J Sports Med* 1995;23:431–435.

Subject Index